DAILY VALUES FOR FOOD LABELS

The Daily Values are standard values developed by the Food and Drug Administration (FDA) for use on food labels. In creating the Daily Values, the FDA first established two sets of reference values. The first set, the Reference Daily Intakes (RDI), is for protein, vitamins, and minerals and reflect average allowances based on the RDA. The second set, the Daily Reference Values (DRV), is for nutrients and food components, such as fat and fiber, that do not have an established RDA but do have important relationships with health. Together, the RDI and DRV make up the Daily Values used on food labels.

Reference Daily Intakes (RDI)

Nutrient	Amount
Protein[a]	50 g
Thiamin	1.5 mg
Riboflavin	1.7 mg
Niacin	20 mg NE
Biotin	300 µg
Pantothenic acid	10 mg
Vitamin B_6	2 mg
Folate	400 µg
Vitamin B_{12}	6 µg
Vitamin C	60 mg
Vitamin A[b]	5000 IU
Vitamin D[b]	400 IU
Vitamin E[b]	30 IU
Vitamin K	80 µg
Calcium	1000 mg
Iron	18 mg
Zinc	15 mg
Iodine	150 µg
Copper	2 mg
Chromium	120 µg
Selenium	70 µg
Molybdenum	75 µg
Manganese	2 mg
Chloride	3400 mg

[a]The RDI for protein varies for different groups of people: pregnant women, 60 g; nursing mothers, 65 g; infants under 1 year, 14 g; children 1 to 4 years, 16 g.
[b]The RDI for fat-soluble vitamins are expressed in International Units (IU), an old system of measurement. The current RDA and tables of food composition use a more accurate system of measurement. Equivalent values are as follows: for vitamin A, 875 µg RE; for vitamin D, 10 µg; for vitamin E, 9 mg α-TE.

Daily Reference Values (DRV)

Food Component	DRV	Calculation
Fat	65 g	30% of kcalories
Saturated fat	20 g	10% of kcalories
Cholesterol	300 mg	Same regardless of kcalories
Carbohydrate (total)	300 g	60% of kcalories
Fiber	25 g	11.5 g per 1000 kcalories
Protein	50 g	10% of kcalories
Sodium	2400 mg	Same regardless of kcalories
Potassium	3500 mg	Same regardless of kcalories

Note: The DRV were established for adults and children over 4 years old. The values for energy-yielding nutrients are based on 2000 kcalories a day.

Glossary of Nutrient Measures

kcal: kcalories; a unit by which energy is measured.

g: grams; a unit of weight equivalent to about 0.03 ounces.

mg: milligrams; one-thousandth of a gram.

µg: micrograms; one-millionth of a gram.

mg NE: milligrams niacin equivalents; a measure of niacin activity.

mg α-TE: milligrams alpha-tocopherol equivalents; a measure of vitamin E activity.

µg RE: micrograms retinol equivalents; a measure of vitamin A activity.

IU: international units; an old measure of vitamin activity determined by biological methods (as opposed to new measures that are determined by direct chemical analysis).

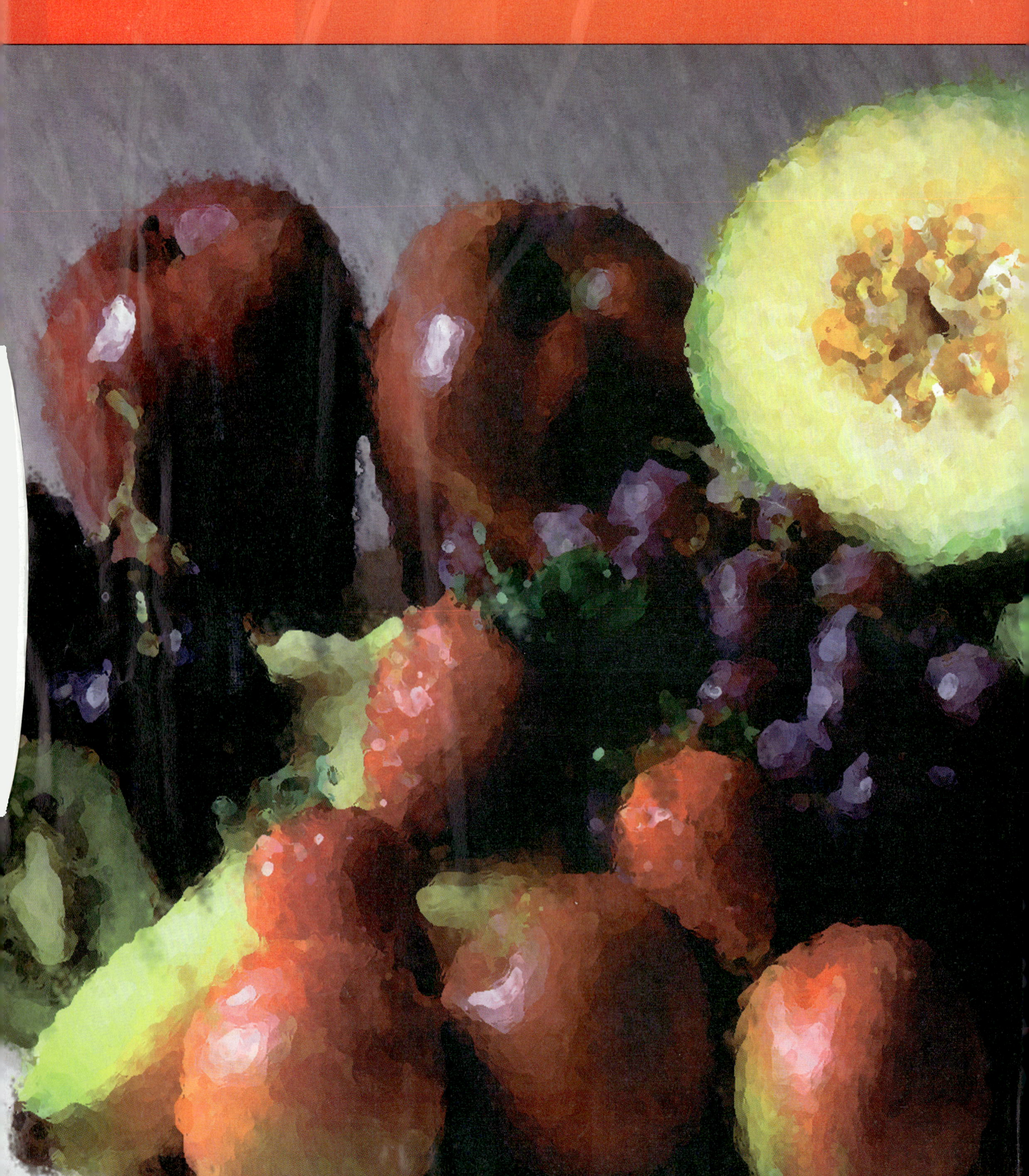

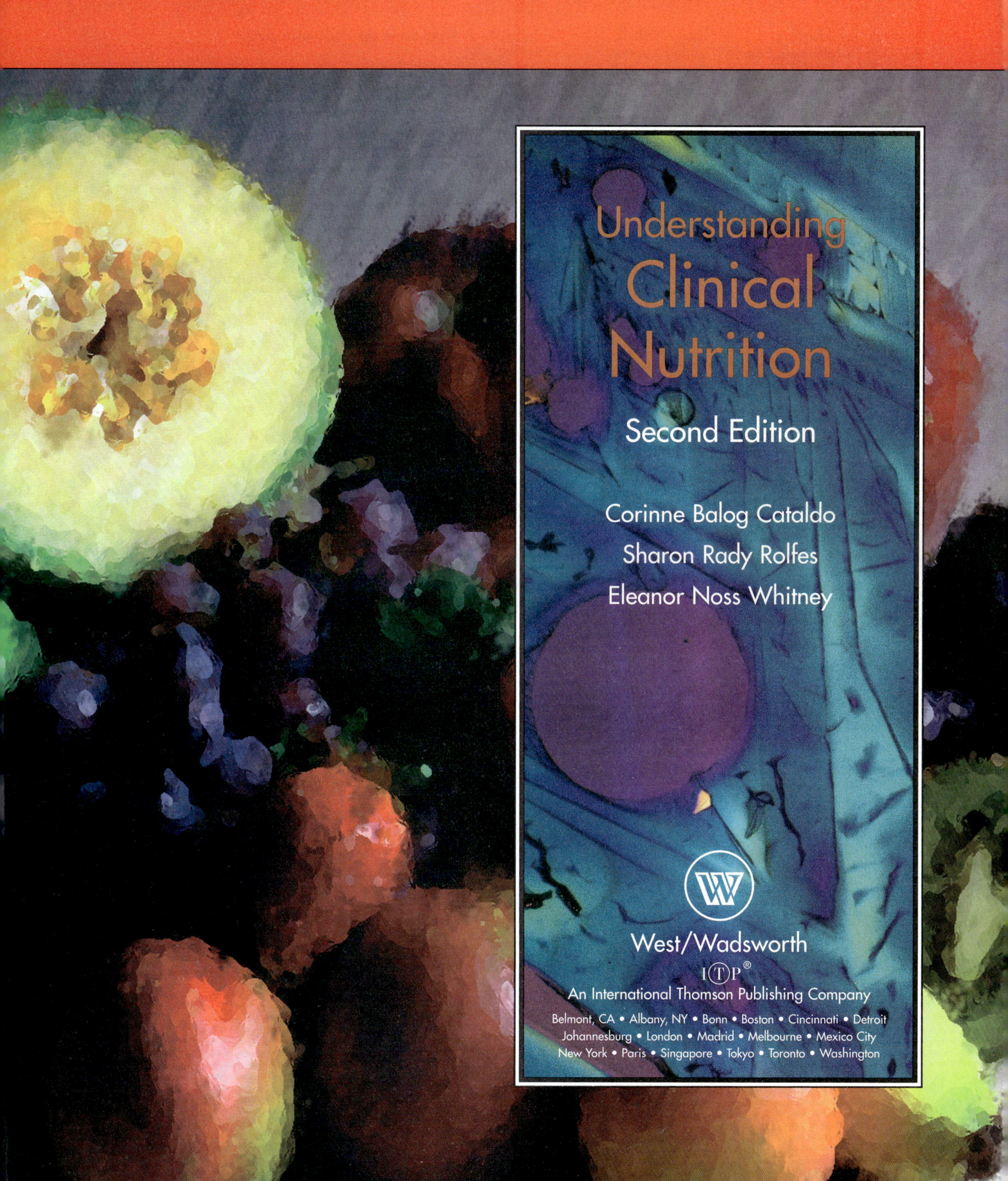
Understanding
Clinical
Nutrition
Second Edition
Corinne Balog Cataldo
Sharon Rady Rolfes
Eleanor Noss Whitney
West/Wadsworth
I(T)P®
An International Thomson Publishing Company
Belmont, CA • Albany, NY • Bonn • Boston • Cincinnati • Detroit
Johannesburg • London • Madrid • Melbourne • Mexico City
New York • Paris • Singapore • Tokyo • Toronto • Washington

Nutrition Publisher: Peter Marshall
Associate Development Editor: Laura Perkinson
Editorial Assistant: Tangelique Williams
Marketing Manager: Becky Tollerson
Project Editor: Sandra Craig
Print Buyer: Barbara Britton
Permissions Editor: Peggy Meehan
Production Coordinator: The Book Company
Text and Cover Design: Janet Bollow
Cover Image: Leptin, © Michael Davidson
Copy Editor: Pat Lewis
Photo Research: Photo Edit, Stephen Forsling
Illustrations: J/B Woolsey and Associates, Todd Smith, Regina Hollistor, Impact Publications
Index: Barbara Farabaugh
Compositor: Parkwood Composition Service
Printer: World Color Book Services/ Taunton

A Word about the Photomicrographs

The chapter opening photomicrographs by Michael Davidson at Florida State University were made of recrystallized vitamins and other nutrients using a variety of different techniques. Many vitamins can be imaged using the melt-recrystallization process where a few milligrams of the chemical are sandwiched between a microscope coverslip and slide, then heated until melted and allowed to slowly recrystallize. Alternately, for vitamin-salts that will not melt, the chemical is dissolved in a suitable solvent (water or alcohol) and a few microliters of solution are allowed to slowly evaporate between a microscope slide and coverslip. Upon recrystallization, the vitamins are viewed in a microscope using cross-polarized illumination where the crystallites diffract light depending both on the molecular orientation within the crystal and the crystal thickness. The colorful patterns illustrated in this text are a manifestation of both molecular orientation and crystal thickness.

Printed in the United States of America
1 2 3 4 5 6 7 8 9 10

For more information, contact Wadsworth Publishing Company, 10 Davis Drive, Belmont, CA 94002, or electronically at http://www.thomson.com/wadsworth.html

International Thomson Publishing Europe
Berkshire House 168-173
High Holborn
London, WC1V 7AA, England

Thomas Nelson Australia
102 Dodds Street
South Melbourne 3205
Victoria, Australia

Nelson Canada
1120 Birchmount Road
Scarborough, Ontario
Canada M1K 5G4

International Thomson Publishing GmbH
Königswinterer Strasse 418
53227 Bonn, Germany

International Thomson Editores
Campos Eliseos 385, Piso 7
Col. Polanco
11560 México D.F. México

International Thomson Publishing Asia
221 Henderson Road
#05-10 Henderson Building
Singapore 0315

International Thomson Publishing Japan
Hirakawacho Kyowa Building, 3F
2-2-1 Hirakawacho
Chiyoda-ku, Tokyo 102, Japan

International Thomson Publishing Southern Africa
Building 18, Constantia Park
240 Old Pretoria Road
Halfway House, 1685 South Africa

Library of Congress Cataloging-in-Publication Data

Cataldo, Corinne Balog.
Understanding clinical nutrition / Corinne Balog Cataldo, Sharon Rady Rolfes, Eleanor Noss Whitney.—2nd ed.
p. cm.
Includes index.
ISBN 0-534-53341-8
1. Diet therapy. 2. Dietetics. I. Rolfes, Sharon Rady.
II. Whitney, Eleanor Noss. III. Title.
RM216.C365 1998
615.8'54--dc21 97–41849

Credits at the end of the book.

To

My son, Adam,
who has been a source
of happiness and pride,
a reminder of the promise
that the future holds,
and a wonderful person
to talk with.
Good luck as you enter
college and begin your life
as an adult.

Mom (Corkie)

To

My loving husband, Tom,
and
our delightful children,
Lyle and Marni.

Sharon

To

Lynn, Liza, and Sally,
all nurturers.
I am proud to call
all three my daughters.

Ellie

About the Authors

Corinne Balog Cataldo, M.M.Sc., R.D., C.N.S.D., received her B.S. in community health nutrition from Georgia State University in 1976 and her M.M.Sc. in clinical dietetics from Emory University in 1979. She has worked in private practice in Atlanta, as a clinical dietitian and metabolic support nutritionist at Georgia Baptist Medical Center in Atlanta, as a faculty member and dietetic internship coordinator at Emory University, and as a nutritionist with the Infant Formula Council. She has made numerous presentations, and in addition to this book, she has written a manual on tube feedings and the books *Nutrition and Diet Therapy*, *Nutrition for Health and Health Care*, and *Understanding Clinical Nutrition*. She is a certified nutrition support dietitian.

Sharon Rady Rolfes, M.S., R.D., received her B.S. in psychology and criminology in 1974 and her M.S. in nutrition and food science in 1982 from Florida State University. She is a founding member of Nutrition and Health Associates, an information resource center that maintains an ongoing bibliographic database that tracks research in over 1000 nutrition-related topics. Her other publications include the textbooks *Understanding Nutrition*, *Understanding Clinical Nutrition*, *Life Span Nutrition: Conception through Life*, and *Nutrition for Health and Health Care* and a multimedia CD-ROM called *Nutrition Interactive*. In addition to writing, she also lectures at universities and at professional conferences and serves as a consultant for various educational projects. She maintains a professional membership in the American Dietetic Association.

Eleanor Noss Whitney, Ph.D., received her B.A. in biology from Radcliffe College in 1960 and her Ph.D. in biology from Washington University, St. Louis, in 1970. Formerly on the faculty at Florida State University, and a dietitian registered with the American Dietetic Association, she now devotes full time to research, writing, and consulting. Her earlier publications include articles in *Science*, *Genetics*, and other journals. Her textbooks include *Understanding Nutrition*, *Nutrition Concepts and Controversies*, *Life Span Nutrition: Conception through Life*, *Nutrition and Diet Therapy*, and *Essential Life Choices* for college students and *Making Life Choices* for high school students. Her most intense interests currently include energy conservation, solar energy uses, alternatively fueled vehicles, and ecosystem restoration.

Contents in Brief

Contents in Brief

Contents

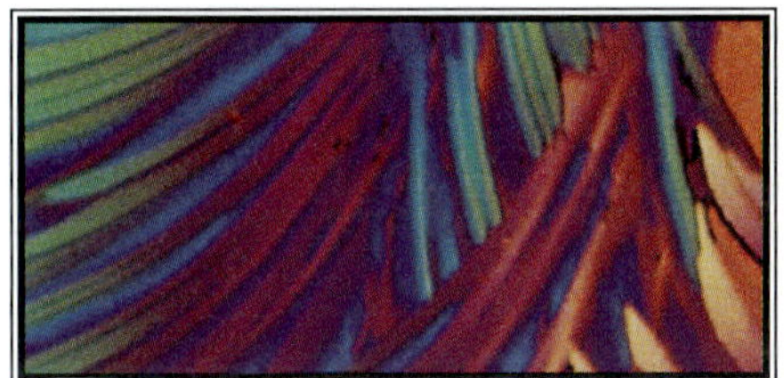

Contents

Chapter 18

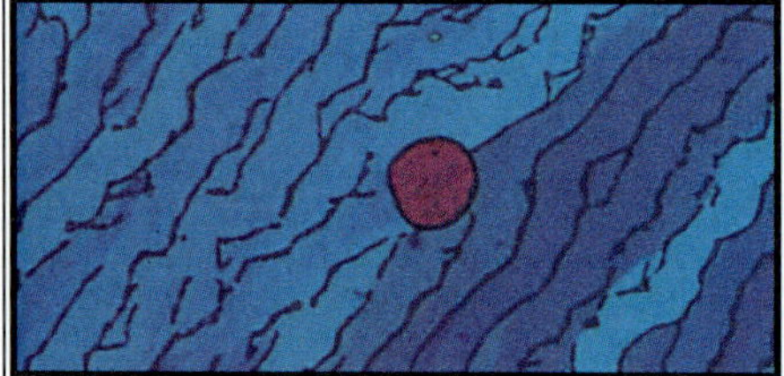

Chapter 19

Chapter 20

Contents

Chapter 21

Chapter 22

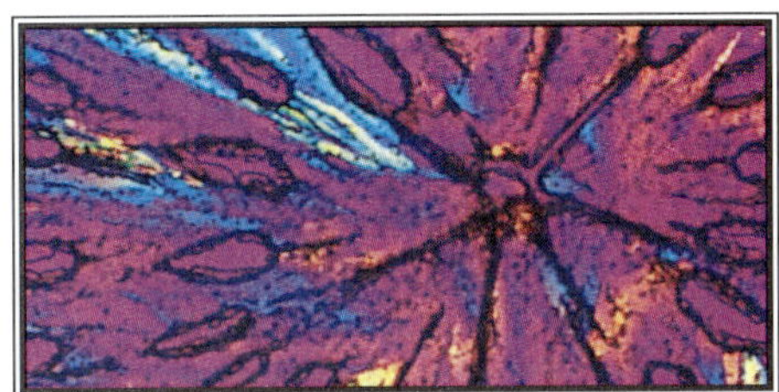

Chapter 23

Chapter 24

Contents

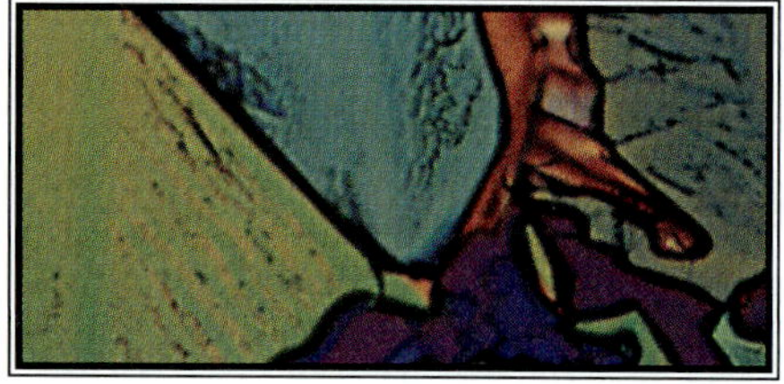

Chapter 25

Chapter 26

Chapter 27

Chapter 28

Contents

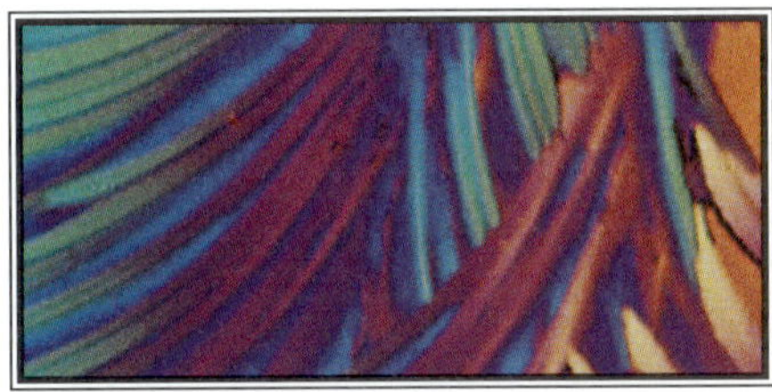

Appendixes

Contents

Glossary

Index

How-To Boxes

Case Studies

Preface

Understanding Clinical Nutrition offers readers the nutrition knowledge they need for their roles as health care professionals. It not only presents the nutrition facts, but also shows readers how to apply these facts to their clinical practice.

This book assumes that readers have had an introductory course in normal nutrition. For many readers, that course was taught using one of our other textbooks—either *Understanding Nutrition* or the first half of *Understanding Normal and Clinical Nutrition*. This text is the second half of *Understanding Normal and Clinical Nutrition*. By presenting just the clinical portion in this book and starting with Chapter 15 on p. 518, we have been able to provide a four-color, high-quality text at a reasonable cost.

The first three chapters describe how health care professionals assess a client's nutrition status and use this information to make plans for the client's nutrition care. Chapter 15 focuses on how health care professionals use health, drug, socioeconomic, and diet histories and physical findings to help pinpoint nutrition problems. Chapter 16 then examines how anthropometric data and biochemical tests help complete the assessment process. Chapter 17 shows how health care professionals integrate assessment data into a plan that meets the client's nutrient and nutrition education needs.

The text continues with an emphasis on conditions that alter nutrient needs. Chapters 18, 19, and 20 present the special needs of people throughout the life cycle—pregnancy and lactation; infancy, childhood, and adolescence; and the later years. The remaining chapters explore how diseases, their symptoms, and their treatments influence nutrient needs and how meeting those needs can enhance recovery. The path of exploration follows the course that foods take as they are ingested, digested, metabolized, distributed, and excreted by the body. Thus Chapters 21 and 22 examine the upper and lower GI tract, and Chapters 23 and 24 describe special ways of feeding people who cannot eat conventional foods. Chapters 25 through 27 delve into disorders whose primary effects are on metabolism—severe stresses, liver disorders, and diabetes and hypoglycemia. Chapter 28 looks at disorders of the heart, blood vessels, and lungs, which affect the distribution of nutrients and oxygen to the cells. Chapter 29 describes kidney disorders, which affect the excretion of nutrients. Finally, Chapter 30 examines cancer and HIV infections—disorders that often lead to wasting and have multiple effects on nutrition status.

To the person reading this text, it will be obvious that, like most sciences, nutrition possesses no absolute certainties. Nutrition scientists simply do not have all the answers; in some cases, we have not even asked all the questions. This is true in virtually all areas of nutrition; it is a young, growing science dating only from around the turn of the century. One of the missions of this text is to show readers how to ascertain the "facts"—a skill vital to developing sound clinical judgment.

In seeking nutrition facts, many people turn to the Internet. In recent years, the number of websites on the Internet has grown exponentially. For this reason, it may be appropriate to comment on the use of the Internet in the study of nutrition (or any subject for that matter). The Internet offers endless opportunities to obtain high-quality information. Unfortunately, it also delivers an abundance of incomplete, misleading, or inaccurate information. Simply put: anyone can publish anything. To distinguish a credible and helpful source from all the others, users must adopt standards similar to those used for printed publications. They must consider whether the author's educational degrees, credentials, and affiliations qualify him or her to speak authoritatively on nutrition. They also need to determine whether the information is based on valid scientific research and note whether credible references are provided. To explore several credible nutrition websites on the Internet, start with a visit to our website:

http://www.wadsworth.com/nutrition

Highlights on current issues of interest alternate with the chapters. Each highlight provides readers with a brief look at a topic that relates to the companion chapter. New highlights in this edition explore nutrition and diagnostic tests, childhood obesity and its influence on the early development of chronic diseases, alternative therapies, foodservice in hospitals, and possible diet-related risk factors for atherosclerosis. The highlights on living with diabetes and cost-conscious health care have been updated.

The appendixes are valuable references for a number of purposes. Appendix A summarizes background information on the hormonal and nervous systems, complementing Appendixes B and C on basic chemistry, the chemical structures of nutrients, and the major metabolic pathways. Appendix D assists readers with calculations and conversions, and Appendix E provides additional information regarding nutrition assessments. Appendix F lists book and journal recommendations and addresses for many nutrition resources including dozens of Internet addresses. Appendix G presents the Recommended Dietary Allowances (1989 RDA), the nutrition-related priorities of Healthy People 2000, the United States Exchange System, and recommendations from the World Health Organization. Appendix H is a 2000-item food composition table compiled from the latest nutrient database assembled by ESHA Research, Inc., of Salem, Oregon. Appendix I presents information for Canadians: the Recommended Nutrient Intakes (1990 RNI), the Choice System, and instructions on reading food labels. Appendix J describes measures of protein quality, and Appendix K offers information on enteral formula products.

We have tried to keep the number of notes to a minimum. Many statements that appeared in the previous edition with notes now appear without them, but every statement is backed by research, and the authors will supply references upon request. We have not provided a separate list of suggested readings, but have tried to include references that will provide readers with additional details or a good overview of the subject.

Preview of Text Elements

How to Calculate the Nutrient Content of IV Solutions

You can have confidence in IV solutions if you know what they contain. The basic thing to remember is that the percentage of a substance in solution tells ... liters. For ... trose per ... grams of a ... tion cont...

Suppos... taining 1... percent a...

How to Help Clients Accept Oral Formulas

People on enteral formulas are often quite ill and frequently have poor appetites. Even when a person enjoys a formula, palatability can become a problem after a while. Hydrolyzed formulas are often less palatable than standard formulas, and clients may find them difficult to accept. Caring professionals can help by using these suggestions:

- Ask the dietitian to let the client try both different flavors and differ-

Figure A How-To Boxes

Many of the chapters in this edition include "How To" skill boxes that guide readers through problem-solving tasks. These boxes demonstrate how to perform mathematical calculations or how to apply nutrition or nutrition-related information in practical terms.

Health care professionals use the nutrition care process to systematically assess, analyze, plan, implement, and evaluate their clients' nutrition and nutrition education needs. The contributions of all members of the health care team enhance the accuracy and effectiveness of the nutrition care plan.

Figure B Summary Paragraphs

New to this edition are summary paragraphs, marked with a thin blue bar in the margin. These paragraphs review the contents of the previous sections.

Nutrition Assessment Checklist
For People Receiving Tube Feedings

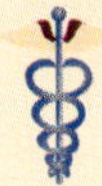

Medical Review the client's medical record for the information necessary to select the appropriate feeding site (gastric versus intestinal), insertion procedure (transnasal or enterostomy), and formula. The development of undesirable symptoms associated with the client's medical condition, therapy (especially drug), or formula selection requires prompt intervention.

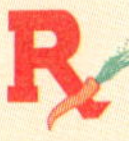

Drug Review the client's drug therapy for possible drug-nutrient interactions and GI side effects that may affect the client's tolerance for the tube feeding. If the feeding tube is used to deliver drugs, follow the precautions on pp. 769–771.

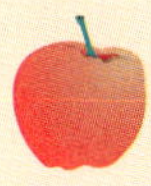

Nutrient Intake Ensure that formula is being delivered as prescribed, and take corrective actions as needed (see p. 774). For clients beginning to eat, determine the degree to which nutrient needs are being met by table foods or formula taken orally, and reduce the volume of the tube feeding accordingly.

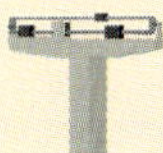

Anthropometric Assess the client's weight daily to make sure that the client is meeting nutrition goals.

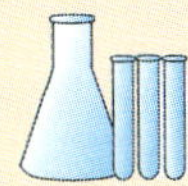

Laboratory Monitor serum and urine lab values for signs of fluid and electrolyte imbalances and glucose intolerance. Check serum protein levels to ensure that they are improving or being maintained. When available, assess nitrogen balance to determine if the tube feeding is meeting the client's protein needs.

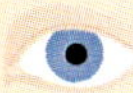

Physical Check gastric residual for signs of delayed gastric emptying to prevent GI complications and reduce the risk of aspiration. Check tube placement and gravity drip rate or infusion pump drip rate as needed (see Table 23–4). Assess blood pressure, temperature, pulse, and respiration every 4 hours. Look for physical signs of malnutrition or dehydration.

Figure C Nutrition Assessment Checklists

New to this edition are the nutrition assessment checklists. The checklists help readers determine the impact of various disorders on nutrition status by highlighting the medical, drug, nutrient intake, anthropometric, laboratory, and physical findings that are particularly relevant to a specific group of clients.

Figure D Study Questions

Each chapter closes with study questions. These offer readers the opportunity to review the major concepts presented in the chapter. Most chapters also include case studies and clinical applications.

Study Questions

1. List conditions of the mouth that can affect the ability to chew foods. What diet would you advise in each case?
2. Discuss ways to stimulate the appetite for people on pureed diets.
3. What is dysphagia, and how is the diet managed to ease its symptoms? Why does dysphagia often go unrecognized? What are its potential consequences?
4. What is reflux esophagitis, and what are its primary symptoms? Why is reflux more likely to occur in people with hiatal hernias?
5. What advice can you give the person with reflux to prevent and treat its symptoms? What long-term complications can result from chronic reflux esophagitis?
6. Under what circumstances can indigestion, nausea and vomiting present a risk to nutrition status?
7. What is gastritis? Describe the role of diet therapy in acute and chronic gastritis.
8. Discuss the therapy for peptic ulcers.
9. What are the possible nutrition consequences of gastric surgery? Describe the relationship of gastric surgery to these consequences. What dietary interventions might help to prevent these consequences?
10. Discuss the dietary recommendations, and the rationale behind them, for a person who undergoes gastric partitioning for clinically severe obesity.

Figure E Case Studies

Case studies guide readers in translating what they have learned about a disorder to a situation involving an actual client.

Case Study Truck Driver with NIDDM

Mr. Evans, a truck driver, was 52 years old when he was first diagnosed with NIDDM. He visited his physician after experiencing excessive thirst, excessive urination, and excessive appetite. Mr. Evans, who stands 5 feet 11 inches tall and currently weighs 200 pounds, experienced a 30-pound weight gain over the past two years. His fasting blood glucose is 235 milligrams per 100 milliliters. His fasting triglycerides and cholesterol are also elevated.

The diabetes health care team members have evaluated Mr. Evans's case. They are eager to help him achieve the first goal of diabetes management—to bring his blood glucose under control. The team has helped Mr. Evans plan a diet and physical activity program that considers the nature of his job and life on the road.

Mr. Evans is concerned about his health. He is worried that he may need insulin injections and overwhelmed by all the information presented to him over the past few days.

What are the differences between NIDDM and IDDM? Describe the factors in Mr. Evans's history that might have predisposed him to NIDDM. Can you explain to Mr. Evans why he will not need insulin injections at this time?

What will be the primary objective of the diet therapy for Mr. Evans? Determine Mr. Evans's desirable body weight, and describe two diet plans that might help him control both his blood glucose and his lipids. Select one of these diet plans and plan Mr. Evans's diet using the information in the box on pp. 855–856. Suggest some types of physical activities that might be appropriate for Mr. Evans. Remember that he travels frequently and needs a plan he can follow regularly. In what ways do diet and physical activity plans benefit clients with NIDDM?

What alternative treatments might Mr. Evans's physician consider if diet and physical activity fail to control his blood glucose?

Consider Mr. Evans's emotional health. How can the health care team help him during this difficult period?

Figure F Clinical Applications

Clinical applications may ask the reader to perform mathematical calculations, synthesize information from previous chapters, or demonstrate the impact of nutrition care on health care professionals or clients.

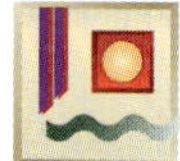

Clinical Applications

1. Using the box on pp. 855–856, plan a diet using the exchange lists for a sedentary woman with IDDM who is 5 feet 9 inches tall and weighs 160 pounds. Assume that the distribution of kcalories will be 55 percent from carbohydrate, 20 percent from protein, and 25 percent from fat. Round off kcalories to develop a sample diet pattern.
2. An important part of learning is being able to apply knowledge and guidelines to real-life situations. Using Table 27–5 as a guide, think about the possible remedies for either hyper- or hypoglycemia. Describe at least one situation when it might be preferable to alter the insulin dose and one situation when it might be preferable to alter the carbohydrate intake.
3. Take a trip to a pharmacy and price these items: blood glucose meter, test strips for the meter selected, glucose test strips for use without a meter, lancets, insulin, and syringes. Determine the approximate cost of insulin injections for a person who uses 14 units of regular insulin and 26 units of NPH insulin daily (don't forget to include the cost of the syringes). Then estimate the cost of testing blood glucose four times daily. How does the cost of using a blood glucose meter compare to the cost of regular blood glucose test strips? How much do lancets add to the total daily cost? Consider how an external pump might affect the total cost of managing diabetes. How does the need for a balanced diet influence the cost of diabetes care? If intensive therapy requires more expenditures for insulin injections, blood glucose testing, and medical checkups than does traditional therapy, how might the added costs be justified?

Menu

Breakfast
1 egg, fried with
1 tbs margarine
1 slice toast
2 tsp margarine
Jelly

Lunch
Sandwich with
2 oz turkey
2 slices bread
1 tbs mayonnaise
Lettuce leaf

Supper
3 oz roast beef
½ c rice
2 tsp margarine
½ c mushrooms sautéed
in 2 tsp olive oil and

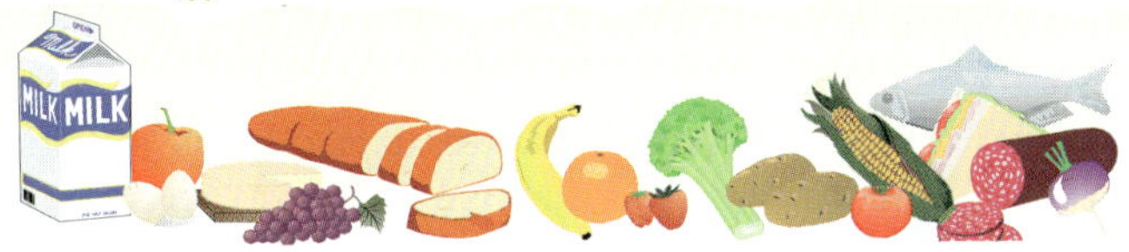

Figure G Menus

Throughout these clinical nutrition discussions are sample menus and prescription pads. The sample menus show readers how the diet order translates into a typical day's meals.

℞ PRESCRIPTION PAD

Drugs used in the treatment of cardiovascular disease may include:

- Anticoagulants (including aspirin)
- Antihypertensives
- Antilipemics
- Diuretics (isosorbide nitrate)
- Nitroglycerin (to ease angina)

See Appendix E for timing with meals and nutrition-related side effects.

Figure H Prescription Pads

The prescription pads list the major classes of drugs used in the treatment of specific disorders and refer readers to a table in Appendix E that explains the timing of food intake with drug administration and lists common nutrition-related side effects.

What Is Available Along with the Textbook?

For the Student

DIET ANALYSIS PLUS SOFTWARE VERSION 3.0 (WINDOWS, DOS, OR MAC)

This software (based on award-winning ESHA Food Processor Software) calculates personal RDA or RNI (for Canadians) goal percentages for fats, carbohydrates and proteins. The software allows you to adjust for personal recommended kcaloric levels by factoring in exercises, and/or choosing a weight loss or weight gain plan. You may then compare your actual diet to these recommendations by entering the foods you eat for up to 7 days. A total of 4,000 foods are available via onscreen lookup, and up to 30 more foods (WIN and DOS versions only) may be added to personalize the database. See your results in spreadsheet and graphic formats. This is software that can be used for a lifetime.

NUTRITION INTERACTIVE CD-ROM

This CD-ROM includes animations, video, and interactive computer exercises which help to bring nutrition to life. For example, after having explored the workings of the digestive tract on the CD-ROM, you will be ready to test your knowledge of common GI problems by identifying their symptoms and preventive strategies. The 25 individual modules cover the body, metabolism, the energy nutrients, vitamins and minerals, fitness, diet choices, medical concerns, life span, health promotion and more.

STUDENT STUDY GUIDE

This study aid is designed to reinforce the key concepts that are presented in the text and to prepare students for exams. The study guide is three-hole punched and perforated, and makes a handy, easy-to-carry review tool!

This Study Guide includes material on both normal and clinical nutrition. The material in chapters 15–30 of the Study Guide match this text exactly.

The Student Study Guide contains:

Chapter Objectives define the essential concepts for each chapter.

Assignments provide study questions, terms to be defined, short answer questions, and problems to solve.

Sample Test Questions offer multiple-choice questions similar to questions instructors are likely to ask on exams.

Nursing Exam Review Questions (for chapters 15–17 and 21–30) review questions to help students prepare for the NCLEX-RN.

Discussions of Clinical Application Questions and Case Studies encourage students to apply knowledge gained from each chapter to hypothetical situations.

Answers to the chapter study questions, problems, and short-answer, sample test, and nursing exam review questions are found at the end of each chapter.

For the Instructor

- ACETATE OVERHEADS *or* ELECTRONIC OVERHEADS* include figures from the text along with enrichments from other sources.

- SOFTWARE includes Computerized Testing* and complimentary Diet Analysis Plus version 3.0 (Windows, DOS, or MAC). See "For the Student".

- INSTRUCTOR'S MANUAL WITH TEST BANK

- CNN/WEST NUTRITION CHRONOLOG QUARTERLY* (exclusive to West/Wadsworth) updates viewers four times per year on important issues in the nutrition field. Each video presents the best of CNN's broadcast coverage which ties into issues and concepts being explored in today's nutrition classrooms.

- NUTRITION VIDEO LIBRARY* includes selected videos on topics such as eating disorders, digestion, metabolism, and more!

- NUTRITION RESOURCE CENTER links you to other nutrition resources via www.wadsworth. com/nutrition

*Please check with your local ITP representative for qualification details.

Acknowledgments

To produce a book requires the coordinated efforts of a team of people—and, no doubt, each team member has another team of support people as well. We salute, with a big round of applause, everyone who has worked so diligently to ensure the quality of this book.

We thank Yvonne Jones for her valuable contributions to the hunger highlight and Margaret Hedley for her assistance in keeping the Canadian information current. A million thank yous to Sally Mayo for her patient attention to manuscript preparation and a multitude of other daily tasks. Thanks also to Laura Perkinson for her help in securing permissions. We also thank the many people who have prepared the ancillaries that accompany this text: Harry Sitren and Melaney Jones for writing and enhancing the Test Bank; Lori Turner, Melaney Jones, and Margaret Hedley for preparing the Instructor's Manual; and Lori Turner and Jana Kicklighter for preparing the Student Study Guide. A big thank you to Elizabeth Hands, Bob Geltz, and their staff at ESHA for their meticulous work in creating the food composition appendix, verifying the data in figures and tables, and developing the computerized data analysis program that accompanies this book. Our special thanks to the editorial team of Peter Marshall, Becky Tollerson, Jane Bass, Laura Perkinson, Sandra Craig, and Dusty Davidson for their conscientious coordination of reviews and production. We also thank John Woolsey and his associates for creating accurate and attractive artwork to complement our writing; Michael Davidson for transforming nutrients into outstanding works of art that grace the cover and chapter opening pages; Tom Harm and Tom Peterson for photographing foods beautifully; and Pat Lewis for copyediting thousands of pages of manuscript. To the many others involved in designing, indexing, typesetting, dummying, and marketing, we tip our hats in appreciation.

We are especially grateful to our associates, friends, and families for their continued encouragement and support. We also thank our many reviewers for their comments and contributions.

We hope our informal, conversational writing style makes the study of nutrition an enjoyable experience. Nutrition is a fascinating subject, and we hope our enthusiasm for it comes through on every page.

Corinne Balog Cataldo
Sharon Rady Rolfes
Eleanor Noss Whitney
August 1997

Reviewers of Understanding Clinical Nutrition

Sara Long Anderson,
Southern Illinois University at Carbondale

Wayne Billon,
University of Southern Mississippi

M. Brian-Keber,
University of San Francisco

Eileen Monahan Chopnick,
Widener University School of Nursing

Beth Clark,
University of Maine at Augusta

Colleen Duggan,
Johnson Community College

Carmen Edwards,
Midland College

Amelia C. Finan,
Anne Arundel Community College

Denise T. Garner,
York College of Pennsylvania

Judith Harr,
University of San Francisco

Irene Langille,
Southern Alberta Institute of Technology

Dawna Torres Mughal,
Gannon University

Amy R. Pemberton,
Lamar University

Tonia Reinhard,
Wayne State University

Marilyn Tapia,
Montana State University at Billings

Connie B. Till,
Orangeburg-Calhoun Technical College

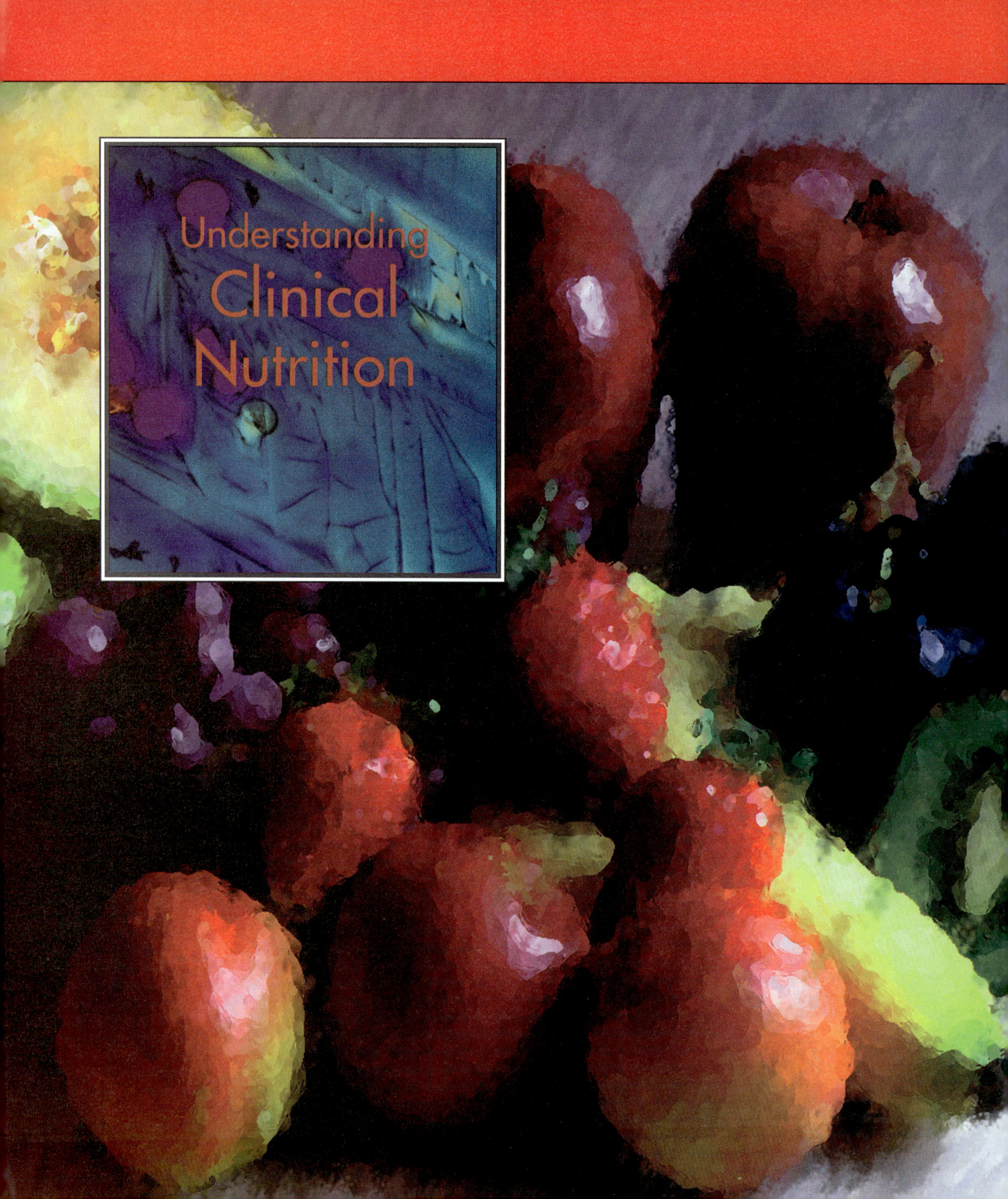
Understanding
Clinical
Nutrition

Chapter 15

The Nutrition Care Process: Assessing Historical and Physical Data

CONTENTS

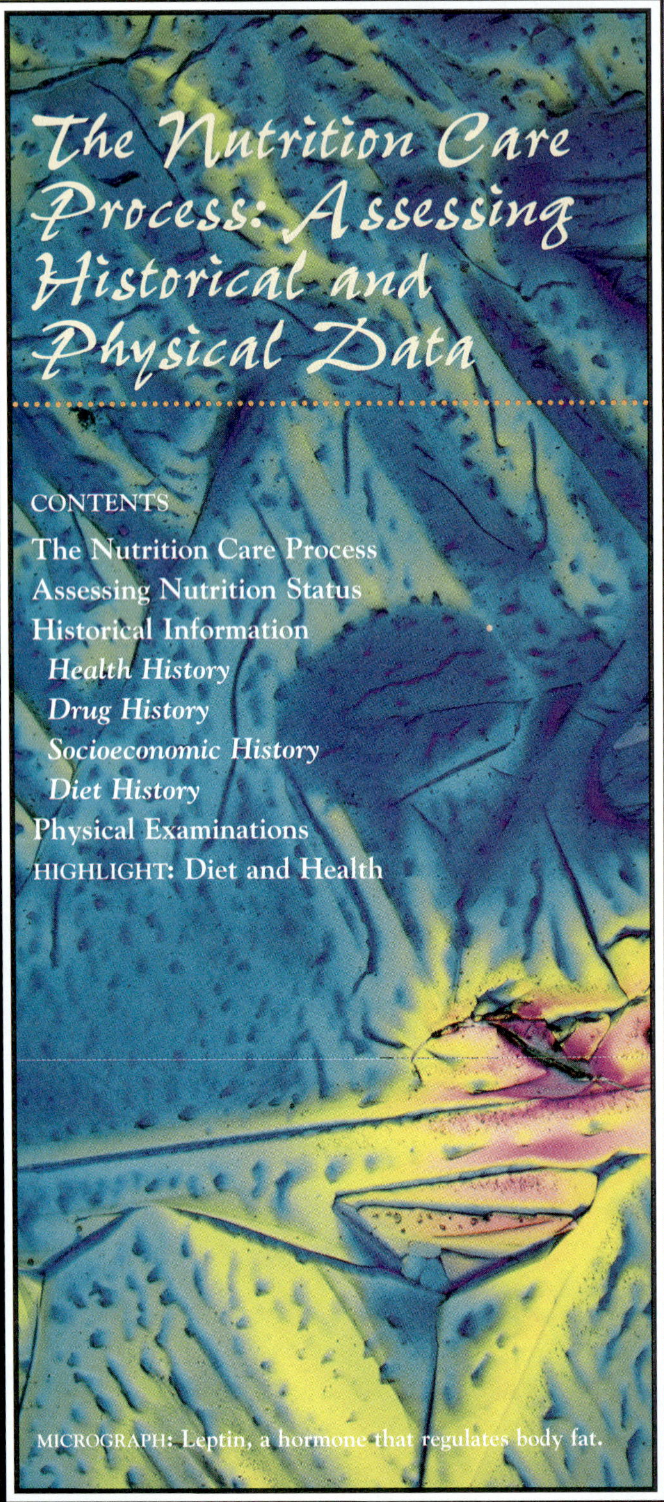

MICROGRAPH: Leptin, a hormone that regulates body fat.

The earlier chapters of this book have shown how a physically fit body and an alert mind depend on good nutrition. Turning now to clinical nutrition, the remaining chapters show how poor nutrition can accelerate the development of certain degenerative diseases and how nutrition therapy can improve the quality of life for people who have become ill.

Health care professionals who recognize the indispensable roles nutrition plays in supporting health make a conscientious effort to think "nutrition." They bridge the gap between knowledge and action by carefully identifying nutrition needs and developing realistic plans of action. This chapter defines the nutrition care process, emphasizing the use of histories and physical examinations in assessing nutrition status. The next chapter shows how anthropometric and biochemical findings complete the assessment process and explains how assessment data then provide the foundation upon which to build nutrition care plans.

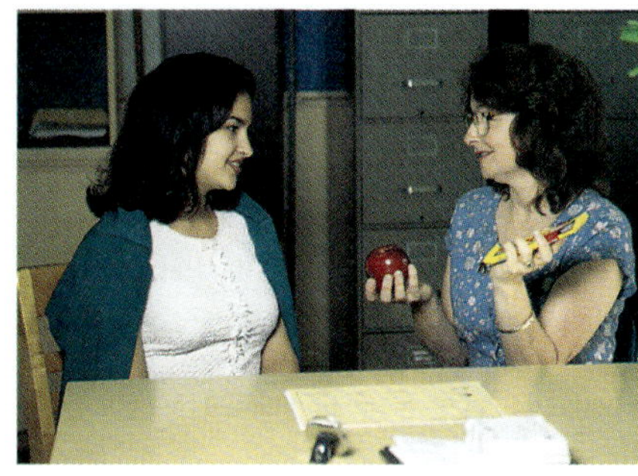

Health care professionals develop nutrition care plans to meet clients' nutrition and nutrition education needs.

The Nutrition Care Process

The nutrition care process is a systematic and logical approach used to identify and meet each person's nutrient and nutrition education needs. Appropriate medical nutrition therapy and skillful communication are two complementary parts of effective nutrition care.

The nutrition care process consists of five steps:

1. Assess nutrition status.
2. Analyze assessment data to determine nutrient requirements.
3. Develop a plan of action for meeting nutrition needs, including client education.
4. Implement the nutrition care plan.
5. Evaluate the effectiveness of the nutrition care plan through ongoing assessment and make changes as needed.

The dietitian has the primary responsibility for assessing nutrition status and developing and implementing nutrition care plans. The physician, nurse, dietetic technician, social worker, pharmacist, physical therapist, and occupational therapist also make valuable contributions (see Highlight 17). To the extent that all of these people apply their nutrition knowledge, technical skills, and interpersonal skills, the care plan will be realistic and attainable.

To ensure the success of the nutrition care process, health care professionals should make sure that, whenever possible, the client is an active participant in the process. In cases where active participation is not possible, such as for infants and young children, people who are very ill or unconscious, people with mental disabilities, or people who are uncooperative, health care professionals can enlist the involvement of family members or other support people.

nutrition care process: an organized approach to nutrition intervention that consists of five steps (assessing, analyzing, planning, implementing, and evaluating). The nutrition care process parallels the *nursing care process* except that it focuses on nutrition concerns.

medical nutrition therapy: a term introduced by the American Dietetic Association in 1994 to emphasize the role of nutrition in medical care. In this book, the terms *medical nutrition therapy* and *diet therapy* are used interchangeably.

nutrition care plan: a plan that translates nutrition assessment data into a strategy for meeting a client's nutrient and nutrition education needs.

Health care professionals use the nutrition care process to systematically assess, analyze, plan, implement. and evaluate their clients' nutrition and nutrition education needs. The contributions of all members of the health care team enhance the accuracy and effectiveness of the nutrition care plan.

health care team: a group of professionals representing several disciplines who work together to resolve their clients' medical problems; see Highlight 17.

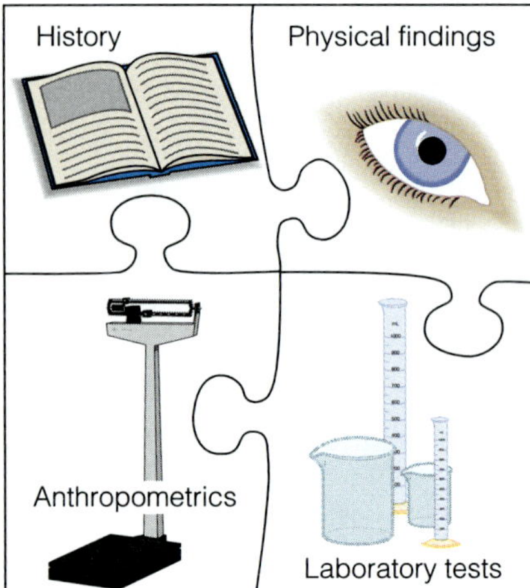

Taken as a whole, the information gathered during a nutrition assessment helps define a person's nutrition status.

nutrition assessment: the evaluation of many factors that influence or reflect nutritional health; the tools used for nutrition assessment include historical information, physical examinations, anthropometric findings, and biochemical analyses.

Nurses and registered dietetic technicians are the professionals who most often assist dietitians in completing nutrition assessments.

Assessing Nutrition Status

Nutrition assessment provides the information needed to determine how well a client's nutrient needs are being met. From the information, the assessor can develop a plan of action to prevent or correct any imbalances. The assessor, usually a registered dietitian assisted by other qualified health care professionals, relies on many sources of data including:

- Historical information.
- Physical examinations.
- Anthropometric data.
- Biochemical analyses (laboratory tests).

By accurately gathering this information and carefully interpreting each finding in relation to the others, the assessor obtains the basis for a meaningful evaluation. Assessors frequently use computer programs to perform many of the mathematical calculations required and to check the results against standards.

The following sections describe many techniques for assessing nutrition status. Using every technique for each assessment is not practical or necessary. Instead, health care professionals determine which techniques to use for different clients and different situations. Chapter 16 provides more information about screening clients for risk factors that suggest the need for a complete nutrition assessment.

A thorough nutrition assessment provides the basis for a nutrition care plan. This chapter and the next emphasize the four components of nutrition assessments: histories, physical examinations, anthropometric data, and biochemical analyses.

Historical Information

Table 15–1 sums up the types of historical data that may provide clues to nutrition status. Form 15–1 shows the data typically collected in recording a client's history. A thorough history alerts the assessor to potential problems that can be further investigated using other assessment techniques.

Table 15–1

Historical Data Used in Nutrition Assessments

Type of History	What It Identifies
Health history	Health factors that affect nutrition status
Drug history	Medications and nutrient supplements that affect nutrition status
Socioeconomic history	Personal, financial, and environmental influences on food intake, nutrient needs, and diet therapy options
Diet history	Nutrient intake excesses or deficiencies and the reasons for imbalances

Form 15–1 Historical Data

Name____________________ Date ____________________
Address____________________ Date of last medical checkup ____________________
____________________ Age __________ Sex __________
____________________ Height __________ Weight __________
Phone____________________ Usual weight ____________________
Reason for admission____________________ Desirable weight range ____________________
____

Health History

1. Have you been told that you have (check any that apply):
   - ☐ Diabetes
   - ☐ GI disorders
   - ☐ High blood pressure
   - ☐ Hardening of arteries
   - ☐ Heart disease
   - ☐ Lung disease
   - ☐ Kidney disease
   - ☐ Liver disease
   - ☐ Ulcers
   - ☐ Cancer
   - ☐ Other ____________________
2. Do you have complaints about any of the following:
   - ☐ Lack of appetite
   - ☐ Difficulty chewing or swallowing
   - ☐ Constipation
   - ☐ Diarrhea
   - ☐ Indigestion
   - ☐ Fever
   - ☐ Nausea
   - ☐ Vomiting
   - ☐ Other
3. Do you use tobacco in any way?____ How much?____________________
4. For females:
   Are you pregnant?__________ How many months?__________
   How many pregnancies have you carried to term? __________
   When was your last child born? __________
   Are your menstrual periods normal? _____If not, please explain: ____________________

Drug History

1. Do you take medication, either prescribed by a doctor or over-the-counter?

Name of drug	Reason for taking	Dose	Frequency	Duration of intake
__________	__________	__________	__________	__________
__________	__________	__________	__________	__________
__________	__________	__________	__________	__________

2. Have you noticed any side effects from taking these medications?_____ If so, please explain: ____________________
3. Do you take vitamins or any kind of supplements?_____ Which ones? ____________________
   How often? __________For what reason? ____________________

Socioeconomic History

1. Last grade of school completed __________Still in school?__________
2. Are you employed? _____Occupation ____________________
3. Does someone else live with you?_____ Who? ____________________
4. Do you regularly eat alone or with others?____________________
5. Do you have a refrigerator?__________Stove?__________
6. How often do you shop for food?__________ Where? __________

Diet History

1. Have you recently lost or gained more than 10 lb? ________ If yes, explain the surrounding circumstances (including associated illness, dietary changes, and time frame): ____________________
2. Do you eat at regular times each day? ________ How many times per day? ____________________
3. Where do you eat most of your meals? ____________________
4. Do you usually eat snacks? ________When? ____________________
5. What foods do you particularly like? ____________________
6. Are there foods you don't eat for other reasons? ____________________
7. Do you have difficulty eating? ____________________
8. How would you describe your feelings about food? ____________________
9. Do your eating habits change when you are emotionally upset? ____________________ How? ________
10. Are you, or any member of your family, on a special diet? _____ If yes, who and what kind? ____________________
11. Do you drink alcohol? __________ How much? __________ How often? __________
12. How would you describe your exercise habits?__________ Type of exercise __________
    Intensity__________ Duration __________Frequency __________
13. Are there any other facts about your lifestyle that you think might be related to your nutritional health? __________
    Explain ____________________

Note: Use the appropriate form to record food intake data (Forms 15–2 and 15–3).

How to Conduct Successful Interviews

To solicit accurate and reliable information from clients, the successful interviewer respects, and shows genuine concern for, the individual. Techniques to help clients feel comfortable and communicate openly and freely include:

- Each time you visit a client, introduce yourself, verify the client's name, and explain the purpose of your visit. In so doing, you confirm that you are talking with the right person, you set the tone for the discussion, and you let the person know who you are and what to expect.
- Arrange for privacy and reassure the client that all the information provided will be treated confidentially.
- Be sure that the client is comfortable and that the physical environment is conducive to an interview. If the client is in pain or is tired, it may be best to arrange another time for the interview. To facilitate communication, you might modify the physical environment by, for example, adjusting the lighting, turning off the television, changing the temperature in the room, providing a glass of water, or repositioning the client.
- Position yourself so that you are comfortable and can maintain eye contact. To do so, you may have to sit down. If you are uncomfortable or if you stand while the client sits or lies in bed, you may nonverbally communicate an unfriendly, overpowering, or hurried feeling.
- Allow adequate time for the interview. Hurrying through an interview conveys to the client that your discussion is not very important and that you really do not care enough to get all the facts.
- Allow others to be themselves. In other words, accept and value people for who and what they are. If an interviewer reacts with advice, criti-

An adept history taker uses the interview not only to gather facts, but also to establish rapport with the client and to assess motivation, education, and ability level. Interviewers who establish a caring and trusting relationship while they gather information are best equipped to deliver effective care. The interviewer must obtain personal facts and information about lifelong habits that are influenced by complex medical, social, cultural, psychological, religious, and economic factors. No one would share this much without trusting that the interviewer truly cared and would accept the information, whatever it might be. The accompanying box provides pointers for conducting successful interviews.

health history: an account of the client's current and past health status and risk factors for disease. Traditionally, the health history has been called the *medical history*. The term *health history* now seems more appropriate, however, since the contents describe the client's health status, and current trends in the medical profession now emphasize health promotion and disease prevention.

HEALTH HISTORY

Physical and mental health both affect and reflect nutrition status; the history taker makes note of all conditions that increase the risk of malnutrition (see Table 15–2). Figure 15–1 on p. 525 illustrates some of the relationships between illness and nutrition.

An assessor is wise to review the client's health, or medical, history before visiting the client. During the interview, the assessor can then keep in mind the factors that may affect the person's nutrition status. Conversations with the client cism, or judgment, the client may withhold important information, not wanting to risk belittlement. To avoid such pitfalls, use open-ended questions, which allow a wide choice of answers. In contrast, closed-ended questions narrowly limit a client's responses. For example, if you ask a client if she prefers orange juice or tomato juice, you aren't giving her an opportunity to say she'd really rather have grapefruit juice or a slice of melon.

- Be an active listener. Let the client do most of the talking and control the direction of the conversation. Don't interrupt the person's thoughts. Try not to follow a set guide for asking important questions; rather, use forms as guides, and ask questions based on the client's responses.
- Avoid giving diet advice when seeking information. If a person tells you he eats a candy bar for breakfast, and you react with advice about better choices for breakfast, the client may be hesitant to tell you he eats two more candy bars before going to bed. Reserve nutrition education sessions for a later time.
- Regularly provide the client with feedback to make sure you understand each other correctly. Repeat key phrases and ask for further information when clarity is needed.
- Prior to ending an interview, let the client know what to expect next. For example, "I'll come back tomorrow to talk with you about your eating plan."

While interviews serve as a tool for gathering information, they also provide an opportunity for establishing a relationship with the client. That relationship will influence all future communications with the client.

Open-versus closed-ended questions:
- *Open-ended:* What is the first time you usually eat during the day?
- *Closed-ended:* What do you usually eat for breakfast?
- *Open-ended:* What foods do you usually eat at that time?
- *Closed-ended:* Do you usually have cereal or eggs for breakfast?

can also uncover valuable health-related information that might otherwise be overlooked because no one thought to ask.

Appetite and Food Intake Loss of appetite commonly accompanies illness. A child with a fever frequently is unable to eat; so is an adult with cancer. Nausea, mouth dryness, problems with chewing or swallowing, and obstructions in the digestive tract can all lead to malnutrition.

The secondary effects of illness can also affect nutrient intake. Pain and anxiety associated with illness can make it difficult or impossible to eat; pain in the mouth or throat is especially problematic. Anxiety stimulates stress hormone activity and suppresses digestive activity, making clients lose their appetites. Medical treatments and procedures may require that a person not eat at the very time when nutrient needs are especially high due to illness.

Digestion and Absorption Illnesses that interfere with digestion or absorption usually affect several nutrients and can cause nutrition status to deteriorate rapidly. Examples include cystic fibrosis, pancreatitis, and inflammatory bowel diseases. (Chapter 22 describes these disorders in more detail.)

Table 15–2

Health Factors That Can Affect or Reflect Nutrition Status

- Acquired immune deficiency syndrome (AIDS)
- Alcoholism
- Alzheimer's disease
- Anorexia (lack of appetite)
- Anorexia nervosa
- Bulimia
- Cancer
- Chewing or swallowing difficulties (including poorly fitted dentures, dental caries, missing teeth, and mouth ulcers)
- Chronic obstructive pulmonary disease
- Circulatory problems
- Constipation
- Crohn's disease
- Decubitus ulcers
- Dementia
- Depleted blood proteins
- Diabetes mellitus
- Diarrhea
- Diseases of the GI tract
- Drug addiction
- Dysphagia
- Failure to thrive
- Fever
- Heart disease
- HIV infection
- Hormonal imbalance
- Hyperlipidemia
- Hypertension
- Infection
- Kidney disease
- Liver disease
- Lung disease
- Malabsorption
- Mental illness
- Mental retardation
- Multiple pregnancies
- Nausea
- Neurologic disorders
- Organ failure
- Overweight
- Pancreatic insufficiency
- Paralysis
- Physical disability
- Pneumonia
- Pregnancy
- Radiation therapy
- Recent major illness
- Recent major surgery
- Recent weight loss or gain
- Surgery of the GI tract
- Tobacco use
- Trauma
- Ulcerative colitis
- Ulcers
- Underweight
- Vomiting

Metabolism Illnesses can directly alter metabolism (Chapters 25 and 30) and change nutrient needs. They can also alter organ function and thereby alter metabolism indirectly; examples are liver disease (Chapter 26), diabetes (Chapter 27), renal failure (Chapter 29), cancer (Chapter 30), and AIDS (also in Chapter 30).

Excretion Illnesses can also interfere with the excretion of nutrients. The result can be either excessive retention of nutrients, as in renal failure (Chapter 29), or excessive loss of nutrients, as in diarrhea (Chapter 22) or nephrotic syndrome (Chapter 29).

Highlight 7 describes nutrition concerns associated with alcohol abuse (one type of substance abuse), and Highlight 9 explores eating disorders and their nutrition consequences.

Emotional and Mental Health Emotional and nutritional health go together. Emotionally healthy people have the capacity to feed themselves well. Well-nourished people experience none of the nutrient deficiencies that might impair mental health. Malnourished people, on the other hand, may suffer the mental symptoms of nutrient deficiencies. People with B vitamin deficiencies, for example, often exhibit "mental" symptoms ranging from confusion, apathy, fatigue, and irritability to delirium and psychoses.

The effects of mental illnesses on nutrition status may be less readily apparent than those of physiological illnesses, but are no less important. Mental illnesses frequently alter emotional health and may lead to anxiety, depression, and severe mood swings, which, in turn, impair nutritional health. People with mental illnesses characterized by illogical thinking or dementia may have little interest in food or may be unable to make appropriate food choices. Those who are paranoid may believe that foods are being used to poison them. People suffering from

Figure 15–1

Relationships between Illness and Nutrition
(Nutrition for people with cancer is discussed in Chapter 30.)

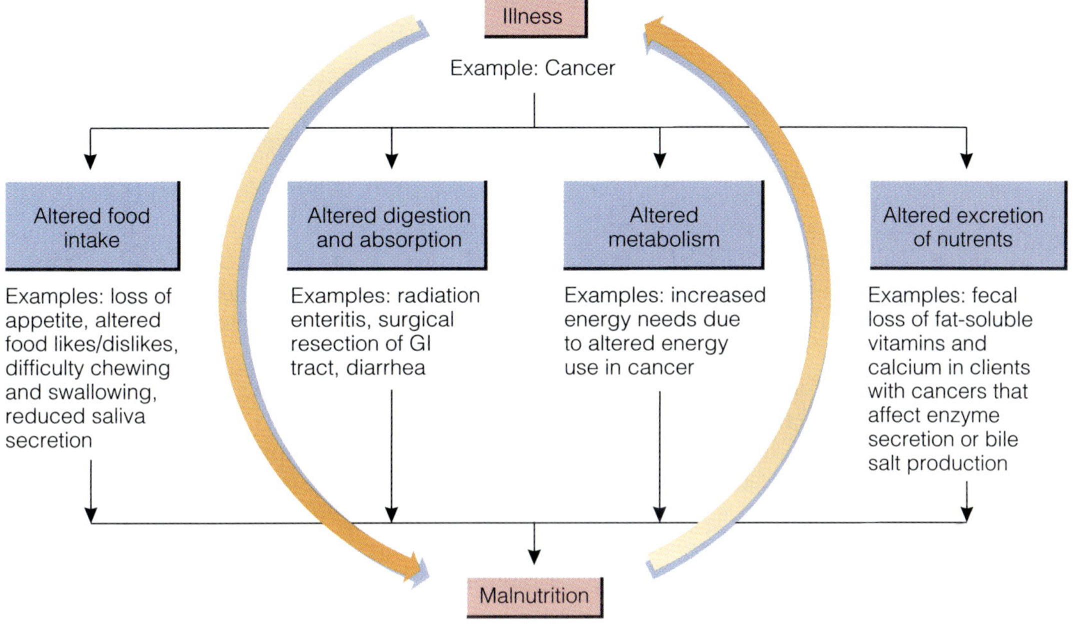

delusions may attribute magical powers to certain foods and insist on eating only those foods. Drugs used to treat mental illnesses can also affect nutrition status. (Drug interactions are described later in this chapter.)

To reflect on the interrelationships between mental, emotional, and nutritional health, consider a typical scenario of an elderly woman who lives alone. Over the years she may have become increasingly isolated from family and friends. As her loneliness progresses, she may become depressed and begin to eat less. Her malnutrition worsens the apathy she feels from the loneliness. Consequently, she has even less energy with which to feed herself. Watch for such a downward spiral in all people who are lonely, especially the elderly or those who have recently lost a loved one.

DRUG HISTORY

Medical drugs are often involved in the treatment of illness, and nearly every drug affects nutrition status to some degree. Therefore, obtaining a drug history is an important part of the assessment process. All medications are of interest: prescription drugs, nonprescription or over-the-counter (OTC) drugs, illicit drugs, and even nutrient supplements. If a person is taking any medication routinely, the assessor records the name of the medication or supplement with the dose, frequency, and duration of intake; the reason for taking the medication; and signs of any adverse or positive effects (see Form 15–1).

drug history: a record of all the medications, over-the-counter and prescribed, that a person takes routinely.

The trend toward making formerly prescription drugs available over-the-counter underscores the need to ask clients about all nonprescription medications they may be taking.

Hundreds of medications and nutrients interact, which can lead to imbalances or interfere with drug effectiveness.[1] This discussion focuses on medical drugs. Adverse drug-nutrient interactions are most likely to occur if medications

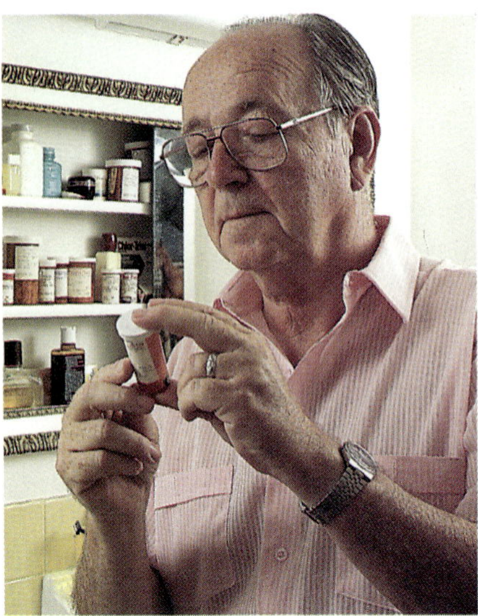

Taking several medications over long periods intensifies the risk of drug-nutrient interactions.

are taken over long periods, if several medications are taken, or if nutrition status is poor or deteriorating. Understandably, then, elderly people with chronic diseases and people with illnesses that dramatically raise nutrient needs are most at risk. Studies of institutionalized elderly people suggest that multiple medication use may significantly affect nutrition status in this population.[2]

Nutrients and medications may interact in many ways:

- Medications can alter food intake and the absorption, metabolism, and excretion of nutrients.
- Foods and nutrients can alter the absorption, metabolism, and excretion of medications.

Table 15–3 lists the general classes of medications notable for their interactions with nutrients. The following sections describe these interactions, and Table 15–4 summarizes this information and provides specific examples. Table E–1 in Appendix E provides details on specific interactions, drug by drug.

Medications and Food Intake Many medications can lead to malnutrition by interfering with food intake. Amphetamines used to treat hyperactivity in children provide an example: they may effectively improve behavior, but they also suppress appetite, alter taste perceptions, dry the mouth, and cause nausea. Conversely, some medications stimulate the appetite and lead to undesirable weight gain. An example is astemizole (Hismanal), an antihistamine used by some people to relieve allergy symptoms.

Absorption and Medications Laxatives provide an example of how medications can interfere with nutrient absorption. Laxatives cause foods to move so rapidly through the intestine that many vitamins do not have enough time to be absorbed. The use of mineral oil as a laxative robs the person of the fat-soluble vitamins, notably vitamin D. The vitamins from foods dissolve in the indigestible oil and are excreted; calcium, too, is excreted. A person who uses laxatives daily for a long time may find that the intestines can no longer function without them. This dependence can lead to malnutrition.

Table 15–3

Classes of Medications That Can Affect Nutrition Status

- Amphetamines and other stimulants
- Analgesics
- Antacids
- Antibiotics
- Anticonvulsants
- Antidepressants
- Antidiabetic agents
- Antidiarrheals
- Antihyperlipemics
- Antihypertensives
- Antineoplastics
- Antiulcer agents
- Catabolic steroids
- Diuretics
- Hormonal agents
- Immunosuppressive agents
- Laxatives
- Oral contraceptives
- Vitamin and other nutrient preparations

Note: Specific examples, drug by drug, appear in Appendix E, Table E–1.

Table 15–4

Mechanisms and Examples of Food-Medication Interactions

Drugs Can Alter Food Intake by:

- Altering the appetite (amphetamines suppress the appetite).
- Interfering with taste or smell (methotrexate changes taste perceptions).
- Inducing nausea or vomiting (digitalis can do both).
- Changing the oral environment (phenobarbital can cause dry mouth).
- Irritating the GI tract (cyclophosphamide induces mucosal ulcers).
- Causing sores or inflammation of the mouth (methotrexate can cause painful mouth ulcers).

Drugs Can Alter Nutrient Absorption by:

- Changing the acidity of the digestive tract (antacids can interfere with iron absorption).
- Altering digestive juices (cimetidine can improve fat absorption).
- Altering motility of the digestive tract (laxatives speed motility, causing the malabsorption of many nutrients).
- Inactivating enzyme systems (neomycin may reduce lipase activity).
- Damaging mucosal cells (chemotherapy can damage mucosal cells).
- Binding to nutrients (some antacids bind phosphorus).

Foods Can Alter Drug Absorption by:

- Changing the acidity of the digestive tract (candy can change the acidity, thereby causing slow-acting asthma medication to dissolve too quickly).
- Stimulating secretion of digestive juices (griseofulvin is absorbed better when taken with foods that stimulate the release of digestive enzymes).
- Altering rate of absorption (aspirin is absorbed more slowly when taken with food).
- Binding to drugs (calcium binds to tetracycline, limiting drug absorption).
- Competing for absorption sites in the intestines (dietary amino acids interfere with levodopa absorption this way).

Drugs and Nutrients Can Interact and Alter Metabolism by:

- Acting as structural analogs (as anticoagulants and vitamin K do).
- Competing with each other for metabolic enzyme systems (as phenobarbitol and folate do).
- Altering enzyme activity and contributing pharmacologically active substances (as monoamine oxidase inhibitors and tyramine do).

Drugs Can Alter Nutrient Excretion by:

- Altering reabsorption in the kidneys (some diuretics increase the excretion of sodium and potassium).
- Displacing nutrients from their plasma protein carriers (aspirin displaces folate).

Foods Can Alter Drug Excretion by:

- Changing the acidity of the urine (vitamin C can alter urinary pH and limit the excretion of aspirin).

A classic example of how foods can interfere with medication absorption is the interaction between the antibiotic tetracycline and the minerals calcium and iron. When calcium and tetracycline, or iron and tetracycline, are taken at the same time, they bind to each other, thus reducing the absorption of both. Clients are therefore instructed not to take tetracycline with milk, milk products, or calcium-containing antacids (such as Tums). Similarly, clients must take their iron supplements two hours apart from their tetracycline doses.

Another example is the interaction between acidic foods and the nicotine gum that is used to help people quit smoking cigarettes. Certain acid-containing foods and beverages interfere with the absorption of nicotine through the lining of the mouth into the blood. For maximum effectiveness, people should refrain from ingesting foods and beverages for 15 minutes before, and while, chewing the gum. When a food or beverage blocks nicotine's absorption from the mouth, the person swallows the nicotine, and this may cause nausea and hiccups as well as interfere with the drug's effectiveness.

Some medications are absorbed better with foods than without them. For this reason, the antifungal drug griseofulvin is always given with meals. In many cases, though, foods delay the rate at which medications are absorbed. In some instances this, too, can be helpful. An aspirin taken on an empty stomach works faster than when it is given with food, but because aspirin can irritate the GI tract, taking it with food can reduce nausea.

Metabolism and Medications To appreciate how drug-nutrient interactions can affect metabolism, consider medications that resemble vitamins in structure. Vitamin K and the anticlotting medication warfarin (Coumadin) provide an example. Warfarin opposes clotting by interfering with vitamin K. To be clinically effective, the warfarin dose must be large enough to counteract whatever vitamin K is in the person's diet. If a person's vitamin K intake increases, as it may in summer when lettuces and greens are in season, then the physician has to increase the medication dose. Another example is methotrexate, which is used to treat certain cancers and rheumatoid arthritis; methotrexate is structurally similar to folate and can cause severe folate deficiencies (see Figure 15–2).

Aspirin can also alter folate metabolism but in a different way. Aspirin competes with folate for its protein carrier, thus hindering the body's use of the vitamin. When aspirin is used over long periods of time, health care professionals should ensure that either the diet or supplements supply sufficient folate to meet the added demands.

The effects of tyramine provide another example of a substance in foods that alters a medication's action. Tyramine is a substance found in some foods, and it interacts with monoamine oxidase inhibitors (MAO inhibitors), which are prescribed to treat certain forms of severe depression. Normally, a certain enzyme in the brain inactivates tyramine, but the MAO inhibitors block the action of that enzyme. When people take the medication, the enzyme fails to act. Thus tyramine remains active and stimulates the release of the neurotransmitter norepi-

Figure 15–2

Folate and Methotrexate

Methotrexate (an antineoplastic drug) is structurally similar to the vitamin folate. When this medication is used, it competes for the enzyme that normally activates folate, creating a secondary deficiency of folate.

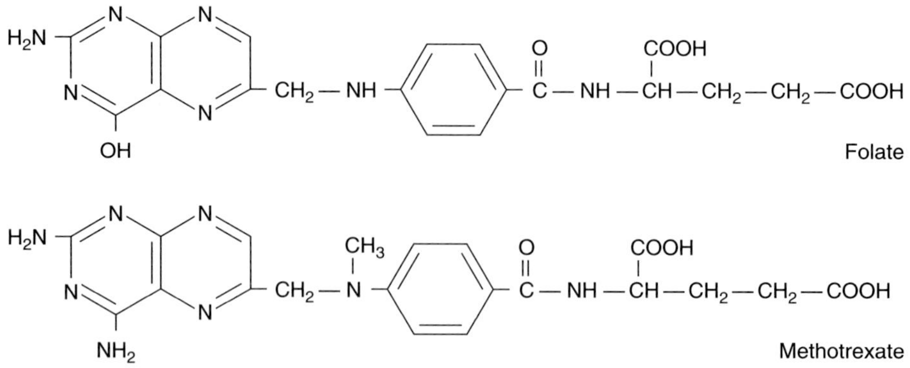

Folate

Methotrexate

nephrine. This action can lead to severe hypertension and headaches. If blood pressure rises high enough, it can be fatal. For this reason, people taking MAO inhibitors must restrict their intakes of foods rich in tyramine (see Table 15–5).

Excretion and Medications Urinary acidity affects drug reabsorption from the kidneys back into the blood. An acidic urine limits the excretion of acidic drugs like aspirin. Large doses of vitamin C given with aspirin increase the urine's acidity, and aspirin remains in the blood longer.

Medications can also alter urinary excretion of nutrients. For example, some diuretics accelerate the excretion of the minerals calcium, potassium, magnesium, and zinc.

Other Ingredients in Medications Besides the active ingredients, medications may contain other substances such as sugar, sorbitol, sodium, alcohol, and caffeine. For most people who use medications on occasion and in small amounts, such ingredients pose no problem. When medications are taken regularly or in large doses, however, people on special diets may need to be aware of these additional ingredients and their effects.

Many liquid preparations contain sugar or sorbitol to make them taste better. For people who must regulate their intakes of simple sugars, such as people with diabetes, the amount of sugar in medications must be considered. Large doses of liquids containing sorbitol may result in diarrhea.

Antibiotics and antacids often contain sodium. People who take Alka Seltzer may not realize that a single 2-tablet dose may exceed their safe sodium intakes for a whole day. Another antacid (Tums) contains a considerable amount of cal-

Table 15–5

Foods Restricted in a Tyramine-Controlled Diet

Beverages:	Red wines including chianti, sherry[a]
Cheeses:	Aged cheeses, American, camembert, cheddar, gouda, gruyère, mozzarella, parmesan, provolone, romano, roquefort, stilton[b]
Meats:	Liver; dried, salted, smoked, or pickled fish; sausage; pepperoni; salami; dried meats
Vegetables:	Fava beans; Italian broad beans; sauerkraut; snow peas; fermented pickles and olives
Other:	Brewer's yeast;[c] all aged and fermented products; soy sauce in large amounts; cheese-filled breads, crackers, and desserts; salad dressings containing cheese

Note: The tyramine contents of foods vary from product to product depending on the methods used to prepare, process, and store the food. In some cases, as little as 1 ounce of cheese can cause a severe hypertensive reaction in people taking monoamine oxidase inhibitors. In general, the following foods contain small enough amounts of tyramine that they can be consumed in small quantities: ripe avocado, banana, yogurt, sour cream, acidophilus milk, buttermilk, raspberries, and peanuts.

[a]Most wine and domestic beer can be consumed in small quantities.

[b]Unfermented cheeses, such as ricotta, cottage cheese, and cream cheese, are allowed.

[c]Products made with baker's yeast are allowed.

cium. Although Tums are sometimes recommended as a calcium supplement, they are less than ideal for this purpose. For one, the form of calcium in Tums is poorly absorbed. For another, antacids neutralize stomach acid, on which the absorption of many nutrients (possibly including calcium itself) depends. Taking any antacid regularly will reduce the absorption of many nutrients.

Medications given by vein provide water and frequently provide sodium, potassium, and other electrolytes, or dextrose (a form of sugar). Assessors must consider these contributions when clients' diets must be modified in any of these nutrients. Administering medications through a feeding tube requires additional precautions (see Chapter 23).

A Note to Assessors Hundreds of drug-nutrient interactions have been identified, and information continues to accumulate. It would be difficult, if not impossible, to remember all the potential effects of drug-nutrient interactions on nutrition status. Instead, assessors serve their clients best if they:

- Keep in mind that drug-nutrient interactions can and do occur, especially when the medication use is long term.
- Record the complete drug and diet histories of clients; review these histories with potential interactions in mind. Keep a reference handy, such as Table E–1 in Appendix E, and check it frequently.
- Be aware of groups of people who are likely to develop drug-related nutrient deficiencies, and be prepared to look up the nutrition effects of medications these clients are taking.
- Reassess nutrition status frequently for high-risk clients.
- Become familiar with the nutrient interactions of the medications commonly used to treat the disorders of their clients. For example, nurses working with people who have heart disease should become familiar with the nutrition effects of medications used to treat that condition.

socioeconomic history: a record of a person's social and economic background, including such factors as education, income, and ethnic identity.

SOCIOECONOMIC HISTORY

Socioeconomic factors can profoundly affect nutrition status and food choices (see Table 15–6 and Form 15–1). Age affects both nutrient requirements and food choices (see Chapters 18–20). Infants and children depend on caregivers to provide nutritious and acceptable foods; so do adults who are unable to care for themselves. Therefore, assessors must sometimes evaluate caregivers as well as clients.

A person's occupation provides clues to the person's education and income. It can also reveal certain eating habits and physical activity levels. One job, for example, may entail desk work and eating out; another may require vigorous physical activity and only a short lunch break.

The ethnic background, religious affiliation, and educational level of both the client and the other members of the household often influence food availability and food choices. These factors also suggest how the interviewer should word questions, interpret answers, and plan for nutrition education. The community environment may also influence the client's nutrition status. The interviewer should be familiar with the food habits of the major ethnic and religious groups within the locale, regional food preferences, local crops, and nutrition resources

Table 15–6

Socioeconomic Factors That Can Affect Food Choices

- Access to grocery stores
- Activities
- Age
- Education
- Ethnic identity
- Income
- Geographical area
- Kitchen facilities
- Number of people in household
- Occupation
- Religious affiliation

and programs available in the community. Local health departments and social agencies can often provide such information.

Income level also influences the diet. In general, diet quality declines as income falls; an inadequate income puts an adequate diet out of reach. Agencies use poverty indexes to identify people at risk for poor nutrition and to qualify people for government food assistance programs. Highlight 18 addresses additional issues regarding poverty and hunger.

Low income affects not only the power to purchase foods but also the ability to shop for, store, and cook them. A skilled assessor will note whether the person has transportation to a grocery store that sells a sufficient variety of low-cost foods and whether the person has access to a refrigerator and stove.

Table 15–7

Dietary Factors That Can Affect Nutrition Status

- Deficient or excessive food intake
- Frequently eating out
- Intravenous fluids (other than total parenteral nutrition) for 7 or more days
- No intake for 7 or more days
- Omission from diet of any food group (for example, vegetables)
- Poor appetite
- Restrictive or fad diets
- Monotonous diet (lack of variety)

DIET HISTORY

A diet history provides a record of eating habits and food intake and can help identify possible nutrient imbalances (see Table 15–7) and factors that affect food intake. Information about the person's eating habits also provides the background for developing realistic and attainable nutrition goals.

Constructing an accurate diet history requires skill. Eating habits are an important part of lifestyle and often reflect a person's philosophy. The assessor who makes nonjudgmental responses and asks open-ended questions about eating habits and food intake encourages trust and enhances the likelihood of obtaining accurate information.

diet history: a record of eating behaviors and the foods a person eats.

Judgmental versus nonjudgmental responses:

- *Helper:* Do you take any type of vitamin or mineral supplements?
- *Client:* I take a vitamin E capsule and 2 grams of vitamin C every day.
- *Judgmental helper response:* You know, of course, that there is no reason for taking these vitamin supplements.
- *Nonjudgmental helper response:* For what reasons do you take these vitamin supplements?

Form 15–1 (on p. 521) shows questions about eating habits and lifestyle that can clue assessors to possible nutrient imbalances and factors that affect food intake. In addition to determining food habits, assessors can evaluate food intake using various tools such as the 24-hour recall, the usual intake record, the food frequency checklist, the food record, and direct observation of food intake. The assessor relies on clinical judgment to select the best tool or tools to obtain the needed information about nutrient intake or food habits. Each tool depends on an accurate account of portion sizes and food composition.[3] Food models or photos and measuring devices can help clients identify the types of foods and quantities consumed. The assessor also needs to know how the foods are prepared and when they are eaten. In addition to asking about foods, assessors ask about beverage consumption, including beverages containing alcohol or caffeine.

24-Hour Recall The 24-hour recall provides data for one day only and is commonly used in nutrition surveys to obtain estimates of the typical food intakes for a population. For individuals, the assessor uses the 24-hour recall to get an idea of general eating habits and meal times. The assessor asks the client to recount everything eaten or drunk in the past 24 hours or for the previous day. Form 15–2 shows a typical 24-hour recall form.

24-hour recall: a record of foods eaten by a person for one 24-hour period.

An advantage of the 24-hour recall is that it is easy to obtain. It is also more likely to provide accurate data, at least about the past 24 hours, than estimates of average intakes over long periods. It does not, however, provide enough information to allow accurate generalizations about an individual's usual food intake. Only when 24-hour recalls are collected on several nonconsecutive days, including both weekdays and weekend days, is this limitation overcome.

Form 15–2 Food Intake for a 24-Hour Recall or Usual Intake Pattern

Name and address ______________________________ Date __________

____

____

Did or do you take vitamin-mineral supplements? ______________________________

If yes, what kind?______________________________ Dose __________

Please record the type and amount of foods and beverages consumed today. [Or: Please record the types and amounts of foods and beverages you typically consume each day.]

Time of Day	Food	Amount (c, tbs, or piece)	Description (how cooked, how served)

Usual Intake To obtain data about a person's usual intake, an inquiry might begin with "What is the first thing you usually eat or drink during the day?" Similar questions follow until a typical daily intake pattern emerges. This method uses the same form as the 24-hour recall (Form 15–2), and can be useful, especially in verifying food intake when the past 24 hours have been atypical. It also helps the assessor verify ususal eating habits. For example, one person may always eat an afternoon snack; another may never eat breakfast. A person whose intake varies widely from day to day, however, may find it difficult to answer such general questions, and in such a case, another food intake tool should be used to estimate nutrient intake.

food frequency checklist: a checklist of foods on which a person can record the frequency with which he or she eats different types of foods.

Food Frequency Checklist A less common approach is to use a food frequency checklist to ascertain how often an individual eats a specific type of food. This information helps pinpoint food groups, and therefore nutrients, that may be excessive or deficient in the diet. That a person ate no vegetables yesterday may not seem particularly significant, but never eating vegetables is a warning sign of possible nutrient deficiencies. When used with the usual intake or 24-hour recall approach, the food frequency record enables the assessor to double-check the accuracy of the information obtained. Form 15–3 (on pp. 534–535) is a food frequency checklist.

Food Records A food record maintained over several days can be a valuable tool for gathering food intake data. The assessor instructs the person keeping the record to write down all foods and beverages consumed, the time of day, the amounts consumed, and methods of preparation. Often the person must record other information as well, depending on the purpose of the food record. When the purpose of the record is to help a person change eating behaviors and lose weight, the record might also include information about the person's mood, the occasion (party, holiday, family meal), behaviors associated with eating food (watching TV, driving in the car on the way to work, sitting at the table with the family), and physical activity. When the purpose of the food record is to establish blood glucose control (see Chapter 27), records include details of drug administration, physical activity, and the results of blood glucose monitoring. When the purpose of the record is to establish food tolerances (such as the amount of lactose a person can handle), food records also include symptoms associated with eating (for example, cramps, diarrhea, nausea, or hives).

food record: an extensive, accurate log of all foods eaten over a period of several days or weeks.

Food records, when carefully kept, provide an accurate account of food intake, food behaviors, and food tolerances. The assessor can use the record to identify problem food behaviors and find solutions. The record keeper assumes an active role and may learn to take responsibility for personal food choices and eating habits.

Observing Food Intake Direct observation of clients' food intakes is possible in health care facilities such as hospitals or nursing homes. Dietitians, dietetic technicians, and nurses frequently work together to keep records of the kinds and quantities of foods a client both receives and leaves on the plate. From these records, the dietitian deduces what has been eaten and estimates nutrient intakes as described in the next section. Often, direct observations are used to estimate a client's current energy and protein intake, and the procedure is simply called a *kcalorie count*.

Analysis of Food Intake Data After collecting food intake data, the assessor estimates nutrient intakes, either informally by using food guides or formally by using food composition tables. Food intakes are then compared with standards, usually nutrient recommendations or dietary guidelines to determine how closely a diet meets the standards. Are the types and amounts of proteins, carbohydrates (including fiber), and fats (including cholesterol) appropriate? Are all food groups included in appropriate amounts? Is caffeine or alcohol consumption excessive? Are intakes of any vitamins or minerals (such as sodium or iron) excessive or deficient? An informal evaluation is possible only if the assessor has enough prior experience with formal calculations to "see" nutrient amounts in reported food intakes without calculations. Assessors often use the exchange system, described in Chapter 17, to estimate nutrient intake. Even then, such an informal analysis is best followed by actual calculations to spot-check for key nutrients.

Formal calculations can be performed either manually (by looking up each food in a table of food composition, recording its nutrients, and adding them up) or by using a computer diet analysis program. The assessor then compares the intakes with standards such as the RDA.

Form 15–3 Food Frequency Checklist

The assessor helps the client estimate portion sizes and frequency of use.

	Number of Servings	*Frequency*[a]
1. How often do you eat the following foods?		
Bread, toast, rolls, muffins	______	______
Cereal (type?) ______	______	______
Rice or other cooked grains	______	______
Noodles (macaroni, spaghetti)	______	______
Pancakes or waffles	______	______
Crackers or pretzels	______	______
Fruits or fruit juices	______	______
Vegetables other than potatoes	______	______
Vegetable juice	______	______
Potatoes	______	______
Dried beans and peas	______	______
Beef	______	______
Pork or ham	______	______
Veal	______	______
Poultry	______	______
Fish	______	______
Organ meats (such as liver)	______	______
Bacon	______	______
Sausage	______	______
Lunch meat	______	______
Hot dogs	______	______
Other meats (type?) ______	______	______
Eggs	______	______
Peanut butter or nuts	______	______
Milk (including on cereal)	______	______
Cheese or cheese dishes	______	______
Yogurt or tofu	______	______
Other milk products (type?) ______	______	______
Butter or margarine (type?) ______	______	______
Salt pork	______	______
Mayonnaise or salad dressing (type?) ______	______	______
Oil (type?) ______	______	______
Cream	______	______
Sugar, jam, jelly, syrup, honey	______	______
Bakery goods (type?) ______	______	______
Candy	______	______
Soft drinks (types?) ______	______	______
Potato or snack chips (type?) ______	______	______
Coffee or tea (type?) ______	______	______
Alcoholic beverages (type?) ______	______	______
Fast foods eaten out (type?) ______	______	______
TV dinners, pot pies, other prepared meals (type?) ______	______	______
Instant meals such as breakfast bars or diet meal beverages (type?) ______	______	______

Form 15–3 (continued)

2. What specific kinds of the following foods do you eat? Include the name of the food; whether it is fresh, canned, or frozen; and how it is prepared.
   Fruits and fruit juices __________
   Vegetables __________
   Milk and milk products __________
   Meats and meat alternates __________
   Breads and cereals __________
   Desserts __________
   Snack foods __________
3. Please list the names of any liquid, powder, or pill forms of vitamin or mineral products you take, and state how often you take them. Please also list any diet supplement you use (such as protein milk shakes or brewer's yeast), how much you use, and how often you use it. __________
4. Is there anything else you can relate about your food/nutrient intake? __________

[a]Number of servings per day, week, month, or year.

Limitations of Food Intake Analysis Food intake data can be informative, but the skillful assessor also keeps their limitations in mind. For example, a computer diet analysis tends to imply greater accuracy than is possible to obtain from data as uncertain as the starting information. Nutrient contents of foods listed in tables of food composition or stored in computer databases are averages and, for some nutrients, are incomplete. In addition, the available data on nutrient contents of foods do not reflect the amounts of nutrients a person actually absorbs. Iron is a case in point: its availability from a given meal may vary from as high as 50 percent to below 2 percent, depending on the person's iron status; the relative amounts of heme iron, nonheme iron, vitamin C, meat, fish, and poultry eaten at the meal; and the presence of inhibitors of iron absorption such as tea, coffee, and nuts. (Chapter 13 explains how to calculate iron absorption from a meal.)

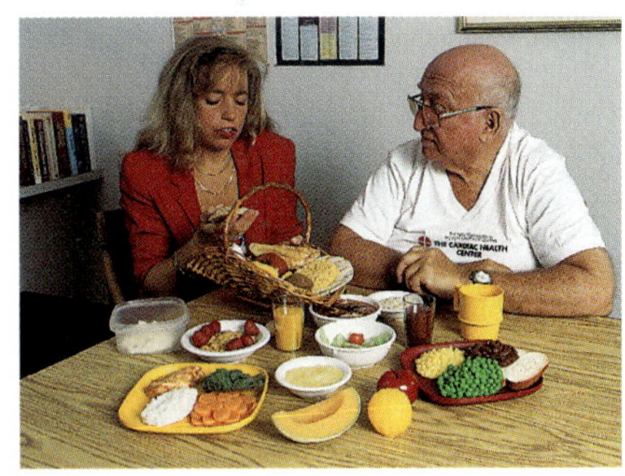

Help clients estimate food sizes by using food models and measuring utensils. When these items are not available, provide comparisons. For example, a small chicken leg is about 2 oz; a slice of luncheon meat is about 1 oz.

Furthermore, reported portion sizes may not be correct. The person who reports eating "a serving" of greens may not distinguish between ¼ cup and 2 whole cups. Children tend to remember the serving sizes of foods they like as being larger than serving sizes of foods they dislike.

Interpretation of Food Intake Data The assessor must remember that adequate nutrient *intakes* do not guarantee adequate nutrient *status* for an individual. Likewise, insufficient intakes do not always indicate deficiencies, but instead alert the assessor to possible problems. Each person digests, absorbs, metabolizes, and excretes nutrients in a unique way; individual needs vary. Intakes of nutrients identified by diet histories are only pieces of a puzzle that must be put together with other indicators of nutrition status in order to extract meaning.

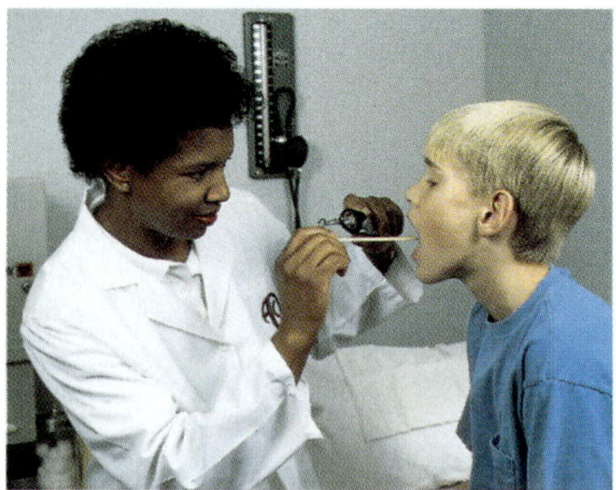

A physical examination provides valuable clues about a person's nutrition status.

Histories alert health care professionals to potential nutrition problems. Diet and socioeconomic histories pinpoint food intake, eating behaviors, and factors that influence food choices and food habits. Medical and drug histories identify health factors and drugs that can alter nutrient requirements. To substantiate findings, other assessment tools including physical examinations (described next) and anthropometric and biochemical measurements (described in the next chapter) are useful.

Physical Examinations

One clinician astutely summarized the role of the physical examination in nutrition assessment this way: "To me, physical examination proves the saying 'A picture is worth a thousand words.' "[4] Indeed, health care professionals can simply look at people to see if they are overweight, underweight, lethargic, confused, or unable to feed themselves, to give a few examples.

With closer examination, a skilled assessor can use a physical examination to search for signs of nutrient deficiency or toxicity. Many tissues and organs can reflect signs of malnutrition. Malnutrition appears most rapidly in parts of the body where cell replacement occurs at a high rate, such as the hair, skin, and digestive tract (including the mouth and tongue). The summary tables in Chapters 10 through 13 list physical signs of vitamin and mineral malnutrition.

Table 15–8

Physical Signs of Dehydration and Fluid Retention

Dehydration
- Sunken eyes
- Hollow cheekbones
- Dry mucous membranes
- Loss of skin turgor (elasticity)[a]
- Weak cry[b]
- Depression of the anterior fontanel[b]
- Deep, gasping respirations
- Weak, rapid pulse
- Thirst
- Reduced urinary output
- Weight loss

Fluid retention
- Edema
- Ascites (abdominal fluid retention)
- Elevated blood pressure
- Increased urinary output
- Weight gain

[a]May not be a useful parameter in the elderly.
[b]Findings specific to infants.

Fluid Balance Among the most useful physical signs of nutrition status are those that reflect dehydration and fluid retention. As Chapter 16 describes, to interpret laboratory tests and anthropometric measurements accurately, the assessor must consider the state of hydration. In addition, many conditions significantly upset fluid balances, and attention to physical signs and laboratory tests that reflect fluid balance help guide therapy. Table 15–8 lists physical signs that may occur in dehydration and fluid retention. Considering the causes of fluid imbalances vary, however, the clinical manifestations vary as well.

Limitations of Physical Findings Like the other assessment methods, such an examination requires knowledge, skill, and clinical judgment. Many physical signs are nonspecific; they can reflect any of several nutrient deficiencies as well as conditions not related to nutrition (see Table 15–9). For example, cracked lips may be caused by sunburn, windburn, dehydration, or any of several B vitamin deficiencies. For this reason, physical findings are most valuable for revealing problems for other assessment techniques to confirm or for confirming other assessment measures. A diet history can provide further support for a suspected vitamin deficiency, for example. Weight and height meaurements (anthropometric measurements) can confirm that a person is underweight and quantify the degree of underweight. Laboratory data can help verify a person's state of hydration or vitamin-mineral status.

Together with historical information, physical examinations provide important clues to a person's nutrition status. The next chapter describes anthropometric and biochemical measurements that further define nutrition status.

Table 15–9

Physical Findings Used in Nutrition Assessments

Body System	Acceptable Findings	Malnutrition Findings	What the Findings Reflect
Hair	Shiny, firm in the scalp	Dull, brittle, dry, loose; falls out	PEM
Eyes	Bright, clear pink membranes; adjust easily to light	Pale membranes; spots; redness; adjust slowly to darkness	Vitamin A, the B vitamins, zinc and iron status
Teeth and gums	No pain or caries, gums firm, teeth bright	Missing, discolored, decayed teeth; gums bleed easily and are swollen and spongy	Mineral and vitamin C status
Face	Clear complexion without dryness or scaliness	Off-color, scaly, flaky, cracked skin	PEM, vitamin A, and iron status
Glands	No lumps	Swollen at front of neck	PEM and iodine status
Tongue	Red, bumpy, rough	Sore, smooth, purplish, swollen	B vitamin status
Skin	Smooth, firm, good color	Dry, rough, spotty; "sandpaper" feel or sores; lack of fat under skin	PEM, essential fatty acid deficiency, vitamin A, the B vitamins, and vitamin C status
Nails	Firm, pink	Spoon-shaped, brittle, ridged, pale	Iron status
Internal systems	Regular heart rhythm, heart rate, and blood pressure; no impairment of digestive function, reflexes, or mental status	Abnormal heart rate, heart rhythm, or blood pressure; enlarged liver, spleen; abnormal digestion; burning, tingling of hands, feet; loss of balance, coordination; mental confusion, irritability, fatigue	PEM and mineral status
Muscles and bones	Muscle tone; posture, long bone development appropriate for age	"Wasted" appearance of muscles; swollen bumps on skull or ends of bones; small bumps on ribs; bowed legs or knock-knees	PEM, mineral, and vitamin D status

Study Questions

1. What are the steps in the nutrition care process?
2. What two services should the nutrition care plan deliver to the client?
3. Identify the four components of nutrition assessment.
4. How can a client's health history affect nutrition status?
5. What factors in a client's drug history suggest a likelihood of drug-nutrient interactions? Describe the mechanisms by which medications and nutrients can interact.
6. In what ways do socioeconomic factors affect nutrition status and food choices?
7. List two important uses for diet histories.
8. Describe ways of gathering food intake data and suggest uses for each method.
9. Itemize the major limitations of two methods of analyzing food intake data.
10. What is the primary use of the physical examination in nutrition assessment?

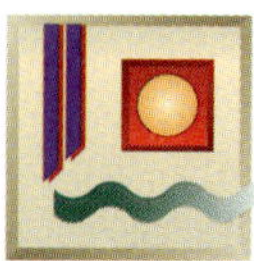

Clinical Applications

1. Considering the many factors that can affect nutrient intake addressed in this chapter, explain why it is important to follow a systematic approach to nutrition care. Describe some ways in which a physician, nurse, dietetic technician, pharmacist, and social worker might assist the dietitian in the assessment process.
2. Describe the possible nutrition implications of these findings from a client's history and physical examination: age 73, lives alone, recently lost spouse, uses a walker, no teeth, pale skin, lack of energy, history of hypertension and diabetes, several medications prescribed.
3. Nurses and nurse's aides often shoulder much of the responsibility for collecting food intake data for kcalorie counts because they often deliver food trays and snacks and later retrieve them. Why is it important for a nurse or aide to verify and record both what the client receives (both the foods and the amounts) and the foods that remain uneaten? When might clients be enlisted to aid in the collection of food intake data, and when might such a course be unwise?
4. During an initial nutrition assessment of a hospitalized client, the dietitian noted that the client appeared to be pale, thin, weak, and apathetic. Upon follow-up two weeks later, the dietitian noted that although the client was still quite thin, her color looked better and she appeared more energetic and talkative. The nurses noted that the client had been eating better and her weight had increased by two pounds. Does the dietary and weight information confirm or contradict the dietitian's observations?

Notes

1. J. A. Thomas, Drug-nutrient interactions, *Nutrition Reviews* 53 (1995): 271–282.
2. C. W. Lewis, E. A. Frongillo, and D. A. Roe, Drug-nutrient interactions in long-term care facilities, *Journal of the American Dietetic Association* 95 (1995): 309–315; R. N. Varma, Risk for drug-induced malnutrition is unchecked in elderly patients in nursing homes, *Journal of the American Dietetic Association* 94 (1994): 192–194.
3. L. R. Young and M. Nestle, Portion sizes in dietary assessment: Issues and policy implications, *Nutrition Reviews* 53 (1995): 149–158.
4. K. Hammond, Nutrition focused physical assessment, *Support Line,* August 1996, pp. 1–4.

Diet and Health

A century ago, our ancestors feared infectious and communicable diseases such as smallpox—diseases that claimed many children's lives and limited the average life expectancy of adults. Today far fewer infectious diseases threaten us, thanks to medial science's ability to identify disease-causing microorganisms and develop vaccines and effective treatments. In developed nations, immunizations protect individuals from some infections, purification of water prevents the spread of infection, and antimicrobial drugs successfully treat infections.

Although some infectious diseases remain serious threats in developed countries, most of today's life-threatening diseases develop and become chronic as a result of physiological deterioration of the body induced by such factors as genetics, age, gender, lifestyle, and environment. Diet is one of many lifestyle factors that influence the risks of developing chronic diseases, and dietary factors that advance or prevent the progression of chronic disease are the focus of this highlight.

MAJOR CHRONIC DISEASES AND THEIR RISK FACTORS

Table H15–1 lists the ten leading causes of death in the United States.[1] Four of these causes, including the top three, have some relationship with diet. Taken together, these four conditions account for two-thirds of the nation's 2 million deaths each year. Earlier chapters described individual nutrients' connections with diseases and may

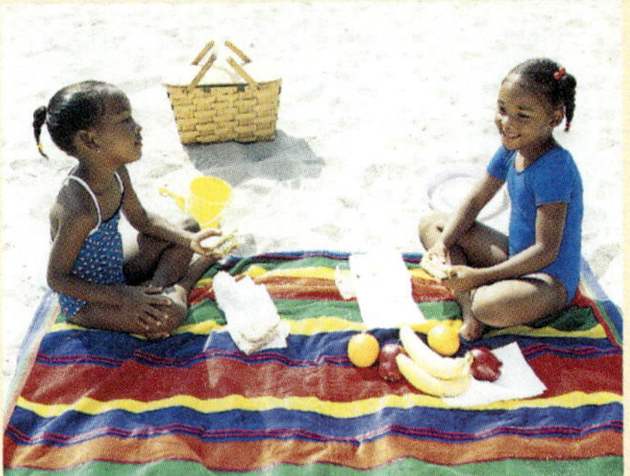

Establishing healthful habits in childhood lowers the risk of developing chronic diseases in adulthood.

have left the mistaken impression that these relationships can be described in terms of "one disease–one nutrient."[2] Indeed, valid links do exist between fat and heart disease, calcium and osteoporosis, and antioxidant vitamins and cancer, but to focus just on these links oversimplifies the story. In reality, each nutrient may have connections with several diseases because its role in the body is not specific to a disease, but to a body function. For example, vitamin C—because it acts as an antioxidant—helps prevent both cancer and heart disease. Furthermore, each of the chronic diseases develops in response to multiple factors, including many nondietary factors such as genetics, physical activity, and smoking. An integrated and balanced approach to disease prevention therefore includes attention to all factors involved. Figure H15–1 on p. 540 illustrates some of the relationships between risk factors and degenerative diseases.

Table H15–1

Ten Leading Causes of Death in the United States

1. **Heart disease.**
2. **Cancers.**
3. **Strokes.**
4. Chronic obstructive lung disease.
5. Unintentional injuries.
6. Pneumonia and influenza.
7. **Diabetes mellitus.**
8. HIV infection.
9. Suicide.
10. Homicide.

Note: The diseases in bold type have documented relationships with diet.

RECOMMENDATIONS FOR POPULATIONS VERSUS INDIVIDUALS

Most chronic diseases that are influenced by diet are also influenced by genetics. Hypertension, obesity, high blood lipids, atherosclerosis, diabetes, and some types of cancer are common in families primarily for genetic reasons. Just as people's hereditary susceptibility to diseases varies, so do their responses to dietary measures. Logically, therefore, preventive efforts may be most beneficial for persons with strong family histories of disease, and health care professionals should single those people out for treatment. In reality, though, such a person-to-person approach is not feasible.

To determine whether dietary recommendations may be important to you personally, examine your family history to see which diseases are common to your parents and grandparents (see Figure H15–2 on p. 542 for a hypothetical "medical family tree"). In addition to family history,

Figure H15–1

Diet/Lifestyle Risk Factors and Degenerative Diseases

The chart at the top shows that the same risk factor can affect many chronic diseases. Notice, for example, how many diseases have been linked to a high-fat diet. The chart also shows that a particular disease, such as atherosclerosis, may have several risk factors.

The flow chart at the bottom shows that many of these conditions are themselves risk factors for other chronic diseases. For example, a person with diabetes is likely to develop atherosclerosis and hypertension. These two conditions, in turn, worsen each other. Notice how all of these diseases are linked to obesity.

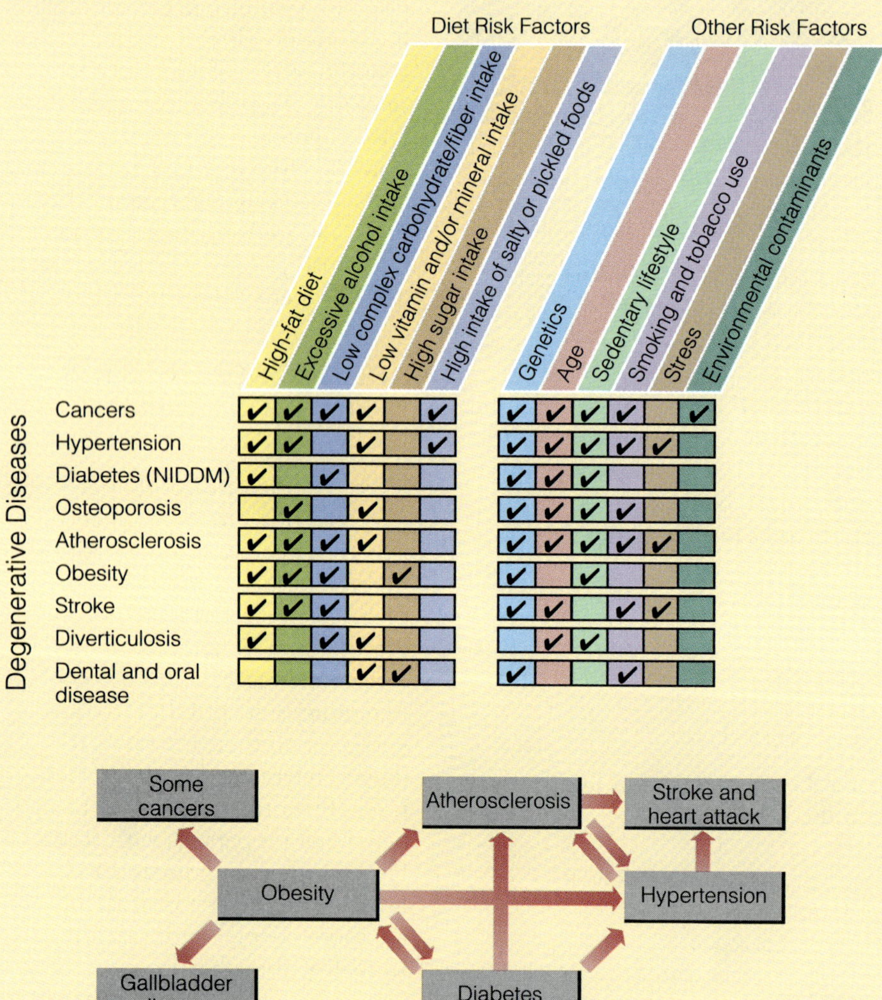

personal history is also important: take note of your own medical problems, weight, blood pressure, blood test results, and lifestyle habits such as smoking and physical activity.

Table H15–2 applies information from the *Dietary Guidelines for Americans* (see p. 541) and shows the medical risk factors that alert people to the personally relevant ones.

PUTTING IT ALL TOGETHER

Dietary excesses, particularly excess food energy and fat intakes, increase the likelihood of all of today's major diseases. Several of the recommendations are aimed at weight control: cut fat, add complex carbohydrates, and balance food intake with activity. The problems of overweight people multiply when medical problems develop. Overweight people with diabetes usually have hypertension and high blood lipids as well. Such a combination of problems may require only one treatment: lose the excess weight by adopting a healthful diet combined with regular physical activity.

Dietary deficiencies, particularly deficiencies in fiber, vitamin, and mineral intakes, also increase the likelihood of the major diseases. Following the recommendation to eat a variety of foods and to include plenty of grains, fruits, and vegetables in the diet addresses this concern.

Not all recommendations apply equally to all of the diseases or to all people with the disease (salt has a special relationship with hypertension in some cases, for example), but fortunately for the consumer, the dietary recommendations to help prevent these diseases do not contradict one another. Thanks to the fruits of recent research, healthy adults have a great opportunity: they can employ the benefits of a nutritious diet to help preserve their health into their later years.

NOTES

1. Centers for Disease Control, Mortality patterns—United States, 1989, *Morbidity and Mortality Weekly Report* 41 (1992): 121–125.

2. W. Mertz, A balanced approach to nutrition for health: The need for biologically essential minerals and vitamins, *Journal of the American Dietetic Association* 94 (1994): 1259–1262.

Table H15–2

Nutrition Recommendations and Health Risks

Nutrition Changes Recommended for Most People	This Is Especially Important if Your Family Health History Indicates:	And/or if Your Personal Health History Indicates:
Energy, energy nutrients, and weight control: • Achieve and maintain a healthy body weight.[a] • Reduce consumption of total fat, saturated fat, and cholesterol.[b] • Increase consumption of complex carbohydrates and fibers.[c]	Obesity, diabetes, cancer, or any form of cardiovascular disease	Unhealthy weight, glucose intolerance, elevated blood cholesterol or triglycerides, hypertension, other cardiovascular disease
Salt/sodium: Reduce intake of salt/sodium.[d]	Hypertension, diabetes, or any form of cardiovascular disease	Hypertension, glucose intolerance
Alcohol: • Take alcohol only in moderation, if at all.[e]	Alcohol abuse or osteoporosis	Unhealthy weight, glucose intolerance, elevated blood cholesterol and triglycerides, any sign of adult bone loss
• Abstain from alcohol.		Pregnancy, alcohol abuse, liver disease, pancreatitis

[a]To achieve and maintain desirable body weight, choose a dietary pattern in which food energy intake matches energy expenditure. To reduce energy intake, limit foods relatively high in kcalories, fats, and sugars and minimize alcohol consumption. Increase energy expenditure through regular and sustained physical activity.

[b]Choose foods relatively low in fats and cholesterol, such as vegetables, fruits, whole-grain foods, fish, poultry, lean meats, and low-fat dairy products. Use food preparation methods that add little or no fat.

[c]To increase consumption of complex carbohydrates and fiber, eat more whole-grain foods and cereal products, vegetables, dried beans and peas, and fruits.

[d]To reduce intake of salt/sodium, choose foods relatively low in sodium, and limit the amount of salt added in food preparation and at the table.

[e]To exercise moderation in the use of alcohol, research suggests that men take no more than two to six drinks per week and that women take no more than one to three drinks per week (see Highlight 28). Avoid drinking any alcohol before or while driving, operating machinery, taking medications, or engaging in any other activity requiring judgment.

Figure H15–2

Hypothetical Medical Family Tree

A "medical family tree" notes the types of diseases family members have had, their ages at the times of major medical events or death, and their pesonal medical histories.

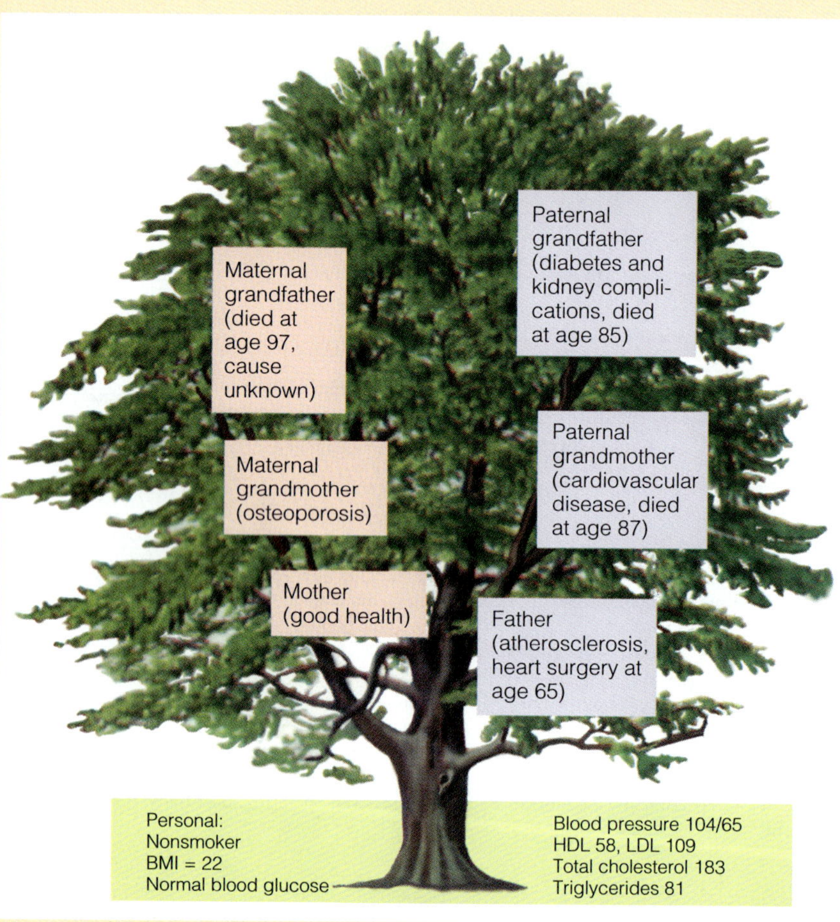

Chapter 16

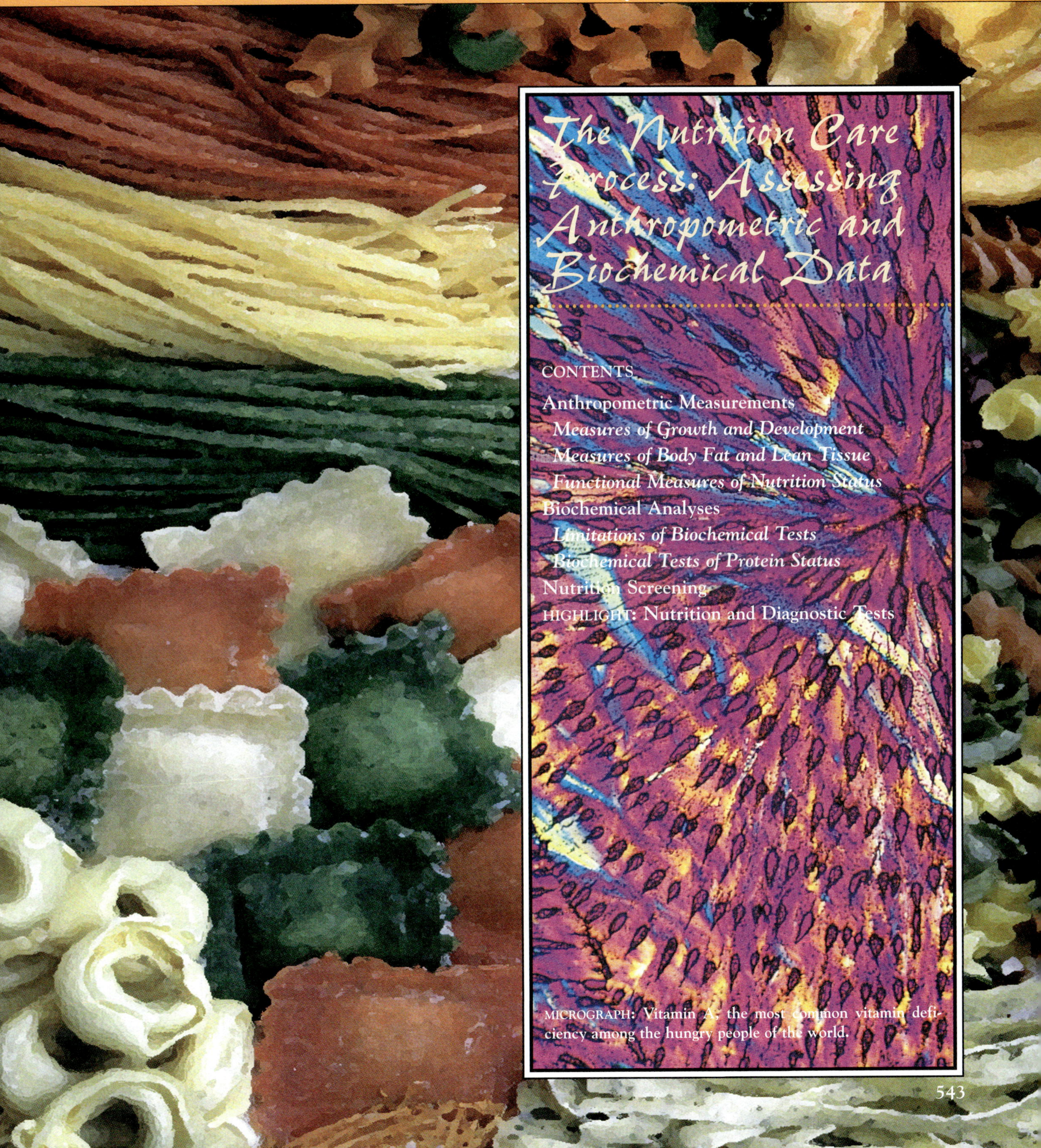

The Nutrition Care Process: Assessing Anthropometric and Biochemical Data

CONTENTS

MICROGRAPH: Vitamin A: the most common vitamin deficiency among the hungry people of the world.

Chapter 15 introduced the nutrition care process and nutrition assessments and showed how the assessor can use historical information and physical examinations to look for signs of nutrient imbalances. This chapter shows how physical and biochemical measurements complete the assessment process.

Anthropometric Measurements

anthropometric: relating to measurement of the physical characteristics of the body, such as height and weight.
anthropos = human
metric = measure

Anthropometrics are physical measurements that provide an indirect assessment of body composition and development (see Table 16–1 on p. 546). They serve three main purposes: first, to evaluate the progress of growth in pregnant women, infants, children, and adolescents; second, to detect undernutrition and overnutrition in all age groups; and third, to measure changes in body composition over time.

Assessors compare anthropometric measurements taken on an individual with population standards specific for gender and age to see how body composition compares to norms. Assessors may also take measurements periodically and compare them with previous measurements to reveal changes in an individual's status.

Height and weight are well-recognized anthropometrics; others include fatfold measurements and various measures of lean tissue. Still other measures are useful in specific situations. For example, a head circumference measurement may help to assess brain development in an infant, and an abdominal girth measurement supplies information about abdominal fluid retention or enlargement of abdominal organs.

Mastering the techniques for taking anthropometric measurements requires proper instruction and practice to ensure reliability. Once the correct techniques are learned, taking the measurements is easy and generally requires minimal equipment.

MEASURES OF GROWTH AND DEVELOPMENT

Height and weight are among the most common and useful anthropometric measurements. Length measurements for infants and children up to age three and height measurements for children over three are particularly valuable in assessing growth, which depends on adequate nutrition. Poor growth in children is an important indicator of malnutrition. For adults, height measurements alone do not reflect current nutrition status but help to estimate desirable weight, to interpret other assessment data, and to estimate energy needs. Once adult height has been reached, changes in body weight may reveal either overnutrition or undernutrition.

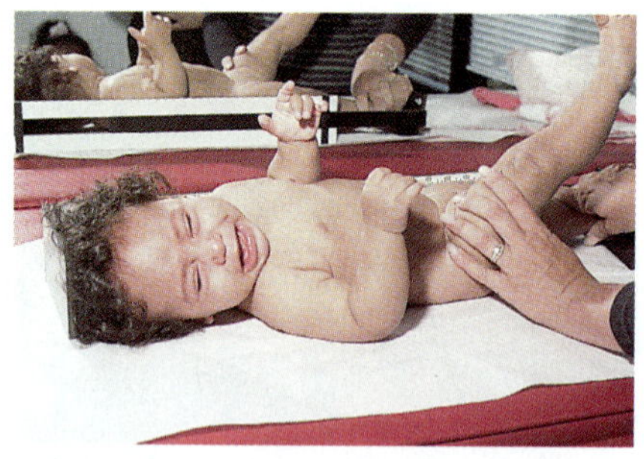

Lying still with legs straight for a length measurement can be a trying experience.

Height For infants and children younger than three, health care professionals may use special equipment to measure length. The assessor lays the barefoot infant on a measuring board that has a fixed headboard and movable footboard attached at right angles to the surface. Often two people are needed to obtain an accurate measurement: one to hold the infant's head against the headboard and keep the legs straight, and the other to do the measuring. This method provides the most accurate measure possible, but many health care professionals use a less exacting method. They may simply hold the infant straight with its head against the headboard or other vertical support, mark the blanket with a chalk or pen at the infant's heel, and then measure the distance from the headboard to the mark. Even more informally and less accurately, they may lay the infant on a flat surface and extend a nonstretchable measuring tape along the infant's side from the top of the head to the heel of the foot.

The procedure for measuring a child who can stand erect and cooperate is the same as for an adult. The best way to measure standing height is with the person's back against a flat wall to which a nonstretchable measuring tape or stick has been fixed. The person stands erect, without shoes, with heels together. The person's line of sight should be horizontal, with the heels, buttocks, shoulders, and head touching the wall. The assessor places a ruler, book, or other stiff object on top of the head at a right angle to the wall, carefully checks the height measurement, and records it immediately in either inches or centimeters. Immediate recording prevents the assessor from forgetting the correct measurement.

The measuring rod of a scale is commonly used to measure height, but is less accurate because of its movability. The assessor follows the same general procedure, asking the person to face away from the scale and to stand erect.

Many health care professionals merely ask clients how tall they are rather than measuring their height. Self-reported height is often inaccurate and should be used only as a last resort when measurement is impractical, as in the case of an uncooperative client or an emergency admission.

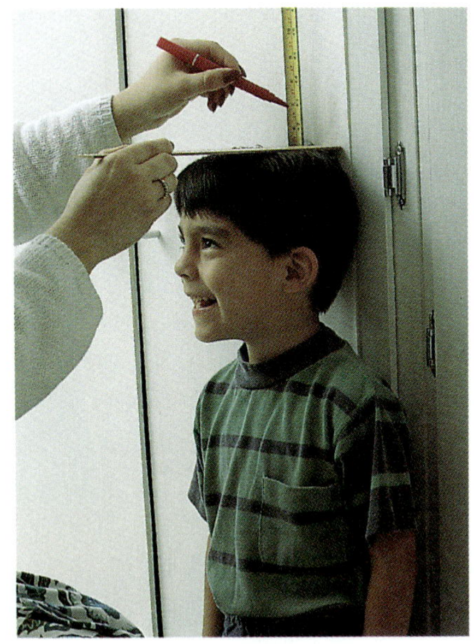

Standing "at attention" allows for an accurate height measurement.

Weight Valid weight measurements require functional scales that have been carefully maintained, calibrated, and checked for accuracy at regular intervals. Beam balance and electronic scales are the most accurate types of scales. Special scales and hospital beds with built-in scales are available for weighing people who are bedridden. Bathroom scales are inaccurate and inappropriate for use in professional settings.

To measure an infant's weight, assessors use special scales that allow infants to lie or sit. Weighing infants naked, without diapers, is standard procedure. Children who can stand are weighed in the same way as adults. Standardized conditions are necessary if repeated measures are to be useful. Each weighing should take place at the same time of day (preferably before breakfast), in the same amount of clothing (without shoes), after the person has voided, and on the same scale. As with all measurements, the assessor records observed weight immediately in either pounds or kilograms.

Head Circumference Assessors may also measure head circumference to confirm that infant growth is proceeding normally or to help detect protein-energy malnutrition (PEM) and evaluate the extent of its impact on brain size. To measure head circumference, the assessor places a nonstretchable tape so that it encircles the largest part of the infant's head: just above the eyebrow ridges, just above the point where the ears attach, and around the occipital prominence at the back of the head. To ensure accurate recording, the assessor immediately notes the measure in either inches or centimeters.

Analysis of Measures in Infants and Children Health professionals evaluate physical development by monitoring the growth rate of a child and comparing this rate with standard charts (see Appendix E for more information).

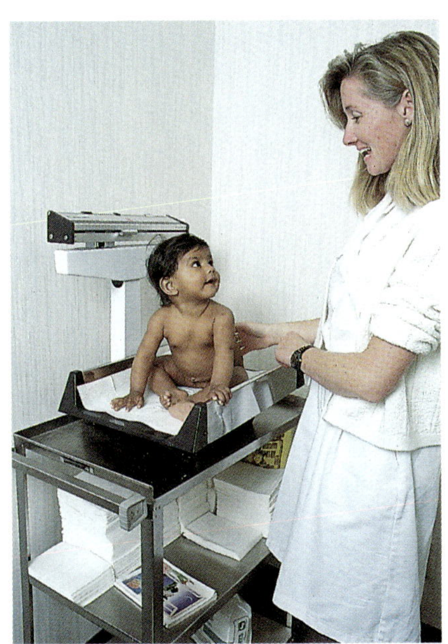

Special scales allow infants to sit and watch while they are being weighed.

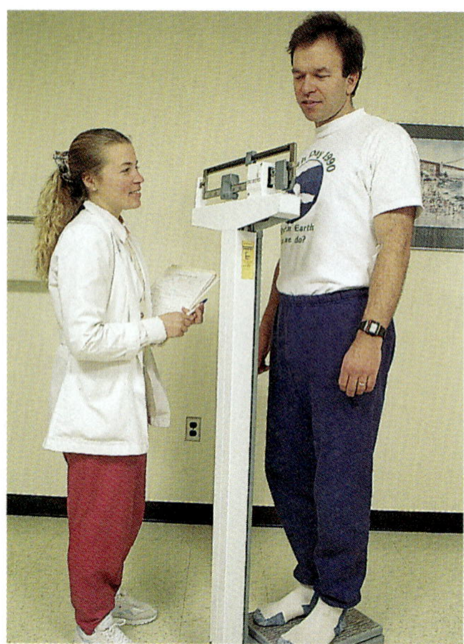

Beam balance scales provide accurate weight measurements for adults.

Table 16–1

Anthropometric Measurements Used in Nutrition Assessments

Type of Measurement	What It Reflects
Abdominal girth measurement	Abdominal fluid retention
Height-weight	Overnutrition and undernutrition; growth in children
Head circumference	Brain growth and development in infants and children under two
Fatfold	Subcutaneous and total body fat
Midarm muscle circumference	Muscle mass (i.e., protein status)

Standard growth charts compare weight to age, height to age, and weight to height; ideally, height and weight are in roughly the same percentile. Although individual growth patterns may vary, a child's growth curve will generally stay at about the same percentile throughout childhood. Measurements below standard for height, weight, or head circumference in infants and young children indicate growth retardation, which is an important sign of malnutrition. (Chapter 19 describes the expected growth patterns and consequences of malnutrition for infants and children.)

In children whose growth has been retarded, nutrition rehabilitation will ideally induce height and weight to increase to higher percentiles. Obesity is also an important sign requiring intervention. In overweight children, the goal is for weight to remain stable as height increases, until weight becomes appropriate for height.

Head circumference is a useful indicator of brain growth in children under two years of age. Since the brain grows rapidly before birth and during early infancy, extreme and chronic malnutrition during these times can impair brain development, curtailing the number of brain cells and the head circumference. Head circumference percentiles should be similar to the child's weight and height percentiles. Nonnutritional factors, such as certain disorders and genetic variation, can also influence head circumference.

Reminder: The *body mass index (BMI)* is an index of a person's weight in relation to height, determined by dividing the weight in kilograms by the square of the height in meters:

$$\text{BMI} = \frac{\text{weight (kg)}.}{\text{height (m)}^2}$$

Analysis of Measures for Adults Chapter 8 (pp. 268–271) discussed healthy body weight and described the controversies regarding weight standards for adults. Health care professionals typically compare weights with weight-for-height standards. Each facility or practitioner decides which standard to use based on review of the literature and clinical judgment. The commonly used standards for nutrition assessment include:

1. The body mass index (BMI) and tables based on the BMI observed to be consistent with health (see pp. 270–271 and inside back cover).
2. The Metropolitan Life Insurance weight-for-height tables (see Appendix E).
3. A quick method of estimating desirable body weight described in the accompanying box.

How to Quickly Estimate Ideal Body Weight

In the health care setting, professionals may bypass standard height and weight tables and simply use a rule of thumb to estimate an "ideal" weight based on height and gender. The assessor considers 106 pounds a reasonable weight for a man who is 5 feet tall and then adds 6 pounds for each inch over 5 feet (or subtracts 6 pounds for each inch under 5 feet). For example, the calculation for a man who is 5 feet 8 inches tall would be:

5 ft = 106 lb.
8 in = 48 lb (8 in × 6 lb).
5 ft 8 in = 154 lb.

A reasonable estimate, then, for this man is 154 pounds. Large-framed individuals may need to add 10 percent, whereas small-framed individuals may need to subtract 10 percent. Thus the range for men of this height is 139 to 169. Compared with the range of 125 to 164 pounds listed in the standard "suggested weights" table found on p. 269, this estimated range is close enough for most purposes.

Similarly, the assessor considers 100 pounds a reasonable weight for a woman who is 5 feet tall and than adds 5 pounds for each inch over 5 feet (or subtracts 5 pounds for each inch under 5 feet). The calculation for a woman who is 5 feet 5 inches tall would be:

5 ft = 100 lb.
5 in = 25 lb (5 in × 5 lb).
5 ft 5 in = 125 lb.

A reasonable estimate for this woman is 125 pounds. Because large-framed individuals may need to add 10 percent, and small-framed individuals may need to subtract 10 percent, the estimated range for women of this height is 112 to 138. Again this range is similar to the suggested range of 114 to 150 (p. 269).

Reminder: Height and weight tables suggest a weight range, rather than pinpointing one ideal weight—a helpful reminder that no weight is perfect for everyone.

The assessor can compare the standard chosen with the person's actual weight to generate a figure known as the percent ideal body weight (%IBW). Current weight can also be compared to usual body weight to generate the percent usual body weight (%UBW), which considers what is normal for a particular individual. The client, family, friends, and older medical records can provide information about usual body weight. The %UBW is particularly useful for evaluating weight changes in cases where an individual has weighed considerably more or less than average throughout life. Additionally, in cases where an overweight individual becomes acutely ill and is rapidly losing weight, the health care professional relying on the %IBW may inadvertently overlook malnutrition. The rate of any recent weight change is important—a 5 percent weight loss within a month might be significant, yet the same loss over five months might not be. The box on p. 549 and Table 16–2 show how to calculate and evaluate the %IBW and the %UBW.

Table 16–2

Weight as an Indicator of Nutrition Status

%IBW	%UBW	Nutrition Status
>120	—	Obese
110–120	—	Overweight
90–109	—	Adequate
80–89	85–95	Mildly underweight
70–79	75–84	Moderately underweight
<70	<75	Severely underweight

Weight Change during Pregnancy One of the anthropometric measures most predictive of an infant's birthweight is the mother's amount and pattern of weight gain or loss during pregnancy. Chapter 18 describes normal weight gains related to pregnancy, and Appendix E provides an example of a chart used to monitor weight gain during pregnancy. Patterns of weight gain that deviate from these require further investigation.

MEASURES OF BODY FAT AND LEAN TISSUE

Isotope studies, ultrasonography, and computerized axial topography (CAT scan) are other methods that have been used to determine body composition. The expense of these tests limits their clinical use, although they are useful in specific situations and in research.

Appendix E shows the proper techniques for measuring triceps fatfold and provides standards for comparison.

Significant weight changes in both children and adults can reflect overnutrition or undernutrition with respect to energy and protein. To estimate the degree to which fat stores or lean tissues are affected by weight changes, several anthropometric measurements are useful.

Body Fat As Chapter 8 explained, both the amount and the distribution of body fat are important. Body fat measurements include fatfold measures, waist-to-hip ratios, hydrodensitometry, and bioelectrical impedance, all described in Chapter 8. Another anthropometric measurement—the midarm muscle circumference—provides information about skeletal muscle mass.

Midarm Muscle Circumferences Just as subcutaneous fat provides an indirect estimate of total body fat, measurable muscles provide an indirect measure of the protein status of muscular organs such as the heart. To determine whether a person has a depleted muscle mass, an indirect measure of arm muscle size is useful: the *midarm muscle* circumference. This measure is estimated by subtracting the amount of fat on the arm from the total area (derived from the arm's circumference). Appendix E shows how this is done and presents standards for comparison.

Cautious Interpretation of Measures The reliability of anthropometric measurements is limited by the skills of the measurer and the accuracy of the equipment used for measuring. Sometimes taking measurements is difficult for physical reasons, such as when a person cannot be moved to be weighed or measured for height. Triceps fatfolds and arm circumferences are sometimes difficult to measure in people with wounds or loose, hanging skin on their arms. In the elderly, the distribution of fat and the compressibility of the skin change, complicating the measurement and interpretation of fatfolds.

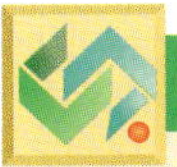

How to Estimate %IBW and %UBW

To estimate %IBW, compare the individual's current weight with the ideal body weight from standard height and weight tables:

$$\%\text{IBW} = \frac{\text{actual weight}}{\text{ideal weight}} \times 100.$$

For example, to calculate %IBW in a man who is 5 feet 8 inches tall and weighs 115 pounds, follow these steps. For ideal weight, use the midpoint of the weight range in Table 8–5 on p. 269. In this example, the ideal weight is 144 pounds.

$$\%\text{IBW} = \frac{115 \text{ lb}}{144 \text{ lb}} \times 100 = 80\%.$$

The man in this example is at 80 percent of his ideal body weight. Look to Table 16–2 to find that 80 percent IBW indicates that he is mildly underweight.

This man has lost 15 pounds in the last month. To calculate %UBW for this man, follow these steps:

$$\%\text{UBW} = \frac{\text{actual weight}}{\text{usual weight}} \times 100.$$

Calculate the usual weight (130 pounds) by adding the weight loss (15 pounds) to the current body weight (115 pounds).

$$\%\text{UBW} = \frac{115 \text{ lb}}{130 \text{ lb}} \times 100 = 88\%.$$

The man is at 88 percent of his usual body weight. A look at Table 16–2 reveals that a person at 88 percent UBW is mildly underweight. Based on %UBW, the degree of underweight is less severe than the %IBW implied, because the person has consistently weighed less than standard weight. Nevertheless, his recent rate of weight change is significant: he lost almost 4 pounds per week.

Even when measurements are taken accurately, interpreting them can present problems. A person's state of hydration, for example, significantly influences anthropometric measurements, because body composition reflects total body water as well as lean body mass and body fat. Diseases or medications that cause fluid retention can mask significant weight loss. Dehydration affects measurements of weight, fatfolds, and midarm muscle circumference. Besides the state of hydration, exercise alters anthropometric measurements. Exercise enhances muscle size, and lack of exercise may diminish muscle mass, independently of nutrition factors.[1]

Accurate interpretations of anthropometric measurements are also confounded by problems with the standards used for comparison. The controversies surrounding weight standards have already been described in Chapter 8. Another difficulty is that fatfold and muscle circumference standards were devel-

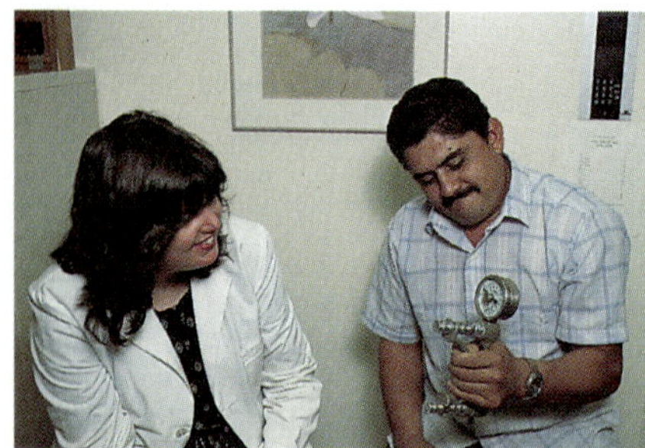
An instrument called a dynamometer measures hand grip strength.

oped for specific populations, often of healthy people in their middle years of life. The application of such standards to people who are sick or who are not within the age groups studied requires cautious clinical judgment.

Another limitation of anthropometrics is their inability to describe small changes in body composition that occur over short periods of time. Thus anthropometrics are of limited value in quantifying the effects of acute illnesses on nutrition status. Furthermore, research is needed to determine if internal fat stores change at the same rate as subcutaneous fat during illnesses that markedly raise the metabolic rate (see Chapter 25).

FUNCTIONAL MEASURES OF NUTRITION STATUS

Two tests of nutrition status, hand grip strength and skin tests, measure the function of organ systems, rather than a specific body compartment. Technically, these tests are not anthropometric measurements, but they both require physical measurements and so are described here.

Hand Grip Strength The measurement of hand grip strength is a practical and inexpensive tool for assessing nutrition status that relates changes in body composition to organ function. The assessor asks the person to grip an instrument (called a dynamometer) as tightly as possible. Low grip strength (weak muscle function) indicates risk for poor nutrition status, which must be confirmed by other tests. People with severe arthritis or muscular disorders may have low grip strengths unrelated to nutrition status.

induration: a raised, hardened area of skin.
durus = hard

Conditions other than PEM that can affect skin tests include metabolic stress, liver disease, kidney disease, and the use of many drugs including corticosteroids and general anesthesia.

Skin Tests Just as hand grip strength measures muscle function, antigen skin tests measure immune function. Organisms (usually three or four kinds) that produce an immune reaction in most people are injected just under the skin.* Raised, hardened areas (induration) appear after 24 to 48 hours in well-nourished people, but are minimal or absent in people with PEM. Many factors other than nutrition interfere with immune responses, however, and skin testing alone cannot identify PEM.

Anthropometric measurements, including height, weight, fatfolds, muscle circumference, and others, provide valuable information regarding body weight and composition. Hand grip strength reflects muscle function and skin tests reflect immune function; poor nutrition may be responsible for test results, but these tests alone may not be conclusive. Anthropometric measurements require properly working equipment and trained assessors to render accurate results that can then be compared to standards for interpretation. Biochemical tests, described next, help define nutrition status, organ function, body composition, and response to medical nutrition therapy.

Biochemical Analyses

All of the approaches to nutrition assessment discussed so far are external approaches. Biochemical analyses or laboratory tests help to determine what is

*Typical antigens include *Candida*, mumps, purified protein derivative (PPD), streptokinase-streptodornase (SK-SD), and *Monilla*.

happening to the body internally. Common tests are based on analysis of blood and urine samples, which contain nutrients, enzymes, and metabolites. Some directly reflect nutrition status. Other tests, such as serum glucose or tests that define fluid and electrolyte balance, acid-base balance, and organ function, help pinpoint disorders or problems with nutrition implications. Table 16–3 identifies some biochemical tests with nutrition implications and shows what these tests reflect. Tests important in specific disorders will be discussed in the appropriate chapters.

The taking of several measurements during a single blood test is referred to as **SMA (simultaneous multiple analysis).** SMA is followed by a number (for example, SMA-12) that indicates how many tests will be run.

The **serum** is the watery portion of the blood that remains after removal of the cells and clot-forming material; **plasma** is the fluid that remains when unclotted blood is centrifuged. In most cases, serum and plasma concentrations are similar. Lab technicians usually prefer serum samples because plasma samples occasionally clog mechanical blood analyzers.

Recall that lab tests that confirm dehydration or fluid retention, including sodium, BUN (blood urea nitrogen), hemoglobin, and hematocrit, alert the assessor to interpret anthropometric measurements cautiously.

LIMITATIONS OF BIOCHEMICAL TESTS

The interpretation of biochemical data requires skill. The person's state of hydration greatly influences laboratory values, and indeed, laboratory tests are often used to detect dehydration and fluid retention. With dehydration, lab results may be deceptively high; with overhydration, lab results may be deceptively low.

No single test is sufficient to diagnose nutrient deficiencies because many factors influence test results. The low blood concentration of a nutrient may reflect a primary deficiency of that nutrient, but it may also be secondary to the deficiency of one or several other nutrients or to a factor unrelated to nutrition. Nutrient concentrations in the blood and urine sometimes reflect recent intakes rather than long-term intakes. Thus blood concentrations of a nutrient may be normal, even when tissue levels are deficient. Assessors who keep these limitations in mind and use lab tests along with other assessment data, however, can create a total picture that becomes clear with careful interpretation.

It is beyond the scope of this text to describe all lab tests used to assess nutrition status, define organ function, and develop nutrition care plans. Instead, the emphasis is on lab tests used to evaluate protein status. Appendix E provides tables of lab tests useful in detecting various vitamin and mineral deficiencies, including nutrition–related anemias.

BIOCHEMICAL TESTS OF PROTEIN STATUS

Protein is found in skeletal muscles, serum, and internal organs. Muscle proteins perform the physical work of the body, and serum and organ proteins maintain fluid balances, synthesize enzymes and hormones, mount immune responses, heal wounds, and much more. When the body is deprived of adequate energy to use as fuel, protein is sacrificed to make glucose. If energy deprivation continues long enough, the function of muscular organs such as the heart and organs that depend on muscles such as the lungs is compromised. Eventually, protein is unavailable to maintain these vital body functions.

While anthropometric measurements and hand grip strength evaluate skeletal muscle mass, lab tests of serum proteins and skin tests help evaluate internal proteins. Serum proteins are synthesized in the liver, and serum levels can reflect liver function, the availability of amino acids (protein intake), the distribution of proteins (proteins may shift from the blood to the intravascular or intracellular compartments, for example), and the rate of protein use by the body. Therefore, when evaluating serum proteins, assessors must consider disorders of metabolism and organ function, the body's rate of use of each protein, and protein status. Table 16–4 provides standards for evaluating the serum proteins most widely used in nutrition assessments. Other biochemical tests useful in assessing protein status include the total lymphocyte count, a measure of immune

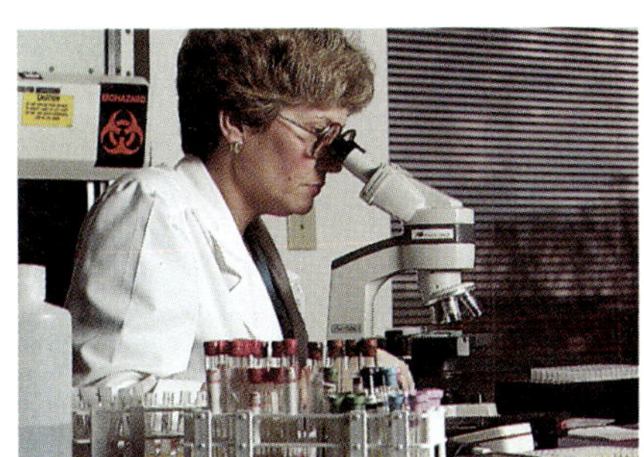

Blood and urine samples offer valuable clues for assessing nutrition status.

Table 16–3

Routine Hospital Laboratory Tests

Test	Uses
HEMATOLOGY	
Hemoglobin (Hg)	To detect anemia and determine state of hydration.
Hematocrit (Hct)	To detect anemia and determine state of hydration.
White blood cells (WBC)	To detect infection and determine total lymphocyte count.
Mean corpuscular volume (MCV)	To detect anemia and determine its causes.
Mean corpuscular hemoglobin (MCH)	To detect anemia and determine its causes.
Mean corpuscular hemoglobin concentration (MCHC)	To detect anemia and determine its causes.
BLOOD CHEMISTRY	
Proteins	
Total protein[a]	To detect PEM and various nutrient imbalances.
Albumin	To detect PEM and determine state of hydration.
Transferrin	To detect PEM and monitor response to feeding.
Prealbumin	To detect PEM and monitor response to feeding.
Electrolytes	
Sodium	To check state of hydration.
Potassium	To monitor acid-base balance and renal function and detect imbalances.
Chloride	To monitor acid-base balance and detect GI losses of chloride (from vomiting or nasogastric suctioning).
Carbon dioxide	To monitor acid-base balance.
Other	
Glucose	To detect diabetes mellitus, pancreatic tumors, and hypoglycemia and monitor glucose intolerance.
Blood urea nitrogen	To monitor renal function and determine state of hydration.
Calcium	To detect hormonal imbalances, certain malignancies, and steatorrhea (malabsorption).
Phosphorus	To detect hormonal imbalances and PEM and monitor renal function and response to feeding.
Magnesium	To monitor renal function and response to feeding and detect PEM.
Cholesterol	To assess risk of heart disease and possibility of obstructive jaundice.
Uric acid	To detect gout and determine state of hydration.
Serum creatinine	To monitor renal function and determine state of hydration.
Serum enzymes	
Creatinine phosphokinase (CPK)	To monitor heart function and muscle damage.
Lactic dehydrogenase (LDH)	To monitor heart and renal function.
Alanine transaminase (ALT, formerly SGPT)	To monitor heart and liver function.
Aspartate transaminase (AST, formerly SGOT)	To monitor heart and liver function.
Alkaline phosphatase	To monitor liver function.
Serum amylase	To monitor pancreatic function.
Serum lipase	To monitor pancreatic function.

Note: This table presents a partial listing of the major uses of certain commonly performed lab tests that have implications for nutrition.
[a]More than half of the total protein is albumin.

Table 16–4

Relationship between Degree of Undernutrition and Serum Proteins

Indicator	Degree of Depletion			
	NORMAL	MILD	MODERATE	SEVERE
Albumin (g/100 ml)	≥3.5	2.8–3.4	2.1–2.7	<2.1
Transferrin (mg/100 ml)	>200	150–200	100–149	<100
Prealbumin (mg/100 ml)	16–30	10–15	5–9	<5
Retinol-binding protein[a] (mg/100 ml)	2.6–7.6	—	—	—

Note: To convert albumin (g/100 ml) to standard international units (g/L), multiply by 100. To convert transferrin (mg/100 ml) to standard international units (g/L), multiply by 0.01.
[a]Levels less than normal suggest compromised protein status. The actual degree of depletion (mild, moderate, and severe) has not been defined.

function; urinary nitrogen, used to evaluate nitrogen balance; and urinary creatinine, a measure of skeletal muscle mass.

Serum Albumin Albumin accounts for over 50 percent of the total serum proteins. Serum albumin is slow to reflect changes in nutrition status because it is plentiful in the body and breaks down slowly.* Therefore, low serum albumin reflects prolonged protein depletion. Likewise, albumin concentrations increase slowly with appropriate nutrition support, so measuring albumin as an indicator of response to nutrition therapy is of limited value. Serum albumin levels appear to correlate well with survival among people in the hospital.[2]

Note that albumin concentrations can be depressed by many conditions besides malnutrition, including liver disease, kidney disease (nephrotic syndrome), eclampsia, and disorders that can markedly raise the metabolic rate (metabolic stress) including infection, cancer, and burns.

Serum Transferrin Transferrin is a protein that transports iron; consequently, its concentrations reflect both protein and iron status. Interpreting transferrin levels as an indicator of protein status is difficult when an *iron* deficiency is present. Transferrin rises as iron deficiency grows worse and falls as iron status improves. Markedly reduced transferrin levels indicate severe PEM; in mild-to-moderate PEM, transferrin levels may vary, limiting their usefulness.[3] Although transferrin breaks down in the body more quickly than albumin, it is still relatively slow to respond to changes in protein intake. Thus it is not a sensitive indicator of response to medical nutrition therapy.†

Conditions other than protein status that lower transferrin concentrations include liver disease, kidney disease (nephrotic syndrome), and metabolic stress. Pregnancy, iron-deficiency anemia, hepatitis, blood loss, and the use of oral contraceptive agents can elevate transferrin levels.

Prealbumin is also known as *thyroxin-binding prealbumin* or *transthyretin*.

Conditions other than protein status that can lower prealbumin levels include metabolic stress, hemodialysis, and hypothyroidism; levels may be elevated in kidney disease and with the use of corticosteroids.

Prealbumin and Retinol-Binding Protein Prealbumin and retinol-binding protein†† respond quickly to changes in protein intake, and both measure response to nutrition therapy.[4] Lab tests of prealbumin and retinol-binding protein are more expensive than the relatively inexpensive test of serum albumin,

*The half-life of albumin is about 20 days, an indication of a slow degradation rate.

†Transferrin has a half-life of 4 to 8 days.

††The half-lives of prealbumin and retinol-binding protein are 2 days and 12 hours, respectively.

Conditions other than protein status that can lower retinol-binding protein levels include vitamin A deficiency, metabolic stress, hyperthyroidism, liver disease, and cystic fibrosis; levels may be elevated in kidney disease.

Somatomedin-C is also known as **insulin-like growth factor** *(IGF-1)*.

which is routinely available. Therefore, tests of prealbumin and retinol-binding protein are often reserved for clients with disorders that markedly change metabolic rates and can rapidly and profoundly affect nutrition status.

Other Serum Proteins Other serum proteins that may be useful in protein assessment include serum somatomedin-C and fibronectin. These indicators of protein status are less practical and more expensive to measure than the other serum proteins used in nutrition support and are not in common use.

Conditions other than protein status that affect the total lymphocyte count include metabolic stress (including infection) and the use of chemotherapy, immunosuppressives, and corticosteroids.

Total Lymphocyte Count PEM compromises the immune system, reducing the number of white blood cells (lymphocytes), which are important in resisting and fighting infections. The total lymphocyte count, derived from the number of white blood cells and the percentage of lymphocytes (see the box below), is inexpensive and easy to obtain, but the many variables that affect the levels of the total lymphocyte count limit its value in nutrition assessment.[5]

Appendix E shows the equations used for calculating nitrogen balance and the creatinine height index.

Urinary Tests of Protein Status Two biochemical tests of protein status—urinary urea nitrogen (UUN) and urinary creatinine excretion—require the collection of urine over a 24-hour period. Both tests require normal kidney function for accurate results. Assessors use the 24-hour UUN measurement, along with an accurate record of the client's energy and protein intake during the same period, to calculate nitrogen balance (see p. 194). Results of nitrogen balance studies determine whether protein intake is adequate to meet needs.

Urinary creatine excretion provides an indirect measure of skeletal muscle mass. By comparing urinary creatinine excretion to standards for sex and height (creatinine height index), assessors determine if muscle mass is adequate or depleted.

Twenty-four-hour urine collections are invalid if even one urine specimen is discarded or if samples are not stored properly. Nitrogen balance studies further

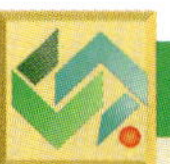

How to Calculate the Total Lymphocyte Count

To calculate the total lymphocyte count (TLC), look at the laboratory report and find the complete blood count (CBC). Two figures from this report, the number of white blood cells (WBC) in cubic millimeters (mm^3) and the percentage of lymphocytes are used to determine the total lymphocyte count:

$$\text{TLC (mm}^3) = \text{WBC (mm}^3) \times \text{\% lymphocytes.}$$

A person with a WBC count of 7500 mm^3 with 15 percent lymphocytes would have a total lymphocyte count of:

$$\text{TLC (mm}^3) = 7500\ \text{mm}^3 \times 0.15 = 1125\ \text{mm.}^3$$

The standard lymphocyte count is 2500 mm^3. Values below 1500 mm^3 suggest mild depletion; below 1200 mm^3, moderate depletion; and below 800 mm^3, severe depletion. In the example, then, a TLC of 1125 mm^3 suggests moderate depletion.

require careful measurement of the food portions presented to and eaten by the client. Such difficulties explain why these tests are not routinely performed in most facilities. Nevertheless, nitrogen balance studies are very useful for evaluating protein needs for clients with severe metabolic stresses.

Laboratory tests help to define protein status, vitamin-mineral status, and alterations of metabolism or organ function with nutrition implications. The most common laboratory tests of protein status include serum levels of albumin, transferrin, prealbumin, and retinol-binding protein; the total lymphocyte count; and urinary urea nitrogen and creatinine. Compared to the serum proteins albumin and transferrin, which reflect long-term protein status, serum prealbumin and retinol-binding protein and urinary urea nitrogen respond more quickly to changes in diet. Urinary creatinine indirectly reflects skeletal muscle mass. The many variables that affect each laboratory test, however, remind assessors to ascertain findings using other assessment techniques.

Nutrition Screening

The numerous markers of nutrition status described in this chapter and the last provide clinicians with a variety of tools for evaluating malnutrition, the risk of malnutrition, and the response to diet therapy. Cost considerations, staffing, and individual preferences determine which tests are routinely available in different facilities and which will be used under specific circumstances. For a person with an elevated cholesterol detected during a routine physical, the assessor might measure height and weight, take a diet history to determine current eating habits, and repeat laboratory tests periodically to evaluate the nutrition care plan. A client admitted to the hospital who is suffering a hypermetabolic stress needs a more detailed assessment. Some hospitals may routinely measure serum albumin; others may not. One approach, the Subjective Global Assessment (SGA), relies on historical, anthropometric, and physical findings to assess nutrition status.[6] Often facilities use readily available information from histories and routine laboratory tests to identify high-risk clients and reserve in-depth assessments for individuals as needed.

Nutrition-screening policies vary from facility to facility but typically include the following:[7]

nutrition screening: the use of routine nutrition assessment procedures to identify people who are malnourished or are at risk for malnutrition.

- *Assessment of health history*. Does the person's health history reveal risk factors for poor nutrition status (review Table 15–2)? Do the current medical problems include metabolic stress, malabsorption, depressed appetite, swallowing problems (dysphagia), or altered organ function?
- *Assessment of diet history*. Do the person's intake data reveal the exclusion of food groups or poor eating habits? Are certain food groups routinely excluded? Has the person been following an extremely restrictive diet?
- *Assessment of height and weight data*. Is the person's weight for height adequate, but not excessive? Has the person lost or gained weight? How much? How fast?
- *Physical assessment*. Does the individual appear to have obvious muscle wasting? Excessive weight? Fluid retention?
- *Assessment of available lab reports*. Do serum albumin and total lymphocyte count suggest malnutrition?

In addition to these screening procedures, health care professionals can use other techniques to screen clients including:

- Check the client's tray to see if food is being eaten.
- If the client is to receive no food or is unable to eat, how long has it been since the client has eaten? Ask if the client is expected to be able to eat soon.
- If the client is unable to eat, determine whether adequate nutrients are being delivered by tube or by vein. (Chapter 24 shows how to calculate the nutrient content of intravenous solutions.)

Regardless of the health care setting in which the client is seen, communicate any problems that you discover and follow up to make sure the problem is being addressed. Always record problems in the medical record to ensure that whoever cares for a particular client will be alert to the problem. A dietitian will perform a more in-depth nutrition assessment if a problem is detected. Be persistent if you suspect that a problem is being ignored.

Nutrition screening provides a cost-effective method for identifying clients who need in-depth nutrition assessments using selected tools described in this chapter and the last. The case study that follows shows how the assessor uses assessment data.

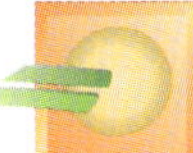

Case Study Nutrition Assessment of a Computer Scientist Following a Car Accident

Ms. Green, a 38-year-old computer scientist, was admitted to the hospital for surgery to repair a broken hip following a car accident. Other injuries included a wound over her left eye and bruises on her arm. After screening her health record, the physician referred Ms. Green to a dietitian for further nutrition assessment. Before visiting the client, the dietitian reviewed the medical record and noted the following:

- Ms. Green has been in good health over the past ten years, although she has experienced a gradual weight gain (height, 5 feet 7 inches; current weight, 150 pounds). She is in stable condition following surgery.
- Prior to hospitalization, Ms. Green was taking one multivitamin-mineral supplement daily and no medications. Morphine sulfate is now being administered for pain.
- Available information from the lab report shows a mildly depleted serum albumin (3 g/100 ml) and a moderately depleted total lymphocyte count (1000 mm^3).

From this information the dietitian keeps these points in mind before visiting the client:

- Even though Ms. Green is overweight, her nutrient requirements are temporarily increased.
- Pain mediation may make it difficult for Ms. Green to provide a detailed diet history.

Once in the client's room, the dietitian confirms Ms. Green's identity, introduces himself, and states the purpose of his visit. He takes time to establish rapport and get a sense of the client's ability to answer questions. Ms. Green appears to be alert, and the dietitian learns that she lives alone. Her busy schedule seldom leaves time for her to prepare meals. Using a usual food intake, the dietitian finds that Ms. Green usually skips breakfast and often eats out. She enjoys foods from all food groups, although she seldom eats the recommended amounts from the fruits and vegetable groups. For the past three weeks, she has been trying to lose weight, and her intake has been less than usual. She has lost 10 pounds during this time. Money for food and facilities for food preparation are not a problem. She appears to be overweight and pale.

Reviewing the elements of typical nutrition-screening procedures described on p. 555, what factors might have alerted the health care team to the need for a complete nutrition assessment? What factors in Ms. Green's health, drug, socioeconomic, and diet histories or physical findings suggest malnutrition?

Determine Ms. Green's ideal body weight and calculate her percent ideal body weight and percent usual body weight. Consider Ms. Green's recent weight change. What is a safe rate of weight loss (see p. 547)? How does Ms. Green's weight loss compare with the safe rate? Does her recent weight change increase her risk of poor nutrition status? What do Ms. Green's lab values indicate with respect to her protein status? What factors besides malnutrition need to be considered when interpreting Ms. Green's lab test results?

Study Questions

1. How do anthropometric measurements help define nutrition status? What anthropometric measurements are frequently used in nutrition assessments? Describe the limitations of anthropometric measurements.
2. How do lab tests help define nutrition status? What factors influence lab test results?
3. Describe the lab tests used to uncover PEM.
4. What is the purpose of nutrition screening? List various screening techniques.

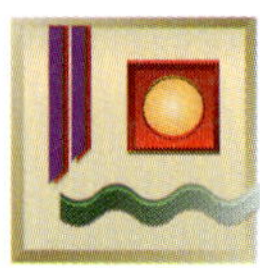

Clinical Applications

1. Calculate percent ideal body weight and percent usual body weight for a man who is 5 feet 11 inches tall with a current weight of 160 pounds and a usual body weight of 180 pounds. Select a weight standard for comparison and briefly defend your choice. What additional information will be important for you to find out about this man's weight loss?
2. Recall that serum proteins are influenced by metabolic stresses. With this in mind, what possible explanations can you suggest for these findings from a nutrition screening: client suffering a metabolic stress, 15-pound weight loss over the last four months (unintentional), depleted serum albumin, elevated serum transferrin, elevated total lymphocyte count. How might one sort through the possible explanations?

Notes

1. K. N. Jeejeebhoy, A. S. Detsky, and J. P. Baker, Assessment of nutrition status, *Journal of Parenteral and Enteral Nutrition* (supplement) 14 (1990): 193–196.
2. J. P. Doweiko and D. J. Nompleggi, The role of albumin in human physiology and pathophysiology, Part III: Albumin and disease states, *Journal of Parenteral and Enteral Nutrition* 15 (1991): 476–483.
3. A. Spiekerman, Proteins used in nutritional assessment, *Clinical Laboratory Medicine* 13 (1993): 353–369.
4. P. Charney, Nutrition assessment in the 1990s: Where are we now? *Nutrition in Clinical Practice* 10 (1995): 131–195; M. Russell, Serum proteins and nitrogen balance: Evaluating response to nutrition support, *Support Line*, February 1995, pp. 3–7.
5. Charney, 1995.
6. A. S. Detsky and coauthors, What is Subjective Global Assessment of nutrition status? *Journal of Parenteral and Enteral Nutrition* 11 (1987): 8–13.
7. Charney, 1995.

Nutrition and Diagnostic Tests

Chapter 16 introduced the laboratory tests that help diagnose malnutrition. Laboratory tests also play a pivotal role in the identification and treatment of many other disorders. Diagnostic tests include laboratory analysis of the blood, stool, urine, and breath and other procedures such as X rays, endoscopy, and other imaging techniques. Nutrition may influence the results of these tests and their interpretations. As you read through the examples presented in this highlight, keep in mind that the concepts introduced may apply to other tests as well.

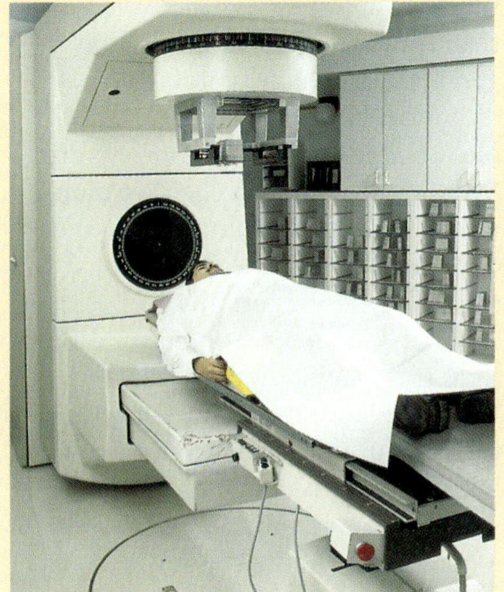

Clients must often adjust their diets in preparation for diagnostic tests.

EFFECTS OF FOODS ON LABORATORY VALUES

After a meal, the concentration of nutrients in the blood rises—a reflection of recent nutrient absorption. These levels may affect the test results for some blood constituents directly; for example, vitamin and mineral tests often reflect recent intake.

In some cases, the expected effect of a food on a lab value is known, and it may even be desirable to study that effect. Such is the case with a glucose tolerance test—a test of glucose metabolism. A person is given a dose of dietary glucose, and blood glucose is checked at regular intervals. By looking at the person's response to the glucose load, the clinician can tell if the person is metabolizing glucose normally. To improve the validity of the test, the person needs to receive a diet adequate in kcalories and protein, and at least 150 grams of carbohydrate, for at least 3 days before the test.[1]

Another test requiring that a set amount of a nutrient be consumed is that for fat malabsorption. To diagnose fat malabsorption, clinicians aim to provide about 100 grams (900 kcalories) of fat per day for 2 to 3 days; during the same period, the person's stools are collected.[2] Some people, however, simply cannot eat that much fat, particularly when they are ill. In those cases, diets can be planned to include from 60 to 80 grams of fat, and different standards are used to determine malabsorption.

Alternatively, some blood tests require that people fast for 8 to 12 hours before blood is drawn. After a meal, triglyceride levels rise and cause the blood sample to become cloudy. The cloudiness interferes with many chemical reactions that affect test results.[3] Fasting blood samples are often recommended when multiple tests will be performed on one blood sample.

Sometimes, tests require specific dietary restrictions to obtain valid results. One example is a stool test used to detect GI bleeding, an aid to the detection of cancer of the colon. The person often takes this test at home as part of a routine physical examination. For 48 to 72 hours before the test, and during the times stools are collected, the person should follow a high-fiber diet and eat no red meats, poultry, fish, turnips, and horseradish. The high-fiber foods speed up intestinal transit time and maximize the likelihood of detecting significant blood loss if it is present. Omitting the red meats and other foods listed above helps prevent false positive results—that is, results that suggest significant GI blood loss, when in fact there was none.

Vitamin C and iron supplements are also restricted during this GI test. Vitamin C supplements (more than 500 milligrams per day) can cause falsely normal test results, even when the person is experiencing significant GI bleeding. In contrast, iron supplements may produce GI bleeding in some people, even though there is no lesion.

A urinary test that requires a restrictive diet is used to detect certain tumors by looking for a compound called 5-hydroxyindoleacetic acid (5-HIAA) in the urine. If present, 5-HIAA signifies abnormal production of the brain neurotransmitter serotonin. Some foods contain significant amounts of serotonin and can interfere with test results. For the 24 hours preceding the test, clients are instructed not to eat avocado, bananas, kiwi, pineapple, plantain, plums, eggplant, tomatoes, butternuts, pecans, and walnuts. Clients must also abstain from alcohol because it suppresses 5-HIAA levels.

Even breath tests can be affected by diet. An analysis of hydrogen in the breath is used to detect lactose intolerance. Breads and pastas made from wheat flour and legumes can contribute significant quantities of hydrogen in the breath, so the person is cautioned not to eat these foods the day before the test. The person must fast from at least midnight until the next morning when breath hydrogen is collected to obtain a baseline hydrogen level; then the person is given an oral dose of lactose. Breath hydrogen is measured thereafter at intervals.

So far, all of the diagnostic tests described have been laboratory tests. X rays, endoscopy, and other imaging techniques may also require special dietary restriction. X rays of the intestinal tract, for example, may require that the person fast from midnight the day before the test. Likewise, endoscopy procedures frequently require fasting.

ASSURING DIET COMPLIANCE

To assure that clients receive appropriate diets for diagnostic tests depends on cooperation and communication between various health care professionals. First, the physician ordering the test must specify the test diet. The diet order may read simply, "diet for breath hydrogen test." In the hospital, the dietary department is then responsible for sending the appropriate diet, which is specified in the diet manual. The nurse working with the client can check the diet manual to see what the diet entails and instruct the client, explaining how long the special diet (or fast) will last. The laboratory analyzing the test may also provide information about testing procedures. To make sure the test is valid, clients are advised to eat only those foods provided by the health care facility.

For tests that require ingestion of a certain amount of a nutrient, such as the fat malabsorption tests, nurses and dietitians frequently share responsibility for monitoring and recording the client's intake. The dietitian is often responsible for calculating expected fecal fat excretion when intakes fall below desirable levels. Nurses are responsible for stool and urine collections; laboratory technicians draw blood for blood tests.

Extra care must be taken when clients are being tested in an outpatient setting. Clients who are at home during the test period have free access to a wide variety of foods, nutrient supplements, and drugs. Like foods and nutrients, drugs can interfere with some test results. The dietitian or nurse is wise to provide oral and clearly written instructions about foods, nutrients, and drugs that may affect test results. Clients may be instructed to keep food and drug records, so that their test results can be assessed.

Finally, it is important to note that diagnostic procedures change from time to time. When new tests are developed, precautions needed earlier may not apply. Regular communication between the department performing the test and the physician, nursing service, and dietary departments can help keep everyone up to date.

NOTES

1. A. Ateshkadi and coauthors, *Basic Skills in Interpreting Laboratory Data* (Bethesda, Md.: American Society of Health-System Pharmacists, 1996), p. 259.
2. J. K. Nelson and coauthors, *Mayo Clinic Diet Manual* (St. Louis: Mosby, 1994), p. 413.
3. *Diagnostic Tests Handbook* (Springhouse, Pa.: Springhouse Corporation, 1993), p. XVI.

Chapter 17

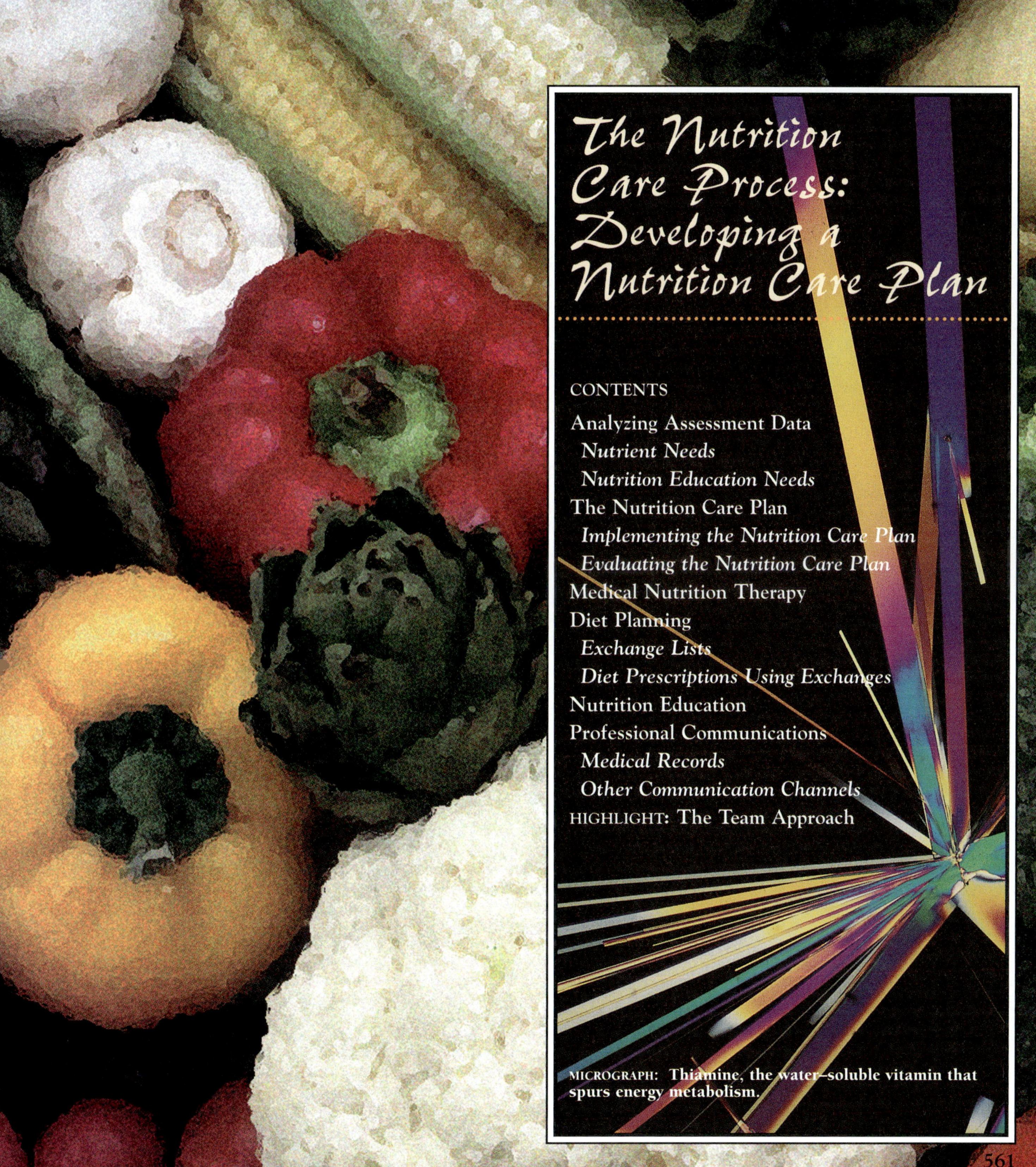

The Nutrition Care Process: Developing a Nutrition Care Plan

CONTENTS

MICROGRAPH: Thiamine, the water-soluble vitamin that spurs energy metabolism.

This chapter describes the process used to analyze assessment data and correct nutrition problems. Because meeting a person's nutrient and nutrition education needs is a key part of this process, this chapter also describes medical nutrition therapy, diet planning, and nutrition education.

Analyzing Assessment Data

The next step following nutrition assessment is to study the accumulated data. What are the potential nutrition problems? Is body weight appropriate? Are lab values within normal limits? Are there physical signs of malnutrition? Are nutrient needs altered due to growth or illness? Will long-term dietary adjustments be necessary? Answers to questions like these enable the assessor to generate a nutrition problem list—the basis of the nutrition care plan. The problems may be past, present, or future conditions that may impair nutrition status or alter nutrient needs. The dietitian then considers nutritional solutions to these problems, estimating nutrient needs, determining the best diet to meet those needs, and making plans for nutrition education.

The word **illness** as used in this book refers to any medical condition that alters nutrient needs. Not all such conditions are diseases. For example, major surgery is a metabolic stress that can alter nutrient needs even though it is not a disease.

The nutrition problem list is to the nutrition care process what the *nursing diagnosis* is to the nursing care process.

NUTRIENT NEEDS

The RDA provide an estimate of energy, protein, vitamin, and mineral intakes for healthy people throughout life. They do not apply to people with health problems. When an illness requires supplemented or restricted intakes, dietitians must make educated estimates of the client's nutrient needs. Always keep in mind that these estimates are just that—estimates. An individual's response to the nutrition care plan reveals the person's needs better than estimates can.

Energy Needs If an adult has maintained a desirable weight over a period of time, then that person's energy needs can be estimated from habitual food intake. The person is already consuming the amount of energy needed. For otherwise healthy individuals who are not at a desirable weight, energy needs can be calculated using the basal metabolic rate as detailed in Chapter 8 on pp. 265–268. As for infants, pregnant and lactating women, children, and others, the chapters that follow describe their changing energy needs. Later chapters describe energy needs imposed by various illnesses.

Protein, Vitamin, and Mineral Needs For people who are ill, especially those with severe stress, protein needs can be estimated by conducting nitrogen balance studies or monitoring the response of serum proteins such as prealbumin and retinol-binding protein. Exact vitamin and mineral needs during illness are largely unknown and can only be estimated. Protein, vitamin, and mineral needs vary among individuals and change in different stages of the life cycle and for different medical conditions, as later chapters describe.

NUTRITION EDUCATION NEEDS

Dietitians use assessment data not only to determine nutrient needs, but also to plan for nutrition education. Information gathered during the interview helps the dietitian determine the best way to present nutrition information, the amount of information the client will be able to handle, and the client's level of interest in nutrition and health. Such plans are estimates as well. The dietitian must be flexible and adjust the nutrition education plan based on the client's goals and understanding of, and motivation to practice, the information presented.

The dietitian analyzes assessment data to generate a problem list, estimate nutrient needs, evaluate the need for nutrition education, and determine the appropriate education strategies. The analysis of assessment data provides the foundation for the nutrition care plan.

The Nutrition Care Plan

Once nutrient needs have been assessed and analyzed, the dietitian develops a plan of action that clearly identifies the client's immediate and long-term nutrition needs and sets forth a strategy for meeting those needs. The plan specifies the objectives of dietary recommendations, the content of counseling sessions, and a tentative time frame for accomplishing each objective.

The nutrition care plan specifies:

- The objectives (to meet the client's nutrition needs and needs for nutrition information).
- The areas of content.
- The tentative time frame.

The dietitian considers the client's nutrient requirements, the appropriate way to deliver the nutrients, and the client's nutrition education needs. For each nutrition problem, the dietitian must first identify the cause, if known, and then may specify one or several strategies to tackle it. Consider, for example, a problem of diarrhea. If a medication is causing the diarrhea, an appropriate strategy might be to prevent dehydration by giving ample fluids and electrolytes while the physician tries substituting other drugs. The client should be informed of this plan. If the diarrhea is caused by a milk allergy, then the problem-solving strategy is to eliminate milk and milk products from the diet. Part of the plan will include nutrition education. The dietitian will plan nutrition counseling sessions to provide the client with instructions and suggestions for a nutritionally adequate diet that eliminates milk and milk products.

If, for another example, a client needs to lose weight, the dietitian might set a goal of one pound a week for three months. Identification of a specific goal guides the design of the weight-loss program. The plan might specify that the diet provide 500 kcalories less than the client's calculated energy needs each day, that the diet will be low in fat, and that each day will include an aerobic activity. The dietitian may plan one counseling session to discuss the nutrition care plan with the client, several sessions to instruct the client about the diet, and another session to evaluate the client's understanding and determine if further action is necessary. The plan is continuously revised to reflect changes in growth, health and nutrition status, and the client's individual responses to the plan.

The dietitian relies on nutrient intake data and food histories to identify food habits and socioeconomic factors that must be considered in devising realistic care plans. Form 17–1 provides a sample nutrition assessment and care plan summary.

IMPLEMENTING THE NUTRITION CARE PLAN

Once a care plan is developed, the next step is to implement it by providing both the appropriate diet and education. In an in-patient health care facility (such as a hospital, nursing home, or in-patient mental health facility), the diet part

Form 17–1 Sample Nutrition Assessment and Care Plan Summary

After analyzing the assessment data, the health care professional summarizes significant findings and key points of the care plan using a form such as this one.

Client: ______________________ Diet order: ______________________

Assessment Summary

Anthropometric data: ______________________

____

Biochemical data: ______________________

____

Health history data: ______________________

____

Socioeconomic history data: ______________________

____

Drug-nutrient interactions: ______________________

____

Dietary intake data: ______________________

____

Recommend additional screening: yes/no ______________________

Problem List:

1. ______________________
2. ______________________
3. ______________________
4. ______________________
5. ______________________

Nutrition Care Plan Summary

Plan of nutrition care: ______________________

____

Other therapy: ______________________

____

Education: ______________________

____

Compliance/understanding: ______________________

____

Follow-up: ______________________

Date: ______________________ Dietitian: ______________________

appears deceptively simple: appropriate foods are delivered to clients. Behind the scenes, however, the dietitian carefully plans the diet for each client, and the foodservice department assures that appropriate foods are carefully prepared and delivered. Highlight 25 describes how foodservice systems operate. Equally important, once delivered, the food must be eaten by the client. Dietitians counsel clients throughout their stay so that they will understand their diets and continue to comply at home, if necessary.

Nurses, thanks to their frequent daily contact with clients, can offer important support in the educational aspect of client care. Clients often think of questions long after the dietitian has left, and they ask the next person who walks into the room—most often, the nurse. The nurse who is confident of the answers should provide them. If not sure of the answers, the nurse should express honest uncertainty and reassure the client that the information will be provided. Then inform the dietitian that the client needs a follow-up visit. Highlight 17 shows more ways that health care team members work together to improve nutrition care.

EVALUATING THE NUTRITION CARE PLAN

While the planned strategies are being implemented, the dietitian must keep track of how they are working. If, for example, a client on a weight-reduction diet fails to lose weight, a change may be needed. Is the client eating too much? Is the client too inactive? Perhaps the client should keep a detailed food and activity record to help identify problems with the weight-loss plans.

If a client's situation changes, so may nutrition status and nutrient needs. Dietitians must keep adjusting care plans to meet changing needs. For example, when a pregnant woman delivers her baby, she will need instructions on how to feed her infant. She will also need information on how to revise her diet to support lactation (if she is breastfeeding) or to return to a healthy weight (if she is bottle feeding). The accompanying case study affords an opportunity to apply some of the planning principles introduced here.

A care plan may be ideal, but will fall short of meeting goals if a client is unable or unwilling to comply with it. If the client is unable to comply, reassessing communication techniques may help. Perhaps the level of instruction needs to be simplified or cultural differences addressed. If the client is unwilling, despite the best efforts of health care professionals, little can be done except to try later when the client may be more receptive.

Once nutrient and nutrition education needs have been identified, the dietitian develops a nutrition care plan to meet those needs. Once implemented, the plan must be carefully evaluated to ensure that it meets the client's needs. Medical nutrition therapy, described next, forms the basis of the nutrition care plan. Later chapters of this book offer details of specific diets.

Medical Nutrition Therapy

An essential component of every nutrition care plan is medical nutrition therapy. Medical nutrition therapy strives to provide the appropriate amounts of energy, protein, carbohydrate, fat, vitamins, major minerals, trace elements, and water in whatever form best meets the client's needs. For example, a person who cannot chew needs soft foods; a person who is in a coma may need to have a formula delivered by tube into the GI tract; a person with diabetes mellitus needs a special diet.

Each prescribed diet has its own purpose and rationale. In one case, the *purpose* of weight reduction may be to improve self-image, and in another case, it may be to improve blood glucose regulation. The *rationale* of a weight-

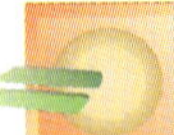

Case Study Computer Scientist with Car Accident Injuries

To practice using nutrition assessment data to develop a nutrition care plan, answer the questions that follow drawing upon the information presented about Ms. Green in the case study on p. 557. Upon completing Ms. Green's nutrition assessment, the dietitian analyzes the assessment data. The dietitian determines that Ms. Green's current medical status indicates a need for sufficient kcalories and protein to minimize weight loss and the breakdown of serum proteins. Once Ms. Green's medical condition has stabilized and she has recovered from her injuries, he will confer with Ms. Green's physician about providing instructions for a safe weight-loss plan.

Contrast Ms. Green's current nutrient needs to her long-term nutrient needs. How will the nutrition care plan reflect these changing needs? Describe methods the dietitian can use to determine if the nutrition care plan is effective while Ms. Green is in the hospital.

Think ahead to Ms. Green's nutrient needs once she goes home from the hospital. What factors in Ms. Green's history need to be considered in devising a realistic plan? Other than adjusting total kcalories, should the dietitian recommend any changes in Ms. Green's usual eating habits?

Once Ms. Green is discharged from the hospital, it is unlikely that she will see the hospital dietitian again. Consider ways the dietitian might arrange for follow-up care.

reduction diet is to provide limited food energy so that the person will use stored body fat and lose weight. Often, medical nutrition therapy complements other therapies. For example, a weight-reduction diet is usually accompanied by a physical activity plan. A diet plan for an individual with insulin-dependent diabetes mellitus (IDDM) is coordinated with meals and the insulin-delivery schedule.

diet order: a physician's written statement in the medical record of what diet a client should receive.

Diet Orders In facilities that serve food, the physician prescribes the client's diet and writes the diet order into the medical record. The dietary department then receives the order from the nursing station. The physician often relies on the dietitian or health care team to suggest a diet prescription or make recommendations when changes in the diet orders appear warranted or when clarity seems to be lacking.

To avoid confusion, physicians should provide clear and precise diet instructions. For example, a "low-sodium diet" order should specify the amount of sodium; otherwise, it could be interpreted as referring to any amount of sodium from 500 to 4000 milligrams. For uncomplicated diets, such as a low-sodium diet, the dietary department often sends a preselected diet to the client until unspecified orders are clarified. Once the dietitian assesses the client's needs, the level of restriction is recorded in the medical record. For more complicated diets, such as a renal diet, meals will not be sent until the order is clarified.

An order to give a client nothing orally (including food, beverages, and medications) reads "NPO." **NPO** stands for *nil per os*, which means "nothing by mouth." On the other hand, **PO** stands for *per os*, which means "by mouth" or "orally."

Occasionally, diet orders may be inappropriate. For example, a physician may describe an obese individual as "well-nourished" and order a regular diet. If this occurs, the dietitian may not see the client, and the client will receive an inappropriate diet and no nutrition advice. As another example, a physician may order that a client receive no food or fluids after midnight for a lab test to be conducted in the morning. The doctor assumes that the order will be discontinued after the test, but it may not be. The client may miss several meals before someone notices the error. These examples illustrate situations where communication between health care professionals can make a difference in client care. Whenever you notice inappropriate diet orders, contact the dietitian or alert the physician.

Diet Manuals The exact foods excluded from or included on a specific modified diet, and even the name given to the same diet, may differ among health care facilities, generally in minor ways. These variations reflect different schools of thought regarding diet; institutional diet manuals are consulted as a standard of practice.

In large hospitals, the staff of dietitians usually compiles a diet manual, subject to approval by the hospital administrator, several physicians, and representatives of the nursing service. A small hospital or clinic may adopt the diet manual of another hospital or an organization such as a state dietetic association. The diet manual describes the foods allowed and not allowed on each diet, outlines the rationale and indications for use of each diet, provides information on the nutritional adequacy of the diets, and offers sample menus. The dietary department uses the manual to design menus for each diet.

diet manual: a book that describes the foods allowed and restricted on a diet, outlines the rationale and indications for use of each diet, and provides sample menus.

Standard and Modified Diets *Standard* or *regular diets* include all foods and provide all the nutrients in amounts appropriate for healthy people. Modified diets are used when standard diets fail to meet the specific needs of clients. Modifying the standard diet is much like tailoring a suit. A tailored suit is the same suit after alterations—only it fits better. In the case of a modified diet, the tailoring may involve changing the consistency; adjusting the amounts of individual nutrients, energy, or fluid; altering the number or size of meals; or eliminating certain foods. Highlight 25 shows how a hospital menu can be modified for different diets. Table 17–1 on pp. 568–569 gives examples of modified diets used to treat diseases involving different organ systems. These diets are described further in later chapters.

standard diet: a *regular diet*—that is, one that includes all foods and meets the nutrient needs of normal, healthy individuals.

modified or therapeutic diet: a regular diet that is adjusted to meet special nutrition needs. Such diets can be adjusted in consistency, in level of energy and nutrients, in amount of fluid, in number of meals, or by the elimination of certain foods.

It is helpful to think about modified diets in terms of the symptoms or conditions they relieve rather than in terms of disorders. Two people with the same disorder may need two different diets. Conversely, people with two different disorders may benefit from the same diet. Consider two people with cancer: one may need a diet that will help control nausea; the other may need a high-kcalorie diet. Now consider a pregnant woman with nausea. She may benefit from the same recommendations as those for the first person with cancer.

Putting the principles of medical nutrition therapy into practice requires careful planning. The therapy must provide the appropriate nutrients and dietary components in a form the client can utilize. Dietitians frequently rely on food group plans and exchange systems to plan menus and educate clients.

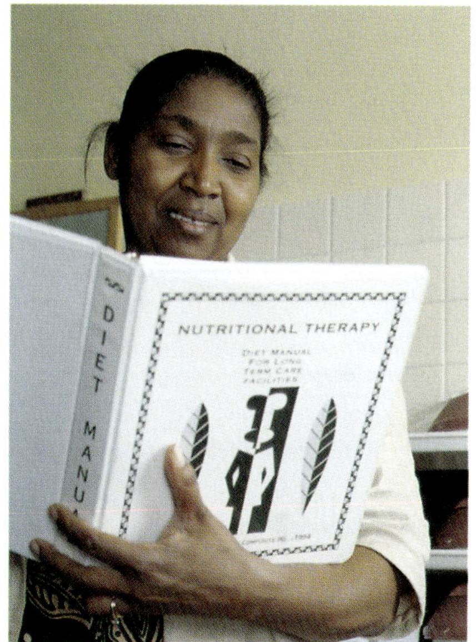

The diet manual specifies which foods to exclude from or include on various modified diets.

Diet Planning

Once diet therapy is prescribed, the dietitian translates the prescription into a diet plan. As later chapters show, diet plans for people who are at their desirable weights and who require either the addition or elimination of certain foods are often based on the food group plans described in Chapter 2. Thus the diet plan for people who need to increase their fiber intakes would recommend the number of servings from each food group with the best sources of fiber within each food group highlighted.

Table 17–1

Summary of Modified Diets by Organ System

Disorders	Possible Diet Modifications[a]
CONDITIONS AFFECTING OR INVOLVING THE GI TRACT, LIVER, AND EXOCRINE PANCREAS[b]	
Blind loop syndrome	Fat-restricted, fluid and electrolyte replacement
Broken jaw	Mechanical soft; liquid
Celiac disease	Gluten-restricted
Cirrhosis	Protein-restricted, sodium-restricted, fluid-restricted
Constipation	High-fiber, increased fluids
Cystic fibrosis	High-kcalorie, high-protein
Delayed gastric emptying	Liquid, low-fiber, tube feeding, total parenteral nutrition (TPN)
Dental caries	Mechanical soft
Diarrhea	Liquid, low-fiber, lactose-free, regular, fluid and electrolyte replacement
Difficulty swallowing (dysphagia)	Mechanical soft, tube feeding, TPN
Diverticulitis	Low-fiber
Diverticulosis	High-fiber
Dry mouth	Mechanical soft
Dumping syndrome	Carbohydrate-restricted, no concentrated sugars, frequent small feedings, fluid and electrolyte replacement
Gastritis	Low-fiber, bland
Hepatic coma	Protein-restricted, sodium-restricted, fluid-restricted
Hepatitis	Regular, high-kcalorie, high-protein
Hiatal hernia	Frequent small feedings, fat-restricted, bland, kcalorie-restricted
Ill-fitting dentures	Mechanical soft
Indigestion (dyspepsia)	Low-fiber, bland, frequent small feedings
Inflammatory bowel disease	Low-fiber, fat-restricted, high-kcalorie, high-protein, fluid and eletrolyte replacement, lactose-restricted, tube feeding, TPN
Irritable bowel syndrome	High-fiber, fat-restricted
Lactose intolerance	Lactose-restricted
Malabsorption	Fat-restricted, high-kcalorie, high-protein, fluid and electrolyte replacement
Missing teeth	Mechanical soft
Nausea	Low-fiber, bland, frequent small feedings, no liquids with meals
Oral surgery	Mechanical soft
Pancreatitis	Fat-restricted, regular, frequent small feedings, tube feeding, TPN
Peptic ulcer	Bland
Periodontal disease	Mechanical soft
Plastic surgery of head or neck	Mechanical soft, tube feeding, TPN
Reflux esophagitis	Frequent small feedings, fat-restricted, bland, kcalorie-restricted
Short bowel syndrome	Fat-restricted, high-kcalorie, high-protein, fluid and electrolyte replacement
Ulcers of mouth or gums	Mechanical soft, avoid spicy foods and foods with seeds
Vomiting	Fluid and electrolyte replacement; NPO

[a]Diet modifications vary for each disease and sometimes depend on medical therapy.
[b]The pancreas produces both external (exocrine) and internal (endocrine) secretions. The external secretions (enzymes) play an important role in the digestion of food; the internal secretions (insulin and other hormones) play a primary role in the regulation of glucose metabolism.

CONDITIONS AFFECTING THE ENDOCRINE PANCREAS[a]	
Diabetes mellitus	Carbohydrate-controlled, kcalorie-controlled, fat-restricted, high-fiber, sodium-restricted
Hypoglycemia	Carbohydrate-controlled, limited simple sugars, frequent small feedings
CONDITIONS AFFECTING THE BLOOD VESSELS, HEART, AND LUNGS	
Atherosclerosis	Fat-restricted, low-cholesterol, kcalorie-restricted, sodium-restricted, high-fiber
Congestive heart failure	Sodium-restricted, kcalorie-restricted, low-fiber, bland, frequent small feedings, fluid-restricted, caffeine-restricted
Coronary heart disease	Fat-restricted, low-cholesterol, kcalorie-restricted, sodium-restricted, high-fiber
Hypertension	Sodium-restricted, kcalorie-restricted, high-potassium, fat-restricted
Myocardial infarction	Sodium-restricted, kcalorie-restricted, bland, frequent small feedings, moderate-temperature foods, fat-restricted, caffeine-restricted
Pulmonary disease	High-kcalorie, high-protein
CONDITIONS AFFECTING THE KIDNEYS	
Acute renal disease	Protein-restricted, high-kcalorie, fluid-controlled, sodium-controlled, potassium-controlled, fat-restricted, carbohydrate-controlled
Chronic renal disease	Protein-restricted, low-sodium, fluid-restricted, potassium-restricted, phosphorus-restricted, fat-restricted
Kidney stones	Increased fluid intake, calcium-controlled, oxalate-restricted, purine-restricted, methionine-restricted
Nephrotic syndrome	High-kcalorie, protein-restricted, sodium-restricted
CONDITIONS AFFECTING MANY ORGAN SYSTEMS	
Acquired immune deficiency syndrome (AIDS)	High-kcalorie, high-protein, fat-restricted, fluid and electrolyte replacement, lactose-restricted, caffeine-restricted, mechanical soft, tube feeding, TPN (see also specific related conditions such as *Ulcers of the mouth*)
Burns	High-kcalorie, high-protein, increased fluid intake
Cancer	High-kcalorie, high-protein (see also specific related conditions such as *Nausea*)
Food sensitivities	Elimination of offending substance
Galactosemia	Galactose-restricted
Obesity, overweight	kcalorie-restricted, fat-restricted, high-fiber
Phenylketonuria (PKU)	Phenylalanine-restricted
Stroke	Mechanical soft, regular, tube feeding, fat-restricted, low-sodium, high-potassium
Surgery	Regular, high-kcalorie, high-protein, increased fluids
Underweight	High-kcalorie, high-protein

exchange lists: diet-planning tools that organize foods by their proportions of carbohydrate, fat, and protein. Foods on any single list can be used interchangeably.

Appendix G gives complete details of the major exchange system used in the United States, and Appendix I provides details of the exchange system used in Canada.

An exchange system:

- Names the foods on each list.
- Specifies portion sizes.
- States the amounts of carbohydrate, protein, fat, and kcalories each portion contributes.

For clients whose diet prescriptions include kcalorie, protein, carbohydrate, or lipid modifications, dietitians often individualize diet plans using exchange lists. The exchange system described here was originally developed for people with diabetes, but is now widely used for evaluating food intakes and planning many types of diets.

EXCHANGE LISTS

Unlike the Daily Food Guide, which sorts foods primarily by their protein, vitamin, and mineral contents, the exchange system sorts foods into three main groups by their proportions of carbohydrate, fat, and protein. The foods in these three groups—the carbohydrate group, the fat group, and the meat and meat substitute group (protein)—are then organized into several exchange lists.

The carbohydrate group includes these exchange lists:

- Starch (cereals, grains, pasta, breads, crackers, snacks, starchy vegetables, and dried beans, peas, and lentils).
- Fruit.
- Milk (nonfat, low-fat, and whole).
- Other carbohydrates (desserts and snacks with added sugars and fats).
- Vegetables.

The fat group includes this exchange list:

- Fats.

The meat and meat substitute group (protein) includes these exchange lists:

- Meat and meat substitutes (very lean, lean, medium-fat, and high-fat).

The Foods on the Lists Foods are not always on the exchange list where you might first expect them to be because they are grouped according to their energy-nutrient contents rather than by their food group. For example, cheeses are grouped with meats in the exchange system because, like meats, cheeses contribute energy from protein and fat but provide negligible carbohydrate. (In the food group plans presented in Chapter 2, cheeses are classed with milk because they are milk products with a comparable calcium content.)

For similar reasons, starchy vegetables such as corn, green peas, and potatoes are listed on the starch list in the exchange system, rather than with the vegetables. Likewise, olives are not classified as a "fruit" as a botanist would claim; they are classified as a "fat" because their fat content makes them more similar to butter than to berries. These groupings permit you to see the characteristics of foods that are significant to energy intake.

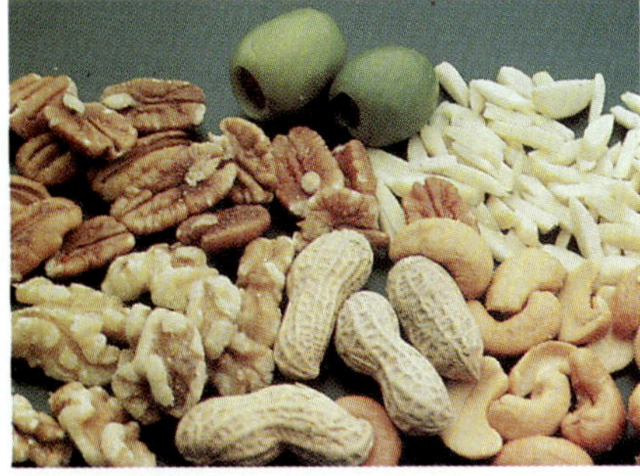

Nuts and olives are so high in fat that they are listed with butter, mayonnaise, and bacon in the fat exchange list.

The exchange lists make it easy for planners to control both the amount and the type of fat in a diet. By allocating items like bacon and avocados to the fat list, the exchange system alerts users to foods that are unexpectedly high in fat. The fat lists also shows which fats are monounsaturated, polyunsaturated, and saturated so that anyone using the list can easily plan a lipid-lowering diet. The starch list specifies which grain products contain added fat (such as biscuits, muffins, and waffles). In addition, the exchange system encourages users to think of nonfat milk as milk and of whole milk as milk with added fat; and to think of very lean meats as meats and of lean, medium- and high-fat meats as meats with added fat. To that end, foods on the milk and meat lists are separated into categories based on their fat contents. Meat exchanges that are particularly high in cholesterol are noted.

Portion Sizes By strictly defining portion sizes, all of the foods in a given exchange list provide approximately the same amounts of energy nutrients (carbohydrate, fat, and protein) and the same number of kcalories. Any food on a list can then be exchanged, or traded, for any other food on that same list without affecting a plan's balance or total kcalories.

To apply the system successfully, users must become familiar with portion sizes. Although this may be quite a task at first, the exchange system is so widely used in diet planning that users quickly become familiar with the contents and portion sizes of each list. A convenient way to remember the portion sizes and energy values is to keep in mind a typical item from each list (see Table 17–2 below). Figure 17–1 (on pp. 572–573) shows the foods on each of the exchange lists and their accurate portion sizes.

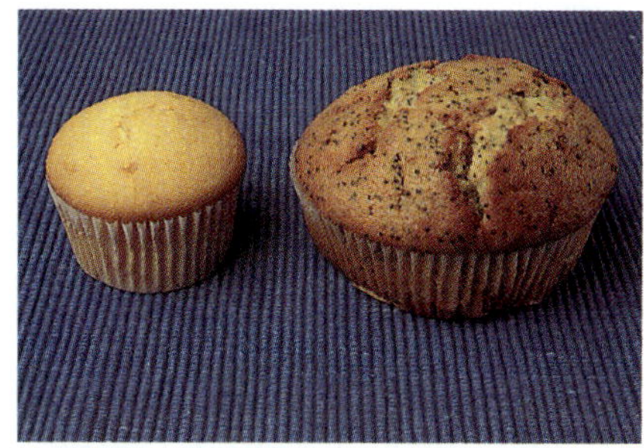

It may look like *one*, but the large muffin counts as *two* servings.

Table 17–2

The Exchange Lists

Group/Lists	Typical Item/Portion Size	Carbohydrate (g)	Protein (g)	Fat (g)	Energy[a] (kcal)
CARBOHYDRATE GROUP					
Starch[b]	1 slice bread	15	3	1 or less	80
Fruit	1 small apple	15	—	—	60
Milk					
Nonfat	1 c nonfat milk	12	8	0–3	90
Low-fat	1 c low-fat milk	12	8	5	120
Whole	1 c whole milk	12	8	8	150
Other carbohydrates[c]	2 small cookies	15	varies	varies	varies
Vegetable	½ c cooked carrots	5	2	—	25
MEAT AND MEAT SUBSTITUTE GROUP[d]					
Meat					
Very lean	1 oz chicken (white meat, no skin)	—	7	0–1	35
Lean	1 oz lean beef	—	7	3	55
Medium-fat	1 oz ground beef	—	7	5	75
High-fat	1 oz pork sausage	—	7	8	100
FAT GROUP					
Fat	1 tsp butter	—	—	5	45

Note: The complete details of the U.S. exchange system are provided in Appendix G. Those of the Canadian system are shown in Appendix I.

[a]The energy value for each exchange list represents an approximate average for the group and does not reflect the precise number of grams of carbohydrate, protein, and fat. For example, a slice of bread contains 15 grams carbohydrate (that's 60 kcalories), 3 grams protein (that's another 12 kcalories), and a little fat—rounded up to 80 kcalories for ease in calculating. A half-cup of vegetables (not including starchy vegetables) contains 5 grams carbohydrate (20 kcalories) and 2 grams protein (8 more), which has been rounded down to 25 kcalories.

[b]The starch list includes cereals, grains, breads, crackers, snacks, starchy vegetables (such as corn, peas, and potatoes), and legumes (dried beans, peas, and lentils).

[c]The other carbohydrates list includes foods that contain added sugars and fats such as cakes, cookies, doughnuts, ice cream, potato chips, pudding, syrup, and frozen yogurt.

[d]The meat and meat substitutes list includes legumes, cheese, and peanut butter.

Figure 17–1 The Exchange System: Examples of Foods, Portion Sizes, and Energy-Nutrient Contributions

THE CARBOHYDRATE GROUP

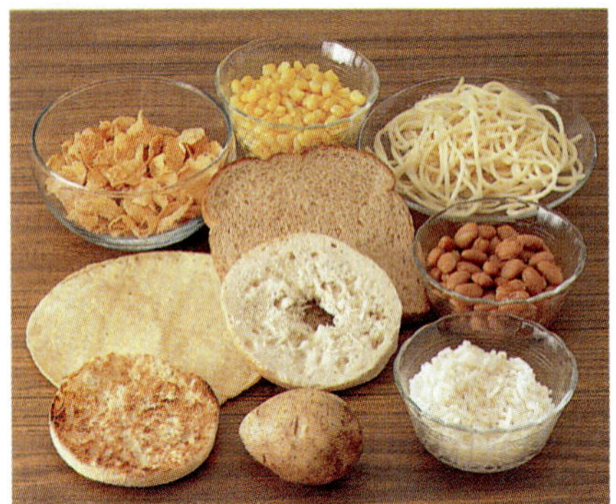

Starch
1 starch exchange is like:
1 slice bread.
¾ c ready-to-eat cereal.
½ c cooked pasta.
⅓ c cooked rice.
½ c cooked beans.[a]
½ c corn, peas, or yams.
1 small (3 oz) potato.
½ bagel, English muffin, or bun.
1 tortilla, waffle, or roll.
(1 starch = 15 g carbohydrate, 3 g protein, 0–1 g fat, and 80 kcal.)
[a]½ c cooked beans = 1 very lean meat exchange *plus* 1 starch exchange.

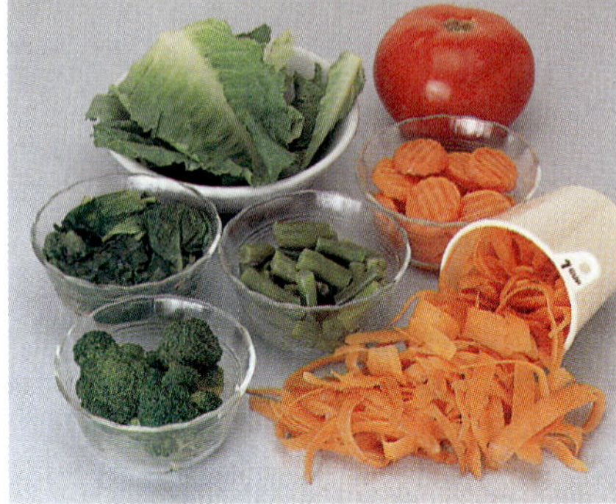

Vegetables
1 vegetable exchange is like:
½ c cooked carrots, greens, green beans, brussels sprouts, beets, broccoli, cauliflower, or spinach.
1 c raw carrots, radishes, or salad greens.
1 lg tomato.
(1 vegetable = 5 g carbohydrate, 2 g protein, and 25 kcal.)

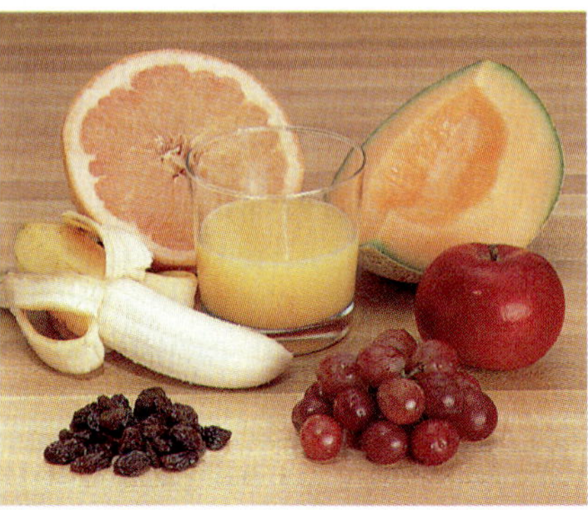

Fruits
1 fruit exchange is like:
1 small banana, nectarine, apple, or orange.
½ large grapefruit or pear.
½ c orange, apple, or grapefruit juice.
17 small grapes.
⅓ cantaloupe (or 1 c cubes).
2 tbs raisins.
(1 fruit = 15 g carbohydrate and 60 kcal.)

THE MEAT AND MEAT SUBSTITUTES GROUP (PROTEIN)

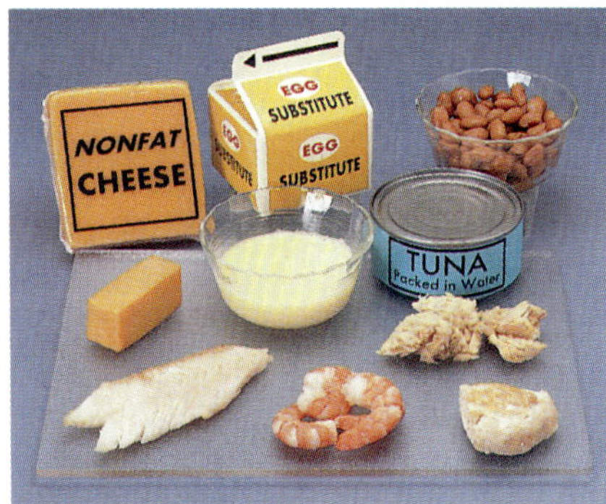

Meat and substitutes (very lean)
1 very lean meat exchange is like:
1 oz chicken (white meat, no skin).
1 oz cod, flounder, or trout.
1 oz tuna (canned in water).
1 oz clams, crab, lobster, scallops, shrimp, or imitation seafood.
1 oz fat-free cheese.
½ c cooked beans, peas, or lentils.
¼ c nonfat or low-fat cream cheese.
2 egg whites (or ¼ c egg substitute).
(1 very lean meat = 7 g protein, 0–1 g fat, and 35 kcal).

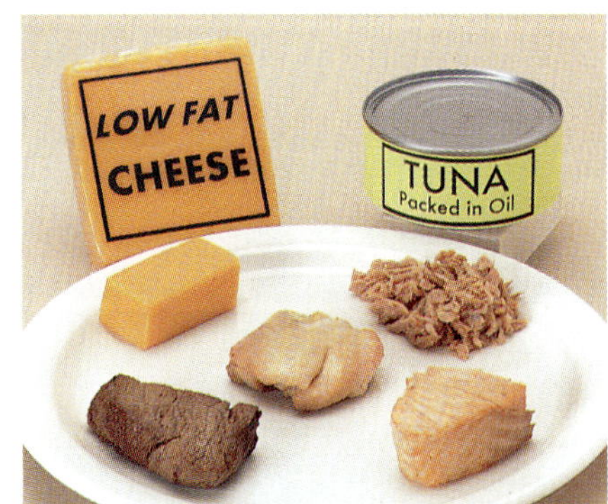

Meats and substitutes (lean)
1 lean meat exchange is like:
1 oz beef or pork tenderloin.
1 oz chicken (dark meat, no skin).
1 oz herring or salmon.
1 oz tuna (canned in oil, drained).
1 oz low-fat cheese or luncheon meats.
(1 lean meat = 7 g protein, 3 g fat, and 55 kcal.)

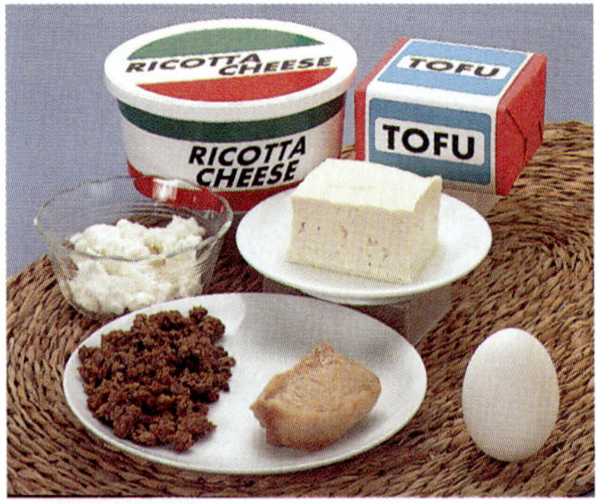

Meats and substitutes (medium-fat)
1 medium-fat meat exchange is like:
1 oz ground beef.
1 oz pork chop.
1 egg.
¼ c ricotta cheese.
4 oz tofu.
(1 medium-fat meat = 7 g protein, 5 g fat, and 75 kcal.)

Figure 17–1 *(continued)*

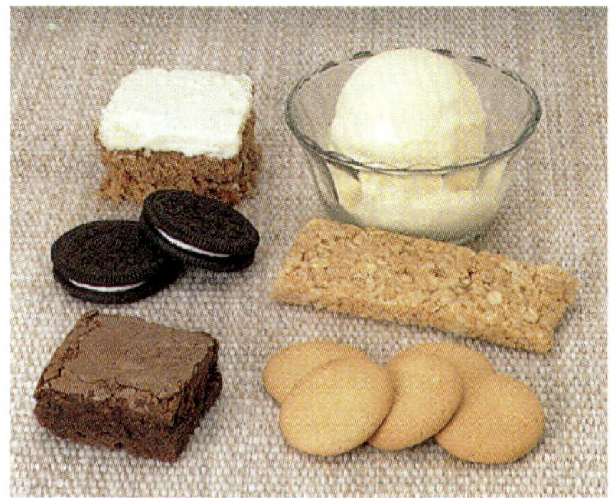

Other carbohydrates
1 other carbohydrates exchange is like:
2 small cookies.
1 small brownie or cake.
5 vanilla wafers.
1 granola bar.
½ c ice cream.
(1 other carbohydrate = 15 g carbohydrate and may be exchanged for 1 starch, 1 fruit, or 1 milk. Because many items on this list contain added sugar and fat, their fat and kcalorie values vary and their portion sizes are small.)

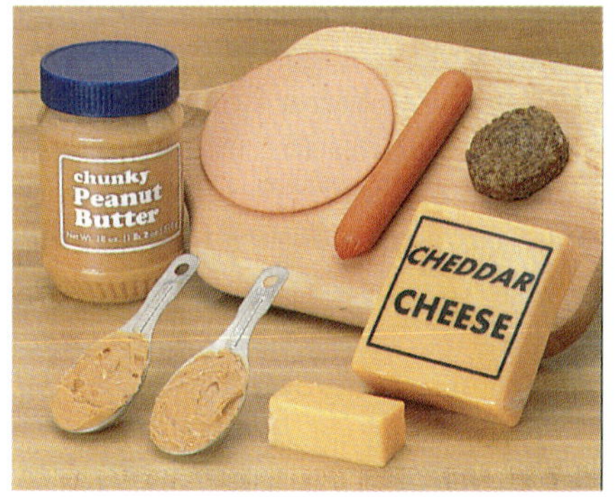

Meats and substitutes (high-fat)
1 high-fat meat exchange is like:
1 oz pork sausage.
1 oz luncheon meat (such as bologna).
1 oz regular cheese (such as cheddar or swiss).
1 small hot dog (turkey or chicken).[b]
2 tbs peanut butter.[c]
(1 high-fat meat = 7 g protein, 8 g fat, and 100 kcal.)

[b]A beef or pork hot dog counts as 1 high-fat meat exchange *plus* 1 fat exchange.

[c]Peanut butter counts as 1 high-fat meat exchange *plus* 1 fat exchange.

Milks (nonfat and very-low fat)
1 nonfat milk exchange is like:
1 c nonfat milk.
¾ c nonfat yogurt, plain.
1 c nonfat or lowfat buttermilk.
½ c evaporated nonfat milk.
⅓ c dry nonfat milk.
(1 nonfat milk = 12 g carbohydrate, 8 g protein, 0–3 g fat, and 90 kcal.)

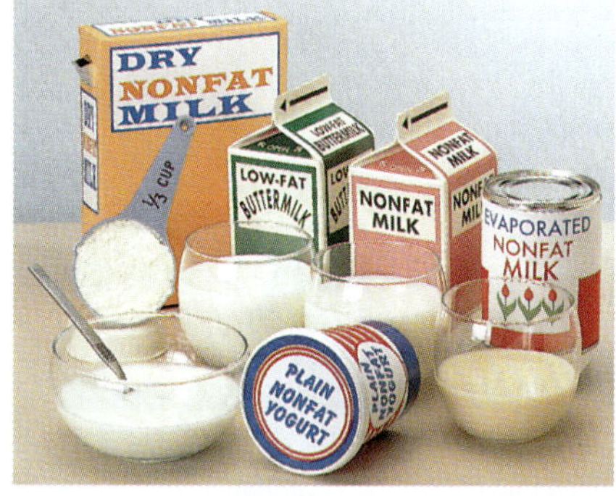

Milks (low-fat)
1 low-fat milk exchange is like:
1 c 2% milk.
¾ c low-fat yogurt, plain.
(1 low-fat milk = 12 g carbohydrate, 8 g protein, 5 g fat, and 120 kcal.)

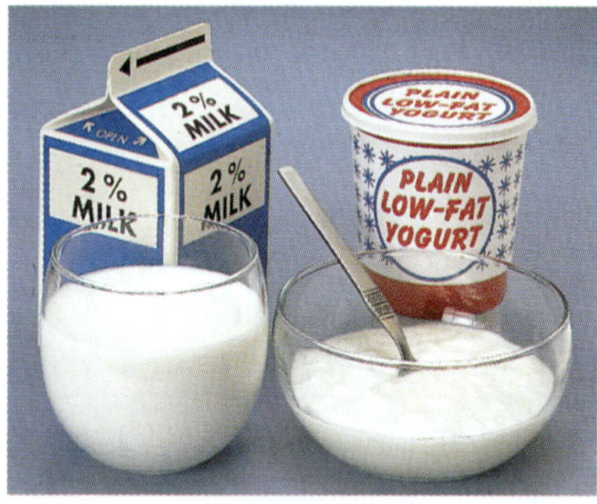

Milks (whole)
1 whole milk exchange is like:
1 c whole milk.
½ c evaporated whole milk.
(1 whole milk = 12 g carbohydrate, 8 g protein, 8 g fat, and 150 kcal.)

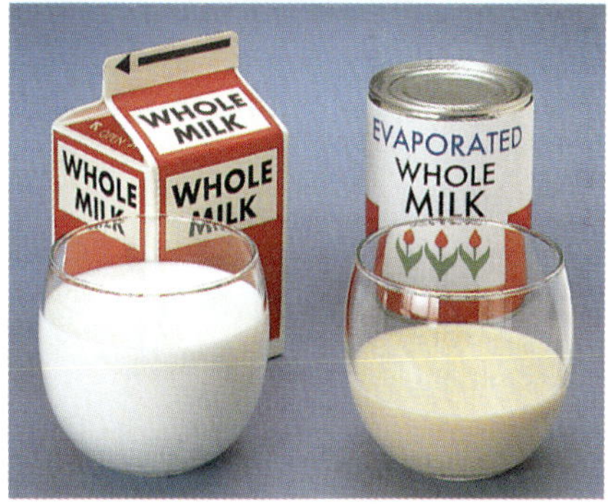

THE FAT GROUP

Fats
1 fat exchange is like:
1 tsp butter.
1 tsp margarine or mayonnaise (1 tbs reduced fat).
1 tsp any oil.
1 tbs salad dressing (2 tbs reduced fat).
8 large black olives.
10 large peanuts.
⅛ medium avocado.
1 slice bacon.
2 tbs shredded coconut.
1 tbs cream cheese (2 tbs reduced fat).
(1 fat = 5 g fat and 45 kcal.)

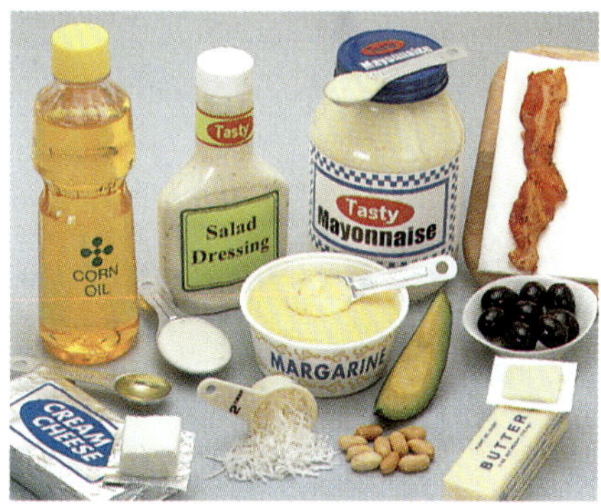

Note: Health recommendations urge people to limit their intakes of saturated fats; butter, bacon, coconut, and cream cheese contain saturated fat.

Figure 17–2

Using Labels to Calculate Exchanges

Home Taste
Lasagna
WITH MEAT SAUCE
Nutrition Facts
Serving size 10 1/2 oz (298 g)
Servings per Package 1
Amount per serving
Calories 361 Calories from Fat 117
% Daily Value*
Total Fat 13 g 20%
Saturated Fat 8 g 40%
Cholesterol 87 mg 29%
Sodium 860 mg 36%
Total Carbohydrate 37 g 12%
Dietary fiber 0 g
Sugars 8 g
Protein 26 g

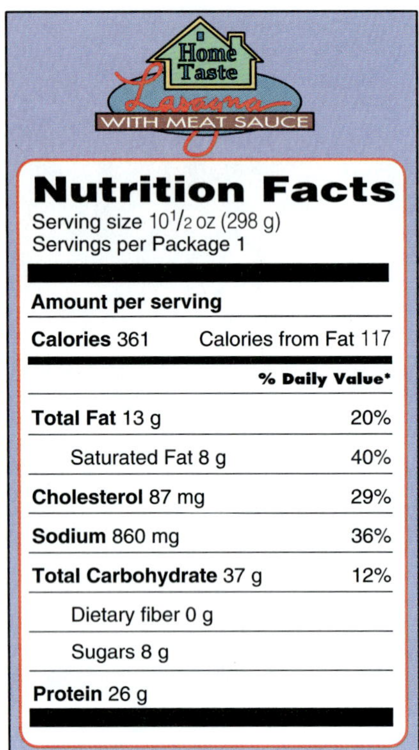

Can you "see" these exchanges in the label above?

Exchange	Carbohydrate	Protein	Fat
2 starches	**30 g**	**6 g**	—
1 vegetable	**5 g**	**2 g**	—
3 medium-fat meats	—	**21 g**	**15 g**
Total	**35 g**	**29 g**	**15 g**

Note that a *portion* in the exchange system is not the same as a *serving* in the Daily Food Guide, especially when it comes to meats. The exchange system lists meats and most cheeses in single ounces; that is, 1 *portion* (or *exchange*) of meat is 1 ounce, whereas one *serving* is 2 to 3 ounces. Thus, if a person's diet plan allows for 3 ounces of meat at dinner, the diet plan would specify 3 meat exchanges. Taking actual portion sizes into account is pivotal to the successful use of the diet.

Food Mixtures Users of the exchange lists learn to view mixtures of foods, such as casseroles and soups, as combinations of foods from different exchange lists. They also learn to interpret food labels with the exchange system in mind (see Figure 17–2). Knowing that foods on the starch list provide 15 grams of carbohydrate and those on the vegetable list provide 5, you can count a lasagna dinner that provides 37 grams of carbohydrate as "2 starches and 1 vegetable"; knowing that foods on the meat list provide 7 grams of protein, you might count it as "3 meats"; the grams of fat suggest that the meat (and cheese) is probably medium-fat.

DIET PRESCRIPTIONS USING EXCHANGES

Once the dietitian has determined the total energy and the percentage of kcalories from carbohydrate, protein, and fat to be included in a client's diet, the next step is to translate the prescription into exchange lists. Table 17–3 provides examples of sample diets at different kcalorie levels. (The box in Chapter 27 shows the steps a dietitian uses to derive such a pattern of exchanges for a client with diabetes.)

Combining Food Group Plans and Exchange Lists Although exchange systems make excellent diet-planning tools, they do not guarantee adequate intakes of vitamins and minerals. Food group plans work better from that standpoint because the food groupings are based on similarities in vitamin-mineral content. To take advantage of the strengths of both exchange patterns and food group plans, diet planners check the exchange pattern to ensure that the diet contains adequate servings from each food group.

Table 17–3

Diet Patterns for Different Energy Intakes

	Energy Level (kcal)						
Exchange	**1200**	**1500**	**1800**	**2000**	**2200**	**2600**	**3000**
Starch/bread	6	7	8	9	11	13	15
Meat (lean)	4	5	6	6	6	7	8
Vegetable	3	4	5	5	5	6	6
Fruit	2	3	4	4	4	5	6
Milk (nonfat)	2	2	2	3	3	3	3
Fat	3	5	6	7	8	10	12

Note: These patterns follow the Daily Food Guide plan and supply less than 30 percent of kcalories as fat.

Translating Exchanges into Meals The next step in diet planning is to assign the exchanges to meals and snacks. The final plan for a 2000-kcalorie diet might look like the one in Table 17–4. The person uses the plan by filling in real foods to create a menu (use Figure 17–1 and Appendix G). For example, the breakfast plan calls for 2 starches, 1 fruit, 1 nonfat milk and 2 fats. A person might select a bowl of shredded wheat with banana slices and milk (1 cup shredded wheat = 2 starches, 1 small banana = 1 fruit, and 1 cup nonfat milk = 1 milk) and save the fat for another meal; or a bagel with two teaspoons of margarine and a bowl of cantaloupe pieces topped with yogurt (1 bagel = 2 starches, ⅓ cantaloupe melon = 1 fruit, and ¾ cup nonfat plain yogurt = 1 milk, 2 teaspoons margarine = 2 fat). Alternatively, the person could have pancakes with strawberries and milk (4 small pancakes = 2 starches plus 2 fats, 1 ¼ cup strawberries = 1 fruit, and a cup of nonfat milk = 1 milk). Then the person could move on to complete the menu for lunch, dinner, and snacks.

Exchange list systems provide a practical tool for diet planning and estimating nutrient intakes. Unlike food group plans, foods on exchange lists are divided by their energy, protein, carbohydrate, and lipid contents. Once the dietitian designs a diet and meal plan for a client, the next step is to explain the diet plan to the client and caregivers.

Nutrition Education

Nutrition education is a continuous process that requires active participation between the dietitian and client. For temporary dietary adjustments (such as a diet for a diagnostic test), the dietitian, dietetic technician, or nurse describes the foods allowed and not allowed on the diet, the length of time the diet will be necessary, and the reasons for the diet. For long-term dietary adjustments, more extensive counseling is required. In such cases, nutrition education is best accomplished in stages, allowing time for the client to assimilate information, ask questions, and recognize potential obstacles in following the diet.

Table 17–4

A Sample 2000-kCalorie Diet Plan

Exchange	Breakfast	Lunch	Snack	Dinner	Evening Snack
9 starch	2	2	1	3	1
6 vegetable		3		3	
5 fruit	1	1	1	1	1
5 lean meat		2		3	
3 nonfat milk	1	1			1
6 fat	2	2		2	

Note: This diet plan is one of many possibilities. It follows the number of servings suggested by the Daily Food Guide and meets dietary recommendations to provide 55 to 60 percent of its kcalories from carbohydrate, 15 to 20 percent from protein, and less than 30 percent from fat.

Responsibility for Nutrition Education In health care facilities that employ dietitians, the primary responsibility for nutrition education lies with the dietitian, but physicians, nurses, and dietetic technicians can help to reinforce and clarify nutrition information. For example, while helping a client prepare for breakfast, a nurse listens as the client comments that breakfast just isn't the same without milk for his cereal now that he is on a low-fat diet. The nurse acknowledges that things will be a bit different, thus reinforcing the importance of making the necessary changes in accordance with the low-fat diet. The nurse adds, however, that the client need not do without milk altogether, but instead can include nonfat and some low-fat milks. Because the nurse sees that the client is confused about his diet, she asks the dietitian to talk with the client again.

In some outpatient clinics, nursing homes, and other facilities, dietitians are not available to provide nutrition education. In these facilities, the nurse or physician most often assumes the responsibility.

Application of Nutrition Education Our abundant knowledge of the relationships between diet and health is purely academic until people can apply that knowledge to their lives. Successful counselors gather thorough client histories and use the information wisely to plan diets and provide diet and health information in a way that helps clients integrate the needed changes into their lifestyles. Just as important, if not more so, successful counselors motivate clients to make the needed changes. Although it is beyond the scope of this text to provide all the details of nutrition counseling, the following paragraphs highlight some key points. The checklist in Table 17–5 shows measures that can facilitate successful counseling.

Establish a caring relationship.

Establishing a Caring Relationship Counselors who show they care about their clients are more likely to gain their clients' trust. A trusting client will provide honest feedback, which is essential to successful nutrition education. To promote trust, work on establishing rapport and empathy. To establish rapport, spend a little time expressing your interest in and concern for your client. To establish empathy, put yourself in your client's shoes: this will lay the foundation for developing understanding between the two of you.

Positive feelings foster learning.

A caring counselor realizes that the client is a whole person and that nutrition is only a part of that person's life. Major life stresses, pain, anger, and resentment may interfere with a client's motivation to change and may block messages from getting through. In some cases, the counselor may fare better by rescheduling a session than by forcing information on an unwilling learner.

Encouraging Behavior Changes Changing behaviors is difficult to say the least. Consider that for most of their lives, clients select foods based on taste, socioeconomic factors, convenience, and persuasive messages from friends and advertisers. Then one day, a nutrition counselor advises a client to make most food selections based on health. To accomplish this goal every time the choice arises—and it arises every time the person eats—requires an incredibly strong commitment.

Changing long-term behaviors takes time, and a person's level of motivation often progresses in stages. A small change that produces a positive result may motivate the person to make further changes. Thus successful counselors plan for several counseling sessions. They present information in a way their client can

Table 17–5

Nutrition Counseling Checklist

PREPARATION

Successful communication begins with adequate preparation. Before beginning a counseling session, be sure to:

- *Assess your client's needs*—nutritional, educational, and motivational. This information allows you to make the information relevant to, and appropriate for, each individual client.
- *Assess your own knowledge* of the diet, medical condition, and treatment plans of your client. Gather the information you might need and be prepared, but don't worry that a client might ask a question or two that you can't answer.
- *Develop objectives* for meeting your client's needs. Define specific, realistic objectives in terms of behaviors that can be observed and measured.
- *Determine the content* of (the type and amount of information to present), as well as the methods used for the counseling session (for example, a filmstrip, a diet booklet, food models, practice menus, or a food record). Let the client's level of interest, motivation, and education guide you in these decisions. For example, an illiterate adult or a child might appreciate diet instructions in picture form. One person may find the in-depth details about the body's response to diet fascinating, whereas another person wants just the diet without the background.
- *Establish a time frame* for accomplishing objectives. The time frame can be tentative and somewhat flexible to reflect the client's needs.
- *Arrange for appropriate others* to be present at the session.

IMPLEMENTATION

When counseling, remember to establish a caring environment, allow others to be themselves, be a good listener, use familiar language and appropriate nonverbal gestures, and maintain eye contact. You will also want to use open-ended questions, center the session around the client, provide positive feedback, and summarize your discussion. In addition, be sure to:

- *Establish rapport* by spending a little time creating a trusting and caring atmosphere before beginning diet instructions.
- *Identify and communicate the objectives* of counseling clearly. If clients know, for example, that they will be told how dietary changes will improve their health, they may listen more closely to the explanation of the diet. Furthermore, this gives the client an opportunity to modify your expectations.
- *Discuss the rationale for diet changes* and show your clients how nutrition supports recovery. Clients who do not understand the benefits will not be motivated to change.
- *Answer all questions accurately*, even if you must explain that you will check on the information and convey it at a later time. This action clearly surpasses giving incorrect advice or ignoring a question.
- *Stress to clients that they carry the responsibility* for their health and for making the necessary diet changes.
- *Encourage client participation* in the counseling session. You will often hear statements such as "You need to talk to my wife; she does the cooking." It does help if the family member who prepares the food participates in the counseling session and understands the diet. However, clients must accept that they—not their spouses and not the counselor—need to accept the responsibility for their diets.
- *Be realistic* when applying principles of diet to lifestyle. Be sure that the person can actually apply the changes. The busy executive who frequently eats restaurant meals must know how to make appropriate food choices in restaurants. A person with a low income may need help with incorporating lower-cost food items into the diet, as well as tips on shopping economically. A person who follows a strictly kosher diet must know how to plan meals around the Jewish dietary laws (see Highlight 2).
- *Make diet instructions relevant* to clients by using many examples consistent with their own eating habits. Do this by becoming familiar with diet histories, having clients plan personal menus, asking them to tell you what they would select in a restaurant, or observing them make selections from the hospital cafeteria line.
- *Encourage active participation* in the sessions and allow clients to arrive at conclusions on their own.
- *Reinforce all positive responses* and acknowledge your client's cooperation during the session.
- *Arrange for follow-up* if needed.

EVALUATION

When a counseling session is complete, consider whether:

- The objectives have been met.
- The content and methods of instruction were appropriate. Ask yourself which methods worked well and which were less effective.
- The time was adequate and whether additional counseling is needed.
- The client's needs have changed.
- Your counseling skills were effective. Ask yourself how you can improve your instructional techniques for future counseling sessions.

A little information remembered and applied is better than a lot of information forgotten and disregarded.

understand, and they limit the amount of information they present at any one session. At each session, the nutrition counselor assesses the client's level of motivation and understanding, sets goals that realistically reflect the client's commitment and knowledge, and modifies the goals as the client's progress indicates.[1]

Counseling Limitations As described, nutrition education to promote long-term behavior changes is most likely to succeed when clients can proceed at their own pace. Unfortunately, many clients receive nutrition education under less than ideal circumstances. In the hospital, for example, dietitians must often begin counseling clients when they are still ill and overwhelmed with a diagnosis and its implications. Even if clients learn to make proper food selections from the hospital menu, they may feel lost when it comes to planning a menu at home. Furthermore, after the immediate danger of illness has passed, the person may lose the motivation to keep following nutrition advice. For these reasons, it is advisable for the dietitian to provide follow-up in any way possible—personally through a phone call, home visit, or scheduled visit by the client to the counselor or through the client's physician.

Whether nutrition counseling is effective depends on the extent to which clients change their eating habits in response to it. Clearly, nutrition counselors face a challenge; they need to use both their nutrition knowledge and their counseling skills. Counseling skills improve with practice, but even the best counselor experiences some failures. In the end, the client, not the counselor, must accept responsibility for making the necessary diet changes.

Professional Communications

Maintaining strong professional communication networks benefits both health care professionals and their clients. Conversely, miscommunication between professionals can result in inappropriate therapy with serious consequences for clients' health. Professionals communicate through the medical record and other written records. In addition, many opportunities exist for professionals to discuss clients' medical conditions, concerns, and progress.

MEDICAL RECORDS

medical record: a continuous written account of a client's health history, diagnosis, therapy, and prognosis.

diagnosis: the disease a person has or is thought to have.
dia = through
gnosis = knowing

prognosis: the predicted course and outcome of a disease.
pro = ahead of time, before

Medical records are legal documents that record a client's history, the assessment and diagnosis of medical problems, the measures being taken to treat those problems, and the results of tests and therapy. Reading the medical record at regular intervals allows health care professionals to continuously assess the client's condition and response to therapy. Writing in the medical records allows health care professionals to document the actions taken to comply with physicians' orders, the client's responses to those actions, and recommendations.

Medical records can be organized in many ways. Most commonly, health care professionals use the problem-oriented medical record (POMR) approach. In this approach, health care team members list each of the client's problems to generate a problem list. Subsequently, each entry in the record addresses the actions being taken to deal with a problem. As new problems arise, they are added to the list.

The Medical Record and Nutrition Care Learn how to effectively use the record in the facility where you work. Regardless of the type of medical record approach used, be sure the client's medical record includes important nutrition-related information. Examples of important information include:

- Evaluation of the client's current diet.
- Nutrition assessment data.
- Recommended medical nutrition therapy.
- The client's acceptance and tolerance of the diet.
- Problems with the client's food intake.
- Documentation of diet counseling.
- Any planned follow-up or referral to another person or agency.
- The client's response to nutrition care.
- The client's response to diet counseling.

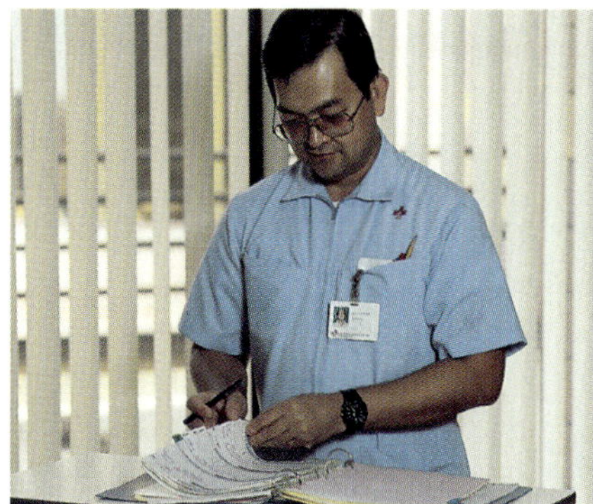
Take time to record important nutrition information in the client's medical record.

Other Records In addition to the formal medical record, various health care professionals keep records of their own. For example, nurses keep nursing care plans, just as dietitians keep the nutrition care plans described earlier. These records contain some of the same information that is in the formal medical record, but they also include more detailed plans and notes specifically pertinent to the individual health team member. For example, a nutrition care plan may have details about a client's reaction to a diet, which the dietitian will later use in preparation for diet counseling. Nursing care plans often contain information that relates to nutrition care. A nurse caring for a client may note that a client isn't eating, is having problems chewing foods, or needs assistance while eating. In the course of a busy day, these problems may not be communicated to the physician or dietitian. The dietitian who reads these notes, however, can initiate actions to correct the problems.

OTHER COMMUNICATION CHANNELS

Opportunities for communication other than by way of written records also exist among health team members. Health team members in a hospital often phone or page each other when they identify problems or when questions arise. Outside the hospital, health team members may be reached in their offices or through their answering services.

Bedside rounds provide an ideal opportunity for professional communication (see Highlight 17). Use these discussions to call attention to nutrition-related problems, recommend changes, or exchange information about clients' concerns and attitudes.

Nurses also report to one another at the end of each shift. Use this time to pass along information about clients' special nutrition and diet needs and requests.

Effective nutrition care addresses the unique needs of the individual, framing nutrient needs in the context of the person's educational, socioeconomic, and medical needs. This chapter has described techniques for building effective nutrition care plans. Later chapters describe how nutrient needs change due to illness and how therapeutic diets can meet them.

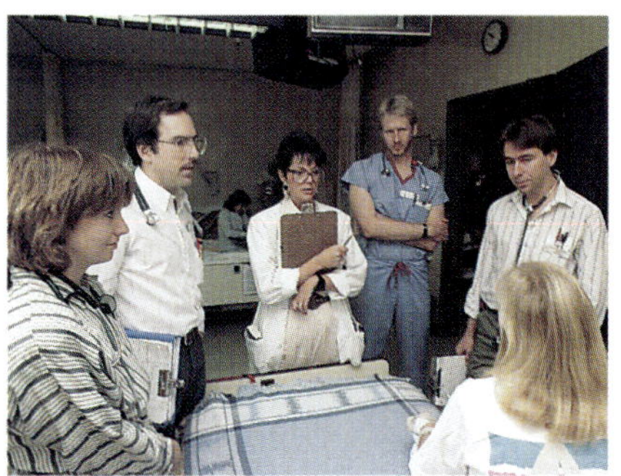
Bedside rounds provide an excellent opportunity to discuss your concerns regarding a person's nutrition status.

Study Questions

1. How does the analysis of assessment data contribute to the nutrition care plan?
2. What are the parts of a nutrition care plan? What two services should the plan deliver to a client? Why must the plan be evaluated from time to time?
3. What is medical nutrition therapy? In what ways can diets be modified to meet individual needs?
4. Describe the exchange lists used for diet planning. How do exchange lists differ from food group plans? What are the strengths of each system? How can the strengths of the two systems be combined?
5. Why is it important to present nutrition information in stages when a client must be on a special diet for a long time? Who is responsible for nutrition education? Describe some of the ways in which counselors can motivate clients to make diet changes.
6. How can you use the medical record to communicate a client's nutrition needs to other health care professionals? What kinds of information about nutrition should you record? Where else can you find written information about a client's nutrient or nutrition education needs?
7. Discuss some other ways that health care professionals can share concerns about a client's nutrition needs.

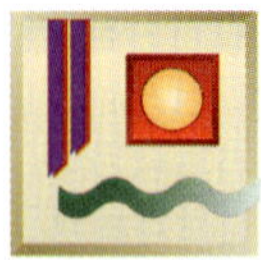

Clinical Applications

1. Refer to the case study about Ms. Green on p. 566. The physician prescribes a weight-loss diet for Ms. Green, and the dietitian plans a 1200-kcalorie, weight-reduction diet. Using Table 17–3 and the exchange lists in Appendix G, plan menus for one day's meals.
2. You are nurse visiting a client who recently suffered a heart attack and is now on a special diet. The client tells you that the dietitian has talked to him about his diet and he is totally confused. He confides in you that the diet is the last thing on his mind right now. What actions should you take?
3. A client has been losing weight while in the hospital, and the physician orders a kcalorie count. The physician's written order is recorded in the medical record, as is a note from the dietitian verifying the details of the procedure. Considering the communications channels described in this chapter, what steps might the dietitian take to ensure that the client's intake will be recorded through all shifts?

Note

1. American Diabetes Association and American Dietetic Association, *Facilitating Lifestyle Change: A Resource Manual* (The American Diabetes Association, Inc., and The American Dietetic Association, 1996), pp. 2–3.

The Team Approach

Human beings depend on one another to accomplish many tasks in everyday life. When several people work together, ideas flow and tasks become manageable. Consider a group of citizens planning a relief effort to deliver food and clothes to victims of a devastating tornado. After discussing the many tasks to be completed, the members of the committee decide how each of them can best contribute to accomplishing their goal. One person volunteers to make flyers to pass out—she has access to a copying machine. Another offers storage space for collecting goods—his business recently expanded and he has some extra space. Still another will call the local radio stations to ask them to make public service announcements. Another knows the owner of a trucking company who can lend a truck for transporting the food and clothes to the areas where they are needed. Working together, the committee members complete a large project efficiently. In much the same way, health care professionals can work together, sharing their unique expertise and skills to benefit their clients' health. Fortunately, the value of the health care team is increasingly being recognized. This highlight illustrates the principles of the team approach and describes some of the responsibilities of health care team members.

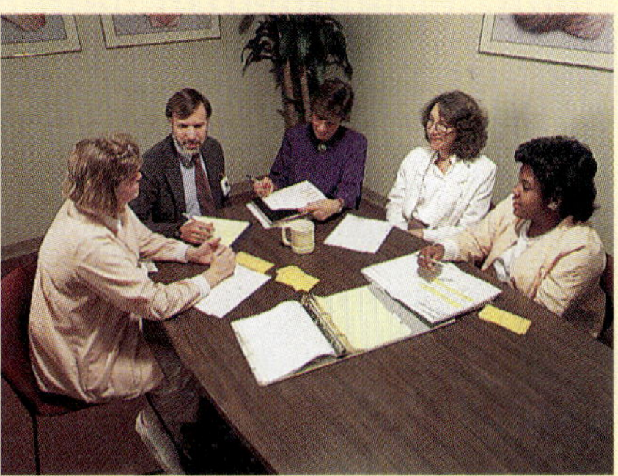

The team approach helps to ensure safe and effective nutrition support.

HEALTH CARE TEAMS

The number and types of health care teams vary from institution to institution. A health care team consists of a group of professionals specializing in a particular medical specialty. For example, the cardiac rehabilitation team works with clients recovering from heart attacks or cardiac surgery. Many health care teams include physicians, nurses, dietitians, pharmacists, and mental health workers among their core members. Other members vary according to the team specialty. A respiratory therapist would be a primary member of a pulmonary rehabilitation team, for example. Physical therapists and occupational therapists frequently participate on rehabilitation or burn teams. Social workers provide solutions to financial problems and coordinate home care programs.

Dietitians participate on health care teams that recognize medical nutrition therapy as essential to client care. Some examples include teams that specialize in disorders of the heart, blood vessels, lungs, endocrine system (such as diabetes mellitus), gastrointestinal tract, liver, and kidneys. Dietitians also serve on teams in cases where multiple organ systems may be involved such as severe trauma, burns, acquired immune deficiency syndrome (AIDS), cancer, and metabolic disorders.

Additionally, many institutions have nutrition support teams that develop protocols for nutrition screening and nutrition assessment, identify people who have nutrition problems, and oversee the care of people who must be fed by tube or by vein (Chapters 23 and 24) either in the hospital or at home.[1] Figure H17–1 shows the core members of the nutrition support team and illustrates how team members interact. Members of the nutrition support team share many of the responsibilities for client care, but each one also provides unique services. By working together, team members integrate their knowledge and provide the client with the benefits of their combined expertise. Team members also benefit—by learning how the others contribute to the care process, they learn to delegate responsibilities to the person who can do each job most effectively.

RESPONSIBILITIES OF TEAM MEMBERS

Team members maintain records and, both individually and as a team, review the progress of each client in their care. They often serve as consultants to the rest of the hospital staff, providing information, answering questions, and solving problems that arise in client care. Team members also carry responsibility for keeping abreast of new developments in their respective fields. They analyze new products, review current research, and communicate their findings to other team members.

The team physician assumes primary responsibility for client care:

Figure H17–1

The Nutrition Support Team

The physician
- Diagnoses medical problems
- Performs medical procedures
- Coordinates and prescribes therapy
- Directs and supervises team
- Approves guidelines and protocols
- Consults with other physicians

The nurse
- Assesses nursing needs
- Performs direct client care
- Explains medical procedures and treatment plans
- Instructs clients regarding medical care
- Acts as a liaison between team and nursing staff
- Coordinates discharge plans

All team members
- Review current research
- Analyze new products
- Develop guidelines
- Provide in-service training
- Monitor clients
- Correct problems
- Educate clients
- Evaluate the outcome of the care provided

The dietitian
- Assesses nutrition status
- Determines clients' nutrient needs
- Recommends appropriate diet therapy
- Reevaluates clients regularly
- Instructs clients about their diets
- Acts as a liaison between the team and the dietary department

The pharmacist
- Recommends appropriate drug therapy
- Identifies drug-drug and drug-nutrient interactions
- Identifies drug-related complications
- Educates clients about their medications
- Acts as a liaison between the team and the pharmacy

diagnosing the client's medical problems, performing medical procedures, and coordinating and prescribing appropriate therapy. The physician frequently supervises the activities of other team members, monitors any complications that may arise, and makes the final decision on what steps to take to correct problems.

Team physicians also direct the development and approval of guidelines and protocols pertinent to the team's area of specialization. They oversee in-hospital educational and training programs for the professional staff and act as consultants to other physicians who require their professional expertise.

The team nurse plays a central role in client care management and communications with the client, caregivers, and nursing staff. The nurse often explains medical procedures and treatment plans to clients and their caregivers. In addition, the team nurse supervises other nurses who care for each client to assure that they are delivering optimal care. The team nurse teaches staff nurses, as a group and individually, the rationales for various procedures and the appropriate administration techniques. The nurse also assists in training physicians and other health care professionals.

The team nurse often coordinates the client's discharge from the hospital. Discharge responsibilities include discussing with clients any steps they will need to follow at home, making sure they have written instructions, providing appropriate supplies and equipment, and arranging for follow-up care.

The dietitian, as the team's nutrition expert, assesses the client's nutrition status, determines nutrient requirements, recommends appropriate diet therapy, and translates diet orders into foods or formulas. Dietitians calculate nutrient intake data and nitrogen balance. The dietitian also instructs clients about their diets and prepares them to follow special diets at home.

Team dietitians provide in-service training on nutrition-related topics in their specialty areas for other dietitians, nurses, or other health care professionals. If particular nutrition problems arise, dietitians actively investigate the cause, devise solutions, and see that they are carried out. The team dietitian also acts as a liaison between the team and the dietary department.

The pharmacist assists the health care team in managing the client's drug therapy; alerts team members to interactions of drugs with other drugs, nutrients, or nutrient solutions; and identifies complications that may be drug related. The pharmacist may recommend an optimal drug administration schedule and educates clients about the proper use of their medications. The pharmacist also serves as a liaison between the pharmacy and the health care team.

HOW THE TEAM APPROACH WORKS

Team members communicate with each other both informally and formally. They may share office space and see each other throughout the day, but their primary avenue for managing team responsibilities is during rounds, when the entire team discusses each client in the team's care. During rounds, the physician oversees the discussions and takes recommendations for changes. For example, the dietitian may express concern for a client who is unable to eat dinners because painful treatments have been scheduled just prior to dinner. The pharmacist recommends pain medication that will be effective through dinner to help alleviate this problem. The physician and pharmacist see no problem with adding this drug to the client's therapy, and the physician writes the medication order. The nurse makes sure that staff nurses working with the client understand the rationale for the new drug therapy and the importance of its timing. Working together, the team has efficiently identified and solved a problem that might otherwise go unresolved.

Team rounds also serve as an avenue of communication for general problems that affect more than one client's care. For example, while discussing a client who has undergone a nitrogen balance study, the physician mentions that problems have occurred repeatedly with this procedure in the last month. The nurse recalls that many of the new nurses are having difficulty with the procedure and suggests an in-service training session on the proper techniques for nitrogen balance studies. The nurse and dietitian agree to jointly conduct the in-service training.

During rounds, team members may bring up current research that may affect the care they give clients, or they may share information about new products they wish to evaluate for use with their clients. The team then decides if further action is warranted.

In these ways, health care teams contribute to optimal client care by combining and coordinating the expertise of various health care professionals. In addition, health care teams can effectively reduce hospital costs by providing the most efficient use of personnel and supplies.

To appreciate the team approach, remember the old adage, "Two heads are better than one." In this case, several heads are better still. Clients benefit when they have many eyes noting problems and many brains searching for solutions. In short, teamwork works.

NOTE

1. J. R. Wesley, Nutrition support teams: Past, present, and future, *Nutrition in Clinical Practice* 10 (1995): 219–228.

Chapter 18

Life Cycle Nutrition: Pregnancy and Lactation

CONTENTS

MICROGRAPH: Folate, a B vitamin critical in preventing birth defects

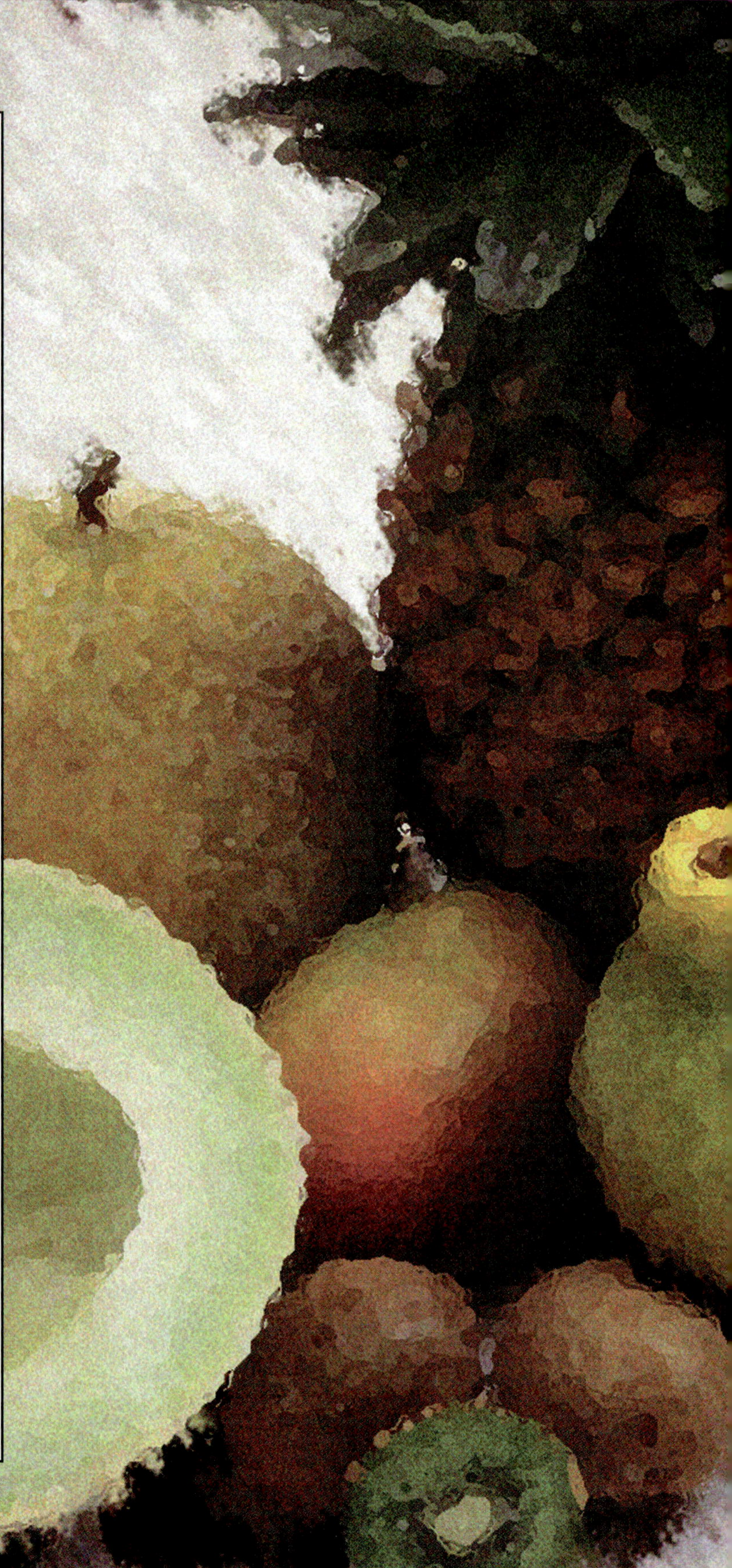

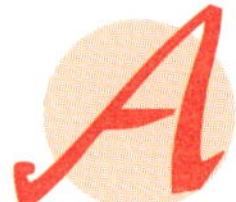
All people need the same nutrients, but the amounts needed vary depending on the stage of life. This chapter focuses on nutrition in preparation for, and support of, pregnancy and lactation.

Growth and Development during Pregnancy

A whole new life begins at conception. Organ systems develop rapidly, and nutrition plays many supportive roles. This section describes placenta and fetal development, paying close attention to times of intense activity.

PLACENTAL DEVELOPMENT

In the early days of pregnancy, a new organ develops within the uterus—the placenta, shown in Figure 18–1. Two associated structures also form. One is the amniotic sac, a fluid-filled balloonlike structure that houses the developing fetus. The other is the umbilical cord, a ropelike structure containing fetal blood vessels that extends through the fetus's "belly button" (the umbilicus) to the placenta. These three structures serve crucial roles during the pregnancy and then are expelled from the uterus following childbirth.

The placenta is composed of spongy tissue in which fetal blood and maternal blood flow side by side, each in its own vessels. The maternal blood transfers oxygen and nutrients to the fetus's blood and picks up fetal waste products. By exchanging oxygen, nutrients, and waste products, the placenta performs the respiratory, absorptive, and excretory functions that the fetus's lungs, digestive system, and kidneys will provide after birth.

The placenta is a versatile, metabolically active organ. Like all body tissues, the placenta uses energy and nutrients to support its work. Like a gland, it produces an array of hormones that maintain pregnancy and prepare the mother's breasts for lactation (making milk). A healthy placenta is essential for normal fetal development.

FETAL GROWTH AND DEVELOPMENT

Fetal development begins with the fertilization of an ovum by a sperm. Three stages follow: the zygote, the embryo, and the fetus.

The Zygote The newly fertilized ovum, or zygote, begins as a single cell and divides to become many cells during the days after fertilization. Within two weeks, the zygote embeds itself in the uterine wall—a process known as implantation. Cell division continues—each set of cells divides into many other cells. Later in gestation, as development proceeds, the zygote becomes an embryo.

The Embryo The embryo accomplishes amazing developmental feats. The number of cells at first doubles approximately every 24 hours; later the rate slows, and only one doubling occurs during the final ten weeks of pregnancy. The embryo's size changes very little, but at eight weeks, the 1¼-inch embryo has a complete central nervous system, a beating heart, a digestive system, well-defined fingers and toes, and the beginnings of facial features.

uterus (YOU-ter-us): the muscular organ within which the infant develops before birth; the womb.

placenta (plah-SEN-tuh): the organ that develops inside the uterus early in pregnancy, in which maternal and fetal blood circulate in close proximity so that materials can be exchanged between them. The fetus receives nutrients and oxygen across the placenta; the mother's blood picks up carbon dioxide and other waste products to be excreted.

amniotic (am-nee-OTT-ic) **sac:** the "bag of waters" in the uterus, in which the fetus floats.

umbilical (um-BILL-ih-cul) **cord:** the ropelike structure through which the fetus's veins and arteries reach the placenta; the route of nourishment and oxygen into the fetus and the route of waste disposal from the fetus. The scar in the middle of the abdomen that marks the former attachment of the umbilical cord is the **umbilicus** (um-BILL-ih-cus), commonly known as the "belly button."

ovum: the female reproductive cell, capable of developing into a new organism upon fertilization; commonly referred to as an egg.

sperm: the male reproductive cell, capable of fertilizing an ovum.

zygote (ZY-goat): the product of the union of ovum and sperm; so-called for the first two weeks after fertilization.

implantation: the stage of development in which the zygote embeds itself in the wall of the uterus and begins to develop; occurs during the first two weeks after conception.

gestation (jes-TAY-shun): the period from conception to birth; for human beings gestation lasts from 38 to 42 weeks. Pregnancy is often divided into thirds, called **trimesters**.

embryo (EM-bree-oh): the developing infant from two to eight weeks after conception.

Figure 18–1

The Placenta and Associated Structures

To understand how placental villi absorb nutrients without maternal and fetal blood interacting directly, think of how the intestinal villi work. The GI side of the intestinal villi is bathed in a nutrient-rich fluid (chyme). The intestinal villi absorb the nutrient molecules and release them into the body via capillaries. Similarly, the maternal side of the placental villi is bathed in nutrient-rich maternal blood. The placental villi absorb the nutrient molecules and release them to the fetus via fetal capillaries.

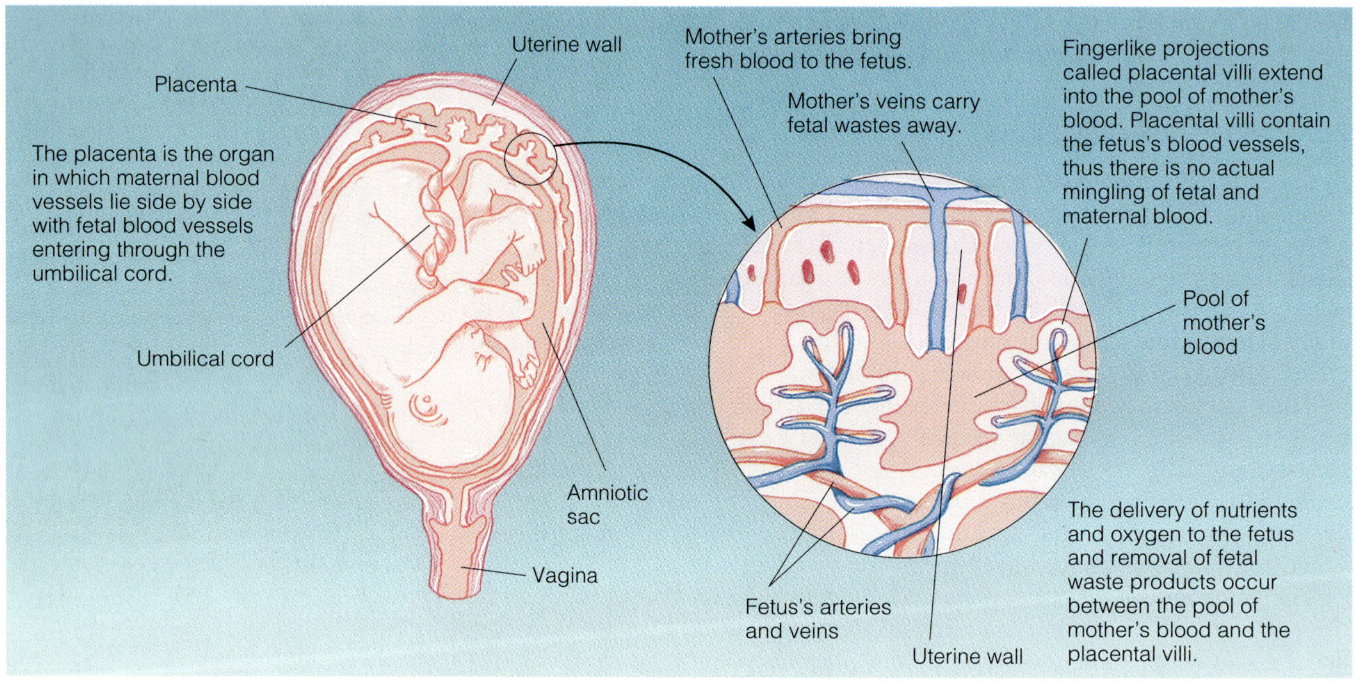

fetus (FEET-us): the developing infant from eight weeks after conception until term.

The Fetus During the next seven months, each organ grows to maturity on its own schedule. As Figure 18–2 shows, fetal growth is phenomenal: weight increases from less than a gram to about 3500 grams (7½ pounds).

CRITICAL PERIODS

critical periods: finite periods during development in which certain events may occur that will have irreversible effects on later developmental stages. In a body organ, a critical period is usually a period of rapid cell division.

The neural tube forms the beginnings of the brain and spinal cord, key structures in the central nervous system.

Times of intense development and rapid cell division are called critical periods—critical in the sense that the events scheduled for those times can occur only then, not later. If cell division and the final cell number achieved in an organ are limited during a critical period, full recovery will not occur (see Figure 18–3 on p. 588).

Each organ and tissue is most vulnerable to adverse influences during its own critical period. The critical period for neural tube development, for example, is from 17 to 30 days gestation.[1] Consequently, neural tube development is most vulnerable to nutrient deficiencies or toxins during this time—a time most women do not even realize that they are pregnant. Any abnormal development of the neural tube or its failure to close completely can produce major defects in the central nervous system, causing serious disabilities and infant death.

Figure 18–2

Stages of Embryonic and Fetal Development

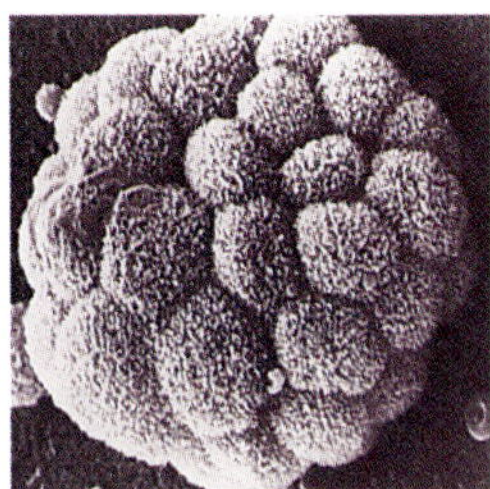

1. A newly fertilized ovum is about the size of the period at the end of this sentence. This zygote at less than one week after fertilization is not much bigger and is ready for implantation.

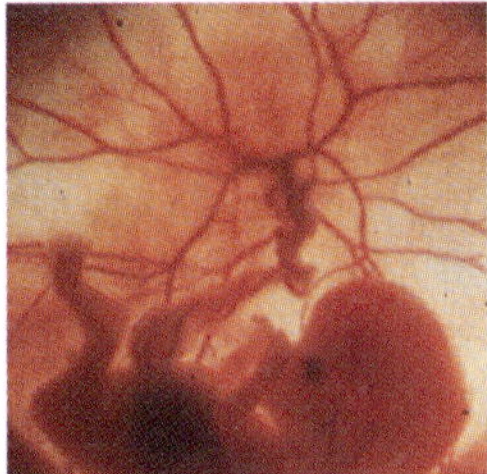

2. After implantation, the placenta develops and begins to provide nourishment to the developing embryo. An embryo five weeks after fertilization is about ½ inch long.

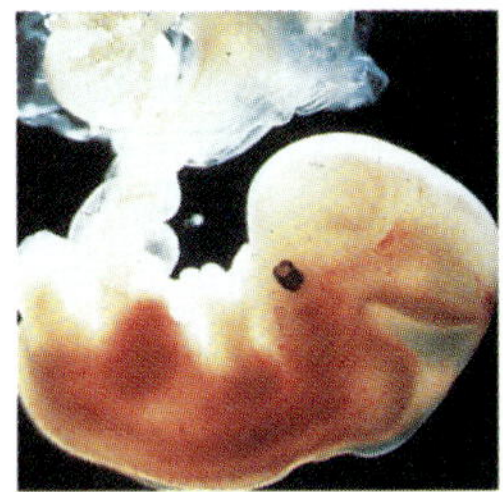

3. A fetus after 11 weeks of development is just over an inch long. Notice the umbilical cord and blood vessels connecting the fetus with the placenta.

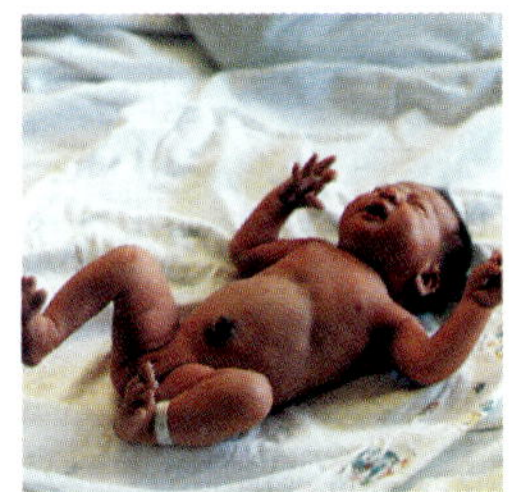

4. A newborn infant after nine months of development measures close to 20 inches in length. From eight weeks to term, this infant grew 20 times longer and 50 times heavier.

Spina Bifida One of the most common types of neural tube defects is spina bifida, a disorder characterized by incomplete closure of the spinal cord and its bony encasement. The membranes covering the spinal cord often protrude as a sac, which may rupture and lead to meningitis, a life-threatening inflammation of the membranes. Spina bifida is accompanied by varying degrees of paralysis, depending on the extent of spinal cord damage. Mild cases may not even be noticed, but severe cases lead to death. Common problems include clubfoot, dislocated hip, kidney disorders, curvature of the spine, muscle weakness, mental handicaps, and motor and sensory losses.

In the United States, approximately 1 of every 1000 newborns has a neural tube defect; some 2500 to 3000 infants are affected each year.* Many other pregnancies with neural tube defects end in abortion or stillbirths.

Folate Supplementation Chapter 10 described how folate supplements taken one month before conception and continued throughout the first trimester can prevent neural tube defects.[2] For this reason, the Public Health Service recommends that all women of childbearing age who are capable of becoming pregnant take 0.4 milligrams of folate daily. This amount of folate is easy to obtain from a diet that includes plenty of fruits and vegetables, but supplements offer women a convenient way to ingest sufficient folate regularly and continuously enough to benefit pregnancy. Most over-the-counter multivitamin supplements contain 0.4 milligrams of folate; prenatal supplements usually contain at least 0.8 milligrams. A woman who has previously had an infant with a neural tube defect may be advised by her physician to take folate supplements in doses

Folate RDA:

- For women: 180 µg (0.18 mg)/day.
- During pregnancy: 400 µg (0.4 mg)/day.

*Worldwide, some 300,000 to 400,000 infants are born with neural tube defects each year.

Figure 18–3

The Concept of Critical Periods

Critical periods occur early in development. An adverse influence felt early can have a much more severe and prolonged impact than one felt later on.

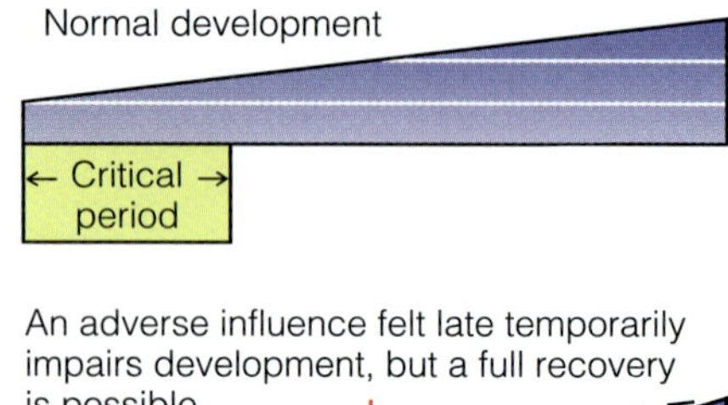

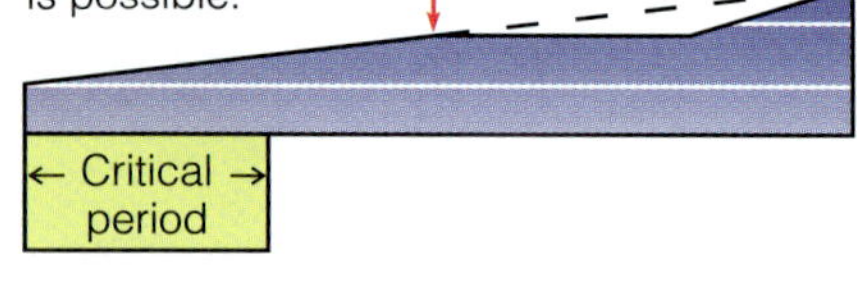

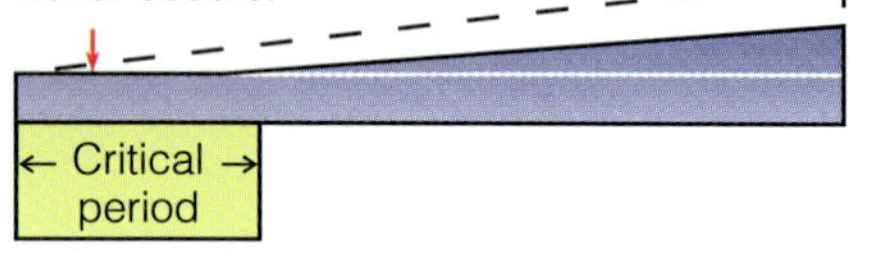

ten times larger—4 milligrams daily. The risks associated with high doses of folate are not all known, but they can mask the pernicious anemia of a vitamin B_{12} deficiency. For this reason, quantities of 1 milligram or more require a prescription.

To deliver folate to the U.S. population, the Food and Drug Administration (FDA) has mandated fortification of grain products. In making this decision, the agency carefully weighed the benefits of fortification against the risks of overconsumption. On the one hand, an adequate folate intake is expected to reduce the incidence of neural tube defects by 50 percent. On the other hand, if vitamin B_{12} deficiency is masked by folate and left untreated, irreversible nerve damage may occur. The FDA regulation requires manufacturers to fortify foods to provide 140 micrograms of folate per 100 grams of foods, which should increase average daily intakes by 100 micrograms. Fortified foods include cereal, pasta, flour, rolls, buns, farina, grits, cornmeal, and rice.

Maternal nutrition before and during pregnancy affects both the mother's health and the infant's growth. As the infant develops through its three stages—the zygote, embryo, and fetus—its organs and tissues grow, each on its own schedule. Times of intense development are critical periods that depend on nutrients to proceed smoothly. Without folate, for example, the neural tube fails to develop completely during the first month of pregnancy, prompting recommendations for all women of childbearing age to take folate daily.

Because critical periods occur throughout pregnancy, a woman should continuously take good care of her health. That care should include, first, achieving and maintaining a healthy body weight and, then, gaining sufficient weight to support a healthy pregnancy.

Maternal Weight

Birthweight is the most reliable indicator of an infant's health. In general, higher birthweights present lower risks for infants. Two characteristics of the mother's weight influence an infant's birthweight: her weight for height prior to conception and her weight gain during pregnancy.

WEIGHT FOR HEIGHT PRIOR TO CONCEPTION

A woman's weight for height prior to conception influences fetal growth. Even with the same weight gain during pregnancy, underweight women tend to have smaller babies than heavier women.

Underweight is defined as BMI <19.8.

preterm (infant)**:** an infant born prior to the 38th week of pregnancy; also called a **premature** infant. A **term** infant is born between the 38th and 42nd week of pregnancy.

Underweight An underweight woman has a high risk of having a low-birthweight infant, especially if she is unable to gain sufficient weight during pregnancy. In addition, the rates of preterm births and infant mortality are higher for underweight women. An underweight woman improves her chances of having a healthy infant by gaining sufficient weight prior to conception or by gaining extra pounds during pregnancy. To increase food energy intake, an underweight woman can follow the dietary recommendations for pregnant women (described in Table 18–3 on p. 593).

Overweight Like underweight women, overweight women face problems related to pregnancy and childbirth. Overweight women face an especially high risk of medical complications such as hypertension, gestational diabetes, and postpartum infections. Compared with other women, overweight women are also more likely to require induced labor and cesarean section.

Infants of overweight women are likely to be born post term and to weigh more than 9 pounds. Overweight women are unlikely to have premature infants, but if they do, the infants may be large for their gestational age. Weight-loss dieting during pregnancy is never advisable, however. An overweight woman should try to achieve a healthy body weight before becoming pregnant, avoid excessive weight gain during pregnancy, and postpone weight loss until after childbirth. Weight loss is best achieved by eating moderate amounts of nutritious foods and exercising to lose body fat.

Overweight is defined as BMI >26.0 to 29.0, which corresponds with 20% over the reference weight in standard weight-for-height tables. Obese is defined as BMI >29.0.

cesarean section: a surgically assisted birth involving removal of the fetus by an incision into the uterus, usually by way of the abdominal wall.

post term (infant): an infant born after the 42nd week of pregnancy.

WEIGHT GAIN AND EXERCISE DURING PREGNANCY

All women must gain weight during pregnancy—fetal growth and maternal health depend on it. Maternal weight gain during pregnancy correlates closely with infant birthweight, and as mentioned earlier, infant birthweight is a strong predictor of the health and subsequent development of the infant.

Recommended Weight Gains The recommended gain for a woman who begins pregnancy at a healthy weight and is carrying a single fetus is 25 to 35 pounds.[3] An underweight woman needs to gain between 28 and 40 pounds; and an overweight woman, between 15 and 25 pounds. Some women should strive for gains at the upper end of the target range, notably, adolescents who are still growing themselves. Short women (5 feet 2 inches and under) should strive for gains at the lower end of the target range. Women who are carrying twins should aim for a weight gain of 35 to 45 pounds. For the normal-weight woman, weight gain ideally follows a pattern of about 5 pounds during the first trimester, and about 1 pound per week thereafter. Health care professionals monitor weight gain using charts; Appendix E presents a prenatal weight gain grid.

Weight-gain recommendations:

- Underweight women: 28 to 40 lb (12.5 to 18 kg).
- Normal-weight women: 25 to 35 lb (11.5 to 16 kg).
- Overweight women: 15 to 25 lb (7 to 11.5 kg).
- Obese women: 13 lb minimum (6 kg minimum).

If a woman gains more than is recommended early in pregnancy, she should not restrict her energy intake later in order to lose weight. To be a little overweight is healthier than to be underweight. A sudden large weight gain, however, may be the first sign of preeclampsia, a serious medical complication discussed later.

Components of Weight Gain Women often express concern about the weight gain that accompanies a healthy pregnancy. They may find comfort in a reminder that most of the gain supports the growth and development of the placenta, uterus, blood, and breasts, as well as an optimally healthy 7½-pound infant. A small amount goes into maternal fat stores, and even that fat is there for a special purpose: to provide energy for labor and lactation. Table 18–1 shows the components of a typical 30-pound weight gain.

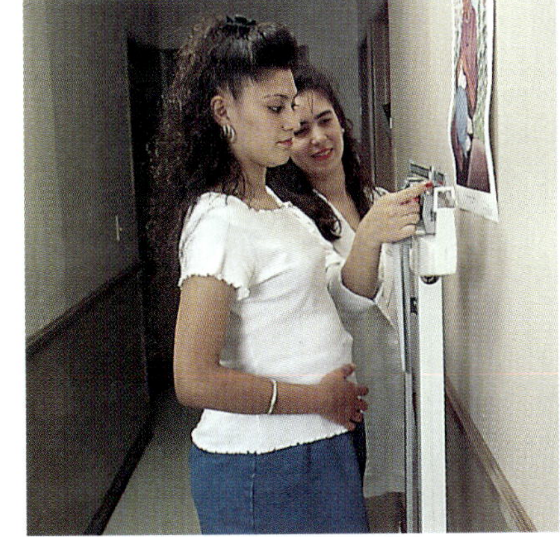

Fetal growth and maternal health depend on a sufficient weight gain during pregnancy.

Weight Loss after Pregnancy The pregnant woman loses some of the weight at delivery. In the following weeks, she loses more as her blood volume returns to normal and she sheds accumulated fluids. The typical woman does not, however, return to her prepregnancy weight. In general, the more weight a woman gains beyond what she needs for pregnancy, the more she will retain.

Table 18–1

Components of Weight Gain during Pregnancy

Development	Weight Gain (lb)
Infant at birth	7½
Placenta	1½
Increase in mother's blood volume to supply placenta	4
Increase in mother's fluid volume	4
Increase in size of uterus and supporting muscles	2
Increase in size of mother's breasts	2
Fluid to surround infant in amniotic sac	2
Mother's fat stores	7
Total	30

Source: ACOG *Guide to Planning for Pregnancy, Birth, and Beyond* (Washington, D.C.: The American College of Obstetricians and Gynecologists, 1990), p. 109.

Even with an average weight gain, though, most women tend to retain a couple of pounds with each pregnancy.[4]

Pregnant women should consult with their health care provider before beginning a fitness program.

Exercise The active, physically fit woman experiencing a normal pregnancy can continue to exercise throughout pregnancy, adjusting the duration and intensity as the pregnancy progresses. Staying active can improve fitness, prevent gestational diabetes, facilitate labor, and reduce stress.[5] It also maintains the habits that help a woman lose excess weight and get back into shape after the birth. A pregnant woman should avoid sports in which she might fall or be hit by other people or objects. For example, playing tennis with one person on each side of the net is safer than a fast-moving game of racquetball in which the two competitors can collide. Swimming is ideal because it allows the body to remain cool and move freely with the water's support. Table 18–2 provides some guidelines for exercise during pregnancy.[6] Several of the guidelines listed are aimed at

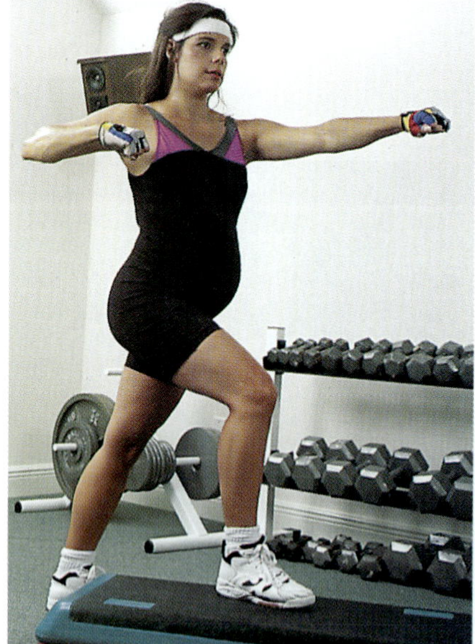

Pregnant women can enjoy the benefits of exercise.

Table 18–2

Exercise Guidelines for Pregnancy

- Exercise regularly (at least three times a week), not intermittently.
- Avoid standing motionless for long periods or lying on the back after the first trimester (the enlarged uterus can obstruct the vena cava and cut off the blood flow to the fetus).
- Lower the intensity of activity or stop exercising when tired or uncomfortable; do not work to exhaustion. Heart rate should not exceed 140 beats per minute.
- Avoid activities that involve the potential for even mild abdominal trauma.
- Eat enough to support the additional needs of both pregnancy and physical activity.
- Drink plenty of fluids before and after exercise; wear appropriate clothing; and avoid physical activity in hot, humid weather.
- After the birth, resume prepregnancy levels of intensity and duration gradually.

preventing excessively high internal body temperature and dehydration, both of which can harm fetal development. To this end, pregnant women should also stay out of saunas, steam rooms, and hot whirlpools.

A healthy pregnancy depends on a sufficient weight gain. Women who begin their pregnancies at a healthy weight need to gain about 30 pounds, which covers the growth and development of the placenta, uterus, blood, breasts, and infant.

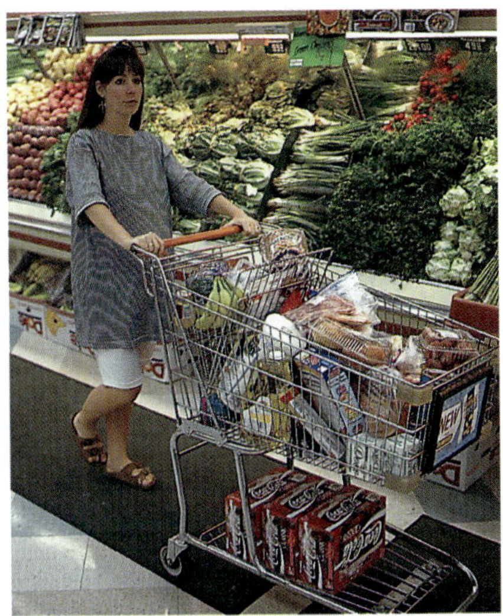

A pregnant woman's nutrition choices support both her health and her infant's growth and development.

Nutrition during Pregnancy

A woman's body changes dramatically during pregnancy. Her blood volume expands; her uterus and its supporting muscles increase in size and strength; her joints become more flexible in preparation for childbirth; her feet swell in response to high concentrations of the hormone estrogen, which promotes water retention and helps to ready the uterus for delivery; and her breasts grow in preparation for lactation. The hormones that mediate all these changes may influence her mood. She can best prepare to handle these changes given a nutritious diet, regular physical activity, plenty of rest, and caring companions. This section highlights the role of nutrition.

ENERGY AND NUTRIENT NEEDS DURING PREGNANCY

From conception to birth, all parts of the infant—bones, muscles, organs, blood cells, skin, and other tissues—are made of nutrients from maternal stores and diet. For most women, nutrients needs during pregnancy and lactation are higher than at any other time (see Figure 18–4).

The RDA table (inside front cover, left) provides separate listings for women during pregnancy and lactation, reflecting their heightened nutritional needs.

Energy Nutrients A pregnant woman needs extra food energy, but only a little extra—300 kcalories above the allowance for nonpregnant women—and only during the second and third trimesters. A woman can easily get 300 kcalories by taking just one extra serving from each of the five food groups—a slice of bread, a serving of vegetables, an ounce of lean meat, a piece of fruit, and a cup of nonfat milk (see Table 18–3 and the sample menu on p. 593). Pregnant teenagers, underweight women, and exceptionally active women may require more.

Energy RDA during pregnancy (2nd and 3rd trimesters):
+300 kcal/day.
Canadian RNI during pregnancy:
+100 to 300 kcal/day.*

For women of average size and moderate physical activity, 300 kcalories represent only 15 percent more food energy than before pregnancy. Nutrient needs expand more than this, however, so nutrient-dense foods should supply the 300 kcalories: foods such as nonfat milk; lean meats, fish, and poultry; eggs; legumes; dark green vegetables; citrus fruits; and whole-grain breads and cereals. Ample carbohydrate is needed to spare the protein for growth.

Protein RDA during pregnancy:
+10 g/day.
Canadian RNI during pregnancy:
+5 to 24/g day.†

Protein The RDA for pregnancy is 10 grams per day higher than for nonpregnant women. Because people in the United States typically exceed the

*For all Canadian RNI values during pregnancy, the lower value indicates recommendations for the first trimester, and the higher value indicates those for the second and third trimesters.

†For the first trimester, the RNI is an additional 5 grams/day; for the second trimester, it is an additional 20 grams/day; and for the third trimester, it is 24 grams/day.

Figure 18–4

Comparison of Nutrient RDA of Nonpregnant, Pregnant, and Lactating Women

For actual values, turn to the table on the inside front cover, left.

[a]Reflect DRI values.

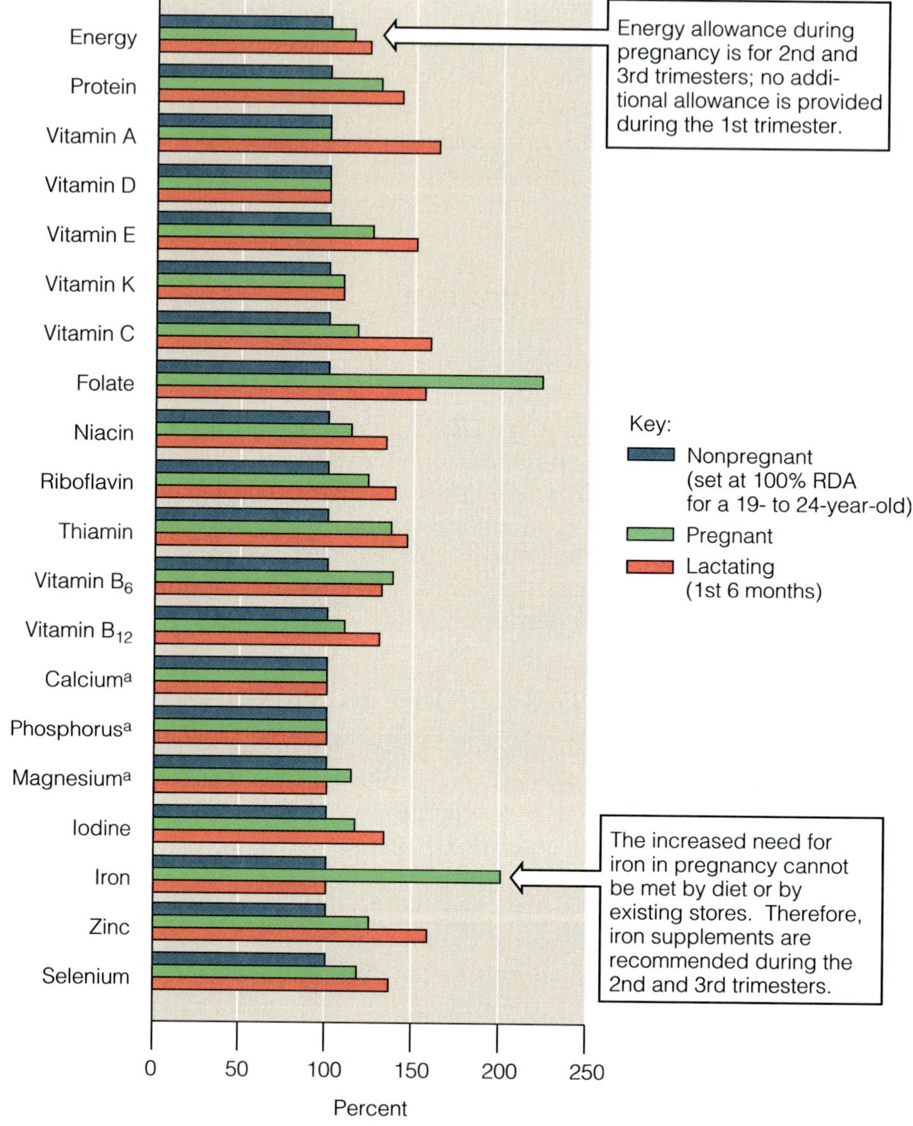

Thiamin RDA during pregnancy: 1.5 mg/day.
Canadian RNI during pregnancy: +0.1 mg/day.

Riboflavin RDA during pregnancy: 1.6 mg/day.
Canadian RNI during pregnancy: +0.1 to 0.3 mg/day

Niacin RDA during pregnancy: 17 mg NE/day.
Canadian RNI during pregnancy: +1 to 2 NE/day.

RDA, most women need not add the full 10 grams to their diets. In fact, pregnant women in the United States—even those with low incomes who are not participating in food assistance programs—generally receive between 75 and 110 grams of protein a day.[7] Pregnant vegetarian women who meet their energy needs by eating ample servings of protein-containing plant foods such as legumes, whole grains, nuts, and seeds meet their protein needs as well. Use of high-protein supplements during pregnancy can be harmful and is discouraged.

B Vitamins Associated with Energy Intake Extra B vitamins are needed in proportion to the increase in energy requirements. The Committee on Dietary Allowances recommends a slight increase above the nonpregnant woman's RDA for thiamin, riboflavin, and niacin. The usual intake of these nutrients is adequate for most pregnant women in the United States.

Table 18–3

Daily Food Choices for Pregnant and Lactating Women

Food Group	Number of Servings	
	ADULT	PREGNANT OR LACTATING WOMEN
Breads/cereals	6 to 11	7 to 11
Vegetables	3 to 5	4 to 5
Fruits	2 to 4	3 to 4
Meat/meat alternatives	2 to 3	3
Milk/milk products	2	3 to 4

Note: Figure 2–1 in Chapter 2 provides a detailed summary of the Daily Food Guide.

Vitamin B_6 Associated with Protein Intake Vitamin B_6 recommendations rise in parallel with protein recommendations. The RDA provides enough additional vitamin B_6 to cover the protein recommendation.

Vitamin B_6 RDA during pregnancy: 2.2 mg/day.
Canadian RNI during pregnancy: 0.015 mg/g dietary protein.

Folate and Vitamin B_{12} for Blood Production and Cell Growth New cells are laid down at a tremendous pace as the fetus grows and develops. At the same time, the mother's red blood cell mass expands, so the RDA for folate more than doubles during pregnancy. It is possible to obtain sufficient folate, without supplements, from a diet that includes fruits, juices, green vegetables, and whole-grain or fortified cereals. When dietary folate is inadequate, daily supplementation is recommended.

Folate RDA during pregnancy: 400 µg/day.
Canadian RNI during pregnancy: +200 µg/day.

Menu

Breakfast
2 medium bran muffins
2 tsp butter/margarine
1 c vanilla yogurt
½ c fresh strawberries
1 c orange juice

Midmorning snack
1 medium apple

Lunch
Sandwich (2 oz ham, 1 oz swiss cheese, 2 slices rye bread, 2 tsp mayonnaise, lettuce)
1 ¼c salad (lettuce, tomatoes, carrots)
1 tbs salad dressing
1 c low-fat milk

Afternoon snack
1 c low-fat milk
3 oatmeal cookies

Dinner
Chicken cacciatore
4 oz chicken
¾ c stewed tomatoes
1 c rice
¾ c summer squash
1 ½ c salad (spinach, mushrooms, onions)
1 tbs salad dressing
2 slices Italian bread
2 tsp butter/margarine
1 c low-fat milk

Sample Menu for Pregnant and Lactating Women
This sample meal plan follows the Daily Food Guide for pregnant and lactating women and provides about 2500 kcalories (50 percent from carbohydrate, 20 percent from protein, and 30 percent from fat).

Vitamin B_{12} RDA during pregnancy: 2.2 μg/day.
Canadian RNI during pregnancy: +0.2 μg/day.

The pregnant woman also has a slightly greater need for the B vitamin that activates folate—vitamin B_{12}. Generally, even modest amounts of meat, fish, eggs, or milk products together with body stores easily meet the need for vitamin B_{12}. Strict vegetarians who exclude all foods of animal origin, however, may need daily supplements to prevent deficiency.

Vitamin D and Calcium for Bone Development Vitamin D and the bone-building minerals calcium, phosphorus, and magnesium are in great demand during pregnancy. Insufficient intakes may produce abnormal fetal bones and teeth.

Reminder: *Osteomalacia* is the vitamin D–deficiency disease characterized by softening of the bones.

Vitamin D DRI during pregnancy: 5 μg/day.

Vitamin D plays a vital role in calcium absorption and utilization. Consequently, maternal vitamin D deficiency is associated with underdeveloped tooth enamel in the fetus and osteomalacia in the mother. Exposure to sunlight and vitamin D–fortified milk is usually sufficient to provide the recommended amount of vitamin D during pregnancy. Routine supplementation is not recommended because of the toxicity risk. Vegetarians who avoid milk, eggs, and fish may receive enough vitamin D from daily exposure to sunlight or from fortified soy milk.

Calcium absorption more than doubles early in pregnancy, and the mother's bones store the mineral. Whether calcium added to the mother's bones early in pregnancy is withdrawn to provide sufficient calcium to the fetus later in gestation is unclear.[8] During the last trimester, as the fetal bones begin to calcify, a dramatic shift of calcium across the placenta occurs. In the final weeks of pregnancy, over 300 milligrams are transferred to the fetus every day. An adequate calcium intake during pregnancy helps conserve maternal bone while meeting fetal needs.

Calcium DRI during pregnancy:
1300 mg/day (14 to 18 yr).
1000 mg/day (19 to 50 yr).

Most pregnant women drink more milk than other women, but still their calcium intakes typically fall below recommendations. Because a woman under 25 may still be actively depositing minerals in her own bones, adequate calcium is especially important for young women. Pregnant women under age 25 who receive less than 600 milligrams of dietary calcium daily need to increase their consumption of milk, cheese, yogurt, and other calcium-rich foods. Alternatively, and less preferably, they may need a daily supplement of 600 milligrams of calcium.

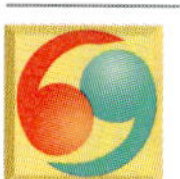

HEALTHY PEOPLE 2000: Increase calcium intake so at least 50% of pregnant and lactating women consume three or more servings daily of foods rich in calcium.

Iron The body makes several adaptations to help meet iron needs during pregnancy. Menstruation, the major route of iron loss in women, ceases, and iron absorption nearly triples due to a rise in blood transferrin, the body's iron-absorbing and iron-carrying protein. Still, iron stores dwindle during pregnancy.

Iron RDA during pregnancy: 30 mg/day.
Canadian RNI during pregnancy: +0 to 10 mg/day.

A pregnant woman needs iron to support her enlarged blood volume and to provide for placental and fetal needs. The developing fetus draws on maternal iron stores to create stores of its own to last through the first four to six months after birth when iron-poor milk will be its sole food. Also, the blood losses inevitable at birth, especially during a cesarean delivery, can drain the mother's supply.*

Few women enter pregnancy with adequate iron stores, so a daily iron supplement is recommended during the second and third trimesters for all pregnant

*The average blood loss during a cesarean delivery is almost twice that occurring during the average vaginal delivery of a single fetus.

women.[9] To enhance absorption, the supplement should be taken between meals or at bedtime on an empty stomach and with liquids other than milk, coffee, or tea, which inhibit iron absorption.[10] Vitamin C does not enhance iron absorption from supplements as it does from foods; supplemental iron is already in the ferrous form.

Zinc RDA during pregnancy: 15 mg/day.
Canadian RNI during pregnancy: +6 mg/day.

Zinc Zinc is required for DNA and RNA synthesis and thus for protein synthesis and cell development. Low blood zinc is a significant predictor of low birthweight.[11] Typical zinc intakes are lower than recommendations, but routine supplementation is not advised.[12] Large doses of iron interfere with the body's absorption and use of zinc, so women taking iron supplements (more than 30 milligrams per day) may need zinc supplementation.

Table 18–4

Nutrient Supplements during Pregnancy[a]

Nutrient	Amount
Folate	300 μg
Vitamin B_6	2 mg
Vitamin C	50 mg
Vitamin D	5 μg
Calcium	250 mg
Copper	2 mg
Iron	30 mg
Zinc	15 mg

[a]For pregnant women at nutritional risk (see Table 18–5).

Source: Reprinted with permission from *Nutrition during Pregnancy* © by the National Academy of Sciences. Published by the National Academy Press, Washington, D.C., 1990.

Nutrient Supplements A balanced diet can meet most of a pregnant woman's nutrient needs, except for iron. As mentioned, iron supplements (30 milligrams per day) are recommended during the second and third trimesters of pregnancy. Daily multivitamin-mineral supplements are recommended for women who do not eat adequately and for those in high-risk groups: women carrying multiple fetuses, cigarette smokers, and alcohol and drug abusers. Table 18–4 lists recommended amounts for supplements.

The nutrients mentioned earlier are those most intensely involved in blood production, cell growth, and bone growth. Of course, other nutrients are also needed during pregnancy. Without adequate nutrient and energy intakes, the growth and health of both fetus and mother may be compromised. Even with adequate nutrition, repeated pregnancies less than a year apart deplete nutrient reserves: fetal growth may be protected, but maternal health may decline.[13]

COMMON NUTRITION-RELATED CONCERNS OF PREGNANCY

Nausea, constipation, heartburn, and food sensitivities are common nutrition-related concerns during pregnancy. A few simple strategies can help avert them.

To alleviate the nausea of pregnancy:
- On waking, arise slowly.
- Eat dry toast or crackers.
- Chew gum or suck hard candies.
- Eat small, frequent meals.
- Avoid foods with offensive odors.
- When nauseated, do not drink citrus juice, water, milk, coffee, or tea.

Nausea Many women have uneasy stomachs in the early months of pregnancy. The nausea of "morning" (actually, anytime) sickness ranges from mild queasiness to debilitating nausea and vomiting. Severe and continued vomiting, known as hyperemesis, may require hospitalization if it results in acidosis, dehydration, or excessive weight loss. The hormonal changes of early pregnancy seem to be responsible for a woman's sensitivities to a food's appearance, texture, or smell. Traditional strategies for quelling nausea are listed in the margin, but some women benefit most from simply eating the foods they want when they feel like eating.[14]

To prevent or alleviate constipation:
- Eat foods high in fiber.
- Exercise daily.
- Drink at least 8 glasses of liquids a day.
- Respond promptly to the urge to defecate.
- Use laxatives only as prescribed by a physician; do not use mineral oil because it impairs fat-soluble vitamin absorption.

Constipation and Hemorrhoids As the hormones of pregnancy alter muscle tone and the growing infant crowds intestinal organs, an expectant mother may experience constipation. She may also develop hemorrhoids (swollen veins of the anus and rectum). These can be painful, and straining during bowel movements makes them worse. The strategies listed in the margin may provide relief.

To prevent or relieve heartburn:
- Eat small, frequent meals.
- Drink liquids between meals.
- Avoid spicy or greasy foods.
- Sit up while eating.
- Wait an hour after eating before lying down.
- Wait 2 hours after eating before exercising.

Heartburn Heartburn is another common complaint during pregnancy. As the growing fetus puts increasing pressure on a woman's stomach, acid may back up and create a burning sensation in the lower esophagus near the heart. Tips to help relieve heartburn are listed in the margin on p. 595.

food craving: a deep longing for a particular food.

food aversion: a strong desire to avoid a particular food.

Reminder: The craving for a nonfood item such as clay, ice, and cornstarch is known as *pica*.

Food Cravings and Aversions Some women develop cravings for, or aversions to, some foods and beverages during pregnancy. These cravings do not seem to reflect real physiological needs. A woman who craves pickles does not necessarily need salt, nor does a woman who craves chocolate need caffeine or fat. Cravings for ice cream are common in pregnancy, but do not signify calcium deficiencies. Food cravings and aversions that arise during pregnancy are probably due to hormone-induced changes in sensitivity to taste and smell.

In summary, energy and nutrient needs are high during pregnancy. A balanced diet that includes an extra serving from each of the five food groups can usually meet these needs, with the exception of iron (supplements are recommended). The nausea, constipation, and heartburn that sometimes accompany pregnancy can usually be averted with a few simple strategies; food cravings do not typically reflect physiological needs.

high-risk pregnancy: a pregnancy characterized by indicators that make it likely the birth will be surrounded by problems such as premature delivery, difficult birth, retarded growth, birth defects, and early infant death.

High-Risk and Low-Risk Pregnancies

Some pregnancies are risky to the life and health of the mother and baby. Table 18–5 identifies several characteristics of "high-risk" pregnancies. A woman with

Table 18–5

High-Risk Pregnancy Factors

Factor	Condition That Raises Risk
Maternal weight	
Prior to pregnancy	Prepregnancy BMI either <19.8 or >26.0
During pregnancy	Insufficient or excessive pregnancy weight gain
Maternal nutrition	Nutrient deficiencies or toxicities; eating disorders
Socioeconomic status	Poverty, lack of family support, low level of education, limited food available
Lifestyle habits	Smoking, alcohol or other drug use
Age	Teens 15 years or younger; women 35 years or older
Previous pregnancies	
Number	Many previous pregnancies (3 or more to mothers under age 20; 4 or more to mothers age 20 and older)
Interval	Short intervals between pregnancies (<1 yr)
Outcomes	Previous history of problems
Multiple births	Twins or triplets
Birthweight	Low- or high-birthweight infants
Maternal health	
High blood pressure	Development of pregnancy-related hypertension
Diabetes	Development of gestational diabetes
Chronic diseases	Diabetes; heart, respiratory, and kidney disease; certain genetic disorders; special diets and drugs

Food Assistance Programs for Pregnant Women, Infants, and Children

WIC (the Special Supplemental Food Program for Women, Infants, and Children) provides nutrition education and nutritious foods to low-income pregnant women and their children. WIC provides eggs, milk, cereal, juice, cheese, legumes, peanut butter, and infant formula to infants, children up to age five, and pregnant and breastfeeding women who qualify financially and are at medical or nutritional risk. The program is both remedial and preventive: services include health care referrals, nutrition education, and food packages or vouchers for specific foods to supply nutrients known to be lacking in the diets of the target population. Prenatal WIC participation can effectively reduce low birthweight and newborn medical costs.[a] For every dollar spent on WIC, an estimated three dollars are saved. In 1992, participation in WIC reduced first-year medical expenses for infants by $1.19 billion.[b]

[a]P. A. Buescher and coauthors, Prenatal WIC participation can reduce low birth weight and newborn medical costs: A cost-benefit analysis of WIC participation in North Carolina, *Journal of the American Dietetic Association* 93 (1993): 163–166.

[b]S. Avruch and A. P. Cackley, Savings achieved by giving WIC benefits to women prenatally, *Public Health Reports* 110 (1995): 27–34.

WIC emphasizes foods rich in:

- Protein.
- Vitamin C.
- Calcium.
- Iron.

Currently, the U.S. Department of Agriculture (USDA) funds WIC, and state health departments administer the program. As Congress considers various cost-cutting measures, this arrangement may be revised.

none of these risk factors is said to have a low-risk pregnancy. The more factors that apply, the higher the risk. High-risk pregnancies need special management, including intervention to correct malnutrition. The accompanying box describes government efforts to provide assistance to pregnant women in the United States.

low-risk pregnancy: a pregnancy characterized by indicators that make a normal outcome likely.

MALNUTRITION AND PREGNANCY

Good nutrition clearly supports a pregnancy. In contrast, malnutrition interferes with the ability to conceive, the likelihood of implantation, and the subsequent development of a fetus should these events occur.

Malnutrition and Fertility The nutrition habits and lifestyle choices people make can influence the course of a pregnancy they are not even planning at the time. Malnutrition and food deprivation can reduce fertility: women may develop amenorrhea, and men may lose their ability to produce viable sperm. Furthermore, men and women lose their interest in sex during times of starvation. Starvation arises predictably during famines, wars, and droughts, but can also occur amidst peace and plenty. Many women who diet excessively and exercise intensely are starving and amenorrheic.

fertility: the capacity of a woman to produce a normal ovum periodically and of a man to produce normal sperm; the ability to reproduce.

Reminder: Women who are *amenorrheic* have a temporary or permanent absence of menstrual periods. Amenorrhea is normal before puberty, after menopause, during pregnancy, and during lactation; otherwise it is abnormal.

Malnutrition and Early Pregnancy If a malnourished woman does become pregnant, she faces the challenge of supporting both the growth of a baby and her own health with inadequate nutrient stores. Malnutrition prior to and around conception prevents the placenta from developing fully.[15] A poorly developed placenta cannot deliver optimum nourishment to the fetus, and the infant will be born small and possibly with physical and cognitive abnormalities.

If this small infant is a female, she may develop poorly and in turn will have an elevated risk of having a poor pregnancy outcome. Thus a woman's malnutrition during or even before her pregnancy can adversely affect not only her children but her *grandchildren*.

Malnutrition and Fetal Development Without adequate nutrition during pregnancy, fetal growth and infant health are compromised. In general, consequences of malnutrition during pregnancy include:

- Fetal growth retardation.
- Congenital malformations (birth defects).
- Spontaneous abortion and stillbirth.
- Premature birth.
- Low infant birthweight.

Of these, birthweight is most frequently used as a predictor of an infant's survival and health. Malnutrition coupled with low birthweight contributes to more than half of all deaths of children under five worldwide.

THE INFANT'S BIRTHWEIGHT

low birthweight (LBW): a birthweight of 5½ lb (2500 g) or less; indicates probable poor health in the newborn and poor nutrition status in the mother during pregnancy, before pregnancy, or both. Normal birthweight for a full-term baby is 6½ to 8¾ lb (about 3000 to 4000 g).

Some preterm infants are of a weight **appropriate for gestational age (AGA)**; others are **small for gestational age (SGA)**, often reflecting malnutrition. The latter type are also called **small-for-date** babies.

The most common outcome of a high-risk pregnancy is low birthweight. Low-birthweight infants, defined as infants who weigh 5½ pounds or less, are classified according to gestational age. Preterm, or premature, infants are born before they are fully developed; they are often underweight and have trouble breathing because their lungs are immature. Preterm infants may be small, but if their size and weight are appropriate for their age, they can catch up in growth given adequate nutrition support. In contrast, small-for-gestational-age infants have suffered growth failure in the uterus and do not catch up as well. For the most part, survival improves with increased gestational age and birthweight.[16]

Low-birthweight infants are more likely to experience complications during delivery than normal-weight babies. They also have a statistically greater chance of having physical and mental birth defects, contracting diseases, and dying early in life. Of infants who die before their first birthdays, about two-thirds are low-birthweight babies.

A strong relationship has been established between socioeconomic disadvantage and low birthweight. Low socioeconomic status impairs fetal development by causing stress and by limiting access to medical care and to nutritious foods. Low socioeconomic status often accompanies teen pregnancies, smoking, and alcohol and drug abuse—all predicators of low birthweight.

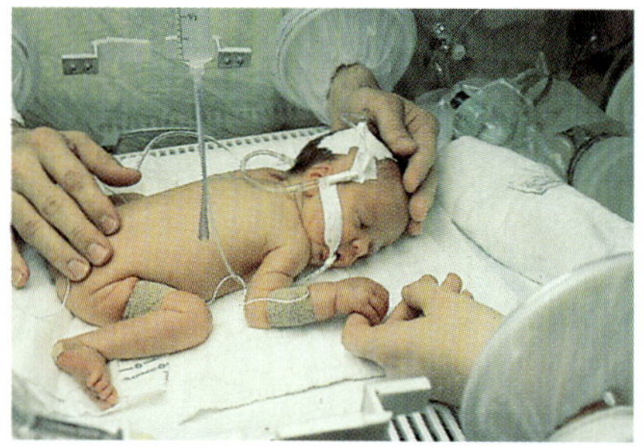

Low-birthweight babies need special care and nourishment.

THE MOTHER'S HEALTH STATUS

Normal weight gain and adequate nutrition support the health of the mother and growth of the infant. Conversely, maternal diseases detract from growth and health. If discovered early, many diseases can be controlled—another reason early prenatal care is recommended.

Preexisting Diabetes The extent to which diabetes presents risks depends on how well it is controlled before and during pregnancy. Without proper management, women with diabetes face an exceptionally high infertility rate, and those who do conceive may experience episodes of severe hypoglycemia or hyperglycemia, spontaneous abortions, and pregnancy-related hypertension. Ideally, a woman with diabetes will have it under control before becoming pregnant and will be able to maintain glucose control throughout pregnancy.

Gestational Diabetes Placental hormones elevate blood insulin and alter insulin resistance during pregnancy. In some women, this can precipitate a condition known as gestational diabetes. Gestational diabetes usually develops during the second half of pregnancy, with subsequent return to normal glucose tolerance after childbirth. In about one-third of such cases, however, women develop diabetes (NIDDM) within five years. To ensure that the problems of gestational diabetes are dealt with promptly, health care professionals look for the risk factors listed in the margin.[17] Gestational diabetes requires dietary management just as other forms of diabetes do. Diet alone may control gestational diabetes, but insulin therapy may be required if blood glucose fails to normalize.

gestational diabetes: the appearance of abnormal glucose tolerance during pregnancy, with subsequent return to normal postpartum.

Risk factors for gestational diabetes:

- Previous gestational diabetes.
- History of large infants (9 lb or more).
- Age 30 or older.
- Obesity or excessive weight gain.
- Complications in previous pregnancies.
- Symptoms of diabetes.
- Family history of diabetes.

Preexisting Hypertension Hypertension complicates pregnancy. In addition to the threats hypertension always carries (such as heart attack and stroke), high blood pressure raises the risks of having a low-birthweight baby or of having the placenta detach from the wall of the uterus before the birth, resulting in stillbirth. Ideally, before a woman with hypertension becomes pregnant, her blood pressure will be normalized by diet, weight loss, and possibly medication.

Transient Hypertension of Pregnancy Some women first develop hypertension during the second half of pregnancy.* Most often, the rise in blood pressure is mild and does not affect the pregnancy adversely.[18] Blood pressure usually returns to normal during the first few weeks after childbirth. This transient hypertension of pregnancy differs from the pregnancy-induced hypertension that accompanies preeclampsia.†

pregnancy-induced hypertension (PIH): high blood pressure that develops in the second half of pregnancy.

Preeclampsia Hypertension may signal the onset of preeclampsia, a condition characterized not only by high blood pressure but by protein in the urine and fluid retention (edema). Preeclampsia usually occurs with first pregnancies after 20 weeks gestation, most often near term. Symptoms typically regress within two days of delivery. The edema of preeclampsia is a whole-body edema, distinct from the localized fluid retention women normally experience late in pregnancy. Preeclampsia affects almost all of the mother's organs—the circulatory system, liver, kidneys, and brain.

Blood flow through the vessels that supply oxygen and nutrients to the placenta diminishes. For this reason, preeclampsia often retards fetal growth. In some cases, the placenta separates from the uterus, resulting in stillbirth.

preeclampsia: a condition characterized by hypertension, fluid retention, and protein in the urine.

The normal edema of pregnancy responds to gravity; fluid pools in the ankles. The edema of preeclampsia is a generalized edema. The differences between these two types of edema help with the diagnosis of preeclampsia.

---

*Blood pressure of 140/90 millimeters mercury during the second half of pregnancy in a woman who has not previously exhibited hypertension indicates high blood pressure. So does a rise in systolic blood pressure of 30 millimeters or in diastolic blood pressure of 15 millimeters on at least two occasions more than six hours apart. By this rule, an apparently "normal" blood pressure of 120/85 would be high for a woman whose normal value was 90/70.

†The Working Group on High Blood Pressure in Pregnancy, convened by the National High Blood Pressure Education Program of the National Heart, Lung, and Blood Institute, has suggested abandoning the term "pregnancy-induced hypertension" because it fails to differentiate between the mild, transient hypertension of pregnancy and the life-threatening hypertension of preeclampsia.

eclampsia: a condition characterized by convulsions and coma that develops in some women with untreated preeclampsia.

Warning signs of preeclampsia:

- Hypertension.
- Protein in the urine.
- Upper abdominal pain.
- Severe and constant headaches.
- Swelling, especially of the face.
- Dizziness.
- Blurred vision.
- Sudden weight gain (1 lb/day).

Preeclampsia can progress rapidly to eclampsia—a condition characterized by convulsions and coma. Maternal mortality during pregnancy and childbirth is extremely rare in developed countries, but eclampsia is a common cause.

Preeclampsia demands prompt medical attention. Treatment focuses on regulating blood pressure and preventing convulsions. If preeclampsia develops early and is severe, induced labor or cesarean birth may be necessary. The infant will be preterm, with all of the associated problems, including poor lung development, and will need special care.

Several approaches have been proposed to prevent preeclampsia, including salt restriction, calcium supplementation, and low-dose aspirin therapy. Salt restriction does not improve the incidence or severity of preeclampsia and is not a part of treatment until and unless the kidneys prove unable to handle sodium.

Several studies have reported an inverse relationship between calcium intake and preeclampsia.[19] Furthermore, research has determined that calcium supplementation during pregnancy can lower high blood pressure.[20] In a group of over 1000 pregnant women given either a calcium supplement or a placebo during the second half of pregnancy, the women who received calcium supplements (2000 milligrams per day) had a reduced risk of hypertensive disorders.[21] Such findings are promising, but at this time evidence is insufficient to recommend routine supplementation; furthermore, calcium supplementation may create risks of its own, including the development of kidney stones.[22]

Another promising option is the use of low doses of aspirin (60 to 100 milligrams a day). Low-dose aspirin appears to reduce the incidence of preeclampsia, and some clinicians recommend its use in high-risk pregnancies (women with a history of preeclampsia, fetal death, or placental insufficiency).[23]

PREGNANCY IN ADOLESCENCE

Most adolescents become sexually active before age 19, and one million adolescent girls face pregnancies each year in the United States. About half of them continue their pregnancies. Put another way, about one out of every five babies is born to a teenager, and more than a tenth of these mothers are age 15 or younger. Clearly, teenage pregnancy is a major public health problem. Even when not pregnant, a teenage girl has difficulty meeting her nutrient needs. Nourishing a growing fetus adds to her burden. The competition between maternal and fetal needs places both mother and infant at risk. Simply being young increases these risks independently of important socioeconomic factors.[24]

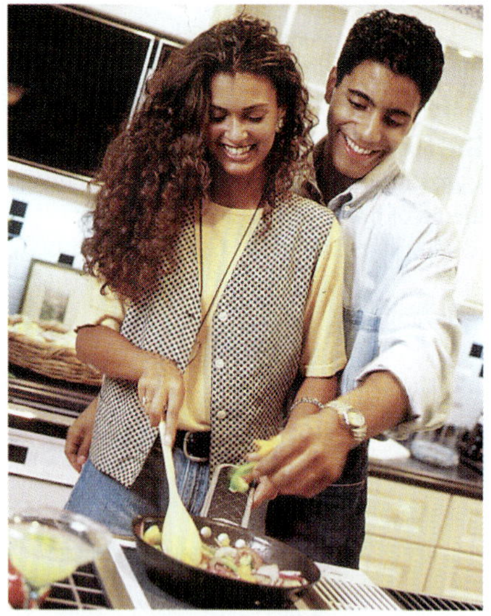

Young adults can prepare themselves for a healthy pregnancy by taking care of themselves today.

To support the needs of both mother and fetus, young teenagers (13 to 16 years old) are encouraged to strive for the highest weight gains recommended for pregnancy. For a teen who enters pregnancy at a healthy body weight, a weight gain of approximately 35 pounds is recommended; this minimizes the risk of delivering a low-birthweight infant.[25] Gaining less may limit fetal growth.[26] Pregnant and lactating teenagers can use the Daily Food Guide presented in Table 18–3 (on p. 593), making sure to select at least 4 servings of milk or milk products daily.

Pregnant adolescents have unique economic, psychosocial, and physical vulnerabilities that jeopardize a healthy pregnancy.[27] To improve their chances for a successful pregnancy and healthy infant, they must seek prenatal care. WIC helps pregnant teenagers obtain adequate food to support a reasonable weight gain.

PREGNANCY IN OLDER WOMEN

In the last three decades, as many women have pursued their education and careers, they have delayed childbearing. As a result, the number of first births to women 35 and older has increased dramatically.

Each year, 994 out of 1000 pregnant women over the age of 35 have healthy pregnancies.[28] Most of the complications associated with later childbearing reflect chronic conditions such as hypertension and diabetes. These complications often result in a cesarean delivery, which is twice as common in women over 35 as among younger women. For all these reasons, maternal mortality rates are higher in women over 35 than in younger women.

The babies of older mothers face problems of their own. Because 1 out of 50 pregnancies in older women produces an infant with genetic abnormalities, obstetricians routinely screen women older than 35. Birth defects, preterm births, growth retardation, and death are common among infants born to women over 35. For a 40-year-old mother, the risk of having a child with Down syndrome, for example, is about 1 in 100 compared with 1 in 300 for a 35-year-old and 1 in 10,000 for a 20-year-old. Fetal mortality is twice as high for women 35 years and older than for younger women.[29] Why this is so remains a bit of a mystery. One possibility is that the uterine blood vessels of older women cannot fully adapt to the increased demands of pregnancy.

Down syndrome: a genetic abnormality that causes mental retardation, short stature, and flattened facial features.

FETAL ALCOHOL SYNDROME

Drinking alcohol during pregnancy endangers the fetus. Alcohol crosses the placenta freely and deprives the developing fetal brain of both nutrients and oxygen. The result may be fetal alcohol syndrome (FAS), a cluster of symptoms that includes:[30]

- Prenatal and postnatal growth retardation.
- Impairment of the brain and nerves, with consequent mental retardation, poor coordination, and hyperactivity.
- Abnormalities of the face and skull (see Figure 18–5).
- Increased frequency of major birth defects: cleft palate, heart defects, and defects in ears, genitals, and urinary system.

Tragically, the damage evident at birth persists: children with FAS never fully recover.[31]

Of every 10,000 children born in the United States some 6 or 7 suffer health problems because their mothers drank alcohol during pregnancy—a sixfold increase over the past 15 years.[32] In addition, many infants are born with the less serious, yet still significant, damage some clinicians describe as fetal alcohol effects (FAE).[33] Some children with FAE have no outward signs; others may be short or have only minor facial abnormalities. Often children with FAE go undiagnosed even when problems develop in the early school years: learning disabilities, behavioral abnormalities, motor impairments, and more.

The surgeon general states that pregnant women should drink absolutely no alcohol. Abstinence from alcohol is the best policy for pregnant women both because alcohol consumption during pregnancy has such severe consequences, and because FAS can only be prevented—it cannot be treated.[34] And because

See Highlight 7 for additional alcohol-related information.

fetal alcohol syndrome (FAS): the cluster of symptoms seen in an infant or child whose mother consumed excess alcohol during pregnancy, including retarded growth, impaired development of the central nervous system, and facial malformations.

fetal alcohol effects (FAE): a subclinical version of FAS, with hidden defects including learning disabilities, behavioral abnormalities, and motor impairments; also called **alcohol-related birth defects (ARBD).**

Figure 18–5

Typical Facial Characteristics of FAS

The severe facial abnormalities shown here are just outward signs of the severe mental impairments within. The internal organs also suffer irreversible damage that, while hidden, may create major problems for a child's health.

Source: Adapted from J. O. Beattie, Alcohol exposure and the fetus, *European Journal of Clinical Nutrition* 46 (1992): S7–S17.

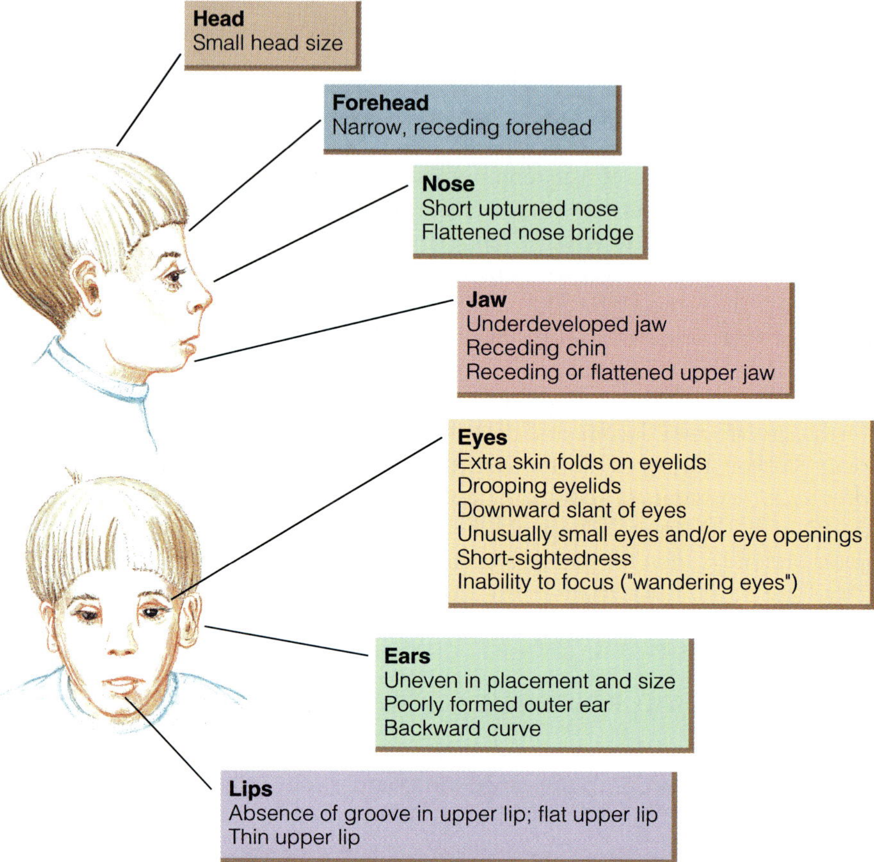

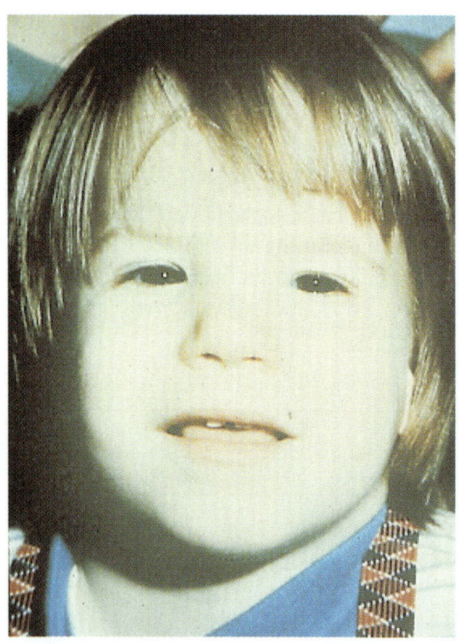

The most obvious symptoms of FAS are the abnormal facial features, but the most tragic ones are the mental disabilities.

the most severe damage occurs around the time of conception—*before a woman may even realize that she is pregnant*—even a woman planning to conceive should abstain.

Drinking during Pregnancy When a woman drinks during pregnancy, she causes damage in two ways: directly, by intoxication, and indirectly, by malnutrition. Prior to the complete formation of the placenta (approximately 12 weeks), alcohol diffuses directly into the tissues of the developing embryo, causing incredible damages. When alcohol crosses the placenta, fetal blood alcohol rises until it reaches an equilibrium with maternal blood alcohol. The mother may not even appear drunk, but the fetus may be poisoned. The fetus's body is small, its detoxification system is immature, and alcohol remains in fetal blood long after it has disappeared from maternal blood. Alcohol interferes with many developmental events, reducing the number of cells produced and damaging those that are produced.

Alcohol also impairs maternal nutrition status. People who abuse alcohol often are malnourished, and as described earlier, maternal malnutrition impedes fetal development. Even if the mother eats well and maintains adequate nutrient stores, alcohol damages the placenta, and so interferes with the transport of nutrients to the fetus, causing fetal malnutrition.

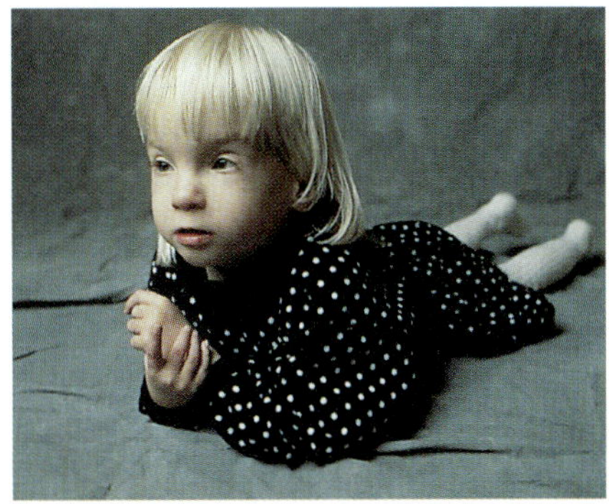

Characteristic facial features may diminish with time, but children with FAS typically continue to be short and underweight for their age.

How Much Alcohol Is Too Much? Alcohol damages the fetus to an extent that correlates directly with the quantity the mother consumes: the number of defects rises with increasing amounts of alcohol. A pregnant woman need not have an alcohol-abuse problem to give birth to a baby with FAS. She need only drink in excess of her liver's capacity to detoxify alcohol. About four drinks a day dramatically worsens the risk of having physical malformations. Even one to two drinks a day threatens to retard growth.

Does this mean that drinking, say, one drink every day or so might be safe? Probably not, for researchers have not yet defined the relationship between alcohol consumption and damage that precisely, nor do they agree on the criteria used to define safety. Although some of alcohol's effects are obvious (such as the physical malformations), others are more subtle (the neurological defects) and often become evident only after several years. Even with those ambiguities resolved, researchers could not specify an amount that would be safe for every woman because individuals respond differently to varying levels of alcohol intake.

In addition to total alcohol intake, drinking patterns play an important role. Most FAS studies report their findings in terms of average intake per day, but people usually drink more heavily on some days than on others. For example, a woman who drinks an *average* of 1 ounce of alcohol (2 drinks) a day may not drink at all during the week but then have 14 drinks on Saturday night, exposing the fetus to highly toxic quantities of alcohol. Whether drinking a certain number of drinks during binges or spreading them out over several days causes more damage depends on the frequency of the binges, the quantity consumed, and the stage of fetal development at the time of each drinking episode.

An occasional drink may be innocuous, but researchers are unable to say how much alcohol is safe to consume during pregnancy. For this reason, health care professionals urge women to stop drinking alcohol as soon as they realize they are pregnant, or better, as soon as they *plan* to become pregnant.[35] Why take any risk? Only the woman who abstains is sure of protecting her infant from FAS.

When Is the Damage Done? The type of abnormality observed in an FAS infant depends on the developmental events occurring at the times of alcohol exposure. During the first trimester, developing organs such as the brain, heart, and kidneys may be malformed. During the second trimester, the risk of spontaneous abortion increases. During the third trimester, body and brain growth may be retarded.

In experiments on laboratory animals, the effects of alcohol on fetal development are most marked when the female takes alcohol during the earliest period—that of organ formation. Effects also appear when the female takes alcohol just *prior* to conception. Studies on human beings also find that alcohol is most potent in causing birth defects within the first eight weeks of gestation.

Male alcohol ingestion may also affect fertility and fetal development. Animal studies have found smaller litter sizes, lower birthweights, reduced survival rates, and impaired learning ability in the offspring of males consuming alcohol prior to conception.[36] One human study found an association between paternal alcohol intake one month prior to conception and low infant birthweight.[37] (Paternal alcohol intake was defined as an average of two or more drinks daily or at least five drinks on one occasion.) This relationship was independent of either parent's smoking and of the mother's use of alcohol, caffeine, or other drugs.

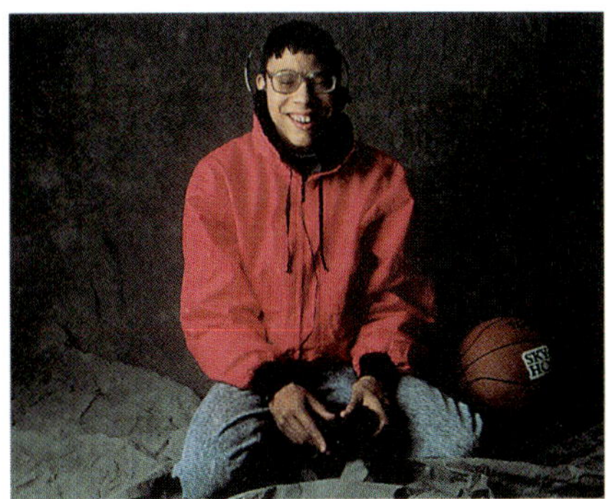

Children born with FAS must live with the long-term consequences of prenatal brain damage.

In view of these findings, it is important to advise women not to drink during pregnancy. Everyone should know of the potential dangers. Heavy drinkers who are sexually active urgently need effective contraception to prevent pregnancy.

All containers of beer, wine, and liquor carry the warning: "Drinking during pregnancy may cause mental retardation and other birth defects. Avoid alcohol during pregnancy." Everyone should hear the message loud and clear: Don't drink alcohol prior to conception or during pregnancy. Once present, FAS has no cure.

OTHER PRACTICES INCOMPATIBLE WITH PREGNANCY

Besides malnutrition and alcohol consumption, which present many hazards to pregnancy, a variety of other lifestyle factors can have adverse impacts; and some may be teratogenic. People who are planning to have children need to know what practices to avoid.

teratogenic (ter-AT-oh-jen-ik): causing abnormal fetal development and birth defects.

terato = monster

genic = to produce

Medicinal Drugs Drugs other than alcohol can also cause complications during pregnancy, problems in labor, and serious birth defects. For these reasons, pregnant women should not take any medicines without consulting their physicians. Drug labels warn: As with any drug, if you are pregnant or nursing a baby, seek the advice of a health professional before using this product. For aspirin and ibuprofen, an additional warning immediately follows: It is especially important not to use aspirin (or ibuprofen) during the last three months of pregnancy unless specifically directed to do so by a doctor because it may cause problems in the unborn child or (excessive bleeding) during delivery.

Fetal effects of abused drugs:

- Amphetamines: Suspected nervous system damage; behavioral abnormalities.
- Barbiturates: Drug withdrawal symptoms in the newborn, lasting up to six months.
- Cocaine (including "crack"): Uncontrolled jerking motions; paralysis; permanent mental and physical damage.
- Marijuana: Short-term irritability at birth.
- Opiates (including heroin): Drug withdrawal symptoms in the newborn; permanent learning disability (attention deficit disorder).

Smoking during pregnancy increases the risk of:

- Fetal growth retardation.
- Low birthweight.
- Complications at birth.
- Mislocation of the placenta.
- Premature separation of the placenta.
- Vaginal bleeding.
- Spontaneous abortion.
- Fetal death.
- SIDS.

Illicit Drugs The recommendation to avoid drugs during pregnancy includes illicit drugs, of course. Unfortunately, use of illicit drugs, such as cocaine and marijuana, is common among pregnant women. One study of over 700 pregnant women found that 15 percent of them tested positive for illicit drugs—regardless of race or socioeconomic status.[38]

Drugs of abuse, such as cocaine, pass easily through the placenta and impair fetal development.[39] Furthermore, they are responsible for preterm births, low-birthweight infants, and sudden infant deaths.[40] If these newborns survive, their cries and behaviors at birth are abnormal, and their cognitive development later in life is impaired.[41] They may be hypersensitive or underaroused; those who test positive for drugs suffer the greatest effects of toxicity and withdrawal.[42]

Smoking and Chewing Tobacco Smoking and chewing tobacco at any time exerts harmful effects, and pregnancy dramatically magnifies the hazards of these practices. Smoking restricts the blood supply to the growing fetus and so limits oxygen and nutrient delivery and waste removal. Also, smokers tend to eat less nutritious foods during their pregnancies than do nonsmokers, which in turn impairs fetal nutrition.[43]

Of all preventable causes of low birthweight in the United States, smoking has the greatest impact. The more a mother smokes, the smaller her baby will be. Furthermore, smoking causes death in otherwise healthy fetuses and newborns. There is a positive relationship between sudden infant death syndrome (SIDS) and both cigarette smoking during pregnancy and postnatal exposure to passive smoke.[44] Smoking during pregnancy may even harm the intellectual and behavioral development of the child later in life.[45] Infants of mothers who chew tobacco also have lower birthweights and higher rates of fetal deaths than infants born to women who do not use tobacco.

The prevalence of smoking in pregnancy is an estimated 20 percent, with higher rates for unmarried women, teenagers, and those who lack education. A woman who smokes and is considering pregnancy or who is already pregnant should try to quit or at least cut back on the number of cigarettes smoked.

sudden infant death syndrome (SIDS): the unexpected and unexplained death of an apparently well infant; the most common cause of death of infants between the second week and the end of the first year of life; also called *crib death*.

Environmental Contaminants Evidence of exposure to environmental contaminants such as lead and mercury has been detected in the amniotic fluid of pregnant women.[46] Infants and young children of these mothers show signs of impaired cognitive development.[47] For this reason, it is particularly important that pregnant women receive foods and beverages grown and prepared in environments free of contamination.

Highlight 13 describes how lead toxicity impairs a child's development.

Vitamin-Mineral Megadoses The pregnant woman who is trying to eat well may mistakenly assume that more is better when it comes to vitamin-mineral supplements. This is simply not true; many vitamins are toxic when taken in excess, and the minerals are even more so, some at levels not far above recommendations. A pregnant woman can obtain most of the vitamins and minerals she needs by eating whole foods and should take supplements only on the advice of a registered dietitian or physician.

Caffeine Pregnant women may wonder whether they should give up coffee, tea, and colas because of their caffeine contents. Research studies have not proven that caffeine (even in high doses) causes birth defects in human babies (as it does in animal studies), but limited evidence suggests that moderate-to-heavy use may lower infant birthweight.[48] All things considered, it might be most sensible to limit caffeine consumption to the equivalent of a cup of coffee or two 12-ounce cola beverages a day.

The caffeine contents of selected beverages, foods, and drugs are listed on p. H–3 of Appendix H.

Weight-Loss Dieting Weight-loss dieting, even for short periods, is hazardous during pregnancy. Low-carbohydrate diets or fasts that cause ketosis deprive the fetal brain of needed glucose and may impair its development. Such diets are also likely to lack other nutrients vital to fetal growth. Regardless of prepregnancy weight, pregnant women should never intentionally lose weight.

Sugar Substitutes Artificial sweeteners have been extensively investigated and found to be safe for use during pregnancy.[49] (Women with phenylketonuria should not use aspartame, as Highlight 4 explains.) It would be prudent for pregnant women to use sweeteners in moderation and within an otherwise nutritious and well-balanced diet.

To recap, high-risk pregnancies, especially for teenagers, threaten the life and health of both mother and infant. Proper nutrition and abstinence from smoking, alcohol, and other drugs improve the outcome. In addition, prenatal care includes monitoring pregnant women for gestational diabetes and preeclampsia.

Nutrition during Lactation

For infants, breastfeeding:

- Prevents a variety of infections.
- Protects against some chronic diseases, such as NIDDM.
- Makes food allergies less likely.

For mothers, breastfeeding:

- Contracts the uterus.
- Lengthens birth intervals.
- Conserves iron stores (amenorrhea).
- Reduces risk of breast cancer.
- Protects bone density.
- Saves money and offers convenience.

Before the end of her pregnancy, a woman will need to consider whether to feed her infant breast milk, infant formula, or both. These options are the only recommended foods for an infant during the first four to six months of life.

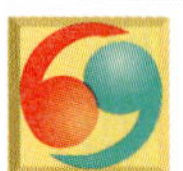

HEALTHY PEOPLE 2000: Increase to at least 75% the proportion of mothers who breastfeed their babies in the early weeks and to at least 50% the proportion who continue breastfeeding until their babies are five to six months old.

Breastfeeding offers many benefits to both mother and infant, and every pregnant woman should seriously consider it. Still, there are valid reasons for not breastfeeding, and formula-fed infants grow and develop into healthy children. After all, the primary goal is to provide the infant with optimal nourishment in a relaxed and loving environment.

To learn about breastfeeding, a pregnant woman can read at least one of the many books available. Appendix F provides a list of other nutrition resources, including La Leche League International.

Some hospitals employ *certified lactation consultants* who specialize in helping new mothers to establish a healthy breastfeeding relationship with their newborns. These consultants are often registered nurses with specialized training in breast and infant anatomy and physiology.

BREASTFEEDING: A LEARNED BEHAVIOR

In many countries around the world, a woman breastfeeds her newborn without considering the alternatives or consciously making a decision. In other parts of the world, a woman feeds her newborn formula simply because she knows so little about breastfeeding. She may have misconceptions or feel uncomfortable about a process she has never seen or experienced.

Although lactation is an automatic physiological process, breastfeeding is a learned behavior that is most successful in a supportive environment. Health care professionals play an important role in providing encouragement and accurate information on breastfeeding. Of women who do breastfeed, 25 to 50 percent stop within the first month, and 50 to 70 percent stop by four months; those who receive early and repeated information and support breastfeed their infants longer than other breastfeeding women.

Fathers also play an important role in encouraging breastfeeding.[50] One study reported that most of those fathers whose partners planned to breastfeed supported that decision and respected breastfeeding women. By comparison, those whose partners planned to bottle feed believed that breastfeeding would make the breasts ugly and interfere with sex. Clearly, educating fathers could change attitudes and promote breastfeeding.

In societies where few women breastfeed, appropriate breastfeeding etiquette remains undefined. A woman faces conflict, confusion, and frustration. Must she retreat to a private place to nurse? What if she cannot find such a place in a public setting? A hungry infant is impatient, and a mother must act quickly. As role models become more numerous, a consensus will develop as to what behaviors are accepted and will provide nursing mothers with more guidance and confidence. Many public buildings now provide "baby rooms" with tables for changing diapers and comfortable chairs for nursing.

Parents in today's society also have to coordinate work and family. All mothers are working women—many of them with jobs outside the home. A social system that provides extended, paid maternity leaves, breaks on the job to nurse infants or pump breasts, and job-site child care promotes breastfeeding as a feasible option.

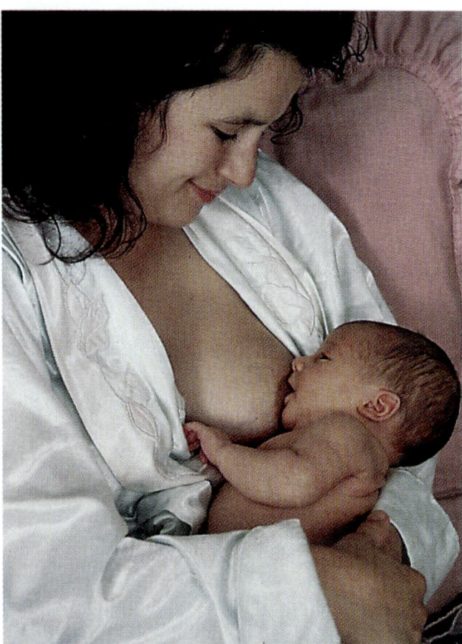

Breastfeeding is a natural extension of pregnancy—of the mother's body nourishing the infant.

Most healthy women who want to breastfeed can do so with a little preparation; physical obstacles to breastfeeding are rare. Successful breastfeeding requires adequate nutrition and rest. This, plus the support of all who care, will help to enhance the well-being of mother and infant.

THE MOTHER'S NUTRIENT NEEDS

By continuing to eat nutrient-dense foods throughout lactation, the mother who chooses to breastfeed her infant will be nutritionally prepared to do so. An adequate diet is needed to support the stamina, patience, and self-confidence that nursing an infant demands.

lactation: production and secretion of breast milk for the purpose of nourishing an infant.

Energy Intake and Exercise A nursing mother produces about 25 ounces of milk a day, with considerable variation from woman to woman and in the same woman from time to time, depending primarily on the infant's demand for milk.[51] To produce milk, a woman needs extra food energy–almost 650 kcalories a day above her regular need during the first six months of lactation. To meet this energy need, the woman is advised to eat an extra 500 kcalories of food each day and let the fat reserves she accumulated during pregnancy provide the rest. Some research suggests that many women need less energy for milk production; other research findings confirm current recommendations.[52] Severe energy restriction, however, hinders milk production.

Energy RDA during lactation: +500 kcal/day (1800 kcal/day minimum).
Canadian RNI during lactation: +450 kcal/day.

After the birth of the infant, many women are in a hurry to lose the extra body fat they accumulated during pregnancy. One study reports that the amount of weight lost does not depend on whether a woman breastfeeds her infant.[53] Another study suggests that breastfeeding enhances weight loss initially, especially fat loss from the lower body, but not thereafter.[54] Still another study indicates that weight loss is significant only if breastfeeding continues for at least six months.[55] A woman who breastfeeds her infant will gradually lose weight if she chooses nutrient-dense foods, even though her energy intake may be greater than normal. Most women lose 1 to 2 pounds a month during the first four to six months of lactation; some may lose more, and others may maintain or even gain weight.[56] Regardless of a woman's prepregnancy weight, the more weight she gains during pregnancy, the more weight she loses following delivery (when measured at six weeks and one year).[57]

Women often exercise to reduce body fat and improve fitness, and this is compatible with breastfeeding.[58] Studies have found that lactating women who exercise compensate for their high energy expenditures by increasing their energy intakes.[59] Intense exercise can raise the lactic acid concentration of breast milk, which influences the milk's taste. Infants appear to prefer milk produced prior to exercise (which has a lower lactic acid content).[60] For this reason, mothers may want to breastfeed their infants before exercise or express their milk before exercise for use afterward.

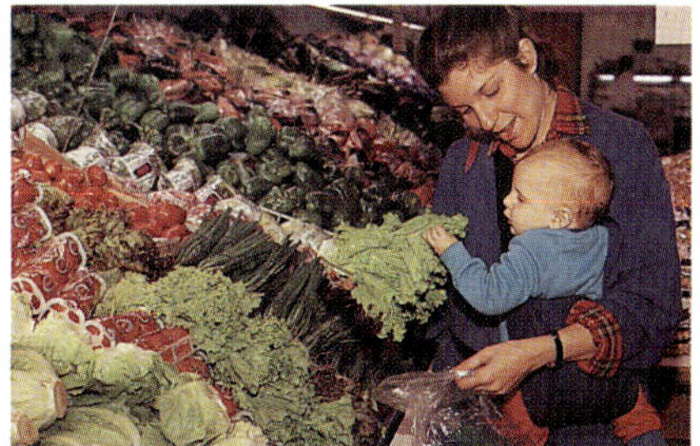

Nutritious foods support successful lactation.

Vitamins and Minerals In addition to providing energy, the foods consumed by the nursing mother should offer abundant nutrients and plenty of fluid. Review Figure 18–4 (on p. 592) to compare a lactating woman's nutrient needs with those of pregnant and nonpregnant women.

A question often raised is whether a mother's milk may lack a nutrient if she fails to get enough in her diet. The answer differs from one nutrient to the next,

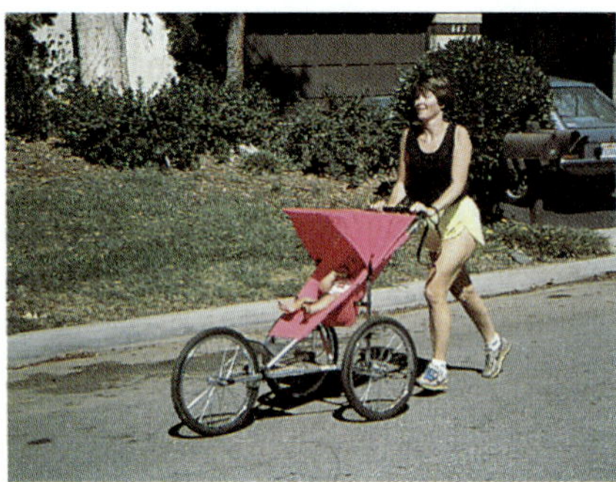

A brisk walk through the neighborhood offers a refreshing opportunity for physical activity and fresh air.

but in general, nutritional inadequacies reduce the *quantity,* not the *quality,* of breast milk. Women can produce milk with adequate protein, carbohydrate, fat, and most minerals, even when their own supplies are limited.[61] For these nutrients and for folate as well, milk quality is maintained at the expense of maternal stores. Nutrients in breast milk are most likely to decline in response to prolonged inadequate intakes of the vitamins—especially vitamins B_6, B_{12}, A, and D.[62]

Water A lactating woman needs to drink plenty of fluids to protect herself from dehydration. A sensible rule of thumb is to drink a glass of milk, juice, or water at each meal and each time the baby nurses. Despite previous misconceptions, a mother who drinks more fluid does not produce more breast milk.[63]

Supplements Most lactating women can obtain all the nutrients they need from a well-balanced diet without taking vitamin-mineral supplements; some, however, may need iron supplements. Maternal iron stores dwindle during pregnancy, when the fetus takes iron to meet its own needs during the first four to six months after birth. In addition, childbirth may have incurred blood losses. A woman may therefore need iron supplements during lactation, not to augment the iron in her breast milk, but to refill her depleted iron stores.

Particular Foods Foods with strong or spicy flavors (such as garlic) may alter the flavor of breast milk.[64] A sudden change in the taste of the milk may annoy some infants. Infants who are sensitive to particular foods such as cow's milk protein may become uncomfortable when the mother's diet includes these foods. Only a few infants exhibit this sensitivity, so only a few nursing mothers need avoid cow's milk. Generally, nutrients from milk products support both the infant's and the mother's health.

In general, a nursing mother can eat whatever nutritious foods she chooses. If she suspects a particular food is causing the infant discomfort, her physician may recommend a dietary challenge: eliminate the food from the diet to see if the infant's reactions subside; then return the food to the diet, and again monitor the infant's reactions. If a food must be eliminated for an extended time, appropriate substitutions must be made to ensure nutrient adequacy.

CONCERNS OF BREASTFEEDING MOTHERS

Some substances impair milk production or enter breast milk and interfere with infant development. Some medical conditions prohibit breastfeeding. This section describes these effects.

Alcohol Alcohol easily enters breast milk. One study showed that the alcohol concentration of breast milk peaks within one hour after ingestion.[65] In this study, even small amounts of alcohol (equivalent to a can of beer) consumed by lactating women significantly reduced their infants' intakes of breast milk. The researchers suggest three possible reasons, acting separately or together. For one, the alcohol may have altered the flavor of the breast milk and thereby the infants' acceptance of it. For another, because infants metabolize alcohol inefficiently, even low doses may be potent enough to suppress their feeding behavior. Third, the alcohol may have reduced the women's milk production.

In the past, alcohol has been recommended to mothers to facilitate lactation despite a lack of scientific evidence that it does so. The research summarized here suggests that alcohol actually hinders breastfeeding. An occasional glass of wine or beer is considered within safe limits, but in general, lactating women should consume little or no alcohol.

Caffeine Caffeine taken during lactation may make a breastfed infant irritable and wakeful. As during pregnancy, caffeine consumption should be moderate—say, one to two cups of coffee a day. Larger doses of coffee may interfere with the availability of iron from the milk and impair the infant's iron status.

Smoking Cigarette smoking reduces milk volume, so smokers may produce too little milk to meet their infants' energy needs. One study of lactating women found that infants of smoking mothers gained less weight than infants of nonsmoking mothers.[66] Furthermore, infant exposure to passive smoke negates the protective effect breastfeeding offers against SIDS and increases the risks dramatically.[67]

Medical Considerations If a woman has an ordinary cold, she can go on nursing without worry. If susceptible, the infant will catch it from her anyway. (Thanks to immunological protection, a breastfed baby may be less susceptible than a formula-fed baby would be.) If a woman has a communicable disease such as tuberculosis or hepatitis that could threaten the infant's health, then mother and baby have to be separated; mothers can pump their breasts several times a day and feed breast milk by bottle.

For mothers with HIV infections, advice differs depending on the context.[68] Where safe alternatives are available, the Centers for Disease Control and the American Academy of Pediatrics recommend that HIV-positive women not breastfeed their infants. In developing countries, however, the feeding of inappropriate or contaminated formulas is the cause of 1.5 million infant deaths each year, so WHO and UNICEF urge mothers to breastfeed irrespective of HIV infection.

Women with chronic diseases such as diabetes (IDDM) may need careful monitoring and counseling to ensure successful lactation.[69] Women with IDDM need to adjust their energy intakes and insulin doses to meet the heightened needs of lactation. Maintaining good glucose control helps to initiate lactation and support milk production.[70]

Many drugs are compatible with breastfeeding, but some medicines are contraindicated, either because they suppress lactation or because they are secreted into breast milk and can harm the infant.[71] As a precaution, a nursing mother should consult with her physician prior to taking any drug. Illicit drugs, of course, are harmful to the physical and emotional health of both the mother and the nursing infant. Breast milk can deliver such high doses of illicit drugs as to cause irritability, tremors, and hallucinations in infants.

Women who breastfeed experience prolonged postpartum amenorrhea. Absent menstrual periods, however, do not protect a woman from pregnancy. To prevent pregnancy, a couple must use some form of contraception—but not oral contraceptive agents. Standard oral contraceptives contain estrogen, which reduces milk volume and the protein content of breast milk.[72]

postpartum amenorrhea: the normal temporary absence of menstrual periods immediately following childbirth.

Some women fear that breastfeeding will cause their breasts to sag. The breasts do swell and become heavy and large immediately after the birth, but even when they are producing enough milk to nourish a thriving infant, they eventually shrink back to their prepregnant size. Given proper support, diet, and exercise, breasts often return to their former shape and size after weaning. Breasts change their shape as the body ages, but breastfeeding does not accelerate this process.

Environmental Contaminants Environmental contaminants, such as DDT, PCBs, and methylmercury can find their way into breast milk. Inuit mothers living in Arctic Québec who eat seal and beluga whale blubber have concentrations of DDT and PCBs in their breast milk two to ten times greater than those found in breast milk from women in southern Québec.[73] The impact of contaminated breast milk on infant development is unclear, however. Preliminary studies indicate the children of these Inuit mothers are developing normally. Researchers speculate that the abundant omega-3 fatty acids of the Inuit diet may protect against damage to the central nervous system.

In summary, the lactating woman needs extra fluid and enough energy and nutrients to produce about 25 ounces of milk a day. Alcohol, other drugs, smoking, and contaminants may impair milk production or enter breast milk and impair infant development.

This chapter has focused on the nutrition needs of the mother during pregnancy and lactation. The next chapter explores the dietary needs of infants, children, and adolescents.

Study Questions

1. Describe the placenta and its function.
2. Describe the normal events of fetal development. How does malnutrition impair fetal development?
3. Define the term *critical period.* How do adverse influences during critical periods affect later health?
4. Explain why women of childbearing age need folate in their diets. How much is recommended, and how can women ensure that these needs are met?
5. How does nutrition *prior* to conception influence a pregnancy?
6. What is the recommended pattern of weight gain during pregnancy for a woman at a healthy weight? For an underweight woman? For an overweight woman?
7. What does a pregnant woman need to know about exercise?
8. Which nutrients are needed in the greatest amounts during pregnancy? Why are they so important? Describe wise food choices for the pregnant woman.
9. Define low-risk and high-risk pregnancies. What is the significance of infant birthweight in terms of the child's future health?
10. Describe some of the special problems of the pregnant adolescent. Which nutrients are needed in increased amounts?
11. What practices should be avoided during pregnancy? Why?
12. How do nutrient needs during lactation differ from nutrient needs during pregnancy?

Notes

1. Committee on Nutritional Status during Pregnancy and Lactation, *Nutrition during Pregnancy* (Washington, D.C.: National Academy Press, 1990), pp. 412–419.
2. American Academy of Pediatrics, Committee on Genetics, Folic acid for the prevention of neural tube defects, *Pediatrics* 92 (1993): 493–494.

3. Committee on Nutritional Status during Pregnancy and Lactation, 1990, p. 10.
4. Committee on Nutritional Status during Pregnancy and Lactation, 1990, p. 229.
5. K. G. Dewey and M. A. McCrory, Effects of dieting and physical activity on pregnancy and lactation, *American Journal of Clinical Nutrition* (supplement) 59 (1994): 446S–453S.
6. ACOG *Technical Bulletin 189: Exercise during Pregnancy and the Postpartum Period* (Washington, D.C.: The American College of Obstetricians and Gynocologists, 1994).
7. Committee on Nutritional Status during Pregnancy and Lactation, 1990, p. 384.
8. Committee on Dietary Reference Intakes, *Dietary Reference Intakes for Calcium, Phosphorus, Magnesium, Vitamin D, and Fluoride* (Washington, D.C.: National Academy Press, 1997), 4–38.
9. Committee on Nutritional Status during Pregnancy and Lactation, 1990, pp. 272–298.
10. Committee on Nutritional Status during Pregnancy and Lactation, 1990 pp. 285–293.
11. Y. H. Neggers and coauthors, A positive association between maternal serum zinc concentration and birth weight, *American Journal of Clinical Nutrition* 51 (1990): 678–684.
12. Committee on Nutritional Status during Pregnancy and Lactation, 1990, pp. 299–317.
13. K. Merchant, R. Martorell, and J. D. Haas, Consequences for maternal nutrition of reproductive stress across consecutive pregnancies, *American Journal of Clinical Nutrition* 52 (1990): 616–620.
14. M. Erick, Battling morning (noon and night) sickness: New approaches for treating an age-old problem, *Journal of the American Dietetic Association* 94 (1994): 147–148.
15. Transplacental nutrient transfer and intrauterine growth retardation, *Nutrition Reviews* 50 (1992): 56–57.
16. D. L. Phelps and coauthors, 28-day survival rates of 6676 neonates with birth weights of 1250 grams or less, *Pediatrics* 87 (1991): 7–17.
17. ACOG *Guide to Planning for Pregnancy, Birth, and Beyond* (Washington, D.C.: The American College of Obstetricians and Gynecologists, 1990), pp. 128–140.
18. F. G. Cunningham and M. D. Lindheimer, Hypertension in pregnancy, *New England Journal of Medicine* 326 (1992): 927–932.
19. Calcium supplementation prevents hypertensive disorders of pregnancy, *Nutrition Reviews* 50 (1992): 233–236.
20. K. B. Knight and R. E. Keith, Calcium supplementation on normotensive and hypertensive pregnant women, *American Journal of Clinical Nutrition* 55 (1992): 891–895; J. R. Repke and J. Villar, Pregnancy-induced hypertension and low birth weight: The role of calcium, *American Journal of Clinical Nutrition* 54 (1991): 237S–241S.
21. J. M. Belizan and coauthors, Calcium supplementation to prevent hypertensive disorders of pregnancy, *New England Journal of Medicine* 325 (1991): 1399–1405.
22. T. F. Ferris, Pregnancy, preeclampsia, and the endothelial cell, *New England Journal of Medicine* 325 (1991): 1439–1440.
23. F. G. Cummingham and N. F. Gant, Prevention of preeclampsia —A reality? *New England Journal of Medicine* 321 (1989): 606–607.
24. A. M. Fraser, J. E. Brockert, and R. H. Ward, Association of young maternal age with adverse reproductive outcomes, *New England Journal of Medicine* 332 (1995): 1113–1117.
25. M. L. Hediger and coauthors, Rate and amount of weight gain during adolescent pregnancy: Associations with maternal weight-for-height and birth weight, *American Journal of Clinical Nutrition* 52 (1990): 793–799.
26. Committee on Nutritional Status during Pregnancy and Lactation, 1990, pp. 1–23; J. M. Rees and coauthors, Weight gain in adolescents during pregnancy: Rate related to birth-weight outcome, *American Journal of Clinical Nutrition* 56 (1992): 868–873.
27. Position of The American Dietetic Association: Nutrition care for pregnant adolescents, *Journal of the American Dietetic Association* 94 (1994): 449–450.
28. F. G. Cunningham and K. J. Leveno, Childbearing among older women—The message is cautiously optimistic, *New England Journal of Medicine* 333 (1995): 1002–1004.
29. R. C. Fretts and coauthors, Increased maternal age and the risk of fetal death, *New England Journal of Medicine* 333 (1995): 953–957.
30. Committee on Substance Abuse and Committee on Children with Disabilities, American Academy of Pediatrics, Fetal alcohol syndrome and fetal alcohol effects, *Pediatrics* 91 (1993): 1004–1006; J. O. Beattie, Alcohol exposure and the fetus, *European Journal of Clinical Nutrition* 46 (1992): S7–S17.
31. H. L. Spohr, J. Willms, and H. C. Steinhausen, Prenatal alcohol exposure and long-term developmental consequences, *Lancet* 341 (1993): 907–910.
32. Update: Trends in fetal alcohol syndrome—United States, 1979–1993, *Morbidity and Mortality Weekly Report* 44 (1995): 249–251.
33. J. M. Aase, K. L. Jones, and S. K. Clarren, Do we need the term "FAE"? *Pediatrics* 95 (1995): 428–430.
34. Committee on Nutritional Status during Pregnancy and Lactation, *Nutrition during Pregnancy* (Washington, D.C.: National Academy Press, 1990), pp. 390–411.
35. Committee on Substance Abuse and Committee on Children with Disabilities, 1993; *The Surgeon General's Report on Nutrition and Health* (Washington, D.C.: Government Printing Office, 1988), p. 72.
36. When dad drinks: Can his liquor intake impair his future offspring? *Scientific American*, February 1990, p. 23; L. F. Soyka and J. M. Joffe, Male mediated drug effects on offspring, *Progress in Clinical and Biological Research* 36 (1980): 49–66.
37. R. E. Little and C. F. Sing, Father's drinking and infant birth weight: Report of an association, *Teratology* 36 (1987): 59–65.
38. I. J. Chasnoff and coauthors, The prevalence of illicit-drug or alcohol use during pregnancy and discrepancies in mandatory

reporting in Pinellas County, Florida, *New England Journal of Medicine* 322 (1990): 1202–1206.
39. D. B. Petitti and C. Coleman, Cocaine and the risk of low birth weight, *American Journal of Public Health* 80 (1990): 25–28; S. Parker and coauthors, Jitteriness in full-term neonates: Prevalence and correlates, *Pediatrics* 85 (1990): 17–23; M. van de Bor, F. J. Walther, and M. Ebrahimi, Decreased cardiac output in infants of mothers who abused cocaine, *Pediatrics* 85 (1990): 30–32; B. Zuckerman and coauthors, Effects of maternal marijuana and cocaine use on fetal growth, *New England Journal of Medicine* 320 (1989): 762–768.
40. W. T. Weathers and coauthors, Cocaine use in women from a defined population: Prevalence at delivery and effects on growth in infants, *Pediatrics* 91 (1993): 350–354.
41. S. D. Azuma and I. J. Chasnoff, Outcome of children prenatally exposed to cocaine and other drugs: A path analysis of three-year data, *Pediatrics* 92 (1993): 396–402; M. J. Corwin and coauthors, Effects of in utero cocaine exposure on newborn acoustical cry characteristics, *Pediatrics* 89 (1992): 1199–1203; L. N. Eisen and coauthors, Perinatal cocaine effects on neonatal stress behavior and performance on the Brazelton Scale, *Pediatrics* 88 (1991): 477–480; M. Mirochnick and coauthors, Circulating catecholamine concentrations in cocaine-exposed neonates: A pilot study, *Pediatrics* 88 (1991): 481–485.
42. Corwin and coauthors, 1992; L. C. Mayes and coauthors, Neurobehavioral profiles of neonates exposed to cocaine prenatally, *Pediatrics* 91 (1993): 778–783.
43. F. M. Haste and coauthors, Nutrient intakes during pregnancy: Observations on the influence of smoking and social class, *American Journal of Clinical Nutrition* 51 (1990): 29–36.
44. H. S. Klonoff-Cohen and coauthors, The effect of passive smoking and tobacco exposure through breast milk on sudden infant death syndrome, *Journal of the American Medical Association* 273 (1995): 795–798; E. A. Mitchell and coauthors, Smoking and the sudden infant death syndrome, *Pediatrics* 91 (1993): 893–896; K. C. Schoendorf and J. L. Kiely, Relationship of sudden infant death syndrome to maternal smoking during and after pregnancy, *Pediatrics* 90 (1992): 905–908; M. G. Bulterys, S. Greenland, and J. F. Kraus, Chronic fetal hypoxia and sudden infant death syndrome: Interaction between maternal smoking and low hematocrit during pregnancy, *Pediatrics* 86 (1990): 535–540; B. Haglund and S. Cnattingius, Cigarette smoking as a risk factor for sudden infant death syndrome: A population-based study, *American Journal of Public Health* 80 (1990): 29–32.
45. D. L. Olds, C. R. Henderson, Jr., and R. Tatelbaum, Intellectual impairment in children of women who smoke cigarettes during pregnancy, *Pediatrics* 93 (1994): 221–227; D. M. Fergusson, L. J. Horwood, and M. T. Lynskey, Maternal smoking before and after pregnancy: Effects on behavioral outcomes in middle childhood, *Pediatrics* 92 (1993): 815–822.
46. M. Lewis and coauthors, Prenatal exposure to heavy metals: Effect on childhood cognitive skills and health status, *Pediatrics* 89 (1992): 1010–1015.
47. Lewis and coauthors, 1992; M. W. Shannon and J. W. Graef, Lead intoxication in infancy, *Pediatrics* 89 (1992): 87–90.
48. Committee on Nutritional Status during Pregnancy and Lactation, 1990, pp. 397–399.
49. Position of The American Dietetic Association: Use of nutritive and nonnutritive sweeteners, *Journal of the American Dietetic Association* 93 (1993): 816–821.
50. G. L. Freed, J. K. Fraley, and R. J. Schanler, Attitudes of expectant fathers regarding breast-feeding, *Pediatrics* 90 (1992): 224–227.
51. K. G. Dewey and coauthors, Maternal versus infant factors related to breast milk intake and residual milk volume: The DARLING Study, *Pediatrics* 87 (1991): 829–837; Committee on Nutrition Status during Pregnancy and Lactation, *Nutrition during Lactation* (Washington, D.C.: National Academy Press, 1991), pp. 1–19.
52. M. A. Guillermo-Tuazon and coauthors, Energy intake, energy expenditure, and body composition of poor rural Philippine women throughout the first 6 mo of lactation, *American Journal of Clinical Nutrition* 56 (1992): 874–880; C. Frigerio and coauthors, A new procedure to assess the energy requirements of lactation in Gambian women, *American Journal of Clinical Nutrition* 54 (1991): 526–533; J. M. A. van Raaij and coauthors, Energy cost of lactation, and energy balances of well-nourished Dutch lactating women: Reappraisal of the extra energy requirements of lactation, *American Journal of Clinical Nutrition* 53 (1991): 612–619.
53. S. Potter and coauthors, Does infant feeding method influence maternal postpartum weight loss? *Journal of the American Dietetic Association* 91 (1991): 441–446.
54. F. M. Kramer and coauthors, Breast-feeding reduces maternal lower-body fat, *Journal of the American Dietetic Association* 93 (1993): 429–433.
55. K. G. Dewey, M. J. Heinig, and L. A. Nommsen, Maternal weight-loss patterns during prolonged lactation, *American Journal of Clinical Nutrition* 58 (1993): 162–166.
56. Committee on Nutritional Status during Pregnancy and Lactation, 1991, pp. 1–19.
57. Potter and coauthors, 1991.
58. Dewey and McCrory, 1994; K. G. Dewey and coauthors, A randomized study of the effects of aerobic exercise by lactating women on breast-milk volume and composition, *New England Journal of Medicine* 330 (1994): 449–453.
59. Dewey and coauthors, 1994; C. A. Lovelady, B. Lonnerdal, and K. G. Dewey, Lactation performance of exercising women, *American Journal of Clinical Nutrition* 52 (1990): 103–109.
60. J. P. Wallace, G. Inbar, and K. Ernsthausen, Infant acceptance of postexercise breast milk, *Pediatrics* 89 (1992): 1245–1247.
61. Committee on Nutritional Status during Pregnancy and Lactation, 1991, p. 140.
62. Committee on Nutritional Status during Pregnancy and Lactation, 1991, p. 140.

63. L. B. Dusdieker and coauthors, Prolonged maternal fluid supplementation in breast-feeding, *Pediatrics* 86 (1990): 737–740.
64. J. A. Mennella and G. K. Beauchamp, Maternal diet alters the sensory qualities of human milk and the behavior of the nursing infant, *Pediatrics* 88 (1991): 737–747.
65. J. A. Mennella and G. K. Beauchamp, The transfer of alcohol to human milk: Effects on flavor and the infant's behavior, *New England Journal of Medicine* 325 (1991): 981–985.
66. F. Vio, G. Salazar, and C. Infante, Smoking during pregnancy and lactation and its effects on breast-milk volume, *American Journal of Clinical Nutrition* 54 (1991): 1011–1016.
67. Klonoff-Cohen and coauthors, 1995.
68. R. F. Black, Transmission of HIV-1 in the breast-feeding process, *Journal of the American Dietetic Association* 96 (1996): 267–274.
69. A. M. Ferris and E. A. Reece, Nutritional consequences of chronic maternal conditions during pregnancy and lactation: Lupus and diabetes, *American Journal of Clinical Nutrition* (supplement) 59 (1994): 465S–473S; A. M. Ferris and coauthors, Perinatal lactation protocol and outcome in mothers with and without insulin-dependent diabetes mellitus, *American Journal of Clinical Nutrition* 58 (1993): 43–48.
70. C. M. van Beusekom and coauthors, Milk of patients with tightly controlled insulin-dependent diabetes mellitus has normal macronutrient and fatty acid composition, *American Journal of Clinical Nutrition* 57 (1993): 938–943.
71. American Academy of Pediatrics, Committee on Drugs, The transfer of drugs and other chemicals into human milk, *Pediatrics* 93 (1994): 137–150.
72. American Academy of Pediatrics, Committee on Drugs, Transfer of drugs and other chemicals into human milk, *Pediatrics* 84 (1989): 924–936.
73. E. Dewailly and coauthors, Inuit exposure to organochlorines through the aquatic food chain in Arctic Québec, *Environmental Health Perspectives* 101 (1993): 618–620.

Highlight 18

Hunger and Global Environmental Problems

In the early 1990s, one person in every ten worldwide was experiencing hunger—not the healthy hunger we all feel, which leads us to sit down and eat a hearty meal, but the chronic, painful hunger people feel when no food is available. Today, hundreds of millions of people are suffering from chronic hunger, both in the developing world and at home in the United States. Many are dying of starvation: tens of thousands each day, one every two seconds.[1] Many are children. Tragic scenes of people starving in drought- and flood-stricken areas are a familiar sight on television. Some of the causes (such as war) are obvious, but the environmental factors that often underlie these situations are less apparent.

This highlight examines hunger in the United States and around the world and discusses how environmental problems contribute to world hunger. Aside from the constant struggle to overcome the devastation wrought by civil unrest and wars, the ultimate solutions to the problem of world hunger involve both large- and small-scale choices made with an awareness of environmental consequences. The objective is to identify sustainable ways of doing things (the glossary below defines sustainable and other terms). Sustainable development permits economic growth without environmental destruction. Sustainable use consumes resources at a rate that nature, forestry, or agriculture can replace. Numerous examples of environmentally conscious choices related to food consumption are presented at the end of this highlight.

Glossary

cash crops: crops grown for cash, as opposed to crops grown for food; examples include cotton and tobacco.

food insecurity: intermittent hunger caused by lack of money or lack of control over other resources needed to assure a reliable food supply; the predominant form of hunger in the United States today.

Food Stamp Program: a federal food assistance program. The USDA issues food stamp coupons through state social services or welfare agencies to households—people who buy and prepare food together. The number of stamps a household receives depends on the household's size and income. Recipients may use the coupons like cash to purchase food and seeds, but not to buy tobacco, cleaning items, alcohol or other nonfood items.

fossil fuel: coal, oil, and natural gas; these are nonrenewable fuels that pollute. (Renewable or alternative fuels, such as solar and wind energy, pollute less or not at all.)

sustainable: able to continue indefinitely. Here, the term means the use of resources at such a rate that the earth can keep on replacing them—for example, cutting trees no faster than new ones grow and producing pollutants at a rate with which the environment and human cleanup efforts can keep pace, so that no net accumulation of pollution occurs.

HUNGER IN THE UNITED STATES

Much as it should surprise us, even in the United States, hunger is a problem. It is estimated that 30 million Americans, including 12 million children, cannot afford to buy enough food to maintain good health.[2] Soup kitchens are numerous and are needed as badly in some regions of the country as were the bread lines of the Great Depression in the 1930s. The prevalence of malnutrition and other health problems associated with chronic hunger—stunted growth, failure to thrive, low-birthweight babies, infant mortality, and anemia—is declining more slowly than in earlier decades; some problems are growing worse. Some studies show that one of every five children in the United States is chronically hungry; these children live in families that do not know where their next meal is coming from or when it will come.[3] Their hunger stems, not from the lack of available food, but from the lack of money with which to buy it.[4]

Who Are the Hungry in the United States?

Hunger is not always easy to recognize. The accompanying box shows

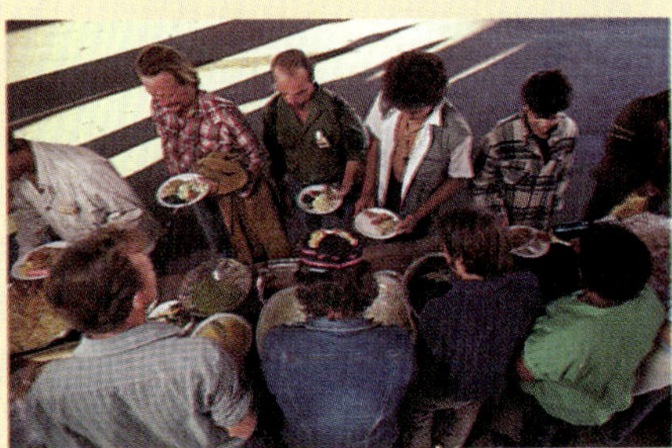

Feeding the hungry—in the United States.

How to Identify Food Insecurity in a U.S. Household

Questions like these are asked on surveys to determine the extent of food insecurity in a household. The more questions that receive a "Yes" answer, the more intense the hunger the household is experiencing.

- Do you usually have enough food to eat? If you don't have enough food to eat, is it because:
  - **a.** you sometimes run out of money to buy food?
  - **b.** you do not have transportation?
  - **c.** you do not have working appliances (stove, refrigerator)?
- Do you ever rely on nutritionally inferior foods to feed yourself or your children because you lack any of these resources?
- Do you ever eat less than you feel you should because you lack any of these resources?
- Do you ever skip meals or cut the size of meals because you lack any of these resources?
- Do you ever rely on neighbors, friends, relatives, or schools to feed any of your children because there is not enough food in the house?
- Do your children ever say they are hungry because there is not enough food in the house?
- Do you or any of your children ever go to bed hungry because there is not enough food in the house?

Sources: Adapted from C. A. Wehler, R. I. Scott, and J. J. Anderson, The Community Childhood Hunger Identification Project: A model of domestic hunger—demonstration project in Seattle, Washington, *Journal of Nutrition Education* (1 supplement) 24 (1992): 29S–35S; R. R. Briefel and C. E. Woteki, Development of food sufficiency questions for the Third National Health and Nutrition Examination Survey, *Journal of Nutrition Education* (1 supplement) 24 (1992): 24S–28S.

how national surveys identify "food insecurity" and hunger in the United States. Questions like these provide crude, but necessary, data to estimate the degree of hunger in this country.

Hunger has many causes, but a major one is poverty. Other causes that contribute to hunger are abuse of alcohol and other drugs; physical and mental illness; lack of awareness of available food assistance programs; and the reluctance of people, particularly the elderly, to accept what they perceive as "welfare" or "charity."[5] Still, poverty remains the major cause of hunger, and solving the poverty problem would do a lot to solve the hunger problem.

In the United States, poverty and hunger reach into all segments of society, affecting not only the chronic poor (migrant workers, the unskilled and unemployed, the homeless, and some elderly) but also the so-called new poor. Some are displaced farm families. Some are former blue-collar and white-collar workers forced out of their trades and professions into minimum-wage jobs. These people outnumber the chronic poor, and they are not on welfare; they have jobs, but the pay is low. Families with incomes below a certain level are simply unable to buy sufficient amounts of nourishing foods, even if they are wise food shoppers.

Assistance Programs Aimed at Hunger and Malnutrition

At present, many programs aimed at preventing or remediating domestic malnutrition and hunger are in effect in the United States. To what extent these federal programs will continue to feed those who are hungry is unknown, given the current political climate; many federal programs are being targeted in cost saving measures.

Several food assistance programs are described in other chapters: the school lunch, breakfast, and child care food programs for children; the WIC program for low-income pregnant women, mothers, and their young children; and food assistance

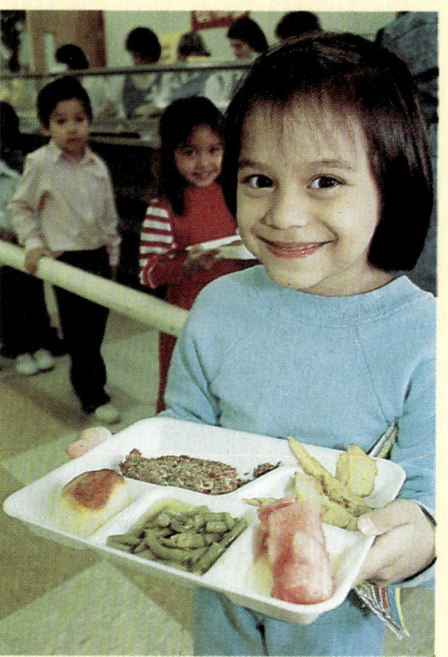

School lunches provide children with nourishment at little or no charge.

programs for older adults such as congregate meals and Meals on Wheels. Another program aimed directly at the poor is the Food Stamp Program, administered by the U.S. Department of Agriculture (USDA). The Food Stamp Program is the largest of the federal food assistance programs, both in amount of money spent and in number of people participating. Over 27 million people in the United States receive food stamps at a budget cost of over $22 billion per year.[6] Over 80 percent of food stamp recipients are families with children.[7]

These federal programs support both health and well-being. For example, children in Project Head Start, an educational program that includes breakfast, are twice as likely to graduate from high school and to become employed as their peers in the same circumstances who do not participate.[8]

Although these programs reach millions of people daily with life-sustaining foods, hunger continues to plague the United States. Of the estimated 2 million homeless people in the United States who are eligible for food assistance, only 15 percent of single adults and 50 percent of families receive food stamps.

To supplement federal programs and reach those who are still hungry, private efforts have sprung up in many communities, where concerned citizens work through local agencies and churches to feed the hungry. Community-based soup kitchens and shelters generally provide good-quality meals. The meals often average 1000 kcalories each, but most homeless people receive fewer than 1½ meals a day, so many are inadequately nourished.[9] Table H18–1 shows how individuals can assist in local hunger relief efforts; it presents a 14-step program for developing a hunger-free community.

WORLD HUNGER

In developing countries, which face more extreme hunger problems than the United States, the causes of hunger are more diverse. Again, the primary cause of hunger is poverty, but the poverty is more extreme. Most people would find it almost impossible to comprehend the

Table H18–1

Fourteen Ways Communities Can Address Their Hunger Problems

1. Establish a community-based emergency food delivery network.
2. Assess community hunger problems and evaluate community services. Create strategies for responding to unmet needs.
3. Establish a group of individuals, including low-income participants, to develop and implement policies and programs to combat hunger and the threat of hunger; monitor responsiveness of existing services; and address underlying causes of hunger.
4. Participate in federally assisted nutrition programs that are easily accessible to targeted populations.
5. Integrate public and private resources, including local businesses, to relieve hunger.
6. Establish an education program that addresses the food needs of the community and the need for increased local citizen participation in activities to alleviate hunger.
7. Provide information and referral services for accessing both public and private programs and services.
8. Support programs to provide transportation and assistance in food shopping, where needed.
9. Identify high-risk populations and target services to meet their needs.
10. Provide adequate transportation and distribution of food from all resources.
11. Coordinate food services with parks and recreation programs and other community-based outlets to which residents of the area have easy access.
12. Improve public transportation to human service agencies and food resources.
13. Establish nutrition education programs for low-income citizens to enhance their food purchasing and preparation skills and make them aware of the connections between diet and health.
14. Establish a program for collecting and distributing nutritious foods—either agricultural commodities in farmers' fields or prepared foods that would have been wasted.

Source: House Select Committee on Hunger, legislation introduced by Tony P. Hall, excerpted in *Seeds*, Sprouts edition, January 1992, p. 3 with permission, © SEEDS Magazine, P.O. Box 6170, Waco, TX 76706. For more guidance on developing a hunger-free community, write: Hunger Free, House Select Committee on Hunger, 505 Ford House Office Building, Washington, DC 20515.

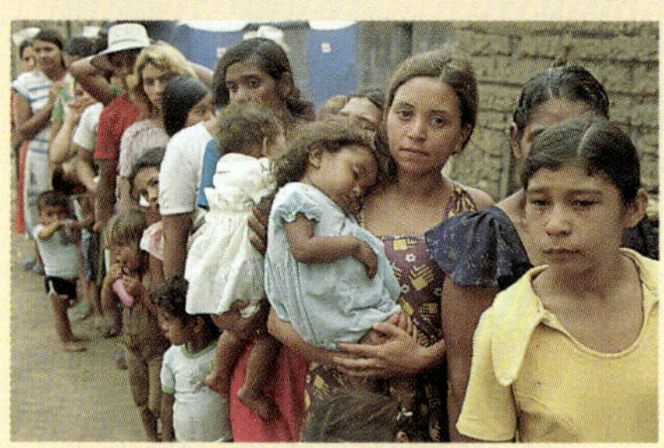
Feeding the hungry—in Nicaragua.

severity of poverty in the developing world. One-fifth of the world's 5 billion people have no land and no possessions *at all*. They survive on less than one dollar a day each, they lack water that is safe to drink, and they cannot read or write.[10] The average U.S. housecat eats twice as much protein every day as one of these people, and the cost of keeping that cat is greater than such a person's annual income.[11]

When we think of world hunger, most frequently we visualize the victims of famine. However, the natural causes of famine—drought, flood, and pests—have become less important in recent years than the social causes. Widespread hunger and starvation can occur even when food is available, if people have lost their ability to obtain that food. Thus a sudden increase in food prices, a drop in workers' incomes, or a change in government policy can create hunger for millions even in the absence of the more familiar obstacles of drought, flood, disease, or even war and civil unrest. Between 15 and 30 million people died during the Chinese famine of 1959 through 1961, the worst famine of this century; it was primarily a result of government policies associated with the "great leap forward," which devastated the Chinese agricultural system.[12]

In the 1990s, armed conflict has become the dominant cause of famine worldwide. In all of the countries that have reported famine so far in the 1990s—Angola, Ethiopia, Liberia, Mozambique, Somalia, and Sudan—armed conflict has been a major cause. Not only do armed conflicts create famines, but they often are the key obstacle preventing famine relief by destroying or blocking food supplies from getting to those in need. The world continues to struggle to find a middle ground between respecting the sovereignty of nations and refusing to allow any nation to prevent humanitarian assistance from reaching its people.

Although we usually associate world hunger with famine, the numbers affected by famine are relatively small compared with those suffering less acute forms of hunger. Nearly 800 million people in developing countries suffer from chronic malnutrition.[13] In addition, one child in six in the world is born underweight, and almost two in five children are underweight by the age of five. Around 2 billion people, mostly women and children, are deficient in one or more of these nutrients: iron, iodine, and vitamin A.[14]

Tens of thousands die each day as a result of malnutrition. Many are children afflicted by the diseases of poverty: parasitic and infectious diseases such as dysentery, whooping cough, measles, tuberculosis, cholera, and malaria. These diseases interact with poor nutrition in a vicious cycle that leads to death—at the rate of one every two seconds. Because of poverty, infection, and malnutrition, the life expectancy in some African countries averages 50 years; in Uganda it is only 38 years, half of the U.S. life expectancy.[15]

Until 1988, the world celebrated an increase nearly every year in its reserves of stored grain, an index of the sufficiency of the world food supply. The often-repeated statement that "We have enough food to feed everyone" was true. Efforts at relieving hunger focused on transporting food to where it was needed and on improving storage. Also, because in many developing countries most of the men were involved in producing cash crops for export, hunger-relief efforts focused on educating and empowering women to grow and use nutritious food to feed their families. These efforts were addressing the causes of the world's hunger problem and were expected to solve it.

Since 1988, however, the situation has changed. The world's population is growing at the rate of about 90 million persons each year, and food production is no longer keeping pace. In recent years, grain reserves have fallen to dangerously low levels (see Figure H18–1). Current grain reserves are estimated to be sufficient to feed the world for only 50 to 60 days.[16] Further growth in the world's food output is being slowed by environmental degradation.

Figure H18–1

World Grain Carryover Stocks, 1961–1995

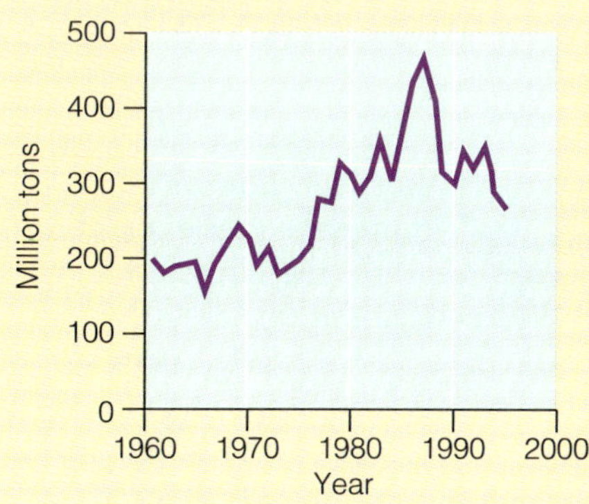

ENVIRONMENTAL DEGRADATION AND HUNGER

Today, environmental degradation is beginning to threaten the world's ability to produce enough food to feed its people. Not only are we losing our resources, but we are losing our ability to compensate for the losses.

Environmental Problems and Food Production

One element of environmental degradation is soil erosion, which is occurring in every nation and is resulting in crop losses estimated at 6 percent per year.[17] Other environmental problems slowing food outputs are deforestation, air pollution, climate change, water scarcity, deterioration of rangelands, and declining fisheries.

Deforestation Deforestation along the watersheds of the Blue Nile led to erosion and during just nine years laid down so much silt behind the Roseires Reservoir dam in Sudan, which supplies irrigation water for the dry season, that one-third of its capacity was lost.[18] In Sierra Leone, where 60 percent of the land was primarily rainforest in 1961, only 6 percent is now.[19] For the world as a whole, if present rates continue, by 2010 per capita forested area will have dropped 30 percent.[20]

Air Pollution Damage to crops from air pollution is now measurable in the car-centered societies of Western Europe, the United States, and Canada and in societies that burn coal to generate electricity—notably, Eastern Europe and China. In the United States, according to a seven-year study by two government agencies, the most damaging air pollutants are ozone, sulfur dioxide, and nitrous oxide, which come from the burning of fossil fuels. Crops are especially sensitive to ground-level ozone concentrations, which increasingly are detected and measured in rural as well as urban areas in ranges that reduce crop yields. An estimate puts the increase in annual crop losses ascribable to ozone pollution at 1 percent per year.

Not only is ground-level ozone pollution reducing agricultural outputs, but outer-atmosphere ozone depletion is doing so, too—especially to radiation-sensitive crops such as soybeans. For each 1 percent loss of outer-atmosphere ozone, the amount of damaging ultraviolet radiation reaching the earth increases by 2 percent. Based on studies of experimental plots, soybean yields fall 1 percent for each 1 percent rise in radiation. Soybeans are the world's leading protein crop, and at last report, no one was monitoring radiation-induced losses.

Climate Change Crop yields may also be affected by climate change caused by increased atmospheric concentrations of heat-trapping, carbon dioxide, produced by fossil fuels. At whatever rate climate change is occurring, it is potentially disruptive. If summers become hotter, droughts during the growing season may become more common. An unusually hot and dry summer in 1988 pushed the U.S. grain harvest below consumption for the first time in history. In 1994, new heat records were set throughout the western United States, northern Europe, the Baltic, and Japan.[21] A rise of only a degree or so in average global temperature may reduce soil moisture, impair pollination of major food crops such as rice and corn, slow growth, weaken disease resistance, and disrupt many other factors affecting crop yields.

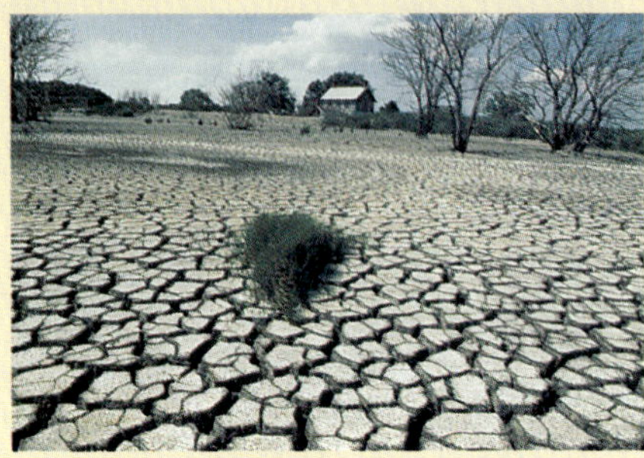
As groundwater is used up, deserts spread.

Water Scarcity Water supplies, too, are becoming limited. Decreases in available water result in reduced crop yields, most obviously on irrigated cropland. Two-thirds of all water taken from rivers and underground aquifers is used for irrigation.[22] Agricultural lands that require irrigation water play a disproportionate role in meeting the world's food needs. Although they account for only one-sixth of total cropland, irrigated croplands yield more than one-third of the total global harvest. The amount of irrigated land per capita, however, peaked in 1978 and has fallen almost 6 percent since then.[23]

Deteriorating Rangelands Grazing land is decreasing along with agricultural cropland. Grasslands for raising beef are already being fully used or misused on every continent. One-fifth of the world's land area is rangeland, twice as much area as is farmed. This land supports most of the world's 3.2 billion cattle, sheep, and goats.[24] Although world beef and mutton production per capita increased 37 percent between 1950 and 1972, more recent yields have dropped.[25] These decreases reflect deterioration in the condition of the rangelands due to environmental problems and extensive overgrazing. The feed needs of livestock in nearly all developing countries now exceed the capacity of their rangelands. In Africa, where this problem is most visible, the annual loss of rangeland productivity is estimated at $7 billion, more than the gross national product of Ethiopia and Uganda combined.[26]

Diminishing Fisheries The yield of fish from the oceans is also declining, for the first time in history, due to overfishing and pollution. Big fish, such as tuna, swordfish, and shark, are becoming threatened because they are being overfished. Atlantic stocks of the heavily fished bluefin tuna have dropped by 94 percent.[27] Cod are rapidly disappearing off the New England coast and are almost gone farther north.

Inland fisheries have also suffered tremendous drops in yield as a result of environmental damage. The Aral Sea, located between Kazakhstan and Uzbekistan, yielded 40,000 tons of fish per year in 1960 and today is biologically dead. As water was diverted for irrigation over the last 30 years, the sea became increasingly salty until finally fish could no longer live in it.[28] Acidification has also taken a toll on inland fisheries. In Canada, 14,000 lakes are considered biologically dead as a result of acid rain.[29]

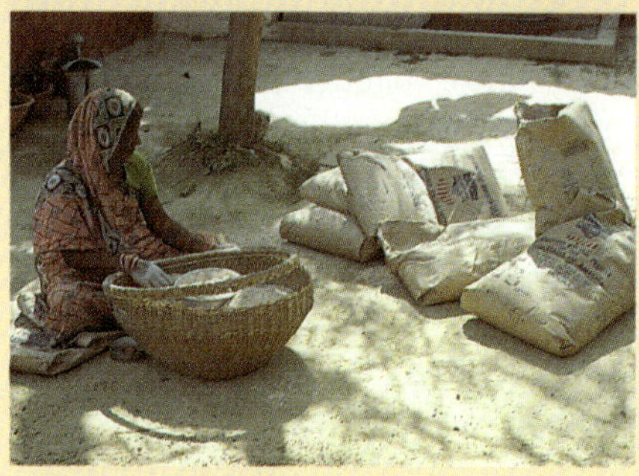

International efforts help to relieve hunger and poverty around the world.

Limitations in Food Production

All in all, then, environmental problems are reducing the world's ability to feed its people. With fish yields and rangelands decreasing, can advances in agriculture compensate for the losses caused by environmental degradation? Historically, agriculture has improved yields by making greater investments in irrigation, fertilizer, and improved genetic strains. Today, however, the contributions these measures can make are reaching limits for the first time in history: the improvements are leveling off. Irrigation can no longer compensate by improving crop yields because almost all the land that can benefit from irrigation is already receiving it. In fact, rising concentrations of salt in the soil—a by-product of irrigation—are *lowering* yields on close to a quarter of the world's irrigated cropland. Nor can fertilizer use enhance agricultural production much. Much of the fertilizing that can be done is being done—and with great effect; fertilizer use supports some 40 percent of the world's total crop yields. Adding more fertilizer, however, brings no further rise in yield. As for the development of high-yielding strains of crops, some advances have been dramatic, but they show little potential to change the overall trends described here. Furthermore, the raw materials necessary for developing new crops are becoming less and less available as genetic variety is lost due to the extinction of many plant species. Of the 5000 food plants used throughout the world a few centuries ago, only 150 are grown in modern agriculture today. Most of the world's population relies on only five cereals, three legumes, and three root crops to meet their energy needs. Even among these, valuable strains are vanishing.[30]

Estimates are that the world grain harvest can be increased by no more than 1 percent a year. The increase might be higher, but for the many forms of environmental degradation described earlier. Meanwhile, the world's population is rising at the rate of at least 2 percent per year.[31] Many authorities in many fields—and more every year—are calling for a reduction in the growth rate of the world's population as the only way to enable the world's food output to keep pace with people's growing numbers.

The world still produces enough food to feed all its people, and the problem of hunger today remains a problem of unequal distribution of resources. If present trends continue, however, the time is approaching when there will be an absolute deficit of food. This conclusion seems inescapable. The world's increasing population threatens the world's capacity to produce adequate food. Population control has become one of the most pressing needs of this time in history. Until the nations of the world resolve the population problem, they can neither support the lives of people already born nor remedy global trends toward environmental deterioration. And to resolve the population problem, a necessary first step is to remedy the poverty problems, for reasons discussed next. Of the 90 million people being added to the population each year, the vast majority are in the most poverty-stricken areas of the world.

POVERTY AND OVERPOPULATION

Population growth is one of many factors contributing to poverty and hunger. The reverse is also true: poverty and hunger contribute to population growth.

Population Growth Leads to Hunger and Poverty The first of these cause-effect relationships is easy to understand. Population growth contributes to poverty and hunger, for the more mouths there are to feed, the worse poverty and hunger become. The sheer magnitude of our annual population increase of 90 million people is difficult to comprehend. Each month the world adds the equivalent of another New York City.[32] During six months of the terrible 1992 famine in Somalia, an estimated 300,000 people starved to death. Yet it took the world only 29 *hours* to replace their numbers! Ninety million people a year, spread over 365 days, comes to a quarter-million people a day—or just over 10,000 people born every hour.[33]

Population growth also contributes to hunger indirectly by preempting good agricultural land for growing cities and industry and forcing people onto marginal land, where they cannot produce sufficient food for themselves. The world's poorest people live in the world's most damaged and inhospitable environments. There they experience, daily, tens of thousands of early deaths from malnutrition and disease.

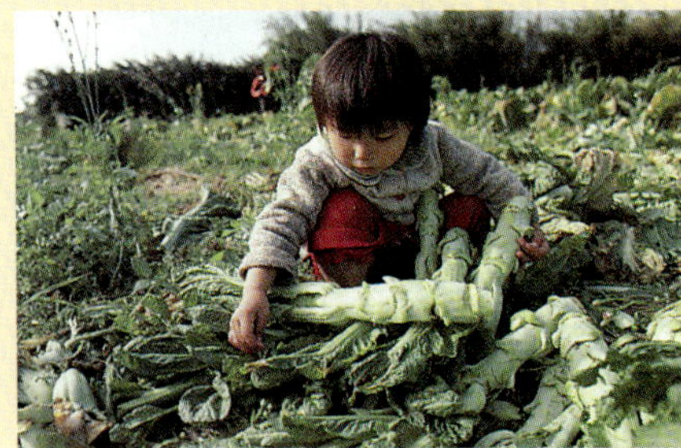

Families in developing countries depend on their children to help provide for daily needs.

Hunger and Poverty Lead to Population Growth Overpopulation, then, together with the environmental degradation that it causes, worsens poverty. How, though, does poverty lead to overpopulation? Poverty and hunger are believed to exert an ironic effect on people, making them bear more children. Poverty and hunger typically go hand in hand with ignorance, including ignorance of how to control family size. Also, a family depends on its children to farm the land, haul water, and care for adults in their old age. If a family faces ongoing poverty with its associated high rates of childhood disease and mortality, the parents will choose to have many children to ensure that some will survive to adulthood. People are willing to risk having fewer children only if they are sure that their children will live.

Relieving poverty and hunger, then, may be a necessary first step in curbing population growth. When people attain better access to health care, education, and family planning, the death rate falls. At first there is a "bulge" in the population, because births outnumber deaths, but as the standard of living continues to improve, families become willing to risk having fewer children. Then the birth rate falls. Thus, after a short but necessary lag time, improvements in economic status help stabilize the population.

The link between improved economic status and slowed population growth has been demonstrated in country after country.[34] Sustainable development is central to this success and must include not only economic growth, but a sharing of resources among all groups. In parts of Sri Lanka, Taiwan, Malaysia, and Costa Rica, where this has happened, population growth has slowed the most. Where economic growth has occurred but only the rich have grown richer, population growth has remained high. Examples include Brazil, Mexico, the Philippines, and Thailand, where large families continue to be a major economic asset for the poor.

SOLUTIONS

Both the poor and the rich nations must contribute to solving the world's hunger, environmental, and poverty problems, but in different ways. The poor nations need to gain control of their rampaging population growth and to slow and reverse the destruction of their environmental resources: forests, waterways, and soil. To do this, they must, among other things, find ways to relieve their people's poverty. The rich nations need to stem their wasteful and polluting uses of resources and energy, which are contributing to global environmental degradation. They also must become willing to help relieve the debtor nations of their poverty in ways that effectively reach the poor.

Sustainable Development Worldwide

Many nations now recognize that improving all nations' economies is a prerequisite to meeting the world's other urgent needs: relief of hunger, population stabilization, arrest of environmental degradation, and sustainable treatment of resources. An important step was taken when a

United Nations convention on the Rights of the Child was ratified by over 100 nations. Significantly, for the first time in world history, the convention cited *nutrition* as an internationally recognized human right.[35]

Another important step was taken in 1992, when more than 100 nations met for the Earth Summit in Rio de Janeiro, Brazil, and discussed the relationship of the environment to poverty and hunger.* At this meeting, many nations agreed for the first time to 27 principles of sustainable development, which the conferees defined as development that would equitably meet both the economic and the environmental needs of present and future generations.

Participants discussed climate change and the possibility of setting legally binding targets and timetables for every nation to cut its emissions of global-warming gases. They began to approach agreement on this issue. They also signed agreements to protect the earth's remaining species of plants and animals and to preserve the world's forests.

The Earth Summit's discussions opened vistas of hope. Much remains to be done, and all nations have major parts to play. For our part, in the United States, the challenges are many. Can we reduce our consumption of fossil fuel and thereby our disproportionate contribution to global environmental degradation? The willingness of U.S. consumers to take responsibility for their individual shares in solving global problems could make a substantial contribution to the quality of life for future generations. Our decision to use fewer goods, devour fewer resources, create less pollution, and consume less energy would go a long way toward remedying global environmental problems and conditions that contribute to world hunger. In addition, the United States can help directly by supporting international moves to relieve poverty and environmental degradation worldwide. The following steps have been recommended:

- First, the developing countries need to be relieved of the gigantic interest payments they have been making to U.S. and international banks.
- Second, the debt relief needs to reach those within the countries who need it, and not just the wealthy.
- Third, rather than emphasizing *technology*-intensive methods of *harvesting* their resources, developing countries might shift toward *labor*-intensive means of *maintaining* their resources.
- Fourth, to account for the great value of environmental resources, soil, water, and trees should be counted in economic balance sheets.

The United States can exert international leadership by adopting these strategies and encouraging other developed nations to support similar measures. The idea behind all these measures is that relieving poverty will help relieve environmental degradation and hunger. To rephrase a well-known adage: If you give a man a fish, he will eat for a day. If you teach him to fish and enable him to buy and maintain his own gear and bait, he will eat for a lifetime and help to feed others. Unlike food giveaways and money doles, which are only stop-gap measures, social programs that will permanently better the lot of the poor can permanently solve the hunger problem.

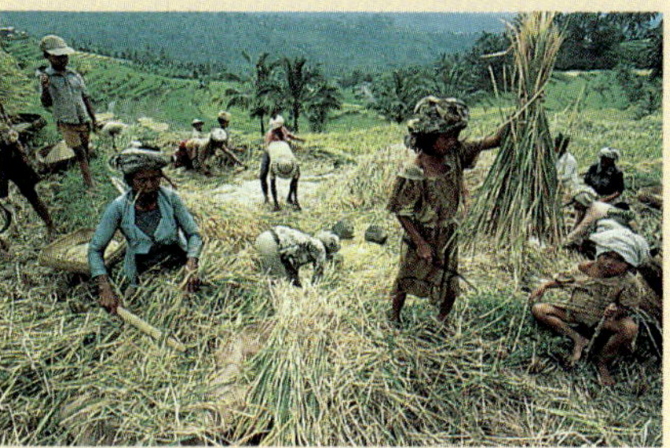

Labor-intensive technology is most often the appropriate technology in developing countries.

Activism and Simpler Lifestyles at Home

Every segment of our society can have a place in the fight against hunger, poverty, and environmental degradation. The federal government, the states, local communities, big business and small companies, educators, and all individuals, including dietitians and foodservice managers, have many opportunities to forward the effort.

Government Action Government policies can change to promote sustainability. For example, the government can stop using tax money to pay for the wasteful use of fossil fuels and of fertilizers and pesticides made from them. Instead, it can pay for energy conservation services and crop protection. Tax laws could be revised to reward energy conservation efforts, which would have a major impact on the research and development of conservation industries and sustainable agriculture. All of these actions are possible, but they depend on the support of elected officials. Keep in

*The formal name of the summit was the United Nations Conference on Environment and Development: UNCED, for short.

mind that you can affect the direction of such government actions by voting and writing letters that express your views on hunger, poverty, and environmental degradation.

Business Involvement Businesses can take initiative to help; some already have. Several large corporations are currently major supporters of antihunger programs. Many grocery stores and restaurants give their out-of-date and leftover food to hunger organizations such as Third Harvest, which then distribute the food where needed in the community.

Education Educators, including nutrition educators, can teach others about the underlying social and political causes of poverty, the root cause of hunger. At the college level, they can teach the relationship between hunger and population, hunger and environmental degradation, hunger and the status of women, and hunger and the global debt crisis. They can advocate legislation to address these problems. They can teach the poor to develop and run nutrition programs in their own communities and to fight on their own behalf for antipoverty, antihunger legislation.

Foodservice Efforts Dietitians and foodservice managers have a special role to play. Their professional organization, the American Dietetic Association (ADA), is urging them to promote the saving of resources by reuse, recycling (including composting), energy conservation, and water conservation, in both their professional and their personal lives. In addition, the ADA urges its members to work for policy changes in private and government food assistance programs, to intensify education about hunger, and to be advocates on the local, state, and national levels to help end hunger in the United States.[36]

Other Opportunities Individuals can support organizations that lobby for the needed economic policy changes toward developing countries. They can join and work for international hunger relief organizations. Appendix F includes some of the major ones.

Most importantly, at every level, individuals can try to make lifestyle choices that consider the environmental consequences. Several possible choices relating to typical U.S. foodways are presented in Table H18–2. These suggested lifestyles changes can easily be extended from food to other areas. All aspects of our lifestyles relate to global problems. Recommendations include personal actions: reduce, reuse, recycle, and cut energy use. Admittedly, these approaches to solving today's global problems seem simplistic, but because we number 5 billion plus, individual actions can add up to exert an immense impact. The problems are complex, they are not fully understood, and high-level scientific research is needed to solve them. But even as that research is being done and the world's best minds are translating the results into recommended actions, individuals can be doing what they already know how to do. As Margaret Mead said, "Never doubt that a small group of thoughtful, committed people can change the world. Indeed, it is the only thing that ever has."

Emphasis on personal lifestyle choices is important because it raises awareness and paves the way for larger actions. Individual choices are, however, only part of the solution to today's problems. Institutional changes are the other part—changes in the way agriculture, industry, and governments do their business domestically and internationally. Students can become involved in promoting both kinds of change: make personal lifestyle changes and then vote for government changes.

"Be part of the solution, not part of the problem," an adage says. In other words, don't waste time or energy moaning and groaning about how tough things are; do something to improve them. This adage is as applicable to today's global environmental problems as it is to an unwashed dish in the kitchen sink. They are our problems: human beings created them, and human beings must solve them.

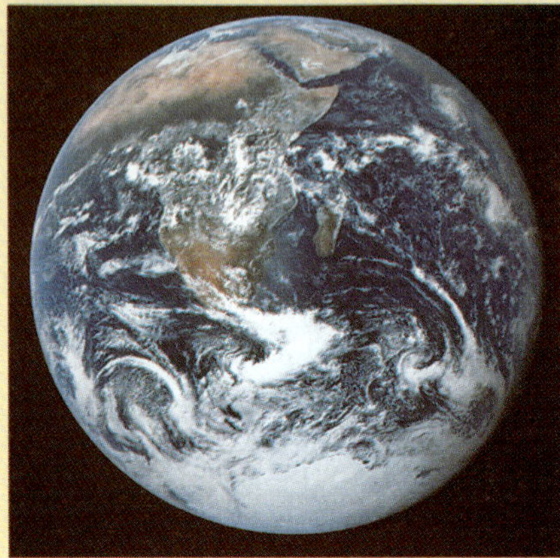
Good planets are hard to find.

NOTES

1. L. N. Burby, *World Hunger* (San Diego, Calif.: Lucent Books, 1995), pp. 13–16; P. L. Kutzner, *World Hunger: A Reference Handbook* (Santa Barbara, Calif.: ABC–CL10, 1991) pp. 158–159.

2. *Tallahassee Democrat,* October 14, 1994; P. Univ, The state of world hunger, *Nutrition Reviews* 52 (1994): 151–161.

Table H18–2

Environmentally Conscious Foodways

Food production taxes environmental resources and causes pollution. Consumers can make environmentally conscious choices at every step from food shopping to cooking and use of kitchen appliances to serving, cleanup, and waste disposal.

Food Shopping

Transportation:
- Whenever possible, walk or ride a bicycle; use car pools and mass transit.
- Shop only once a week, share trips, or take turns shopping for each other.
- When buying a car, choose an energy-efficient one.

Food choices:
- Eat low on the food chain; that is, eat plants, rather than animals that eat plants (this suggestion complements the Food Guide Pyramid recommendations for eating for good health).
- Avoid buying canned beef products (many of these foods come at the expense of cleared rainforest land).
- Eat small portions of meat; select range-fed beef, buffalo, poultry, and fish.
- Select local foods (they are transported shorter distances and less fuel is required to pack them, label them, and keep them cold if they are fresh).

Food packages:
- Whenever possible, select foods with no packages; next best are minimal, reusable, or recyclable ones.
- Buy juices and sodas in large glass or recyclable plastic bottles (not small individual cans or cartons); grains in bulk (not separate little packages); and eggs in pressed fiber cartons (not foam, unless it is recycled locally).
- Carry reusable shopping bags; alternatively, ask for plastic bags if they are recyclable.

Cooking Food

- Cook foods quickly in a pressure cooker or microwave oven.
- When using the oven, bake a lot of food at one time and keep the door closed tightly.
- Refuse throwaway utensils.
- Avoid spray products.

Kitchen Appliances

- Do without small electrical appliances such as can openers, mixers, knife sharpeners, and food processors.
- When buying a refrigerator, choose an energy-efficient one.
- Consider the possibility of using solar energy to meet home electrical needs.
- Set the water heater at 130°F (54°C), no hotter; put it on a timer; wrap it and the hot-water pipes in insulation; install water-saving faucets.

Food Serving, Dish Washing, and Waste Disposal

- Use "real" plates, cups, and glasses instead of disposable ones.
- Use cloth towels and napkins, reusable storage containers with lids, and dishcloths instead of paper towels, plastic wrap, plastic storage bags, and sponges.
- Run the dishwasher only when it is full.
- Recycle all glass, plastic, and aluminum.
- Compost all vegetable scraps, fruit peelings, and leftover plant foods.

3. *Fact Sheet on Childhood Hunger and Poverty*, (c. 1992), available from Bread for the World, 802 Rhode Island Avenue NE, Washington, DC 20018.

4. S. Lewis, Food security, environment, poverty, and the world's children, *Journal of Nutrition Education* (1 supplement) 24 (1992): 3S–5S.

5. L. D. McBean, ed., with D. Derelian, R. J. Fersh, and L. Parker, Hunger and undernutrition in America, *Dairy Council Digest*, March/April 1992.

6. U.S. Department of Commerce, *Statistical Abstract of the United States, 1994* (Washington, D.C.: Bureau of the Census, 1994), p. 386.

7. Food Research and Action Center, *Community Childhood Hunger Identification Project: A Survey of Childhood Hunger in the United States*, Executive Summary (Washington, D.C.: Food Research and Action Center, March 1991), as cited in McBean, 1992.

8. *Fact Sheet on Childhood Hunger and Poverty*, c. 1992.

9. J. C. Wolgemuth and coauthors, Wasting malnutrition and inadequate nutrient intakes identified in a multiethnic homeless population, *Journal of the American Dietetic Association* 92 (1992): 834–839; M. A. Drake, The nutritional status and dietary adequacy of single homeless women and their children in shelters, *Public Health Reports* 107 (1992): 312–319; B. E. Cohen, N. Chapman, and M. R. Burt, Food sources and intake of homeless persons, *Journal of Nutrition Education* (1 supplement) 24 (1992): 45S–51S.

10. World Bank, *World Development Report 1991* (New York: Oxford University Press, 1991); S. Postel, Denial in the decisive decade, in L. R. Brown and coauthors, *State of the World 1992* (New York: W. W. Norton, 1992), pp. 3–8.

11. L. Timberlake, *Only One Earth*, cited in Food for thought, *Seeds*, Sprouts edition, 1988.

12. R. W. Kates, Ending deaths from famine: The opportunity in Somalia, *New England Journal of Medicine* 328 (1993): 1055–1057.

13. *Tallahassee Democrat*, October 14, 1994.

14. Kates, 1993.

15. U.S. Department of Commerce, 1994, pp. 854–855.

16. L. R. Brown and coauthors, *State of the World 1995* (New York: W. W. Norton, 1995), p. 11; *Tallahassee Democrat*, June 10, 1995.

17. L. R. Brown and J. E. Young, Feeding the world in the nineties, in L. R. Brown, *State of the World 1990* (New York: W. W. Norton, 1990).

18. J. W. Clay and coauthors, *The Spoils of Famine: Ethiopian Famine Policy and Peasant*

Agriculture (Cambridge, Mass.: Cultural Survival, 1988), as cited in L. R. Brown and H. Kane, *Full House* (New York: W. W. Norton, 1994), pp. 146–157.

19. R. D. Kaplan, The coming anarchy, *Atlantic Monthly*, February 1994, pp. 44–76.
20. L. R. Brown and coauthors, *State of the World, 1994* (New York: W. W. Norton, 1994), p. 202.
21. Brown and coauthors, 1995, p. 191.
22. Brown and coauthors, 1995, p. 192.
23. Brown and coauthors, 1994, p. 201.
24. FAO, *FAO Production Yearbook 1992* (Rome: 1993); FAO, *FAO Production Yearbook 1991* (Rome: 1992); FAO, *1948–1985 World Crop and Livestock Statistics* (Rome: 1987), as cited in L. R. Brown and H. Kane, *Full House* (New York: W. W. Norton, 1994), pp. 89–95.
25. U.S. Department of Agriculture (USDA), *Dairy, Livestock, and Poultry: World Livestock Situation* (Washington, D.C.: October 1993), as cited in L. R. Brown and H. Kane, *Full House* (New York: W. W. Norton, 1994), pp. 89–95.
26. H. Dregne and coauthors, A new assessment of the world status of desertification, *Desertification Control Bulletin* 20 (1991), as cited in L. R. Brown and H. Kane, *Full House* (New York: W. W. Norton, 1994), pp. 89–95.
27. FAO, cited in World Resources Institute (WRI), *World Resources 1992–93* (New York: Oxford University Press, 1992); bluefin tuna figure from D. Meadows and coauthors, *Beyond the Limits* (Post Mills, Vt.: Chelsea Green Publishing Company, 1992), as cited in L. R. Brown and H. Kane, *Full House* (New York: W. W. Norton, 1994), pp. 75–88.
28. L. Brown, The Aral Sea: going, going . . ., *World Watch*, January/February 1991.
29. Government of Canada, *The State of Canada's Environment* (Ottawa: 1991).
30. K. Dixit, The shrinking pool, *New Internationalist*, March 1991, p. 20.
31. Brown and Young, 1990, pp. 64–65.
32. Population Reference Bureau (PRB), *1993 World Population Data Sheet* (Washington, D.C.: 1993), as cited in L. R. Brown and H. Kane, *Full House* (New York: W. W. Norton, 1994), pp. 49–61.
33. Centers for Disease Control, Population based mortality assessment: Baidoa and Afgoi, Somalia, 1992, *Journal of the American Medical Association* (1993), as cited in L. R. Brown and H. Kane, *Full House* (New York: W. W. Norton, 1994), pp. 49–61.
34. P. S. Dasgupta, Population, poverty and the local environment, *Scientific American*, February 1995, pp. 40–45.
35. Lewis, 1992.
36. Position of The American Dietetic Association: Environmental issues, *Journal of the American Dietetic Association* 93 (1993): 589–591; Position of The American Dietetic Association: Domestic hunger and inadequate access to food, *Journal of the American Dietetic Association* 90 (1990): 1437–1441.

Chapter 19

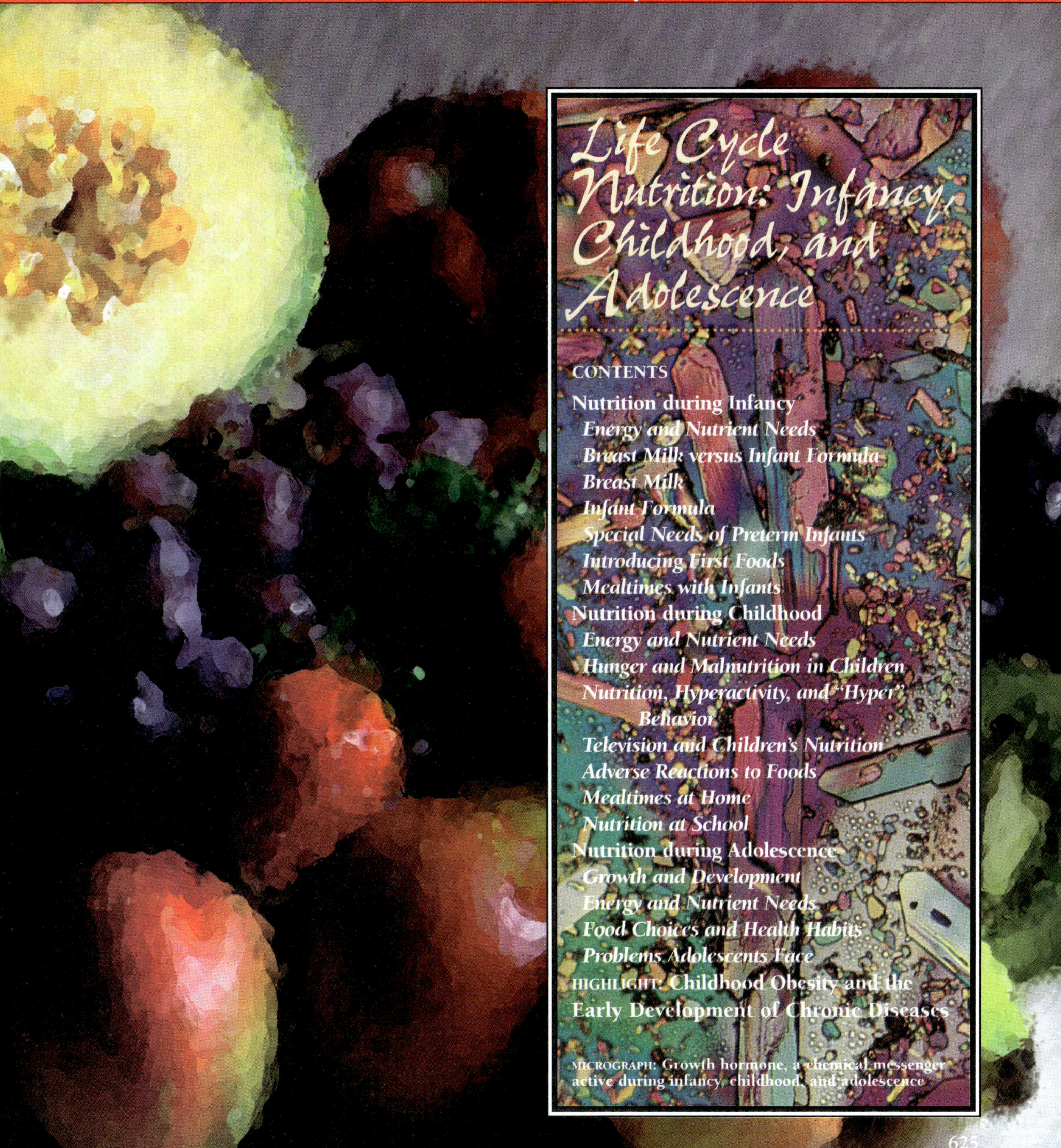

Life Cycle Nutrition: Infancy, Childhood, and Adolescence

CONTENTS

MICROGRAPH: Growth hormone, a chemical messenger active during infancy, childhood, and adolescence

The first year of life is a time of phenomenal growth and development. After the first year, a child continues to grow and change, but more slowly. Still, the cumulative effects over the next decade are remarkable. Then, as the child enters the teen years, the pace toward adulthood accelerates dramatically. This chapter examines the special nutrient needs of infants, children, and teenagers.

Figure 19–1

Weight Gain of Human Infants in Their First Five Years of Life
In the first year, an infant's birthweight may triple, but over the following several years, the rate of weight gain gradually diminishes.

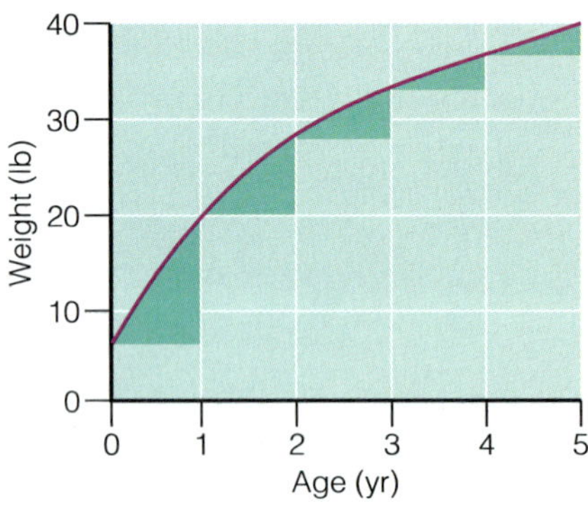

Nutrition during Infancy

For a while, the infant drinks only breast milk or formula, but later begins to eat some foods, as appropriate. Trends change and experts argue about the fine points, but properly nourishing a baby is relatively simple overall. Common sense in the selection of infant foods and a nurturing, relaxed environment go far to promote an infant's health and well-being.

ENERGY AND NUTRIENT NEEDS

An infant grows faster during the first year than ever again, as Figure 19–1 shows. Growth directly reflects nutrient intake and is an important parameter in assessing the nutrition status of infants and children. Health care professionals measure the heights and weights of infants and children at intervals and compare measures both with standard growth curves for sex and age and with previous measures of each child (see Figure 19–2).

Energy Intake and Activity A healthy infant's birthweight doubles by about four months of age and triples by the age of one year, typically reaching 20 to 25 pounds. (If an adult were to do this, a person weighing 150 pounds would increase to 450 pounds in a single year.) By the end of the first year, infant growth slows considerably; an infant gains less than 10 pounds during the second year.

A newborn baby requires about 650 kcalories per day, whereas most adults require about 2000 kcalories per day. In comparison to body weight, the difference is remarkable.

Recommended water intake for infants:
1.5 mL/kcal energy expenditure.
For example, a six-month-old infant who expends 850 kcal a day needs:

1.5 mL/kcal × 850 kcal = 1275 mL, or about 5 c of water/day.

Not only do infants grow rapidly, but their basal metabolic rate is remarkably high—about twice that of an adult, based on body weight.[1] Infants require about 100 kcalories per kilogram of body weight per day, whereas most adults need fewer than 40. (A 170-pound adult who tried to eat like an infant would have to ingest over 7000 kcalories a day.) After six months, metabolic needs decline as the growth rate slows down, but some of the energy saved by slower growth is spent in increased activity.

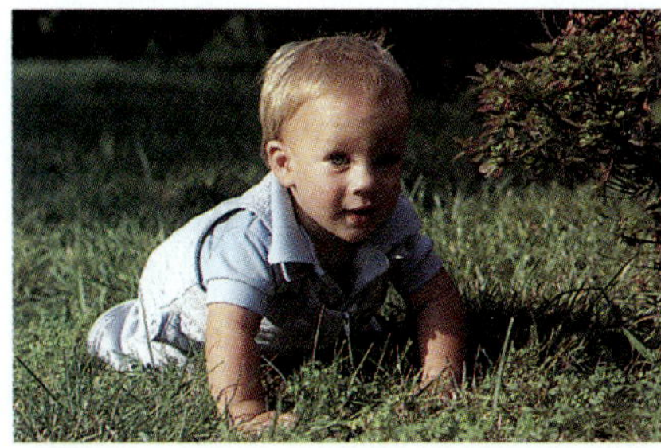

After six months, energy saved by slower growth is spent in increased activity.

Vitamins and Minerals Vitamin and mineral recommendations are based on the contents of human milk, which seems appropriate considering that neither deficiencies nor toxicities develop when infants receive these amounts.[2] Figure 19–3 (on p. 628) compares a five-month-old infant's needs per unit of body weight with those of a man and shows that some of the differences are extraordinary.

Water An important nutrient for infants, as for everyone, is the one easiest to forget: water. The younger the infant, the greater the percentage of body weight that is present as fluids between the cells and in the vascular space—fluids *outside* the cells that are easy to lose. Breast milk or infant formula normally provides enough water to replace a healthy infant's fluid losses, but an infant who is exposed to hot weather, has diarrhea, or vomits repeatedly needs supplemen-

Figure 19–2

Examples of Growth Charts

These two charts are used for girls from birth to 36 months. The first chart gives percentiles for length and weight for age; the other, percentiles for head circumference for age and weight for length. Appendix E describes how to monitor growth and provides these and six other growth charts for both boys and girls of various ages.

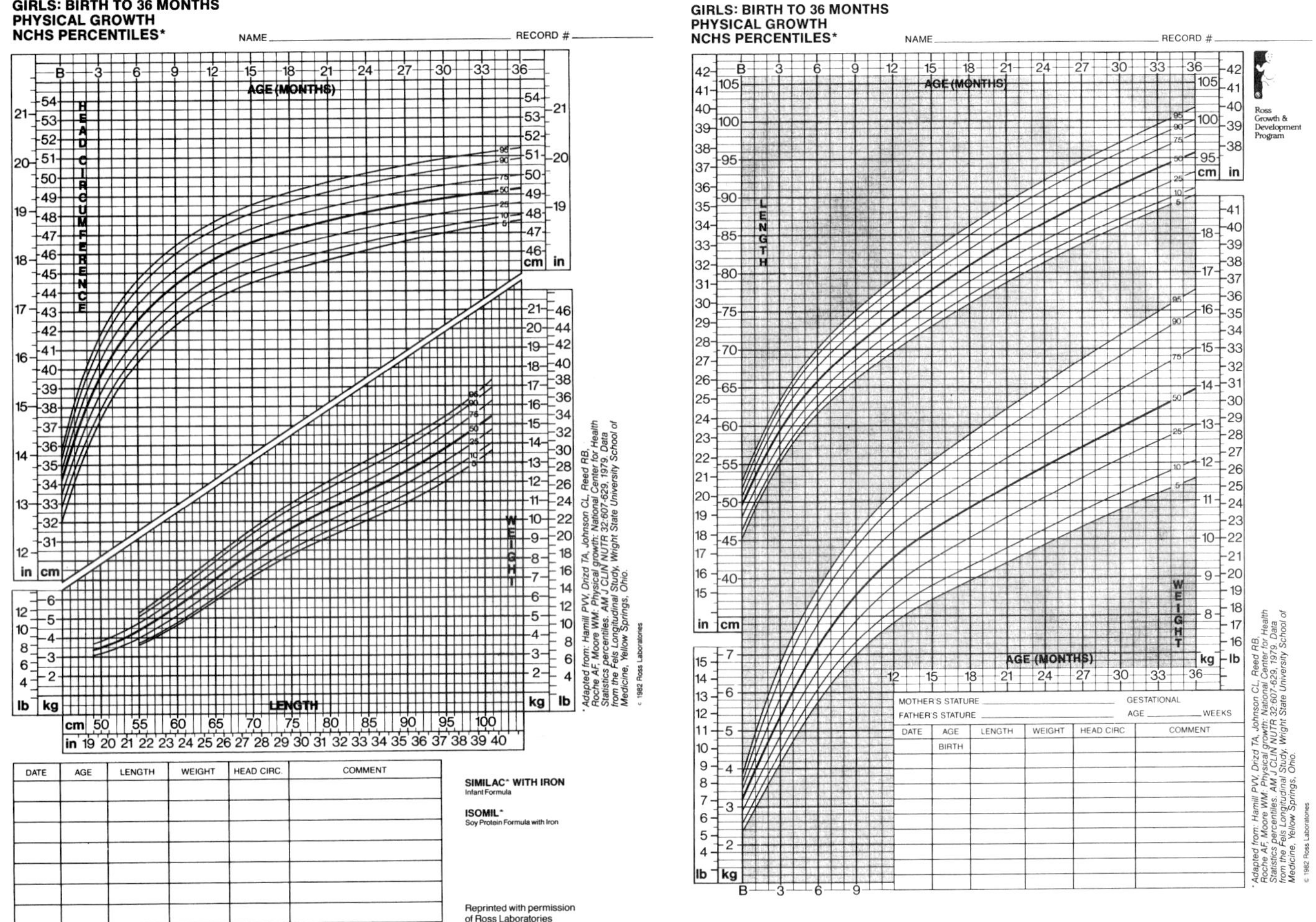

tal water to prevent life-threatening dehydration.[3] Infants cannot explain why they are crying; adults must remember that an infant may need water, and then provide as much as the infant will drink.

BREAST MILK VERSUS INFANT FORMULA

The American Academy of Pediatrics recommends that infants receive breast milk for the first 6 to 12 months.[4] The American Dietetic Association also advocates breastfeeding because of its many benefits to both infant and mother.[5] Breast milk's unique nutrient composition and protective factors promote optimal infant health and development. Experts add, though, that iron-fortified for-

Figure 19–3

Nutrient RDA of a Five-Month-Old Infant and an Adult Male Compared on the Basis of Body Weight

Because infants are small, they need smaller total amounts of the nutrients than adults do, but when comparisons are based on body weight, infants need over twice as much of many nutrients. Infants use large amounts of energy and nutrients, in proportion to their body size, to keep all their metabolic processes going.

Infant's metabolism:

- Heart rate: 120 to 140 beats per minute.
- Respiration rate: 20 per minute.
- Energy needs: 45 kcalories per pound (100 kcalories per kilogram) body weight.

Adult's metabolism:

- Heart rate: 70 to 80 beats per minute.
- Respiration rate: 12 to 14 per minute.
- Energy needs: <18 kcalories per pound (<40 kcalories per kilogram) body weight.

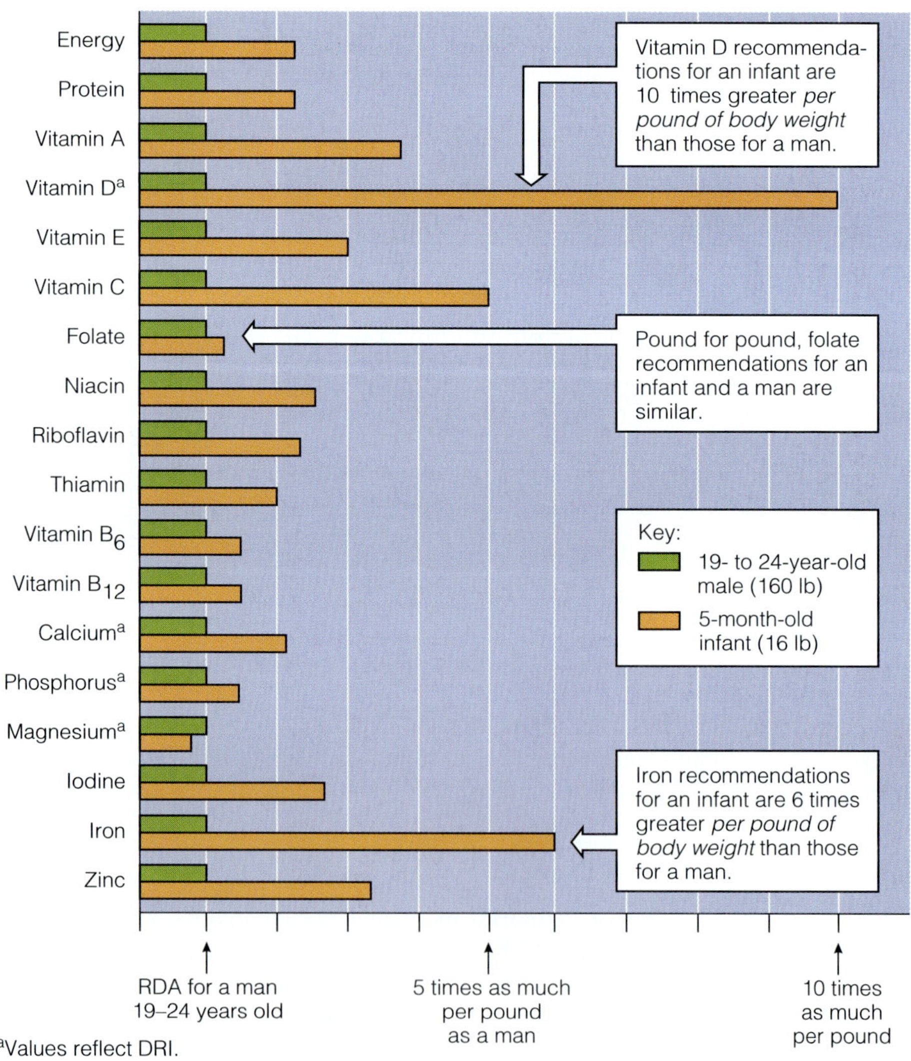

[a]Values reflect DRI.

mula is an acceptable alternative to breast milk, for it imitates the composition of breast milk as closely as possible.

Even two or three months of breastfeeding give the infant immunological protection and other special advantages during the most critical period after birth—protection that persists beyond the breastfeeding period itself.[6] The mother can then shift to formula, if necessary, knowing she has given her infant those benefits.

In the United States and Canada, the two dietary practices that have the most effect on an infant's nutrition status are, first, the milk the infant receives, and second, the age at which solid foods are introduced. The next sections are devoted to feeding the infant and identifying common nutrient deficiencies.

BREAST MILK

Breast milk excels as a source of nutrients for the young infant.[7] The American Academy of Pediatrics and the Canadian Pediatric Society have issued this joint statement: "Breastfeeding is strongly recommended for full-term infants, except in the few instances where specific contraindications exist."

Breastfed infants generally gain weight at about the same rate as formula-fed infants during the first two or three months, even though they usually drink less milk and therefore have lower energy intakes.[8] For the next six months, breastfed infants tend to gain slightly less weight than formula-fed infants, but then resume gaining at a similar rate again.[9]

With the possible exception of vitamin D, breast milk provides all the nutrients a healthy infant needs for the first four to six months of life. Breast milk also confers immunological protection, described later.

Figure 19–4

Percentages of Energy-Yielding Nutrients in Human Milk and in Recommended Adult Diets

The proportions of energy-yielding nutrients in human breast milk differ from those recommended for adults.

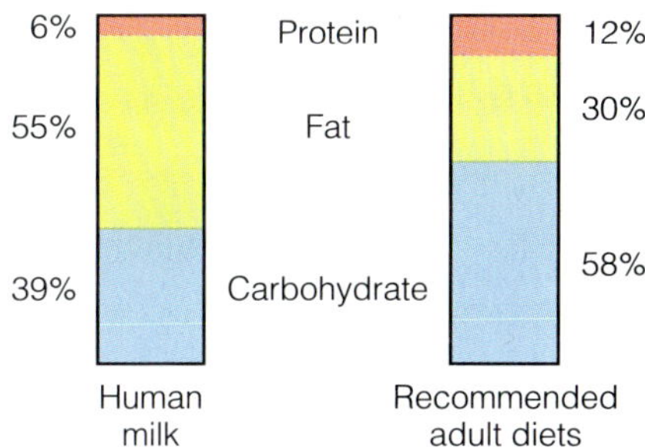

Energy Nutrients The energy-nutrient composition of breast milk differs dramatically from the dietary recommendations for adults (see Figure 19–4). Yet for infants, breast milk is the most nearly perfect food, proving that people at different stages of life really do have different nutrient needs.

Breast milk's carbohydrate is lactose, which enhances calcium absorption. Breast milk's fat offers a generous proportion of the essential fatty acid linoleic acid. The total protein in breast milk is less than in cow's milk, which is good because it places less stress on the infant's immature kidneys to excrete the major end product of protein metabolism, urea. The main protein in breast milk is alpha-lactalbumin, which is easy for infants to digest.

alpha-lactalbumin (lact-AL-byoo-min): the chief protein in human breast milk, as opposed to casein (CAY-seen), the chief protein in cow's milk.

Vitamins With the possible exception of vitamin D, the vitamins in breast milk are ample to support infant growth. Even vitamin C, for which cow's milk is a poor source, is abundant in the breast milk of a well-nourished mother. The vitamin D in breast milk is low, however, and vitamin D deficiency impairs bone mineralization in infants and children.[10] Manufacturers fortify cow's milk and infant formulas with vitamin D, and physicians may prescribe vitamin D supplements for breastfed infants who do not receive sufficient exposure to sunlight.

Infants who are exposed to sunlight regularly can make enough vitamin D to meet their needs. The amount formed depends on skin color, exposure time, atmospheric pollution, time of year, and latitude. Vitamin D deficiency is a risk for infants who are not exposed to sunlight daily, who receive breast milk without supplementation, and who have darkly pigmented skin.

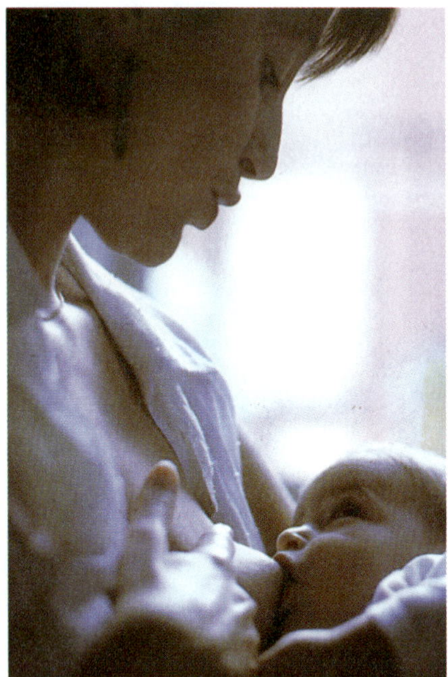

Women are encouraged to breastfeed whenever possible because breast milk offers infants many nutrients and health advantages.

Minerals The calcium-to-phosphorus ratio of breast milk is ideal for calcium absorption. The iron in breast milk is highly absorbable, as is the zinc, thanks to the presence of a zinc-binding protein. Breast milk is low in sodium, another benefit for immature kidneys.

Fluoride is not an essential nutrient, but it does help to prevent dental caries. Breast milk provides little fluoride, regardless of the mother's intake.

Supplements Breastfed newborns usually require no supplements, with the possible exception of vitamin D. At six months, depending on food and water intake, infants may require iron and fluoride supplements (see Table 19–1).

All newborns receive a single dose of vitamin K at birth.

Immunological Protection Breast milk offers unsurpassed protection against infection during a time when an infant's immune system is not fully functional. It contains antiviral agents such as immunoglobulins, antibacterial agents such as lactoferrin, and other infection inhibitors.

During the first two or three days of lactation, the breasts produce colostrum, a premilk substance containing antibodies and white cells from the mother's blood. Because it contains maternal immune factors, colostrum helps protect the newborn from infections the mother has developed immunity against. These diseases are the ones in her environment and are precisely those against which the infant needs protection. The maternal antibodies swallowed with the milk inactivate disease-causing bacteria within the digestive tract before they can start infections. This explains, in part, why breastfed infants have fewer intestinal infections than formula-fed infants. Later, breast milk also delivers antibodies, although not as many as colostrum.

colostrum (co-LAHS-trum): a milklike secretion from the breast, present during the first day or so after delivery before milk appears; rich in protective factors.

Table 19–1

Supplements for Full-Term Infants

	Vitamin D[a]	Iron[b]	Fluoride[c]
Breastfed infants:			
Birth to six months of age	✓		
Six months to one year	✓	✓	✓
Formula-fed infants:			
Birth to six months of age			
Six months to one year		✓	✓

[a]Vitamin D supplements are recommended only for as long as breast milk is the infant's major milk.

[b]Infants four to six months of age need additional iron, preferably in the form of iron-fortified cereal for both breastfed and formula-fed infants and iron-fortified infant formula for formula-fed infants.

[c]The Committee on Nutrition of the American Academy of Pediatrics recommends initiating fluoride supplements at six months of age for breastfed infants, formula-fed infants who receive ready-to-use formulas (these are prepared with water low in fluoride), and those who receive formula mixed with water that contains little or no fluoride (less than 0.3 ppm).

Sources: Adapted from Committee on Nutrition, American Academy of Pediatrics, Vitamin and mineral supplement needs of normal children in the United States, in *Pediatric Nutrition Handbook*, 3rd ed., ed. L. A. Barness (Elk Grove Village, Ill.: American Academy of Pediatrics, 1993), pp. 34–42; American Academy of Pediatrics, Committee on Nutrition, Fluoride supplementation for children: Interim policy recommendations, *Pediatrics* 95 (1995): 777.

In addition to antibodies, colostrum and breast milk provide other powerful agents that help to fight against bacterial infection. Among them are bifidus factors, which favor the growth of the "friendly" bacterium *Lactobacillus bifidus* in the infant's digestive tract, so that other, harmful bacteria cannot gain a foothold there. An iron-grabbing protein in breast milk, lactoferrin, keeps bacteria from getting the iron they need to grow, helps absorb iron into the infant's bloodstream, and kills some bacteria directly. Also present is a growth factor that stimulates the development and maintenance of the infant's digestive tract and its protective factors. Several breast milk enzymes, hormones, and lipids also help protect the infant against infection. Much remains to be learned about the composition and characteristics of human milk, but clearly it is a very special substance.

bifidus (BIFF-id-us, by-FEED-us) **factors:** factors in colostrum and breast milk that favor the growth of the "friendly" bacterium *Lactobacillus* (lack-toh-ba-SILL-us) *bifidus* in the infant's intestinal tract, so that other, less desirable intestinal inhabitants will not flourish.

lactoferrin (lack-toh-FERR-in): a factor in breast milk that binds iron and keeps it from supporting the growth of the infant's intestinal bacteria.

INFANT FORMULA

Breastfeeding offers many benefits to both mother and infant, and every woman should seriously consider it. Still, there are valid reasons for not breastfeeding, and formula-fed infants grow and develop into healthy children. The mother who chooses to feed formula to her infant can offer the same closeness, warmth, and stimulation during feedings as the breastfeeding mother can. Other family members can help with feedings, thus allowing the mother additional time to rest.

Formula preparation:

- Liquid concentrate (inexpensive, relatively easy)—mix with equal part water.
- Powdered formula (cheapest, lightest for travel)—read label directions.
- Ready-to-feed (easiest, most expensive)—pour directly into clean bottles.
- Whole milk—do not use during first year.

Appropriate Uses of Formula A woman who breastfeeds for a year can wean her infant to cow's milk, bypassing the need for infant formula. Many breastfeeding women use some infant formula, however. Some substitute formula for breastfeeding on occasion. Some wean from breast milk to formulas within the first year. And some women, of course, feed formula to their infants from birth. Whatever the case, a woman who uses formula must select an appropriate formula and learn to prepare it.

wean: to gradually replace breast milk with infant formula or other foods appropriate to an infant's diet.

Infant Formula Composition Formulas made from cow's milk closely resemble human milk in nutrient content. Figure 19–5 illustrates the energy-nutrient balance of both, and Table 19–2 compares breast milk, cow's milk, and a standard infant formula.

The American Academy of Pediatrics recommends iron-fortified infant formula for all formula-fed infants. The increasing use of iron-fortified formulas during the past few decades is a major reason for the decline in iron-deficiency anemia among U.S. infants.

Infant formulas contain no protective antibodies for infants, but in general, vaccinations, clean water, and clean environments in the developed countries make this deficit less important than in the past. Formulas can be prepared safely by following the rules of proper food handling and using water that is sanitary and free of contamination. Lead-contaminated water is a major source of lead poisoning in infants (see Highlight 13).[11]

Figure 19–5

Percentages of Energy-Yielding Nutrients in Human Milk and in Infant Formula

The proportions of energy-yielding nutrients in human breast milk and formula differ slightly.

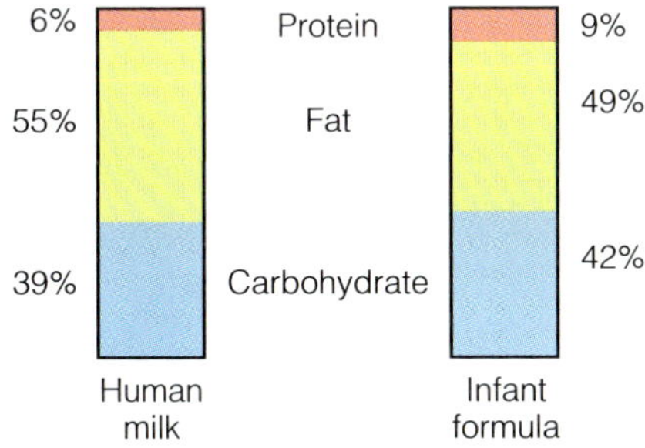

Risks of Formula Feeding In developing countries and in poor areas of this country, formula may be unavailable or may be prepared with contaminated water or overdiluted in an attempt to save money. More than 1.2 billion people in developing countries have no safe drinking water. Contaminated formulas often cause infections, leading to diarrhea, dehydration, and failure to absorb

Table 19–2

Comparison of Human Milk, Cow's Milk, and Infant Formula

Nutrient (per 100 mL)	Human Milk	Cow's Milk	Infant Formula[a]
ENERGY-YIELDING NUTRIENTS			
Energy (kcal)	64	66	67
Protein (g)	0.9	3.4	1.5
Fat (g)	3.4	3.7	3.7
Carbohydrate (g)	6.6	4.9	7.1
MINERALS			
Sodium (mg)	17	58	20
Potassium (mg)	55	138	68
Chloride (mg)	43	103	43
Calcium (mg)	26	125	47
Phosphorus (mg)	14	96	35
Magnesium (mg)	4	12	5
Iron (mg)	0.5	0.5	1.2[b]
Zinc (mg)	0.2	0.4	0.5
Copper (mg)	0.04	0.01	0.06
VITAMINS			
Vitamin A (IU)	190	103	255
Thiamin (μg)	16	44	63
Riboflavin (μg)	36	175	110
Vitamin B_6 (μg)	10	64	41
Niacin (μg)	159	93	700
Pantothenic acid (μg)	198	352	277
Biotin (μg)	1	4	1.4
Folate (μg)	5	5	9
Vitamin B_{12} (μg)	0.04	0.04	0.14
Vitamin C (mg)	4.6	1.2	5.6
Vitamin D (IU)	2.2	3.4	41
Vitamin E (IU)	0.2	0.04	1.7
Vitamin K (μg)	1.5	6.0	5.7
Inositol (μg)	37	17	3
Choline (μg)	6	20	10

[a]Values represent the average for three major commercial products: (1) Similac, Ross Laboratories; (2) Enfamil, Mead-Johnson Laboratories; and (3) SMA, Wyeth Laboratories.

[b]The value represents formulas with iron fortification. The value for unfortified formula is 0.1 milligram.

Source: Adapted with permission from K. J. Motil, Breast-feeding: Public health and clinical overview, in *Pediatric Nutrition*, eds. R. J. Grand, J. L. Sutphen, and W. H. Dietz, Jr. (Boston: Butterworths, 1987), pp. 251–263.

nutrients. Without sterilization and refrigeration, bottles of formula are an ideal breeding ground for bacteria. Whenever such risks are present, breastfeeding can be a life-saving option. Wherever sanitation is poor, breastfeeding is preferred: breast milk is sterile, and its antibodies enhance an infant's resistance to disease. An infant who lives in a house without indoor plumbing and is not breastfed is twice as likely to die early in life as a breastfed infant who lives in a house with good sanitation.

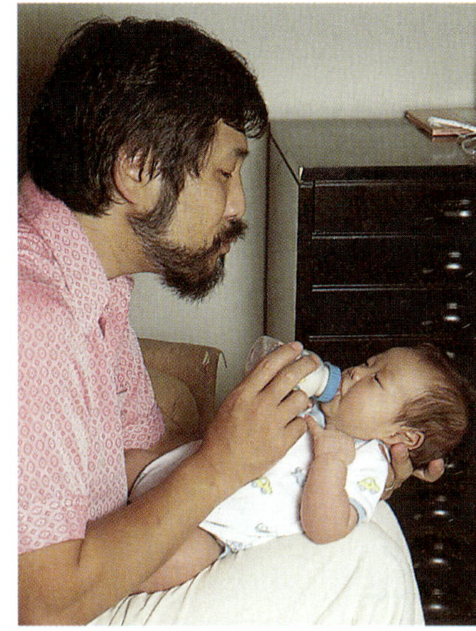

The infant thrives on infant formula offered with affection.

Infant Formula Standards National and international standards have been set for the nutrient contents of infant formulas. U.S. standards are based on American Academy of Pediatrics recommendations, and the Food and Drug Administration (FDA) mandates quality control procedures to ensure that they are met. All formulas that meet the standards are nutritionally similar; small differences are sometimes confusing, but usually not important unless infants have special needs.

Special Formulas Standard formulas are inappropriate for some infants. For example, infants with inherited diseases may need special formulas. Special formulas based on soy protein are available for infants allergic to milk protein. Soy formulas are usually lactose-free, and so can be used for infants with lactose intolerance as well. Other variations have been formulated for infants with other special needs.

Inappropriate Formulas Caretakers must use only products designed for infants; soy *beverages*, for example, are nutritionally incomplete and inappropriate for infants.[12] Goat's milk is also inappropriate for infants because of its low folate content. An infant receiving goat's milk is likely to develop "goat's milk anemia," an anemia characteristic of folate deficiency.

nursing bottle tooth decay: extensive tooth decay due to prolonged tooth contact with formula, milk, fruit juice, or other carbohydrate-rich liquid offered to an infant in a bottle.

Nursing Bottle Tooth Decay Dentists advise against putting a baby to bed with a bottle. Salivary flow, which normally cleanses the mouth, diminishes as the baby falls asleep. Sucking for long times pushes the jawline out of shape and causes a bucktoothed profile, with protruding upper and receding lower teeth. Furthermore, prolonged sucking on a bottle of formula, milk, or juice bathes the upper teeth in a carbohydrate-rich fluid that nourishes decay-producing bacteria. (The tongue covers and protects most of the lower teeth, but they, too, may be affected.) The result is extensive and rapid tooth decay. To prevent it, no child should be put to bed with a bottle of nourishing fluid. If a bottle is given, it should contain water. In fact, caregivers are wise to offer infants water after each feeding to rinse the mouth.

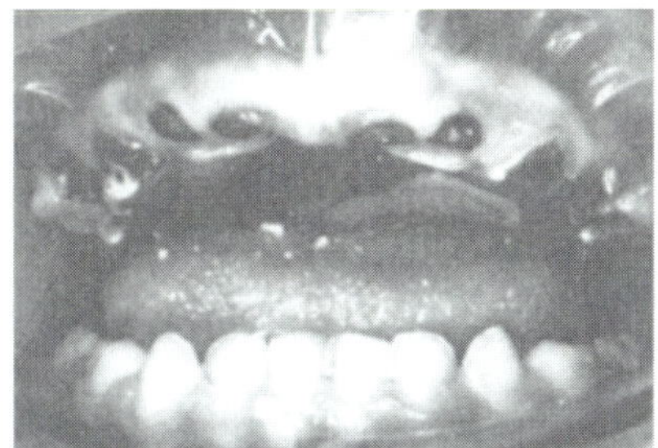

An extreme example of nursing bottle tooth decay. This child was frequently put to bed sucking on a bottle filled with apple juice, so that the teeth were bathed in carbohydrate for long periods of time—a perfect medium for bacterial growth. The upper teeth have decayed all the way to the gum line.

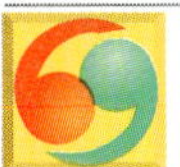

HEALTHY PEOPLE 2000: Increase to at least 75% the proportion of parents and caregivers who use feeding practices that prevent nursing bottle tooth decay.

SPECIAL NEEDS OF PRETERM INFANTS

The terms *preterm* and *premature* imply incomplete fetal development, or immaturity, of many body systems. The preterm infant faces physical independence before some of the organs and tissues are ready. The fastest fetal weight gain occurs during the last trimester of gestation, so a preterm infant is most often a low-birthweight infant. With a premature birth, the infant is forced to endure the time of maximal growth without the continued nutritional support of the placenta.

The last trimester of gestation is also a time when nutrients are stored for later use. Having limited nutrient stores intensifies the precarious situation for premature infants, and their metabolic immaturity further compromises their nutrition status. Their absorption of nutrients, especially of fat and calcium, is also limited. Preterm, low-birthweight infants are likely candidates for nutrient deficiencies.

Infants who are born eight to ten weeks prior to term have acquired only about 30 percent as much calcium as full-term infants, so their calcium requirements are high. They miss out on the normal mineralization of bone that takes place during the last trimester of gestation. As a result, they often develop the metabolic bone disease osteopenia, the rickets of prematurity. Susceptibility to osteopenia varies directly with the infant's weight: the smaller the infant, the greater the risk.

osteopenia: a metabolic bone disease common in preterm infants; also called **rickets of prematurity**

Preterm infants often receive both breast milk and formula. Breast milk provides protection against infection, and its composition is excellent for the immature intestine, kidneys, and liver. Breast milk cannot, however, fully meet the calcium and phosphorus needs of the preterm infant. Formulas for preterm infants contain more highly concentrated calcium and phosphorus than standard formulas, and breastfed preterm infants receive human milk supplemented with these minerals.[13] Special formulas designed for preterm infants offer the advantages of known composition and precise measurement of intake.

INTRODUCING FIRST FOODS

Changes in body organs during the first year affect the baby's readiness to accept solid foods. For example, the stomach and intestines can easily digest the milk sugar lactose at birth, but they cannot digest starch for several months. One reason why breast milk or formula is the ideal first food is that its easily digested carbohydrate can best supply energy for the baby's intense growth and activity. Breast milk or infant formula should therefore be the baby's major food, at first. Cow's milk is inappropriate during the first year because it provides insufficient vitamin C and iron and excessive sodium and protein. If introduced too soon, cow's milk displaces iron-fortified formula or breast milk and causes GI blood loss in many infants.

Supplemental, or weaning, foods are sometimes called beikost (BYE-cost).

When to Introduce Solid Food In addition to formula or breast milk, an infant needs to begin eating other foods around four to six months. Infants who do not receive solid foods before the end of the first year may suffer delayed growth.

Physical readiness for solid foods develops in small steps. Teeth begin to erupt, and the infant develops the ability to swallow solid foods at around four to six months. Offering food by spoon and liquids by cup helps an infant learn to swallow. At nine months to a year, a baby can sit up and handle objects; at that time, hard crackers and other finger foods can help the infant develop manual dexterity and control of the jaw muscles.

Table 19–3

First Foods for the Infant

Breast milk or iron-fortified formula is the only source of nourishment for the first 4 to 6 months. Throughout the first year, the infant's intake of breast milk or iron-fortified formula will gradually decline as solid food intake increases.

Age (mo)	Addition
4 to 6	Iron-fortified rice cereal, followed by other single-grain cereals, mixed with breast milk, formula, or water Pureed vegetables and fruits, one by one (perhaps vegetables before fruits, so the baby will learn to like their less sweet flavors)
6 to 8	Infant breads and crackers Mashed vegetables and fruits, and their juices[a]
8 to 10	Breads and cereals from the table Soft, cooked vegetables and fruit from the table Finely cut meats, fish, chicken, casseroles, cheeses, yogurts, tofu, eggs, and legumes
10 to 12	Continue to introduce a variety of nutritious foods

[a]All baby juices are fortified with vitamin C. Orange juice may cause allergies; apple juice may be a better juice to feed first. Dilute juices with water and offer in a cup to prevent nursing bottle tooth decay.

Source: Adapted in part from Committee on Nutrition, American Academy of Pediatrics, *Pediatric Nutrition Handbook*, 3rd ed., ed. L. A. Barness (Elk Grove Village, Ill.: American Academy of Pediatrics, 1993), pp. 23–33.

Infants differ, and each program of adding foods should depend on the infant, not on a rigid schedule. Indications of readiness for solid foods include:

- The infant's birthweight has doubled.
- The infant can sit with support and can control head movements.
- The infant is four to six months old.

Table 19–3 presents a suggested sequence for adding foods to the infant's diet.

Some parents want to feed solids at an earlier age on the mistaken belief that "stuffing the baby" at bedtime promotes sleeping through the night. On the average, babies start to sleep through the night at about three to four months, regardless of when solid foods are introduced.

The Need for Water An infant's kidneys are unable to concentrate waste efficiently, so the infant must excrete relatively more water than an adult to carry off a comparable amount of waste. When solid foods are introduced, the risk of dehydration becomes greater, and infants may require supplemental water.

Allergy-Causing Foods New foods should be introduced singly and at intervals spaced to permit detection of allergies. For example, when cereals are introduced, rice cereal is offered first for several days because it is least likely to cause an allergy. When it is clear that rice cereal is not causing an allergy, another grain is introduced. Wheat cereal is offered last because it is the most common

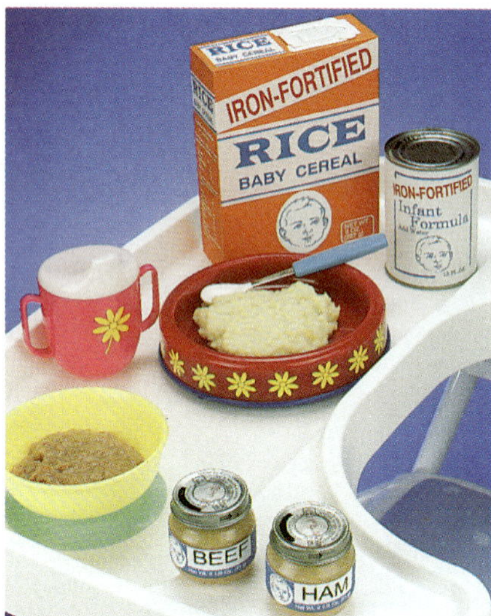

Foods such as iron-fortified cereals and formulas, mashed legumes, and strained meats provide iron.

offender. If a cereal causes an allergic reaction such as skin rash, digestive upset, or respiratory discomfort, its use should be discontinued before introducing the next food. A later section in this chapter offers more on food allergies.

Choice of Infant Foods Commercial baby foods in the United States and Canada are generally safe, nutritious, and of high quality. They contain little or no salt, less sugar than in the past, and few or no additives. Except for mixed dinners and heavily sweetened desserts, commercial baby foods typically have high nutrient density. Alternatively, parents who want to feed the baby family foods can follow safe food handling practices, cook foods without salt, and "blenderize" small portions at each meal. The foods offered should include good sources of iron and vitamin C.

Foods to Provide Iron Iron deficiency is common in children throughout the world, especially between six months and three years when they are growing fast and milk, which is a poor source of iron, has a large place in their diets. The iron an infant stored during gestation typically runs out after the birthweight doubles, long before the end of the first year.

In addition to breast milk or formula with iron, infants can receive iron from iron-fortified cereals and, later, from meat or meat alternates such as legumes. Iron-fortified cereals contribute a significant amount of iron to an infant's diet, but the iron's bioavailability is poor. Consequently, cereal alone, or in combination with cow's milk, is insufficient to meet iron needs.[14] During the first year, cereals should be mixed with iron-fortified formula, breast milk, or water rather than cow's milk. Parents or caretakers can enhance iron absorption from iron-fortified cereals by selecting vitamin C–rich foods to go with meals.

Foods to Provide Vitamin C The best sources of vitamin C are fruits and vegetables. Some authorities suggest that an infant who is introduced to fruits before vegetables may develop a preference for sweets and find the vegetables less palatable. To prevent this, introduce vegetables first, fruits later.

Fruit juices should be diluted and served in a cup, not a bottle. They should also be served in reasonable quantities as part of a balanced selection of foods. Cases have been reported of children failing to grow and thrive because they were drinking such large amounts of juice daily that other more energy- and nutrient-dense foods were displaced from their diets.[15] Such findings prove that any one food—even a healthful and nutritious one—can create nutrient imbalances and impair growth when consumed in excess.

Foods to Omit Sweets of any other kind, including baby food "desserts," have no place in an infant's diet. They convey no nutrients to support growth, and the extra food energy can promote obesity. Canned vegetables are also inappropriate for infants, as they often contain too much sodium. Honey and corn syrup should never be fed to infants because of the risk of botulism.* Babies and even young children cannot safely chew and swallow popcorn, whole grapes,

botulism (BOT-chew-lism): an often fatal food-borne illness caused by the ingestion of foods containing a toxin produced by bacteria that grow in improperly canned acidic foods (see Chapter 14 for details).

*In infants, but not in older individuals, ingestion of *Clostridium botulinum* spores can cause illness when the spores germinate in the intestine and produce toxin, which is absorbed. Symptoms include poor feeding, constipation, loss of tension in the arteries and muscles, weakness, and respiratory compromise. Infant botulism has been implicated in 5 percent of cases of sudden infant death syndrome (SIDS).

Menu

Breakfast
½ c whole milk
3 tbs cereal
1 to 2 tbs fruit
Teething crackers

Morning snack
½ c whole milk
1 to 2 tbs fruit
Teething crackers

Lunch
1 c whole milk
2 to 3 tbs vegetables
2 tbs chopped meat or well-cooked, mashed legumes

Afternoon snack
½ c whole milk
Teething crackers
1 tbs peanut butter

Dinner
1 c whole milk
1 egg
2 tbs cereal or potato
2 to 3 tbs vegetables
2 to 3 tbs fruit

Sample Menu for a One-Year-Old

Note: Fruit choices need to include citrus fruits, melons, and berries and vegetable choices need to include dark green, leafy and deep yellow vegetables.

whole beans, hot dog slices, hard candies, and nuts; they can easily choke on these foods, a risk not worth taking.

Foods at One Year At one year of age, whole cow's milk becomes the primary source of most of the nutrients an infant needs; 2 to 3½ cups a day meets those needs sufficiently. More milk than this displaces foods necessary to provide iron and can lead to milk anemia. Children one to two years old should drink whole milk, not low-fat or nonfat milk. If they use powdered milk, it should be one of the fat-containing varieties. Other foods—meats, iron-fortified cereals, enriched or whole-grain breads, fruits, and vegetables—should be supplied in variety and in amounts sufficient to round out total energy needs. Ideally, a one-year-old will sit at the table, eat many of the same foods everyone else eats, and drink liquids from a cup, not a bottle. The accompanying menu shows a sample meal plan that meets a one-year-old's requirements.

milk anemia: iron-deficiency anemia that develops when an excessive milk intake displaces iron-rich foods from the diet.

MEALTIMES WITH INFANTS

The wise parent of a one-year-old offers nutrition and love together. "Feeding with love" produces better growth and brain development than feeding the same food without love.

The person feeding a one-year-old has to be aware that exploring and experimenting are normal and desirable behaviors at this time in a child's life. The child is developing a sense of autonomy that, if fostered, will provide the foundation for later confidence and effectiveness as an individual. The child's impulses, if consistently denied, can turn to shame and self-doubt. In light of the developmental needs of one-year-olds and their often willful behavior, a few

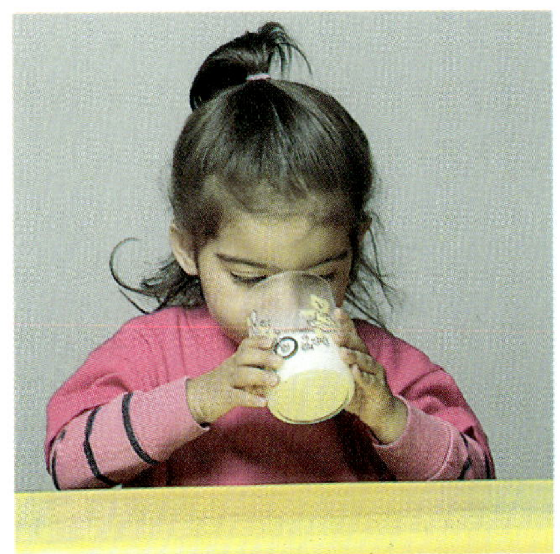

Toddlers need vitamin A– and vitamin D–fortified whole milk.

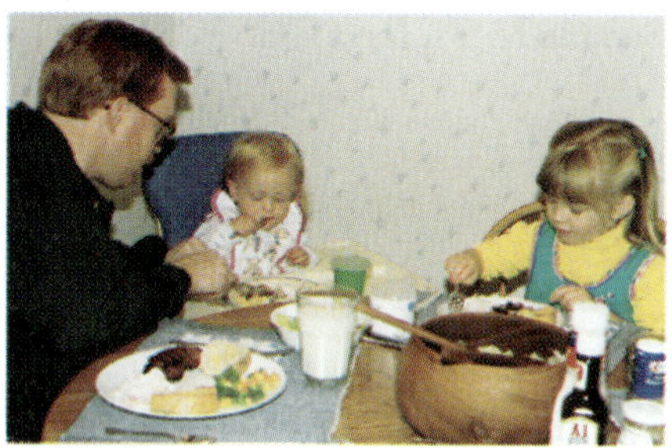

Ideally, a one-year-old eats many of the same foods as the rest of the family.

feeding guidelines may be helpful:

- Discourage unacceptable behavior, such as standing at the table or throwing food, by removing the child from the table to wait until later to eat. Be consistent and firm, not punitive. The child will soon learn to sit and eat.
- Let the child explore and enjoy food, even if this means eating with fingers for a while. Use of the spoon will come in time.
- Don't force food on children. Rejecting new foods is normal; acceptance is more likely as infants and children become familiar with new foods through repeated opportunities to taste them.[16]
- Provide children with nutritious foods, and let them choose which ones and how much they will eat. Gradually, they will acquire a taste for different foods.
- Limit sweets. Infants have little room in their daily energy allowance for empty-kcalorie foods. Do not use sweets as a reward for eating meals.
- Don't turn the dining table into a battleground. Make mealtimes enjoyable. Teach children healthy food choices and eating habits in a pleasant environment.

These recommendations reflect the spirit of tolerance that best serves the emotional and physical interests of the young child.

To recap, the primary food for infants during the first 6 to 12 months is either breast milk or iron-fortified formulas. In addition to nutrients, breast milk also offers immunological protection. At about 4 to 6 months, infants should gradually begin eating solid foods so that by 1 year, they are drinking from a cup and eating many of the same foods as the rest of the family.

Nutrition during Childhood

Each year from age one to adolescence, a child typically grows taller by 2 to 3 inches and heavier by 5 or so pounds. Growth charts provide valuable clues to a child's health. Weight gains out of proportion to height gains may reflect overeating and inactivity, whereas measures significantly below the standard suggest malnutrition.

Increases in height and weight are only two of the many developmental changes occurring during childhood. At age one, children can stand alone and are learning to toddle; by two, they can walk and are learning to run; by three, they can jump and are climbing with confidence. Bones and muscles increase in mass and density to make these accomplishments possible. Thereafter, further lengthening of the long bones and increases in musculature proceed, unevenly and more slowly, until adolescence.

ENERGY AND NUTRIENT NEEDS

Children's appetites begin to diminish around one year, consistent with the slowing of growth. Thereafter, children spontaneously vary their food intakes to coincide with their growth patterns; they demand more food during periods of rapid growth than during slow periods. At times they seem to be insatiable, and at other times they seem to live on air and water.

Although children's energy intakes may vary widely from meal to meal, their total daily intakes are remarkably constant.[17] If children eat less at one meal, they typically eat more at the next, and vice versa. Overweight children are an exception: they do not always adjust their energy intakes appropriately and may eat in response to external cues, disregarding appetite-regulation signals.

Energy Intake and Activity A one-year-old child needs perhaps 1000 kcalories a day; a three-year-old needs only 300 kcalories more. By age ten, a child needs about 2000 kcalories a day. Total energy needs increase slightly with age, but energy needs per kilogram body weight actually decline gradually.

Individual children's energy needs vary widely, depending on their physical activity. Inactive children can become obese even when they eat less food than the average. They would do well to learn to enjoy physical play and exercise.

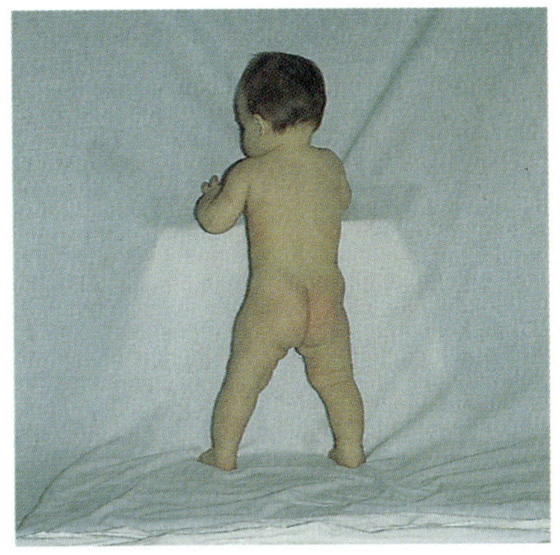

The body shape of a one-year-old (above) changes dramatically by age two (below). The two-year-old has lost much of the baby fat; the muscles (especially in the back, buttocks, and legs) have firmed and strengthened; and the leg bones have lengthened.

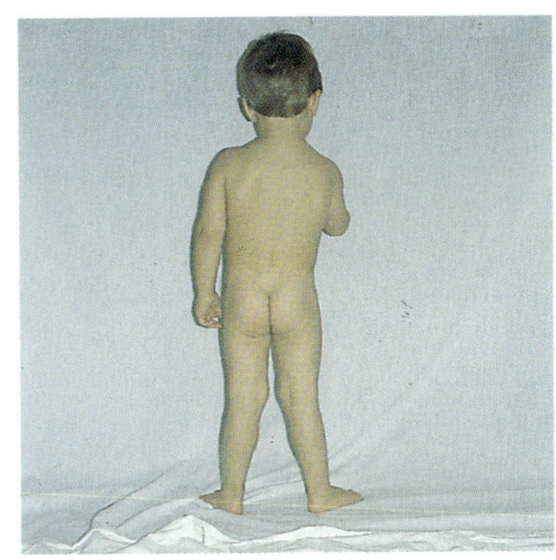

Vitamins and Minerals Steady growth during childhood implies gradually increasing needs of all nutrients. Before adolescence, children accumulate stores of nutrients. Then, when they take off on the adolescent growth spurt and their nutrient intakes cannot meet the demands of rapid growth, they draw on those stores. This is especially true of calcium; the denser the bones grow in childhood, the better they can support teen growth and still withstand the inevitable bone losses of later life. The way preteen children eat, then, influences their nutritional health during childhood, during their teen years—and in their old age.

Planning Children's Meals To provide all the needed nutrients, children's meals should include a variety of foods from each food group—in amounts suited to their appetites and needs. Serving sizes increase with age. A portion of meat, grains, fruits, or vegetables for children is loosely defined as 1 tablespoon per year. Thus, at four years of age, a portion is about 4 tablespoons, or ¼ cup. This rule of thumb applies until they reach the teen years. Table 19–4 offers a daily food pattern for children.

To ensure that children have healthy appetites and plenty of room for nutritious foods when they are hungry, parents and teachers must limit access to candy, cola, and other concentrated sweets. If such foods are permitted in large quantities, the only possible outcomes are nutrient deficiencies, obesity, or both. The preference for sweets is innate; most children do not naturally select nutritious foods on the basis of taste. In one study, when children were allowed to create meals freely from a variety of foods, they selected foods that provided 25 percent of the kcalories from sugar.[18] When their parents were watching, or even when they thought their parents were watching, the children improved their selections. Overweight children, especially, need help in sticking to nutrient-dense foods that will meet their nutrient needs within their energy allowances.

Sweets need not be banned altogether. Children who are exceptionally active can enjoy high-kcalorie foods such as ice cream or pudding from the milk group or pancakes or cookies from the bread group. These foods carry valuable nutrients and bring pleasure. As for sedentary children, they need to become more active, and then they, too, can enjoy some of these foods without unhealthy weight gain.

Table 19–4

Children's Daily Food Patterns for Good Nutrition

Food Group	Servings per Day	Average Size of Serving		
		1 TO 3 YEARS	4 TO 6 YEARS	7 TO 12 YEARS
Bread and cereals (whole grain or enriched)[a]	6 or more	½ slice	1 slice	1 to 2 slices
Vegetables[b]	3 or more	2–4 tbs or ½ c juice	¼–½ c or ½ c juice	½–¾ c or ½ c juice
Fruits[b]	2 or more	2–4 tbs or ½ c juice	¼–½ c or ½ c juice	½–¾ c or ½ c juice
Meat and meat alternates[c]	2 or more	1–2 oz	1–2 oz	2–3 oz
Milk and milk products[d]	3 to 4	½–¾ c	¾ c	¾–1 c

[a]1 slice bread = ¾ c dry cereal, ½ c cooked cereal, ½ c potato, rice, or noodles.

[b]Vitamin C source (citrus fruits, berries, tomatoes, broccoli, cabbage, cantaloupe) daily; vitamin A source (spinach, carrots, squash, tomato, cantaloupe) 3 to 4 times weekly.

[c]1 oz meat, fish, poultry = 1 egg, 1 frankfurter, 2 tbs peanut butter, ½ c cooked legumes.

[d]½ c milk = ½ c cottage cheese, pudding, yogurt; ¾ oz cheese; 2 tbs dried milk.

Source: Adapted from P. M. Queen and R. R. Henry, Growth and nutrient requirements of children, in *Pediatric Nutrition*, eds. R. J. Grand, J. L. Sutphen, and W. H. Dietz, Jr. (Boston: Butterworths, 1987), p. 347.

HUNGER AND MALNUTRITION IN CHILDREN

Highlight 18 examines the causes and consequences of hunger in the United States and around the world.

Most U.S. and Canadian children are well nourished. Their average energy intakes are sufficient to support normal growth, and their average nutrient intakes, except for iron, meet or exceed recommendations. Some low-income children, however, are malnourished and have suffered growth retardation. An estimated 11 million U.S. children under age 12 are hungry and living in poverty.

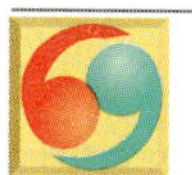

HEALTHY PEOPLE 2000: Reduce growth retardation among low-income children aged five years and younger to less than 10%.

Malnutrition and Health When hunger is chronic, children become malnourished. Worldwide, malnutrition takes a devastating toll on children, contributing to nearly half of the deaths of children under four years old. Vitamin A deficiency afflicts more than 5 million children worldwide, inducing blindness, stunted growth, and infections. Zinc deficiency also retards growth and typically accompanies protein-energy malnutrition and vitamin A deficiency.

Hunger and Behavior Even when hunger is temporary, as when a child misses one meal, behavior and academic performance are affected. Children who eat nutritious breakfasts function better than their peers who do not. Young children who participate in the federally funded School Breakfast Program improve their scores on achievement tests and are tardy or absent significantly less often than children who qualify for the program, but do not participate. Without breakfast, children perform poorly in tasks requiring concentration, their attention spans are shorter, and they even show lower IQs on testing than their well-fed peers; malnourished children are particularly vulnerable. Common sense dictates that it is unreasonable to expect anyone to learn and perform work when no fuel has been provided. By late morning, discomfort from hunger may become distracting even if a child has eaten breakfast.

The problem children face when attempting morning schoolwork on an empty stomach appears to be at least partly due to low blood glucose. The average child up to age ten or so needs to eat every four to six hours to maintain a blood glucose concentration high enough to support the activity of the brain and nervous system. A child's brain is as big as an adult's, and the brain is the body's chief glucose consumer. A child's liver is much smaller than an adult's, however, and the liver is the organ responsible for storing glucose as glycogen and releasing it into the blood as needed. A child's liver can store only about four hours' worth of glycogen—hence the need to eat fairly often. Teachers aware of the late-morning slump in their classrooms wisely request that midmorning snacks be provided; snacks improve classroom performance all the way to lunchtime. For the child who hasn't had breakfast, the morning's lessons may be lost altogether.

Eating breakfast also helps children to meet their nutrient needs each day. Children who skip breakfast typically do not make up the deficits at later meals—they simply have lower intakes of energy, vitamins, and minerals than those who eat breakfast.[19]

The brain uses about three times as much glucose per day as the rest of the body.

Table 19–5

Iron-Rich Foods Children Like[a]

Breads, cereals, and grains
- Canned macaroni (½ c)
- Canned spaghetti (½ c)
- Cream of wheat (¼ c)
- Fortified dry cereals (1 oz)[b]
- Noodles, rice, or barley (½ c)
- Tortillas (1 flour, 2 corn)
- Whole-wheat, enriched, or fortified bread (1 slice)
- Bran muffins

Vegetables
- Baked flavored potato skins (½ skin)
- Cooked mushrooms (½ c)
- Cooked mung bean sprouts or snow peas (½ c)
- Green peas (½ c)
- Mixed vegetable juice (1 c)

Fruits
- Apple juice (1 c)
- Canned plums (3 plums)
- Cooked dried apricots (½ c)
- Dried peaches (4 halves)
- Raisins (1 tbs)

Meats and legumes
- Bean dip (¼ c)
- Canned pork and beans (⅓ c)
- Mild chili or other bean/meat dishes (¼ c) such as burritos
- Liverwurst (½ oz)
- Meat casseroles (½ c)
- Peanut butter and jelly sandwich (½ sandwich)
- Lean roast beef or cooked ground beef (1 oz)
- Sloppy joes (½ sandwich)

[a]Each serving provides at least 1 milligram iron, or one-tenth of a child's RDA for iron. Vitamin C–rich foods included with these snacks increase iron absorption.

[b]Some fortified breakfast cereals contain more than 10 milligrams iron per half-cup serving (read the labels).

Iron Deficiency Iron-deficiency anemia is a major problem worldwide, as well as being the most prevalent nutrient deficiency among U.S. and Canadian children. The high iron needs of growth combined with typically low iron intakes leave many children with marginal iron status. Reducing iron deficiency among young children is one of the foremost health priorities in the United States.[20] Internationally, the World Health Organization is collaborating with a United Nations subcommittee on nutrition to develop a ten-year plan to eliminate iron deficiency.[21]

HEALTHY PEOPLE 2000: Reduce iron deficiency to less than 3% among children aged one through four years.

To prevent iron deficiency, children's foods must deliver approximately 10 milligrams of iron per day. To achieve this goal, snacks and meals should include the iron-rich foods listed in Table 19–5, and milk should be limited to 3 or 4 cups a day, so that it will not displace lean meats, fish, poultry, eggs, legumes, and whole-grain or enriched products.

Iron Deficiency and Behavior Iron deficiency has well-known and widespread effects on children's behavior. In addition to carrying oxygen in the blood, iron transports oxygen within cells, which use it to help produce energy. Iron is also used to make neurotransmitters—most notably, those that regulate the ability to pay attention, which is crucial to learning. An iron deficiency not only causes an energy crisis but also directly affects mood, attention span, and learning ability.

Iron deficiency is usually diagnosed by a deficit of iron in the *blood*, after the deficiency has progressed all the way to anemia. A child's *brain*, however, is sensitive to low iron concentrations long before the blood effects appear. Research has shown that iron deficiency lowers the "motivation to persist in intellectually

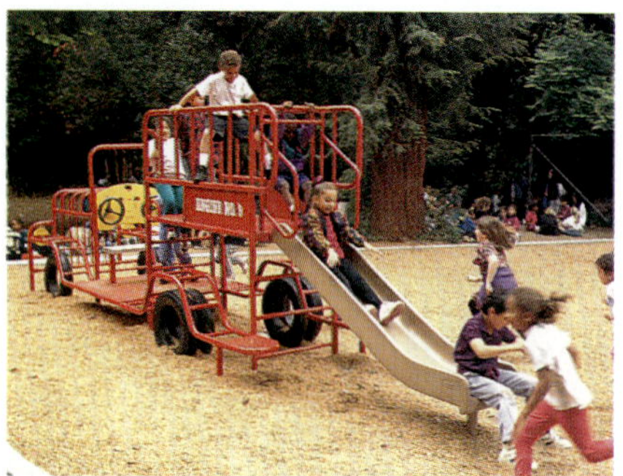
Healthy, well-nourished children are alert in the classroom and energetic at play.

challenging tasks," shortens the attention span, and impairs overall intellectual performance. Anemic children perform less well on tests and are more disruptive than their nonanemic classmates. At least one study found that children who had had iron-deficiency anemia *as infants* still continued to perform poorly at age five compared with their peers, even though they had regained excellent iron status.[22] The long-term damaging effects on mental development make prevention of iron deficiency during infancy and early childhood a high priority.[23]

Other Nutrient Deficiencies and Behavior Iron is not the only nutrient that can be displaced from a diet by nutrient-poor foods. Several dozen other nutrients may be lacking as well, causing both physical and behavioral symptoms.

A child with nutrient deficiencies may be irritable, aggressive, disagreeable, or sad and withdrawn. Such a child may be labeled "hyperactive," "depressed," or "unlikable," when in fact these traits may arise from simple, even marginal, malnutrition. In any such case, inspection of the child's diet by a qualified health care professional is clearly in order. Should suspicion of dietary inadequacies be raised, no matter what causes may be implicated, the people responsible for feeding the child should take steps to correct those inadequacies promptly.

Lead Toxicity and Malnutrition Malnutrition is quite often a complex condition involving multiple nutrients and other environmental factors. An example of a possible complicating factor is lead poisoning. Lead toxicity can cause iron deficiency, and iron deficiency can impair the body's defenses against lead absorption. Highlight 13 describes the mental, behavioral, and other health problems associated with lead toxicity. Such problems are important to investigate, but even before they have been identified, the child should be fed properly.

Parents and medical practitioners often overlook the possibility that malnutrition may account for abnormalities of appearances and behavior. Any departure from normal healthy appearance and behavior is a sign of possible poor nutrition (see Table 19–6).

NUTRITION, HYPERACTIVITY, AND "HYPER" BEHAVIOR

Because malnutrition can impair children's functioning in many ways, people tend to look to food habits for explanations of hyperactivity. Hyperactivity is not caused by a poor diet, but a poor diet may be part of a cluster of factors seen in a hyperactive child's life.

tension-fatigue syndrome: apparent hyperactivity produced in a child by the combination of lack of sleep, overstimulation, and anxiety.

Tension-Fatigue Syndrome Children can become excitable, rambunctious, and unruly out of a desire for attention, lack of sleep, overstimulation, too much television, or a lack of physical activity. Together, these factors produce the tension-fatigue syndrome, which suggests that more consistent care, and not just better food, is needed. It helps most to insist on regular hours of sleep, regular mealtimes, and regular outdoor activity.

hyperactivity: a condition of excessive activity. When hyperactivity is accompanied by an inability to pay attention and poor impulse control, professionals call this syndrome **attention deficit hyperactivity disorder (ADHD)**

Hyperactivity Hyperactivity is a condition that may affect behavior and learning in about 5 percent of young school-age children. Left untreated, hyperactivity can interfere with a child's social development and ability to learn. Treatment focuses on relieving the symptoms and controlling the associated problems; there is no cure.

Table 19–6

Physical Signs of Health and Malnutrition in Children

	Healthy	Malnourished
Hair:	Shiny, firm in the scalp	Dull, brittle, dry, loose; falls out
Eyes:	Bright, clear pink membranes; adjust easily to darkness	Pale membranes; spots; redness; adjust slowly to darkness
Teeth and gums:	No pain or cavities, gums firm, teeth bright	Missing, discolored, decayed teeth; gums bleed easily and are swollen and spongy
Face:	Good complexion	Off-color, scaly, flaky, cracked skin
Glands:	No lumps	Swollen at front of neck and cheeks
Tongue:	Red, bumpy, rough	Sore, smooth, purplish, swollen
Skin:	Smooth, firm, good color	Dry, rough, spotty; "sandpaper" feel or sores; lack of fat under skin
Nails:	Firm, pink	Spoon-shaped brittle, ridged
Behavior:	Alert, attentive, cheerful	Irritable, apathetic, inattentive, hyperactive
Internal systems:	Heart rate, heart rhythm, and blood pressure normal; normal digestive function; reflexes and psychological development normal	Heart rate, heart rhythm, or blood pressure abnormal; liver and spleen enlarged; abnormal digestion; mental irritability, confusion; burning, tingling of hands and feet; loss of balance and coordination
Muscles and bones:	Good muscle tone and posture; long bones straight	"Wasted" appearance of muscles; swollen bumps on skull or ends of bones; small bumps on ribs; bowed legs or knock-knees

Note: The physical signs shown here are consistent with malnutrition but not diagnostic of it.

Physicians often manage hyperactivity through behavior modification, special educational techniques, psychological counseling, and drug therapy. The drugs most commonly prescribed are stimulants. Normally, stimulants speed up people's activity, but they have a paradoxical effect on hyperactivity: they normalize it by stimulating control centers in the brain. If a child calms down when given stimulant drugs, the response indicates that the drugs may be correcting a biochemical imbalance in the nervous system and can help control the behavior.

Many parents mistakenly believe a solution may lie in manipulating the diet—most commonly, by eliminating sugar or food additives. Diet is one area of a child's life in which parents feel they can exert some control. If problems can be solved by adding carrots or eliminating candy, then parents are eager to give diet advice a try. While nutrition should be considered whenever a person's health is less than optimal, it is unwise to jump at appealing solutions that are unfounded. Several studies have found no convincing evidence that sugar causes hyperactivity or worsens behavior.[24] Recommendations to restrict sugar in children's diets to prevent or treat behavior problems are groundless. Sugar can influence children's behavior only by displacing nutritious foods and contributing to nutrient deficiencies.

Caffeine and Behavior Caffeine is often overlooked as a source of "hyper" behavior in children, but it is a matter of some concern to pediatricians. A 12-

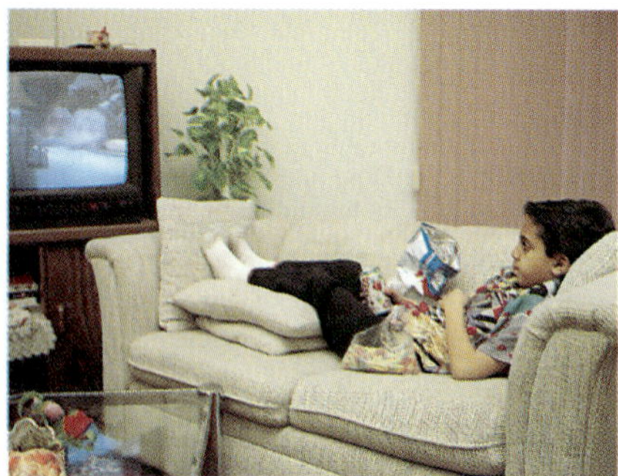

Television watching influences children's eating habits and activity patterns.

ounce cola beverage may contain as much as 50 milligrams caffeine; in the body of a 60-pound child, two or more such beverages are equivalent to the caffeine in 8 cups of coffee for a 175-pound adult. Children who are troubled by sleeplessness, restlessness, and irregular heartbeats may need to limit their caffeine consumption. Children not accustomed to caffeine who are given doses equivalent to about two cola beverages a day become noticeably inattentive and restless. As long as children are surrounded by attractive temptations such as cola beverages, adults must prevent abuse until the children learn to control consumption themselves. (Appendix H presents a table that lists the caffeine contents of foods, beverages, and medicines.)

TELEVISION AND CHILDREN'S NUTRITION

The average child watches 5000 hours of television before the end of preschool and has seen 19,000 hours by the end of high school.[25] Watching programs or videos on television is second only to sleeping among children's uses of time.

Besides contributing to tension-fatigue syndrome, watching television adversely affects children's nutritional health in several ways. As Chapter 9 reported, studies have found that the prevalence of obesity increases with each hour of television viewed; even daydreaming appears to use more energy than watching television.[26] Children who watch more than two hours of television per day also have higher serum cholesterol than do more active children.

TV fosters obesity because it:

- Requires no energy beyond basal metabolism.
- Replaces vigorous activities.
- Encourages snacking.
- Promotes a sedentary lifestyle.

Playing computer games influences activity patterns similarly.

The average child sees an estimated 10,000 commercials a year—almost all luring viewers to purchase sugar-coated breakfast cereals, candy bars, chips, fast foods, and carbonated beverages. These foods add sugar, fat, and salt to the diet and displace foods that provide needed nutrients. Many parents and pediatricians believe that food ads aimed at children should be banned because they support corporate profits rather than children's health. Alternatively, parents can teach their children how to evaluate food ads and make healthful choices.

ADVERSE REACTIONS TO FOODS

adverse reactions: unusual responses to food (including intolerances and allergies).

Adverse reactions to foods can threaten nutritional health to varying extents, depending on the severity and duration of the reactions and the foods they involve. Temporary reactions may lead to permanent avoidance of foods; permanent reactions, if not detected and treated, can cause chronic illness.

food intolerances: adverse reactions to foods that do not involve the immune system.

Food Intolerances Not all adverse reactions to foods are food allergies, although even physicians may describe them as such. Signs of adverse reactions to foods include stomachaches, headaches, pain, rapid pulse rate, nausea, wheezing, hives, bronchial irritation, coughs, and other such discomforts. Among the causes may be reactions to chemicals in foods, such as the flavor enhancer monosodium glutamate (MSG), the natural laxative in prunes, or the mineral sulfur; digestive diseases, such as obstructions or injuries; enzyme deficiencies, such as lactose intolerance; and even psychological aversions. These reactions involve symptoms but no antibody production. Therefore, they are food intolerances, not allergies.[27]

food allergies: adverse reactions to foods that involve an immune response; also called *food-hypersensitivity reactions*.

Food Allergies A true food allergy occurs when a whole food protein or other large molecule enters the body and elicits an immunologic response. (Recall that large molecules of food are normally dismantled in the digestive tract to smaller ones that are absorbed without such a reaction.) The body's immune system reacts to a large food molecule as it does to other antigens—by producing antibodies, histamines, or other defensive agents.

Allergies may have one or two components. They always involve antibodies; they may or may not involve symptoms. This means that allergies can be diagnosed only by testing for antibodies. Even symptoms exactly like those of an allergy may not be caused by one.

For help with food allergies, call the Food Allergy network at (800) 929-4040.

histamine (HISS-tah-mean, or HISS-tah-men)**:** a substance produced by cells of the immune system as part of a local immune reaction to an antigen; participates in causing inflammation.

A person who produces antibodies *without* having any symptoms has an **asymptomatic allergy**; a person who produces antibodies *and* has symptoms has a **symptomatic allergy**.

Allergic reactions to food may be immediate or delayed. In both cases, the antigen interacts immediately with the immune system, but the timing of symptoms varies from minutes to 24 hours. Identifying the food that causes an immediate allergic reaction is easy because the symptoms correlate closely with the time of eating the food. Identifying the food that causes a delayed reaction is more difficult because the symptoms may not appear until a day later. By this time, many other foods have been eaten, complicating the picture.

Almost 75 percent of adverse reactions are caused by three major foods—eggs, peanuts, or milk.[28] Allergic reactions to single foods are common. Reactions to multiple foods are the exception, not the rule.

Identifying a true food allergy requires a thorough health history, physical examination, and diagnostic tests to eliminate other diseases.[29] Skin pricks with food extracts are one of the most common tests for food allergies, even though the high incidence of false positive results can complicate diagnosis. Physicians also conduct dietary trials that first eliminate the offending food and then reintroduce it in small quantities to substantiate that reactions occur only when that particular food is eaten.[30] Once a food allergy has been diagnosed, therapy requires strict elimination of the offending food.

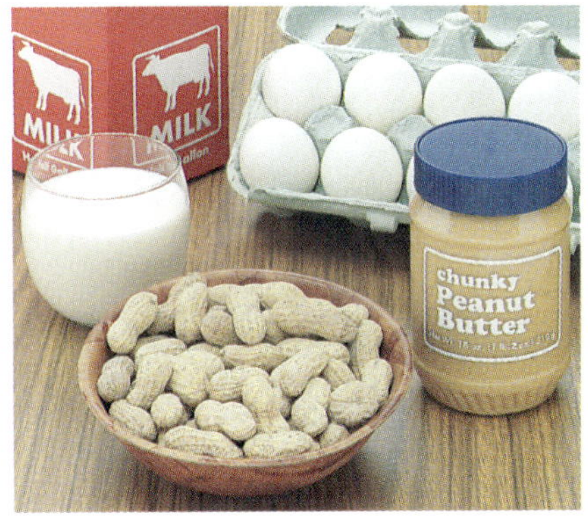

Eggs, peanuts, and milk are most likely to induce symptoms in people with food allergy.

Food allergies are most common during the first few years of life, but then children typically outgrow (become tolerant to) their hypersensitivity. Between 2 and 8 percent of young children are allergic to certain foods, whereas only 2 percent of adults have food allergies.[31] Tolerance is most likely if the offending food can be identified and eliminated from the diet for at least a year or two.[32]

When parents stop serving a suspected food to their child, they risk the child's suffering nutrient deficiencies. They should be sure to include other foods that offer the same nutrients as the omitted food. Children with allergies, like all children, need all their nutrients.

Healthful food choices and regular physical activity both promote growth and help prevent the degenerative diseases of later life—cardiovascular disease, cancer, diabetes, and osteoporosis. In contrast, poor food choices and lack of exercise can lead to obesity, elevated cholesterol levels, and hypertension—major risk factors for degenerative diseases. The highlight that follows this chapter describes how behaviors during the childhood and teen years influence disease in adulthood. The next two sections examine how children's eating behaviors are shaped both at home and at school.

MEALTIMES AT HOME

The childhood years represent a parent's best, and maybe last, chance to influence food choices. Parents are gatekeepers; they determine what foods and activities will be available in their children's environments. Then the children make their own selections. One survey reports that 65 percent of fourth through eighth graders choose their own breakfasts, 46 percent select their lunches, and 74 per-

gatekeepers: with respect to nutrition, key people who control other people's access to foods and thereby exert profound impacts on their nutrition. Examples are the spouse who buys and cooks the food, the parent who feeds the children, and the caretaker in a day-care center.

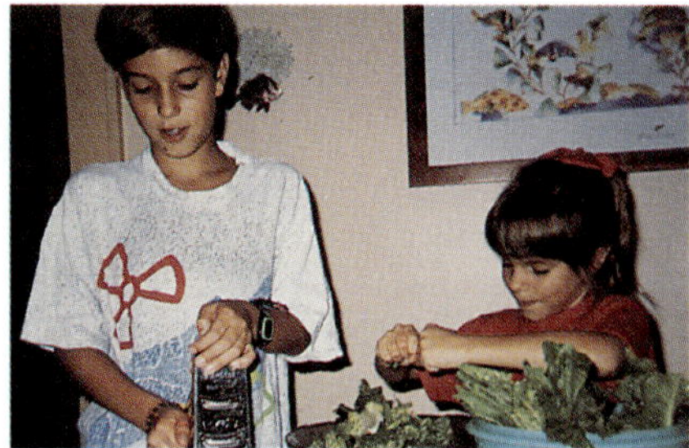

Children enjoy eating the foods they help to prepare.

cent select their snacks.[33] Gatekeepers who want to promote nutritious choices and healthful habits provide access to nutrient-dense, delicious foods and opportunities for active play at home.

- Child feeding pointer: Provide child-sized portions and utensils.
- Child feeding pointer: Serve vegetables raw or slightly undercooked and crunchy.

Honoring Children's Preferences Little children like to eat at little tables and to be served little portions of food. They also like to eat with other children, and they tend to eat more in the company of their peers. Children also more easily overcome their prejudices against foods when they see their peers eating them.

Children usually like raw vegetables better than cooked ones, so it is wise to offer vegetables that are raw or slightly undercooked and crunchy, served separately, and easy to eat. Foods should be warm, not hot, because a child's mouth is much more sensitive than an adult's. The flavor should be mild because a child has more taste buds, and smooth foods such as mashed potatoes or pea soup should contain no lumps (a child wonders, with some disgust, what the lumps might be). Children prefer foods that are familiar, so offer various foods regularly.

- Child feeding pointer: Encourage children to help plan and prepare meals.

Learning through Participation Helping to plan and prepare family meals can be an enjoyable learning experience. Children are also more likely to eat the foods they have prepared. Vegetables are pretty, especially when fresh, and provide opportunities for children to learn about color, about growing things and their seeds, and about shapes and textures—all of which are fascinating to young children. Measuring, stirring, washing, and arranging vegetables are skills that even a young child can practice with enjoyment and pride.

- Child feeding pointer: Offer children nutritious foods, but don't insist that they eat.

Avoiding Power Struggles When introducing new foods at the table, parents are advised to offer them one at a time and only in small amounts at first. The more often a food is presented to a young child, the more likely the child will like that food. Whenever possible, offer the new food at the beginning of the meal, when the child is hungry, and allow the child to make the decision to accept or reject it. Never make an issue of food acceptance, not even to reward acceptance. Children who are pushed to try new foods are less likely to try those foods again than children who are left to decide for themselves. The parent is responsible for *what* the child is offered to eat, but the child is responsible for *how much* and even *whether* to eat.

A bright, unhurried atmosphere free of conflict is conducive to good appetite. Parents who serve meals in a relaxed and casual manner, without anxiety, provide a climate that minimizes a child's negative emotions. Unaware parents can promote conflicts, despite their good intentions. Parents who beg, cajole, and demand that their children eat deny opportunities to develop self-control. Instead, the children engage in battles that take on more importance than their own hunger. A power struggle almost invariably results in a confirmed pattern of resistance and a permanently closed mind on the child's part.

- Child feeding pointer: To prevent choking, watch children eat and enforce a "sit-down" rule.

Young children can easily choke on:

- Popcorn.
- Whole grapes.
- Whole beans.
- Hot dog slices.
- Hard candies.
- Nuts.

Choking Prevention Parents must always be alert to the dangers of choking. A choking child is a silent child, and an adult should be present whenever a child is eating. Serve foods cut into small bite-size pieces and encourage children to sit when eating; choking is more likely when a child is running or falling. (Highlight 3 describes the Heimlich maneuver for children.)

- Child feeding pointer: Play first, then eat.

Play First Ideally, each meal is preceded, not followed, by fun activities. A number of schools have discovered that children eat a much better lunch if recess occurs before, rather than after, the meal—otherwise children "hurry up and eat" so that they can go play.

Snacks Parents may find that their children snack so much that they aren't hungry at mealtimes. Instead of teaching children *not* to snack, parents might be wise to teach them *how* to snack. Provide snacks that are as nutritious as the foods served at mealtime. Snacks can even be mealtime foods served individually over time, instead of all at once on one plate. When providing snacks to children, a smart parent thinks of the food groups and offers such snacks as pieces of cheese, tangerine slices, carrot sticks, and peanut butter on whole-wheat crackers. Snacks need to be easy to prepare, especially for children who arrive home from school before parents.

• Child feeding pointer: Provide healthful snacks.

Preventing Dental Caries Children frequently snack on sticky, sugary foods that stay on the teeth and provide an ideal environment for the growth of bacteria that cause dental caries. Teach children to eat sweets at mealtimes, to brush and floss after meals, to brush or rinse after eating snacks, to avoid sticky foods, and to select crisp or fibrous foods instead. Table 19–7 lists food suggestions for controlling dental caries.

Serving as Role Models In an effort to practice these many tips, parents may overlook perhaps the single most important influence on their children's food habits—themselves. Parents who don't eat carrots shouldn't be surprised when their children refuse to eat carrots. Likewise, parents who dislike the smell

• Child feeding pointer: Set a good example—enjoy nutritious foods.

Table 19–7

Food Suggestions for Controlling Dental Caries

Food Group	Frequent Use Recommended	Infrequent Use Suggested[a]
Milk/ milk products	Milk, cheese, plain yogurt	Chocolate milk, ice cream, ice milk, milk shakes, fruited yogurt
Meat/meat alternates	Lean meat, fish, poultry; eggs; legumes	Peanut butter with added sugar, lunch meats with added sugar, meats with sugared glazes
Fruits	Fresh or packed in water	Dried, packed in syrup or juice, jams, jellies, preserves, fruit juices or drinks
Vegetables	Salad greens, cauliflower, cucumbers, radishes, carrots, celery	Candied sweet potatoes, glazed carrots
Bread/cereal	Popcorn, soda crackers, toast, hard rolls, pretzels, corn chips, pizza	Cookies, sweet rolls, pies, cakes, potato chips, ready-to-eat sweetened cereals as between-meal snacks
Other	Sugarless gum	Sugared soft drinks, candy, fudge, caramels, honey, sugars, syrups

[a]It is particularly important to brush, floss, and rinse after eating these foods.

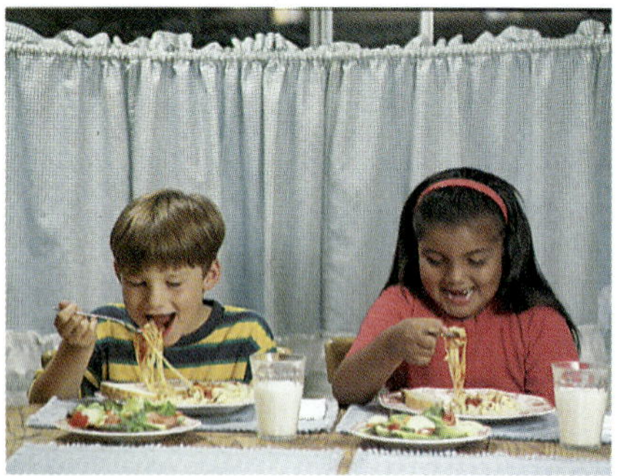

Eating is more fun when your friends are there.

of brussels sprouts may not be able to persuade children to try them. Children learn much through imitation. Parents and older siblings set an irresistible example by enjoying nutritious foods.

While serving and enjoying food, caretakers can promote both physical and emotional growth at every stage of a child's life. They can help their children to develop both a positive self-concept and a positive attitude toward food. If the beginnings are right, children will grow without the conflicts and confusions over food that can lead to nutrition and health problems.

NUTRITION AT SCHOOL

While parents are doing what they can to establish good eating habits in their children at home, child-care centers and schools are introducing foods prepared and served by others. In addition, children begin to learn about food and nutrition in the classroom. Meeting the nutrition and education needs of children is critical to supporting their healthy growth and development.[34]

School Meals The U.S. government funds several programs to provide nutritious meals for children at school. Both the School Breakfast Program and the National School Lunch Program provide meals at a reasonable cost to children from families with the financial means to pay. Meals are available free or at reduced cost to children from low-income families. (School lunches in Canada are administered locally and therefore vary from area to area.) Several studies have reported that children who participate in school food programs show improvements in learning. The accompanying box describes food programs for children, and Table 19–8 shows school lunch patterns for children of different ages.

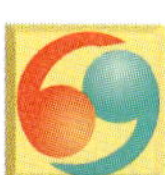

HEALTHY PEOPLE 2000: Increase to at least 90% the proportion of school lunch and breakfast services and increase to at least 50% the proportion of child-care foodservices with menus that are consistent with the nutrition principles in the *Dietary Guidelines for Americans*.

Table 19–8

School Lunch Patterns for Different Ages

Food Group	Preschool (Age)		Grade School through High School (Grade)		
	1 TO 2	3 TO 4	K TO 3	4 TO 6	7 TO 12
Meat or meat alternate					
1 serving:					
Lean meat, poultry, or fish	1 oz	1½ oz	1½ oz	2 oz	3 oz
Cheese	1 oz	1½ oz	1½ oz	2 oz	3 oz
Large egg(s)	1	1½	1½	2	3
Cooked dry beans or peas	½ c	¾ c	¾ c	1 c	1½ c
Peanut butter	2 tbs	3 tbs	3 tbs	4 tbs	6 tbs
Vegetable and/or fruit					
2 or more servings, both to total	½ c	½ c	½ c	¾ c	¾ c
Bread or bread alternate					
Servings	5 per week	8 per week	8 per week	8 per week	10 per week
Milk					
1 serving of fluid milk	¾ c	¾ c	1 c	1 c	1 c

Food Assistance Programs for Children

The federal School Lunch and School Breakfast Programs assist schools financially so that every student can receive a nutritious lunch, breakfast, or both. These programs enable schools to provide low-income students with meals at no cost while charging other students somewhat less than the full costs of their meals. In addition, schools that participate in the programs can obtain food commodities. Nationally, the U.S. Department of Agriculture (USDA) administers the programs; on the state level, state departments of education operate them (although Congress may change this arrangement in its efforts to cut federal spending). The programs usually cost school districts little.

Nearly 25 million children receive lunches through the National School Lunch Program—half of them at a free or reduced price. School lunches are designed to provide at least a third of the RDA for each of many nutrients and must include specified numbers of servings of milk, protein-rich foods (meat, poultry, fish, cheese, eggs, legumes, or peanut butter), vegetables, fruits, and breads or other grain foods.

The School Breakfast Program is available in slightly more than half of the nation's schools, and about 5 million children participate in it. The school breakfast must provide at least a fourth of the RDA for each of many nutrients and contain at least one serving of milk; one serving of fruit, juice, or vegetable; and either two servings of bread (or bread alternates), two servings of meat (or meat alternates), or one serving of each.

Another federal program, the Child Care Food Program, operates similarly and provides funds to organized child-care programs. All eligible children, centers, and family day-care homes have the right to participate. Meal reimbursements cover most of the meal and administration costs. Sponsors may also receive USDA commodity foods.

School lunches offer a variety of food choices and are available to most children. To their credit, these lunches help our nation's children meet at least one-third of their daily RDA. These lunches are supposed to meet the *Dietary Guidelines*, but unfortunately, almost all of the participating schools exceed recommendations for fat, saturated fat, and sodium and fall short on recommendations for carbohydrate.[35] Yet given the choice, many children will select low-fat meals.[36] Schools that have made special efforts to lower fat in school lunches typically have trouble providing enough energy and nutrients, especially iron, to meet the RDA specifications. The American Dietetic Association (ADA) advocates the development of dietary guidelines specifically for children to ensure that school lunches will both provide adequate energy and nutrients and support health.[37] According to the ADA, the guidelines currently used may be appropriate for adults, but may not be adequate to meet children's unique needs.

Nutrition Education at School Coincident with the school breakfast and lunch programs is a program of nutrition education and training (NET) in all the public schools. This program is minimally funded, but program administrators are ingenious and creative in accomplishing its highest-priority objectives. Children need to be fed well *and* learn enough about nutrition to make healthful food choices when the choices become theirs to make.

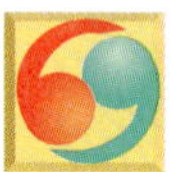

HEALTHY PEOPLE 2000: Increase to at least 75% the proportion of the nation's schools that provide nutrition education from preschool through grade 12, preferably as part of quality school health education.

In summary, children's appetites and nutrient needs reflect their stage of growth. Those who are chronically hungry and malnourished suffer growth retardation; when hunger is temporary and nutrient deficiencies are mild, the problems are usually more subtle—such as poor academic performance. Iron deficiency is widespread and has many physical and behavioral consquences. "Hyper" behavior is not caused by poor nutrition, but may reflect too much caffeine and inconsistent care, including too much television watching, which can contribute to obesity by promoting inactivity and an overconsumption of snack foods. Adults at home and at school need to provide children with nutrient-dense foods and teach them how to make healthful choices.

Nutrition during Adolescence

adolescence: the period from the beginning of puberty until maturity.

Nutrient needs are greater during adolescence than at any other time of life, except for pregnancy and lactation. In general, nutrient needs rise throughout childhood and then level off or even diminish slightly as the adolescent passes into adulthood.

Teenagers make many more choices for themselves than they did as children. They are not fed, they eat; they are not sent out to play, they choose to go. At the same time, social pressures thrust choices at them: whether to drink alcoholic beverages and whether to develop their bodies to meet extreme ideals of slimness or athletic prowess.

Adolescents learn about nutrition—both valid information and misinformation—from personal, immediate experiences. They are concerned with how diet can improve their lives now—they engage in crash dieting in order to buy a new bathing suit, avoid greasy foods in an effort to clear acne, or eat a pile of spaghetti to prepare for a big sporting event. The person concerned with the nutrition and health of adolescents, then, must learn about these subjects of interest and show the relationships with nutrition.

GROWTH AND DEVELOPMENT

The steady growth of childhood speeds up abruptly and dramatically with the onset of adolescence, and female and male growth patterns become distinct. A female's adolescent growth spurt begins at age 10 or 11 and reaches its peak at 12. A male's growth spurt begins at 12 or 13 and peaks at 14.

Gender differences become apparent in the skeletal system, lean body mass, and fat stores. In females, fat becomes a larger percentage of the total body weight, and in males, the lean body mass—muscle and bone—becomes much greater. On the average, males grow 8 inches taller during the growth spurt;

females, 6 inches. Males add approximately 45 pounds to their weight; females, about 35 pounds. Hormonal changes profoundly affect every organ of the body, including the brain, and within two or three years, physically mature adults emerge.

Teenagers' rates and patterns of growth exhibit such wide variations that growth charts used for children must be abandoned when the signs of puberty begin to appear. Age in years indicates little about development; one way to be sure a teenager is growing normally is to compare his or her height and weight with previous measures. To record developmental changes during puberty, health care professionals use standard rating scales based on stages of adolescent development.[38]

puberty: the period in life in which a person becomes physically capable of reproduction.

ENERGY AND NUTRIENT NEEDS

As children become adults, they change in many ways. Their physical changes make their nutrient needs high, and their emotional, intellectual, and social changes make meeting those needs a challenge.

Energy Intake and Activity The energy needs of adolescents vary to a great extent, depending on the current rate of growth, body size, and physical activity. Boys' energy needs may be especially high; they grow faster and, as mentioned, develop more lean body mass. An active boy of 15 may need 4000 kcalories or more a day just to maintain his weight. Girls start growing earlier than boys and attain lower body weights, so their energy needs peak sooner and decline more quickly than those of their male peers. An inactive girl of 15 whose growth is nearly at a standstill may need fewer than 2000 kcalories a day if she is to avoid excessive weight gain. Thus adolescent girls need to pay special attention to being physically active and selecting foods of high nutrient density in order to meet their nutrient needs without exceeding their energy needs.

The insidious problem of obesity becomes apparent in adolescence and often continues into adulthood; it occurs mostly in females, especially in African-American females.[39] Young women who become interested in nutrition may make choices that will benefit their fitness, or they may become unhealthily obsessed with weight control (see Highlight 9).

Iron Iron remains a nutrient of special concern. Iron needs increase in females as they start to menstruate and in males as their lean body mass develops. Adolescent iron intakes often fail to keep pace with increasing needs, especially for females, who typically consume less iron-rich meat and fewer total kcalories than males.[40]

Iron RDA during adolescence:
12 mg/day (males).
15 mg/day (females).

Calcium Adolescence is a crucial time for bone development, and the requirement for calcium reaches its peak during these years.[41] Unfortunately, many adolescents have calcium intakes below current recommendations.[42] Low calcium intakes during the adolescent growth spurt, especially if paired with physical inactivity, may compromise the development of peak bone mass. As emphasized earlier, the attainment of maximal bone mass is considered the best protection against age-related bone loss and fractures.[43] Once again, teenage girls are at greatest risk, for their milk—and therefore calcium—intakes begin to decline at the time when their calcium needs are greatest.

Calcium DRI during adolescence:
1300 mg/day.

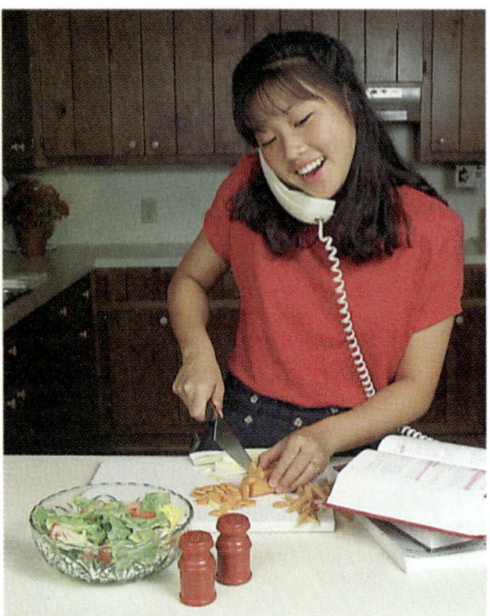

Nutritious snacks play an important role in an active teen's diet.

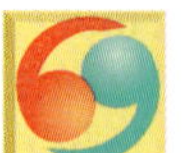

HEALTHY PEOPLE 2000: Increase calcium intake, so that at least 50% of youth aged 12 through 24 years consume three or more servings of calcium-rich foods daily.

FOOD CHOICES AND HEALTH HABITS

Teenagers come and go as they choose and eat what they want when they have time. With a multitude of after-school, social, and job activities, they almost inevitably fall into irregular eating habits. The teenage snacker who finds only nutritious foods around the house is well provided for.

Snacks Snacks typically provide at least a fourth of the average teenager's daily food energy intake. Snacks often fail to provide enough calcium, iron, vitamin A, and folate. Many adolescents need to eat a greater variety of foods to obtain these nutrients. Table 19–9 shows how to combine foods from different food groups to create healthy snacks. Most vending machines offer few nutrient-dense options, and nutrition information alone does not convince people to make healthy choices.[44]

The nutritive values of selected fast foods are presented in Appendix H.

Eating Away from Home Inevitably, adolescents do a lot of eating away from home, and their nutritional welfare is enhanced or hindered by the choices they make. A lunch of a hamburger, a chocolate shake, and french fries supplies substantial quantities of many nutrients, as shown in Table 19–10, at a kcalorie cost of 800, an energy cost many adolescents can afford. When they eat this sort of lunch, teens can balance their diets by adjusting their breakfast and dinner choices. They need to select fruits and vegetables for vitamins A, C, folate, and fiber, and lean meats for iron and zinc at their other meals.

Table 19–10

Selected Nutrients in a Hamburger, Chocolate Shake, and Small Serving of French Fries

Nutrient	Male[a] % RDA	Female[a] % RDA
Energy	30	35
Protein	47	64
Fat[b]	26	31
Calcium[c]	35	35
Iron	30	24
Zinc	16	20
Vitamin A	9	11
Thiamin	41	48
Riboflavin	42	49
Niacin	35	41
Folate	18	20
Vitamin C	7	7
Sodium[b]	34	34

[a]RDA for a 15- to 18-year-old, moderately active person of average height and weight.
[b]Daily Values used for fat and sodium.
[c]Reflects DRI value.

Peer Influence Many of the food and health choices adolescents make reflect the opinions and actions of their peers. When others perceive milk as "babyish," a teen will choose soft drinks instead; when others skip lunch and hang out in the parking lot, a teen may join in for the camaraderie, regardless of hunger. Adults need to remember that teenagers have the right to make their own decisions—even if they are contrary to the adults' views. Gatekeepers can set up the environment so that nutritious foods are available and can stand by with reliable nutrition information and advice, but the rest is up to the adolescents. Ultimately, they make the choices. Highlight 9 examines the influence of social pressures on the development of eating disorders.

PROBLEMS ADOLESCENTS FACE

Physical maturity and growing independence present adolescents with new choices to make. The consequences of those choices will influence their nutritional health both today and throughout life. Some teenagers begin using drugs, alcohol, and tobacco; others wisely refrain. Information about the use of these substances is presented here because most people are first exposed to them during adolescence, but it actually applies to people of all ages.

Marijuana Three of every five high school seniors report that they have at least tried an illicit drug, most commonly marijuana. The body processes all sub-

Table 19–9

Healthful Snack Ideas—Think Food Groups, Alone and in Combination

Selecting two or more foods from different food groups adds variety and nutrient balance to snacks. The combinations are endless, so be creative.

Grain Products

Grain products are filling snacks, especially when combined with other foods:
- Cereal with fruit and milk.
- Crackers and cheese.
- Wheat toast with peanut butter.
- Popcorn with grated cheese.
- Oatmeal raisin cookies with milk.

Vegetables

Cut-up fresh, raw vegetables make great snacks alone or in combination with foods from other food groups:
- Celery with peanut butter.
- Broccoli, cauliflower, and carrot sticks with a flavored cottage cheese dip.

Fruits

Fruits are delicious snacks and can be eaten alone—fresh, dried, or juiced—or combined with other foods:
- Apples and cheese.
- Bananas and peanut butter.
- Peaches with yogurt.
- Raisins mixed with sunflower seeds or nuts.

Meats and Meat Alternates

Meat and meat alternates add protein to snacks:
- Refried beans with nachos and cheese.
- Tuna on crackers.
- Luncheon meat on wheat bread.

Milk and Milk Products

Milk can be used as a beverage with any snack, and many other milk products, such as yogurt and cheese, can be eaten alone or with other foods as listed above.

stances, and marijuana is no exception. The active ingredients are rapidly and almost completely absorbed from the lungs.* Then, being fat soluble, these substances are packaged in lipoproteins before traveling in the blood to the various body tissues. The liver and other tissues metabolize these substances, and their remnants linger in the body for several days, being gradually excreted for a week or more after the smoking of a single marijuana cigarette. With repeated exposure, these substances accumulate in body fat, the lungs, the liver, the reproductive organs, and the brain.

---

*The active ingredient of marijuana, which is primarily responsible for its intoxicating effects, is delta-9-tetrahydrocannabinol, or THC.

Smoking a marijuana cigarette seems to enhance the enjoyment of eating, especially of sweets, a phenomenon commonly known as "the munchies." Why or how this effect occurs is not known; it may be a social effect induced by suggestibility, or it may be that the drug stimulates appetite. Prolonged use of the drug does not seem to bring about a weight gain.

Marijuana users may think that because they usually smoke fewer marijuana cigarettes in a day than they would tobacco cigarettes, their lungs will incur fewer harmful, long-term effects. This is a myth. One marijuana cigarette is as bad for the body as four or five tobacco cigarettes, because people who smoke marijuana inhale more smoke and hold it in their lungs longer. People who regularly smoke several marijuana cigarettes a day face the same risk of lung cancer as people who smoke a pack of tobacco cigarettes a day.[45]

Reminder: *Euphoria* is an inflated sense of well-being and pleasure brought on by some drugs; popularly called a *high*.

Cocaine One in 20 high school seniors reports having used cocaine at least once.[46] Cocaine elicits diverse effects: intense euphoria, restlessness, heightened self-confidence, irritability, insomnia, and loss of appetite. Weight loss is common, and cocaine abusers often develop eating disorders. Notably, the craving for cocaine replaces hunger; rats given unlimited cocaine will choose it over food until they starve to death. Thus, unlike marijuana use, cocaine use has major nutritional consequences.

Cocaine can cause rapid and irregular heartbeats, heart attacks, and even death. Its use continues to escalate as cheaper and more addictive forms become available. In its smokable form, crack cocaine is more addicting than any other drug. One former crack addict tells of holding a gun to his brother's head to steal money for his next drug purchase.

Nutrition problems of drug abusers:

- They buy drugs with money that could be spent on food.
- They lose interest in food during "highs."
- Some drugs depress appetite.
- Their lifestyle fails to promote good eating habits.
- If they use intravenous (IV) drugs, they may contract AIDS, hepatitis, or other infectious diseases, which increase their nutrient needs. Hepatitis also causes taste changes and loss of appetite.
- Medicines used to treat drug abusers may alter their nutrition status.

Drug Abuse, in General The effects of other addictive drugs vary in degree but are similar in kind to those caused by cocaine. Drug abusers face the multiple nutrition problems listed in the margin. During withdrawal from drugs, an important part of treatment is to identify and correct these nutrition problems.

Alcohol Abuse Sooner or later all teenagers face the decision whether to drink alcohol. The law forbids the sale of alcohol to people under a specific age, but most adolescents who seek alcohol find it easy to obtain.

Many adolescents find that alcohol and marijuana serve similar purposes, and the pattern of substance use indicates parallel consumption, not a displacement of one by the other. Some adolescents use alcohol as an escape or for support—an ineffective way to cope with problems that leads to greater problems. Dependency on any drug severely impairs development and deserves attention, but is beyond the scope of this text.

Highlight 7 describes how alcohol affects nutrition status. To sum it up, alcohol is an empty-kcalorie beverage that can displace nutritious foods from the diet. It alters nutrient absorption and metabolism, so that imbalances develop. People who cannot keep their alcohol use moderate must abstain to maintain their health.

Tobacco Cigarette smoking is a pervasive health problem causing thousands of people to suffer from cancer and diseases of the cardiovascular, digestive, and respiratory systems. These effects are beyond the scope of nutrition, but smoking cigarettes does influence hunger, body weight, and nutrient status. Links between nutrients and lung cancer are also known.

Smoking a cigarette eases feelings of hunger. When smokers receive a hunger signal, they can quiet it with cigarettes instead of food. Such behavior ignores body signals and postpones energy and nutrient intake. Studies on rats confirm that nicotine reduces food intake, causing weight loss.[47]

Indeed, smokers tend to weigh less than nonsmokers and to gain weight when they stop smoking.[48] Weight gain is often a concern for people contemplating giving up cigarettes. They should know that the average person who quits smoking gains less than 10 pounds. Smokers wanting to quit need to prepare for this possibility and adjust their diet and activity habits so as to maintain weight during and after quitting. Smoking cessation programs need to include strategies for weight management.

Nutrient intakes of smokers and nonsmokers differ. Smokers tend to have lower intakes of dietary fiber, vitamin A, beta-carotene, folate, and vitamin C.[49] The association between smoking and low vitamin intake may be noteworthy, considering the altered metabolism of vitamin C in smokers and the protective effect of vitamin A and beta-carotene against lung cancer.

Research shows that compared to nonsmokers, smokers require almost twice as much vitamin C to maintain steady body pools. Oxidants in cigarette smoke accelerate vitamin C metabolism and deplete smokers' body stores of this antioxidant; this depletion is even evident to some degree in nonsmokers who are exposed to passive smoke.[50]

The vitamin C RDA for people who regularly smoke cigarettes is 100 mg/day. The Canadian RNI suggests smokers should add 50% to the vitamin C recommendation.

Beta-carotene enhances the immune response and protects against some cancer activity.[51] Specifically, the risk of lung cancer is greatest for smokers who have the lowest intakes of carotene. Of course, such evidence should not be misinterpreted. It does not mean that as long as people eat their carrots, they can safely use tobacco. Smokers are ten times more likely to get lung cancer than nonsmokers. Both smokers and nonsmokers can, however, reduce their cancer risks by eating fruits and vegetables rich in carotene (see Highlight 11 for details on antioxidant nutrients and disease prevention).

To review, nutrient needs rise dramatically as children enter the rapid growth phase of the teen years. The busy lifestyles of teenagers add to the challenge of meeting their nutrient needs—especially for iron and calcium. In addition to making wise foods choices, teenagers need to refrain from using substances that will impair their health—including illicit drugs, tobacco, and alcohol.

The nutrition and lifestyle choices people make as children and teenagers have long-term, as well as immediate, effects on their health. Highlight 19 describes how sound choices and good habits during childhood can help prevent disease later in life.

Study Questions

1. Describe some of the nutrient and immunological attributes of breast milk.
2. What are the appropriate uses of formula feeding? What criteria would you use in selecting an infant formula?
3. Why are solid foods not recommended for an infant during the first few months of life? When is an infant ready to start eating solid food?
4. Name foods that are inappropriate for infants and explain why they are inappropriate.

(continued on the next page)

5. What nutrition problems are most common in children? What strategies can help prevent them?
6. Describe the relationships between nutrition and behavior. How does television influence nutrition?
7. Describe a true food allergy. Which foods most often cause allergic reactions? How do food allergies influence nutrition status?
8. List strategies for introducing nutritious foods to children.
9. What impact do school meal programs have on the nutrition status of children?
10. Describe the changes in nutrient needs from childhood to adolescence. Why is a teenaged girl more likely to develop an iron deficiency than is a boy?
11. How do teen eating habits influence their nutrient intakes?
12. How does the use of illicit drugs influence nutrition status?
13. How do the nutrient intakes of smokers differ from those of nonsmokers? What impacts can those differences exert on health?

Notes

1. P. S. W. Davies, Energy requirements and energy expenditure in infancy, *European Journal of Clinical Nutrition* (supplement 4) 46 (1992): S29–S35.
2. H. L. Greene and coauthors, Vitamins for newborn infant formulas: A review of recommendations with emphasis on data from low birth-weight infants, *European Journal of Clinical Nutrition* 46 (1992): S1–S8.
3. Committee on Nutrition, American Academy of Pediatrics, *Pediatric Nutrition Handbook,* 3rd ed., ed. L. A. Barness (Elk Grove Village, Ill.: American Academy of Pediatrics, 1993), pp. 23–33.
4. American Academy of Pediatrics, Committee on Nutrition, The use of whole cow's milk in infancy, *Pediatrics* 89 (1992): 1105–1109.
5. Position of The American Dietetic Association: Promotion and support of breast feeding, *Journal of the American Dietetic Association* 93 (1993): 467–469.
6. J. S. Forsyth, Is it worthwhile breast-feeding? *European Journal of Clinical Nutrition* (supplement 1) 46 (1993): 519–525.
7. A. C. Goedhart and J. G. Bindels, The composition of human milk as a model for the design of infant formulas: Recent findings and possible applications, *Nutrition Research Reviews* 7 (1994): 1–23.
8. N. F. Butte, E. O. Smith, and C. Garza, Energy utilization of breast-fed and formula-fed infants, *American Journal of Clinical Nutrition* 51 (1990): 350–358.
9. M. J. Heinig and coauthors, Energy and protein intakes of breast-fed and formula-fed infants during the first year of life and their association with growth velocity: The DARLING Study, *American Journal of Clinical Nutrition* 58 (1993): 152–161.
10. Committee on Nutritional Status during Pregnancy and Lactation, *Nutrition during Lactation* (Washington, D.C.: National Academy Press, 1991), pp. 155–156.
11. M. W. Shannon and J. W. Graef, Lead intoxication in infancy, *Pediatrics* 89 (1992): 87–90.
12. D. Stehlin, Soy beverages not complete formulas, *FDA Consumer,* September 1990, p. 29.
13. S. Ryan, Bone mineralization and growth, *European Journal of Clinical Nutrition* 46 (1992): S41–S44.
14. T. Walter and coauthors, Effectiveness of iron-fortified infant cereal in prevention of iron deficiency anemia, *Pediatrics* 91 (1993): 976–982; G. J. Fuchs and coauthors, Iron status and intake of older infants fed formula vs cow milk with cereal, *American Journal of Clinical Nutrition* 58 (1993): 343–348.
15. M. M. Smith and F. Lifshitz, Excess fruit juice consumption as a contributing factor in nonorganic failure to thrive, *Pediatrics* 93 (1994): 438–443.
16. S. A. Sullivan and L. L. Birch, Infant dietary experience and acceptance of solid foods, *Pediatrics* 93 (1994): 271–277.
17. L. L. Birch and coauthors, Effects of a nonenergy fat substitute on children's energy and macronutrient intake, *American Journal of Clinical Nutrition* 58 (1993): 326–333; S. Shea and coauthors, Variability and self-regulation of energy intake in young children in their everyday environment, *Pediatrics* 90 (1992): 542–546; L. L. Birch and coauthors, The variability of young children's energy intake, *New England Journal of Medicine* 324 (1991): 232–235.
18. R. E. Klesges and coauthors, Parental influence on food selection in young children and its relationships to childhood obesity, *American Journal of Clinical Nutrition* 53 (1991): 859–864.
19. T. A. Nicklas and coauthors, Breakfast consumption affects adequacy of total daily intake in children, *Journal of the American Dietetic Association* 93 (1993): 886–891.
20. P. L. Splett and M. Story, Child nutrition: Objectives for the decade, *Journal of the American Dietetic Association* 91 (1991): 665–668.
21. N. S. Scrimshaw, Iron deficiency, *Scientific American,* October 1991, pp. 46–52.
22. B. Lozoff, E. Jimenez, and A. W. Wolf, Long-term developmental outcome of infants with iron deficiency, *New England Journal of Medicine* 325 (1991): 687–694.

23. F. A. Oski, Iron deficiency in infancy and childhood, *New England Journal of Medicine* 329 (1993): 190–193; S. J. Fairweather-Tait, Iron deficiency in infancy: Easy to prevent—or is it? *European Journal of Clinical Nutrition* (supplement 4) 46 (1992): S9–S14.
24. D. A. Gans, Sucrose and unusual childhood behavior, *Nutrition Today*, May/June 1991, pp. 8–14; E. H. Wender and M. V. Solanto, Effects of sugar on aggressive and inattentive behavior in children with attention deficit disorder with hyperactivity and normal children, *Pediatrics* 88 (1991): 960–966; J. A. Bachorowshi and coauthors, Sucrose and delinquency: Behavioral assessment, *Pediatrics* 86 (1990): 244–253.
25. R. Zoglin, Is TV ruining our children? *Time*, October 15, 1990, p. 75.
26. R. C. Klesges, M. L. Shelton, and L. M. Klesges, Effects of television on metabolic rate: Potential implications for childhood obesity, *Pediatrics* 91 (1993): 281–286.
27. H. A. Sampson and D. D. Metcalfe, Food allergies, *Journal of the American Medical Association* 268 (1992): 2840–2844.
28. S. A. Bock and F. M. Atkins, Patterns of food hypersensitivity during sixteen years of double-blind, placebo-controlled food challenges, *Journal of Pediatrics* 117 (1990): 561–567.
29. Sampson and Metcalfe, 1992.
30. V. L. Olejer, Food hypersensitivities, *Handbook of Pediatric Nutrition* (Gaithersburg, Md.: Aspen Publishers, 1993), pp. 206–231.
31. A. T. Hingley, Food allergies: When eating is risky, *FDA Consumer*, December 1993, pp. 27–31.
32. Sampson and Metcalfe, 1992.
33. National Center for Nutrition and Dietetics, International Food Information Council, Kids at the table: Who's placing the orders? (Chicago: American Dietetic Association, 1991).
34. Position of The American Dietetic Association: Nutrition standards for child care programs, *Journal of the American Dietetic Association* 94 (1994): 323.
35. K. Schuster, Feds put schools on a lowfat diet, *Food Management* 29 (1994): 78–84; J. Burghardt and B. Devaney, The School Nutrition Dietary Assessment Study: Summary of findings, Food and Nutrition Service, U.S. Department of Agriculture, October 1993.
36. R. C. Whitaker and coauthors, An environmental intervention to reduce dietary fat in school lunches, *Pediatrics* 91 (1993): 1107–1111.
37. Timely statement of The American Dietetic Association: Dietary guidance for healthy children, *Journal of the American Dietetic Association* 95 (1995): 370.
38. L. E. Underwood, Normal adolescent growth and development, *Nutrition Today*, March/April 1991, pp. 11–16.
39. T. A. Wadden and coauthors, Obesity in black adolescent girls: A controlled clinical trial of treatment by diet, behavior modification, and parental support, *Pediatrics* 85 (1990): 345–352.
40. J. B. Anderson, The status of adolescent nutrition, *Nutrition Today*, March/April 1991, pp. 7–10.
41. S. M. Ott, Bone density in adolescents, *New England Journal of Medicine* 325 (1991): 1646–1647.
42. S. I. Barr, Associations of social and demographic variables with calcium intakes of high school students, *Journal of the American Dietetic Association* 94 (1994): 260–266, 269.
43. V. Matkovic, Diet, genetics, and peak bone mass of adolescent girls, *Nutrition Today*, March/April 1991, pp. 21–24.
44. S. M. Hoerr and V. A. Louden, Can nutrition information increase sales of healthful vended snacks? *Journal of School Health* 63 (1993): 386–390.
45. T. C. Wu and coauthors, Pulmonary hazards of smoking marijuana as compared with tobacco, *New England Journal of Medicine* 318 (1988): 347–351.
46. American Council on Science and Health, *Cocaine: Facts and Dangers* (New York: American Council on Science and Health, 1990).
47. S. R. Schwid, M. D. Hirvonen, and R. E. Keesey, Nicotine effects on body weight: A regulatory perspective, *American Journal of Clinical Nutrition* 55 (1992): 878–884.
48. D. F. Williamson and coauthors, Smoking cessation and severity of weight gain in a national cohort, *New England Journal of Medicine* 324 (1991): 739–745.
49. T. A. B. Sanders and coauthors, Essential fatty acids, plasma cholesterol and fat-soluble vitamins in subjects with age-related maculopathy and matched control subjects, *American Journal of Clinical Nutrition* 57 (1993): 428–433; A. F. Subar, L. C. Harlan, and M. E. Mattson, Food and nutrient intake differences between smokers and non-smokers in the US, *American Journal of Public Health* 80 (1990): 1323–1329.
50. D. L. Tribble, L. J. Giuliano, and S. P. Fortmann, Reduced plasma ascorbic acid concentrations in nonsmokers regularly exposed to environmental tobacco smoke, *American Journal of Clinical Nutrition* 58 (1993): 886–890.
51. G. van Poppel, S. Spanhaak, and T. Ockhuizen, Effect of β-carotene on immunological indexes in healthy male smokers, *American Journal of Clinical Nutrition* 57 (1993): 402–407; T. V. Ringer and coauthors, Beta-carotene's effects on serum lipoproteins and immunologic indices in humans, *American Journal of Clinical Nutrition* 53 (1991): 688–694.

Highlight 19

Childhood Obesity and the Early Development of Chronic Diseases

When people think of the health problems of children and adolescents, they typically think of measles and acne, not cardiovascular disease (CVD). They think of CVD as the number one killer of adults in the United States and Canada, but CVD begins in childhood.[1]

Much of our knowledge about the early development of CVD comes from the Bogalusa Heart Study, a long-term epidemiological study of some 14,000 young people. For nearly three decades, researchers have been observing how changes in body weight, blood lipids, blood pressure, and individual behaviors correlate with the development of CVD over time—from infancy to childhood through adolescence and into young adulthood. Some major findings have emerged from the research:

- Changes inside the arteries—changes predictive of CVD—are evident in childhood.
- Obesity in children affects these changes.
- Behaviors that influence the development of obesity and of CVD are learned and begin early in life. These behaviors include overeating, eating high-fat foods, physical inactivity, and cigarette smoking.

This highlight focuses on efforts to prevent childhood obesity and CVD, but the benefits extend to cancer, diabetes, and other chronic diseases as well. The years of childhood are emphasized here, for the earlier in life health-promoting habits become established, the better they will stick.

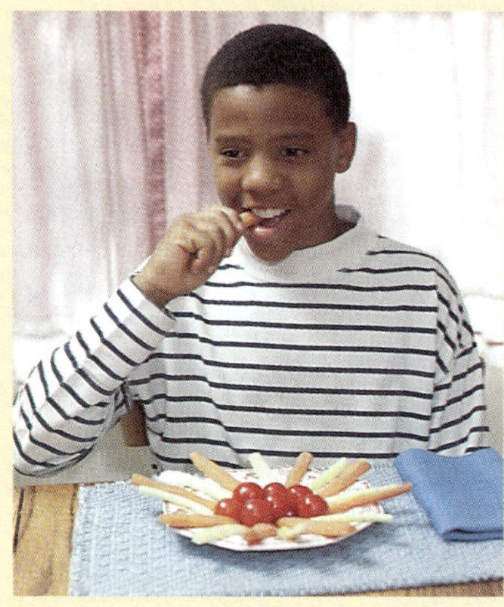

Take care of your body and your body will take care of you.

Invariably, questions arise as to what extent genetics is involved in CVD development. Children who are obese and who have high blood lipids and high blood pressure are often from families with a history of CVD. Genetics does not appear to play a *determining* role in CVD; that is, a person is not simply destined at birth to develop CVD.[2] Instead, genetics appears to play a *permissive* role—the potential is inherited and then will develop, if given a push by poor health choices such as excessive weight gain, poor diet, sedentary lifestyle, and cigarette smoking.

EARLY DEVELOPMENT OF CVD

Most people consider CVD to be an adult disease: its incidence rises with advancing age, and symptoms rarely appear before age 30. The disease process begins much earlier, though.

Atherosclerosis

Most CVD involves atherosclerosis—the accumulation of cholesterol and other blood lipids along the walls of the arteries. Atherosclerosis eventually blocks the flow of blood to the heart and causes a heart attack, or cuts off blood flow to the brain and causes a stroke. Infants are born with healthy, smooth, clear arteries, but within the first decade of life, fatty streaks may begin to appear (see Figure H19–1). During adolescence, these fatty streaks may begin to turn to fibrous plaques. By early adulthood, the fibrous plaques may begin to calcify and become raised lesions, especially in boys and young men.[3] As the lesions grow more numerous and enlarge, the heart disease rate begins to rise, and the rise becomes dramatic at about age 45 in men and 55 in women.[4] From this point on, arterial damage and blockage progress rapidly, and heart attacks and strokes threaten life. In short, the consequences of atherosclerosis, which become apparent only in adulthood, have their beginnings in the first decades of life.[5]

Atherosclerosis is not inevitable; people can grow old with relatively clear arteries. Early lesions may either progress or regress, depending on several factors, many of which reflect lifestyle behaviors. Smoking, for example, is strongly associated

Figure H19–1

The Formation of Plaques in Atherosclerosis

When plaques have covered 60 percent of the coronary artery walls, the critical phase of heart disease begins.

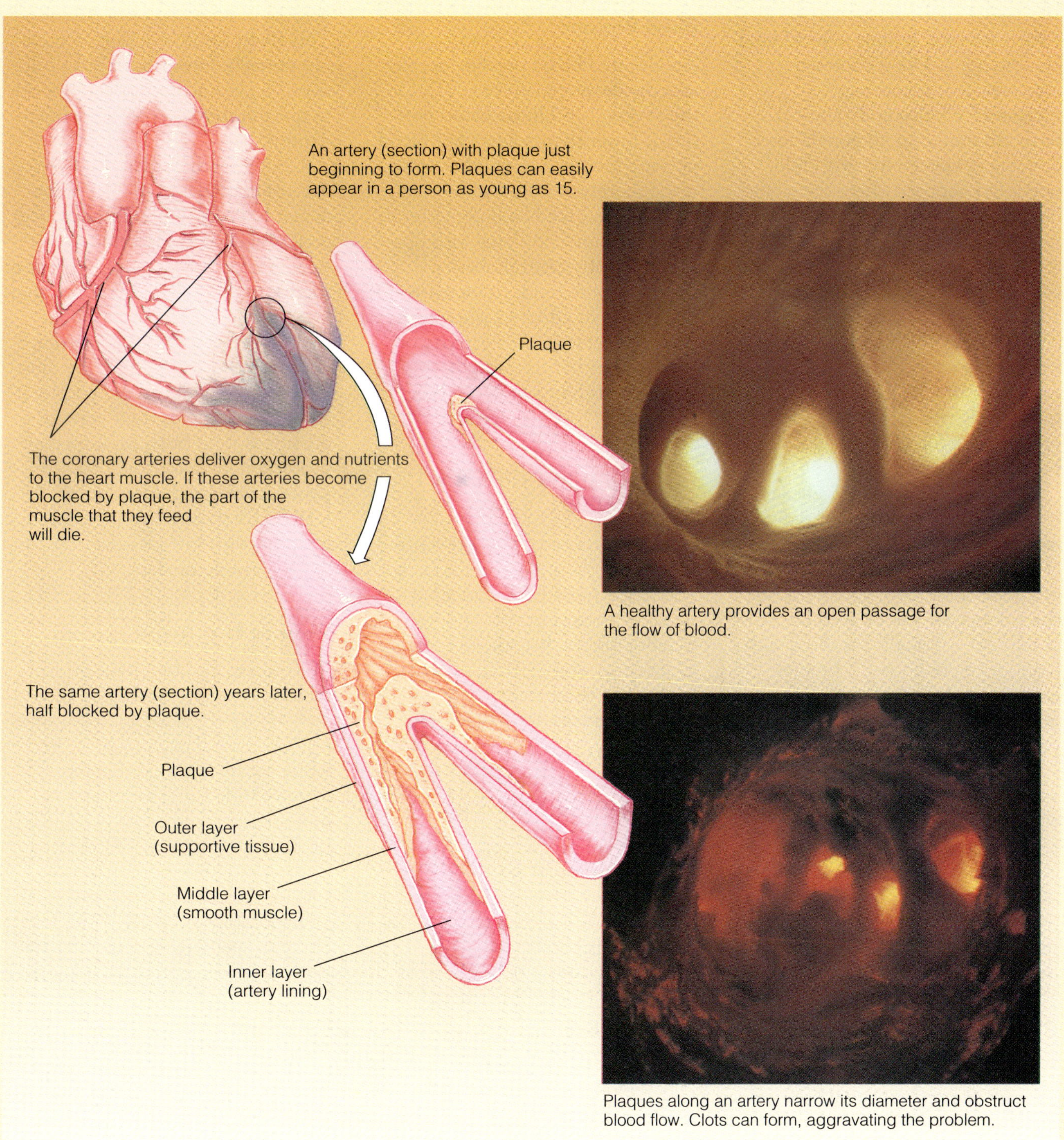

A healthy artery provides an open passage for the flow of blood.

Plaques along an artery narrow its diameter and obstruct blood flow. Clots can form, aggravating the problem.

with the prevalence of raised lesions, even in young adults.[6]

Blood Cholesterol

Atherosclerotic lesions reflect blood cholesterol: as blood cholesterol increases, lesion coverage increases.[7] Cholesterol values at birth are similar in all populations; differences emerge in early childhood. In countries where the adults have high blood cholesterol and high rates of CVD, the children also tend to have high blood cholesterol. Conversely, in countries where the adults have low blood cholesterol and low rates of CVD, the children tend to have low blood cholesterol, suggesting that adult heart disease tracks early trends and that early preventive efforts might reduce the incidence of later CVD.[8]

The studies just described examined population trends; but individual cholesterol status also becomes established in early childhood. At one year, cholesterol values predict the values that will be seen later in childhood, especially for those with high blood cholesterol.[9] Studies examining children for more than a decade have found that the best predictor of their blood cholesterol is earlier baseline values: childhood values correlate with values in young adulthood.[10] Quite simply, if you want to know a child's future cholesterol, measure it now.

Blood cholesterol also correlates with obesity, especially central obesity. LDL cholesterol correlates positively, and HDL negatively.[11] These relationships are apparent throughout childhood, and their magnitude increases with age.

Research has also confirmed an association between blood lipids and physical activity in children similar to that seen in adults.[12] Inactive children have higher total cholesterol and LDL and lower HDL than physically active children.

Blood Pressure

An elevated blood pressure accelerates the development of CVD. On the average, children's blood pressure is lower than adults', but blood pressure increases as children grow, rising sharply at puberty and then leveling off. Like blood cholesterol, blood pressure correlates with obesity, especially central obesity.[13] Blood pressure tends to increase at a slower rate in children who participate in regular aerobic activity or who have either lost weight or maintained their weight as they grew taller.[14]

DEVELOPMENT OF OBESITY IN CHILDREN

Many experts agree that preventing or treating obesity in childhood will reduce the rate of CVD in adulthood. Without intervention, overweight children become overweight adolescents who become overweight adults, and being overweight exacerbates every chronic disease that adults face.[15]

Growing Fatter

Children are heavier today than they were 10 to 20 years ago. On the average, they have gained more than 5 pounds over the past two decades. This pattern is a secular trend—that is, one that cannot be explained by genetics. Diet and physical activity must be responsible.

Not Eating More

Reports from the Bogalusa Heart Study indicate that children's energy intakes have remained relatively stable over the past 15 years. There has even been a slight decline in fat intake, from 38 to 36 percent of kcalories from fat daily.[16] This slight decline in dietary fat is not enough, however, to have influenced body weight, nor is it enough to meet current dietary recommendations.

Children's dietary fat intakes vary, of course, and some children do eat high-fat diets. Children who prefer high-fat foods tend to consume a relatively large percentage of their energy intake from fat.[17] They also tend to be more overweight than their peers. Particularly noteworthy is the finding that the children's fat preferences and consumption correlate with their parents' obesity as well. Such findings confirm the significant roles parents play—teaching children about healthy food choices, providing children with low-fat selections, and serving as role models.

Growing Less Active

Most likely, children have grown more overweight because of their lack of physical activity.[18] An inactive child can become obese even while eating less food than an active child. Today's children are more sedentary and less physically fit than children were 20 years ago.

Watching television accounts for some 24 hours a week of sedentary behavior. Beyond these 24 hours, children spend more sedentary time working at computers and playing video games. As mentioned in earlier chapters, studies have found that both obesity and blood cholesterol correlate with hours of television viewed.[19] TV uses no more energy than it takes to rest, displaces participation in more vigorous activities, and fosters snacking on high-fat foods.

Just as blood cholesterol and obesity track over the years, so does a person's level of physical activity. A study of almost 1000 teenagers reported that over half of those who were initially described as inactive remained inactive six years later.[20] Similarly, almost half of those who were physically active remained so. Compared with inactive teens, those who were physically active weighed less, smoked less, ate a diet lower in saturated fats, and had a better blood lipid profile. The message is clear: physical activity offers numerous health benefits and children who are active today are most likely to be active for years to come.

PREVENTING CHILDHOOD OBESITY

In light of all these findings, parents and teachers of children are encouraged to make major efforts to prevent child obesity. Among directives are the following: encourage children to eat slowly, to pause and enjoy their table companions, and to stop eating when they are full. Teach them how to select low-fat snacks and to serve themselves appropriate portions. Never force children to clean their plates. Encourage physical activity daily to promote strong skeletal, muscular, and cardiovascular development and to instill in children the desire to be physically active throughout life. Physical activity is a natural and lifelong behavior of healthy living.[21] It can be as simple as riding a bike, playing tag, jumping rope, or doing chores. It need not be an organized sport; it just needs to be some activity on a regular basis.

It is important to use sensitivity in teaching children nutrition principles that can help to prevent obesity. Children can easily get the idea that their worth is tied to their body weight. Some parents fail to realize that society's ideal of slimness can be perilously close to starvation, and that a child encouraged to "diet" cannot obtain the energy and nutrients required for normal growth and development. Even healthy children without diagnosable eating disorders have been observed to limit their growth through "dieting."[22] Weight gain in truly overweight children can be controlled safely without compromising growth, but should be overseen by a health care professional.

DEALING WITH CHILDHOOD OBESITY

The child who is already obese needs careful management. Weight loss is not ordinarily recommended because restrictive diets can easily impair growth in children. Instead, aim to maintain a constant weight while the child grows taller. The object is to support normal lean body development, while letting children "grow out" of their obesity.

CHOLESTEROL SCREENING FOR CHILDREN

Many children in the United States are not only overweight but also have high blood cholesterol.[23] The question of whether to screen children for high blood cholesterol is controversial.[24] Currently, selective screening for children and adolescents whose parents or grandparents have CVD is recommended.[25] Since blood cholesterol in children is a good predictor of adult values, however, some experts recommend universal screening to identify all children with high blood cholesterol.[26] They note that many children who have high blood cholesterol do not have family histories of CVD and would be missed under current screening criteria.[27] Opponents argue that some children with high blood cholesterol may reach adulthood with normal blood cholesterol and that treating adults who have high blood cholesterol should be sufficient. They believe screening will create unnecessary anxiety and lead to an overuse of drug therapy and overly restrictive dieting during childhood and adolescence.[28] Furthermore, studies have found that few children follow up with additional testing or dietary changes anyway.[29] Standard values for cholesterol screening in children and adolescents are listed in Table H19–1.

In some cases, parents are too young to have a CVD history. In many other cases, children, or their parents, may not know their family histories. For these reasons, it may be most effective for physicians of adult heart patients to refer the children and grandchildren of these patients for cholesterol screening.[30]

Some research shows that overweight children should also be con-

Table H19–1

Cholesterol Values for Children and Adolescents

Disease Risk	Total Cholesterol (mg/dL)	LDL Cholesterol (mg/dL)
Acceptable	<170	<110
Borderline	170–199	110–129
High	≥200	≥130

Note: Adult values appear in Chapter 28.

sidered for cholesterol screening, even if they do not satisfy the current criteria.[31] The incidence of high blood cholesterol in obese children with no other criteria is similar to that of nonobese children with family histories of CVD.

Considering the many lifestyle factors that accompany the development of CVD, questions regarding a child's health behaviors might also be informative. Health care professionals should determine whether children smoke, and how physically active they are, especially when family history is unknown.[32]

Early—but not advanced—atherosclerotic lesions are reversible, making screening and education a high priority. Both those with family histories of CVD and those with multiple risk factors need intervention. Children with the highest risks of developing CVD are sedentary and obese, with high blood pressure and high blood cholesterol. In contrast, children with the lowest risks of heart disease are physically active and of normal weight, with low blood pressure and favorable lipid profiles. Routine pediatric care should identify these known risk factors and provide education when needed (see Table H19–2).

DIETARY RECOMMENDATIONS FOR CHILDREN

An expert panel on blood cholesterol in children and adolescents recommends that, regardless of family history, all children over age two should eat a variety of foods and maintain desirable weight.[33] Children should receive less than 30 percent of total energy from fat, less than 10 percent from saturated fat, and less than 300 milligrams of cholesterol per day. The American

Table H19–2

Health Professional's Schedule of Cardiovascular Disease Assessment in Children

Birth	• Family history for early heart disease, high blood lipids (if positive, discuss risk factors and refer parents to health care). • Start growth chart. • Parental smoking history (if positive, refer to smoking cessation program).
0–2 years	• Update family history, growth chart. • With introduction of solids, begin teaching about healthy diet (nutritionally adequate, low in salt, low in saturated fats). • Recommend healthy snacks as finger foods. • Change to whole milk from formula or breastfeeding at approximately 1 year of age.
2–6 years	• Update family history, growth chart (review growth chart[a] with family and discuss concept of weight for height). • Introduce moderately low-fat diet. • Change to low-fat milk. • Start blood pressure chart at approximately 3 years of age;[b] review for concept of lower salt intake. • Encourage active parent-child play. • Lipid determination in children with positive family history or with parental cholesterol >240 mg/dl (if abnormal, initiate nutrition counseling).
6–10 years	• Update family history, blood pressure, and growth charts. • Complete cardiovascular health profile with child; determine family history, smoking history, blood pressure percentile, weight for height, fingerstick cholesterol, and level of activity and fitness. • Reinforce low-fat diet. • Begin active antismoking counseling. • Introduce fitness for health and encourage lifelong sport activities for child and family. • Discuss role of watching television in sedentary lifestyle and obesity.
>10 years	• Update family history, blood pressure, and growth charts annually. • Review low-fat diet, risks of smoking, fitness benefits whenever possible. • Consider lipid profile in all patients. • Final review of personal cardiovascular health status.

[a]If weight is >120% of normal for height, diagnosis of obesity should be considered and the subject addressed with the child and family.
[b]If three consecutive interval blood pressure measurements exceed the 90th percentile and blood pressure is not explained by height or weight, diagnosis of hypertension should be made and appropriate evaluation considered.

Source: Adapted with permission from W. B. Strong and coauthors, Integrated cardiovascular health promotion in childhood: A statement for health professionals from the Subcommittee on Atherosclerosis and Hypertension in Childhood of the Council on Cardiovascular Disease in the Young, American Heart Association, *Circulation* 85 (1992): 1638–1650. Copyright 1992 American Heart Association.

Academy of Pediatrics agrees, but cautions against fat intakes of less than 30 percent of total kcalories for growing children.

Not before Two

Recommendations limiting fat and cholesterol are not intended for infants or children under two years old. Infants and toddlers need a higher percentage of fat to support their rapid growth.

Moderation, Not Deprivation

Healthy children over age two can begin the transition to eating according to recommendations. Even then, meals can include moderate amounts of a child's favorite foods, even if they are high-fat selections such as french fries and ice cream.[34] Without such additions, diets might be too low in fat, not to mention unappetizing and boring.

Balanced meals need to provide lean meat, poultry, fish, and vegetable sources of protein; fruits and vegetables; whole grains; and low-fat milk products. Such meals can provide enough food energy and nutrients to support growth and maintain blood cholesterol within a healthy range.[35] Pediatricians warn parents to avoid extremes; they caution that while intentions may be good, excessive food restriction may create nutrient deficiencies and impair growth. Furthermore, parental control over eating may instigate battles and foster attitudes about foods that can lead to inappropriate eating behaviors.

Diet First, Drugs Later

Experts agree that children at high risk should first be treated with diet. If, in children ten years and older, blood cholesterol remains high after 6 to 12 months of dietary intervention, then drugs may be used to lower blood cholesterol.[36] Pharmacological doses of niacin effectively lower LDL cholesterol in children, but adverse effects are common; such treatment should be reserved only for severe cases.[37]

SMOKING

Another risk factor for CVD that starts in childhood and carries over into adulthood is cigarette smoking. Each day 3000 children begin to use tobacco, 40 percent of them in grade school. Among high school students, two out of three have tried smoking, and one in eight smokes regularly. Over half of all adult smokers began smoking before the age of 18.

Efforts to teach children about the dangers of smoking need to be aggressive to compete with the tobacco industry's promotional campaigns. The tobacco industry spends millions of dollars on advertising aimed at young people and makes over $200 million a year on sales to children under 18. Cigarette companies use cartoon characters, advertise in youth-oriented publications, and sponsor sporting events. Children and teenagers are not likely to consider the long-term health consequences of tobacco use. They are more likely to be struck by the immediate health consequences, such as shortness of breath when playing sports, or social consequences, such as having bad breath. Whatever the context, the message to all children and teens should be clear: don't start smoking. If you've already started, quit.

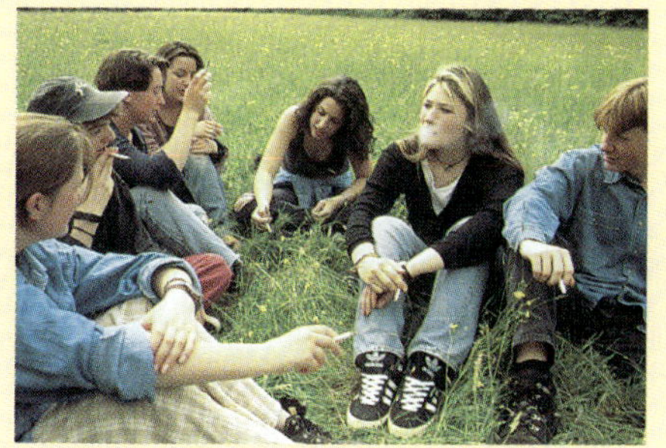

Cigarette smoking is the number-one cause of premature deaths.

In conclusion, *adult* CVD is a major *pediatric* problem. Without intervention, some 60 million children are destined to suffer its consequences within the next 30 years. Optimal prevention efforts focus on children, especially on those who are overweight.

Just as young children receive vaccinations against infectious diseases, they need screening for, and education about, CVD. Many health education programs have been implemented in schools around the country.[38] These programs are most effective when they include education in the classroom, heart-healthy meals in the lunchroom, fitness activities on the playground, and parental involvement at home.

NOTES

1. G. S. Berenson and coauthors, Review: Atherosclerosis and its evolution in childhood, *American Journal of the Medical Sciences* 30 (1987): 429–440; W. B. Strong and coauthors, Integrated cardiovascular health promotion in childhood: A statement for health professionals from the Subcommittee on Atherosclerosis and Hypertension in Childhood of the Council on Cardiovascular Disease in the Young, American Heart Association, *Circulation* 85 (1992): 1638–1650.

2. W. B. Kannel, R. B. D'Agostino, and A. Belanger, Concept of bridging the gap from

youth to adulthood—The Framingham Study, an address presented at the Recognition and Prevention of Heart Disease: State of the Art conference, New Orleans, Louisiana, April 27 and 28, 1994.

3. G. S. Berenson and coauthors, Atherosclerosis of the aorta and coronary arteries and cardiovascular risk factors in persons aged 6 to 30 years and studied at necropsy (the Bogalusa Heart Study), *American Journal of Cardiology* 70 (1992): 851–858.

4. Kannel, D'Agostino, and Belanger, 1994.

5. Committee on Nutrition, Statement on cholesterol, *Pediatrics* 90 (1992): 469–473; National Cholesterol Education Program, Report of the Expert Panel on Blood Cholesterol Levels in Children and Adolescents, Overview and summary, *Pediatrics* (supplement) 89 (1992): 525–527.

6. Pathobiological Determinants of Atherosclerosis in Youth (PDAY) Research Group, Relationship of atherosclerosis in young men to serum lipoprotein cholesterol concentrations and smoking: A preliminary report from the Pathobiological Determinants of Atherosclerosis in Youth (PDAY) Research Group, *Journal of the American Medical Association* 264 (1990): 3018–3024.

7. Pathobiological Determinants of Atherosclerosis in Youth (PDAY) Research Group, 1990.

8. L. Snetselaar and R. M. Lauer, Childhood, diet and the atherosclerotic process, *Nutrition Today*, January/February 1992, pp. 22–28.

9. M. J. T. Kallio and coauthors, Tracking of serum cholesterol and lipoprotein levels from the first year of life, *Pediatrics* 91 (1993): 949–954.

10. S. Guo and coauthors, Serial analysis of plasma lipids and lipoproteins from individuals 9–21 years of age, *American Journal of Clinical Nutrition* 58 (1993): 61–67.

11. W. A. Wattigney and coauthors, Increasing impact of obesity on serum lipids and lipoproteins in young adults: The Bogalusa Heart Study, *Archives of Internal Medicine* 151 (1991): 2017–2022.

12. E. Suter and M. R. Hawes, Relationship of physical activity, body fat, diet, and blood lipid profile in youths 10–15 yr, *Medicine and Science in Sports and Exercise* 25 (1993): 748–754.

13. C. L. Shear and coauthors, Body fat patterning and blood pressure in children and young adults: The Bogalusa Heart Study, *Hypertension* 9 (1987): 236–244.

14. S. Shea and coauthors, The rate of increase in blood pressure in children 5 years of age is related to changes in aerobic fitness and body mass index, *Pediatrics* 94 (1994): 465–470.

15. S. S. Guo and coauthors, The predictive value of childhood body mass index values for overweight at age 35 y, *American Journal of Clinical Nutrition* 57 (1994): 810–819.

16. T. A. Nicklas and coauthors, Secular trends in dietary intakes and cardiovascular risk factors of 10-year-old children: The Bogalusa Heart Study (1973–1988), *American Journal of Clinical Nutrition* 57 (1993): 930–937.

17. J. O. Fisher and L. L. Birch, Fat preferences and fat consumption of 3- to 5-year-old children are related to parental obesity, *Journal of the American Dietetic Association* 95 (1995): 759–764.

18. S. A. Schlicker, S. T. Borra, and C. Regan, The weight and fitness status of United States children, *Nutrition Reviews* 52 (1994): 11–17.

19. E. Obarzanek and coauthors, Energy intake and physical activity in relation to indexes of body fat: The National Heart, Lung, and Blood Institute Growth and Health Study, *American Journal of Clinical Nutrition* 60 (1994): 15–22.

20. O. T. Raitakari and coauthors, Effects of persistent physical activity on coronary risk factors in children and young adults: The Cardiovascular Risk in Young Finns Study, *American Journal of Epidemiology* 140 (1994): 195–205.

21. Committee on Sports Medicine and Fitness, Fitness, activity, and sports participation in the preschool child, *Pediatrics* 90 (1992): 1002–1004.

22. F. Lifshitz and N. Moses, Nutritional dwarfing: Growth, dieting, and fear of obesity, *Journal of the American College of Nutrition* 7 (1988): 367–376.

23. G. S. Berenson, S. R. Srinivasan, and L. S. Webber, Cardiovascular risk prevention in children: A challenge or a poor idea? *Nutrition, Metabolism and Cardiovascular Diseases* 4 (1994): 46–52.

24. S. S. Gidding, The rationale for lowering serum cholesterol levels in American children, *American Journal of Diseases of Children* 147 (1993): 386–392; P. T. Einhorn and B. M. Rifkind, Cholesterol measurement in children, *American Journal of Diseases of Children* 147 (1993): 373–375; G. S. Berenson, Cholesterol: Myth vs reality in pediatric practice, *American Journal of Diseases of Children* 147 (1993): 371–373.

25. Report of the Expert Panel on Blood Cholesterol Levels in Children and Adolescents, *Pediatrics* 89 (1992): entire supplement.

26. Berenson, Srinivasan, and Webber, 1994.

27. S. J. Wadowski and coauthors, Family history of coronary artery disease and cholesterol: Screening children in disadvantaged inner-city population, *Pediatrics* 93 (1994): 109–113; K. Resnicow and D. Cross, Are parents' self-reported total cholesterol levels useful in identifying children with hyperlipidemia? An examination of current guidelines, *Pediatrics* 92 (1993): 347–354.

28. National Cholesterol Education Program, Overview and summary, 1992.

29. C. M. Lannon and J. Earp, Parents' behavior and attitudes toward screening children for high serum cholesterol levels, *Pediatrics* 89 (1992): 1159–1163.

30. L. E. Muhonen and coauthors, Coronary risk factors in adolescents related to their knowledge of familial coronary heart disease and hypercholesterolemia: The Muscatine Study, *Pediatrics* 93 (1994): 444–451.

31. M. S. Glassman and S. M. Schwarz, Cholesterol screening in children: Should obesity be a risk factor? *Journal of the American College of Nutrition* 12 (1993): 270–273.

32. Committee on Nutrition, 1992.

33. NCEP Expert Panel on Blood Cholesterol Levels in Children and Adolescents, National Cholesterol Education Program (NCEP): Highlight of the report of the Expert Panel on Blood Cholesterol Levels in Children and Adolescents, *Pediatrics* 89 (1992): 495–501.

34. N. Sigman-Grant, S. Zimmerman, and P. M. Kris-Etherton, Dietary approaches for reducing fat intake of preschool-age children, *Pediatrics* 91 (1993): 955–960.

35. Timely statement on NCEP report on children and adolescents, *Journal of the American Dietetic Association* 91 (1991): 983; Is there a relationship between dietary fat and stature or growth in children three to five years of age? *Pediatrics* 92 (1993): 579–586.

36. Committee on Nutrition, 1992.

37. R. B. Colletti and coauthors, Niacin treatment of hypercholesterolemia in children, *Pediatrics* 92 (1993): 78–82.

38. A. M. Downey, J. L. Cresanta, and G. S. Berenson, Cardiovascular health promotion in children: "Heart Smart" and the changing role of physicians, *American Journal of Preventive Medicine* 5 (1989): 279–295.

Chapter 20

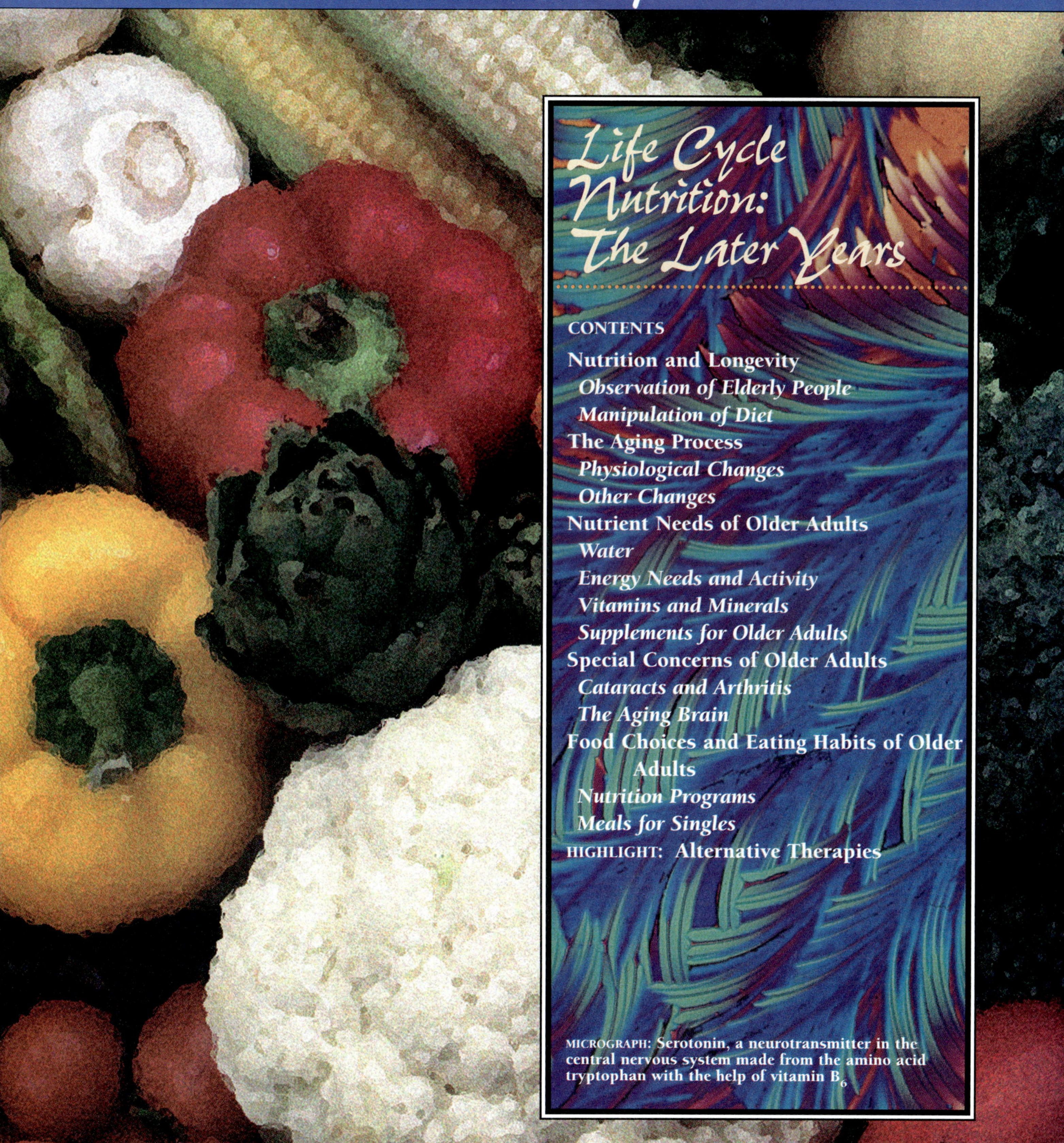

Life Cycle Nutrition: The Later Years

CONTENTS

MICROGRAPH: Serotonin, a neurotransmitter in the central nervous system made from the amino acid tryptophan with the help of vitamin B_6

Wise food choices, made throughout adulthood, can support a person's ability to meet physical, emotional, and mental challenges and to achieve freedom from disease. Three goals inspire adults to take responsibility for their nutritional health: promotion of overall wellness, prevention of disease, and slowing of aging. Much of this text has focused on nutrition to support wellness during adulthood; this chapter presents information on aging and the nutrition needs of older adults.

The U.S. population is "graying." The majority is now middle-aged, and the ratio of old people to young is becoming greater, as Figure 20–1 shows. Our society uses the arbitrary age of 65 years to define the transition point between middle age and old age, but growing "old" happens day by day, with change occurring gradually over time. Since 1950 the population of those over 65 has more than doubled. Remarkably, the fastest-growing age group is people over 85 years (see Figure 20–2).[1]

life expectancy: the average number of years lived by people in a given society.

longevity: long duration of life.

life span: the maximum number of years of life attainable by a member of a species.

The life expectancy for U.S. women is 79 years and for men, 72 years—up from about 47 years in 1900. Advances in medical science—antibiotics and other treatments—are largely responsible for almost doubling the life expectancy in this century. Improved nutrition and an abundant supply of food have also contributed to lengthening life expectancy.[2] Still, there appears to be an upper limit on human longevity that even nutrition cannot extend. The human life span is about 115 years and has not changed much over the years.

Figure 20–1

The Aging of the U.S. Population (= 65 years or older)

In 1940, 6.8 percent of the population was 65 or older. In 1990, 12.7 percent of us had reached age 65, with 1.2 percent of the population 85 years or older; by 2040, 21.7 percent will have reached age 65; and a century from now, nearly one of four Americans will be 65 and older. An estimated 25,000 Americans now living are 100 years old or older.

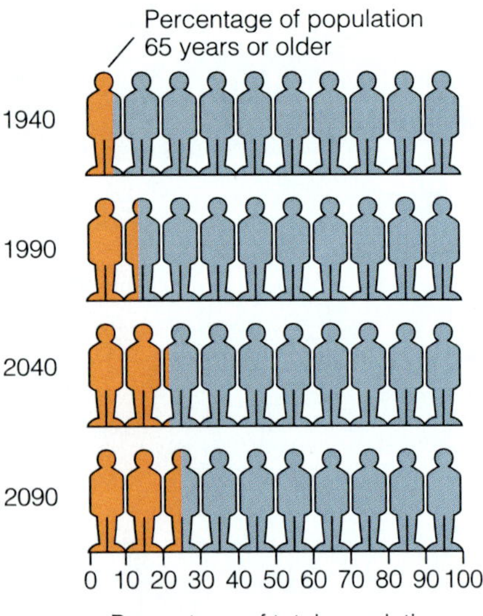

Nutrition and Longevity

Only in this century have human beings achieved a life expectancy that permits science to study aging. Research in the field now is active—and difficult. Researchers are challenged by the diversity of older adults. When older adults experience health problems, it is hard to know whether to attribute them to normal, age-related processes or to other reasons and relationships. If some of the health problems of later life are preventable, then research that focuses on how nutrition and other factors affect aging and disease processes is of great value. The findings will be vital to ensuring that more and more people can look forward to long, healthy lives.

The idea that nutrition can influence the aging process is particularly appealing, because people can control and change their eating habits. Among the questions researchers are asking are:

- To what extent is aging inevitable, and can it be slowed through changes in lifestyle and environment?
- What role does nutrition play in the aging process, and what role can it play in retarding aging?

With respect to the first question, it seems that aging is an inevitable, natural process, programmed into the genes at conception. People can, however, slow the process within the natural limits set by heredity. They need to adopt healthy lifestyle habits such as engaging in physical activity.

With respect to the second question, good nutrition helps to maintain a healthy body and can therefore ease the aging process in many significant ways. Clearly, nutrition can improve the quality of the life in later years.

OBSERVATION OF ELDERLY PEOPLE

One approach researchers use to search out the secret of long life has been to study older people. No doubt, you have noticed that some people are young for their ages, others old for their ages. What makes the difference?

Healthy Habits Six healthy habits seem to have a profound influence on physiological age:[3]

- Abstinence from, or moderation in, alcohol use.
- Regularity of meals.
- Weight control.
- Regular, adequate sleep.
- Abstinence from smoking.
- Regular physical activity.

physiological age: a person's age as estimated from her or his body's health and probable life expectancy.

The effects of all these factors are cumulative—that is, those who follow all of the practices are in better health, even if older in chronological age, than people who fail to do so. In fact, the physical health of people who report all positive health practices is comparable to that of people *30 years younger* who follow few or none. Other studies have confirmed that these health habits both extend longevity and support independence in later life.[4] The findings suggest that even though people cannot alter the years of their births, they can alter the probable lengths and quality of their lives.

chronological age: a person's age in years from his or her date of birth.

Especially Physical Activity Vigorous physical activity and long life seem to go together.[5] Even a moderate amount of physical activity—for example, a brisk 30-minute walk each day—is protective against early mortality. An extensive study of more than 16,000 men demonstrates this clearly.[6] The men were between 35 and 74 years of age and were studied for 12 to 16 years. The group whose members expended 2000 or more kcalories in exercise per week (equal to walking or running about 20 miles per week) had a death rate 25 to 33 percent lower than the less active group's rate. Exercise seemed to affect the risk of death even more than did heredity, smoking, hypertension, or extremes in body weight. Physical activity slows cardiovascular aging and reduces heart disease risks. The numerous benefits derived from regular physical activity emphasize the importance of making it a priority in everyone's life.

Figure 20–2

U.S. Population Growth, 1960 to 1990

The "oldest old"—those 85 years and older—are the fastest-growing age group in the United States. Between 1960 and 1990, the U.S. population grew 39 percent, but the population of those over 85 more than doubled.

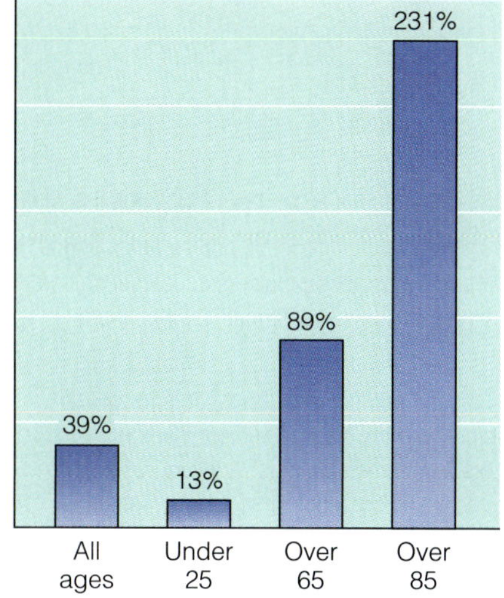

MANIPULATION OF DIET

Another approach researchers use to learn about longevity has been to manipulate animals' diets. This research has given rise to some interesting and suggestive findings.

To extend the life span, rats were restricted to 60 percent of their regular intake.

Energy Restriction in Rats Rats live longer when their food intakes are restricted in the early weeks of their lives or even after they are mature. Extensive research shows that it is the restriction of food energy rather than restriction of a specific nutrient that exerts the antiaging effect.[7]

Several mechanisms to explain how energy restriction prolongs life in rats have been proposed but not proven. Food restriction may extend the life span by delaying age-related diseases, retarding growth and development, reducing body fat, slowing the metabolic rate, controlling blood glucose, and preventing lipid oxidation.[8]

While restricting energy intake is the most effective way to lengthen rats' lives, no evidence suggests that these findings apply to human beings. To apply the results of animal studies to human beings is often unrealistic and, in this case, would even be dangerous. The animals given restricted feedings suffered distinct disadvantages: half of them died *very* early (before 300 days); the surviving animals were retarded and malformed in a number of ways. Extreme starvation to extend life, like any extreme, is probably never worth the price.

Energy Restriction in Human Beings One group of researchers studied the relationship between *moderate* energy restriction and the retardation of aging in human beings.[9] Sixteen middle-aged, nonobese men were studied during 10 weeks of energy restriction (80 percent of their usual weight-maintaining intake). They lost weight, mostly due to loss of fat. Their blood pressures dropped significantly, and their HDL cholesterol concentrations rose significantly. Energy restriction had no adverse effects on their mental and physical performances. For these men, moderate energy restriction favorably changed disease risk factors such as obesity, blood pressure, and blood cholesterol.

In summary, life expectancy in the United States has increased dramatically in the last century. Factors that enhance longevity include limited or no alcohol use, regular balanced meals, weight control, adequate sleep, abstinence from smoking, and regular physical activity. Nutrition alone, even if ideal, cannot guarantee a long and robust life. At the very least, however, nutrition can influence aging and longevity in human beings by helping to prevent disease. Later chapters present the relationships between diet and disease prevention; the focus here is on changes that commonly accompany the aging process.

The Aging Process

stress: any threat to a person's well-being; a demand placed on the body to adapt.

stressor: an environmental element, physical or psychological, that causes stress.

stress response: the body's response to stress, mediated initially by both nerves and hormones; begins with an *alarm reaction*, proceeds through a stage of *resistance*, and then leads to *recovery* or, if prolonged, to *exhaustion*. This three-stage response has also been termed the **general adaptation syndrome**.

As people get older, each person becomes less and less like anyone else. Everyday stresses and habits have had more time to affect the body's health. Both physical stressors, such as alcohol abuse, other drug abuse, smoking, pain, heat, and illness, and psychological stressors, such as exams, divorce, moving, and death of a loved one, elicit the body's stress response. The body responds to such stressors with an elaborate series of physiological steps, using the nervous and hormonal systems to bring about defensive readiness in every body part. The effects all favor physical action—the classic fight-or-flight response. Stress that is prolonged or severe can drain the body of its reserves and leave it weakened, aged, and vulnerable to illness, especially if physical action is not taken. As people age, they lose their ability to adapt to both external and internal disturbances. When disease strikes, the reduced ability to adapt makes the aging individual more vulnerable to death than a younger person.

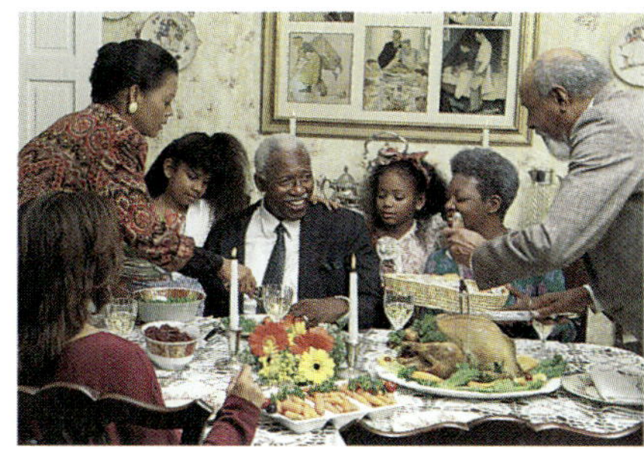

Growing old is enjoyable for people who take care of their health and live each day fully.

PHYSIOLOGICAL CHANGES

As aging progresses, inevitable changes in each of the body's organs contribute to the body's declining function. These physiological changes influence nutrition status, just as growth and development do in the earlier stages of the life cycle.

Body Composition Optimal nutrition and physical activity can minimize the body composition changes associated with aging. In general, though, older people tend to lose bone and lean body mass and gain body fat.[10] Many of these changes in body composition occur because some hormones that regulate metabolism become less active with age while others become more active. The action of insulin, for example, diminishes with age as the pancreas begins to secrete less of the hormone and the cells lose their ability to respond efficiently.*

Immune System Changes in the immune system also bring declining function with age.[11] The immune system is also compromised by nutrient deficiencies, and so the combination of age and malnutrition makes older people vulnerable to infectious diseases.[12] Adding insult to injury, antibiotics often are not effective against infections in people with compromised immune systems.[13] Consequently, infectious diseases are a major cause of death in older adults.

GI Tract In the GI tract, the intestinal wall loses strength and elasticity with age, and this slows motility. Constipation is four to eight times more common in the elderly than in the young.[14] Atrophic gastritis, a condition that affects almost one-third of those over 60, is characterized by an inflamed stomach, abundant bacteria, and a lack of hydrochloric acid—all of which can impair the digestion and absorption of nutrients, most notably, vitamin B_{12}, biotin, calcium, and iron.

Reminder: *Atrophic gastritis* is a condition characterized by chronic inflammation of the stomach accompanied by a diminished size and functioning of the mucosa and glands.

Tooth Loss Tooth loss and gum disease are common in old age, making chewing difficult or painful. Dentures, even when they fit properly, are less effective than natural teeth, and inefficient chewing can cause choking. People with tooth loss, gum disease, and ill-fitting dentures tend to limit their selections to soft foods. If foods such as corn on the cob, apples, and hard rolls are replaced by creamed corn, applesauce, and rice, then nutrition status may not be greatly affected, but when food groups are eliminated and variety is limited, inadequate intakes of vitamins, minerals, and fiber follow.

Sensory Losses A multitude of sensory losses can also interfere with an older person's ability to obtain adequate nourishment. Failing eyesight, for example, can make driving to the grocery store impossible and shopping for food a frustrating experience. It may become so difficult to read food labels and count

*Other examples of hormones that change with age include the growth hormone and androgens, which decline with advancing age, thus contributing to the decrease in lean body mass, and the hormone prolactin, which increases with age, helping to maintain body fat.

money that the person doesn't buy the needed foods. Carrying bags of groceries may be an unmanageable task. Similarly, a person with limited mobility may find cooking and cleaning up too hard to do.

Sensory losses can interfere with a person's ability or willingness to eat. Taste and smell sensitivities tend to diminish with age and may make eating less enjoyable.[15] Loss of vision and hearing may contribute to social isolation.[16]

OTHER CHANGES

In addition to the physiological changes that accompany aging, adults are changing in many other ways that influence their nutrition status. Psychological, economic, and social factors play big roles in a person's ability and willingness to eat.

Psychological Changes Though not an inevitable component of aging, depression is common among older adults. It is frequently accompanied by loss of appetite and of the motivation to cook. These feelings are especially apparent when a person has recently lost a loved one. When a person is suffering the heartache and loneliness of bereavement, cooking meals may not seem worthwhile. The support and companionship of family and friends, especially at mealtimes, can help overcome depression and enhance appetite. In addition to depression, older adults are often troubled by insomnia, worry, anxiety, apathy, and forgetfulness.

Economic Changes Overall, the older population today has a higher income than their cohorts of previous generations. Still, poverty is a major problem for about 20 percent of the people over age 65. Factors such as living arrangements and income make significant differences in the food choices, eating habits, and nutrition status of older adults, especially those over age 80.[17] People of low socioeconomic status are likely to have inadequate food and nutrient intakes. For example, studies report a consistent relationship between low income and low intakes of vitamin B_6.[18]

Social Changes Malnutrition among older adults is most likely to occur among those with the least education, those living alone in federally funded housing (an indicator of low income), and those who have recently experienced a change in lifestyle. The risk of nutrient deficiencies is high among people living alone, especially men.[19] One study of home-delivered meals confirmed that men living alone eat less than men living with others; interestingly, women living alone eat more than women living with others.[20] Adults who live alone do not necessarily make poor food choices, but they often consume too little food: loneliness is directly related to nutritional inadequacies, especially of energy intake.[21]

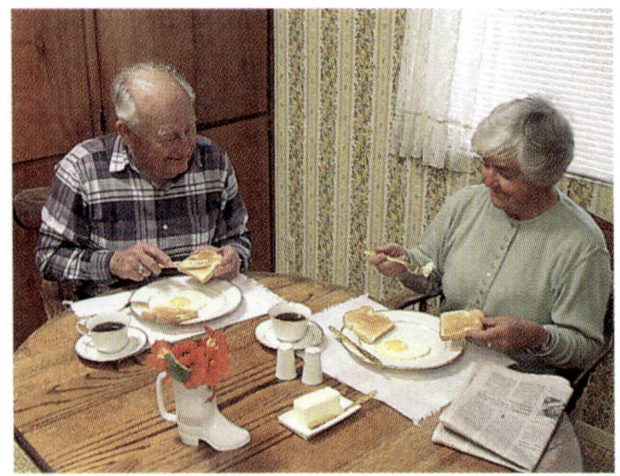

Shared meals can brighten the day and enhance the appetite.

To quickly review, many changes that accompany aging can impair nutrition status. Among physiological changes, hormone activity alters body composition, immune system changes raise the risk of infections, atrophic gastritis interferes with nutrient digestion and absorption, and tooth loss limits food choices. Psychological changes such as depression, economic changes such as loss of income, and social changes such as loneliness contribute to poor food intake.

Nutrient Needs of Older Adults

Knowledge about the nutrient needs and nutrition status of older adults has grown considerably in the last decade or so. The 1989 RDA, however, combine all people over 50 into one group. The 1997 revision split this group into two age categories—one group of 51 to 70 years old and one of 71 and over.[22]* After all, the needs of people 50 to 60 years old may be very different from those of people over 80. The need for more age-specific recommendations is becoming more and more urgent as the population ages.

Setting standards for older people is difficult, though, because individual differences become more pronounced as people grow older. One person may tend to omit vegetables from his diet, and by the time he is old, he will have an associated set of nutrition problems. Another may have omitted milk and milk products all her life—her nutrition problems will be different. Also, as people age, they suffer different chronic diseases and take different drugs—both having impacts on nutrient needs. Even before all this, people start out with different genetic predispositions and ways of handling nutrients, and the effects of these became magnified with the years. Researchers have difficulty even defining "healthy aging," a prerequisite to developing recommendations that are designed to meet the "needs of practically all healthy persons."[23] Still some generalizations are valid, and although new recommendations are needed, the present RDA for adults are of some use. The next sections give special attention to a few nutrients of concern.

WATER

Dehydration is a risk for older adults, who may not notice or pay attention to their thirst, or who find it difficult and bothersome to get a drink or to get to a bathroom. Older adults who have lost bladder control may be afraid to drink too much water. Despite real fluid needs, older people do not seem to feel thirsty or notice mouth dryness.[24] Many nursing home employees say it is hard to persuade their elderly clients to drink enough water and fruit juices.

Total body water also decreases as people age, so that even mild stresses such as fever or hot weather can precipitate rapid dehydration in older adults. Chapter 12 described the importance of water and recommended an intake of 6 to 8 glasses of water a day. Milk and juices may replace some of this water, but beverages containing alcohol or caffeine should be limited because of their diuretic effect.[25]

Water recommendation for adults: 1 to 1½ oz/kg actual body weight.

- Older adult feeding pointer: Drink plenty of water.

ENERGY NEEDS AND ACTIVITY

Energy needs decline with advancing age. As a rule of thumb, adult energy needs decline an estimated 5 percent per decade. For one thing, as people age, they usually reduce their physical activity, although they need not do so. For another, lean body mass diminishes, slowing the basal metabolic rate. The lower energy expenditures require that older adults eat less food energy to maintain their weights. Accordingly, the energy RDA for adults decreases slightly, beginning at

*The Canadian RNI divide older people into two age groups—50 to 74, and 75 and older.

age 51. Energy intakes typically decline in parallel with needs. Still, many older adults are overweight, indicating that their food intakes do not decline enough to compensate for their reduced energy expenditure.[26]

- Older adult feeding pointer: Select nutrient-dense foods low in fats, sugars, and alcohol.

On limited energy allowances, people must select mostly nutrient-dense foods. There is little leeway for sugars, fats, oils, or alcohol. Because overweight creates many health problems and shortens the life span, these seem to be life-sustaining recommendations. The Daily Food Guide (on pp. 42–43) offers a dietary framework for adults of all ages. Those who need additional food energy should choose extra servings from each of the groups listed.[27]

Regular Physical Activity The many and remarkable benefits of regular physical activity are not limited to the young: older adults who are active weigh less and have greater flexibility, more endurance, and better balance than those who are inactive.[28] They reap additional benefits as well; for example, evening exercise helps to eliminate late night trips to the bathroom, and strength training significantly improves mobility and resistance to injury.[29]* In fact, regular physical activity is the most powerful predictor of a person's mobility in the later years.[30]

- Older adult pointer: Exercise to maintain muscle and bone mass.

Activities of all kinds are recommended to maintain and promote health: strength training can build muscles, and aerobic exercise can improve cardiorespiratory endurance and lower blood lipid concentrations.[31] Although aging affects both speed and endurance to some degree, older adults can still train and achieve exceptional performances.

Ideally, physical activity should be part of each day's schedule and should be intense enough to prevent muscle atrophy and to speed up the heartbeat and respiration rate. Healthy older adults who have not been active can ease into a suitable routine. They can start by walking short distances until they can walk at least a mile three times a week; then they can gradually increase their pace to achieve a 20- to 25-minute mile.[32]

Muscle mass and muscle strength tend to decline with aging, making older people vulnerable to falls and immobility. Falls are a major cause of fear, injury, disability, dependence, and even death among older adults. Regular exercise tones, firms, and strengthens muscles, helping to improve confidence, reduce the risk of falling, and minimize the risk of injury should a fall occur. Strength training, even in frail, elderly people over 85 years of age, has been shown to not only improve muscle strength and mobility but to increase energy expenditure and energy intake, thereby enhancing nutrient intakes.[33] This finding highlights another reason to exercise: a person spending energy on physical activity can afford to eat more food and with it, more nutrients. People who are committed to an ongoing fitness program can maintain their body weights and have higher energy and nutrient intakes than more sedentary people.[34]

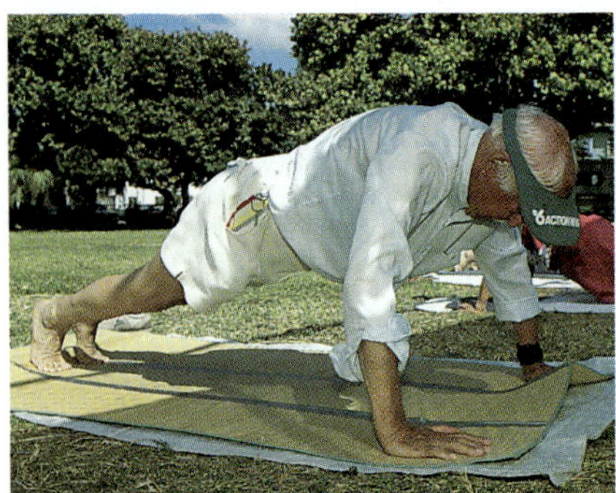

Strength training promotes strong muscles and bones and healthy appetites.

One expert suggests the following physical activity program to maintain good health and function in older adults:[35]

- *Every day.* 60 minutes of some physical activity: gardening, walking, climbing

*Exercising keeps body fluids circulating; when sedentary people lie down, the excess fluid that has pooled in their lower extremities begins to circulate again, creating the need to urinate. Interview with W. E. Wooldridge, MD, professor emeritus of clinical medicine at the University of Missouri in Columbia as reported in *The Physician and Sportsmedicine* 19 (1991): 49.

stairs, or simply moving about. This can be for 5 minutes at a time, 12 times a day; 12 minutes at a time, 5 times a day; or any combination of activity to total 60 minutes.

- *Three days a week.* 30 to 45 minutes of vigorous and continuous physical activity, such as swimming, dancing, rowing, or brisk walking.

With persistence, people can achieve great improvements at any age. Training not only tones, firms, and strengthens muscles but also increases the blood flow to the brain, thereby improving mental ability.

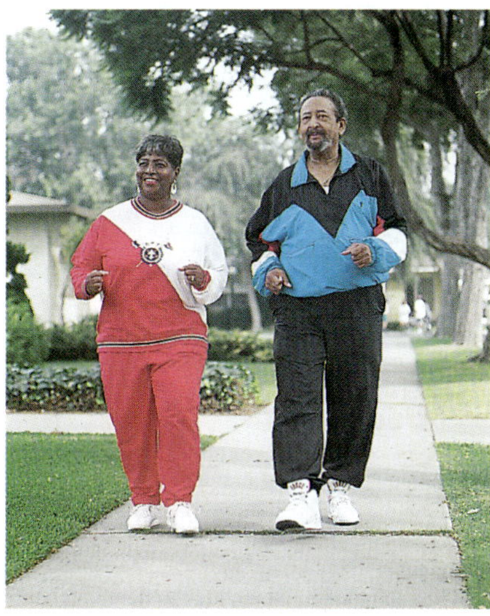

A walk in the neighborhood provides many physical benefits and a time to visit with others.

Protein The protein needs of older adults appear to be about the same as, or even greater than, those of younger people. Since energy needs decrease, however, the protein has to be obtained from low-kcalorie sources of high-quality protein, such as lean meats, poultry, fish, and eggs; nonfat and low-fat milk products; and legumes and grains.

Carbohydrate Abundant carbohydrate is needed to protect protein from being used as an energy source. Complex carbohydrate foods such as vegetables, whole grains, and fruits are also rich in fiber and essential vitamins and minerals.

The combination of ample water and high-fiber foods can alleviate constipation—a condition common among older adults, and especially among nursing home residents. Physical inactivity and medications probably contribute to the high incidence of constipation, but lack of water and fiber does, too, in many cases. In fact, average fiber intakes are lower than current recommendations.

Fat As is true for people of all ages, fat needs to be limited in the diet of most older adults. Cutting fat may help retard the development of cancer, atherosclerosis, and other degenerative diseases. Restricting fat intakes to less than 30 percent of total energy presents a challenge for many older adults, given their limited energy allowances and food intakes. For some older adults, limiting fat intake too severely may lead to nutrient deficiencies and weight loss—two problems that carry greater health risks in the elderly than overweight.[36]

VITAMINS AND MINERALS

Most people can achieve adequate vitamin and mineral intakes simply by including foods from all food groups in their diets, but studies show that older adults often omit fruits and vegetables.[37] About 18 percent of people 60 years and older are reported to eat no vegetables at all, and up to one of every three older adults reports never eating fruit. When almost 500 participants in a meal program were asked about their food likes and dislikes, nine of the ten most-disliked foods were vegetables. Similarly, few older adults consume the recommended amounts of milk products.[38]

Vitamin A Vitamin A stands alone in that it is absorbed and stored more efficiently by the aging GI tract and liver, although its processing within the body slows slightly.[39] Several studies have reported that healthy older adults have normal levels of plasma vitamin A even when their dietary intakes fall below the RDA, suggesting that the current RDA may be too high.[40] The Committee on Dietary Allowances has hesitated in lowering the RDA, recognizing both the need to prevent vitamin A deficiency and the possibility that the vitamin A precursor beta-carotene might delay the onset of some age-related diseases.

Vitamin D Older adults face a greater risk of vitamin D deficiency than younger people do. Only vitamin D–fortified milk provides significant vitamin D, and many older adults drink little or no milk. Consequently, many older adults have vitamin D intakes of less than half of the recommended intake. Further compromising the vitamin D status of many older people, especially those in nursing homes, is their limited exposure to sunlight. Finally, aging reduces the skin's capacity to make vitamin D and the kidneys' ability to convert it to its active form. Not only are older adults not getting enough vitamin D, but they may actually need more than the RDA to maintain bone health.[41] The recommended intake for vitamin D was recently raised from 5 to 10 micrograms daily to prevent bone loss and to maintain vitamin D status in older people, especially in those who engage in minimal outdoor activity.[42]

Vitamin B_6 Studies of vitamin B_6 reveal that its metabolism is altered with age, resulting in a higher requirement. The current RDA for people over 50 may need to be raised.[43]

Vitamin B_{12} People with atrophic gastritis are particularly vulnerable to vitamin B_{12} deficiency for two reasons. First, digestion in the inflamed stomach is inefficient. Second, the abundant bacteria that accompany this condition use the vitamin. Given the devastating effects of a vitamin B_{12} deficiency, an RDA higher than the current one may be appropriate.[44]

Iron Among the minerals, iron deserves first mention. Iron-deficiency anemia is less common in older adults than in younger people, but it still occurs in some, especially in those with low food energy intakes. Aside from diet, other factors in many older people's lives make iron deficiency likely: chronic blood loss from disease conditions and medicines, and poor iron absorption due to reduced stomach acid secretion and antacid use. Anyone concerned with older people's nutrition should keep these possibilities in mind.

Zinc Zinc intake is commonly low in older people. As many as 95 percent of older adults may not get the zinc they need, and many receive less than half of the recommended amount.[45] In addition, older adults may absorb zinc less efficiently than younger people do. A number of different factors, including medications that older adults commonly use, can impair zinc absorption or enhance its excretion and thus lead to deficiency.[46] Older adults who do not make special efforts to eat zinc-rich foods such as meats, fish, and poultry will no doubt fail to meet the zinc RDA. Some of the symptoms of zinc deficiency resemble symptoms associated with aging—for example, decline in taste acuity and dermatitis. Whether these symptoms are attributable to zinc deficiency remains unclear.

Calcium DRI for older adults: 1200 mg/day.

Calcium The appropriate calcium intake for older adults remains controversial. A National Institutes of Health panel has concluded that women over 50 who are not on estrogen replacement therapy and all adults over 65 should receive 1500 milligrams of calcium daily.[47] Recommended intakes for older adults were recently raised from 800 to 1200 milligrams of calcium daily.[48]

While researchers attempt to reach agreement about the calcium requirements of older adults, especially those of women, one thing is clear: the calcium intakes of many people, especially women, in the United States are well below recommendations. If fresh milk causes stomach discomfort, as some older people report, then special efforts should be made to eat other calcium-rich foods. One simple solution is to incorporate dry nonfat milk into recipes; Chapter 12 offers many other strategies.

The importance of abundant dietary calcium throughout life, and especially for women after menopause, to protect against osteoporosis was discussed in Chapter and Highlight 12.

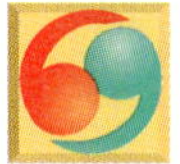

HEALTHY PEOPLE 2000: Increase calcium intake so that at least 50% of people aged 25 years and older consume two or more servings of calcium-rich foods daily.

Malnutrition It has been estimated that as many as 50 percent of nursing home residents may be malnourished and underweight.[49] For these people, a diet that emphasizes fiber-rich foods such as whole grains, fruits, and vegetables may be too low in concentrated protein and energy. Protein- and energy-dense snacks such as hard-boiled eggs, tuna fish and crackers, peanut butter on graham crackers, and homemade soups are valuable additions to the diets of underweight or malnourished older adults. Table 20–1 lists risk factors for malnutrition in elderly people.

Table 20–1

Risk Factors for Malnutrition in Older Adults

Difficulties in chewing or swallowing
Difficulties in procuring or preparing food
Recent loss of spouse
Oral health problems
Poverty
Multiple drug use
Confusion or depression
Neurologic disorders
Chronic lung disease
Eating fewer than three meals per day
Anorexia
Institutionalization
Inability to self-feed
Alcoholism
Altered taste or smell
Recent surgery
Diabetes
Loneliness

Source: Adapted from R. Chernoff, Meeting the nutritional needs of the elderly in the institutional setting, *Nutrition Reviews* 52 (1994): 132–136.

SUPPLEMENTS FOR OLDER ADULTS

Advertisers target older people with appeals to take supplements and eat "health" foods, claiming that these products prevent disease and promote longevity. About half of all women over 65 years of age take some type of nutrient supplement, while about one-fifth of older men do. Quite often those who take supplements are not deficient in the nutrients being supplemented.[50] Certain diseases or health problems may necessitate the taking of supplements, but quite often, supplements have not been prescribed by health care professionals and are inappropriate.

When recommended by a physician, vitamin D and calcium supplements for osteoporosis or iron for iron-deficiency anemia may be beneficial. In most cases, though, the money spent on supplements would be better spent on nutritious foods. Older adults with food energy intakes less than about 1500 kcalories should probably take supplements—not megavitamins, but just the once-daily type of vitamin-mineral supplements.

People with small energy allowances would do well to become more active and earn the right to eat more food. Food is the best source of nutrients for everybody. Supplements are just that—supplements to foods, not substitutes for them. For anyone who is motivated to obtain the best possible health, it is never too late to learn to eat well, drink water, exercise regularly, and adopt other lifestyle changes such as quitting smoking, moderating alcohol use, and the like.

Table 20–2

Summary of Nutrient Concerns in Aging

Nutrient	Effect of Aging	Comments
Energy	Need decreases.	Physical activity moderates the decline.
Fiber	Likelihood of constipation increases with low intakes and changes in the GI tract.	Inadequate water intakes and lack of physical activity, along with some medications, compound the problem.
Protein	Needs stay the same.	Low-fat, high-fiber legumes and grains meet both protein and other nutrient needs.
Vitamin A	Absorption increases.	RDA may be high.
Vitamin D	Increased likelihood of inadequate intake; skin synthesis declines.	Daily limited sunlight exposure may be of benefit.
Water	Lack of thirst and decreased total body water make dehydration likely.	Mild dehydration is a common cause of confusion. Difficulty obtaining water or getting to the bathroom may compound the problem.
Iron	In women, status improves after menopause; deficiencies are linked to chronic blood losses and low stomach acid output.	Adequate stomach acid is required for absorption; antacid or other medicine use may aggravate iron deficiency; vitamin C and meat increase absorption.
Zinc	Often inadequate intakes and reduced absorption; but needs may also decrease.	Medications interfere with absorption; deficiency may depress appetite and sense of taste.
Calcium	Intakes may be low; osteoporosis common.	Stomach discomfort commonly limits milk intake; calcium substitutes are needed.

Table 20–2 summarizes the nutrient concerns of aging. While some nutrients need special attention in the diet, supplements are not routinely recommended. The ever-growing number of older people in the world presents an urgent need to know more about how their nutrient requirements differ from those of younger people and how such knowledge can enhance their health.

Special Concerns of Older Adults

Nutrition through the prime years may play a greater role than has been realized in preventing many changes once thought to be inevitable consquences of growing older. The following discussions of cataracts, arthritis, and the aging brain show that nutrition may provide at least some protection against some of the conditions associated with aging.

CATARACTS AND ARTHRITIS

Two common causes of distress among older people are cataracts and arthritis. Both of these conditions have nutrition links.

cataracts: thickenings of the eye lenses that impair vision and can lead to blindness.

Cataracts Cataracts are age-related thickenings in the lenses of the eye that impair vision. If not surgically removed, they ultimately lead to blindness. Cataracts occur even in well-nourished individuals due to ultraviolet light exposure, free-radical damage, injury, viral infections, toxic substances, and genetic disorders. Many cataracts, however, are vaguely called senile cataracts—meaning "caused by aging." In the United States, some 46 percent of people between the ages of 75 and 85 have cataracts, compared to only 5 percent of those between the ages of 52 and 64.[51]

Reminder: *Free radicals* are highly reactive molecules that arise during oxidative reactions and readily attack other molecules; see Highlight 11 for more details.

Oxidative stress appears to play a significant role in the development of cataracts, and the antioxidant nutrients may help minimize the damage.[52] Studies have reported an inverse relationship between cataracts and dietary intakes of vitamin C, vitamin E, and carotenoids.[53] One study found that people who had no cataracts took significantly more supplements of vitamins C and E than those who had cataracts.[54]

arthritis: a usually painful inflammation of a joint caused by many conditions, including infections, metabolic disturbances, or injury; joint structure is usually altered, with loss of function.

Arthritis Another condition that disables older people is arthritis, a painful swelling of the joints. During movement, the ends of bones are normally protected from wear by cartilage and by small sacs of fluid that act as a lubricant; but with age, bones sometimes disintegrate, and the joints become malformed and painful to move. Arthritis afflicts millions of people around the world, especially the elderly. Nutrition quackery to treat arthritis is abundant, but no known diet prevents, relieves, or cures.

Not effective against arthritis:

- Alfalfa tea.
- Amino acid supplements.
- Blackstrap molasses.
- Burdock root.
- Calcium.
- Celery juice.
- Cod liver oil.
- Copper supplements.
- Dimethyl sulfoxide (DMSO).
- Fasting.
- Fresh fruit.
- Garlic.
- Honey.
- Inositol.
- Kelp.
- Lecithin.
- Para-amino benzoic acid (PABA).
- Raw liver.
- *Aloe vera* liquid.
- Superoxide dismutase (SOD).
- Vitamin D.
- Vitamin megadoses.
- Watercress.
- Yeast.
- 100 other substances.

One possibly valid link between arthritis and diet is through the immune system. Researchers believe that in rheumatoid arthritis, the immune system mistakenly attacks the bone coverings as if they were made of foreign tissue.[55] The integrity of the immune system depends on adequate nutrition, and a poor diet may worsen arthritis. It is also possible that in some individuals, certain foods may stimulate the immune system to attack. For example, milk and milk products seem to aggravate arthritis in some people.[56]

Another nutrient linked to arthritis is the omega-3 fatty acid found in fish oil, EPA. Research shows that the same diet recommended for heart health—one low in saturated fat from meats and milk products and high in oils from fish—helps prevent or reduce the inflammation in the joints that makes arthritis so painful.[57] Researchers theorize that EPA probably interferes with the action of prostaglandins, chemicals involved in inflammation.

Another possible link between nutrition and arthritis involves the lipid peroxidation reaction described in Highlight 11—which vitamin E helps to prevent. Lipid peroxidation of the membranes within joints causes inflammation and swelling.[58] Vitamin E has not improved active cases of arthritis, but this is not surprising since the vitamin's role in lipid peroxidation is preventive, not restorative.

A known connection between arthritis and nutrition is overweight. Weight loss is important for overweight persons with arthritis, partly because the joints affected are often weight-bearing joints that are stressed and irritated by having to carry excess poundage. Interestingly, though, weight loss often relieves the worst of the pain of arthritis in the hands as well, even though they are not weight-bearing joints. Jogging and other weight-bearing exercises do not worsen arthritis, even in marathon runners.

Drugs used to relieve arthritis can impose nutrition risks.[59] Many drugs affect appetite and alter the body's use of nutrients, as Chapter 15 explains.

These brief discussions of cataracts and arthritis show that nutrition may provide at least some protection against certain conditions associated with aging. In fact, it is beginning to look as though nutrition through the prime years may play a greater role than has been realized in preventing many changes once thought to be inevitable consequences of growing older.

THE AGING BRAIN

The brain, like all of the body's organs, responds to both inherited and environmental factors that can enhance or diminish its amazing capacities. One of the challenges researchers face when studying aging of the brain in human beings is to distinguish among normal age-related physiological changes, changes caused by diseases, and changes that result from cumulative, extrinsic factors such as diet.

neuron: a nerve cell; the structural and functional unit of the nervous system. Neurons initiate and conduct nerve transmissions.

cerebral cortex: the outer surface of the cerebrum.

The brain normally changes in some characteristic ways as it ages. For one thing, its blood supply decreases. For another, the number of neurons, the brain cells that specialize in transmitting information, diminishes as people age. When the number of nerve cells in one part of the cerebral cortex diminishes, hearing and speech are affected. Losses of neurons in other parts of the cortex can impair memory and cognitive function. When the number of neurons in the hindbrain diminishes, balance and posture are affected. Losses of neurons in other parts of the brain affect still other functions.

Clinicians now recognize that much of the cognitive loss and forgetfulness generally attributed to aging is due in part to extrinsic, and therefore controllable, factors such as nutrient deficiencies. In some instances, the degree of cognitive loss is extensive and attributable to a specific disorder such as a brain tumor. In cases such as Alzheimer's disease, deterioration may be genetically determined and will not yet yield to external approaches.

senile dementia: the loss of brain function beyond the normal loss of physical adeptness and memory that occurs with aging.

senile dementia of the Alzheimer's type (SDAT): a degenerative disease of the brain involving memory loss and major structural changes in neuron networks; also known as **primary degenerative dementia of senile onset** or **chronic brain syndrome**, but often simply called **Alzheimer's disease**.

Alzheimer's Disease Much attention has focused on the *abnormal* deterioration of the brain called senile dementia of the Alzheimer's type (SDAT), which affects 5 percent of U.S. adults by age 65 and 20 percent of those over 80.[60] Diagnosis of SDAT depends on its characteristic symptoms: the victim gradually loses memory and reasoning, the ability to communicate, physical capabilities, and eventually life itself. Nerve cells in the brain die and communication between the cells breaks down.

To date, the causes of SDAT continue to elude researchers, although genetic factors are apparently involved. Consequently, researchers have yet to find a cure for this devastating degenerative disease. Treatment involves providing care to clients and support to their families. One drug (trade-named Tacrine) seems to slow the advance of the disease in about 20 percent of those who use it, but it does not reverse the damage already done. Meanwhile, some drugs seem to favorably influence the ability to remember and so hold promise for improving the lives of those with Alzheimer's disease. Other drugs may be used to control depression or behavior problems.

Nutrition may be somehow linked to SDAT. For example, as blood flow to the brain diminishes with age, the brain normally compensates by absorbing more glucose and oxygen. In SDAT, no such compensation occurs, so the glucose and oxygen uptake declines. Whether the brain's diminished capacity to take up glucose and oxygen causes or results from SDAT remains unclear.

Reminder: A *neurotransmitter* is a chemical that is released by one nerve cell and acts upon a second nerve cell, altering its electrical state or activity.

Another abnormality of interest involves the extremely low concentrations of the enzyme that makes the neurotransmitter acetylcholine from choline and acetyl CoA. Acetylcholine is essential to memory. To date, supplements of choline (or of lecithin, which contains choline) have had no effect on memory or on the progression of the disease. Trials of lecithin in combination with drugs show some improvement in limited areas of cognitive deficiencies.

Most people have heard of an association between aluminum and the development of SDAT, although a causal connection seems unlikely. Brain concentrations of aluminum in SDAT people exceed normal brain concentrations by some 10 to 30 times, but blood and hair aluminum remains normal, indicating that the accumulation is caused by something in the brain itself, not by an overload of aluminum in the body. Thus the high brain aluminum must be at least partly a result, rather than a cause, of SDAT. Researchers are still investigating the relationship between dietary aluminum and SDAT in individuals, and the question is still open whether aluminum cookware, which slightly increases the aluminum content of foods, significantly affects the progress of SDAT.

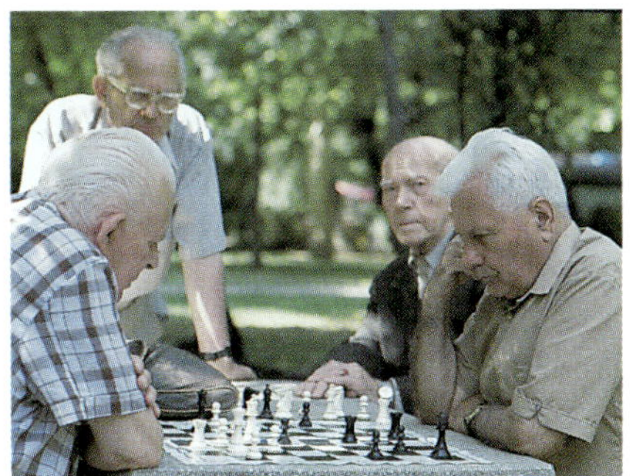

The brain is nourished by both foods and mental challenges.

Maintaining appropriate body weight may be the most important nutrition concern for the person with SDAT. Depression and forgetfulness can lead to poor food intake, and restlessness may increase energy needs. Perhaps the best that a caretaker can do nutritionally for an SDAT client is to supervise food planning and mealtimes. Providing well-liked and well-balanced meals and snacks in a cheerful atmosphere encourages food consumption. To minimize confusion, offer a few ready-to-eat foods, in bite-size pieces, with seasonings and sauces. To avoid mealtime disruptions, control distractions such as television, children, and the telephone.

SDAT is an identifiable disease, the course of which is probably not influenced by nutrition. But poor nutrition in general does affect the brain in other ways.

Nutrient Deficiencies and Brain Function Moderate, long-term nutrient deficiencies may contribute to the loss of memory and cognition that some older adults experience. For example, the ability of neurons to synthesize specific neurotransmitters depends in part on the availability of precursor nutrients that are obtained from the diet. The neurotransmitter serotonin derives from the amino acid tryptophan. To function properly, the enzymes involved in neurotransmitter synthesis require vitamins and minerals. Severe dietary deficiencies of thiamin, vitamin B_6, vitamin B_{12}, folate, and vitamin C impair mental ability, including memory. Trace elements such as iron and zinc also support normal brain function. Table 20–3 summarizes some of the better known connections between impaired brain function and severe nutrient deficiencies. If long-term,

Table 20–3

Summary of Nutrient-Brain Relationships

Brain Function	Inadequate Intake or Deficiency of:
Short-term memory loss	Vitamin B_{12}, vitamin C
Poor performance in problem-solving tests	Riboflavin, folate, vitamin B_{12}, vitamin C
Dementia	Thiamin, zinc
Cognition	Folate, vitamin B_6, vitamin B_{12}, iron
Degeneration of brain tissue	Vitamin B_6

moderate nutrient deficiencies influence the loss of cognitive function that accompanies aging, then the loss may be preventable or at least diminished or delayed through diet.

Senile dementia and other losses of brain function afflict millions of older adults. As the number of people over age 65 continues to grow, the need for solutions to the problems that this major portion of the population faces is becoming urgent. Some problems may be inevitable, but others are preventable.

We can now state with certainty that a person's nutrition status affects the health and functioning of the whole body. Eating a nutritious, balanced diet throughout life seems a small effort in light of the rewards of continued health and enjoyment in later life.

In addition, there is much people can do, besides obtaining adequate nutrition, to support a high quality of life into old age. By practicing stress-management skills, maintaining physical fitness, participating in activities of interest, and cultivating spiritual health, a person can grow old gracefully (see Table 20–4 for some strategies).

Table 20–4

Strategies for Growing Old Gracefully

- Choose nutrient-dense foods.
- Maintain appropriate body weight.
- Reduce stress.
- For women, see a physician about estrogen replacement.
- For people who smoke, quit.
- Expect to enjoy sex, and learn new ways of enhancing it.
- Use alcohol only moderately, if at all; use drugs only as prescribed.
- Take care to prevent accidents.
- Expect good vision and hearing throughout life; obtain glasses and hearing aids if necessary.
- Be alert to confusion as a disease symptom, and seek diagnosis.
- Control depression through activities and friendships.
- Drink 8 glasses of water every day.
- Practice mental skills. Keep on solving math problems and crossword puzzles, playing cards or other games, reading, writing, imagining, and creating.
- Make financial plans early to ensure security.
- Accept change. Work at recovering from losses; make new friends.
- Cultivate spiritual health. Cherish personal values. Make life meaningful.
- Go outside for sunshine and fresh air as often as possible.
- Be physically active. Walk, run, dance, swim, bike, row, or climb for aerobic activity. Lift weights, do calisthenics, or pursue some other activity to tone, firm, and strengthen muscles. Change activities to suit changing abilities and tastes.
- Be socially active—play bridge, join an exercise group, take a class, teach a class, eat with friends, volunteer time to help others.
- Stay interested in life—pursue a hobby, spend time with grandchildren, take a trip, read, grow a garden, or go to the movies.
- Enjoy life.

Food Choices and Eating Habits of Older Adults

Older people are an incredibly diverse group, and for the most part they are independent, socially sophisticated, mentally lucid, fully participating members of society who report themselves to be happy and healthy. Most people over 65 live in their own or relatives' homes; only 5 percent of those 65 to 85, and 20 percent of those over 85, live in facilities such as nursing homes.

Older people spend more money per person on foods to eat at home than other age groups and less money on foods away from home. Manufacturers would be wise to cater to the preferences of older adults by providing good-tasting, nutritious foods in easy-to-open, single-serving packages with labels that are easy to read. Such services enable older adults to maintain their independence; most of them want to take care of themselves and need to feel a sense of control and involvement in their own lives.

- Older adult feeding pointer: Try to maintain independence.

Familiarity, taste, and health beliefs are most influential on older people's food choices. Eating foods that are familiar, especially those that recall family meals and pleasant times, can be comforting. The importance of diet and health beliefs in food selection is evidenced by surveys indicating that older adults are choosing low-fat poultry and fish, low-fat milk and milk products, and high-fiber breads and grains.[61] People 65 and over are less likely to diet to lose weight than younger people are, but are more likely to diet in pursuit of medical goals such as controlling blood glucose, cholesterol, and sodium.

- Older adult feeding pointer: Select familiar foods, especially ethnic favorites.

NUTRITION PROGRAMS

Nutrition services are an integral part of health care, and different subgroups of the aging population need different programs designed to meet their specific needs.[62] People living alone can benefit from congregate meal programs; people confined to their homes need meals delivered. The Nutrition Screening Initiative is part of a national effort to identify and treat nutrition problems in older persons; it uses a screening checklist (see Table 20–5 on p. 682). To *determine* the risk of malnutrition in older clients, health care providers can keep in mind the characteristics listed in the margin.[63]

Risk factors for malnutrition in older adults:

- Disease.
- Eating poorly.
- Tooth loss or oral pain.
- Economic hardship.
- Reduced social contact.
- Multiple medications.
- Involuntary weight loss or gain.
- Needs assistance with self-care.
- Elderly person older than 80 years.

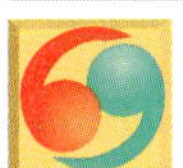

HEALTHY PEOPLE 2000: Increase to at least 80% the receipt of home food-services by people aged 65 and older who have difficulty in preparing their own meals or are otherwise in need of home-delivered meals.

The U.S. government funds programs to provide nutritious meals to older adults at congregate meal sites. These meals are a valuable source of nutrients for many older adults. Like the school lunches, though, congregate meals do not typically meet current dietary recommendations to limit sodium, fat, and cholesterol.[64] The box on p. 683 describes food assistance programs for older adults.

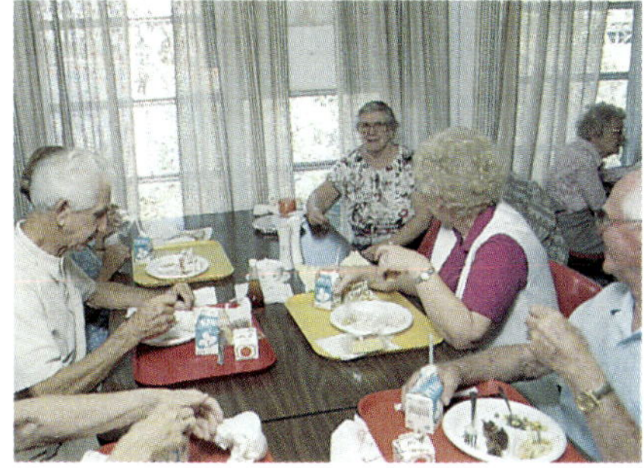

Social interactions at a congregate meal site can be as nourishing as the foods served.

MEALS FOR SINGLES

Singles of all ages face difficulties in purchasing, storing, and preparing food. Large packages of meat and vegetables are often intended for families of four or more, and even a head of lettuce can spoil before one person can use it all. Many

Table 20–5

Nutrition Screening Initiative Checklist

Circle the number to the right if the statement applies to you.

Statement	Yes
I have an illness or condition that made me change the kind and/or amount of food I eat.	2
I eat fewer than 2 meals per day.	3
I eat few fruits or vegetables or milk products.	2
I have 3 or more drinks of beer, liquor, or wine almost every day.	2
I have tooth or mouth problems that make it hard for me to eat.	2
I don't always have enough money to buy the food I need.	4
I eat alone most of the time.	1
I take 3 or more different prescribed or over-the-counter drugs a day.	1
Without wanting to, I have lost or gained 10 pounds in the last 6 months.	2
I am not always physically able to shop, cook, and/or feed myself.	2
Total	

SCORE:

0–2: Good. Recheck your score in 6 months.

3–5: Moderate nutritional risk. Visit your local office on aging, senior nutrition program, senior citizens center, or health department for tips on improving eating habits.

6 or more: High nutritional risk. See your doctor, dietitian, or other health care professional for help in improving your nutrition status.

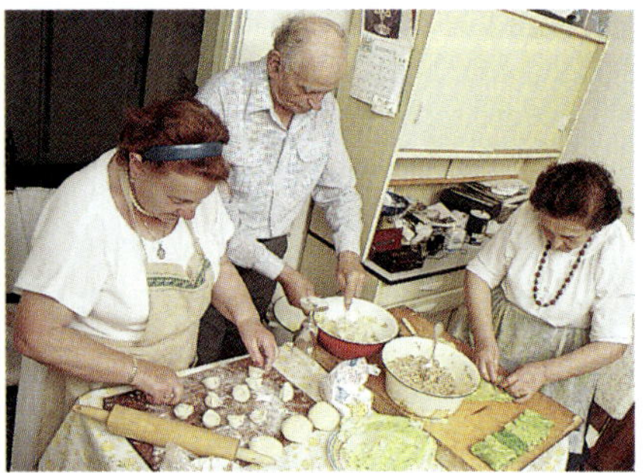

Taking time to nourish your body well is a gift you give yourself.

singles live in small dwellings and have little storage space for foods. A limited income presents additional obstacles. This section presents ideas that can help to solve some of these problems.

Spend Wisely People who have the means to shop and cook for themselves can cut their food bills just by being wise shoppers. The first decision a person with a tight grocery budget must make is where to shop. Large supermarkets are usually less expensive than convenience stores, but the cost of transportation to the market is a consideration. A grocery list helps reduce impulse buying, and specials and coupons can save money when the items featured are those that the shopper needs and uses.

Buy Bulk Many foods that offer a variety of nutrients for practically pennies have a long shelf life and can be purchased in bulk. Staples such as rice, pastas, nonfat dry powdered milk, and dried beans and peas can be stored on a shelf for months at room temperature. Other foods that are usually a good buy include whole pieces of cheese rather than sliced or shredded cheese; fresh produce in season; variety meats such as chicken livers; and cereals that require cooking instead of ready-to-serve cereals.

A person who has ample freezing space can buy large packages of meat, such as pork chops, ground beef, or chicken, when they are on sale. Then, the package

Food Assistance Programs for Older Adults

The federal Nutrition Program for Older Americans (Title III) is intended to improve older people's nutrition status and enable them to avoid medical problems, continue living in communities of their own choice, and stay out of institutions. Its specific goals are to provide low-cost, nutritious meals; opportunities for social interaction; homemaker education and shopping assistance; counseling and referral to social services; and transportation.

Title III provides for congregate meal programs. Administrators try to select sites for congregate meals so as to feed as many eligible people as possible. Volunteers may also deliver meals to those who are homebound either permanently or temporarily; these efforts are known as Meals on Wheels. The home-delivery program ensures nutrition, but its recipients miss out on the social benefit of the congregate meal sites; every effort is made to persuade older people to come to the shared meals, if they can. All persons aged 60 years and older are eligible to receive meals from these programs, regardless of their income. Priority is given to those who are economically and socially needy. These programs provide at least one meal a day that meets a third of the RDA for this age group; they must operate five or more days a week. Many programs voluntarily offer additional services: provisions for therapeutic diets, food pantries, ethnic meals, and delivery of meals to the homeless.

Older adults can learn about the available programs in their communities by looking in the yellow pages of the telephone book under "Social Services" or "Senior Citizens' Organizations." In addition, the local senior center and hospital can usually direct people to programs providing nutrition and other health-related services.

congregate meal sites: nutrition programs that provide food for the elderly in a conveniently located setting such as a community center.

can be immediately divided into individual servings and wrapped in aluminum foil, not freezer paper: the foil can become the liner for the pan in which to bake or broil the meat, thus saving work. All the individual servings can be put in a bag marked appropriately with the contents and the date. The bag will be easy to locate in the freezer, and a person can see when the supply is running low.

Frozen vegetables are more economical in large bags than in small boxes. The amount needed can be taken out, and the bag closed tightly with a rubber band. If the package is returned quickly to the freezer each time, the vegetables will stay fresh for a long time.

Finally, breads and cereals usually must be purchased in larger quantities. Again the amount needed for a few days can be taken out and the rest stored in the freezer.

Buy Small Buying the right amount in order not to waste any food is a challenge for people eating alone. They can buy fresh milk in the size best suited for personal needs. Pint-size and even cup-size boxes of milk are also available and can be stored unopened on a shelf for up to three months without refrigeration.

Boxes of milk kept at room temperature on the shelves of grocery stores have been treated with a process called **ultrahigh temperature (UHT);** the milk is exposed to temperatures above those of pasteurization just long enough to sterilize it.

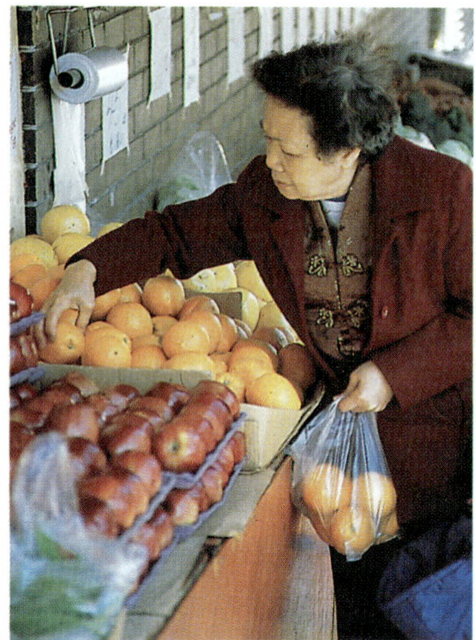
Buy only what you will use.

Grocers will break open a package of wrapped meat and rewrap the portion needed. Similarly, eggs can be purchased by the half-dozen. Eggs do keep for long periods, though, if stored properly in the refrigerator.

Fresh fruits and vegetables can be purchased individually. A person can buy three pieces of each kind of fresh fruit: a ripe one to eat right away, a semiripe one to eat soon after, and a green one to ripen on the windowsill. If vegetables are packaged in large quantities, the grocer can break open the package so that a smaller amount can be purchased. Small cans of fruits and vegetables, even though they are more expensive per unit, are a reasonable alternative, considering that it is expensive to buy a regular-size can and let the unused portion spoil.

Be Creative For times when a person has to buy more food than one person can use, here are a few hints. Mixtures of leftovers can be prepared and served again. A thick stew made from leftover green beans, carrots, cauliflower, broccoli, and any meat with added onion, pepper, celery, and potatoes makes a complete and balanced meal—except for milk, but then powdered milk can be added to the stew.

Glass jars are ideal for storing shelf staple items—rice, tapioca, lentils or other dry beans, flour, cornmeal, nonfat dry milk, macaroni, cereal, and the like. Freezing each filled jar for one night first kills any insect eggs that might be present. The jars will then keep bugs out of the food indefinitely. They make an attractive display and serve to remind the cook of different choices to vary menus. The directions-for-use labels from the packages can be stored in the jars.

Creative chefs think of various ways to use a vegetable when only large amounts are available. For example, a head of cauliflower can be divided into thirds. Then one-third is cooked and eaten hot. Another third is put into a vinegar and oil marinade for use in a salad. And the last third can be used in a casserole or stew.

Also, single people shouldn't hesitate to invite someone to share meals with them whenever there is a lot of food. It's likely that that person will return the invitation, and both parties will get to enjoy companionship and a meal prepared by others.

An occasional frozen TV dinner can also be useful—although expensive—if it makes the difference between a person's eating and not eating. Many such dinners that are now available are low in fat and nutritious. Adding a fresh salad, a whole-wheat roll, and a glass of milk can make a nice meal. Another option for those who can afford it is to eat meals from restaurants. Most restaurants offer take-out meals and many provide delivery services.

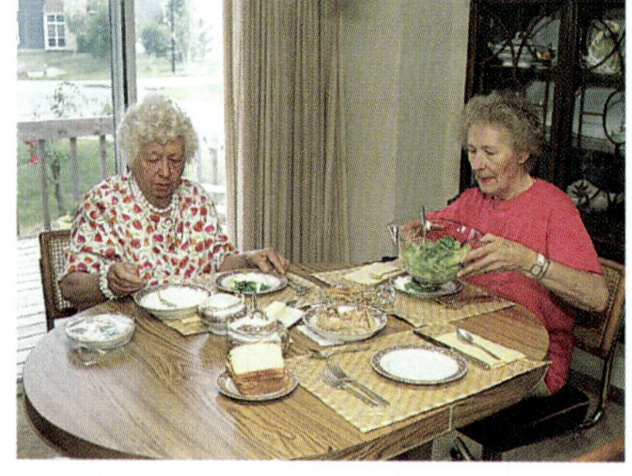
Invite guests to share a meal.

One more suggestion for those who are alone at mealtime is this: make it a special occasion. One way to do this is to set the table with a tablecloth, a napkin, a full set of utensils, and fresh flowers. Set a pot of stew or homemade soup with vegetables and fresh herbs on low heat to cook, and make a salad. Get comfortable in a stuffed chair, and enjoy a book or some soothing music until the rich aroma of a simmering dinner beckons. After serving your plate, light a candle, dim the lights, savor the food, and relish some of the best company you will have—your own.

Study Questions

1. What roles does nutrition play in aging, and what roles can it play in retarding aging?
2. What are some of the physiological changes that occur in the body's systems with aging? To what extent can aging be prevented?
3. Why does the risk of dehydration increase as people age?
4. Why do energy needs usually decline with advancing age?
5. Which vitamins and minerals need special consideration for the elderly? Explain why. Name some factors that complicate the task of setting nutrient standards for older adults.
6. Discuss the relationships between nutrition and cataracts and between nutrition and arthritis.
7. What characteristics contribute to malnutrition in older people?

Notes

1. R. Chernoff, Demographics of aging, in *Geriatric Nutrition: The Health Professional's Handbook*, ed. R. Chernoff (Gaithersburg, Md.: Aspen Publishers, 1991), pp. 1–9.
2. K. G. Kinsella, Changes in life expectancy 1900–1990, *American Journal of Clinical Nutrition* 55 (1992): 1196S–1202S; S. Kobayashi, A scientific basis for the longevity of Japanese in relation to diet and nutrition, *Nutrition Reviews* 50 (1992): 353–359.
3. L. Breslow and N. Breslow, Health practices and disability: Some evidence from Alameda County, *Preventive Medicine* 22 (1993): 86–95.
4. A. Z. LaCroix and coauthors, Maintaining mobility in late life: Smoking, alcohol consumption, physical activity, and body mass index, *American Journal of Epidemiology* 137 (1993): 858–869.
5. R. S. Paffenbarger and coauthors, The association of changes in physical-activity level and other lifestyle characteristics with mortality among men, *New England Journal of Medicine* 328 (1993): 538–545; S. N. Blair and coauthors, Physical fitness and all-cause mortality, *Journal of the American Medical Association* 262 (1989): 2395–2401.
6. R. S. Paffenbarger and coauthors, Physical activity, all-cause mortality, and longevity of college alumni, *New England Journal of Medicine* 314 (1986): 605–611.
7. E. J. Masoro, Retardation of aging processes by food restriction: An experimental tool, *American Journal of Clinical Nutrition* (supplement) 55 (1992): 1250–1252.
8. E. J. Masoro, Assessment of nutritional components in prolongation of life and health by diet, *Proceedings of the Society for Experimental Biology and Medicine* 193 (1990): 31–34; Energy intake restriction and oxidant defense, *Nutrition Reviews* 49 (1991): 278–280.
9. E. J. M. Velthuis-te Wierik and coauthors, Energy restriction, a useful intervention to retard human ageing? Results of a feasibility study, *European Journal of Clinical Nutrition* 48 (1994): 138–148.
10. R. Roubenoff and L. C. Rall, Humoral mediation of changing body composition during aging and chronic inflammation, *Nutrition Reviews* 51 (1993): 1–11.
11. T. Tada, Nutrition and the immune system in aging: An overview, *Nutrition Reviews* 50 (1992): 360.
12. R. K. Chandra, Nutrition and immunity in the elderly, *Nutrition Reviews* 50 (1992): 367–371.
13. K. Hirokawa, Understanding the mechanism of the age-related decline in immune function, *Nutrition Reviews* 50 (1992): 361–366.
14. S. Hosoda and coauthors, Age-related changes in the gastrointestinal tract, *Nutrition Reviews* 50 (1992): 374–377.
15. C. Murphy, Age-associated changes in taste and odor sensation, perception, and preference, in *Nutrition of the Elderly*, eds. H. Munro and G. Schlierf (New York: Raven Press, 1992), pp. 79–87.
16. C. O. Mitchell and R. Chernoff, Nutritional assessment of the elderly, in *Geriatric Nutrition: The Health Professional's Handbook*, ed. R. Chernoff (Gaithersburg, Md.: Aspen Publishers, 1991), pp. 363–395.
17. J. V. White and coauthors, Consensus of the Nutrition Screening Initiative: Risk factors and indicators of poor nutritional status in older Americans, *Journal of the American Dietetic Association* 91 (1991): 783–787.
18. A. K. Kant and G. Block, Dietary vitamin B-6 intake and food sources in the US population: NHANES II, 1976–1980, *American Journal of Clinical Nutrition* 52 (1990): 707–716.
19. M. A. Davis and coauthors, Living arrangements and dietary quality of older U.S. adults, *Journal of the American Dietetic Association* 90 (1990): 1667–1672; I. Darnton-Hill, Psychosocial aspects of nutrition and aging, *Nutrition Reviews* 50 (1992): 476–479.
20. E. Fogler-Levitt and coauthors, Utilization of home-delivered meals by recipients 75 years of age or older, *Journal of the American Dietetic Association* 95 (1995): 552–557.
21. D. Walker and R. E. Beauchene, The relationship of loneliness, social isolation, and physical health to dietary adequacy of independently living elderly, *Journal of the American Dietetic*

Association 91 (1991): 300–304.

22. Committee on Reference Intakes, *Dietary Reference Intakes for Calcium, Phosphorus, Magnesium, Vitamin D, and Fluoride* (Washington, D.C.: National Academy Press, 1997).
23. A. Bendich, Criteria for determining recommended dietary allowances for healthy older adults, *Nutrition Reviews* 53 (1995): S105–S110.
24. B. J. Rolls and P. A. Phillips, Aging and disturbances of thirst and fluid balance, *Nutrition Reviews* 48 (1990): 137–144.
25. Water: The beverage of life (Chicago, Ill.: The American Dietetic Association, 1994).
26. E. T. Poehlman and E. S. Horton, Regulation of energy expenditure in aging humans, *Annual Review of Nutrition* 10 (1990): 255–275.
27. A. Greeley, Nutrition and the elderly, *FDA Consumer,* October 1990, pp. 25–28.
28. L. E. Voorrips and coauthors, The physical condition of elderly women differing in habitual physical activity, *Medicine and Science in Sports and Exercise* 25 (1993): 1152–1157.
29. M. A. Fiatarone and coauthors, High-intensity strength training in nonagenarians: Effects on skeletal muscle, *Journal of the American Medical Association* 263 (1990): 3029–3034; W. E. Wooldridge as cited by *The Physician and Sportsmedicine* 19 (1991): 49.
30. A. Z. LaCroix and coauthors, Maintaining mobility in late life: Smoking, alcohol consumption, physical activity, and body mass index, *American Journal of Epidemiology* 137 (1993): 858–869; Breslow and Breslow, 1993.
31. Fiatarone and coauthors, 1990; D. E. Danforth and coauthors, Report on the fourth conference for federally supported human nutrition research units and centers, *American Journal of Clinical Nutrition* 54 (1991): 164–168; M. Whitehurst and E. Menendez, Endurance training in older women, *The Physician and Sportsmedicine* 19 (1991): 95–102.
32. J. Posner, M. D., professor of medicine and chief of the divisions of Geriatric Medicine at the Medical College of Pennsylvania in Philadelphia, as cited in C. L. Pollock, Breaking the risk of falls, *The Physician and Sports Medicine* 20 (1992): 146–156.
33. M. A. Fiatarone and coauthors, Exercise training and nutritional supplementation for physical fraility in very elderly people, *New England Journal of Medicine* 330 (1994): 1769–1775; W. W. Campbell and coauthors, Increased energy requirements and changes in body composition with resistance training in older adults, *American Journal of Clinical Nutrition* 60 (1994): 167–175.
34. D. E. Butterworth and coauthors, Exercise training and nutrient intake in elderly women, *Journal of the American Dietetic Association* 93 (1993): 653–657.
35. P. Astrand, Physical activity and fitness, *American Journal of Clinical Nutrition* (supplement) 55 (1992): 1231–1236.
36. P. J. Nestel, Dietary fat for the elderly: What are the issues? in *Nutrition of the Elderly,* eds. H. Munro and G. Schlierf (New York: Raven Press, 1992), pp. 119–127.
37. V. Holt, J. Nordstrom, and M. B. Kohrs, Food preferences of older adults, *Journal of Nutrition for the Elderly* 6 (1987): 47.
38. J. G. Fischer and coauthors, Dairy product intake of the oldest old, *Journal of the American Dietetic Association* 95 (1995): 918–921.
39. Processing of dietary retinoids is slowed in the elderly, *Nutrition Reviews* 49 (1991): 116–119.
40. Russell and Suter, 1993.
41. Russell and Suter, 1993.
42. A. R. Webb and coauthors, An evaluation of the relative contributions of exposure to sunlight and of diet to the circulating concentrations of 25-hydroxyvitamin D in an elderly nursing home population in Boston, *American Journal of Clinical Nutrition* 51 (1990): 1075–1081; Committe on Dietary Reference Intakes, 1997.
43. Russell and Suter, 1993.
44. Russell and Suter, 1993.
45. C. A. Swanson and coauthors, Zinc status of elderly adults: Response to supplement, *American Journal of Clinical Nutrition* 48 (1988): 343–349.
46. G. J. Fosmire, Trace mineral requirements, in *Geriatric Nutrition: The Health Professional's Handbook,* ed. R. Chernoff (Gaithersburg, Md.: Aspen Publishers, 1991), pp. 77–105.
47. D. V. Porter, Washington update: NIH consensus development conference statement optimal calcium intake, *Nutrition Today,* September/October 1994, pp. 37–40.
48. Committee on Dietary Reference Intakes, 1997.
49. A. A. Abbase and D. Rudman, Undernutrition in the nursing home: Prevalence, consequences, causes and prevention, *Nutrition Reviews* 52 (1994): 113–122.
50. W. A. McIntosh and coauthors, The relationship between beliefs about nutrition and dietary practices of the elderly, *Journal of the American Dietetic Association* 90 (1990): 671–675; H. Payette and K. Gray-Donald, Do vitamin and mineral supplements improve the dietary intake of elderly Canadians? *Canadian Journal of Public Health* 82 (1993): 58–60.
51. G. E. Bunce, J. Kinoshita, and J. Horwitz, Nutritional factors in cataract, *Annual Review of Nutrition* 10 (1990): 233–254.
52. Bunce, Kinoshita, and Horwitz, 1990; S. D. Varma, Scientific basis for medical therapy of cataracts by antioxidants, *American Journal of Clinical Nutrition* 53 (1991): 335S–345S.
53. P. F. Jacques and L. T. Chylack, Epidemiologic evidence of a role for the antioxidant vitamins and carotenoids in cataract prevention, *American Journal of Clinical Nutrition* 53 (1991): 352S–355S; G. E. Bunce, Antioxidant nutrition and cataract in women: A prospective study, *Nutrition Reviews* 51 (1993): 84–86.
54. J. M. Robertson, A. P. Donner, and J. R. Trevithick, A possible role for vitamins C and E in cataract prevention, *American Journal of Clinical Nutrition* 53 (1991): 346S–351S.
55. E. D. Harris, Rheumatoid arthritis: Pathophysiology and implications for therapy, *New England Journal of Medicine* 322 (1990): 1277–1289.

56. R. S. Panush, Nutritional therapy for rheumatic diseases, *Annals of Internal Medicine* 106 (1987): 619–621.
57. J. M. Kremer and coauthors, Fish-oil fatty acid supplementation in active rheumatoid arthritis: A double-blind, controlled crossover study, *Annals of Internal Medicine* 106 (1987): 497–503.
58. P. Merry and coauthors, Oxidative damage to lipids within the inflamed human joint provides evidence of radical-mediated hypoxic-reperfusion injury, *American Journal of Clinical Nutrition* 53 (1991): 362S–369S.
59. R. Roubenoff and coauthors, Catabolic effects of high-dose corticosteroids persist despite therapeutic benefit in rheumatoid arthritis, *American Journal of Clinical Nutrition* 52 (1990): 1113–1117.
60. R. N. Butler, Senile dementia of the Alzheimer type (SDAT), in *The Merck Manual of Geriatrics* (Rahway, N.J.: Merck & Co., Inc., 1990), pp. 933–938.
61. Are older Americans making better food choices to meet diet and health recommendations? *Nutrition Reviews* 51 (1993): 20–22.
62. Position of The American Dietetic Association: Nutrition, aging, and the continuum of health care, *Journal of the American Dietetic Association* 93 (1993): 80–82.
63. J. Dwyer and coauthors, Screening older Americans' nutritional health: Future possibilities, *Nutrition Today*, September/October 1991, pp. 21–24.
64. M. B. Moran and E. Reed, Are congregate meals meeting clients' needs for "heart healthy" menus? *Journal of Nutrition for the Elderly* 13 (1993): 3–10.

Highlight 20

Alternative Therapies

If you suffered from migraine headaches or severe joint pain, where would you turn for relief? Would you visit a physician? Or are you more likely to go to an herbalist or an acupuncturist? Most physicians diagnose and treat medical conditions in ways that are accepted by the established medical community; by comparison, herbalists and acupuncturists, among others, use unconventional methods that offer alternatives to standard medical practice. Instead of taking two aspirin, for example, you might be advised to chew two fresh leaves of the herb feverfew or to swallow a tincture of white willow bark. Or you might receive a massage and several acupuncture needles.

Alternative therapies have become increasingly popular in recent years. Many consumers have become distrustful of, and feel overwhelmed by, the high-tech diagnostic tests and costly treatments that conventional medicine offers. They want to take more responsibility for maintaining their own health and finding cures for their own diseases, especially when traditional medical therapies prove ineffective. This highlight explores alternative therapies in search of their possible benefits and with an awareness of their potential harms.

DEFINING ALTERNATIVE MEDICINE

By definition, alternative therapies lie outside the realm of conventional medicine. An alternative therapy is any intervention that:

- Is not taught by most medical schools in the United States.

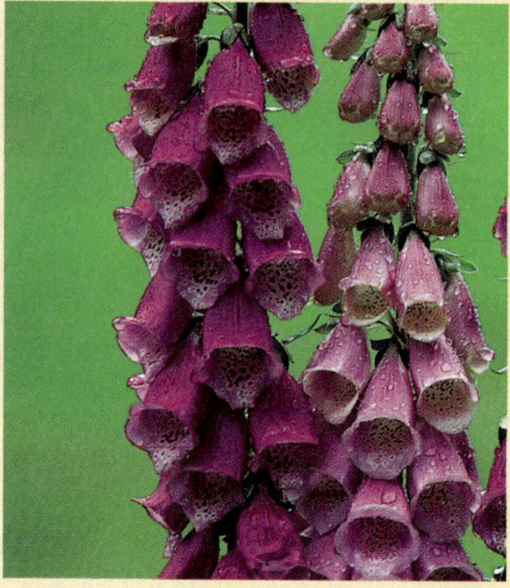

Digoxin, a drug commonly prescribed for abnormal heart rhythms, derives from the foxglove plant.

- Is not reimbursable by most health insurance providers in the United States.
- Is not well supported by scientific tests establishing its safety and effectiveness.

If it is proven safe and effective, an alternative therapy may gradually become part of mainstream conventional medicine. Cancer radiation therapy, for example, was once considered an unconventional therapy, but now is commonly accepted as standard medical practice. In some cases, a therapy that is accepted by traditional medicine for a specific ailment is used for a different purpose in an alternative therapy. For example, chelation therapy, the preferred biomedical treatment for lead poisoning, is a common alternative therapy for cardiovascular disease.

Table H20–1 lists selected fields of alternative medicine, and the accompanying glossary defines terms. Notice that most alternative medicines fall outside the field of nutrition, but that nutrition itself can be an alternative therapy. Furthermore, many alternative therapies prescribe specific dietary regi-

Table H20–1

Fields of Alternative Medicine and Selected Examples

- Mind-body interventions
  - Biofeedback
  - Faith healing
  - Hypnotherapy
  - Imagery
  - Meditation
- Bioelectromagnetic applications in medicine
  - Electroacupuncture
  - Microwave resonance therapy
- Alternative systems of medical practice
  - Acupuncture
  - Ayurveda
  - Homeopathic medicine
  - Naturopathic medicine
- Manual healing methods
  - Biofield therapeutics
  - Chiropractic
  - Massage therapy
- Pharmacological and biological treatments
  - Cartilage therapy
  - Chelation therapy
  - Ozone therapy
- Herbal medicine
- Diet and nutrition in the prevention and treatment of chronic disease
  - Macrobiotic diets
  - Orthomolecular medicine

Source: Alternative Medicine: Expanding Medical Horizons, A report to the National Institutes of Health and Alternative Medical Systems and Practices in the United States (Washington, D.C.: Government Printing Office, 1992).

Glossary

acupuncture (AK-you-PUNK-cher): a technique that involves piercing the skin with long thin needles at specific anatomical points to relieve pain or illness. Acupuncture sometimes uses heat, pressure, friction, suction, or electromagnetic energy to stimulate the points.

alternative therapies: approaches to medical diagnosis and treatment that are not fully accepted by the established medical community; as such, they are not widely taught at U.S. medical schools or practiced in U.S. hospitals; also called *adjunctive*, *unconventional*, or *unorthodox* therapies.

aroma therapy: a technique that uses oil extracts from plants and flowers (usually applied by massage or baths) to enhance physical, psychological, and spiritual health.

ayurveda (EYE-your-VAY-dah): a traditional Hindu system of improving health by using herbs, diet, meditation, massage, and yoga to stimulate the body to make its own natural drugs.

bioelectromagnetic medical applications: the use of electrical energy, magnetic energy, or both to stimulate bone repair, wound healing, and tissue regeneration.

biofeedback: the use of special devices to convey information about heart rate, blood pressure, skin temperature, muscle relaxation, and the like to enable a person to learn how to consciously control these medically important functions.

biofield therapeutics: a manual healing method that directs a healing force from an outside source (commonly God or another supernatural being) through the practitioner and into the client's body; commonly known as "laying on of hands."

cartilage therapy: the use of cleaned and powdered connective tissue, such as collagen, to improve health.

chelation therapy: the use of ethylene diamine tetraacetic acid (EDTA) to bind with metallic ions, thus healing the body by removing toxic metals.

chiropractic (KYE-roe-PRAK-tik): a manual healing method of manipulating vertebrae to relieve musculoskeletal pain suspected of causing problems with internal organs.

DHEA (dehydroepiandrosterone): a hormone secreted by the adrenal glands. DHEA is available without prescription and is sold as an anti-aging remedy to improve energy, strength, and immunity. Proof of safety or effectiveness is lacking.

faith healing: healing by invoking divine intervention without the use of medical, surgical, or other traditional therapy.

garlic oil: extract of garlic; proof of effectiveness is lacking.

hemlock: a poisonous herb having finely divided leaves and small white flowers.

herbal medicine: the use of plants to treat disease or improve health; also known as *botanical medicine* or *phytotherapy*.

homeopathic (home-ee-OP-ah-thick) **medicine:** a practice based on the theory that "like cures like," that is, that substances that cause symptoms in healthy people can cure those symptoms when given in very dilute amounts.
- *homeo* = like
- *pathos* = suffering

hypnotherapy: a technique that uses hypnosis and the power of suggestion to improve health behaviors, relieve pain, and heal.

imagery: a technique that guides clients to achieve a desired physical, emotional, or spiritual state by visualizing themselves in that state.

iridology: the study of changes in the iris of the eye and their relationships to disease.

macrobiotic diet: a diet consisting of brown rice, miso soup, sea vegetables, and other traditional Japanese foods.

massage therapy: a healing method in which the therapist manually kneads muscles to reduce tension, increase blood circulation, improve joint mobility, and promote healing of injuries.

meditation: a self-directed technique of relaxing the body and calming the mind.

melatonin: a hormone secreted by the pineal gland believed to help regulate the body's daily rhythms and promote sleep. Proof of safety or effectiveness is lacking.

naturopathic medicine: a system that integrates traditional medicine with botanical medicine, clinical nutrition, homeopathy, acupuncture, East Asian medicine, hydrotherapy, and manipulative therapy.

orthomolecular medicine: the use of large doses of vitamins to treat chronic disease.

ozone therapy: the use of ozone gas to enhance the body's immune system.

---

mens. The many dietary recommendations presented throughout this text are based on scientific evidence and do *not* fall into the alternative category; strategies that are still experimental, however, do. For example, alternative therapists may recommend megadoses of antioxidant supplements or macrobiotic diets to help prevent chronic diseases, whereas most registered dietitians would advise people to eat at least five servings of vegetables and fruits daily instead.

SOUND RESEARCH, LOUD CONTROVERSY

Most information on alternative therapies comes from folklore, tradition, and testimonial accounts. The clinical trials that have been conducted generally suffer from such poor methodology as to invalidate their findings.[1] In short, scientific evidence proving the safety and effectiveness of alternative therapies is lacking. Some say that alternative therapies simply do not work; others argue that the established medical community has not given these therapies a fair trial.

Sound research would answer two important questions. First, does the treatment offer better results than either doing nothing or giving a placebo? Second, do the benefits clearly outweigh the risks? Each of these points is worthy of elaboration.

Placebo Effect

As Chapter 1 explained, a placebo is an inert, harmless medication used in research studies to control for the beneficial effect that a treatment—even an inactive one—has on recovery. Placebos are inert, but they can also be effective, accounting for an apparent benefit about as often as not.[2] Traditional medicine tends to neglect this most powerful remedy, whereas many alternative therapies embrace it. While health professionals cannot conceal serious illnesses or intentionally deceive a client, they might be wise to provide a caring confidence in the appropriate treatment and likelihood of recovery.

Risks versus Benefits

Ideally, a therapy provides benefits with little or no risk. The use of ginseng as an adjunct in the management of diabetes (NIDDM), for example, correlates with an improved fasting blood glucose and glycated hemoglobin without adverse side effects.[3] Though still in the experimental stage, such findings, if replicated, hold promise that this alternative therapy may one day become accepted medical practice.

Some alternative therapies are innocuous, providing little or no benefit for little or no risk. Sipping a cup of warm tea with a pleasant aroma, for example, won't cure heart disease, but it may improve the person's mood and help release tension. Given no physical hazard and little financial risk, such therapies are acceptable.

In contrast, other products and procedures are downright dangerous, posing great risks while providing no benefits. One example is the folk practice of geophagia (eating earth or clay), which can cause GI impaction and impair iron absorption. Clearly, such therapies are too harmful to be used.

Perhaps most controversial are alternative therapies that may provide benefits, but also carry significant, unknown, or debatable risks. These therapies tend to appeal most to those who are most vulnerable—people with very serious illnesses. Smoking marijuana is a current example of such an alternative therapy: it seems to provide relief from symptoms such as nausea, vomiting, and pain that commonly accompany cancer, AIDS, and other diseases, but also poses risks that some people, including many physicians, consider acceptable and others, mainly politicians, deem intolerable.[4] Physicians have focused on individuals and recognize that marijuana stimulates the appetite in their nauseated clients; politicians and others have focused on society and realize that marijuana is one of many drugs that can be abused. Figure H20–1 summarizes the relationships between risks and benefits.

Funds and Findings

The public's growing interest in unorthodox remedies, coupled with the soaring costs of traditional medical approaches, opened the way for alternative medicine to prove itself. In 1992, Congress passed legislation requiring the National Institutes of Health (NIH) to create an Office of Alternative Medicine. Its task is "to more adequately explore unconventional medical practices."[5]

The use of tax dollars to fund research in alternative therapies has many medical professionals concerned.[6] They claim that establishing a special office lends credibility to these unproven methods of health care. Others demand that these methods be given a fair chance to prove themselves through scientifically valid research. Alternative therapies currently under study include:[7]

- Acupuncture to treat depression, attention deficit hyperactivity disorder, osteoarthritis, and postoperative dental pain.
- Hypnosis to treat chronic low back pain and to speed fracture healing.
- Ayurvedic herbals to treat Parkinson's disease.

Figure H20–1

Risk-Benefit Relationships

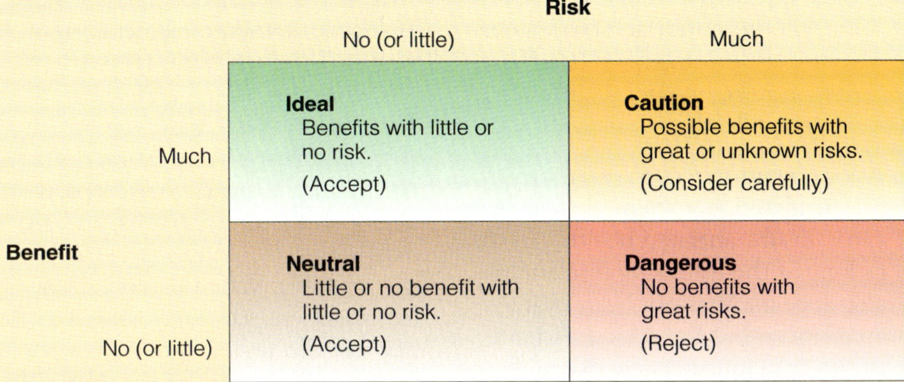

- Biofeedback to treat diabetes, low back pain, and face and mouth pain caused by jaw disorders.
- Electric currents to treat tumors.
- Imagery to treat asthma and breast cancer.

NUTRITION AND HERBAL MEDICINES

Of greatest interest to students of nutrition is the use of foods and herbs to prevent and treat illnesses. With the proliferation of research on antioxidants and disease prevention (see Highlight 11), medical science has begun to accept the health-promoting powers of vitamin-rich vegetables. It is even beginning to consider the possibility that supplementation might someday be an appropriate preventive therapy. Herbs, on the other hand, continue to meet with resistance.[8]

Herbal Traditions

From earliest times, people have used a myriad of herbs and other plants to cure aches and ills with varying degrees of success. Upon scientific study, dozens of these folk remedies reveal their secrets. For example, myrrh, a plant resin used as a painkiller in ancient times, does indeed have an analgesic effect.[9] The herb valerian, which has long been used as a tranquilizer, contains oils that have a sedative effect. Senna leaves, brewed as a laxative tea, produce compounds that act as a potent cathartic drug. The compounds that plants make are so beneficial that today they contribute to more than half of our modern medicines. Once analyzed, the chemicals in plants can be synthesized in pharmaceutical labs, thus cutting costs and conserving endangered species. Without laboratory production, valued plants could quickly disappear; consider that it took all of the bark from one 40-foot-tall, 100-year-old Pacific yew tree to obtain one 300-milligram dose of the anticancer drug paclitaxel (Taxol), until scientists learned how to synthesize it.[10]

Herbal Precautions

Simply because plants are "natural" does not mean that they are beneficial or even safe. Nothing could be more natural—and deadly—than hemlock. Several herbal remedies have toxic effects. The popular Chinese herbal potion Jin Bu Huan, which is used as a pain and insomnia remedy, has been linked with several cases of acute hepatitis. Germanium, an ingredient in many herbal products, has been associated with chronic renal failure. Paraguay tea produces symptoms of agitation, confusion, flushed skin, and fever. Kombucha tea, commonly used in the hopes of preventing cancer, relieving arthritis, curing insomnia, and stimulating hair regrowth, can cause severe metabolic acidosis.[11]

When used to diagnose, treat, or prevent disease, herbs are drugs. Yet few herbalists have the understanding of botany, chemistry, or pharmacology necessary to prescribe plant drugs.[12] Instead, they rely on hearsay and folklore. The herbs they prescribe are not regulated by the Food and Drug Administration (FDA). Under the Dietary Supplement Health and Education Act, rather than the herb manufacturers having to prove the safety of their products, the FDA has the burden of proving that a product is not safe.[13] Because information on the safety and effectiveness of herbs derives largely from users' reports, consumers may lack information about or find discrepancies regarding:

- True identification of herbs. Most mint teas are safe, for instance, but some varieties contain the highly toxic pennyroyal oil. Mistakenly used to treat colic, mint tea laden with pennyroyal has been blamed for the liver and neurological injuries of at least two infants, one of whom died.[14]

- Purity of herbal preparations. Potentially toxic quantities of arsenic and mercury have been detected in traditional Chinese herbal balls used to treat fever, rheumatism, and cataracts.[15] Analysis of one tea prescribed by a Chinese herbalist contained lead at 20,000 times the Environmental Protection Agency's allowable level; arsenic was over 1000 times the allowable level.[16]
- Appropriate uses and contraindications of herbs. Herbal remedies may be appropriate for minor ailments—a cup of chamomile tea to ease gastric discomfort or the gel of an aloe vera plant to soothe a sunburn, for example—but not for major health problems such as cancer.
- Safe dosages of herbs. Herbs that are effective contain active ingredients that need to be administered in proper doses. Each of these active ingredients has a different potency, time of onset, duration of activity, and consequent effects, making the plant itself too unpredictable to be useful. Foxglove leaves, for example, contain dozens of compounds that have an effect on the heart; digoxin, a drug derived from foxglove, offers a standard dosage that allows for a more predictable cardiac response.
- Interactions of herbs with medicines and other herbs. Like drugs, herbs may interfere with, or potentiate, the effects of other herbs and drugs. Chewing foxglove leaves when taking the drug digoxin, for example, could be catastrophic.
- Adverse reactions and toxicity levels of herbs. As is true of all drugs, herbs may produce undesirable reactions. The herb ephedra, commonly known as ma huang and used to promote weight loss, acts as a strong central nervous system stimulant, causing rapid heart rate, nervousness, headaches, insomnia, and even death.

Not only are herbal preparations not regulated, but their labels may carry unsubstantiated health claims as long as the following disclaimer also appears: "has not been evaluated by the Food and Drug Administration." Consumers who decide to use herbs do so at their own risk.

THE CLIENT'S PERSPECTIVE

Health care professionals may quickly dismiss alternative therapies as ineffective and perhaps even dangerous, but their clients think otherwise. In a survey of more than 1500 people, one out of every three had used at least one alternative therapy in the past year for a variety of medical complaints from anxiety and headaches to cancer and tumors.[17] Visits to alternative therapists outnumbered visits to primary care physicians.

Most often, people use alternative therapies in addition to, rather than in place of, conventional therapies. Only a few of the people surveyed saw an alternative therapist without also seeing a physician; all of those with life-threatening conditions such as cancer, diabetes, or lung problems who used alternative therapies saw a medical doctor as well. In fact, most people seem to seek alternative therapies for nonserious medical conditions or health promotion. They simply want to feel better and access is easy. Sometimes their symptoms are chronic and subjective, such as pain and fatigue, and difficult to treat. In these cases, the chances of finding relief are often as good with an alternative therapy as they are with a placebo, standard medical intervention, or even nonintervention.

Consumers spend an estimated $13.7 billion on alternative health services a year.[18] This figure does not include expenditures on products such as herbs, crystals, and aromas, which would raise the total considerably. When revenues soar to this extent, consumers need to beware. (To review how a person can identify health fraud and quackery, turn to pp. 33–34. For a list of credible sources of nutrition information see p. 35.)

THE HEALTH CARE PROFESSIONAL'S PERSPECTIVE

How should health care professionals react to clients who use alternative therapies? Those who condemn alternative therapies risk driving clients away, especially if alternative therapists appear more understanding and less judgmental.[19] When listening to clients, health care professionals will want to:

- Be culturally sensitive; acknowledge and respect the beliefs, attitudes, and lifestyles of their clients.[20]
- Keep an open mind; standard medical treatments simply don't work for some people in some situations.
- Accept and integrate alternative therapies into the care plan if they bring comfort without harm.
- Provide accurate information, not unsubstantiated opinions; an accurate diagnosis and information on all treatment options will

help clients make their health care decisions.

- Discourage practices only if they are harmful.

Some health care professionals have begun to embrace some of the alternative therapies and incorporate them into their medical practice. In much of Europe, biomedicine and alternative therapies have been combined into a system of "complementary medicine," which takes advantage of the best of both approaches. Many practitioners in the United States would like to see such an integrated approach used here as well.[21]

In closing, remember that alternative therapies come in a variety of shapes and sizes. Both their benefits and their risks may be either small, none, or great. Accept the beneficial, or even neutral, practices with an open mind and reject only those practices known to cause harm. Making healthful choices requires knowing what all the choices are.

NOTES

1. J. Kleijnen, P. Knipschild, and G. terRiet, Clinical trials of homeopathy, *British Medical Journal* 302 (1991): 316–323.
2. M. M. Lipman, The power of placebos, *Consumer Reports on Health*, February 1996, p. 23.
3. E. A. Sotaniemi, E. Haapakoski, and A. Rautio, Ginseng therapy in non-insulin-dependent diabetic patients: Effects on psychophysical performance, glucose homeostasis, serum lipids, serum aminoterminalpropeptide concentration, and body weight, *Diabetes Care* 10 (1995): 1373–1375.
4. J. P. Kassirer, Federal foolishness and marijuana, *New England Journal of Medicine* 336 (1997): 366–367.
5. Alternative Medicine: Expanding Medical Horizons, A report to the National Institutes of Health and Alternative Medical Systems and Practices in the United States (Washington, D.C.: Government Printing Office, 1992).
6. M. Larkin, NIH's office of alternative medicine: A wise use of tax dollars? *Priorities*, vol. 6, no. 4, 1994, pp. 32–36.
7. I. B. Stehlin, An FDA guide to choosing medical treatments, *FDA Consumer*, June 1995, pp. 10–14.
8. K. McNutt, Medicinals in food—Part I: Is science coming full circle? *Nutrition Today* 30 (1995): 218–222.
9. P. Lipkin, An ancient salve dampens pain, *Science News* 149 (1996): 20.
10. A photo finish for total taxol synthesis, *Science News* 145 (1994): 223.
11. Unexplained severe illness possibly associated with consumption of kombucha tea—Iowa, 1995, *Journal of the American Medical Association* 275 (1996): 96–98.
12. V. E. Tyler, *The Honest Herbal: A Sensible Guide to the Use of Herbs and Related Remedies* (New York: Pharmaceutical Products Press, 1993).
13. K. McNutt, Medicinals in food: What's new and what's not? *Nutrition Today* 30 (1995): 261–262.
14. J. A. Bakerink and coauthors, Multiple organ failure after ingestion of pennyroyal oil from herbal tea in two infants, *Pediatrics* 98 (1996): 944–947.
15. E. O. Espinoza, M. J. Mann, and B. Bleasdell, Arsenic and mercury in traditional Chinese herbal balls, *New England Journal of Medicine* 333 (1995): 803–804.
16. S. B. Markowitz and coauthors, Lead poisoning due to *Hai Ge Fen:* The prophyrin content of individual erythrocytes, *Journal of the American Medical Association* 271 (1994): 932–934.
17. D. M. Eisenberg and coauthors, Unconventional medicine in the United States: Prevalence, costs, and patterns of use, *New England Journal of Medicine* 328 (1993): 246–252.
18. J. Langone, Challenging the mainstream, *Time*, Fall 1996, pp. 40–43.
19. E. W. Campion, Why unconventional medicine? *New England Journal of Medicine* 328 (1993): 282–283.
20. L. M. Pachter, Culture and clinical care: Folk illness beliefs and behaviors and their implications for health care delivery, *Journal of the American Medical Association* 271 (1994): 690–694.
21. C. Marwick, Complementary medicine congress draws a crowd, *Journal of the American Medical Association* 274 (1995): 106–107.

Chapter 21

Nutrition and Disorders of the Upper GI Tract

CONTENTS

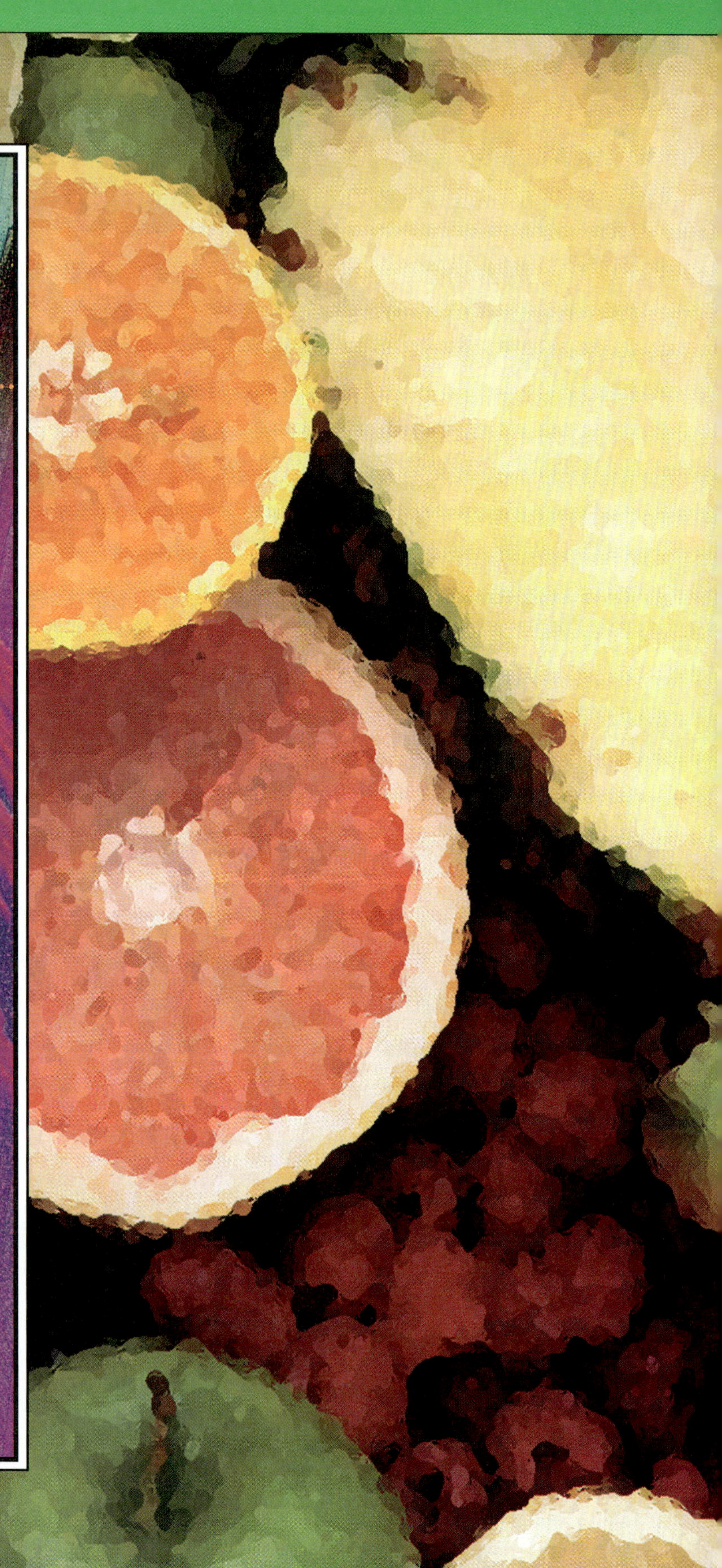

MICROGRAPH: Vitamin B_{12}.

The remarkable GI tract serves as a conduit from the external world to the internal body environment. It wisely distinguishes nutrients from substances for which the body has no use. Over the course of the life cycle, the GI tract undergoes changes that affect the absorption of nutrients and modify nutrient needs. As the healthy newborn's GI tract matures, it progressively allows the body to ingest, digest, and absorb nutrients in many forms—functions essential to life. With aging, the muscular functions of the GI tract gradually decline, and the stomach frequently changes in ways that affect the absorption of several nutrients. By adjusting diets to accommodate these normal physiologic changes, optimal nourishment can be provided. Similarly, dietary adjustments can ease symptoms, prevent malnutrition, and treat disorders that affect the functions of the GI tract. With this chapter, you begin your study of medical nutrition therapy, specifically how diet can aid the treatment of some upper GI tract symptoms and disorders. The next chapter presents disorders of the lower GI tract and their relationships to diet and nutrition status.

Disorders of the Mouth and Esophagus

Figure 21–1 on p. 696 illustrates the upper GI tract and reviews the functions of its various organs and sphincters. In the mouth, the teeth and jaw muscles work together to break down food to a consistency that can be easily swallowed and digested. The upper esophagus assists in the swallowing process, and the remaining esophagus transports food from the mouth to the stomach. The muscles controlling the esophagus push foods down and prevent them from moving back toward the throat.

A variety of dental, medical, and surgical conditions that affect the mouth and esophagus can temporarily or permanently interfere with chewing (see Table 21–1). Without appropriate adjustments in diet, people with these conditions may find eating a difficult or painful experience. They may eat too little, lose too much weight, and suffer the consequences of a deteriorating nutrition status.

The process of chewing is sometimes called **mastication**.

Table 21–1

Conditions That May Interfere with Chewing and Swallowing

Achalasia	Ill-fitting dentures
Acquired immune deficiency syndrome (AIDS)	Missing teeth
	Multiple sclerosis
Alzheimer's disease	Myasthenia gravis
Broken jaw	No teeth
Cancer	Oral Surgery
Chemotherapy	Parkinson's disease
Congenital defects of upper GI tract	Periodontal disease
Dental caries	Radiation therapy of the head and neck
Dryness of mouth	Sensitivity of mouth to hot or cold
Dysphagia	Strokes
Guillain-Barré syndrome	Surgery of the head and neck
Head injury	Ulceration of mouth, gums, or esophagus

Figure 21–1

The Upper GI Tract

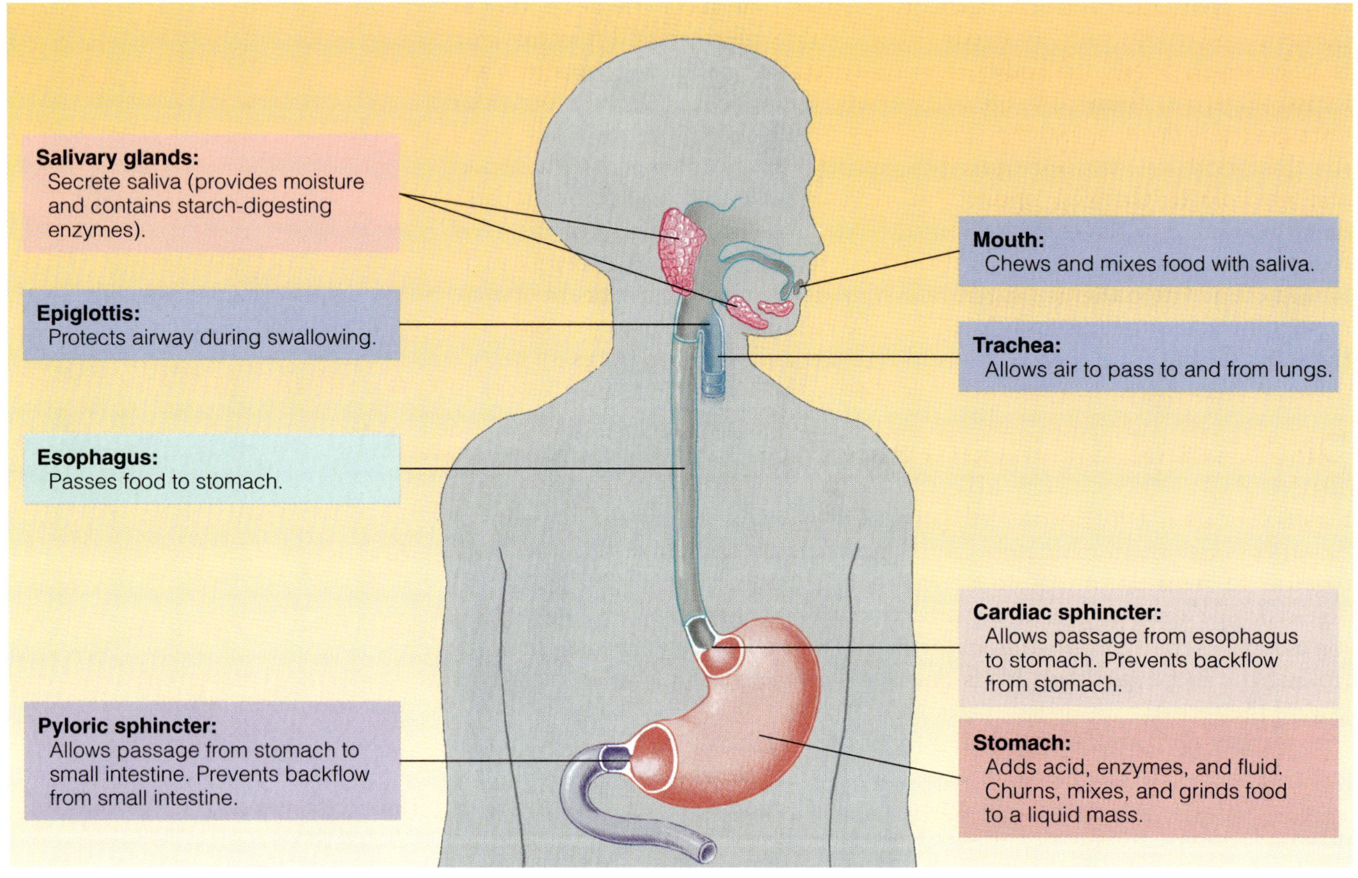

DIFFICULTIES CHEWING

Conditions that interfere with the ability to chew foods include dental problems, surgery involving the mouth and gums, mouth ulcers, and a reduced flow of saliva. A mechanical soft diet that eliminates foods the person cannot easily chew can help ease the problem. All foods and seasonings are permitted on mechanical soft diets, but are prepared in liquid, chopped, tender-cooked, or pureed form.

mechanical soft diet: a diet that excludes all foods that are difficult to chew or swallow; also called a dental soft diet.

pureed foods: foods that have been strained and blenderized to a thickened, near-liquid consistency.

Individualizing the Diet Dietitians work closely with people on mechanical soft diets to identify the types of foods they can tolerate and to encourage them to eat foods as similar as possible to those of a regular diet. This strategy enhances appetite, prevents boredom, and minimizes the likelihood of nutrient deficiencies. The longer the person requires a mechanical soft diet, the more important this strategy becomes.

People's tolerances of food consistencies vary greatly. A person with a newly broken jaw, for example, may be able to consume only liquids; a person without teeth, however, may be able to eat baked chicken or fish, ground beef, and

A person without teeth is edentulous (ee-DENT-you-lus).

casseroles; soft fruits such as peaches, melons, and canned fruits; and soft vegetables such as potatoes, peeled tomatoes, and tender-cooked carrots. Moist, soft-textured foods, such as foods prepared with sauces and gravies, often work well. Drinking liquids along with meals makes it easier to chew and swallow foods.

Pureed Foods When clients can tolerate only pureed foods for long periods of time, the monotony of eating food of the same consistency can create a psychological block to eating, and malnutrition can follow. Foodservice departments in nursing homes, rehabilitation centers, and other long-term care facilities that must provide many clients with pureed foods over long periods of time face a particular challenge. In addition to the problem of accepting pureed diets, clients in long-term care facilities lack the comforts of home and may be overwhelmed by their medical conditions, isolation, and loss of control. Addressing the client's emotional needs is critical to stimulating the appetite.

Preparing pureed foods takes time, and people sometimes substitute baby foods for convenience. Although baby foods are nutritious, they may look and taste bland because manufacturers often prepare them without salt or spices. In addition, baby foods are often so finely pureed that they do not hold their shapes and are difficult to arrange attractively on a plate. The box on p. 698 offers suggestions for improving acceptance of pureed foods and baby foods.

Mouth Ulcers The mechanical soft diet for people with mouth ulcers provides moist, soft-textured foods and eliminates spicy, salty, or acidic foods (such as citrus fruits and juices and tomato products) that may be painful to eat. In addition, nuts or seeds in foods (such as sesame or poppy seeds in breads) can become trapped in mouth ulcers and cause discomfort. Heat may intensify pain, too. Clients with mouth ulcers often prefer cold foods or beverages.

mouth ulcers: lesions or sores in the lining of the mouth. Certain drugs, radiation therapy, and some disorders, such as oral herpes virus infections, can cause mouth ulcers.

Reduced Flow of Saliva Clients with dry mouths due to a reduced flow of saliva often tolerate moist, soft foods. Clients can moisten foods with sauces and gravies. Salty foods and snacks dry the mouth and should be avoided. Encourage these clients to practice good oral hygiene; when salivary flow is reduced, the mouth is poorly defended against dental caries. Clients can increase salivary secretions by sucking on sugarless candy or chewing gum or by using drugs that stimulate the flow of saliva.

DYSPHAGIA

Problems with swallowing, known as dysphagia, can arise from many causes, including aging, nervous system diseases, developmental disabilities, and strokes. A person with dysphagia may be unable to initiate swallowing, to chew foods and mix them with saliva, or to push foods to the back of the throat and into the esophagus. Some forms of dysphagia specifically interfere with the muscular contractions of the esophagus.

dysphagia (dis-FAY-gee-ah): difficulty in swallowing.
dys = bad
phagein = to eat

Dysphagia often goes undiagnosed, especially when associated with aging, because symptoms are not always obvious. Everybody "catches food in the throat" at one time or another, so a person who gradually does this more and more frequently may consider the condition normal and ignore it. The person may gradually eat less and develop nutrient deficiencies.

Dysphagia can be dangerous. Foods that move back into the throat may enter the trachea and pass into the lungs (aspiration), allowing bacteria to multiply

aspiration (as-peh-RAY-shun): to draw in by suction, as may occur when food or liquid is sucked into the lungs.

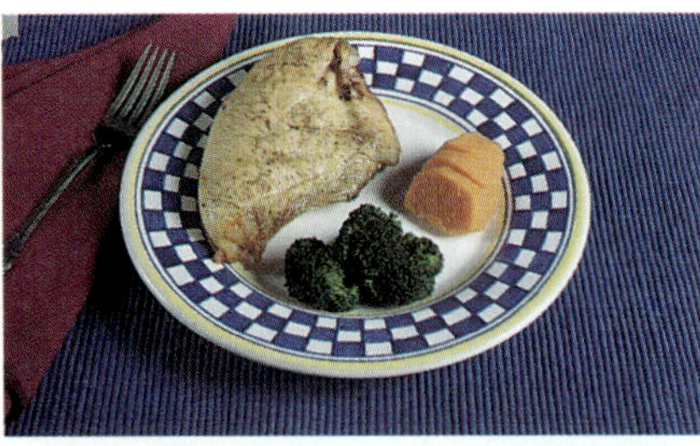

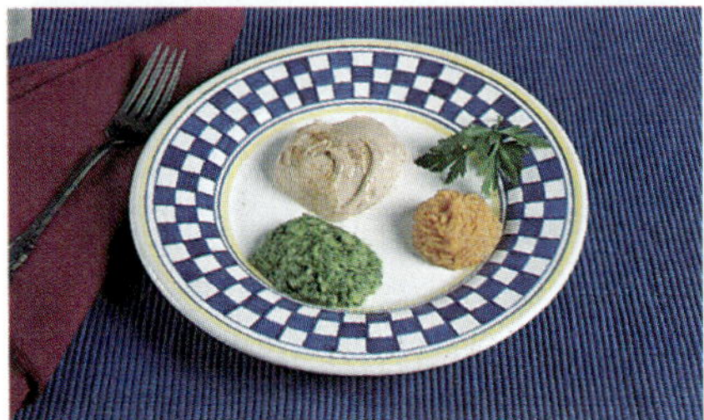

Pureed foods make an appetizing meal when chosen with an eye for color and served attractively.

How to Improve Acceptance of Pureed Diets

Take a moment to think about a pureed diet. A typical dinner of baked chicken, boiled potatoes, and green beans is pureed to white mush, more white mush, and a green blob. The foods may taste great, but on seeing the plate, the person may have a hard time taking the first bite. To stimulate the appetite, use creative techniques for preparing and serving food such as these:

- Encourage clients and their caregivers to prepare a variety of favorite foods and blenderize them to a tolerable consistency. The smells of favorite foods cooking and the thought of consuming a favorite food often stimulate the appetite.
- Consider color when planning meals. The meal of baked chicken, mashed potatoes, and green beans, described above, can be made more appealing by substituting mashed sweet potatoes for the white potatoes. Arranging the foods attractively on a plate with appropriate garnishes also adds color and eye appeal.
- Serve foods at the right temperature and puree them so that they are smooth and thick—not watery and thin. Commercially available thickeners add shape, texture, and even nutrients to food.
- Experiment with seasonings and spices to enliven food flavors, excluding only those that the person cannot tolerate or are not allowed for medical reasons. When clients and their caregivers choose to use baby foods for convenience, seasoning the food to accommodate adult tastes adds flavor and improves the appetite.
- Supplement the diet with nutritious liquids such as milk, instant breakfast drinks, or liquid formulas (described in Chapter 23).

Efforts to improve the acceptance of pureed diets can go a long way toward helping people to eat and maintain or improve their weights.[a] When efforts to improve clients' intakes of pureed foods are unsuccessful, feeding the person by tube becomes an option (see Chapter 23).

[a]D. Cassens, E. Johnson, and S. Keelan, Enhancing taste, texture, appearance, and presentation of pureed food improved resident quality of life and weight status, *Nutrition Reviews* (supplement) 11 (1996): 51–54.

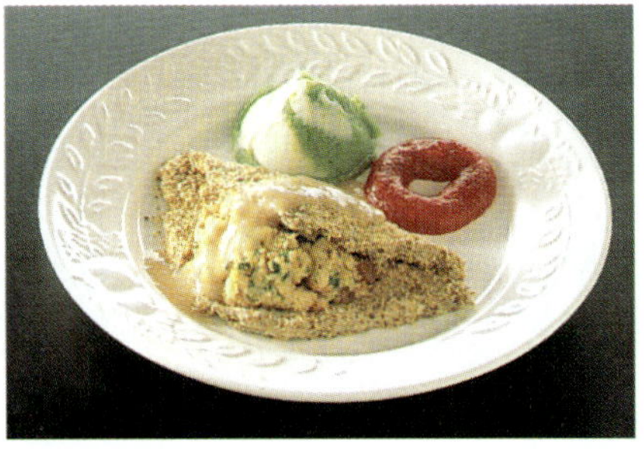

Adding commercial thickeners to pureed foods greatly enhances their appeal.

and causing pneumonia. In healthy people, the presence of food in the trachea elicits a coughing response, which prevents food from entering the lungs. Some people with dysphagia, however, fail to cough when food slips into the trachea. Such "silent" aspiration, which has been observed in people following strokes, carries the risk of serious pneumonia and death.[1]

Reminder: When food becomes lodged in the trachea, *choking* occurs (see pp. 94–96).

Signs of Dysphagia Health care professionals should be alert to subtle symptoms of dysphagia including an unexplained decline in food intake or repeated bouts of pneumonia.[2] Other symptoms include pain upon swallowing, weight loss, a fear of eating certain foods or any food at all, a feeling that food is sticking in the throat, a tendency to hold food in the mouth rather than swallowing it, coughing or choking during meals, frequent throat clearing, drooling, or a change in voice quality. Depending on the cause of dysphagia, the voice may be hoarse, nasal, or have a "wet" sound. Diagnosis is based on extensive testing that may include cranial nerve assessment, X rays, fluoroscopy, and measurements of esophageal sphincter pressure and esophageal peristalsis.

The fear of eating is called sitophobia (SIGH-toe-FOE-bee-ah).
sitos = food
phobos = fear

Conditions that may lead to dysphagia:

- Acquired immune deficiency syndrome (AIDS).
- Aging.
- Alzheimer's disease.
- Brain tumors.
- Cancers of the head and neck.
- Developmental feeding disorders.
- Guilain-Barré syndrome.
- Head injuries.
- Lou Gehrig's disease (amyotrophic lateral sclerosis).
- Multiple sclerosis.
- Myasthenia gravis.
- Parkinson's disease.
- Polio.
- Reflux esophagitis.
- Strokes.

Dietary Interventions for Dysphagia The mechanical soft diet for dysphagia leaves little room for error or experimentation. A person may appear to be tolerating a particular food when, in fact, the food is being aspirated.[3] Speech pathologists, dietitians, physicians, and nurses work together to assess a person's swallowing abilities and design an individualized diet. Often, the person can handle only semisolid foods or thickened liquids, which flow slowly enough to allow time to coordinate swallowing movements. Smooth solids such as puddings, custards, and smooth yogurts are frequently good choices; commercial thickeners, tapioca pudding, or baby cereal can be used to thicken liquids. Many of the suggestions offered in the box on p. 698 apply to diets for dysphagia.

With time, swallowing function may improve. The health care team continuously monitors the person and expands the diet to include additional foods as tolerated. Ideally, the diet is progressed to a solid diet, although this is not always possible.

Tube Feedings Feedings by tube (described in Chapter 23) are necessary only if attempts to feed the person orally are unsuccessful. Tube feedings may be particularly beneficial for severely malnourished individuals who are unable to take adequate nourishment orally and for those whose swallowing function continues to deteriorate. Tube feedings delivered into the stomach, however, may be contraindicated due to the high risk of aspiration pneumonia in people with dysphagia. Intestinal tube feedings often provide a safer alternative.

Many disorders that affect the mouth and esophagus can interfere with chewing and swallowing and may require a modification in food consistency. Dysphagia, a serious swallowing disorder that frequently goes undiagnosed, can lead to repeated bouts of pneumonia and even death. Management includes a highly individualized mechanical soft diet. The nutrition assessment checklist on p. 700 highlights important considerations in maintaining nutrition status for people with chewing and swallowing problems.

Disorders of the Stomach

Once swallowed, food travels down the esophagus into the stomach. The stomach retains the bolus for a while, adding acids, fluids, and enzymes to the mixture before slowly releasing its contents into the intestine. Disorders of the stomach range from occasional bouts of indigestion to serious conditions that require surgical resections.

dyspepsia: vague abdominal pain; a symptom, not a disease.
dys = bad
peptein = to digest

epigastric: the region of the body just above the stomach.
epi = above
gastric = stomach

INDIGESTION AND REFLUX ESOPHAGITIS

Indigestion, or dyspepsia, is a vague term used to describe epigastric pain and fullness, early satiety, and belching. Highlight 3 (pp. 98–99) describes the causes and

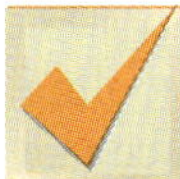

Nutrition Assessment Checklist
For People with Chewing and Swallowing Disorders

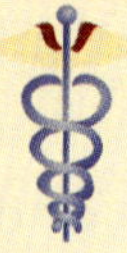

Medical Determine if the client's primary medical condition requires further dietary alterations; treatment of the primary medical condition may ease problems with chewing and swallowing. Healthy people who require short-term modifications (following wisdom tooth extraction, for example) can make up nutrient deficits when they resume their normal diets.

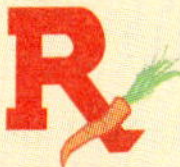

Drug Review the client's drug therapy for possible drug-nutrient interactions.

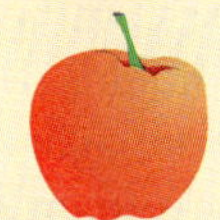

Food Intake Regularly assess the client's intake to pinpoint tolerable food consistencies and quickly address problems with failing appetite and possible nutrient deficiencies.

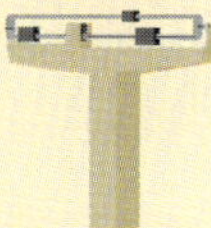

Anthropometric Take accurate baseline height and weight measurements. For people with long-term swallowing disorders, monitor changes in height and weight in children and weight in adults as frequently as possible. Adjust diet to support growth in children and desirable weight in adults.

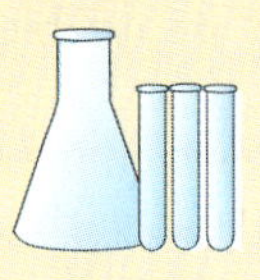

Laboratory Monitor changes in serum albumin. Serum electrolytes and blood urea nitrogen can help detect dehydration, a common problem in people with swallowing disorders. Hemoglobin and hematocrit levels help in detecting dehydration and anemia.

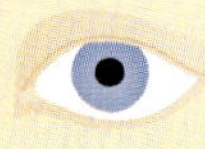

Physical Check for physical signs of nutrient deficiencies and dehydration; assess the client's energy level and emotional state.

consequences of occasional bouts of indigestion including belching, hiccups, heartburn, and regurgitation of the stomach's acid fluids into the mouth. Acid indigestion can become a chronic problem. When the reflux of highly acidic gastric fluids occurs frequently, the esophagus becomes irritated, causing a painful inflammation called reflux esophagitis. Severe inflammation and scarring may narrow the inner diameter of the esophagus. Dysphagia and its potential complications (see p. 697), esophageal ulcers, and bleeding are possible consequences.

Certain drugs, aging, and the use of feeding tubes that pass from the nose through the stomach are associated with an increased risk of reflux esophagitis. Most often, however, reflux esophagitis develops as a consequence of a hiatal hernia.

Hiatal Hernia The esophagus joins the stomach at the cardiac sphincter. Normally, this sphincter sits right in the hiatus of the diaphragm and is reinforced by it. The esophagus lies completely above, and the stomach completely

reflux esophagitis (eh-sof-ah-JYE-tis): the backflow or regurgitation of gastric contents from the stomach into the esophagus, causing inflammation of the esophagus; also called **gastroesophageal reflux, gastric reflux**, or **acid indigestion**.

re = back

fluxus = flow

The continuous reflux of gastric juices may cause scarring of the esophageal mucosa. As scar tissue forms, the diameter of the esophagus narrows, a condition referred to as an **esophageal stricture**.

esophageal ulcers: lesions or sores in the lining of the esophagus.

below, the diaphragm. Sometimes, however, the diaphragm weakens, and a portion of the stomach protrudes up through it, an abnormality called a hiatal hernia. Once a hiatal hernia forms, the cardiac sphincter is no longer reinforced by the surrounding diaphragm, and it becomes easy for gastric juices to reflux into the esophagus. Because reflux occurs more readily in people with hiatal hernias, they frequently suffer from heartburn, acid regurgitation into the mouth, and esophagitis; treatment aims to prevent these consequences. Figure 21–2 shows the normal relationship of the upper GI tract to the diaphragm and the changes that occur with reflux and with a hernia.

The **cardiac sphincter** is also called the **lower esophageal sphincter (LES)** or the **gastroesophageal sphincter**.

hiatus (high-AY-tus): the opening in the diaphragm through which the esophagus passes.
- *hiatus* = to yawn

hiatal hernia: a protrusion of a portion of the stomach through the esophageal hiatus of the diaphragm. There are several types of hiatal hernias, but the *sliding hiatal hernia* is the most common (see Figure 21–2).

Dietary Prevention and Treatment The tips for preventing acid indigestion described in Highlight 3 also apply to people who suffer from reflux esophagitis; the box on p. 702 reviews these suggestions and their rationale. Treatment for active reflux esophagitis aims to alleviate reflux and irritation of the inflamed esophagus by reducing gastric acidity and eliminating foods, substances, and activities that weaken the cardiac sphincter (see Table 21–2).

Figure 21–2

Relationship of the Upper GI Tract to the Diaphragm

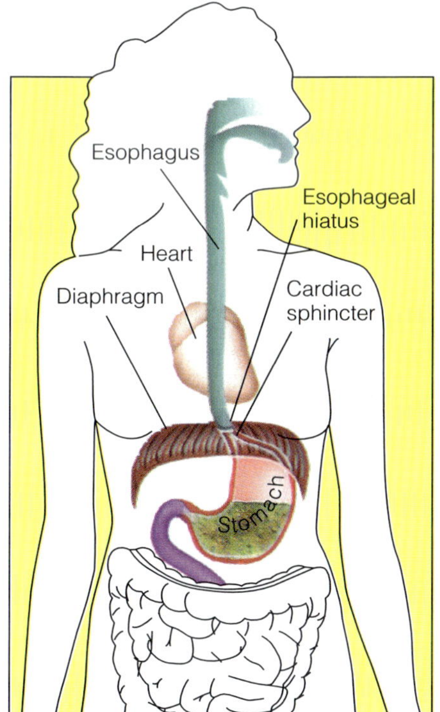

NORMAL
The stomach lies below the diaphragm, and the esophagus passes through the esophageal hiatus. The cardiac sphincter prevents reflux of stomach contents.

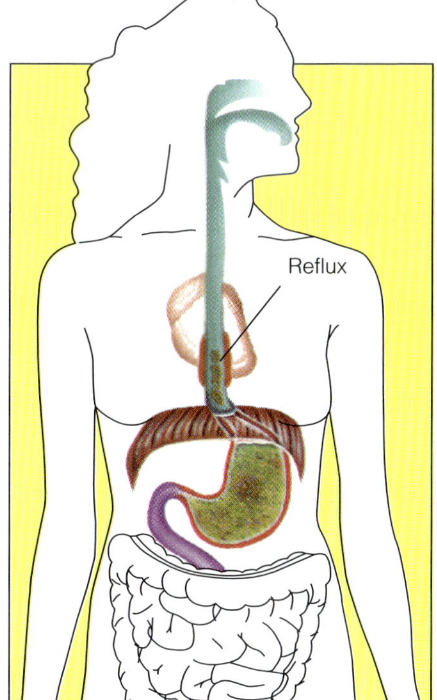

REFLUX
Overeating and overdrinking can increase pressure in the stomach. Whenever the pressure in the stomach exceeds the pressure in the esophagus, there is a greater chance of reflux. The resulting "heartburn" is so-named because it is felt in the area of the heart.

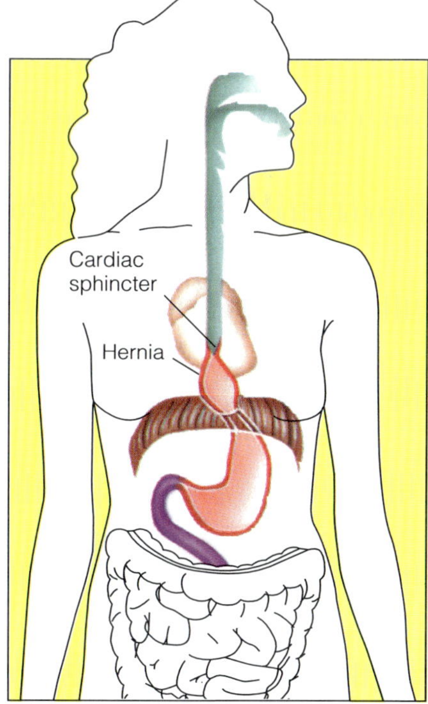

SLIDING HIATAL HERNIA
A sliding hiatal hernia results when part of the stomach, with the cardiac sphincter, slips through the diaphragm. This type of hiatal hernia is the most common.

Table 21–2

Substances That Relax the Cardiac Sphincter

Alcohol
Anticholinergic agents
Calcium channel blockers
Chocolate
Cigarette smoking
Diazepam
Garlic
High-fat foods
Meperidine
Onions
Peppermint and spearmint oils
Theophylline

How to Prevent and Treat Reflux Esophagitis

To prevent and treat reflux esophagitis and its associated discomfort, instruct clients to:

- Eat small meals and drink liquids one hour before or one hour after meals to avoid distending the stomach.
- Relax during mealtimes, eat foods slowly, and chew foods thoroughly to avoid swallowing air and distending the stomach.
- Limit foods that weaken cardiac sphincter pressure or increase gastric acid secretion, including fat, alcohol, caffeine, decaffeinated coffee and tea, chocolate, spearmint, and peppermint.
- Avoid foods and beverages that irritate the esophagus, such as citrus fruits and juices, tomatoes and tomato-based products, pepper, spices, and very hot or very cold foods according to individual tolerances.
- Lose weight, if overweight.
- Refrain from lying down or bending over and from wearing tight-fitting clothing or belts, particularly after eating, to avoid increasing stomach pressure.
- Elevate the head of the bed by 4 to 6 inches. Keeping the chest higher than the stomach helps to prevent reflux.
- Refrain from smoking cigarettes.

Individual tolerances to types and amounts of foods and spices vary markedly. Health care professionals can help clients pinpoint individual intolerances by advising them to record the types and amounts of foods and beverages consumed, the time of consumption, GI symptoms, and time of occurrence. Assessment of the record by a dietitian provides the basis for determining the types and amounts of food or food components that the client can handle without discomfort.

antacids: acid-buffering agents used to counter excess acidity in the stomach.

Most **antiulcer agents** suppress or inhibit gastric acid secretion. Those that do are also classed as **antisecretory agents** or **anti-GERD (GastroEsophageal Reflux Disease)**.

PRESCRIPTION PAD

Drugs used in the treatment of reflux esophagitis may include:

- Antacids
- Antiulcer agents
- Cholinergics (metoclopramide and bethanecol, see *antinauseants*)

See Appendix E for timing with meals and nutrition-related side effects.

Drug Therapy Turn on the television set and quite likely you will see several advertisements touting a new generation of over-the-counter medications that are highly effective in both preventing and relieving indigestion. Physicians frequently prescribe such drugs to ease the discomfort of reflux esophagitis. Antacids neutralize gastric acidity, and antiulcer agents suppress or inhibit gastric acid secretion. Medications that strengthen cardiac sphincter pressure (cholinergics) are used when other measures prove unsuccessful in controlling symptoms. If drug therapy fails, however, surgery may be indicated. The case study provides questions that review the nutrition needs of a client with a hiatal hernia and reflux esophagitis.

NAUSEA AND VOMITING

Nausea, another vague term, is used to describe the feeling that one is about to vomit. The discussion here focuses on prolonged nausea and vomiting, unrelated

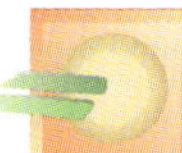

Case Study Accountant with Reflux Esophagitis

Mrs. Scarlatti, a 49-year-old accountant, recently underwent a complete physical examination. She told her physician that she had been feeling fairly well, except for heartburn, which had been occurring with increasing frequency. The attacks usually occurred after she had eaten a large meal, particularly when she lays down after eating. She told the doctor that her life was pretty hectic because it is the middle of the tax season.

Mrs. Scarlatti's past medical history shows no signs of significant health problems. During her last physical, the physician did advise her to stop smoking cigarettes and to lose 20 pounds, which she has yet to do. A diet history taken by the nurse shows that Mrs. Scarlatti usually skips breakfast, eats lunch hurriedly while she continues to work, and eats a large dinner around 8:00 P.M. She generally enjoys one or two alcoholic beverages in the evening before going to sleep. She drinks 6 to 8 cups of coffee during the day. Her current height and weight are 5 feet 6 inches and 170 pounds. After inspecting the interior of her esophagus, stomach, and duodenum with a long tube equipped with a special optical device called a gastroscope, the physician diagnosed a sliding hiatal hernia.

Can you explain to Mrs. Scarlatti what a sliding hiatal hernia is and how its leads to heartburn? Describe the care plan you would develop for Mrs. Scarlatti. What suggestions can you make to help her relieve the symptoms associated with the hernia? What other therapy might her physician prescribe?

to eating habits, which can lead to weight loss and malnutrition. As later chapters show, nausea is a symptom of many medical conditions that arise either within or outside of the GI tract. Nausea is also a common side effect of many drugs and medical treatments. Emotional tension or even the sight or smell of certain foods can precipitate or worsen nausea.

As Highlight 3 describes, simple vomiting is certainly unpleasant and wearying for the nauseated person but is not cause for alarm. Prolonged vomiting, however, can be serious and dangerous enough to require professional medical care. When nausea leads to vomiting, foods and medications fail to reach the intestine and are unavailable to the body. Large amounts of fluids and electrolytes from the body's cells are expelled along with the foods, further increasing the likelihood of dehydration and nutrient deficiencies.

nausea (NAW-see-ah): the feeling that one is about to vomit.

Conditions that can lead to indigestion and nausea include pregnancy, reflux esophagitis, peptic ulcers, gallbladder disorders, pancreatic disorders, kidney disorders, cancer, and delayed gastric emptying.

Treatment of Nausea Treatment of nausea depends on its severity and cause. The longer the person suffers from nausea and the greater its severity, the greater the risk of significant dehydration, weight loss, and malnutrition. Treatment of the related medical condition or a change in drug therapy, if possible, often alleviates the problem. Emotional stresses may require counseling to resolve underlying emotional conflicts. The next box (see p. 704) suggests other measures to ease nausea.

Dietary Interventions for Vomiting Controlling nausea is often successful in preventing vomiting. During episodes of vomiting, foods are withheld. If possible, fluids and electrolytes are replaced orally using clear liquids. If oral liquids cannot be tolerated, intravenous (IV) fluids may be given to provide fluids, glucose, and electrolytes until the vomiting resolves. When vomiting continues for long periods of time, IV fluids that meet all nutrient needs (described in Chapter 24) may be indicated.

intravenous (IV): through a vein.
intra = within
vena = vein

Notice that the suggestions in Chapter 18 for alleviating the indigestion and nausea associated with pregnancy parallel the suggestions provided here.

How to Minimize Nausea

The following suggestions can help alleviate nausea:

- Encourage clients to relax before they eat and to avoid overeating. Eating small meals and saving liquids for between meals prevent distention of the stomach.
- Remind clients to drink liquids between meals, especially when vomiting is a problem. Although individual tolerances vary, many clients tolerate cold or carbonated liquids and juices best.
- Help clients identify individual food intolerances and aromas that precipitate nausea; clients should avoid these foods and aromas, if possible. High-fat foods and highly spiced foods are often poorly tolerated. Cold or room-temperature foods may be better tolerated than hot foods, especially if food aromas trigger nausea. Recommend that others prepare foods for the client, if possible.
- Advise clients who experience nausea to eat carbohydrate-rich, low-fat foods before they get out of bed. Crackers or bread can be kept at bedside.
- Recommend a meal and snack schedule for clients who experience nausea at specific times of the day. Clients should avoid eating or drinking immediately before or during those times.
- Suggest that clients relax after eating, but not lie down. Getting fresh air after meals and wearing nonconstrictive clothing can also help.

Physicians may also prescribe antinauseants or antiemetic drugs to help control nausea and vomiting. Counsel clients to take these drugs at least 30 minutes before eating to ensure effectiveness during mealtimes.

GASTRITIS

gastritis: inflammation of the stomach lining.

Bacterial infection with *Helicobacter pylori* can cause acute or chronic gastritis.

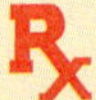

PRESCRIPTION PAD

Drugs used in the treatment of gastritis may include:

- Antacids
- Antibiotics
- Antiulcer agents

See Appendix E for timing with meals and nutrition-related side effects.

Gastritis is a common disorder in which the mucosal lining of the stomach becomes inflamed and painful. The person with gastritis may complain of anorexia, indigestion, nausea, vomiting, and epigastric pain. Although gastritis generally resolves with treatment, unresolved gastritis can lead to hemorrhage, shock, obstruction, perforation, and gastric cancer.

Acute Gastritis Acute gastritis most often follows the repeated use of aspirin or other drugs that irritate the gastric mucosa. Alcohol abuse, food irritants, food allergies, food poisoning, radiation therapy, metabolic stress, and bacterial infection can also cause gastritis.

For the person with gastritis who cannot eat because of nausea or vomiting, foods are generally withheld for a day or two. Then, the diet progresses from liquids to a bland diet as tolerated. Bland diets (see Table 21–3) are highly individualized diets that eliminate foods that stimulate gastric acid secretion or irritate the gastric mucosa. Antacids, antiulcer drugs, and antibiotics may also be prescribed.

Chronic Gastritis Chronic gastritis presents the same symptoms as acute gastritis, but persists over time. Chronic gastritis may be associated with gastric

Table 21–3

The Bland Diet

A bland diet provides three meals a day and includes all foods except those that irritate the gastric mucosa. Substances generally contraindicated on a bland diet include:

- Any foods an individual identifies as irritating to the GI tract.
- Alcohol.
- Caffeine and caffeine-containing beverages (including cola beverages, cocoa, coffee, and tea).
- Decaffeinated coffee and tea.
- Pepper and spicy foods except as tolerated.

Note: The liberal bland diet shown here has replaced the earlier "traditional bland diet," which was invalidated by research.

surgery, chronic diseases of the stomach or liver, bacterial infection, or may have no known cause. It is common in the elderly. As gastritis progresses, the gastric cells atrophy, gastric secretions decline, and the production of intrinsic factor is reduced.

Chronic gastritis requires diagnosis and treatment before damage progresses too far. Interventions need to begin early enough to prevent complications such as dehydration, malnutrition, or damage to the esophagus. An individualized bland diet may help relieve GI symptoms in some cases.

The reduced production of intrinsic factor can result in vitamin B_{12} malabsorption, which can lead to pernicious anemia. When necessary, vitamin B_{12} is given by injection to bypass the need for absorption.

Reminder: *Intrinsic factor* is a glycoprotein made in the stomach that is necessary for the absorption of vitamin B_{12}.

In atrophic gastritis all of the layers of the stomach's mucosal cells are inflamed.

ULCERS

The term *ulcers* brings to mind the image of a frantic businessman rushing through the day with coffee cup in hand, gulping down high-fat, spicy foods, and working until midnight while suppressing the pain of bleeding sores caused by excessive acid in his stomach. But like other aspects of ulcer prevention and treatment, this stereotype has fallen by the wayside. Neither a stressful lifestyle nor male gender typifies the person with ulcers; ulcers occur in stressed and unstressed men and women alike.

Ulcers can develop both inside and outside the body, but the term *ulcer* generally refers to a *peptic ulcer*—an erosion of the top layer of cells from the GI tract lining. This erosion leaves the underlying layers of cells exposed to gastric juices. When the gastric juices reach the capillaries, the ulcer bleeds, and when they reach the nerves, they cause pain.

Causes of Ulcers Highlight 3 introduced the three major causes of ulcers: bacterial infection, the use of certain anti-inflammatory drugs, and disorders that cause excessive gastric acid secretion. One such disorder, the Zollinger-Ellison syndrome, results from a tumor of the pancreas that produces gastrin, which, in turn, stimulates the production of gastric acid. Severe peptic ulcer disease follows.

peptic ulcer: an erosion of the top layer of cells from the mucosa of the stomach (gastric ulcer) or duodenum (duodenal ulcer). Ulcers may also develop in the mouth, esophagus, and intestines and on the skin.

The bacterial infection frequently associated with ulcers is caused by *Helicobacter pylori*, the same bacterium that can cause gastritis. The drugs associated with ulcers are nonsteroidal anti-inflammatory agents such as ibuprofen and naproxen.

Zollinger-Ellison syndrome: marked hypersecretion of gastric acid and consequent peptic ulcers caused by a tumor of the pancreas, which releases gastrin.

℞ PRESCRIPTION PAD

Drugs used in the treatment of ulcers may include:

- Antacids
- Antibiotics
- Antiulcer agents

See Appendix E for timing with meals and nutrition-related side effects.

Therapy for Ulcers As mentioned in Highlight 3, treatment aims at relieving pain, healing the ulcer, and minimizing the likelihood of recurrence. Drug therapy plays the primary role in the treatment; the specific type of drug depends on the cause of the ulcer. Antibiotics are used to treat bacterial infections. Antiulcer drugs may be used to suppress or inhibit gastric acid secretion or otherwise protect the stomach and duodenal wall from acid erosion. As for diet, the client need only eliminate foods that cause pain or discomfort. In rare cases, surgical intervention is necessary.

For clients with Zollinger-Ellison syndrome, surgical removal of the tumor, when possible, reduces gastric acid production. Often surgery is necessary to sever the nerves that stimulate gastric acid production, and in some cases, surgery that removes all or part of the stomach, described next, may be indicated.

GASTRIC SURGERY

In a **subtotal** or **partial gastrectomy,** a portion of the stomach is removed; in a **total gastrectomy,** the entire stomach is removed.

vagotomy: surgery that severs the nerves to the stomach that stimulate gastric acid secretion.

The surgical procedures used in the treatment of obesity are discussed on pp. 298–299.

Several surgical procedures affect the functions of the stomach. During a gastrectomy, the surgeon removes either a portion or all of the stomach. Figure 21–3 illustrates three common gastrectomy procedures. Another type of gastric surgery, pyloroplasty, enlarges the pyloric sphincter (the sphincter that joins the stomach and small intestine) so that the basic intestinal fluids reflux into the stomach and neutralize gastric acidity. During a vagotomy, the surgeon severs the nerves that stimulate gastric acid production. A vagotomy may accompany either a gastrectomy or a pyloroplasty in some cases. In gastric partitioning, a treatment for severe obesity, the stomach remains intact, but all or a portion of the stomach is bypassed. Figure 9–5 on p. 298 shows two gastric partitioning procedures.

Chapter 25 describes nutrition care for surgical clients in general, and those considerations apply to gastric surgery as well. This section addresses nutrition concerns that arise specifically in clients undergoing gastric surgery.

Dumping Syndrome One problem that may occur when the portion of the stomach containing the pyloric sphincter has been removed, bypassed, or disrupted is dumping syndrome (see Figure 21–4). A typical scenario goes something

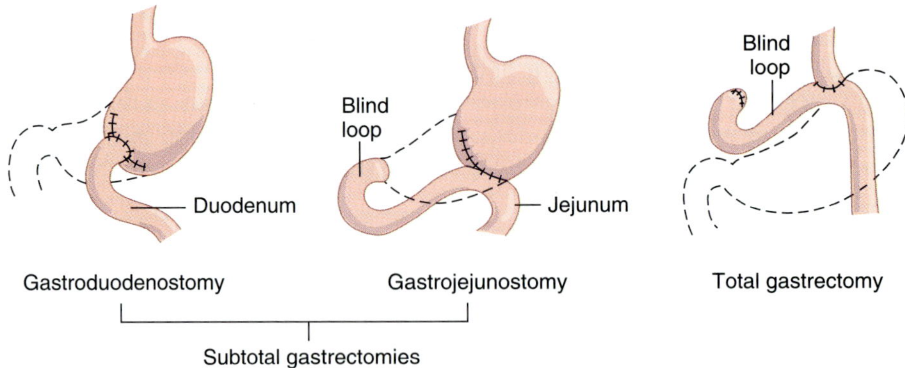

Figure 21–3

Typical Gastric Surgery Resections

In a gastric resection, part, or all, of the stomach is surgically removed. The dashed lines show the removed section.

like this: Mr. Clark had a fairly extensive gastric resection about a week ago and has just begun to eat solid foods. He swallows the food and about 15 minutes later begins to feel weak and dizzy. He looks pale, his heart beats rapidly, and he breaks out in a sweat. Shortly thereafter, he develops diarrhea. What causes this sequence of events?

Mr. Clark has lost an important function of his stomach: its control of the rate at which food empties into the intestine. Now, food gets "dumped" rapidly into the jejunum. (The duodenum is short, and even if it had not been bypassed during surgery, food would still pass quickly through it into the jejunum.) As the mass of food is digested, the intestinal contents rapidly become concentrated

dumping syndrome: the symptoms that result from the rapid emptying of undigested food into the jejunum: sweating, weakness, and diarrhea shortly after eating and hypoglycemia later. Dumping syndrome is common following pyloroplasties, vagotomies, total gastrectomies, and gastric bypass surgery (see Figure 21–3).

Figure 21–4

Dumping Syndrome

When partially digested food rapidly enters the jejunum, it is quickly digested and creates a hyperosmolar load. Fluid from the intestinal capillaries enters the jejunum, diminishing blood volume and stimulating peristalsis. The result: low blood pressure and diarrhea.

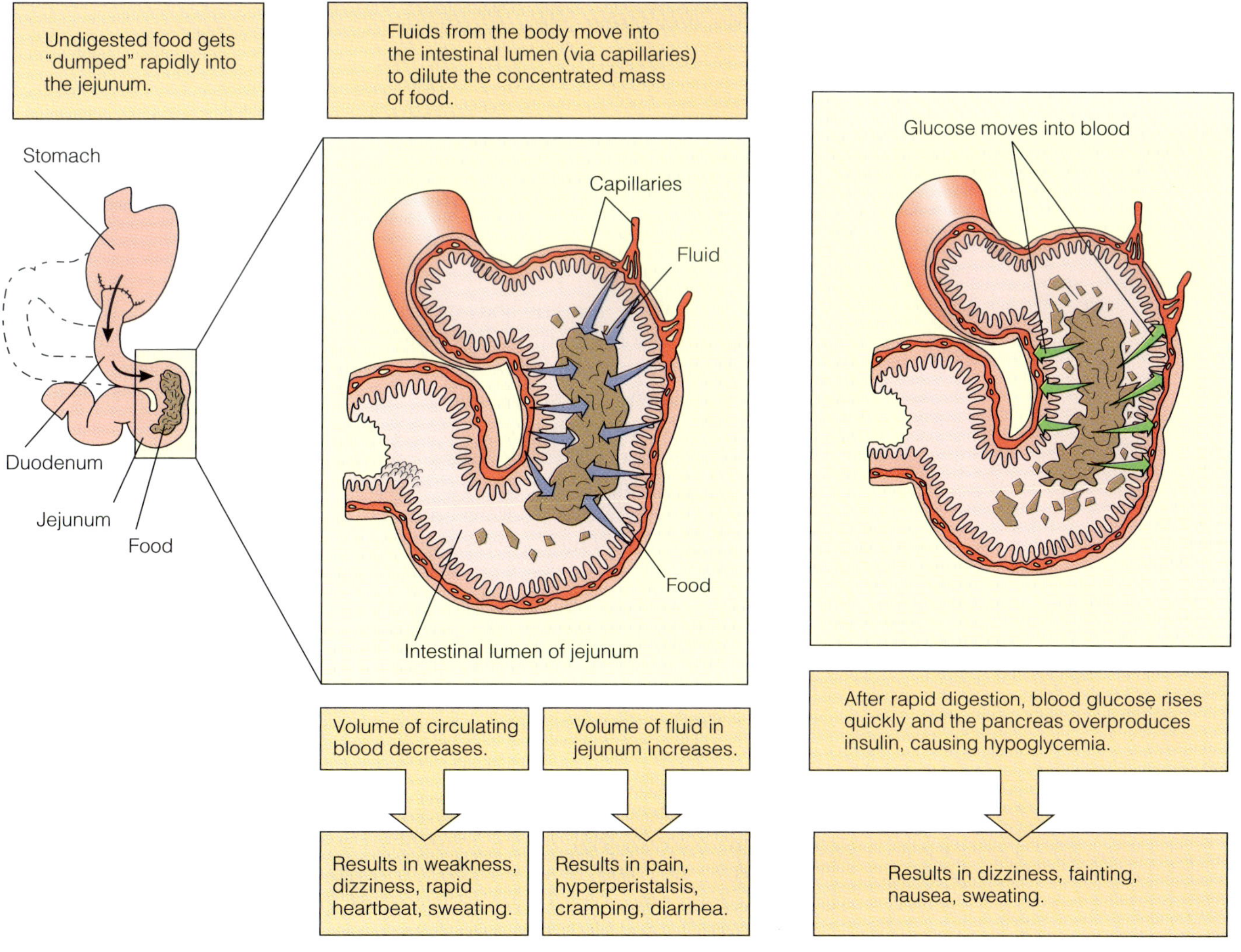

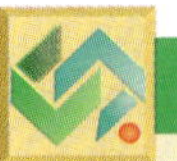

How to Adjust Meals to Prevent Dumping Syndrome

Advice for the person who has had gastric surgery includes the following suggestions:

- Eat no concentrated sweets (sugar, cookies, cakes, pies, or soft drinks) because the body digests these carbohydrates rapidly and breaks them down into many particles that attract fluids into the intestines.
- Eat frequent small meals to fit the reduced storage capacity of the stomach.
- Drink liquids in small amounts about 45 minutes before or after meals, not with them. This precaution prevents overloading the stomach's reduced storage capacity and slows the rate at which food passes from the stomach to the intestine.
- Lie down immediately after eating to help slow the transit of food to the intestine. Clients who experience gastric reflux, however, should not lie down after eating.
- Be aware that lactose intolerance (see Chapter 4) may develop and produce discomfort in response to milk and milk products. Enzyme-treated milk and milk products should also be avoided because the enzymes break down lactose to glucose and galactose, simple sugars that may promote dumping. Discontinue use of these products until recovery is under way. Then reintroduce them gradually in small amounts.

(hypertonic). Water from the body moves into the intestinal lumen to dilute the concentration. Consequently, the volume of circulating blood diminishes rapidly, causing weakness, dizziness, and a rapid heartbeat. The large volume of hypertonic fluid and unabsorbed material in the jejunum causes pain and hyperperistalsis, and diarrhea results.

Two to three hours later, Mr. Clark experiences many of the same symptoms again: dizziness, fainting, nausea, and sweating. This time the cause is different. The intestines efficiently absorbed so much glucose from the meal that blood glucose rose quickly. The pancreas responded by overproducing insulin, which made the blood glucose *fall* quickly. Now, hypoglycemia is causing the symptoms.

The type of hypoglycemia that occurs following gastric surgery is called **alimentary** (AL-ee-MEN-tah-ree) or **postgastrectomy hypoglycemia**. Chapter 27 provides more information about hypoglycemia.

Not all people who have had gastric surgery or vagotomies experience the diarrhea of dumping syndrome. Even fewer develop hypoglycemia. Most people who initially experience dumping syndrome gradually adapt to a fairly regular diet. However, dietary modifications benefit clients during the immediate postsurgical period and in prolonged or severe cases.

postgastrectomy diet: a carbohydrate-controlled diet given to prevent the symptoms of dumping syndrome and hypoglycemia that sometimes follow gastric surgery.

The Postgastrectomy Diet In the immediate postsurgical period, the client receives no foods or fluids by mouth. After several days, liquids and solids are gradually introduced in small amounts. The postgastrectomy diet limits carbohydrates, especially simple sugars, in order to alleviate the symptoms of dumping syndrome. Health care professionals monitor fluid and electrolyte balances carefully, and the physician corrects any imbalances promptly. The diet emphasizes foods containing protein and fat, which are digested more slowly and produce fewer particles than carbohydrates and therefore do not attract fluid as rapidly as carbohydrates do. Table 21–4 on p. 710 lists foods included on, and excluded from, the postgastrectomy diet. Diet advice to offer with the postgastrectomy diet is provided in the box on p. 708 and the sample menu (below) shows a day's meals.

Dietitians carefully tailor the postgastrectomy diet to meet individual needs. Initially, visits to the client after each meal reveal food intolerances. With time, the symptoms of dumping syndrome resolve or improve in most people. Gradually, most people begin to tolerate limited amounts of concentrated sweets, larger quantities of food, and some liquids with meals. Sometimes adding pectin and guar gum (types of dietary fiber) to the diet can help prevent dumping syndrome. If dietary and medical management of dumping syndrome fail to resolve the problem, additional surgery may be necessary.

Unintentional Weight Loss and Malabsorption After gastric surgery, many people experience weight loss and develop nutrient deficiencies. Early satiety, postsurgical pain, and the desire to prevent the symptoms of dumping syndrome often limit food intake. Epigastric pain from reflux esophagitis, and sometimes dysphagia, can further interfere with nutrient intake. Weight loss is the goal for people undergoing gastric partitioning, but people with severe peptic ulcer disease or cancer often suffer significant weight loss before surgery and risk serious malnutrition.

Be aware that protein and fat malabsorption can be a problem for any client who has had a total gastrectomy or who has had the stomach surgically connected directly to the jejunum. Normally, food entering the duodenum triggers the release of the hormones secretin and cholecystokinin. These hormones, in

Rx PRESCRIPTION PAD

Drugs used in the treatment of dumping syndrome may include:

- Anticholinergics (atropine, see *antidiarrheals*)
- Antihistamines (cyprohepatine, see *miscellaneous*)
- Hormones (octreotide, see *miscellaneous*)

See Appendix E for timing with meals and nutrition-related side effects.

Sample Postgastrectomy Diet Menu

Menu

Breakfast	Lunch	Supper
1 scrambled egg	2 oz hamburger patty	2 oz boiled ham
1 slice toast	½ c mashed potatoes	⅓ c rice
1 tsp butter	1 tsp margarine	½ c carrots
Coffee (take 30–60 minutes after meal)	½ small banana	2 tsp butter
	Iced tea (take 30–60 minutes after meal)	¼ c unsweetened peach slices
		Tea (take 30–60 minutes after meal)

Midmorning Snack	Midafternoon Snack	Evening Snack
¼ c cottage cheese	2 tbs peanut butter	¼ c tuna
3 saltine crackers	3 butter crackers	1 tsp mayonnaise
		1 slice bread

Table 21–4

Postgastrectomy Diet[a]

Meat and Meat Alternatives

Any type allowed.

Milk and Milk Products

Withheld initially and then gradually introduced as tolerated.

Grains and Starchy Vegetables

Allowed (up to 5 servings per day): Plain breads, crackers, rolls, unsweetened cereal, rice, pasta, corn, lima beans, parsnips, peas, white potatoes, sweet potatoes, pumpkin, yams, winter squash.

Excluded: Sweetened cereal; cereal containing dates, raisins, or brown sugar.

Nonstarchy Vegetables

Allowed (unlimited): Cabbage, Chinese cabbage, celery, cucumbers, lettuce, parsley, radishes, watercress.

Allowed (up to two ½ c servings per day as individual tolerances permit): Asparagus, bean sprouts, beets, broccoli, brussels sprouts, carrots, cauliflower, eggplant, green pepper, greens, mushrooms, okra, onions, rhubarb, sauerkraut, string beans, summer squash, tomatoes, turnips, zucchini.

Excluded: Vegetables prepared with sugar or creamed.

Fruits

Allowed (up to 3 servings per day): Unsweetened fruits and fruit juices.

Excluded: Sweetened fruits and fruit juices, dates, raisins.

Fats

Any type allowed.

Beverages

Allowed: Coffee, tea, artificially sweetened drinks.

Excluded: Alcohol; sweetened milk, beverages, and fruit drinks; cocoa.

Other

Excluded: Cakes, cookies, ice cream, sherbet, honey, jam, jelly, syrup, and sugar.

[a]Clients with dumping syndrome who are unable to tolerate a sufficient variety or volume of foods over long periods of time often require nutrient supplements.

turn, mediate the secretion of digestive enzymes and bile into the duodenum. When the duodenum is bypassed, these processes are also bypassed and cannot aid fat digestion and absorption as usual. In addition, malabsorption results whenever food passes rapidly through the GI tract.

Reduced gastric acid secretion can also lead to bacterial overgrowth in the stomach or upper small intestine, which results in the malabsorption of fat, fat-soluble vitamins (especially vitamin D), folate, vitamin B_{12}, and calcium. Chapter 22 describes the problems of malabsorption related to bacterial overgrowth, called the *blind loop syndrome*, in greater detail.

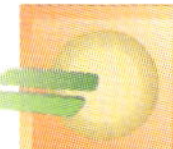

Case Study Commercial Artist Requiring Gastric Surgery

Mr. Miyamotto, a 58-year-old commercial artist, was admitted to the hospital for gastric surgery after numerous attempts to medically manage his severe peptic ulcer disease had failed. A gastrojejunostomy and vagotomy were performed, and Mr. Miyamotto is recovering as expected. The health care team members anticipate nutrition-related problems and are taking measures to prevent them.

Review Figure 21–3 to understand the surgical procedure that Mr. Miyamotto underwent. Consider the possibilities that he might experience early satiety, nausea, vomiting, weight loss, dumping syndrome, malabsorption, anemia, and bone disease. Describe how these conditions might occur.

What type of diet will the physician prescribe for Mr. Miyamotto after he begins eating orally? Describe the diet and how it progresses. What advice can you give Mr. Miyamotto to prevent dumping syndrome?

Discuss the nutrition-related concerns associated with fat malabsorption and anemia. How can these concerns be handled?

Anemia Iron-deficiency anemia is another common problem following gastrectomies and gastric partitioning procedures, although it may take several years to develop. When iron's exposure to gastric acid is limited, less iron is converted to its absorbable form. Furthermore, 50 percent of iron absorption normally takes place in the duodenum. Following gastric surgery, the transit time through the duodenum may be rapid, or the duodenum may be bypassed altogether. Inadequate intake of iron and gastrointestinal blood loss can also contribute to the problem. An iron supplement helps to correct the deficiency.

Inadequate intake and malabsorption can also lead to anemia caused by folate and, less often, vitamin B_{12} deficiencies. To correct deficiencies, clients receive supplements. Use the case study above to review the needs of a client following a gastrectomy.

Although one might expect vitamin B_{12} deficiencies to be common after gastric surgery because intrinsic factor production might be affected, surgeons often avert this problem by leaving intact a small part of the stomach that produces intrinsic factor. This step generally prevents the malabsorption of vitamin B_{12} due to a lack of intrinsic factor.

Reminder: *Osteomalacia* is a bone disease characterized by softening of the bones.

Bone Disease People who experience fat malabsorption following gastric surgery also malabsorb vitamin D and calcium. After many years, a significant number of people who have undergone gastrectomies develop a bone disease similar to osteomalacia.[4] Although the bone disease usually does not respond well to treatment, vitamin D and calcium supplements are often provided.

Gastric Partitioning Unlike other gastric surgeries, weight loss is a goal following gastric partitioning. In addition, diet therapy aims to prevent nutrient deficiencies related to reduced food intake and malabsorption and promote eating and lifestyle habits that will help the client maintain a desirable weight.

The long-term safety and effectiveness of gastric partitioning depend, in large part, on compliance with dietary instructions. Poor dietary habits may prevent weight loss, rupture staples, or obstruct the small passage into the lower stomach. Other postsurgical complications include infections, nausea, vomiting, dehydration, dumping syndrome, esophageal reflux, and, as a result of all this and more, depression. Although the reasons are unclear, clients undergoing gastric bypass surgery frequently say that foods taste sweeter to them than before surgery; others develop an aversion to red meats.[5]

Diet following Gastric Partitioning After surgery, clients initially follow a liquid diet. Liquids reduce the risk of disrupting the line of surgical staples and flow easily through the opening to the lower stomach (or jejunum). Clients gradually begin to eat pureed foods, then soft foods, and then regular foods. Regardless of food consistency, clients can tolerate only small amounts at one time because of the reduced size of the stomach; overeating or overdrinking can cause nausea, reflux, and vomiting. Although individual tolerances vary, most clients can eat regular foods by 12 weeks after surgery, provided they chew foods thoroughly.[6] Foods must be chewed thoroughly to prevent large pieces of food from obstructing the gastric outlet.

Food Selections Clients must understand that their selections of foods and beverages influence the extent of their weight loss. If they drink high-kcalorie liquids or eat high-kcalorie foods all the time, even if only in small quantities, they will not lose weight. Their selections also affect the nutritional quality of the diet. Nutrient deficiencies, particularly of vitamin B_{12}, folate, and iron, are common after gastric bypass surgery. Careful planning, diligent compliance with the prescribed diet, and vitamin-mineral supplements are needed to ensure the adequacy of an energy-restricted diet that strictly limits intake.[7]

Indigestion, reflux esophagitis, nausea, and vomiting are frequent GI problems that can lead to weight loss and malnutrition. When treatment for a medical condition requires gastric surgery, the impact on nutrition status can be severe. The accompanying nutrition assessment checklist reminds health care professionals of factors to assess and monitor for clients with disorders of the upper GI tract.

This chapter has described how problems of the upper GI tract can affect dietary intake and how dietary intake, in turn, can affect these problems. The next chapter examines problems of the lower GI tract.

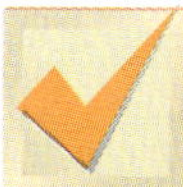

Nutrition Assessment Checklist

For People with Upper GI Tract Disorders

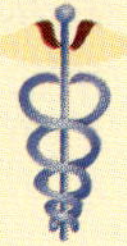

Medical Assess the client's medical history for conditions and treatments that produce symptoms of indigestion, nausea, and vomiting. Medical conditions that are likely to produce severe symptoms for long periods of time alert the assessor to anticipate serious nutrition problems and to work diligently to prevent or correct them.

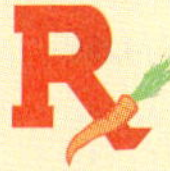

Drug Review the client's drug therapy for possible drug-nutrient interactions. Antacids and antiulcer agents are often used in the treatment of indigestion, reflux esophagitis, gastritis, and ulcers. Aluminum-containing antacids may lead to phosphorus deficiencies. Magnesium-containing antacids may cause diarrhea. Calcium- and sodium-containing antacids contribute calcium and sodium, respectively, to the diet. Some antiulcer agents (cimetidine and omeprazole) may interfere with iron absorption; iron supplements should be given 2 hours before or after taking these medications. Antiemetics may cause mouth dryness.

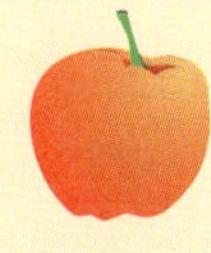

Food Intake Assess food intake to determine individual food tolerances for people with indigestion, nausea, vomiting, or dumping syndrome. Instruct clients to keep records of food intake and GI symptoms to help identify food intolerances. Reassess clients to make sure they are eating sufficiently to maintain nutrition status.

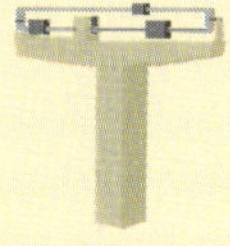

Anthropometric Be alert to unintentional weight loss in people with severe indigestion, early satiety, nausea, vomiting, and dumping syndrome. Clients with reflux esophagitis should lose weight if overweight. Safe weight loss is also the goal for people undergoing gastric partitioning.

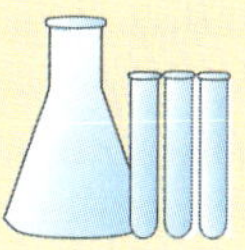

Laboratory Monitor changes in serum albumin. Serum electrolytes, blood urea nitrogen, and hemoglobin and hematocrit can help detect electrolyte imbalances and dehydration, especially important for people with persistent vomiting or dumping syndrome. Anemia is a frequent problem for people with chronic gastritis or following gastric surgery. Hemoglobin and hematocrit help uncover anemia; mean corpuscular volume, serum ferritin, total iron-binding capacity, serum iron, serum folate, serum vitamin B_{12}, and tests of vitamin B_{12} absorption can help differentiate between anemias caused by iron, folate, and vitamin B_{12} deficiencies (see Appendix E).

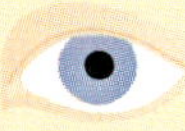

Physical Check for physical signs of dehydration for people experiencing vomiting or dumping syndrome; vitamin B_{12} deficiencies for people with reflux esophagitis, gastritis, and ulcers; and protein-energy malnutrition and vitamin D, folate, iron, and calcium deficiencies for people undergoing gastric surgery.

Study Questions

1. List conditions of the mouth that can affect the ability to chew foods. What diet would you advise in each case?
2. Discuss ways to stimulate the appetite for people on pureed diets.
3. What is dysphagia, and how is the diet managed to ease its symptoms? Why does dysphagia often go unrecognized? What are its potential consequences?
4. What is reflux esophagitis, and what are its primary symptoms? Why is reflux more likely to occur in people with hiatal hernias?
5. What advice can you give the person with reflux to prevent and treat its symptoms? What long-term complications can result from chronic reflux esophagitis?
6. Under what circumstances can indigestion, nausea, and vomiting present a risk to nutrition status?
7. What is gastritis? Describe the role of diet therapy in acute and chronic gastritis.
8. Discuss the therapy for peptic ulcers.
9. What are the possible nutrition consequences of gastric surgery? Describe the relationship of gastric surgery to these consequences. What dietary interventions might help to prevent these consequences?
10. Discuss the dietary recommendations, and the rationale behind them, for a person who undergoes gastric partitioning for clinically severe obesity.

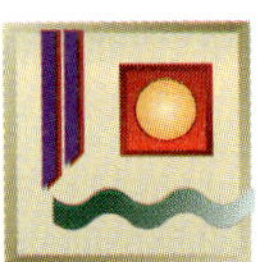

Clinical Applications

1. People on mechanical soft diets differ in the kinds of foods they can handle, in the amounts of time they remain on the diets, and in the help they need from health care professionals. Think about the difference between working with a person who has been edentulous for years and a person who recently had mouth surgery and is just beginning to eat again. Describe some nutrition-related concerns you might have for the person who has been following a mechanical soft diet for years. How would these concerns differ for a person who needs the mechanical soft diet only temporarily? Contrast the amounts of time the nurse or dietitian might spend working with the two clients.
2. Many of the diets described in this chapter are highly individualized. A particular food may give one person indigestion and have no effect on another. One person with a gastrectomy may experience lactose intolerance, while another may not. Describe practical ways to identify food tolerances.
3. Many symptoms and disorders of the upper GI tract are interrelated. Consider, for example, a person with clinically severe obesity who undergoes gastric partitioning. Explain why nausea, vomiting, indigestion, and reflux esophagitis might develop in this person. Consider further how chronic reflux might lead to dysphagia.
4. Review the chapter to find disorders that often occur as a consequence of aging. Referring to Chapter 20, describe the effects of aging on the upper GI tract and relate these changes to the disorders you find.

Notes

1. J. Horner and E. W. Massey, Silent aspiration following stroke, *Neurology* 38 (1988): 317–319.
2. E. M. Pardoe, Development of a multistage diet for dysphagia, *Journal of the American Dietetic Association* 93 (1993): 568–571.
3. Pardoe, 1993.
4. J. Grant, G. Chapman, and M. K. Russell, Malabsorption associated with surgical procedures and its treatment, *Nutrition in Clinical Practice* 11 (1996): 43–52.
5. J. C. Burge and coauthors, Changes in patients' taste acuity after Roux-en-Y gastric bypass for clinically severe obesity, *Journal of the American Dietetic Association* 95 (1995): 666–670.
6. J. K. Nelson and coauthors, *Mayo Clinic Diet Manual*, 7th ed. (St. Louis: Mosby, 1994), p. 198.
7. T. Andersen and U. Larsen, Dietary outcome in obese patients treated with gastroplasty program, *American Journal of Clinical Nutrition* 50 (1989): 1328–1340.

Highlight 21

Living with Feeding Disabilities

Thousands of people face obstacles in the ordinary task of eating. These obstacles can arise at any time in a person's life and from any number of conditions. An infant may be born with a physical impairment such as cleft palate, an adolescent may suffer injuries in a car accident, a middle-aged adult may lose motor control following a stroke, or an older adult may struggle with the pain of arthritis. Table H21–1 lists some of the conditions that might lead to feeding problems.

This highlight deals primarily with the kinds of disabilities that make it difficult for people to eat, although disabilities do have other nutrition-related aspects. As one example, a disability may make it difficult for a person to engage in enough physical activity to support a healthy appetite. As another example, a person who has lost a limb to amputation has altered energy needs. Energy needs are reduced in proportion to the weight and metabolism represented by the missing limb, but may be increased if extra effort is necessary to do ordinary things—such as walking on crutches. As still another example, people with involuntary motor activity may have exceedingly high energy needs.

The dietitian, nurse, and occupational therapist most often become involved with feeding disabilities. They can help people achieve as much independence in eating as possible and can teach caregivers to help.

WAYS DISABILITIES CAN IMPAIR EATING

When you consider the number of individual coordinated motions that are required to get food from the table to the stomach, you may be amazed. Think about what an infant experiences when learning to feed himself. At first, the infant cannot sit upright and finds it impossible even to hold a spoon. Every single little action—from picking up the utensils, to biting and chewing, to swallowing—requires coordinated movements. Any injury or disability that interferes with these movements can lead to feeding problems. Some of the feeding skills that might be affected include:

- Sitting and balancing oneself.
- Moving the head and neck in a coordinated way.
- Moving the jaw, lips, and tongue.
- Sucking, swallowing, chewing, and drinking.
- Employing protective reflexes that prevent choking, cutting oneself, biting one's tongue, and others.
- Moving the eyes and hands.
- Making grasping motions.

Other disabilities do not involve oral-motor skills. For example, a person who has problems with sight, or who cannot drive or walk or carry groceries, or who cannot plan meals and think through what to buy has a disability that affects eating. Disabilities of any type can cause people to have trouble maintaining adequate nutrition status.[1] As you might expect, their number one problem is inadequate food intake, which leads to malnutrition, underweight, and, in children, poor growth.[2] Many conditions that lead to feeding problems also alter metabolism and require medications, which further affect nutrition status.

On top of nutrition-related problems, people who have difficulty eating often encounter emotional and social problems. For example,

Table H21–1

Conditions Leading to Feeding Problems

The following conditions may lead to feeding problems by interfering with a person's ability to suck, bite, chew, swallow, or coordinate hand-to-mouth movements.

- Accidents
- Amputations
- Arthritis
- Birth defects
- Cerebral palsy
- Cleft palate
- Down's syndrome
- Head injuries
- Huntington's chorea
- Hydrocephalia
- Language, visual, or hearing impairment
- Microcephalia
- Multiple sclerosis
- Muscle weakness
- Muscular dystrophy
- Neuromotor dysfunction
- Parkinson's disease
- Polio
- Spinal cord injuries
- Stroke

children fail to receive the social training that mealtimes provide, and older people miss the social stimulation that goes with eating in the company of others.

INDEPENDENT EATING FOR PEOPLE WITH DISABILITIES

The evaluation and treatment of a feeding problem require the joint efforts of several health care professionals, possibly including a dietitian, psychologist, occupational therapist, physical therapist, speech pathologist, dentist, and one or several nurses.[3] Table H21–2 provides a checklist of observations health care professionals use to assess feeding skills and nutrition needs. Because each case is different, it makes sense for everyone on the health care team to be familiar with all of these variables.

The dietitian assesses the client's nutrition status, plans a diet, and provides nutrition counseling. The most valuable assessment tool is observation of the client during mealtimes. While observing the client's feeding skills, the assessor can conduct a complete nutrition assessment and provide appropriate nutrition counseling. The dietitian must also ensure that the diet provides foods appropriate for the client's oral-motor capabilities. For example, people with swallowing problems prefer thickened liquids and pureed foods, which flow slowly enough to allow time to coordinate oral movements (see Chapter 21). If the client's abilities to eat improve, the diet can gradually progress through all stages from pureed foods to a regular diet.[4] The planner faces many challenges in designing a diet that coordinates the client's energy and nutrient needs, stage of development, and personal preferences.[5]

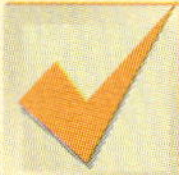

Nutrition Assessment Checklist
For People with Feeding Disabilities

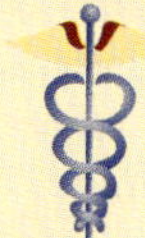

Medical Determine if the client's primary medical problem imposes further dietary changes.

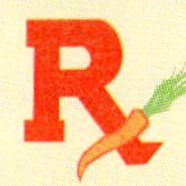

Drug Be aware that anticonvulsant drugs used to treat some disorders may induce folate deficiency, impair vitamin D status, and raise blood cholesterol; drugs prescribed for attention deficit hyperactivity disorder may suppress appetite and slow growth. Remember that some drugs may slow GI tract motility, contributing to constipation; other drugs may cause gastric irritability, drowsiness, nausea, and altered taste sensations—factors that diminish appetite and food intake. Remember that clients on long-term drug therapy and those taking multiple drugs are particularly vulnerable to nutrient imbalances.

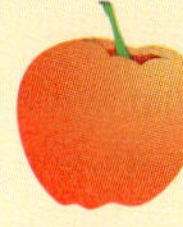

Food Intake When taking a diet history, interview all parents and caregivers responsible for feeding the client. Take into account the differences between food offered and food eaten; spills can contribute to substantial food losses.

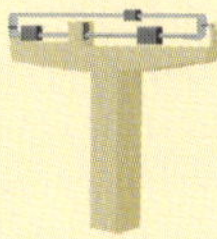

Anthropometric Obtain anthropometric measures as accurately as possible. In cases where standing height cannot be measured, use arm span length instead (measured from the tip of the middle finger on one hand to the tip of the middle finger on the other hand with arms stretched out as far as possible). Use standards specific to the medical disorder if available.

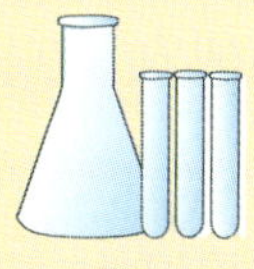

Laboratory Monitor serum albumin to ensure adequate protein status, serum ferritin to detect iron deficiency, and vitamin and mineral status as needed.

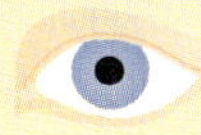

Physical Use Table H21–2 to assess the client's feeding disabilities. Note any dental problems that may interfere with food intake.

But seeing a client's ability to swallow improve due to a change in the diet's texture and consistency can be very rewarding.[6] The accompanying nutrition assessment checklist focuses on topics of notable concern for people with feeding disabilities.

The occupational therapist evaluates oral-motor abilities and feeding skills and then develops a care plan, educates the client, and shows the caregiver, if there is one, ways to implement feeding techniques at home. For example, it may be necessary to teach the client (or caregiver) the proper sitting position for ease of eating. The therapist may instruct the client to sit in a chair with the head and trunk in midline, the back straight and supported, the

Table H21–2

Feeding Evaluation

Oral ability
- Sucking
- Oral prehension
- Swallowing
- Breathing and swallowing coordinated
- Drooling
- Lips
- Tongue size, thrust, mobility
- Biting
- Munching
- Chewing
- Drinking
- Response to input

Dental health
- Structural malformation
- Impaired oral-motor ability
- Delayed weaning
- Use of cariogenic foods or drugs
- Occlusion
- Teeth
- Caries
- Gingiva
- Oral hygiene
- Palate
- Pain on exam
- Hypersensitivity
- Teething stage

Body position
- General tone and movement
- Reflex activity
- Head control
- Sitting balance
- Placement of feet
- Usual feeding position

Hand use
- Palmar grasp
- Pincer grasp
- Opposition finger/thumb
- Hand-to-mouth control

Developmental feeding
- Breast ___ bottle ___ weaned ___
- Baby food ___ junior food ___ mashed table food ___ minced foods ___
- Cut table foods ___ regular table foods ___
- Closes hands in on bottle
- Hand to mouth/sucks on fingers
- Teething biscuit, holds and brings to mouth
- Finger feeds
- Opposes lips to rim of cup
- Attempts to grasp spoon
- Grasps spoon
- Dips spoon in dish
- Brings spoon to mouth
- Holds bottle and drinks independently
- Grasps cup
- Raises cup to mouth
- Lifts cup, drinks, and replaces
- Scoops well with spoon
- Feeds independently with spoon
- Drinks with straw
- Spears with fork
- Spreads with knife

Feeding environment
- Time of feedings (note number and length of feedings)
- Atmosphere of feedings (tense, pleasant, unpleasant)
- Person responsible for feeding
- Parental and/or caregivers' attitude toward feeding
- Past successful and unsuccessful methods
- Identify positive and negative reinforcing behavior
- Behavioral problems

Diet history, including:
- Total fluid intake
- Types of foods consumed
- Method of feeding
- Texture modifications
- Food aversions, intolerances, or allergies
- Use of food as rewards

Medications
- Type
- Dosage
- Time given

Bowel concerns
- Regular
- Constipation
- Diarrhea

Sources: Adapted from J. J. Cafferky, Nutrition assessment of children with developmental disabilities: Special considerations, *Support Line* (a newsletter of Dietitians in Nutrition Support) June 1993; R. B. Howard, Nutritional support of the developmentally disabled child, *Textbook of Pediatric Nutrition*, ed. R. M. Suskind (New York: Raven Press, 1981), pp. 577–582.

Figure H21–1

Examples of Special Feeding Devices

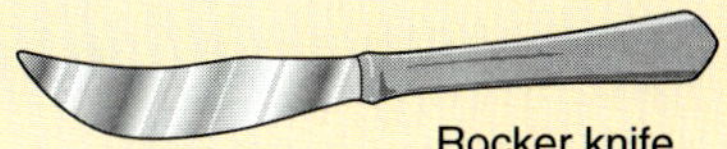

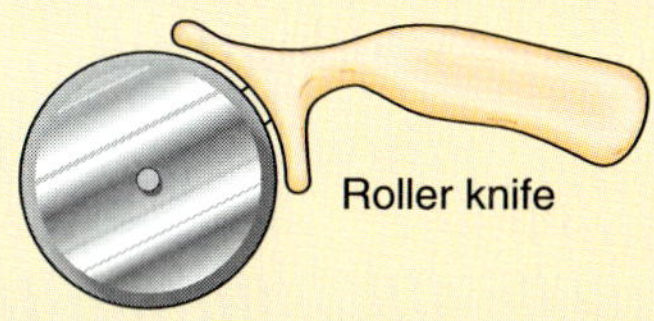

People with only one arm or hand may have difficulty cutting foods and may appreciate using a *rocker knife* or a *roller knife*.

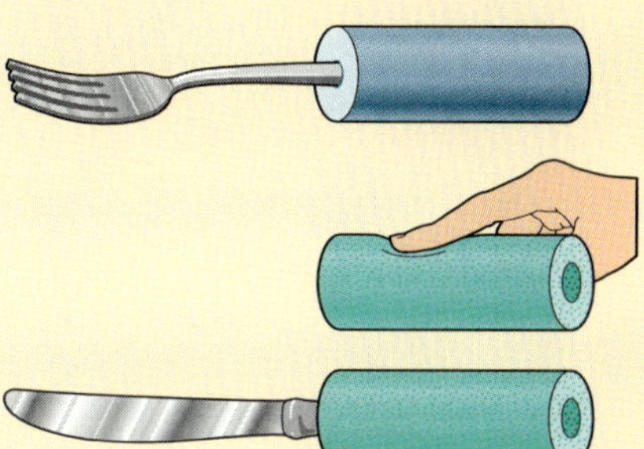

People with a limited range of motion can feed themselves better when they use *flatware with built-up handles*.

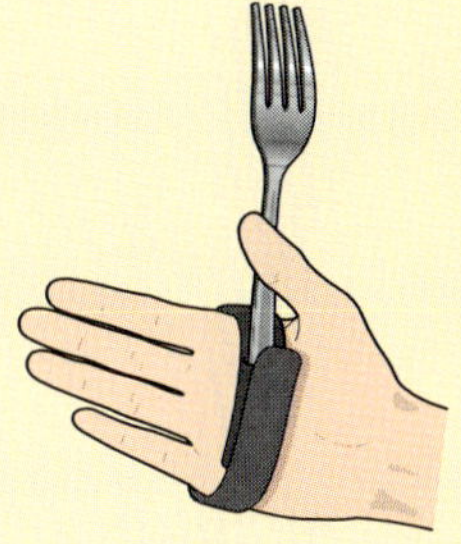

People with extreme muscle weakness may be able to eat with a *utensil holder*.

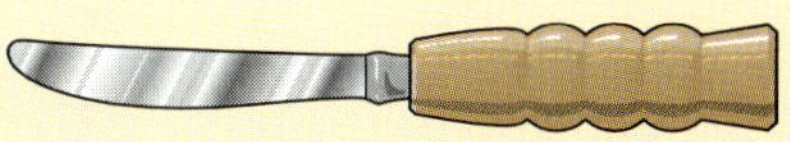

For people with tremors, spasticity, and uneven jerky movements, *weighted utensils* can aid the feeding process.

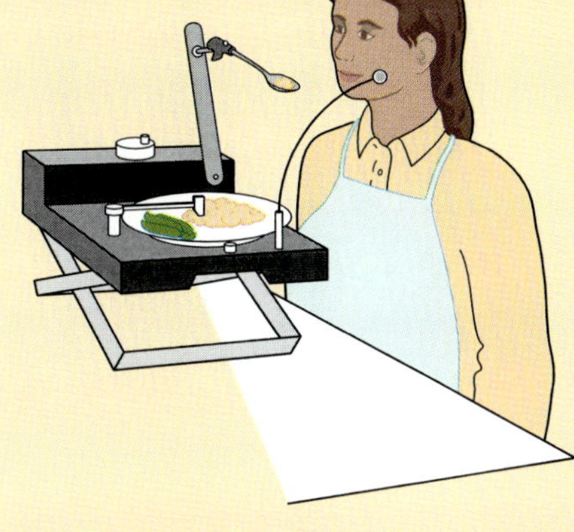

Battery-powered feeding machines enable people with severe limitations to eat with less assistance from others.

Plates

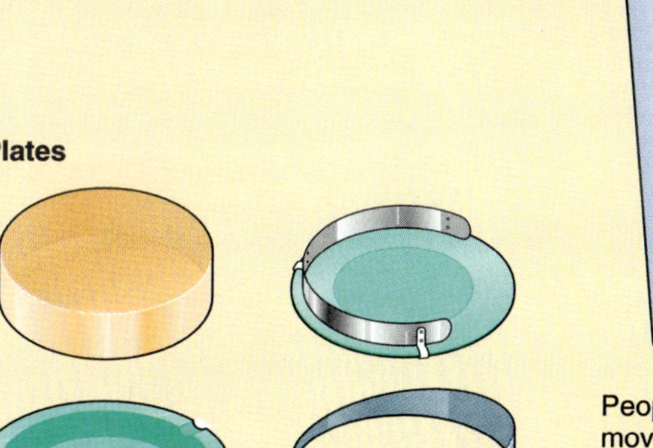

People who have limited dexterity and difficulty maneuvering food find *scoop dishes* or *food guards* useful.

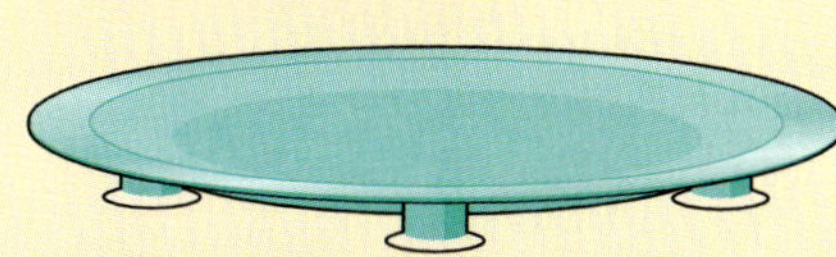

People with uncontrolled or excessive movements might move dishes around while eating and may benefit from using *unbreakable dishes with suction cups*.

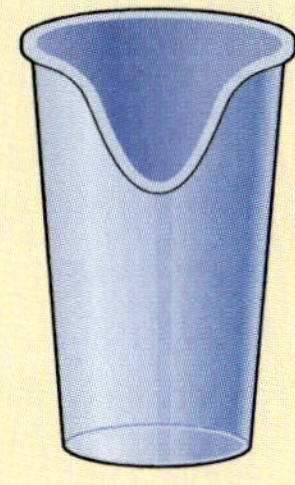

People with limited neck motion can use a *cutout plastic cup*.

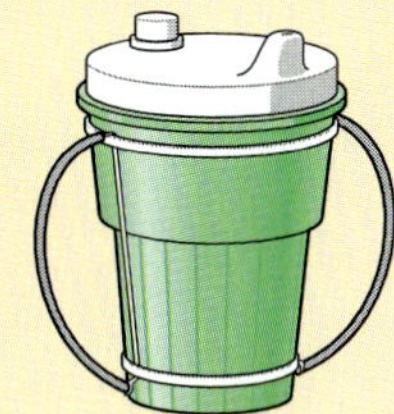

Two-handed cups enable people with moderate muscle weakness to lift a cup with two hands.

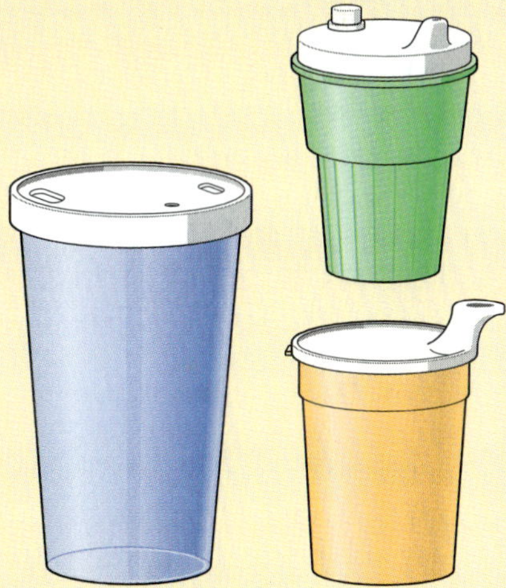

People with uncontrolled or excessive movements might prefer to drink liquids from a *covered cup* or glass with a *slotted opening* or *spout*.

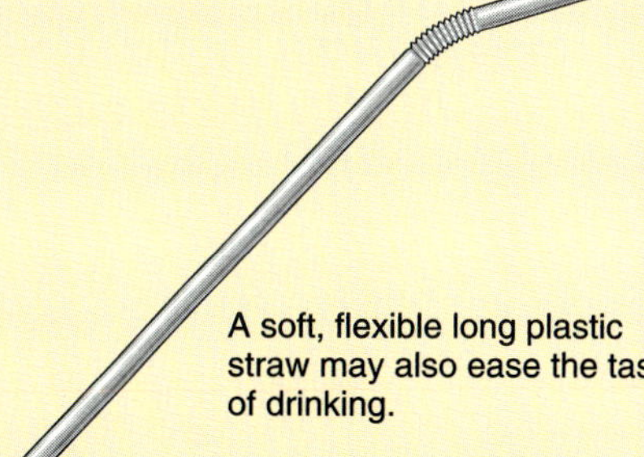

A soft, flexible long plastic straw may also ease the task of drinking.

hips and knees at right angles, and the feet flat and supported on a surface.

Special feeding devices can make a remarkable difference in a person's ability to eat independently. For a person who cannot grasp an ordinary fork, for example, a usable fork may be the key to future health. Becoming independent often improves nutrition status; people who can feed themselves seem to have better appetites and eat more food than those who require assistance.

The occupational therapist selects the appropriate feeding devices and trains the client and caregivers in their use (see Figure H21–1). Everyone on the health care team should be familiar with these devices, however, and should keep track of improved utensils that regularly become available.

Clients may need help in developing eating skills—for example, in learning to swallow. Commonly, a care plan allocates this task to a speech therapist, who trains clients to use the lips, tongue, and throat in both speaking and eating. A dentist may also be needed to evaluate the client's dental health and provide instructions on oral hygiene.

Developing feeding skills requires practice. Helpers can employ strategies such as those listed in Table H21–3 to help clients gain skills. For example, if a hyperreactive child is overly sensitive to oral sensations, an attendant can help by desensitizing the client gradually over time. Start by gently stroking the face with a hand, washcloth, or soft pliable toy. (This can be done playfully, making a game of it.) When the child can tolerate touch on less sensitive areas of the face such as the forehead, cheeks, and lips, then slowly and firmly rub the gums, palate, and tongue.

Table H21–3

Areas of Concern and Suggested Strategies for Developing Feeding Skills

Inability to Suck
• Use cold substances around lips to stimulate sucking. • Use a cloth soaked with water for child to suck. • Try different types of nipples. • As child's ability begins to improve, change to nipple with a smaller hole.
Inability to Chew
• Place a small amount of food between back teeth and move jaw up and down. A mirror may help demonstrate and point out various body parts. • Place foods such as peanut butter on lips and encourage client to wash lips with tongue. Gradually change from pureed foods to solid foods (sprinkle crackers in soup, etc.).
Inability to Swallow
• Close jaw and lips of client together (swallowing is easiest when the mouth is closed). • Stroke throat upward under chin. • Offer next bite of food only after client swallows. • Demonstrate—let client feel *you* swallow.
Inability to Grasp
• Allow client to finger feed. • Guide client in exploring mouth. • Cut food into small pieces. • Place your hand over client's hand and help client grasp spoon. • Use adaptive equipment (plastic spoon, etc.). • Make sure bowl is stabilized (suction, tape). • Use plates with high straight sides, or build higher edge using aluminum foil.
Poor Hand-Mouth Coordination
• Pour sand, etc. • Exercise with ball. • Exercise with push-pull objects. • Study body parts with client, if appropriate.

This discussion of ways to help clients achieve independence in feeding themselves has been brief, but the principles are clear. Accurate identification of the eating-related skills that are impaired leads to appropriate treatment. The treatment can be considered a success if the client becomes independent—that is, able to prepare, serve, and eat nutritionally adequate food daily without help.

THE ROLES OF HELPERS

In the best-case scenario, a person with a disability learns to plan, serve, and eat meals independently. In some cases, however, the person cannot function without help. To ensure that long-term care is successful, the health care team addresses the caregiver's personal needs and develops the caregiver's knowledge and skills.

Impaired Vision
• Place meats and vegetables consistently in same areas of plate.
Overweight
• Cut down snacks and high-kcalorie foods., • Refrain from rewarding with food. • Increase exercise and leisure-time activities.
Underweight
• Increase number of meals per day. • Include high-kcalorie foods, especially liquid supplements. • Encourage proper exercise.
Lack of Nutrition Education
• Work with families. • Stress the importance of proper nutrition for *all* family members. • Teach proper feeding environment (good eating habits, eating positions). • Provide nutrition-instruction materials.

Source: Adapted with permission from S. Calvert and F. Davies, Nutrition of children with handicapping conditions, *Dietetic Currents* 4 (1977): 13–17.

The health care team offers support and encouragement and recognizes that the caregiver's role demands a great deal of responsibility and many personal sacrifices. To learn how to effectively feed another, a caregiver needs training.[7] Training may cover how to prepare and serve foods, as well as what to expect at each level of development in terms of food acceptance, readiness for different textures, correct feeding techniques, messiness, and self-feeding abilities.

The caregiver also needs to learn how to cope with inappropriate feeding behaviors. Otherwise the emotional distress of a difficult situation can escalate during feedings and cause both the person being fed and the caregiver to dislike mealtimes. Negative feelings during mealtimes can hinder efforts to learn appropriate eating behaviors and independent self-feeding.

Consider an example. Children with cerebral palsy can take ten times longer to eat than other children. Some mothers have reported spending up to seven hours a day feeding these children.[8] The caregiver must not only put in this extra time, but ideally also try to establish an emotionally pleasant atmosphere at mealtimes. This means dealing with any feelings of hostility or resentment at other times and places. Psychologists can offer counseling for caregivers; all members of the health care team need to be alert to a caregiver's emotional frustrations.[9]

The basic human drive to eat without assistance supports nutrition adequacy. Fortunately, some people with disabilities can attain this independence with training. In other cases, caregivers can obtain the necessary education and training to provide appropriate support.

The combined efforts of the health care team support both clients and caregivers in achieving feeding independence on every level—physically, mentally, and emotionally. To whatever degree independence can be achieved, it enhances the quality of life.

NOTES

1. Position of The American Dietetic Association: Nutrition in comprehensive program planning for persons with developmental disabilities, *Journal of the American Dietetic Association* 92 (1992): 613–615.
2. M. Thommessen and coauthors, Energy and nutrient intakes of disabled children: Do feeding problems make a difference? *Journal of the American Dietetic Association* 91 (1991): 1522–1525; R. K. Johnson and M. Maeda, Establishing outpatient nutrition services for children with cerebral palsy, *Journal of the American Dietetic Association* 89 (1989): 1504–1507; L. M. Thommessen and coauthors, Nutrition and growth retardation in 10 children with congenital deaf-blindness, *Journal of the American Dietetic Association* 89 (1989): 69–73.
3. L. A. Wodarski, An interdisciplinary nutrition assessment and intervention protocol for children with disabilities, *Journal of the American Dietetic Association* 90 (1990): 1563–1568.
4. E. M. Pardoe, Development of a multistage diet for dysphagia, *Journal of the American Dietetic Association* 93 (1993): 568–571.
5. M. Williams, Dysphagia—the new frontier, *Nutrition Today*, May/June 1992, pp. 26–31.
6. Pardoe, 1993; B. C. Sonies and M. C. Dalakas, Dysphagia in patients with the postpolio syndrome, *New England Journal of Medicine* 324 (1991): 1162–1167.
7. H. N. Sanders, S. B. Hoffman, and C. A. Lund, Feeding strategy for dependent eaters, *Journal of the American Dietetic Association* 92 (1992): 1389–1390.
8. Johnson and Maeda, 1989.
9. Thommessen and coauthors, 1991.

Chapter 22

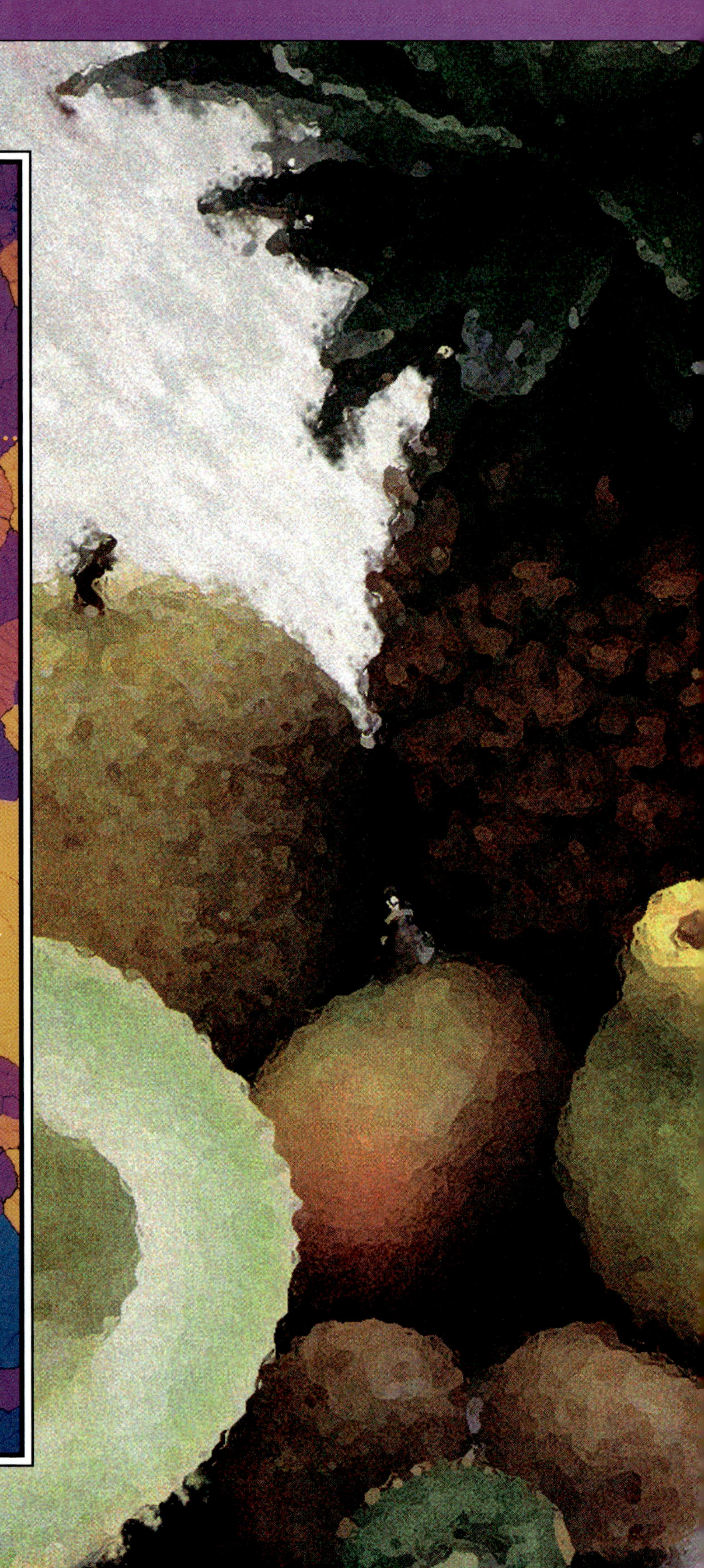

Nutrition and Disorders of the Lower GI Tract

CONTENTS

MICROGRAPH: Vitamin D.

As Chapter 3 noted, the intestine is "the" organ of digestion and absorption. The intestine also provides a physical barrier against invading organisms and contains many immune cells that help protect against disease. (Figure 22–1 shows the intestinal tract and related organs for your review.) Any disorder of the intestine, particularly if it results in malabsorption, can seriously impair nutrition status. This chapter describes disorders of the lower GI tract that either influence nutrition status or are affected by diet. It begins with common disorders, then takes up disorders that cause malabsorption, and finally examines disorders of the large intestine. (Some common digestive problems that do not seriously affect nutrition status, such as gas and short bouts of diarrhea and constipation, were already discussed in Highlight 3.)

Figure 22–1

The Lower GI Tract and Related Organs

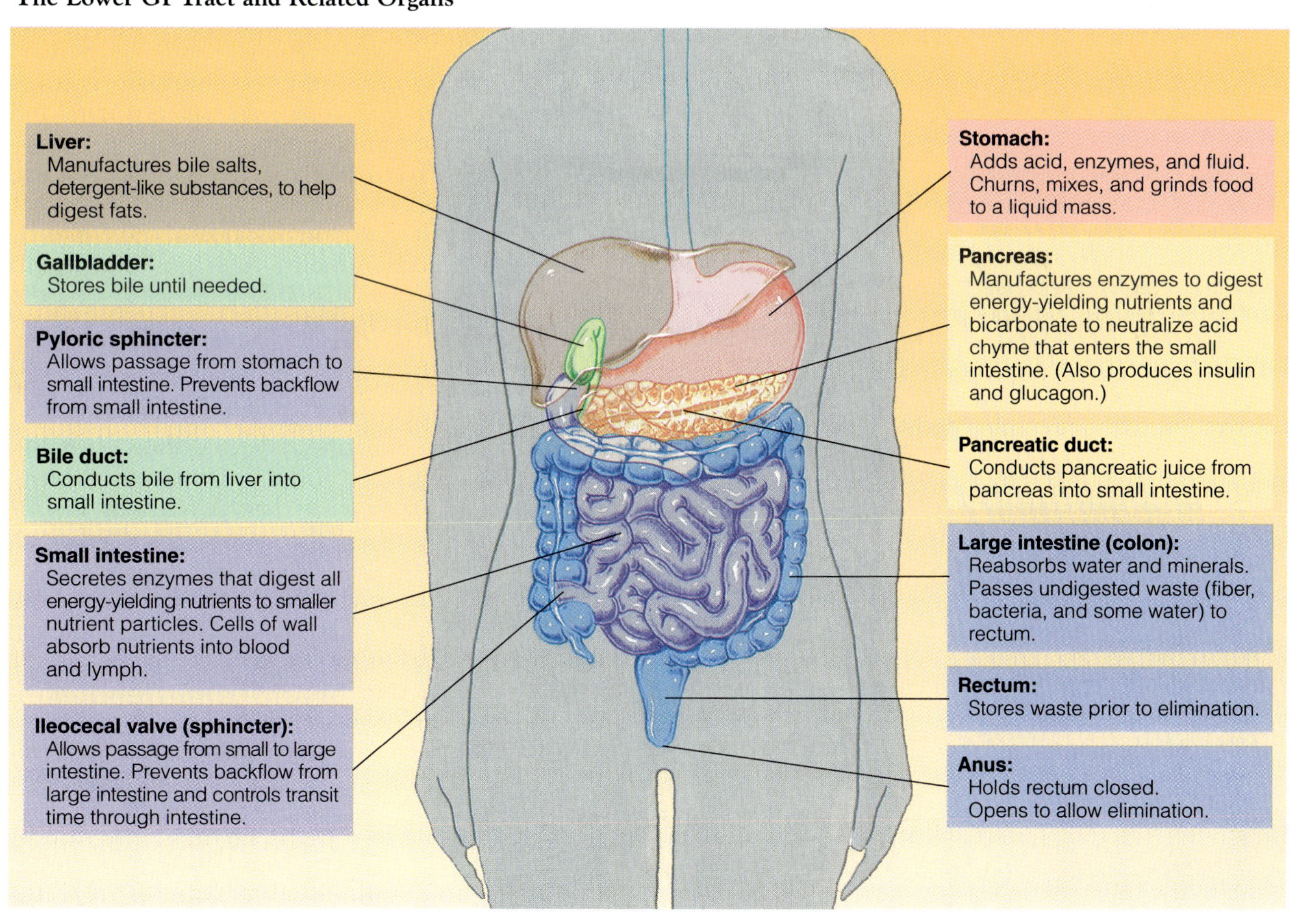

Severe Diarrhea and Irritable Bowel Syndrome

Two common disorders of the GI tract are diarrhea and irritable bowel syndrome. Their causes may not always be known, but nutrition support may help alleviate their symptoms until a diagnosis is made.

DIARRHEA

Diarrhea that results from an accelerated movement of fluids and electrolytes from the intestinal capillaries into the lumen of the intestine is called **secretory diarrhea.**

Diarrhea that results from an increase in the osmolarity of the intestinal contents due to unabsorbed water and electrolytes is called **osmotic diarrhea.**

Severe, chronic diarrhea that does not respond to treatment is often called **intractable diarrhea.**

Permanent and temporary problems with lactose intolerance occur frequently as a consequence of many medical conditions and malabsorption syndromes (see pp. 115–116).

Drugs used to treat diarrhea are called **antidiarrheal agents.** Some antidiarrheal agents include diphenoxylate with atropine sulfate, kaolin- and pectin-containing drugs, loperamide, and tincture of opium. Antidiarrheal agents are generally contraindicated for diarrhea caused by infectious agents, because they slow GI motility and prolong the time that the toxin remains in contact with the GI cells.

Rx **PRESCRIPTION PAD**

Drugs used in the treatment of diarrhea may include:

- Antidiarrheals
- Anti-Infective Agents

See Appendix E for timing with meals and nutrition-related side effects.

Diarrhea refers to an increased frequency or volume of stools. Like other GI complaints, diarrhea is not a disease but a symptom of many medical conditions and treatments. It can be acute, lasting less than 2 weeks, or chronic, lasting longer. Mild diarrhea that remits in 24 to 48 hours is seldom a cause for concern unless the person is already dehydrated. A person with severe, persistent diarrhea may rapidly become dehydrated, lose weight, and develop multiple nutrient deficiencies. A child or infant can lose proportionately more fluid and weight and can develop dehydration and malnutrition in a short time.

Causes of Diarrhea Acute diarrhea that occurs abruptly in a healthy person frequently results from viral, bacterial, or protozoal infections or as a side effect of medications. It can also occur in the person who begins to eat foods or begins a tube feeding after a period of fasting or starvation. Infants often develop diarrhea when given formulas their immature GI tracts cannot handle or when they are ill. When used in large quantities, food ingredients such as sorbitol and olestra may cause diarrhea in some people.

Chronic diarrhea can occur as a result of disorders that alter GI tract motility, such as the irritable bowel syndrome (described next); from any disorder that causes malabsorption (described later); from food intolerances (lactose intolerance, for example); and from some infections, including some parasitic infections and human immunodeficiency virus (HIV). The diarrhea associated with the dumping syndrome was described in the last chapter.

Treatment of Diarrhea The treatment of diarrhea requires treatment of the primary medical condition. If a food is responsible for diarrhea, then that food must be omitted from the diet. If a drug is responsible, a different drug, when possible, or different drug form (injectable versus oral, for example) may alleviate the problem. Infections are treated with appropriate drugs. Drugs that slow GI motility are often recommended along with other therapies to treat diarrhea.

Oral Diets Often people with diarrhea can tolerate regular diets. They may benefit from temporarily avoiding highly seasoned foods, fatty foods, gas-forming foods (see Table 22–1), lactose-containing foods, caffeinated beverages, and any food that aggravates the diarrhea. In other cases, clients may be advised to drink only clear liquids (see Table 22–2 on p. 726) to avoid irritating the GI tract while replacing fluids and electrolytes. For these clients, homemade or commercial oral rehydration formulas—simple solutions of water, salts, and sugar—provide needed fluids and electrolytes. For mild cases of diarrhea, fluids and electrolytes can be replaced using fruit juices, sport drinks, caffeine-free carbonated beverages, tea, and broth with crackers.

Once the diarrhea remits, the client may gradually advance to a regular diet by adding moderately seasoned, low-fiber, low-fat foods as tolerated. Frequent small meals are easiest to tolerate at first. The diet temporarily excludes lactose

Table 22–1

Foods That May Produce Gas

Apples	Garlic
Artichokes, Chinese	Gravy
Asparagus	High-fat meats
Barley	Honey
Beer	Kohlrabi
Bran	Legumes (dried beans and peas)
Broccoli	Mannitol
Brussels sprouts	Milk
Cabbage	Molasses
Carbonated beverages	Nuts
Cauliflower	Onions
Celery	Pastries
Coconut	Prunes
Cream sauces	Radishes
Cucumbers	Raisins
Eggplant	Sorbitol
Eggs	Soybeans
Figs	Wheat
Fish	Yeast
Fried foods	

and any foods believed to have irritated the GI tract. Permanent dietary changes may be necessary for diarrhea caused by food sensitivities or allergies.

The World Health Organization recipe for rehydration in diarrheal disease is: Dissolve 3.5 g sodium chloride (table salt), 2.5 g sodium bicarbonate (baking soda), 1.5 g potassium chloride, and 20 g glucose in enough water to make 1 liter.

Bowel Rest In severe cases of diarrhea, it may become necessary to stop placing demands on the GI tract by withholding all foods and beverages until the diarrhea remits, usually in about 24 to 48 hours. During bowel rest, intravenously administered fluids and electrolytes replace losses. After a day or so of bowel rest, the person tries a clear-liquid diet and then, as tolerance permits, advances to a regular diet as described in the previous paragraph.

Alternative Feedings Clients who are still unable to tolerate adequate amounts of foods after a few days on an oral diet may benefit from nutritionally complete, lactose-free liquid formulas (see Chapter 23) provided orally, if the client can drink them, or by tube, if oral intake remains inadequate. For people with severe diarrhea who are unable to tolerate any type of oral or tube feeding, intravenous nutrition (see Chapter 24) is indicated, and nothing is given by mouth (NPO).

Formulas given by mouth or by tube are called enteral formulas; formulas given by vein are parenteral formulas.

IRRITABLE BOWEL SYNDROME

Irritable bowel syndrome is another common disorder characterized by a disturbance in the motility of the GI tract. The person with irritable bowel syndrome may experience a variety of symptoms including indigestion, nausea, abdominal

Table 22–2

Foods Included on Liquid Diets

Clear-Liquid Diets	Full-Liquid Diets
Bouillon	All clear liquids
Broth, clear	Butter
Carbonated beverages	Cheese, cottage[a]
Coffee, regular and decaffeinated	Commercially prepared liquid formulas (all)
Commercially prepared clear liquid formulas	Cooked cereals, strained
Fruit drinks	Cream
Fruit ices	Custard
Fruit juices, strained	Egg, soft cooked or scrambled[a]
Gelatin	Flavorings
Hard candy	Ice cream, plain
Honey	Instant breakfast drinks
Lemonade	Margarine
Popsicles	Milk, all types
Salt	Potatoes, mashed and diluted in cream soups
Salt substitutes	Pudding
Sugar substitutes	Sherbet
Tea, regular and decaffeinated	Soups, strained vegetables, meat, or cream
	Sugar
	Sour cream
	Vegetable juices, strained
	Vegetable purees, diluted in cream soups
	Yogurt

[a]As tolerated.

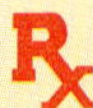

PRESCRIPTION PAD

Drugs used in the treatment of irritable bowel syndrome may include:

- Anticholinergics (to relax GI tract muscles)
- Antidiarrheals
- Antiflatulents (to relieve symptoms due to excess gas)
- Laxatives

See Appendix E for timing with meals and nutrition-related side effects.

pain, bloating, flatulence, diarrhea, constipation, or alternating diarrhea and constipation. Emotional stress may worsen the symptoms, which frequently occur shortly after a person eats and often resolve temporarily following a bowel movement. The next box provides dietary and other suggestions that may help to reduce the symptoms of irritable bowel syndrome.

Dietary adjustments can help ease the symptoms of diarrhea and irritable bowel syndrome. The dietary treatment of diarrhea depends on its medical cause and its severity. Mild diarrhea may remit without treatment, whereas severe diarrhea can lead to dehydration, electrolyte imbalances, and malnutrition. During treatment, diet therapy may range from complete bowel rest to individualized regular diets. Diarrhea is often a symptom of irritable bowel syndrome, a motility disorder that also causes other uncomfortable GI symptoms. Dietary treatment of irritable bowel syndrome hinges on identifying and avoiding individual foods that cause intolerance. For most people, a low-fat diet provided in small meals, with a gradual increase in fiber, is helpful. The next section of this chapter describes malabsorption syndromes, disorders that frequently result in chronic diarrhea and malnutrition.

How to Lessen the Symptoms of Irritable Bowel Syndrome

To reduce the discomforts associated with irritable bowel syndrome, recommend that clients:

- Identify individual food intolerances by keeping a food record that includes symptoms and the time they occur in relation to meals.
- Avoid offending foods or substances. Common intolerances include milk and milk products (lactose), fatty foods, gas-forming foods and beverages (review Table 22–1), caffeine, alcohol, and foods containing large amounts of fructose or sorbitol.
- Eat frequent small meals at a relaxed pace and at regular times.
- Gradually add dietary fiber to the diet by including more whole-grain breads and cereals, fruits and vegetables, dried beans and peas, and nuts. (Table 4–4 on p. 129 shows the fiber content of selected foods.) Because high-fiber foods are often gas producing, add fiber gradually to allow the GI tract time to adapt.
- Drink plenty of fluids. Fiber attracts water as it moves through the GI tract, so more water is needed.
- Get regular physical activity to reduce stress.

Physicians may also recommend bran or hydrophilic colloids to help relieve constipation. Bran is likely to produce gas, so hydrophilic colloids may be a better choice for some people.

hydrophilic colloid: a type of laxative that attracts water in the intestine to form a bulky stool, which then stimulates peristalsis. (Metamucil and Fiberall are examples of hydrophilic colloids.)

Nutrition Consequences of Malabsorption

Many disorders lead to malabsorption, and any nutrient can be involved. Chapter 21 described vitamin B_{12} malabsorption resulting from chronic gastritis and general malabsorption resulting from the dumping syndrome. The lower GI disorders that affect nutrition most profoundly are those that cause fat malabsorption, which consequently affects the absorption and metabolism of many other nutrients. Unabsorbed fat is excreted from the body in the stools, causing the type of diarrhea known as steatorrhea. Protein may also be malabsorbed, although usually to a lesser degree, further contributing to malnutrition.

steatorrhea (stee-ah-toe-REE-ah): fatty diarrhea characteristic of fat malabsorption; stools are loose, foamy, and foul smelling.

FAT MALABSORPTION

The body's process for absorbing fat (see pp. 154–160) depends on lipase from the pancreas and bile from the liver and is more complex than the process for absorbing protein and carbohydrate. Thus malabsorption syndromes affect fat absorption more profoundly than protein and carbohydrate absorption. The loss of fat in the stools means that valuable food energy, fat-soluble vitamins, and some minerals are lost as well (see Figure 22–2). The loss of food energy affects protein metabolism as well; protein will be sacrificed for energy, limiting its availability to maintain its vital functions.

Figure 22–2

The Effects of Fat Malabsorption

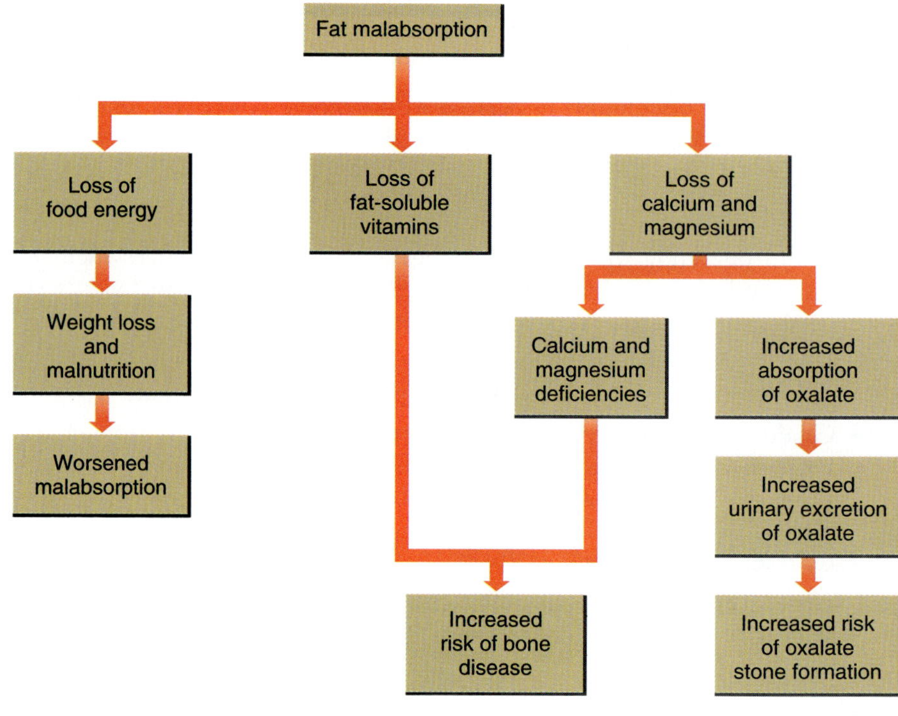

Vitamin and Mineral Malabsorption Fat-soluble vitamins normally travel through the intestine with fat, so they are lost when fat is excreted in steatorrhea. Minerals normally are absorbed in the colon, but when fat malabsorption occurs, unabsorbed fatty acids form soaps with calcium and magnesium and carry these minerals out of the body. Vitamin D losses further aggravate calcium malabsorption.

Oxalate Stones The binding of calcium to fatty acids can cause another problem, enteric hyperoxaluria. Oxalate, which is present in some foods, normally binds with some of the calcium in the gut and is excreted with it. But when fatty acids bind the calcium, the oxalate remains unbound. The intestine absorbs the unbound oxalate, but the body cannot metabolize it and so excretes it in the urine. High urinary oxalate favors the formation of kidney stones (see Highlight 29).

enteric hyperoxaluria (en-TER-ick HIGH-per-oxa-LOO-ree-ah): a condition of excess oxalate absorption that comes about because calcium is unable to bind oxalate in the gut; may lead to kidney stone formation.
enteric = intestinal

As you read through these sections on diets for fat malabsorption syndromes, keep in mind the following diet-planning principles:

- Fat is best tolerated when taken in frequent small meals.
- Part of the fat allowance may be supplied by medium-chain triglycerides (MCT).
- Fat-soluble vitamins may be given in a water-miscible form when malabsorption is severe.

TREATMENTS FOR FAT MALABSORPTION

To treat steatorrhea successfully, the underlying disorder must be diagnosed and treated. Drug therapy, and sometimes surgery, may be necessary. Dietary fat is often restricted; otherwise, enzyme replacements (described later) are provided to aid absorption.

Fat-Restricted Diets Individual tolerances determine the specific amount of fat prescribed, but usually it ranges from 20 to 40 percent of total energy. Typically, the person with malabsorption begins with a diet containing 35 to 45 grams of fat. The person may gradually increase fat intake to provide additional energy as needed. Tolerance improves if fat is consumed in frequent small meals.

Table 22–3

Fat-Restricted Diet (35 grams)

Use:

1. Nonfat milk, cheeses and yogurt made from nonfat milk, sherbet, and fruit ices.
2. Low-fat egg substitutes and up to three regular eggs per week.
3. Up to 6 oz of lean meats and poultry without skin daily.
4. Up to 3 servings of fat daily. One serving is any one of the following:
   1 tsp butter, margarine, shortening, oil, or mayonnaise
   1 strip crisp bacon
   1 tbs salad dressing
   ⅛ avocado
   2 tbs cream (half and half)
   10 small nuts
   8 large olives
   If fat is used to cook or season food, it must be taken from this allowance.
5. All vegetables prepared without fat.
6. All fruits prepared without fat.
7. Plain white or whole-grain bread; nonfat cereals, pasta, rice, noodles, and macaroni.
8. Clear soups.
9. Angel food cake and fruit whips made with gelatin, sugar, and egg-white meringues.
10. Jelly, jam, honey, gumdrops, jelly beans, and marshmallows.

Do Not Use:

1. Whole milk, chocolate milk, whole-milk cheeses, and ice cream.
2. Pastries, cakes, pies, sweet rolls, breads, or vegetables made with fat.
3. More than one egg a day, fried or fatty meats (sausage, luncheon meats, spareribs, frankfurters), duck, goose, or tuna packed in oil (unless well drained).
4. More than 3 servings of fat.
5. Desserts, candy, or anything made with chocolate, nuts, or foods not allowed.
6. Creamed soups made with whole milk.

Suggestions:

1. To make the diet still lower in fat, reduce the fat and meat (and egg) servings.
2. To raise the fat content, give additional fat or meat servings.
3. To improve acceptance of the diet, check the fat content of a well-liked food and allow that food if possible. Use the exchange system fat list for alternate suggestions for fat servings (see Appendix G).

Note: The box on p. 168 provides additional tips for lowering fat in the diet.

Table 22–3 provides instructions for a fat-restricted diet, and a sample fat-restricted diet menu is shown on p. 730.

Medium-Chain Triglycerides Note that the diet is not severely restricted in fat for any longer than is necessary; the person needs food energy. Instead, the diet may provide some fat from medium-chain triglycerides (MCT) rather than long-chain triglycerides (LCT). Products made from MCT oil and formulas con-

Sample Fat-Restricted Diet Menu
All foods are prepared without added fat.

Menu

Breakfast	Lunch	Supper
1 soft-cooked egg	3 oz broiled chicken	3 oz lean roast beef
½ c dry cereal	½ c rice	½ c mashed potatoes
4 oz orange juice	½ c green beans	½ c peas
1 slice whole-wheat toast	1 tsp margarine	1 slice bread
½ tsp margarine	Tossed salad	1 tsp margarine
Nonfat milk	1 tbs low-fat French dressing	Peaches
Coffee, sugar	Fresh apple	Nonfat milk
	Iced tea, sugar	
		Snack
		Fruit ice

Most naturally occurring fats are LCT; LCT contain fatty acid side chains with at least 14 carbon atoms, and they require lipase and bile for absorption. MCT contain fatty acid side chains with 8 to 12 carbon atoms, and they can be absorbed with minimal lipase and bile.

taining MCT supply about as many kcalories as regular fats, but people who cannot digest and absorb LCT can digest and absorb MCT. MCT oil does not contain essential fatty acids, however, so the diet must include some LCT. The accompanying box offers suggestions for improving acceptance of fat-restricted diets and includes tips for using MCT oil.

water-miscible (MISS-ih-bul) **vitamins:** fat-soluble vitamins that readily mix with water and can be absorbed without fat.

Water-Miscible Fat-Soluble Vitamins Most often, the person with malabsorption absorbs enough fat-soluble vitamins so that a standard supplement can be given. For people who fail to maintain adequate vitamin pools, however, fat-soluble vitamins can be supplemented in a water-miscible form that facilitates absorption.

Oxalate-Restricted Diets To reduce the risk of oxalate stones, clients with fat malabsorption may be advised to limit foods high in oxalate. Foods notable for their high oxalate contents include spinach, rhubarb, beets, nuts, chocolate, tea, wheat bran, and strawberries.

enzyme replacements: extracts of pork or beef pancreatic enzymes that are taken as supplements to help with digestion.

Enzyme Replacement Therapy Enzyme replacements are used when the person suffers malabsorption related to chronic and severe damage to the pancreas or whenever steatorrhea is severe. They improve digestion and absorption, thereby helping to control steatorrhea. Enzyme replacements taken with meals may lessen the malabsorption of protein and fat, but may not fully correct it.

Of the energy nutrients, fat undergoes the most complex process of digestion and absorption and, therefore, is the most likely to be affected by disorders that cause malabsorption. The loss of fat in the stools leads to the loss of food energy; the malabsorption of fat-soluble vitamins, calcium, and magnesium; and the

How to Improve Acceptance of Fat-Restricted Diets

Fat-restricted diets can be difficult for people to follow. Fats give flavors to foods—flavors that people may miss. Unlike some diets that can be introduced gradually, a fat-restricted diet must be implemented right away without giving the person time to adapt to the changes. These suggestions may help:

- Provide clients with tips for making foods palatable while lowering the fat intake, such as those found in the box on p. 168.
- Suggest that clients use cookbooks that feature low-kcalorie and low-fat recipes.
- Remind clients that new fat-free and low-fat products appear on market shelves daily, and most people find these products very acceptable.

People who use MCT oil need additional advice:

- Advise clients to add MCT to the diet gradually. Nausea, vomiting, abdominal pain, and distention can result from using too much MCT at once.
- Recommend that clients improve the palatability of MCT oil by substituting it for regular oil in salad dressing and for baking and cooking and by adding it to beverages, desserts, and other dishes.
- Warn clients that MCT products are expensive, and explain that these products can be purchased at pharmacies and may be covered by insurance.

increased absorption of oxalate. Dietary therapy for fat malabsorption may include fat- and oxalate-restricted diets and the use of MCT, water-miscible fat-soluble vitamins, and enzyme replacements. Disorders that result in malabsorption are described next.

Malabsorption Syndromes

Malabsorption syndromes and their treatments profoundly threaten nutrition status and may lead to wasting by reducing nutrient intakes, accelerating nutrient losses, and raising nutrient needs (see Table 22–4). Malabsorption can occur when the flow of enzymes from the pancreas or bile from the liver is disrupted, when the surface area of the bowel is reduced, or when normal mechanisms for absorbing nutrients are impaired. Many drugs and disorders can cause malabsorption; several are discussed throughout the remainder of this chapter, but whatever the cause, malnutrition always threatens.

Because the pancreas is an accessory organ in digestion and absorption, some pancreatic disorders result in malabsorption and cause nutrition consequences similar to those of intestinal disorders and so are described here. Malabsorption caused by other disorders such as liver disease, cancer, and HIV infection, which have additional nutrition consequences, are described in later chapters.

PANCREATITIS

Pancreatic secretions contain many enzymes necessary for the digestion of protein, fat, and carbohydrate, together with bicarbonate-rich juices that provide

Table 22–4

Possible Causes of Wasting in Malabsorption Syndromes

Reduced Nutrient Intake	Excessive Nutrient Losses	Raised Nutrient Needs
Abdominal pain	Blood loss	High basal energy expenditure
Anorexia	Diarrhea	Infection
Bowel rest	Fistulas	Medications
Emotional stress	General malabsorption	Surgery
Food intolerance	Intestinal losses of serum proteins	
Indigestion	Medications	
Medications	Steatorrhea	
Nausea	Vomiting	
Obstructions		

the optimal pH necessary to activate these enzymes. Consequently, pancreatic disorders can impair digestion and result in malabsorption and poor nutrition status.

pancreatitis: inflammation of the pancreas.

Acute Pancreatitis Normally, the pancreas stores digestive enzymes in an inactive form to protect itself from digestion. In pancreatitis, however, digestive enzymes are activated within the pancreas and begin to damage the organ itself. The blood picks up some of these enzymes; thus elevated serum amylase and lipase serve as indicators of pancreatitis. Typical symptoms of pancreatitis include severe abdominal pain, nausea, and vomiting. In some cases, pancreatitis leads to serious complications including reduced blood volume, acute renal failure (see Chapter 29), respiratory failure, pancreatic hemorrhages, fistulas, and abscesses.[1] Pancreatitis most often develops as a consequence of gallstones or alcoholism; sometimes, though, the reasons are unclear because a variety of medical conditions and some drugs can also precipitate pancreatitis.[2]

fistula (FIS-too-lah): an abnormal opening between two organs or from an organ to the skin.
fistula = pipe

abscess: an accumulation of pus, caused by a local infection, that builds up and may eventually burst.

Treatment of Pancreatitis The treatment of acute pancreatitis depends on its severity, although initial therapy in all cases aims to suppress pancreatic secretions. Food is withheld, because food stimulates pancreatic secretions. In some cases, a nasogastric tube is inserted to suction out the stomach's secretions and further reduce stimulation of the pancreas. Edema within the pancreas, losses through nasogastric suction, and lack of oral intake can disrupt fluid and electrolyte balance, making intravenous fluids necessary.

Mild-to-Moderate Pancreatitis In most cases, pancreatitis resolves in less than a week; the person can begin oral intake when abdominal pain subsides and serum amylase levels return to normal or near normal. The diet progresses from a clear-liquid diet to a low-fat diet and, finally, to a regular diet as tolerated. If eating aggravates the pain, or if serum amylase rises, food is withheld; when these signs and symptoms subside, food can again be reintroduced. Clients may tolerate frequent small meals better at first.

If pancreatitis is severe or if complications arise, and if food intake fails to meet nutrient needs for more than a week, tube feeding is indicated.[3] The presence of nutrients in the stomach stimulates pancreatic secretions, but studies suggest that feedings delivered by tube directly into the jejunum do not significantly stimulate pancreatic secretions.[4] Thus people with pancreatitis may benefit from tube feedings of easy-to-absorb formulas delivered into the jejunum. If enteral feedings worsen abdominal pain, edema, or drainage from fistulas, or if vomiting is a problem, intravenous feedings may be necessary.

Chronic Pancreatitis If an acute episode of pancreatitis doesn't subside or if episodes recur at frequent intervals, the pancreatic cells can be permanently destroyed, leading to chronic pancreatitis. Chronic alcohol abuse is the most frequent cause of chronic pancreatitis.

The pancreas normally excretes enzymes far in excess of needs, so even after considerable damage has occurred, digestion may proceed normally. With extensive degeneration of the pancreas and chronic pancreatitis, however, digestion, especially of fat, becomes permanently impaired. Abdominal pain is often severe and unrelenting, vomiting is frequent, and severe weight loss is common.

Nutrition Support The goals of diet therapy in chronic pancreatitis are to maintain optimal nutrition status, reduce steatorrhea (if present), minimize pain, and avoid subsequent attacks of active pancreatitis. Health care professionals recommend a moderate fat-restricted diet; restricting fat too severely makes it difficult for the person to gain or maintain weight. Small meals may be easiest to digest. Absolutely no alcohol is permitted.

Enzyme replacements taken with meals aid in the digestion and absorption of protein and fat. Enzyme replacements, like naturally occurring enzymes, work best in a basic pH. To improve the effectiveness of enzyme replacements, people with pancreatic insufficiency often need to take drugs to limit gastric acid production, because the basic secretions from the pancreas may be reduced.

Complicating Conditions During active attacks of pancreatitis, diet therapy reverts to that described earlier for acute pancreatitis. Sometimes pancreatitis damages the cells that produce the hormones insulin and glucagon. In these cases, clients become glucose intolerant, as in diabetes (see Chapter 27), and must follow a diet for diabetes. Deficiencies of glucagon, which lead to hypoglycemia, complicate the task of regulating blood glucose. The case study on p. 734 provides a review of pancreatitis and its treatment.

Rx PRESCRIPTION PAD

Drugs used in the treatment of pancreatitis may include:

- Analgesics (to relieve pain)
- H2-blockers (to improve efficiency of enzyme replacements)
- Insulin (to control blood glucose levels)
- Pancreatic enzyme replacements

See Appendix E for timing with meals and nutrition-related side effects.

CYSTIC FIBROSIS

People with cystic fibrosis, the most common fatal genetic disorder in North America, produce thick, sticky mucus secretions that may seriously impair the function of many organs, most notably the lungs and pancreas.[5] Just a few decades ago, an infant born with cystic fibrosis seldom survived to adulthood. Today, thanks to advances in medical therapy and nutrition care, the outlook is much brighter, with some surviving into their forties and even fifties.

Cystic fibrosis has three major consequences: chronic lung disease, pancreatic insufficiency, and abnormally high electrolyte concentrations in the sweat. Chronic lung disease develops because the airways in the lungs become

cystic fibrosis: a hereditary disorder characterized by the production of thick mucus that affects many organs, including the lungs, pancreas, liver, heart, gallbladder, and small intestine.

fibrous: composed of fibers. The development of excess fibrous tissue is **fibrosis**.

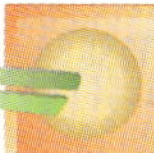

Case Study Homemaker with Pancreatitis

Mrs. Corey is a 52-year-old homemaker who was admitted to the hospital with severe abdominal pain, nausea, and vomiting. Laboratory tests reveal very high serum amylase, low serum albumin, and red blood cell indices consistent with folate-deficiency anemia. Mrs. Corey is diagnosed as having pancreatitis. She is 5 feet 3 inches tall and weighs 100 pounds. Mrs. Corey's family has told her physician that she may have a problem with alcohol abuse. The health care team is concerned not only with the diagnosis of pancreatitis, but also with Mrs. Corey's nutrition status and possible alcohol abuse.

How would you describe pancreatitis to Mrs. Corey? Why is her serum amylase elevated? How can pancreatitis lead to poor nutrition status? Discuss factors in Mrs. Corey's medical history that put her at risk for poor nutrition status. (Assume alcohol abuse for the purposes of this question, and review Highlight 7's description of how alcohol impairs nutrition status.)

Describe when and how Mrs. Corey should be fed. What factors would determine the need for tube feedings or parenteral nutrition?

If Mrs. Corey develops chronic pancreatitis, how should her diet be modified? What other measures should be taken to ensure adequate digestion and absorption?

congested with mucus, causing breathing to be labored. As the thick mucus stagnates in the bronchial tubes, bacteria multiply there. Lung infections are the usual cause of death in people with cystic fibrosis.

Cystic fibrosis probably causes some degree of pancreatic insufficiency in all cases, with about 90 percent of cases serious enough to require enzyme replacement therapy. With aging, damage to the pancreas worsens. The thick mucus obstructs the small pancreatic ducts and interferes with the secretion of digestive enzymes, pancreatic juices, and pancreatic hormones. Eventually, the pancreatic cells are surrounded by mucus and are gradually replaced by fibrous tissues. Malabsorption of many nutrients including fat, protein, vitamins, and minerals often leads to malnutrition. Additionally, the secretion of insulin may be affected resulting in glucose intolerance and diabetes.

Rx PRESCRIPTION PAD

Drugs used in the treatment of cystic fibrosis may include:

- Antibiotics
- Bronchodilators (to ease breathing)
- H2-blockers
- Insulin (to control blood glucose)
- Mucolytics (to thin mucous secretions)
- Pancreatic enzyme replacements

See Appendix E for timing with meals and nutrition-related side effects.

Treatment of Cystic Fibrosis Therapy for cystic fibrosis aims to promote appropriate growth and development and prevent respiratory failure and complications. Treatment includes respiratory, diet, and drug therapy.

Energy and Nutrient Needs Nutrient losses through malabsorption, frequent infections, rapid turnover of protein and essential fatty acids, high protein catabolism, and high basal energy expenditures raise energy needs for people with cystic fibrosis to between 120 and 150 percent of the RDA for sex and age. Extra energy is needed simply to breathe. Dietitians estimate individual energy requirements based on basal metabolic rate, activity level, pulmonary function, and degree of malabsorption.

Obtaining enough energy can be complicated, however, because people with cystic fibrosis frequently experience a loss of appetite that is aggravated by repeated infections, emotional stress, and drug therapy. Coughing to clear the lungs may trigger vomiting or reflux of foods from the stomach. Thus the person with cystic fibrosis finds it difficult to take in enough food energy, protein, and other nutrients to meet needs.

With the widespread use of supplemental vitamins for people with cystic fibrosis, overt vitamin deficiencies are uncommon. Abnormal electrolyte losses through the sweat or from vomiting require replacement.

Diet and Enzyme Replacement Therapy With such high energy needs, fat restrictions are inappropriate; instead, pancreatic enzyme replacements are used to control steatorrhea, relieve abdominal pain, and reduce the mass and frequency of stools passed. To improve the effectiveness of the enzyme replacements, H2-blockers are often provided as well. Even with enzyme replacements, from 10 to 20 percent of food energy is lost in the stools.[6]

Feeding Infants How can the enhanced energy and nutrient needs of infants with cystic fibrosis be met? For some infants with cystic fibrosis, breastfeeding can sustain normal growth, if enzyme replacements are given.[7] These infants must be closely monitored, however, to ensure that they meet their high energy and nutrient needs. Additionally, the breastfed infant with cystic fibrosis needs about ⅛ to ¼ teaspoon of table salt daily, given with water to replace sweat-induced electrolyte losses.[8]

Infants who are not breastfed can usually tolerate regular infant formulas. Infants who cannot tolerate regular formulas often receive special formuals that are easy to digest and absorb. Regardless of the type of feeding—human milk, regular infant formula, or hydrolyzed formula—enzyme replacements are always given as well. As for solid foods, the recommendations for feeding infants and for introducing solid foods during the first year, shown on p. 635, apply to infants with cystic fibrosis.

Formulas that are easy to digest and absorb are called **hydrolyzed formulas** (see Chapter 23).

Feeding Children and Adults A child with cystic fibrosis is weaned from breast milk or infant formula to a high-kcalorie, nutritionally balanced diet carefully tailored to the child's tolerances. Indirect calorimetry may provide a more accurate assessment of energy needs than formula estimates, especially in preadolescent children.[9]

Nutrient Supplementation Carbohydrate supplements, MCT oil and protein powders can be added to foods to boost energy and protein intakes (see Appendix K). Liquid formulas taken orally to improve energy and nutrient intake can also be used.[10]

Multivitamin supplements are prescribed to help meet the high vitamin requirements that a high-energy, high-protein intake demands. As the disorder progresses, fat-soluble vitamins may be given in addition to a multivitamin supplement. For people with severe steatorrhea, the water-miscible vitamin form is appropriate.

As for minerals, as mentioned earlier, abnormally high concentrations of electrolytes (sodium and chloride) in sweat are characteristic of cystic fibrosis. Fever, high environmental temperatures, vomiting, and malabsorption can further deplete electrolytes and lead to dehydration in people with cystic fibrosis. The liberal use of table salt and fluids is encouraged.

Fluids help liquefy thick secretions and prevent dehydration.

Alternate Feedings People with cystic fibrosis need regular nutrition assessments to ensure that their diets are supporting their growth and well-being. Height and weight measurements are particularly relevant. For adults, the goal is

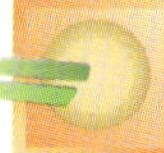

Case Study Child with Cystic Fibrosis

Ryan is a seven-year-old boy diagnosed with cystic fibrosis. Symptoms of steatorrhea and failure to gain weight during infancy prompted tests that led to the diagnosis. Ryan is currently in the hospital to treat a respiratory infection. He has a temperature of 102°F. He is 43½ inches tall and weighs 38 pounds.

Describe the medical consequences of cystic fibrosis. Why are growth failure and repeated respiratory infections hallmarks of the disorder? Look at the growth chart appropriate for Ryan's age and sex in Appendix E. Plot Ryan's height and weight. What does the chart tell you about his growth?

What type of diet should Ryan follow? How can enzyme replacements be used effectively? What important measure should be taken to ensure that Ryan's diet is adequate?

How can the people caring for Ryan and his family offer emotional support?

to maintain a healthy weight for height. For children, every effort should be made to maintain weight at greater than 90 percent of that appropriate for height, gender, and age.[11] If weight falls below 85 percent of standard weight, feeding by tube is indicated.[12] Weight below 75 percent indicates advanced malnutrition that necessitates feeding by tube or by vein. Clients may benefit from home nutrition programs that include oral diets during waking hours and tube feedings or intravenous nutrition during sleep.

Emotional Support People with cystic fibrosis face repeated hospitalizations and often an early death. They, and their caregivers, must deal with many aspects of care important to survival, of which nutrition is only one. They must manage daily respiratory therapy treatments, enzyme replacements, and, often, antibiotics. Caregivers must also help people with cystic fibrosis to adjust to their disease, maintain their social life, keep up with work or schoolwork, and assume as much responsibility for their health as possible. The accompanying case study discusses the needs of a child with cystic fibrosis.

CROHN'S DISEASE

Crohn's disease: inflammation and ulceration along the length of the GI tract, often with granulomas; also called **regional ileitis** (ILL-ee-EYE-tis).

granulomas (gran-you-LOH-mahs): granular tumors or growths.
- *granulum* = little grain
- *oma* = tumor

The two most prevalent disorders that inflame the bowel are Crohn's disease and ulcerative colitis (described later). Inflammatory bowel diseases (IBD) share some clinical features but are distinct conditions. Their causes remain unknown, although heredity, environment, and immune functions are thought to be contributing factors.[13]

In Crohn's disease, cracklike ulcers and many granulomas accompany inflammation of the bowel. Crohn's disease most often affects the ileum and colon, but can affect the entire GI tract and even the liver, kidneys, joints, eyes, and skin. The incidence of Crohn's disease is highest in people from 20 to 40 years of age and in Jews. There is no medical cure for Crohn's disease, and even after acute symptoms resolve, recurrences are likely.

Complications As the disease progresses, fibrous tissue forms in the intestine, reducing its absorptive ability, narrowing the intestinal lumen, and sometimes causing an obstruction. The intestine may also rupture and cause a severe, and sometimes fatal, infection (peritonitis).

Reminder: A *fistula* is an abnormal opening between two organs or from an organ to the skin.

Fistulas may develop if an inflamed loop of intestine sticks to another loop of intestine, to another organ, or to the skin and gradually erodes. If a fistula forms between the stomach or the upper portion of the small intestine and the colon, ingested food is shunted directly into the colon, and further malabsorption results. Bacteria from the colon can then invade the stomach or upper small intestine, contributing to further malabsorption (described next), increasing the risk of serious infections, and causing severe inflammation, nausea, and vomiting. If a fistula forms between the small intestine and the skin, significant malabsorption can occur if large volumes of fluid are lost. Surgery to remove a diseased or obstructed portion of the intestine or to repair a fistula further taxes nutrition status.

Fistulas through which 100 ml or more of fluid per day are lost are called *high-output fistulas*.

Nutrition Status Nutrition status is severely threatened in Crohn's disease. The person with Crohn's disease often experiences emotional stress, anorexia, weight loss, fever, diarrhea, malabsorption, and cramping abdominal pain—all of which can lead to nutrient deficiencies. Oral intake may be withheld so that the bowel can rest, particularly when an obstruction develops or a fistula forms. In addition, bleeding from lesions can lead to anemia, and inflammation can cause the secretion and loss of serum proteins, with resulting hypoalbuminemia.[14] The accompanying drug therapy can further impair nutrition status. If the person requires surgery or develops an infection, nutrient needs become even greater. Because surgery removes a portion of the bowel, the procedure itself may contribute to malabsorption (see "Short-Bowel Syndrome" later in this chapter).

The intestinal loss of serum proteins is called protein-losing enteropathy.

PRESCRIPTION PAD

Drugs used in the treatment of Crohn's disease may include:

- Antibiotics (metronidazole, sulfasalazine)
- Anti-inflammatory agents (prednisone)

See Appendix E for timing with meals and nutrition-related side effects.

Because children with Crohn's disease need additional nutrients to support growth and maturation, nutrition problems are compounded. Growth failure is common and may be the manifestation of the disease that leads to its diagnosis.

Restoring and maintaining nutrition status for the person with Crohn's disease can be a challenging task. Protein-energy malnutrition (PEM) and deficiencies of calcium, magnesium, zinc, iron, vitamin B_{12}, folate, vitamin C, and fat-soluble vitamins are commonly reported. Low serum albumin and multiple nutrient deficiencies threaten immune function and may reduce the effectiveness of drug therapy.

Nutrition Support People with active Crohn's disease benefit from formulas provided by mouth or by tube or total nutrition by vein (see Chapters 23 and 24).[15] Enteral nutrition is the preferred feeding route, and easy-to-absorb (hydrolyzed) formulas may offer some advantages over standard formulas or table foods.[16] Hydrolyzed formulas may be unpalatable to some people, however, and if the formula cannot be taken orally, it may be given by tube. In some cases, feeding tubes can be placed so as to bypass fistulas or partial obstructions, allowing feeding by tube without adding to the risk of complications. Feedings by vein are used to deliver needed nutrients when oral or tube feedings significantly aggravate pain and diarrhea; when the bowel is obstructed or the client is at risk for obstruction; when complete bowel rest might help a fistula to close; or when oral or tube feedings cannot meet nutrient requirements.

Oral Diets As the acute stage of Crohn's disease resolves, the person gradually progresses, as tolerance permits, to an oral diet, often a high-kcalorie, high-protein diet. A fat-restricted diet is necessary for people with fat malabsorption. Low-fiber diets are sometimes recommended for those with partial obstructions of the intestine. Clients may be intolerant to certain foods or food components, including lactose, and these should be identified and eliminated from the diet.

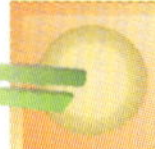

Case Study College Student with Crohn's Disease

Lilinoe, a 19-year-old college student, was first diagnosed with Crohn's disease when she was 18 years old. At that time, she weighed 120 pounds and was 5 feet 7 inches tall. Her normal weight had been 130 pounds until the disease symptoms began to appear. Since then, she has been hospitalized several times for recurrent attacks of Crohn's disease. As anticipated from her weight-loss history, Lilinoe's nutrition assessment shows that she is suffering from severe PEM. In talking with Lilinoe, you discover that she is very particular about the foods she eats and often simply does not eat. Her physician has ordered an easy-to-absorb formula diet to be fed to Lilinoe by tube.

Review Lilinoe's weight history. What is her desirable body weight? What measures could have been taken to avoid weight loss?

What possible benefits might an easy-to-absorb formula offer Lilinoe? Why might the physician prefer a tube feeding rather than oral feedings?

Consider Lilinoe's long-term dietary management. What type of diet should she eventually follow? What goals should be set for weight gain? Why is it important to reassess her nutrition status regularly?

Given Lilinoe's age and stage of development, what emotional concerns might she be experiencing? What interventions might be planned to enhance her sense of hope, self-esteem, and well-being?

Supplemental vitamin-mineral preparations are frequently prescribed. Encourage clients to eat a nutrient-rich, well-balanced diet, and reassess nutrition status frequently to ensure that nutrient needs are being met. Later sections of this chapter describe additional nutrition concerns for clients who have undergone ileostomies, colostomies, or intestinal resections. A case study describing a person with Crohn's disease is presented in the accompanying box.

MALABSORPTION CAUSED BY BACTERIAL OVERGROWTH

Although the colon normally houses a bacterial population, the small intestine is protected from bacterial overgrowth by gastric acid, which kills bacteria, and peristalsis, which flushes microorganisms through the small intestine before they can flourish. Sometimes, however, these protective mechanisms fail, allowing bacteria to thrive in the small intestine. Gastric surgeries, for instance, can interfere with gastric acid secretions and alter peristalsis. In some types of gastric surgery, a portion of the small intestine is bypassed, causing stasis in the intestine and allowing bacteria to flourish. The bypassed portion is called a blind loop, and the symptoms associated with bacterial overgrowth are called the blind loop syndrome. Figure 22–3 on p. 739 shows blind loops created by gastric surgeries.

Bacterial overgrowth can also occur for other reasons besides gastric surgery. Chronic gastritis (see p. 704), drug therapy (antiulcer agents), and HIV infections, for instance, can significantly reduce gastric acid secretions and lead to bacterial overgrowth in the stomach and upper small intestine. Small bowel obstructions and nerve dysfunction associated with diabetes can also lead to bacterial overgrowth by altering peristalsis.

Consequences of Bacterial Overgrowth Bacteria in the small intestine partly dismantle the bile salts, which are essential for fat digestion and absorp-

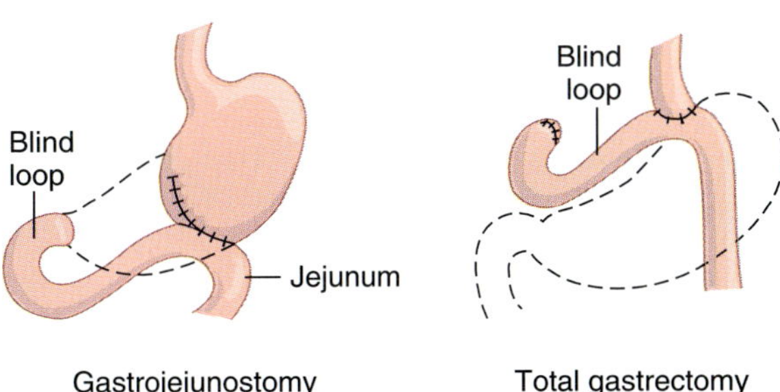

Figure 22–3

Blind Loops Created by Gastric Surgery

In some gastric resections or bypass surgeries, a portion of the intestine is bypassed (the blind loop), peristalsis through the segment is disrupted, and bacteria flourish.

tion. Fat malabsorption and its related consequences occur as a result. Figure 22–4 repeats the figure from Chapter 5 (p. 156) that shows how bile prepares fat for digestion, this time illustrating how bacteria interfere with that process. The bacteria also compete with the body for vitamin B_{12} and folate, limiting the available supply and leading to deficiencies.

Treatment of Bacterial Overgrowth To control bacterial overgrowth, physicians prescribe antibiotics. Along with drug therapy, clients receive fat-restricted diets, parenterally administered vitamin B_{12}, and oral folate supplements. If medical treatment fails, people with surgically created blind loops may need additional surgery to remove the blind loop.

short-bowel or **short-gut syndrome:** severe malabsorption that may occur when the absorptive surface of the small bowel is reduced, resulting in diarrhea, weight loss, bone disease, hypocalcemia, hypomagnesemia, and anemia.

SHORT-BOWEL SYNDROME

Short-bowel, or short-gut, syndrome is characterized by diarrhea, weight loss, muscle wasting, bone disease, protein and fat malabsorption, hypocalcemia,

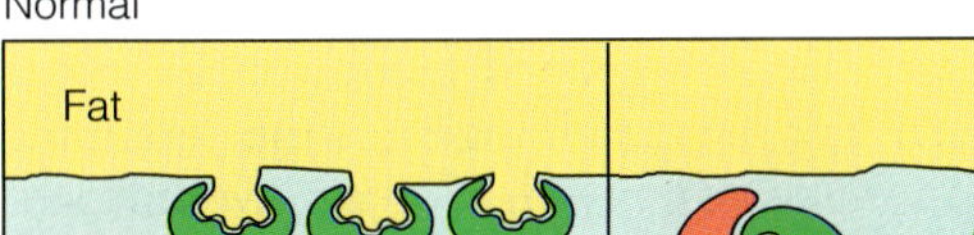

When fat enters the small intestine, bile arrives. Bile has an affinity for both fat and water, so it can bring the fat into solution in the water.

After emulsification, the fat is mixed in the water solution, so the enzymes have access to it.

In blind loop syndrome, bacteria damage the bile, so that it is ineffective in fat digestion and absorption. The result is fat malabsorption and steatorrhea.

Figure 22–4

Bacterial Overgrowth and Steatorrhea

Figure 22–5

Nutrient Absorption and Consequences of Intestinal Surgeries

About 90 to 95 percent of nutrient absorption takes place in the first half of the small intestine. After a resection, nutrient absorption is reduced.

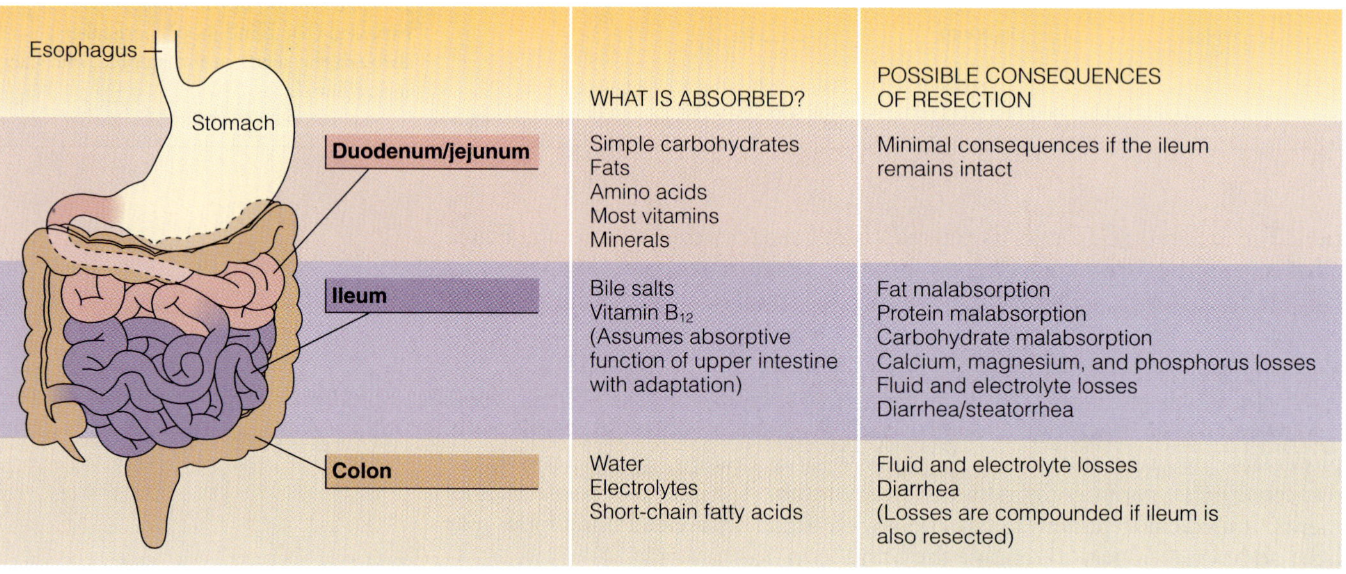

	WHAT IS ABSORBED?	POSSIBLE CONSEQUENCES OF RESECTION
Duodenum/jejunum	Simple carbohydrates Fats Amino acids Most vitamins Minerals	Minimal consequences if the ileum remains intact
Ileum	Bile salts Vitamin B_{12} (Assumes absorptive function of upper intestine with adaptation)	Fat malabsorption Protein malabsorption Carbohydrate malabsorption Calcium, magnesium, and phosphorus losses Fluid and electrolyte losses Diarrhea/steatorrhea
Colon	Water Electrolytes Short-chain fatty acids	Fluid and electrolyte losses Diarrhea (Losses are compounded if ileum is also resected)

hypomagnesemia, and anemia. It can occur whenever the absorptive surface of the small intestine is significantly reduced. Short-bowel syndrome frequently results from surgery to remove a significant portion of the small intestine, which may be necessary for people with inflammatory bowel diseases, cancer of the intestine, obstructions, fistulas, diverticulitis, or impaired blood supply to the intestine. The length, location, and health of the remaining intestine determine the degree to which nutrient absorption is affected. Figure 22–5 reviews nutrient absorption in the GI tract and describes how absorption is affected by different surgical resections.

Extent and Location of the Resection Generally, up to 50 percent of the intestine can be resected without serious nutrition consequences. Remarkably, even resections of up to 80 percent may be well tolerated, provided that the terminal ileum, the ileocecal valve, and the colon remain intact.[17] When the ileum has been resected, however, the absorption of fat, protein, carbohydrate, fat-soluble vitamins, vitamin B_{12}, calcium, and magnesium can be impaired. The ileum is also where bile salts are normally reabsorbed. Without bile salt reabsorption, the body's pool of bile salts diminishes, and fat malabsorption worsens.

The Ileocecal Valve The ileocecal valve controls the rate at which the intestinal contents move from the small to the large bowel. Without the valve, transit time through the small intestine is rapid, and the time available for nutrient absorption is limited. Consequently, the colon receives large volumes of unabsorbed nutrients, fluids, electrolytes, and bile salts. Nutrient absorption is impaired and diarrhea results. If the colon is resected as well, severe fluid and electrolyte imbalances threaten health.

The Colon Recent studies suggest that an intact colon plays a significant role in reducing carbohydrate and, to a lesser extent, protein malabsorption following intestinal resections.[18] Bacteria in the colon salvage energy from some of the unabsorbed carbohydrate by metabolizing it to short-chain fatty acids, which can then be absorbed and utilized for energy. This salvage function appears to be enhanced in people with intestinal resections—a form of adaptation.

Adaptation After an intestinal resection, a remarkable adaptive response occurs in the portion of the intestine that remains: it gets longer, thicker, and wider, and it either absorbs nutrients more efficiently or begins to absorb nutrients it did not absorb before. Maximum bowel adaptation may take as long as one to two years following a resection.[19] The presence of nutrients in the remaining gut appears to stimulate this adaptation—a good reason to begin enteral nutrition as early as possible. Specific dietary constituents, such as the amino acid glutamine, short-chain fatty acids, and fiber, and growth hormone may also aid in this adaptation (see Highlight 22). With an extensive bowel resection, however, even adaptation will fail to compensate for the reduced surface area.

Nutrition Support following Small Bowel Resections Immediately after surgery, the primary nutrition concern is to maintain fluid and electrolyte balance. For resections of less than 50 percent of the intestine, oral nutrition begins a few days after surgery. A moderate fat-restricted diet with supplemental vitamin B_{12} is recommended.[20] For more extensive resections, parenteral nutrition is often provided initially to ensure that nutrient needs are met until adaptation has occurred. Enteral nutrition (usually by tube feeding) is initiated as early as possible to stimulate adaptation. Drugs are also used to treat the disorder.

Once oral intake begins, people whose colons remain intact following surgery benefit from diets that are high in complex carbohydrates (60 percent of kcalories), restricted in fat (20 percent of kcalories), and low in oxalate.[21] With time, fat intake can be liberalized if additional energy is needed and if the fat does not precipitate steatorrhea or diarrhea. People with short-bowel syndrome who do not have intact colons have greater difficulty absorbing energy from either fat or carbohydrates than those with intact colons. These people are more likely to need parenteral nutrition to supply part or all of their nutrient needs.

Rx PRESCRIPTION PAD

Drugs used in the treatment of short-bowel syndrome may include:

- Antidiarrheals
- Calcium carbonate antacids (to bind oxalate)
- H2-blockers

See Appendix E for timing with meals and nutrition-related side effects.

CELIAC DISEASE

Celiac disease provides an example of how food sensitivities can cause malabsorption. Celiac disease is a hereditary disorder with an incidence of about 1 in every 2000 to 3000 births. It alters the intestinal mucosal cells, so that they become sensitive to gliadin, a fraction of the protein gluten, which is found in wheat, oats, rye, and barley. Gliadin acts as a toxic substance, causing the

celiac (SEE-lee-ack) **disease:** a sensitivity to gliadin that causes flattening of the intestinal villi and generalized malabsorption; also called **gluten-sensitive enteropathy** (EN-ter-OP-ah-thee) or **celiac sprue**.

gliadin (GLIGH-ah-din): a fraction of the gluten protein.

gluten (GLUE-ten): a protein found in wheat, oats, rye, and barley. (Remember the acronym "WORB" to recall these grains.)

intestinal villi to atrophy and seriously reducing the absorptive surface of the intestinal tract. The disaccharidases (including lactase) and the carrier molecules normally found on the villi disappear. The result is malabsorption of many nutrients, including fat, protein, carbohydrate, fat-soluble vitamins, iron, calcium, magnesium, zinc, and some water-soluble vitamins.

Nutrition Status The person with celiac disease often experiences steatorrhea, diarrhea, weight loss, and malnutrition. Anemia may occur as a result of iron, folate, or vitamin B_{12} deficiency. Because protein is malabsorbed, serum protein levels can fall dramatically, inducing edema. A vitamin K deficiency may precipitate clotting abnormalities, and the person may bleed easily. Furthermore, calcium deficiency can cause tetany and bone pain.

Treatment of Celiac Disease Unlike most malabsorption syndromes, which often benefit from fat-restricted diets, the malabsorption caused by celiac disease responds to gluten restriction. Once gluten is removed from the diet, the intestinal changes reverse almost completely. Generally, improvement occurs within a few weeks of strict adherence to the diet. Lactase deficiency and lactose intolerance may be permanent. If the person fails to follow the gluten-restricted diet, the symptoms will return.

Gluten-Restricted Diets The treatment of celiac disease sounds deceptively simple: eliminate gluten. Such a diet is easier to prescribe than follow, however, for wheat, oats, rye, and barley are common in many foods, as Table 22–5 shows. In particular, processed foods such as ice cream, salad dressings, and canned foods often use wheat flour as an extender. People with celiac disease and their caregivers need help understanding what foods they can eat and what foods they must avoid. Be sure they understand how to read food labels.

Suggestions Dietitians often suggest the use of corn, potato, rice, and soybean flours as substitutes for wheat flour in recipes. A low-gluten wheat starch flour is also available. People who are lactose intolerant will also need to exclude milk and milk products as discussed on pp. 115–116. A family with a member who has celiac disease needs a lot of support from the health care team. Dietitians can offer tips about support groups, books, recipes, and special food products that can help clients manage their diet restrictions.

Disorders of the Large Intestine

Diverticular disease, ulcerative colitis, and resections of the large intestine are conditions that affect the colon and have nutrition implications. In diverticular disease, described next, diet plays a role in both prevention and treatment.

DIVERTICULAR DISEASE OF THE COLON

Reminder: The outpocketings of the intestinal wall that balloon through the weakened muscles of the intestine are known as *diverticula* (the singular is *diverticulum*).

Sometimes pouches of the intestinal wall (called diverticula) bulge out through the muscles surrounding the large intestine, often at points where blood vessels enter the muscles (see Figure 4–14 on p. 128). Evidence suggests that the pouches result from high pressure in the intestinal lumen combined with weak-

Table 22–5

Gluten-Restricted Diet

Meat and Meat Alternates
Any allowed except those that are breaded, prepared with bread crumbs, or creamed.
Milk and Milk Products
Any allowed if client is not intolerant to lactose except milk mixed with Ovaltine, commercial chocolate milk with a cereal additive, pudding thickened with wheat flour, or ice cream or sherbet containing gluten stabilizers.
Fruits and Vegetables
Any allowed except those that are breaded, prepared with bread crumbs, or creamed.
Starches and Grains
Allowed: Bread, cereal, or dessert products made from cornmeal, soybean flour, rice flour, potato flour, and gluten-free starch; gluten-free macaroni and porridge; tapioca; cornmeal, cornflakes, popcorn, and hominy; rice, cream of rice, puffed rice, and rice flakes; potato chips. *Not allowed:* Bread, cereal, or dessert products made from wheat, rye, oats, or barley; commercially prepared mixes for biscuits, cornbread, muffins, pancakes, buckwheat pancakes, cakes, cookies, or waffles; bran; pasta, macaroni, and noodles; malt; pretzels; wheat germ; doughnuts; ice cream cones; matzo.
Other
Not allowed: Beer; ale; certain whiskeys (Canadian rye); cereal beverages (Postum); root beer; commercial salad dressings that contain gluten stabilizers; soups containing any ingredients not allowed (such as barley or noodles).

ness of the supporting muscles in the intestinal wall. Strong intestinal contractions pinch off segments of the intestine; pressure then builds in these segments and forces parts of the intestinal membrane to balloon outward through the muscle layer. Aging and low-fiber diets (see p. 127) may increase the risk of diverticular disease.

Diverticulosis and Diverticulitis People with diverticulosis are frequently symptom-free and unaware of the disorder. In some people, however, fecal material and bacteria get trapped in the diverticula. A localized area of inflammation and infection develops, a condition called diverticulitis. People with diverticulitis may suffer from abdominal pain, alternating periods of diarrhea and constipation, dyspepsia, flatus, abdominal distention, and fever. Occasionally, a diverticulum ruptures, causing localized or sometimes life-threatening infection (peritonitis). If the diverticula become inflamed repeatedly, the intestinal wall can thicken (fibrosis), narrowing the intestinal lumen and creating an obstruction. An inflamed bowel segment can also stick to other pelvic organs, forming a fistula.

Reminder: The term *diverticulosis* describes the condition of having diverticula. The term *diverticulitis* describes the condition when the diverticula become inflamed.

Nutrition Support Both drugs and diet play a role in the treatment of diverticular disease. For many years, health care professionals advised low-fiber diets

PRESCRIPTION PAD

Drugs used in the treatment of diverticular disease may include:

- Analgesics
- Antibiotics
- Laxatives (bulk-forming agents)

See Appendix E for timing with meals and nutrition-related side effects.

for people with diverticulosis in the belief that fiber tended to become trapped in the diverticula and cause irritation. This advice has changed dramatically. Now, health care professionals believe a high-fiber diet may actually reduce the incidence of diverticulosis by stimulating normal GI action and maintenance. Many people with established diverticular disease have been observed to remain symptom-free while following a high-fiber diet. They may need to avoid foods with seeds such as okra and strawberries, however; the seeds may get trapped in the diverticula and cause irritation.

A high-fiber diet includes generous servings of plant foods: grains, fruits, and vegetables, especially legumes (see Table 4–4 on p. 129). Tips for adapting to a high-fiber diet are provided on p. 128, and a sample high-fiber diet menu is shown below. The accompanying case study presents an example of diverticular disease.

People with diverticular disease benefit from high-fiber diets to help them maintain GI tract function. Although diverticular diseases do not affect the intestine's absorptive functions, ulcerative colitis and intestinal resections can have a serious impact on these functions.

ULCERATIVE COLITIS

ulcerative colitis (ko-LYE-tis): inflammation and ulceration of the colon. See also *Crohn's disease* on p. 736.

Ulcerative colitis is an inflammatory bowel disease that develops in the large intestine. It causes severe diarrhea, rectal bleeding, cramping, abdominal pain, anorexia, and weight loss. Diarrhea can be almost continuous, resulting in malabsorption and major losses of fluids and electrolytes. Anemia may develop due to bleeding and nutrient losses. For people with active ulcerative colitis who fail to respond to medical therapy, surgery to remove the colon and rectum

Sample High-Fiber Diet Menu

Menu

Breakfast	Lunch	Supper
1 c multigrain cereal	1 c black bean soup	3 oz baked fish
½ banana	3 oz broiled chicken	1 baked potato with skin
1 c nonfat milk	½ c steamed broccoli	½ c peas
½ grapefruit	½ c baked sweet potatoes	1 whole-wheat dinner roll
2 slices whole-wheat toast	1 fresh pear	2 tsp margarine
2 tbs peanut butter	1 whole-wheat dinner roll	1 piece carrot cake
1 c coffee	1 tsp margarine	1 c nonfat milk
	Iced tea	
		Snack
		3 c popcorn
		1 c tomato juice

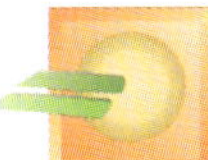

Case Study Retired Schoolteacher with Diverticular Disease

Mr. Stavros is a 69-year-old retired school teacher. He recently told his doctor that he had been experiencing abdominal pain and fever. He also described a change in bowel function: he is frequently constipated, although he occasionally experiences diarrhea. He further complained of indigestion and a bloated feeling. Mr. Stavros was admitted to the hospital. After an examination that included X rays of the intestine, the physician made a diagnosis of diverticulitis, for which Mr. Stavros was treated. No food or drink was allowed by mouth, and a tube was inserted to suction gastric contents. An intravenous (IV) solution of fluid and electrolytes was started to prevent dehydration and maintain electrolyte balance. Antibiotics were given to treat the infection, and analgesics were given for pain and to lower Mr. Stavros's fever. After several days, suction was discontinued, and oral intake was initiated. Once Mr. Stavros was tolerating adequate liquids orally, the IV was discontinued. He is now symptom-free and ready for discharge from the hospital.

Describe diverticular disease to Mr. Stavros. Be sure to distinguish between diverticulosis and diverticulitis. How do diverticula form, and what consequences may follow?

Are Mr. Stavros's symptoms typical of people with diverticulitis? Do all people with diverticular disease have such symptoms?

What diet would you recommend for Mr. Stavros to treat the diverticular disease? What advice can you give him about adjusting to such a diet?

(described in the next section) is often recommended. Unlike intestinal surgery for Crohn's disease, which fails to cure the disorder, removal of the colon and rectum does cure ulcerative colitis.

Nutrition Support For people with active ulcerative colitis, no dietary interventions seem to lessen disease activity. People with severe abdominal pain and diarrhea need complete bowel rest with no enteral stimulation. Parenteral nutrition can help maintain nutrition status, especially when surgery is anticipated.[22] Meanwhile, medications can help to control disease symptoms.

Oral Diets Many of the dietary principles outlined for Crohn's disease apply to ulcerative colitis. A primary concern is to ensure adequate intakes of fluids and electrolytes. The diet often emphasizes high-kcalorie, high-protein foods and restricts fat if the client has symptoms of fat malabsorption. Individual tolerances determine if other foods should be restricted. A low-residue or low-fiber diet is necessary for some clients: others may tolerate a regular diet. Milk and milk products may need to be eliminated if lactose intolerance is present. Supplemental vitamins and minerals may be necessary.

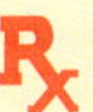

PRESCRIPTION PAD

Drugs used in the treatment of ulcerative colitis may include:

- Analgesics
- Antidiarrheals
- Anti-Infective agents
- Anti-Inflammatory agents

See Appendix E for timing with meals and nutrition-related side effects.

RESECTIONS OF THE LARGE INTESTINE

People with ulcerative colitis or cancer of the colon sometimes need surgery to remove the affected portion of the colon. Resections of the large intestine are less likely to create nutrient deficiencies than resections of the small intestine, because most nutrients are absorbed before the intestinal contents reach the colon. Fluids and electrolytes are normally reabsorbed in the colon, however, so their losses can be a problem.

stoma (STOH-ma): a surgically formed opening. After an ileostomy or colostomy, a stoma is formed from the cutoff end of the intestine and brought out through the abdominal wall, rerouting the excretion of wastes.
stoma = window

In a colostomy, a segment of the colon, rectum, or both is removed. The remaining portion is then brought out through the abdominal wall via a stoma to allow for defecation (see Figure 22–6). In an ileostomy, both the entire colon and the rectum are removed, and the ileum becomes the terminal GI segment. In an alternative to an ileostomy, called the ileal pouch/anal anastomosis, the surgeon removes the diseased colon and rectal tissue and connects the ileum to the anus. Thus defecation can occur through the anus, rather than through a stoma, and a more normal bowel movement results. A temporary ileostomy is made at the time of surgery to give the intestine time to heal. After about two to three months, the ileostomy is closed.

The consistency of the stools following colostomies and ileostomies varies depending on both the length and the portion of the resected bowel. In general, ileostomies result in watery stools and colostomies in more formed stools.

Nutrition Support following Ostomies Once oral intake is permitted following surgery, people who have undergone colostomies or ileostomies often receive low-fiber, bland diets to prevent obstructions, help promote healing of

Figure 22–6

Colostomy and Ileostomy

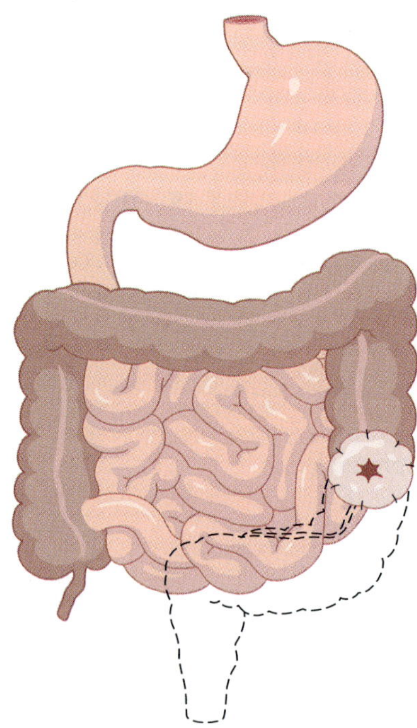

In a colostomy, the rectum and anus are removed, and the stoma is formed from the remaining colon.

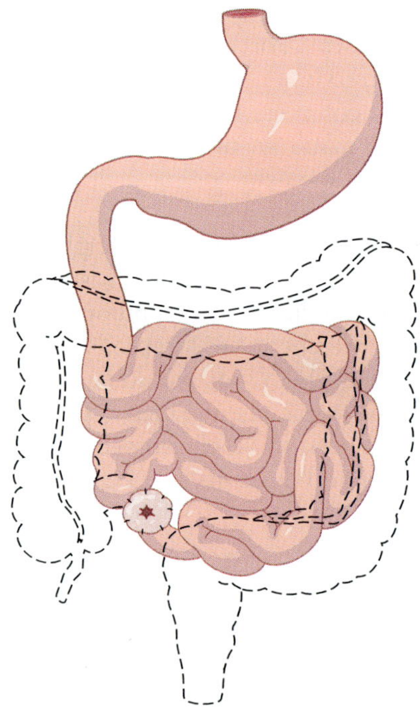

In an ileostomy, the entire colon, rectum, and anus are removed, and the stoma is formed from the ileum.

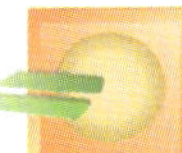

Case Study Accountant with an Ileostomy

Tim is a 24-year-old accountant who recently developed a severe small bowel obstruction secondary to recurrent bouts of Crohn's disease. Medical and dietary management failed, and Tim underwent an ileostomy in which the ileocecal valve remained intact. Tim was malnourished on admission, and he began receiving parenteral nutrition in the immediate postoperative period. After several days, he was placed on an oral diet.

Describe the nutrients most likely to be affected by Tim's surgery.

Tim will be coping with many fears and concerns associated with his ileostomy. How can you help him make the necessary adjustments? Remember that diet is only a small part of that adjustment.

What diet will be appropriate for Tim once he has advanced to a solid diet? What advice can you give him for trying new foods, preventing obstructions, getting enough fluids, controlling diarrhea, and reducing gas and odors? How can he keep track of foods that give him problems?

the stoma, and prevent GI upsets. Encourage people to try other foods as soon as possible, however. They should add foods one at a time and in small amounts so that their effects can be assessed. If a new food presents problems, the person can try it again in a few weeks or months.

Preventing Obstructions Some foods are more likely than others to be incompletely digested and cause obstructions for ostomates. These include stringy foods such as celery, spinach, and bean sprouts; foods with tough skins such as dried fruits, raw apples, and corn; foods with seeds; mushrooms; and nuts. Practitioners report that some of these foods can be used if the client cuts the food into small pieces and chews them thoroughly. An undigested mushroom, for example, may act as a plug and obstruct an ostomy, but it will not be a problem if it arrives in the intestine in very small pieces.

ostomate (OSS-toe-mate): a person who has a surgically formed opening from the bowel to the outside of the body, bypassing the anus. An ileostomate (ILL-ee-OSS-toe-mate) has an ileostomy; a colostomate (ko-LOSS-toe-mate) has a colostomy.

Encouraging Fluids Ostomates need extra fluids because they are absorbing less fluid from the large intestine. They may tend to restrict their fluid intakes, however, for fear of aggravating diarrhea. Explain to ostomates that drinking fluids helps prevent constipation and dehydration, and reassure them that excess fluid taken above and beyond the amount lost through the ostomy will be absorbed by the kidneys and excreted in the urine; it will not aggravate diarrhea.

Controlling Diarrhea Ostomates may benefit from foods that thicken the stool and help control diarrhea. These foods include applesauce, bananas, cheese, creamy peanut butter, and starchy foods such as breads, rice, and potatoes. Foods that may aggravate diarrhea include apple, grape, and prune juices; highly seasoned foods; and caffeine. The foods mentioned here are suggestions only; what works for the individual is determined by trial and error.

Reducing Gas and Odors Ostomates are often concerned about gas and odors associated with eating certain foods. Table 22–1 provides a general list of gas-forming foods, and some ostomates identify the following as particularly bothersome: asparagus, beans, beer, broccoli, brussels sprouts, cabbage, carbon-

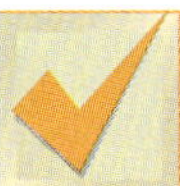

Nutrition Assessment Checklist

For People with Disorders of the Lower GI Tract

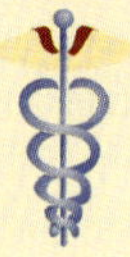

Medical Review the client's medical record daily for test results that pinpoint the cause of diarrhea or malabsorption, improvements in the medical condition, or the development of complications (such as obstructions or fistulas) that might call for dietary adjustments. Review Table 22–4 and make note of any conditions that might affect nutrition status.

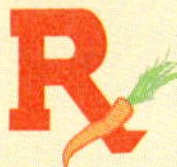

Drug Review the client's drug therapy for possible drug-nutrient interactions. Many anti-infective agents have potential interactions. Anti-inflammatory agents may cause nausea, esophagitis, abdominal pain, fluid retention (may mask weight loss), and glucose intolerance. Laxatives may cause nausea and interfere with the absorption of fat-soluble vitamins. People taking mucolytics need adequate fluids to help liquefy thick mucous secretions.

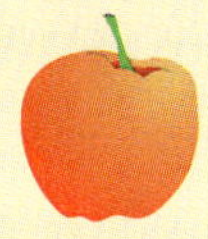

Food Intake Determine if energy and protein intake is adequate to support a desirable weight and maintain protein status. Assess food intake to determine individual tolerances for people with diarrhea, irritable bowel syndrome, Crohn's disease, or ulcerative colitis and for people who have undergone intestinal resections. For people with steatorrhea, fat-restricted diets aim to reduce the frequency and volume of steatorrhea. Individual nutrient deficiencies accompany many of the lower GI tract disorders—assess diet and supplement intake to be sure that these needs are met.

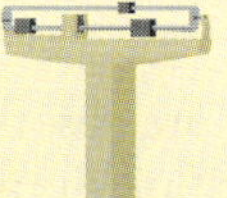

Anthropometric Adjust diet to support growth in children and desirable weight in adults.

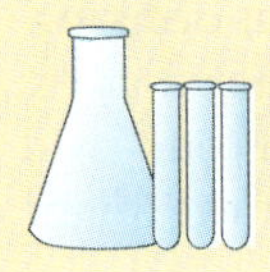

Laboratory Monitor lab values for signs of protein malnutrition (serum albumin), dehydration (electrolytes, blood urea nitrogen, hemoglobin, and hematocrit), anemia (hemoglobin and hematocrit), and serum nutrient levels (as appropriate to the disorder). Table 22–6 shows the laboratory tests useful in detecting fat malabsorption and its severity.

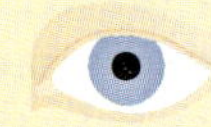

Physical Check for physical signs of nutrient deficiencies, dehydration, and anemia; assess the client's energy level and emotional state.

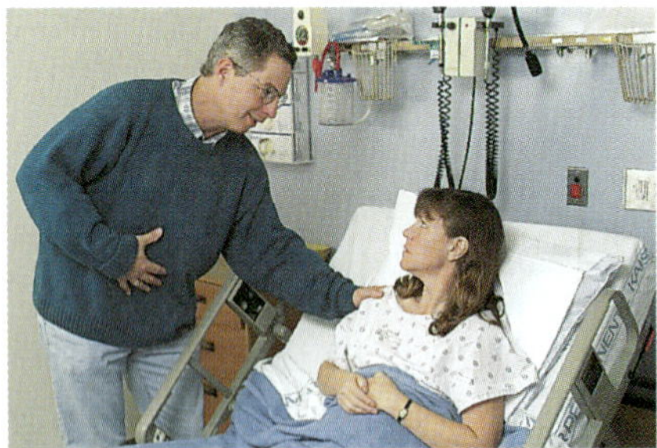

A person who has adjusted to an ostomy can greatly encourage a new ostomy client.

ated beverages, cauliflower, eggs, fish, garlic, and onions. Foods thought to reduce odors include buttermilk, cranberry juice, parsley, and yogurt.

Providing Emotional Support Ostomates will have many adjustments to make after surgery, so emotional support is best begun before surgery occurs. Often ostomates feel they have lost control over a basic and private function.

Table 22–6

Laboratory Tests Useful in Assessing Malabsorption Syndromes

- Direct stool examinations: Stool checked for weight (greater than normal weight suggests malabsorption) and oily materials (excess fat in stool suggests steatorrhea).
- Chemical analysis of fecal fat: Fecal fat of greater than 7 g/day when the diet includes 100 g of fat/day indicates fat malabsorption.
- Serum carotene: Low serum levels accompany steatorrhea.
- Serum calcium: Low levels seen in calcium or vitamin D malabsorption. (Recall that steatorrhea can lead to calcium and vitamin D malabsorption.)
- D-xylose test: Test of carbohydrate absorption.
- Chemical analysis of fecal nitrogen: Normal fecal nitrogen is less than 2 g/day.
- Schilling test: Identifies vitamin B_{12} malabsorption.

The training required to care for the ostomy and maintain bowel function may be difficult. Ostomates may also worry that loved ones, particularly spouses, will find them unattractive. The health care team must work closely with each person and the family to help everyone make the necessary adjustments and resume normal activities.

An **enterostomal** (en-ter-oh-STOME-al) **therapist (ET)** is a health care professional specially educated to assist ostomates in learning the proper methods of caring for ostomy sites and adjusting to the ostomy.

This chapter has shown how diseases of the intestine and their treatments can seriously impair nutrition status. The nutrition assessment checklist provides guidelines for the nutrition care of people with lower GI tract disorders. Careful attention to diet and medical intervention can help people maintain their quality of life and, in some cases, recover from their diseases.

Study Questions

1. Describe the dietary treatment of diarrhea. When is diarrhea a cause for alarm?
2. What is irritable bowel syndrome, and how is diet used to control its symptoms?
3. Discuss various conditions that can lead to malabsorption. Why does fat most frequently cause problems for people with malabsorption? What roles do fat-restricted diets, low-oxalate diets, enzyme replacements, and water-miscible fat-soluble vitamins play in the treatment of fat malabsorption?
4. Recommend ways to improve acceptance of a fat-restricted diet. How should MCT be introduced into the diet?
5. How can pancreatitis lead to the malabsorption of nutrients? Contrast the dietary treatment of the person with acute pancreatitis with the dietary treatment of a person with chronic pancreatitis.
6. What are the nutrition needs of people with cystic fibrosis? How can an infant with cystic fibrosis be fed? What is the optimal diet for a child or adult with cystic fibrosis? How and why are enzyme replacements used in the treatment of cystic fibrosis?
7. What is Crohn's disease? Describe the diet therapy for a person with Crohn's disease. What special concerns arise in children with the disorder?
8. How can bacteria in the stomach or upper intestine lead to fat malabsorption? What are the other nutrition consequences of bacterial overgrowth?
9. Describe short-bowel syndrome and its effect on nutrition status. What factors affect absorption after small bowel surgery?
10. Describe the adaptive process that occurs in the remaining intestine after a portion of the intestine

is resected. What diet is most useful following intestinal resections?

11. What dietary protein and protein fraction are of particular concern in the person with celiac disease? What diet is useful in treatment? Discuss the difficulties involved in following the diet.
12. What theory explains the development of diverticula in the intestine? What dangers are associated with diverticular disease? What diet is useful for treating diverticular disease?
13. What is the recommended diet for a person with ulcerative colitis? What is the primary nutrition concern in this disorder?
14. What is an ileostomy? What is a colostomy? What diet, if any, can benefit the person who has undergone one of these procedures?

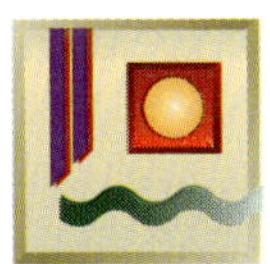

Clinical Applications

1. Using Table 22–3 as a guide, plan a day's menu for a diet containing 35 grams of fat. Take care to make the menu both palatable and nutritious. How can this menu be improved using the suggestions on p. 168?
2. Treatments for a disease often aim to alleviate disease symptoms rather than the disease itself. With this in mind, describe the similarities in the treatments of chronic pancreatitis and cystic fibrosis. In what ways do the treatments differ and why?
3. As stated in this chapter, treatment of celiac disease is deceptively simple—eliminate gluten. Take a trip to the grocery store and randomly select 20 to 25 of your favorite snack and convenience foods. Check the labels of these products and see if they are allowed on gluten-restricted diets. Find acceptable substitutes for the products that are not allowed. No doubt, this will be a tough assignment.

Notes

1. J. Hurst and A. L. Gallagher, Pathophysiology and nutrition management in acute pancreatitis, *Support Line*, December 1994, pp. 6–11.
2. S. Marulendra and D. F. Kirby, Nutrition support in pancreatitis, *Nutrition in Clinical Practice* 10 (1995): 45–53.
3. A.S.P.E.N. Board of Directors, Practice guidelines: Pancreatitis, *Journal of Parenteral and Enteral Nutrition* (supplement) 17 (1993): 16.
4. S. A. McClave and coauthors, Comparison of the safety of early enteral *vs* parenteral nutrition in mild acute pancreatitis, *Journal of the American Society for Parenteral and Enteral Nutrition* 21 (1997): 14–20.
5. M. R. Dambro, *Griffith's 5 Minute Clinical Consult* (Baltimore: Williams & Wilkins, 1995), pp. 278–279.
6. J. Dowsett, Nutrition in the management of cystic fibrosis, *Nutrition Reviews* 54 (1996): 31–33.
7. B. W. Ramsey and coauthors, Nutritional assessment and management in cystic fibrosis: A consensus report, *American Journal of Clinical Nutrition* 55 (1992): 108–116.
8. Ramsey and coauthors, 1992.
9. M. D. Murphy and coauthors, Resting energy expenditures measured by indirect calorimetry are higher in preadolescent children with cystic fibrosis than expenditures calculated from prediction equations, *Journal of the American Dietetic Association* 95 (1995): 30–33.
10. A. L. Rettammel and coauthors, Oral supplementation with a high-fat, high-energy product improves nutritional status and alters serum lipids in patients with cystic fibrosis, *Journal of the American Dietetic Association* 95 (1995): 454–459.
11. Ramsey and coauthors, 1992.
12. A.S.P.E.N. Board of Directors, Practice guidelines: Cystic fibrosis—pediatric, *Journal of Parenteral and Enteral Nutrition* (supplement) 17 (1993): 44.
13. Y. Kim, Can fish oil maintain Crohn's disease in remission? *Nutrition Reviews* 54 (1996): 248–257.
14. M. D. Sitrin, Nutrition support in inflammatory bowel disease, *Nutrition in Clinical Practice* 7 (1992): 53–60.
15. A.S.P.E.N. Board of Directors, Practice guidelines: Inflammatory bowel disease, *Journal of Parenteral and Enteral Nutrition* (supplement) 17 (1993): 18–19.

16. M. H. Giaffer, G. North, and C. D. Holdsworth, Controlled trial of polymeric versus elemental diet in treatment of active Crohn's disease, *Lancet* 335 (1990): 816–819; S. Klein, Elemental versus polymeric feeding in patients with Crohn's disease—Is there really a winner? *Gastroenterology* 99 (1990): 893–894; A.S.P.E.N. Board of Directors, Inflammatory bowel disease, 1993, pp. 18–19.
17. Presented by W. D. Heizer, Short bowel syndrome: Treatment strategies, *Fourth Annual Advances and Controversies in Clinical Nutrition*, sponsored by the Mayo Clinic, Jacksonville, Fla., April 18, 1994.
18. I. Nordgaard, B. S. Hansen, and P. B. Mortensen, Importance of colonic support for energy absorption as small-bowel failure proceeds, *American Journal of Clinical Nutrition* 64 (1996): 222–231.
19. T. A. Byrne and coauthors, A new treatment option for patients with short bowel syndrome: Bowel rehabilitation with growth hormone, glutamine, and a modified diet, *Support Line*, February 1996, pp. 1–7.
20. J. P. Grant, G. Chapman, and M. K. Russell, Malabsorption associated with surgical procedures and its treatment, *Nutrition in Clinical Practice* 11 (1996): 43–52.
21. Byrne and coauthors, 1996.
22. A.S.P.E.N. Board of Directors, Inflammatory bowel disease, 1993, pp. 18–19.

Promoting Intestinal Adaptation

The ability to survive a massive intestinal resection is a relatively recent medical advance spurred largely by the development of techniques for providing all needed nutrients by vein (total parenteral nutrition or TPN) and the adaptation of these techniques for use at home. Early studies report that prior to the availability of TPN, only 20 percent of people who survived the surgery itself lived for more than one year.[1] Currently, estimates suggest that most people who survive the surgery are still living after a year.[2] Without TPN, the medical team could only provide simple intravenous solutions of fluids, electrolytes, and minimal energy and hope that the person would be able to eat before malnutrition was irreversible.

As experience with TPN grew, clinicians began to recognize that although long-term TPN was a lifesaving strategy, it was accompanied by serious complications and extremely high costs. (Chapter 24 discusses these issues in more detail.) While recognizing the limitations to adaptation imposed by the extent and location of the resection, the person's age, and the health of the remaining intestine, clinicians sought ways to foster adaptation to the fullest extent possible.[3] What strategies might improve the likelihood of maintaining nutrition status with an oral diet or minimal TPN? This highlight focuses on research aimed at promoting optimal adaptation in the remaining small bowel, or bowel rehabilitation. Controversies remain, of course, partly because much of the research has been conducted on animals and partly because studies in human beings require further elucidation and confirmation.

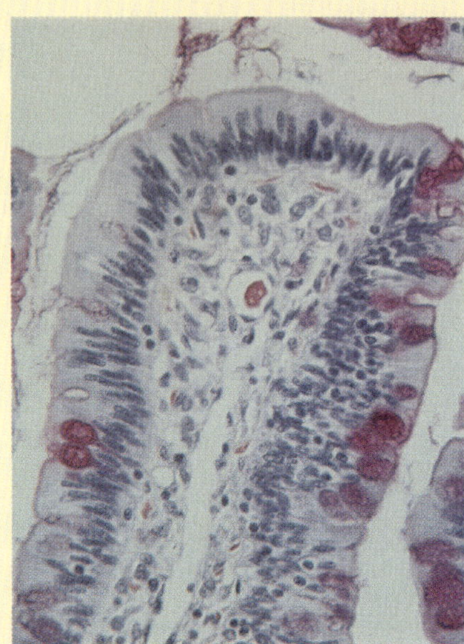

The need for intravenous feedings after extensive intestinal resections may be eliminated or reduced by taking full advantage of the remaining intestinal cells' ability to adapt.

DIETARY FACTORS AND ADAPTATION

For some time, clinicians have accepted that intestinal adaptation can occur only when the GI tract is stimulated by enteral nutrients.[4] Animal studies further suggest that providing enteral nutrients as early as possible after an intestinal resection improves the chances that the person will be able to tolerate enteral nutrition and not be dependent on TPN.[5] Spurred by such findings, researchers and clinicians have begun to identify specific factors, including dietary components, that might optimally stimulate adaptation.

Glutamine

The amino acid glutamine is common in food and is the most abundant amino acid in the blood. Glutamine provides fuel for rapidly dividing cells and is the major fuel for the intestinal cells. After the intestinal cells have metabolized glutamine, the liver uses the end products, alanine and ammonia, to make glucose and urea, respectively. Glutamine is also important for the replication of all body cells, which use it to synthesize purines, pyrimidines, and nucleotides, as well as other amino acids.

In healthy individuals, glutamine is a nonessential amino acid. If food sources fail to meet the body's needs, the body can synthesize more glutamine from the branched-chain amino acids of skeletal muscle. Following an intestinal resection, however, the body may need more glutamine than it receives from typical nutrient sources or than it can synthesize. Under such conditions, glutamine becomes a conditionally essential amino acid.

Various animal studies show that adding glutamine to intravenous feeding solutions helps to promote adaptation following intestinal resections.[6] Animal studies further suggest that enteral, but not parenteral, glutamine facilitates glucose absorption.[7] Human studies suggest that oral glutamine raises growth hormone levels, which may further promote adaptation, as described in a later section.

Short-Chain Fatty Acids

As Chapter 22 noted, bacteria in the colon degrade dietary fibers to short-chain fatty acids. Short-chain fatty acids possess two characteristics that enhance their importance following intestinal resections. First, they stimulate intestinal cell growth, enhance intestinal blood flow, bolster secretion of pancreatic enzymes, and promote sodium and water absorption in the colon.[8] Animal studies show that short-chain fatty acids stimulate intestinal cell growth following resections, even when they are provided intravenously.[9]

Second, short-chain fatty acids provide the body with usable energy. The remarkable capacity of colonic bacteria to salvage energy following extensive small bowel resections has only recently been realized.[10]

In healthy people with full-length intestinal tracts, short-chain fatty acids normally provide about 5 to 10 percent of the total daily energy needs (about 100 to 200 kcalories per day). Following extensive small bowel resections in which the colon remains intact, however, adaptation occurs in the colon so that it assumes a greater role in providing energy. When the bacteria in the colon are confronted with more substrates in the form of dietary fiber, unabsorbed carbohydrate, and, to a lesser extent, unabsorbed protein, they step up production of short-chain fatty acids and can provide about 1000 kcalories per day of usable energy.[11] This contribution represents a substantial source of energy sorely needed by people with malabsorption.

Thus, for people whose colons remain intact following intestinal resections, providing a diet high in complex carbohydrates supports adaptation and improves energy conservation. Because the colonic bacteria cannot convert fat to short-chain fatty acids, unabsorbed fat reaching the colon provides no additional energy and can contribute further to malabsorption as described in Chapter 22.

Researchers have also found that factors unrelated to diet can foster adaptation. Growth hormone and insulin-like growth factor-1 (IGF-1), described next, are two such factors.

HORMONES AND ADAPTATION

Research suggests that both growth hormone and IGF-1 play significant roles in promoting intestinal adaptation.[12] As its name implies, growth hormone stimulates the growth of tissues. It mediates its effects on intestinal cells through the regulation of IGF-1, which appears to directly stimulate intestinal cell growth.[13] Some studies show that IGF-1 stimulates the growth of intestinal cells to a greater degree than diet alone.[14] (Recall that oral glutamine may mediate some of its positive effects on intestinal adaptation by raising growth hormone levels.)

PRACTICAL APPLICATIONS

Following extensive small bowel resections, clinicians strive to promote maximum absorptive capacity in the remaining bowel. The most desirable outcome is for the person to be able to meet all nutrient needs orally. When that is not possible, the goal is to minimize the need for TPN, thus reducing the complications and costs associated with it.

Very impressive results have been obtained from clinical studies designed to assess the effectiveness of a combination therapy in promoting bowel rehabilitation.[15] The therapy consisted of growth hormone administration, glutamine supplementation, and a diet high in complex carbohydrates, low in fat, and supplemented with fiber. Eight clients with severe short-bowel syndrome comprised the first study group; all were believed to be dependent on TPN for life and past the period of intestinal adaptation. They were able to consume oral foods as tolerated but were unable to maintain nutrition status or adequate fluid balance without parenteral nutrition. After only three weeks of treatment, clients showed significant improvements in their energy intake and abilities to absorb protein, carbohydrates, water, and sodium.

The positive study results prompted a subsequent study of 47 clients to determine if the combination therapy could eliminate or reduce TPN requirements.[16] Again, all clients were considered to be dependent on TPN for life and past the period of intestinal adaptation. All clients received the combination therapy for a minimum of 26 days, after which time growth hormone was discontinued. Clients were discharged from the research facility and instructed to continue oral glutamine supplements and the modified diet. After about a year, 40 percent of the clients were able to maintain nutrition status with an oral diet, and another 40 percent were able to reduce their TPN requirements.

The promising results of these studies offer hope of improved treatments and outcomes for people with severe short-bowel syndrome. They also raise questions requiring further research. Would even better results occur if combination therapy was provided soon after surgery, before adaptation has occurred? Might an individual component of the combination therapy prove just as effective as all three in minimizing or reducing the need for TPN?

Medical research is a continuously evolving quest to lengthen life and improve its quality. Often research in one area overlaps with research in another. For example, severe stresses cause atrophy of the intestinal cells and significantly reduce their absorptive capacity. Factors that stimulate intestinal cell growth and adaptation for short-bowel syndrome might also help correct the intestinal atrophy that accompanies stress. Indeed, current research is examining how glutamine and growth hormone might benefit people suffering from severe stresses (Chapter 25).

NOTES

1. H. E. Haymond, Massive resection of the small intestine, *Surgery, Gynecology, and Obstetrics*, 61 (1935): 693–705.
2. G. J. Blatchford, J. S. Thompson, and L. F. Rikkers, Intestinal resection in adults: Causes and consequences, *Digestive Surgery* 6 (1989): 57–61.
3. F. Carbonnel and coauthors, The role of anatomic factors in nutritional autonomy after extensive small bowel resection, *Journal of Parenteral and Enteral Nutrition* 20 (1996): 275–280.
4. T. A. Byrne and coauthors, A new treatment option for patients with short bowel syndrome: Bowel rehabilitation with growth hormone, glutamine, and a modified diet, *Support Line*, February 1996, pp. 1–7.
5. W. D. A. Ford and coauthors, Total parenteral nutrition inhibits intestinal adaptation in young rats: Reversal by feeding, *Surgery* 96 (1983): 527–534.
6. M. C. Gouttebel and coauthors, Influence of N-acetylglutamine or glutamine infusion on plasma amino acid concentrations during the early phase of small-bowel adaptation in the dog, *Journal of Parenteral and Enteral Nutrition* 16 (1992): 117–121; H. Tamada and coauthors, Alanyl glutamine-enriched total parenteral nutrition restores intestinal adaptation after either proximal or distal massive resection in rats, *Journal of Parenteral and Enteral Nutrition* 17 (1993): 236–242.
7. A. Gardemann and coauthors, Increases in intestinal glucose absorption and hepatic glucose uptake elicited by luminal but not vascular glutamine in the jointly perfused small intestine and liver of the rat, *Biochemistry Journal* 283 (1992): 759–765.
8. M. M. Gottschlich, Selection of optimal lipid sources in enteral and parenteral nutrition, *Nutrition in Clinical Practice* 7 (1992): 152–165.
9. S. A. Kripke and coauthors, Stimulation of intestinal mucosal cell growth with intra colonic infusion of short-chain fatty acids, *Journal of Parenteral and Enteral Nutrition* 13 (1989): 109–116; M. J. Koruda and coauthors, Effect of parenteral nutrition supplemented with short-chain fatty acids on adaptation to massive small bowel resection, *Gastroenterology* 95 (1988): 715–720.
10. I. Kelberman and coauthors, Effect of fiber and its fermentation on colonic adaptation after cecal resection in the rat, *Journal of Parenteral and Enteral Nutrition* 19 (1995): 100–106; I. Nordgaard, B. S. Hansen, and P. B. Mortensen, Importance of colonic support for energy absorption as small-bowel failure proceeds, *American Journal of Clinical Nutrition* 64 (1996): 222–231.
11. Nordgaard, Hansen, and Mortensen, 1996.
12. J. A. Vanderhoof, Results of IGF-1 studies show promise in the treatment of intestinal disorders, *Journal of Parenteral and Enteral Nutrition* 20 (1996): 315–316; D. I. Shulman and coauthors, Effects of short-term growth hormone therapy in rats undergoing 75% small intestinal resection, *Journal of Pediatric Gastroenterology and Nutrition* 14 (1992): 3–11; A. B. Lemmey, IGF-1 and the truncated analogue des-(1-3) IGF-1 enhance growth in rats after gut resection, *American Journal of Physiology* 260 (1991): E213–E219.
13. T. Inaba and coauthors, Effects of growth hormone and insulin-like growth factor 1(IGF-1) treatments on nitrogen metabolism and hepatic IGF-1 messenger RNA expression in postoperative parenterally fed rats, *Journal of Parenteral and Enteral Nutrition* 20 (1996): 325–331; K. Chen and coauthors, Insulin-like growth factor-1 prevents gut atrophy and maintains intestinal integrity in septic rats, *Journal of Parenteral and Enteral Nutrition* 19 (1995): 119–124.
14. J. A. Vanderhoof and coauthors, Truncated and native insulin-like growth factors (IGF-1) treatments on the nitrogen metabolism and hepatic IGF-1–messenger RNA expression in postoperative parenterally-fed rats, *Gastroenterology* 102 (1992): 1949–1956.
15. T. A. Byrne and coauthors, Growth hormone, glutamine, and a modified diet enhance nutrient absorption in patients with short bowel syndrome, *Journal of Parenteral and Enteral Nutrition* 19 (1995): 296–302.
16. T. A. Byrne and coauthors, A new treatment for patients with short bowel syndrome: Growth hormone, glutamine and a modified diet, *Annals of Surgery* 222 (1995): 243–255.

Chapter 23

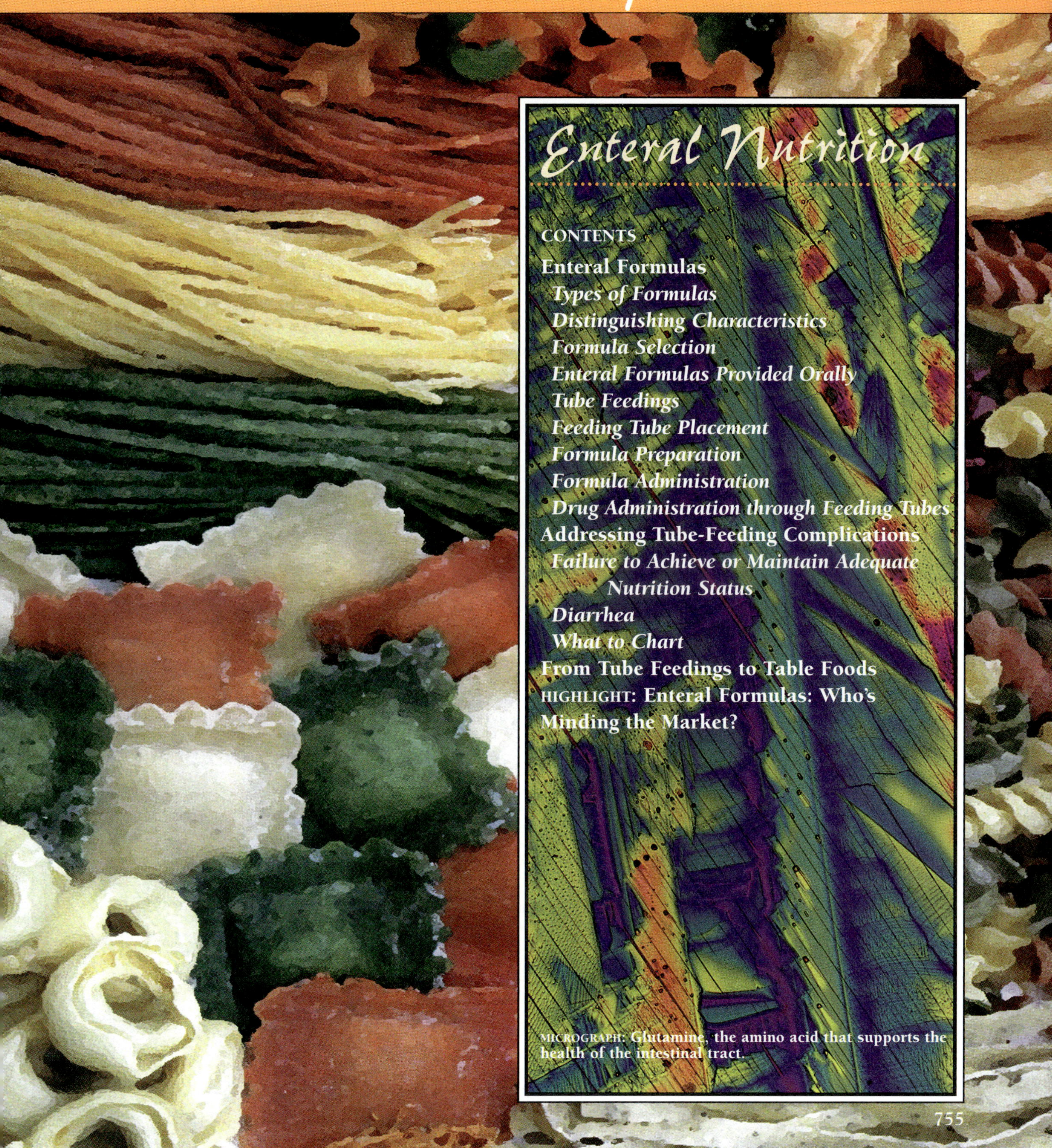

Enteral Nutrition

CONTENTS

MICROGRAPH: Glutamine, the amino acid that supports the health of the intestinal tract.

To meet nutrient needs, a person must be able to eat, digest, and absorb nutrients in the amounts necessary to satisfy metabolic demands. Most people, whether healthy or ill, can meet these needs with conventional foods. Some illnesses, however, interfere with eating, digestion, and absorption, as Chapters 21 and 22 described. Other illnesses raise the metabolic rate to such a degree that conventional foods fail to deliver necessary nutrients. If poor appetite is the primary nutrition problem, health care professionals diligently encourage clients to eat. The accompanying box provides suggestions for helping clients to eat enough foods to meet their needs. Alternatively, liquid formulas, given orally in sufficient amounts, may help meet nutrient needs.

For clients who cannot eat or drink, it may be necessary to deliver nutrients by tube or by vein. Feedings provided either orally or by tube are *enteral* feedings, the subject of this chapter. Enteral feedings can be used whenever a client can digest and absorb nutrients via the GI tract. Otherwise, feedings are given by vein as *parenteral* feedings, the subject of the next chapter. Figure 23–1 summarizes some of the factors involved in deciding the most appropriate way to feed a client.

Enteral Formulas

enteral formulas: liquid diets intended for oral use or for tube feedings.
enteron = intestine

The number of enteral formulas on the market is staggering (several are listed in Appendix K). Most formulas are available in ready-to-use or powered form. They are designed to meet a variety of medical and nutrition needs and can be used

Figure 23–1

Selecting a Feeding Method

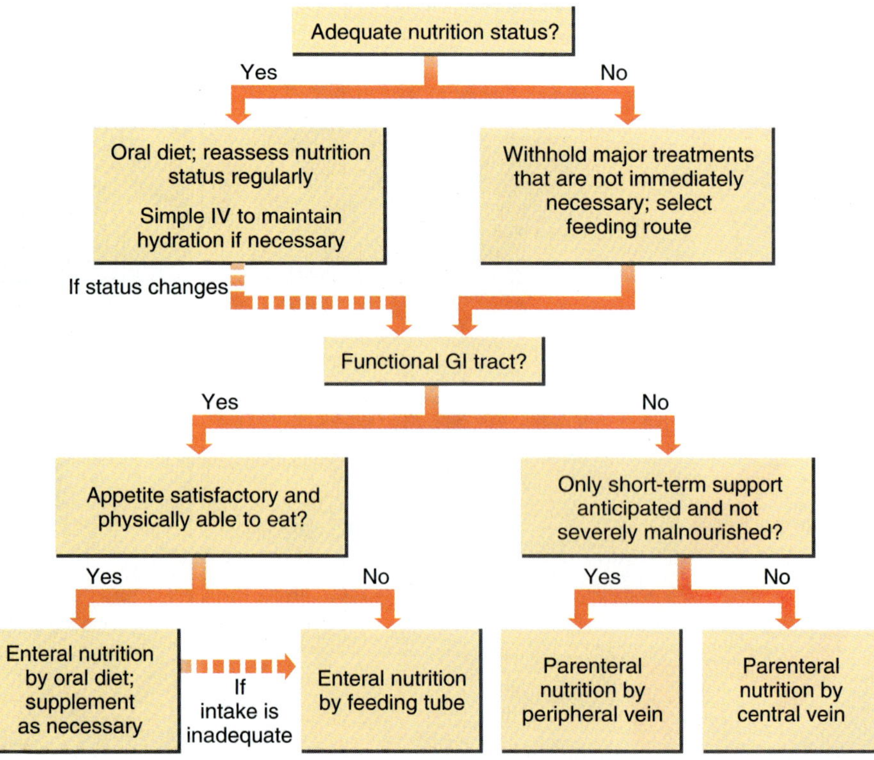

How to Help Clients Meet Nutrient Needs with Ordinary Foods

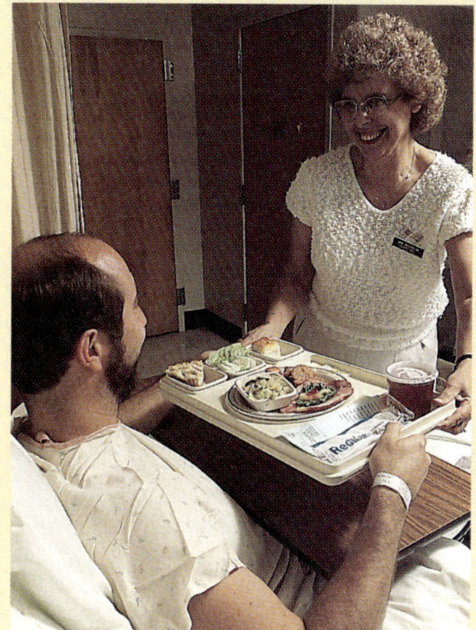
People enjoy eating when they feel comfortable and cared for.

1. Empathize. If the person is frightened, angry, or confused, show that you care and are there to help. Imagine feeling too sick to move or too tired to sit up. Show that you understand how difficult it is to eat.
2. Motivate. Be sure the client understands how important nutrition is to recovery.
3. Help clients select foods they like and mark menus appropriately. Call the dietitian, if the client needs extra help. When appropriate and permissible, let a friend or family member bring in favorite foods from outside the hospital. This may be especially helpful for clients with strong ethnic, religious, or personal food preferences.
4. Solve eating problems. Encourage clients who feel full after a short time to eat the most nutritious foods first and save liquids until after meals. For clients who are weak or tired, suggest foods that require little effort to eat. Eating a roast beef sandwich, for example, requires less effort than cutting and eating a steak; drinking soup is easier than eating it with a spoon. For clients who either fill up quickly when eating or are weak or tired, smaller meals combined with snacks, such as a sandwich at bedtime and milk shakes or instant breakfast drinks between meals, can improve intake considerably.
5. Suggest that clients add extra energy to the foods they eat by using extra sugar or fats. Dry milk powder added to milk-based drinks, soups, and casseroles boosts nutrient intake.
6. Help clients prepare for meals. Encourage clients to wash their hands and faces and to brush their teeth or rinse their mouths before eating. Help them get comfortable, either in bed or in a chair. Adjust the extension table to a comfortable distance and height, and make sure it is clean. A clean, odor-free room also helps. Take these steps before the tray arrives, so the meal can be served promptly and at the right temperature.
7. Check for accuracy and appearance. When the food cart arrives, check the client's tray. Confirm that the client is receiving the right diet, that the foods on the tray are the ones the client marked on the menu, and that the foods look appealing. Order a new tray if foods are not appropriate.
8. Help with eating. Help clients who need assistance in opening containers or cutting meats and those who are unable to feed themselves.
9. Take a positive attitude toward the hospital's food. Never say something like "I couldn't eat this stuff either." Instead, say, "The dietary department really tries to make foods appetizing. Let me call the dietitian. I'm sure we can find a solution."

either alone or given along with foods. The client's specific nutrition needs, identified through a careful medical and nutrition assessment, guides selection of the most appropriate formula. Highlight 23 describes some of the concerns regarding appropriate marketing and use of formulas.

Whenever formula is the primary source of nutrients, complete formulas are necessary. Such is the case when a client is on a tube-feeding or an oral liquid diet for more than a few days. Complete formulas, when provided in appropriate amounts, supply all the nutrients a client needs. Complete formulas can also be (and often are) used in smaller quantities to supplement regular diets.

complete formulas: enteral formulas designed to supply all needed nutrients when given in sufficient volume.

TYPES OF FORMULAS

Formulas are classified in many ways, but for purposes of this book, it is reasonable to think of two major kinds categorized by the type of protein they supply. Standard, or intact, formulas contain complete proteins, whereas hydrolyzed formulas contain small fragments of protein, which may include free amino acids, dipeptides, and tripeptides.

standard formula: a liquid diet that contains complete molecules of proteins; also called **intact** or **polymeric formulas**.

protein isolate: a protein that has been separated from a food. Examples include casein from milk and albumin from egg.

Standard, or Intact, Formulas Standard, or intact, formulas are appropriate for people who are able to digest and absorb nutrients without difficulty; they come as either protein isolate formulas or blenderized formulas. A protein isolate formula contains a purified protein. Blenderized formulas may contain pureed meat, vegetables, fruits, milk, and starches with vitamins and minerals added as necessary; they can be made in a blender or purchased commercially.

hydrolyzed formula: a liquid diet that contains broken-down molecules of protein, such as amino acids and short peptide chains; also called a **monomeric formula**.

Hydrolyzed Formulas To simplify the body's work, a complete protein can be hydrolyzed—that is, partially broken down to yield small peptides. Alternatively, a formula can be made from free amino acids. In this text we call both types *hydrolyzed* for simplicity. Hydrolyzed formulas are often also low in fat because fat is difficult to digest and absorb. People who cannot digest or adequately absorb standard formulas may benefit from hydrolyzed formulas.

modules: formulas or foods that provide a single nutrient and are designed to be added to other formulas or foods to alter nutrient composition; they can also be combined together to create a highly individualized formula.

CAUTION: Although formulas designed to be delivered intravenously can also be delivered enterally, the reverse is not true. Enteral formulas cannot be delivered by vein without serious consequences.

Modular Formulas Unlike complete formulas, a few formulas, called modules, provide essentially a single nutrient (protein, carbohydrate, or fat). In addition to commercial modular formulas, intravenous nutrients can serve as modules; enteral or intravenous modules can be added to enteral formula to alter its nutrient composition (for example, to add kcalories or protein). Modules can also be combined with other modules to construct individualized formulas for clients with unique nutrient needs. Designing, preparing, and delivering such a formula is a challenge that requires an in-depth knowledge of enteral nutrition and the skills of a committed nutrition support team.[1]

DISTINGUISHING CHARACTERISTICS

Formulas vary not only in the form of protein they contain but in other characteristics as well. The physician or dietitian considers these characteristics when selecting a formula for an individual client.

Nutrient Composition The formulas available offer a wide variety of nutrient compositions. These variations allow clinicians to select formulas with particular types or proportions of nutrients to meet the needs of clients with a variety of medical conditions.

For practical purposes, 1 ml (milliliter) is equivalent to 1 cc (cubic centimeter).

Standard formulas provide about 1 kcalorie per milliliter. Formulas containing 1.5 to 2.0 kcalories per milliliter meet energy and nutrient needs in a smaller volume. One formula may provide a higher percentage of energy from fat, another from carbohydrate, and still another from protein. A person with fat malabsorption may need a formula low in fat; a person with constipation may benefit from a formula with part of the carbohydrate derived from fiber. Percentage of vitamins with minerals also vary from one formula to the next.

Formulas also derive their nutrients from different sources. One formula may derive its protein from beef. another from milk, and still another from free amino acids. Some formulas provide all of their fat from long-chain triglycerides (LCT); others provide varying amounts of medium-chain triglycerides (MCT) in addition to LCT. Sources of carbohydrate also vary; one client may benefit from a formula containing fiber, another may prefer the taste of a formula sweetened with simple sugars.[2]

Although formulas differ, many fit into general categories, and some can be used interchangeably. For example, several intact formulas provide similar amounts of kcalories, protein, carbohydrate, fat, and other nutrients. They may derive their protein from different sources, but both sources are high-quality proteins. One may provide more vitamins in a smaller volume, but that may be of little consequence to the person who is receiving a large volume of formula. In some cases, however, such differences can be significant. One client may be allergic to milk protein, for example, and another might be on a fluid-restricted diet and benefit from a formula with a high nutrient density.

Residue and Fiber Residue and fiber contribute to fecal bulk. Low-residue formulas are well tolerated and are useful in the treatment of some GI tract disorders, following surgeries of the GI tract, and as early feedings after GI tract disuse. Since hydrolyzed formulas are almost completely absorbed, they leave little residue in the gut. Most standard formulas have a low-to-moderate residue content.

Adding fiber to a formula adds residue because dietary fibers cannot be digested by enzymes in the human digestive tract. Blenderized formulas contain fiber; other formulas may have fiber added. High-fiber formulas can cause gas and GI upsets in some clients, but help to maintain GI tract integrity in those who can tolerate them. Because formula diets are usually used for relatively short periods, determining which people might benefit from them is difficult.[3] Research suggests that fiber might most benefit people with diarrhea or constipation and those who must have tube feedings for long periods.[4] Fiber is also beneficial when it is degraded to short-chain fatty acids by bacteria in the colon (see Highlight 22). These fatty acids provide fuel to support the growth, maintenance, and repair of the intestinal lining, enabling it to adapt more readily after large portions of the small bowel have been resected.

residue: the total amount of material in the colon; it includes dietary fiber and also undigested food, intestinal secretions, bacterial cell bodies, and cells shed from the intestinal mucosa.

fiber: see pp. 108–111; the portion of the intestinal contents that remains in the colon because people don't have the enzymes to digest it—mostly plant fibers such as cellulose, lignin, and pectin.

Osmolality Osmolality is a measure of the concentration of molecular and ionic particles in a solution. A formula that approximates the osmolality of blood serum (about 300 milliosmoles per kilogram) is referred to as an isotonic formula. A hypertonic formula has a higher osmolality than serum.

Most formulas are isotonic or only moderately hypertonic and are well tolerated by most people. When delivered directly into the intestine, however, hypertonic formulas are initially provided at a slow, even rate to improve tolerance.[5]

Cost Costs of individual products vary greatly in different parts of the country and for different hospitals. As a general rule, however, hydrolyzed formulas and products formulated for specific disorders (renal or respiratory failure, for example) are more expensive than standard formulas.

osmolality: (OZ-mow-LAL-eh-tee): the concentration of particles in a solution, expressed as the number of milliosmoles (mOsm) per kilogram.

isotonic formula: a formula with an osmolality similar to that of blood serum (300 mOsm/kg).

iso = the same
ton = tension

hypertonic formula: a formula with an osmolality higher than that of blood serum.

hyper = greater, more

FORMULA SELECTION

Choosing a formula can be a complicated process. Dietitians and physicians can use a logical approach to simplify the process (see Figure 23–2). In a nutshell, the formula that meets the client's medical and nutrient needs with the lowest risk of complications and at the lowest cost is the best choice. If no formula can be found that meets all of the client's nutrient needs, then modules can be used to construct an appropriate formula.

Digestive and Absorptive Function Most people on tube feedings tolerate standard formulas. Hydrolyzed formulas should be reserved for people with minimal digestive and absorptive capacity. A person whose GI tract is not functioning is not a candidate for an enteral formula.

Nutrient Requirements Nutrient requirements are estimated based on careful nutrition assessment. The client's age, medical condition, nutrition status, and metabolic rate are all important considerations in estimating nutrient requirements. If a nutrient must be restricted, a formula must be selected that delivers no more than the prescribed amount of that nutrient per day. The choice of formulas is narrowed when a person needs a low-residue or high-fiber diet.

Individual Tolerances Food allergies or intolerances sometimes limit formula selection. Lactose-free formulas are frequently selected because temporary and permanent lactose intolerances are common problems following surgery, stress, or long periods of GI tract disuse.

For more information about lactose intolerance, see Chapter 4.

Figure 23–2

Selecting a Formula

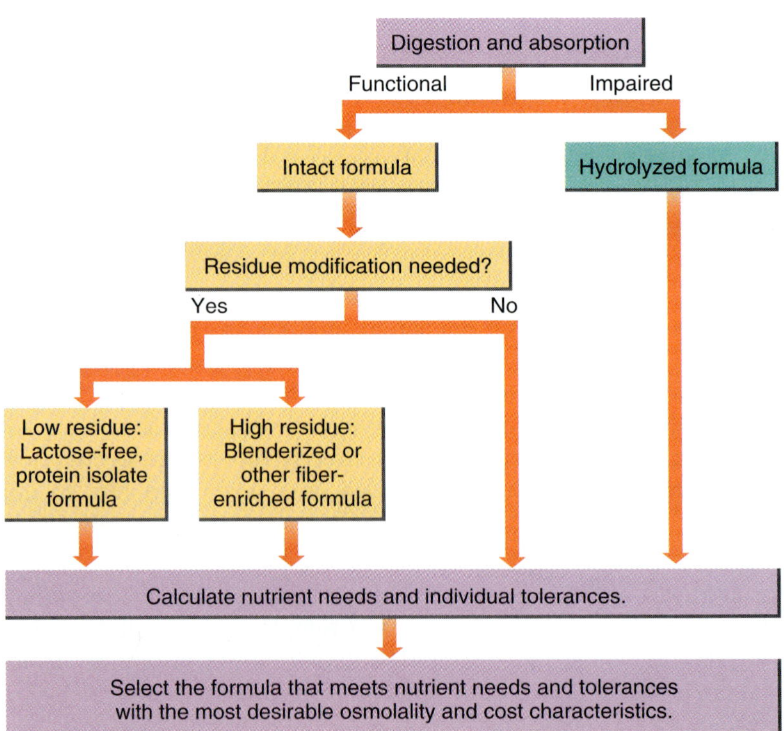

Availability A health care facility cannot stock all of the vast number of formulas available. Instead, the nutrition support team or other qualified professionals review their client's needs and evaluate products to find the most appropriate choices. Then those formulas are kept on hand.

In the final analysis, health care professionals can only make an educated guess about the best formula for an individual. They monitor each person's nutrition status and tolerance to the formula and are prepared to make or recommend changes to help ensure that individual needs are being met.

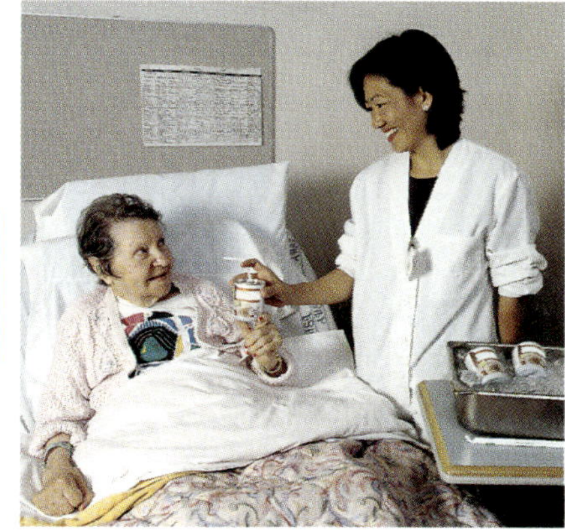

With help from caring professionals, a client can meet nutrient needs with enteral formula supplements.

ENTERAL FORMULAS PROVIDED ORALLY

Sometimes a formula meets nutrient needs in ways foods cannot. For people who can tolerate only liquids for long periods and for those who need hydrolyzed formulas, formulas are the major source of nutrients. If people can drink the formula, and drink enough of it, they can avoid being fed by tube.

More often, formulas are used orally to supplement a conventional diet. Some people can eat table foods, but not in sufficient quantities to meet their nutrient needs. Enteral formulas provide a reliable source of nutrients and work particularly well for adding energy and protein to the diet. Psychologically, liquids seem less filling than foods, and they are easier for debilitated, weak, or tired people to handle.

When used as an oral diet, the formula's taste must be acceptable to the individual. As a general guide, the more hydrolyzed the formula and the lower its fat content, the less tasty it will be. Remember, however, that people's likes and dislikes vary greatly, and what is unpalatable to one person might be acceptable to another. Limited evidence suggests that hydrolyzed formulas may become more acceptable over time.[6] Allowing clients to sample different flavors of formula and select the ones they like best is helpful in promoting acceptance. The box on p. 762 offers suggestions for helping clients accept oral formulas.

TUBE FEEDINGS

Tube feedings are simply complete formulas delivered by tube into the stomach or intestine. A thorough nutrition assessment provides the data needed to plan a successful tube feeding. Based on the assessment, the health care team can evaluate the client's need for a tube feeding, select the formula that will best meet the client's nutrient needs, and choose the tube and method that will deliver nutrients most effectively.

Candidates for Tube Feedings An individual who has a functioning GI tract but is unable to ingest enough nutrients (or the appropriate type of nutrients) by mouth is a candidate for a tube feeding. Such a person may have physical problems that make chewing and swallowing difficult; have no appetite for an extended period of time; have an obstruction, fistula, or altered motility in the upper GI tract; be in a coma; have very high nutrient requirements; or be unable to ingest a hydrolyzed formula orally. Table 23–1 on p. 762 lists indications and contraindications for feeding people by tube.

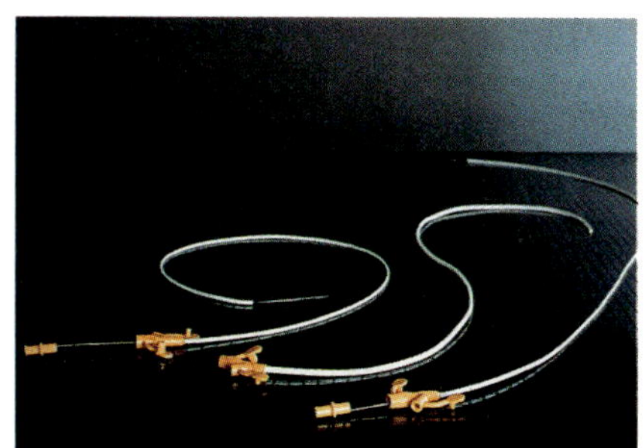

Feeding tubes provide access to the stomach and intestine for clients who cannot eat oral diets.

Advantages of Tube Feedings Tube feedings are always preferred to parenteral nutrition because enteral nutrition helps maintain normal gut function, causes fewer complications, and costs less than feeding by vein (see Highlight

How to Help Clients Accept Oral Formulas

People on enteral formulas are often quite ill and frequently have poor appetites. Even when a person enjoys a formula, palatability can become a problem after a while. Hydrolyzed formulas are often less palatable than standard formulas, and clients may find them difficult to accept. Caring professionals can help by using these suggestions:

- Ask the dietitian to let the client try both different flavors and different formulas appropriate for the client's needs; use those the client likes best.
- Serve formulas attractively and remind clients to drink them. Formulas offered in a glass are more appealing than those served from a can with an unfamiliar name. Some people find the smell of formulas unappealing. Covering the top of the glass with plastic wrap or a lid, leaving just enough room for a straw, can help.
- Provide easy access. Keep the formula close to the client's bed where little effort is required to reach it, and within sight to remind the client to drink it. Clients who are very ill may lack the motivation even to reach for formula, let alone drink it. In such cases, offer the formula ready-to-drink and in small amounts frequently through the day.
- Keep formula in an ice bath, so that it will be cool and refreshing when the client drinks it.
- Ask the dietitian for help if the client stops drinking the formula after a while. The dietitian may be able to recommend different flavors or another formula to help relieve boredom.

30).[7] Enteral feedings can also stimulate intestinal adaptation following intestinal resections or following long periods of GI tract disuse. Evidence also suggests that early enteral feedings during critical illness may speed wound healing, reduce bacterial infections, and reduce the need for intensive care.[8]

FEEDING TUBE PLACEMENT

Feeding tubes are inserted into different locations along the GI tract depending on the client's medical problems and the estimated length of time that the feedings will be required. Figure 23–3 shows various tube feeding placement sites and the glossary describes various feeding tube placement sites (see p. 764).

For infants, feeding tubes are frequently passed from the mouth to the stomach before each feeding and removed after each feeding to allow the infant to breathe easily and reduce the risk of regurgitation.

Insertion Methods When clients are not expected to be on tube feedings for more than about four weeks, feeding tubes are frequently inserted through the nose and passed into the stomach or intestine.[9] The client often remains fully alert during the procedure and helps pass the tube by swallowing. Health care professionals can insert a feeding tube transnasally with minimal discomfort to the client when a tube of the correct size and type is used and the client has been

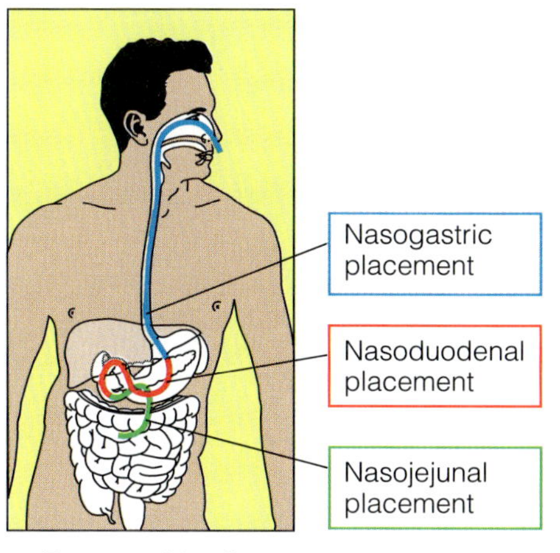

Transnasal feeding tube placements

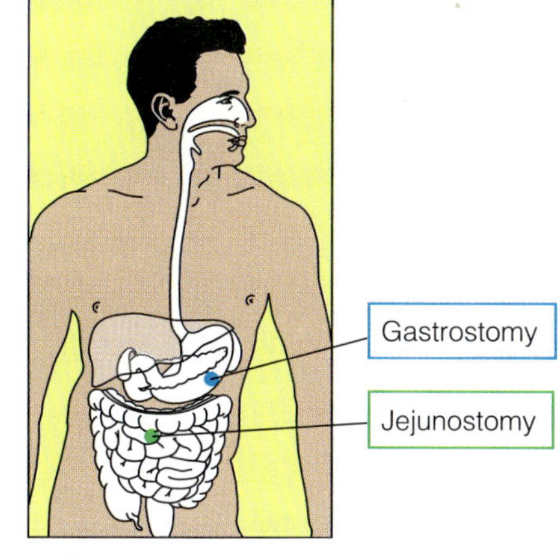

Enterostomies

Figure 23–3

Feeding Tube Placement Sites

Glossary of Feeding Tube Placement Sites

These terms are listed in order from the nose to lower organs of the digestive system.

transnasal: through the nose. A **transnasal feeding tube** is one that is inserted through the nose.

naso = nose

nasogastric (NG): from the nose to the stomach.

nasoenteric: from the nose to the stomach or intestine. *Nasoenteric feedings* include nasogastric, nasoduodenal, and nasojejunal feedings. Most clinicians use *nasoenteric* to refer to nasoduodenal and nasojejunal feedings only.

nasoduodenal (ND): from the nose to the duodenum.

nasojejunal (NJ): from the nose to the jejunum.

orogastric: from the mouth to the stomach. This method is often used to feed infants because they breathe through their noses, and tubes inserted through the nose can hinder the infant's breathing. The tube is inserted before, and removed after, each feeding.

enterostomy (EN-ter-OSS-toe-mee): a gastric or jejunal opening made surgically or under local anesthesia through which a feeding tube can be passed.

gastrostomy (gas-TROSS-toe-mee): an opening in the stomach made surgically or under local anesthesia through which a feeding tube can be passed. The technique for creating a gastrostomy under local anesthesia is called **percutaneous endoscopic gastrostomy**, or **PEG** for short. When the feeding tube is guided from such an opening into the jejunum, the procedure is called **percutaneous. endoscopic jejunostomy (PEJ)**, a misnomer because the enterostomy site is in the stomach.

jejunostomy (JEE-ju-NOSS-toe-mee): an opening in the jejunum made surgically or under local anesthesia through which a feeding tube can be passed. A **duodenostomy** (DEW-odd-eh-NOSS-toe-mee) is not used as a feeding site because the duodenum swings toward the back of the body and is not easily accessible. The technique for creating a jejunostomy under local anesthesia is called a **direct endoscopic jejunostomy (DEJ)**. Note: Some clinicians also refer to this procedure as a PEJ, which is a more accurate use of the term than the more common use described above.

Table 23–1

Indications and Contraindications for the Use of Tube Feedings

Indications
Protein-energy malnutrition with inadequate oral nutrient intake for 5 or more days
Less than 50% of required nutrient intake orally for 7–10 days
Severe dysphasia (difficulty swallowing)
Metabolic stress
Major bowel resections (see Chapter 22) when used along with parenteral nutrition
Low-output fistulas (between the GI tract and the skin)
Contraindications
Intestinal obstruction that prohibits use of the intestine
Paralytic ileus (paralysis of the intestine)
Intractable vomiting
Peritonitis
Severe diarrhea
High-output fistulas between the GI tract and the skin
Severe acute pancreatitis

Note: In all cases, tube feedings are recommended only when the GI tract is functional.

emotionally prepared. Careful procedures must be followed to ensure that the tube is placed in the GI tract rather than in the respiratory tract. A major disadvantage of transnasal tube placement is that a client who is disoriented or uncooperative can easily pull the tube out. Furthermore, if an inappropriate tube is selected, or if feedings continue for long periods, the nasal passages and esophagus can become irritated.

When a client will be on tube feedings for a longer period, or when a feeding tube cannot be passed through the nose, esophagus, or stomach due to an obstruction or for other medical reasons, a feeding tube can be passed through an opening made into the stomach or jejunum. Enterostomies can be made either surgically or nonsurgically using local anesthesia. Surgeons who anticipate the need for a tube feeding during an earlier surgery (intestinal resections, for example) may create a gastrostomy or jejunostomy during the procedure. Gastrostomy and jejunostomy feedings offer advantages for clients receiving long-term tube feedings, because the feeding site is invisible under clothing and feeding tube irritation is eliminated. Friction from the tube and leakage of GI secretions can cause skin irritation, however. Close attention to skin care is usually effective in minimizing skin irritation.

Clinicians may use fluoroscopy, endoscopy, or laparoscopy to guide feeding tubes to their intended location or to make sure tubes have remained in their appropriate location. To help feeding tubes pass into the intestine, some clinicians also use drugs that promote gastrointestinal motility, such as metoclopramide or erythromycin. Table 23–2 on p. 765 compares some of the features of various feeding tube placement sites. The box on p. 766 suggests ways to reduce anxiety for clients beginning a tube feeding.

Table 23–2

Features of Feeding Tube Sites

Site	Insertion	Potential Irritations	Risk of Regurgitation[a]	Long-Term Tolerance	Chance of Removal by Uncooperative Client
Nasogastric	Nonsurgical	Nasal passages, esophagus	High	Fair[b]	Likely
Nasoduodenal	Nonsurgical	Nasal passages, esophagus	Moderate	Fair[b]	Likely
Nasojejunal	Nonsurgical	Nasal passages, esophagus	Low	Fair[b]	Likely
Gastrostomy	Surgery may be required	Skin	Moderate	Good	Unlikely
Jejunostomy	Surgery may be required	Skin	Low	Good	Unlikely

[a]Relative to the other feeding sites. The absolute risk of regurgitation depends on the person's medical condition.
[b]When the appropriate tube and placement site are selected.

Gastric Feedings Using the nasogastric or gastrostomy routes allows the digestive process to begin in the stomach, just as an oral diet does. The stomach empties it contents at a controlled rate and delivers small volumes of nutrients into the intestine. Gastric feedings are not possible for people with gastric obstructions or conditions that significantly interfere with the stomach's ability to empty. A major disadvantage of gastric feedings is that some clients tend to regurgitate them. If regurgitated fluids are inhaled into the lungs, a fatal infection (aspiration pneumonia) may develop. To minimize the risk of aspiration, clinicians may prefer a nasoenteric feeding for clients with a compromised cardiac sphincter or delayed gastric emptying. Alternatively, for clients with a very high risk of aspiration, some clinicians prefer gastrostomies or jejunostomies, which allow the cardiac sphincter to remain tightly closed.

Gastric feedings are contraindicated in clients with gastric outlet obstructions.

aspiration pneumonia: an infection of the lungs caused by inhaling fluids regurgitated from the stomach. Aspiration pneumonia can be a fatal complication of a tube feeding.

Intestinal Feedings Following severe stress (see Chapter 25), GI motility may be temporarily disrupted, but activity resumes more quickly in the small intestine than in the stomach. Thus, after severe stress, the delivery of formulas into the small intestine can be initiated earlier than gastric feedings. Intestinal feedings are also less likely to cause regurgitation of fluids. The fluids are delivered farther down the tract, and both the pyloric and cardiac sphincters are working to keep them there. The major disadvantage of intestinal feedings is loss of the controlled emptying action of the stomach. Assuring passage of the feeding tube into the appropriate location is also more difficult, and placement of the tube must be confirmed before the feeding begins. Formulas must be carefully administered to avoid diarrhea and dehydration.

The final location of the feeding tube determines the type of feeding. If a feeding tube is passed through a gastrostomy into the duodenum or jejunum, the feeding is intestinal rather than gastric.

Transnasal Feeding Tubes Transnasal feeding tubes are soft and flexible and come in a variety of diameters and lengths. Many have characteristics that make them desirable for specific purposes. Some tubes are weighted at one end, for example, to facilitate placement and retention in the intestine, although controversies over the value of such tubes abound.

How to Help Clients Cope with Tube Feedings

The thought of being "force-fed" is frightening to many people. One person may envision a large feeding tube and fear that the procedure will be extremely painful. Another may have heard about tube feedings only from the popular press and associate them with irreversible comas. All clients benefit when they understand the insertion procedure, the expected duration of the tube feeding, and the strategic role that nutrition plays in recovery from disease. These pointers can help health care professionals prepare clients for transnasal tube feedings:

- Allow clients to see and touch the feeding tube. Seeing first hand that the tube is soft and narrow (only about half the diameter of a pencil) often alleviates anxiety. Show clients how the feeding apparatus is attached to the feeding tube and explain how the feeding will work. Use dolls or stuffed toys to demonstrate tube insertion and feeding procedures to a young child.
- Explain that the client remains fully alert during the procedure and helps pass the tube by swallowing. A numbing solution sprayed on the back of the throat minimizes discomfort and prevents gagging during the procedure.
- Tell the client that once the tube has been inserted, most people become accustomed to its presence within a few hours. In most cases, the client can easily swallow foods and liquids with the tube in place. If permitted, favorite foods or beverages can still be enjoyed.
- Assure the client that the tube feeding will be temporary, if such assurance is appropriate.

Although tube feeding may be frightening for some, for others, it is a relief. People who understand that they should eat, but can't, may be relieved to receive sound nutrition without any effort. As they feel better and begin to eat again, the tube feeding can often be reduced or discontinued.

Some people feel a loss of control over their lives; others feel self-conscious about how the feeding tube looks or awkward about moving around with the equipment. A few simple measures can help:

- Involve older children, teens, and adults in the decision-making and care process whenever possible. Clients can help arrange daily feeding schedules, and some can also perform many of the feeding procedures themselves.
- Show clients how to manipulate the feeding equipment so that they can get out of bed and move around.
- Recommend that clients walk around and socialize with other clients, if permissible.
- Recommend that clients maintain contact with friends and keep busy with hobbies and activities they enjoy. This measure is especially important for children, teens, and for those on long-term feedings.
- For infants and children, keep the developmental age of the child in mind and work with parents to ensure that appropriate feeding skills are mastered (see Highlight 21). For infants, providing a pacifier during feedings helps maintain the associations between sucking, swallowing, eating, and fullness. When possible, some of the tube-feeding formula may be provided by bottle or by spoon to further develop skills.

The more complex the procedure that a health care professional is responsible for, the easier it becomes to focus on the procedure and forget about the client's emotions. No matter how many technicalities you have to keep in mind, remember to stay focused on the person receiving your care.

The inner open space of a tube or hollow organ (such as the intestine) is called the **lumen**.

Which feeding tube is appropriate depends on the client's age, how the tube will be placed (for example, nasogastric or gastrostomy), where it will be placed (stomach or intestine), and its inner diameter. Once the appropriate length is selected, the smallest tube through which the formula will flow without clogging is best. Unclogging a tube is a difficult procedure that interrupts the feeding schedule and is frequently unsuccessful.[10] Insertion of a new tube can cause undue stress and anxiety.

Following selection of a feeding site, formula, and tube for a feeding, attention turns to preparing and administering the formula. Thereafter, faithful and frequent monitoring helps ensure success.

FORMULA PREPARATION

Most individuals beginning a tube feeding are seriously ill or malnourished. Many risk developing infections; people with suppressed immune systems are particularly vulnerable to infection from food-borne illness.[11] Unfortunately, bacterial contamination of formulas is commonly reported, opening the way for more serious illness. To prevent contamination, all personnel involved in preparing or delivering formulas should handle them only in clean environments, using clean equipment and clean hands.

At the Preparation Site Formulas that must be mixed or diluted are most often prepared and packaged in the dietary department or pharmacy. Once a formula has been mixed or diluted, the container is labeled with the client's name, room, date, and time of preparation and sent to the nursing station. Ready-to-use cans of formulas are often sent unopened to the nursing station; they, too, should be labeled with the client's name and room number.

At the Nursing Station Once a formula reaches the nursing station, the nursing staff assumes responsibility for its safe handling. The following steps reduce the likelihood of formula contamination:

- Before opening a can of formula, carefully clean the lid. If you do not use the entire can at one feeding, label the can with the time it was opened.
- Cover opened cans. Store mixed or diluted formulas in clean, closed containers. Refrigerate the unused portion of formula promptly.
- Discard unlabeled or improperly labeled containers and all opened containers of formula not used within 24 hours.

At Bedside Prevent the risk of bacterial contamination by following these procedures:

- Before adding formula to the feeding bag or bottle, rinse the feeding container and the attached tubing with water and allow them to air dry. Never add fresh formula to formula still in the container.
- Flush the feeding tube with water before and after each use.
- Change the feeding bag or bottle and the attached tubing (except the feeding tube itself) every 12 to 24 hours.

Tube feedings sometimes come prepackaged in closed containers that can be connected directly to the feeding tube without having to be transferred to another feeding container. Such systems save nursing time and significantly reduce the risk of bacterial contamination.

FORMULA ADMINISTRATION

Recommended formula administration schedules vary between institutions, and many protocols are based on clinical judgment rather than research. Most people can receive undiluted formula (either isotonic or hypertonic) at the start of a feeding.[12] People under severe stress, those who have not eaten for several weeks, or those receiving intestinal feedings, however, may not be able to tolerate large volumes of hypertonic formulas initially. In such cases, formulas may need to be given slowly at first, at about 25 to 50 milliliters per hour. If the person tolerates the formula, the rate can be increased by about 25 milliliters per hour every 4 to 12 hours (see the margin note), depending on the location of the feeding tube (gastric, duodenal, or jejunal) as well as the person's medical condition. If the new rate is not tolerated, back up and proceed more slowly, giving the person more time to adapt. In a few cases, formulas may need to be diluted at first, the strength increased gradually, and then the rate advanced.

As an example of volume progression for a tube feeding, start the feeding at 50 ml/hour at full strength and then progress as follows:

- After 6 hours: 75 ml/hour.
- After 12 hours: 100 ml/hour.
- After 18 hours: 125 ml/hour.

For infants, the formula's concentration, infusion rate, and volume must be changed one by one and in small increments. Infants' stomachs are very small, their rate of gastric emptying is slow, and their immature GI tracts are highly sensitive to even minor changes in formula composition.

Delivery Techniques When people are receiving formula, they should not be lying flat; the risk of aspiration is too great. Instead, elevate the client's upper body to at least a 30-degree angle during, and for at least 30 minutes after, a feeding, whenever possible.

A day's volume of formula can be given either intermittently or continuously over a period of 8 to 24 hours. Each method has its specific uses, advantages, and disadvantages.

A can of ready-to-feed formula typically contains 240 ml of formula, and feedings are often divided so that one can of formula can be given at each feeding.

Intermittent Feedings Intermittent feedings are best tolerated when they are delivered into the stomach and no more than 250 to 400 milliliters is given in 20 to 30 minutes using the gravity drip method or an infusion pump. The larger the volume of formula required to meet nutrient needs, the more frequently feedings are delivered. (People who have very high nutrient needs benefit from either high–nutrient density formulas or large volumes of formula delivered continuously.) Rapid delivery (in 10 minutes or less) of a large volume of formula (300 to 400 milliliters)—called a bolus feeding—often leads to complaints of abdominal discomfort, nausea, fullness, and cramping. This makes sense. After all, people do not gobble down a meal in just a few minutes, especially when they are not feeling well.

Delivery of no more than 250 ml of formula over 30 minutes is sometimes called an **intermittent feeding**.

Delivery of about 300 to 400 ml of formula over 10 minutes or less is called a **bolus feeding**.

Nurses measure gastric residuals to ensure that the stomach is emptying properly and to prevent nausea, vomiting, and possible aspiration of formula into the lungs. For intermittent feedings, the gastric residual is measured before each feeding and should not exceed 100 milliliters. If the residual is excessive, the feeding is withheld for about an hour, and then the residual is rechecked. If excessive residuals persist, the physician may withhold the feeding, reduce the rate of administration, or begin drug therapy to stimulate gastric emptying.

gastric residual: the volume of formula that remains in the stomach from a previous feeding. It is measured by gently withdrawing the gastric contents through the feeding tube using a syringe. If the measured gastric residual is acceptable, the residual is returned to the client through the feeding tube.

Intermittent feedings work well for clients able to tolerate them. Often clients gradually adapt to larger volumes of formula given over shorter periods of time. Such feedings mimic the usual pattern of eating and allow clients freedom of movement between meals. They also require less time, making them less costly and easier for people to use at home.

Continuous Feedings Continuous feedings are delivered slowly and in constant amounts over a period of 8 to 24 hours. Such feedings benefit people who

How to Plan a Tube-Feeding Schedule

After selecting a formula that meets the client's medical and nutrient needs, the planner, usually a dietitian, determines the volume of formula per day that meets those needs. Consider a client who needs 2000 milliliters of formula per day. If the client is to receive the formula intermittently six times a day, he needs about 330 milliliters of formula at each feeding (2000 ml ÷ 6 feedings = 333 ml/feeding). Alternatively, if he is to receive the same volume of formula eight times a day, then he needs 250 milliliters (or about one can of ready-to-feed formula) at each feeding (2000 ml ÷ 8 feedings = 250 ml/feeding). He will probably tolerate this volume of formula best if it is given to him over 20 to 30 minutes at each feeding. If the client is to receive the formula continuously over 24 hours, he needs 85 milliliters of formula each hour (2000 ml ÷ 24 hr = 83 ml/hr).

have received no food through the GI tract for a long time, those who are hypermetabolic, and those receiving intestinal feedings. Infusion pumps help ensure accurate and constant flow rates. Gastric residuals for people receiving continuous feedings are measured every 4 to 6 hours and should not exceed the volume of formula infused during the preceding 2 hours. The accompanying box explains several ways to schedule tube feedings.

CAUTION: Young children may be attracted to the bright lights, interesting sounds, and many controls of an infusion pump. Keep infusion pumps at a safe distance to prevent children from changing the flow rate or toppling the infusion pump or intravenous pole and possibly injuring themselves or damaging the pump.

Supplemental Water In addition to the formula itself, water can also be provided through the feeding tube. Using water to flush the feeding tube before and after a feeding or when the feeding apparatus is being changed helps prevent clogged feeding tubes and keeps the client hydrated. (Water can also be given orally if the person can drink it.) Supplemental water is often needed to meet the client's daily fluid requirements. As a guideline, adults require about 2000 milliliters (approximately 2 quarts) of water daily. Fever, excessive sweating, severe vomiting, diarrhea, blood loss, and burns raise water requirements. In kidney, liver, and heart diseases, water may need to be restricted.

Formulas themselves contain considerable amounts of water. A standard formula (1.0 kcal/ml) contains about 850 ml of water per liter of formula. Higher-kcalorie formulas contain less water: formulas that contain 1.5 kcal/ml or 2.0 kcal/ml provide about 775 ml and 600 ml of water per liter of formula, respectively.

Attention to indicators of body water balance can help determine how much additional water an individual needs. In alert adults, thirst is a good indicator of water needs; a person complaining of thirst generally needs water. In the elderly, however, thirst may be slow to develop in response to dehydration. Other clues to dehydration include unexplained weight loss, high serum electrolytes or hematocrit, and low blood pressure.

CAUTION: Fluid needs must be carefully monitored in infants, the elderly, and people who are unconscious.

DRUG ADMINISTRATION THROUGH FEEDING TUBES

Clients receiving tube feedings are usually quite ill and are also likely to be receiving numerous medications. Often these medications are delivered through feeding tubes, and in some cases, complications can occur.

Keep in mind that enteral formulas can interact with drugs in the same ways that foods can. The health care team must consider the effects of drug therapy on nutrient requirements, the effects of the formula on drug absorption, the effects of drugs on formulas, and the prevention of tube-feeding complications.

Drug Forms A drug may come in any of several forms including tablet, liquid, injectable, and intravenous. People on tube feedings have functioning GI tracts, and oral drugs are less costly and easier to deliver than injectable or intravenous forms. Thus clinicians often prefer to use oral drugs for clients on tube feedings. The following guidelines may be helpful in preventing drug-drug interactions, drug-formula interactions, or clogged feeding tubes when drugs are delivered through feeding tubes:

- Give the medication orally whenever possible.
- Do not mix medications together or mix medications with the formula. Instead, stop the feeding temporarily and give each drug individually. Flush the feeding tube with warm water before and after administering each drug.
- Deliver liquid drugs through the tube using a syringe, if possible. If liquid medications are thick or sticky, dilute them with water first.
- Consider using the injectable or intravenous form if the drug is not available in liquid form. Ideally, tablets should not be crushed and administered through feeding tubes. If using tablets is unavoidable, crush the tablets to a *fine* powder and mix them with water before administering them. Do not crush tablets or capsules intended to release their contents slowly; in these cases, another drug form must be given.
- Avoid drugs known to be incompatible with formulas, such as those listed in Table 23–3.

Additional Considerations The location of the feeding tube (whether gastric or intestinal) is also relevant to drug administration. Some drugs are designed to dissolve in the stomach's acidic environment. Such drugs may not be readily

Table 23–3

Selected Drugs That Are Incompatible with Some Formulas

Aluminum hydroxide	MCT oil
Chlorpromazine concentrate	Mellaril concentrate
Cibalith-S syrup	Mellaril oral solution
Cimetidine	Paregoric elixir
Dimetane elixir	Potassium chloride
Dimetapp elixir	Reglan syrup
Feosol elixir	Riopan
Fleet's phosphosoda	Robitussin expectorant
Gevrabon liquid	Sudafed syrup
Klorvess syrup	Throazine concentrate
Mandelamine Forte suspension	Zinc sulfate capsules

Note: These substances may be compatible with some formulas and not others.

Sources: P. E. Burns, L. McCall, and R. Wirsching. Physical compatibility of enteral formulas with various common medications, *Journal of the American Dietetic Association* 88 (1988): 1094–1096; A. J. Cutle, E. Altman, and L. Lenkel, Compatibility of enteral products with commonly employed drug additives, *Journal of Parenteral and Enteral Nutrition* 7 (1983): 186–191; Z. M. Pronsky, *Food-Medication Interactions*, 9th ed. (Pottstown, Pa.: Food-Medication Interactions, 1995).

absorbed if delivered directly to the duodenum or jejunum. Similarly, a drug that is optimally absorbed in the duodenum may be poorly absorbed in the jejunum. In such cases, oral, intravenous, or injectable forms of the drug should be used.

In some cases, formulas alter drug absorption. One example is phenytoin, a drug used to control seizures. Absorption of phenytoin may be markedly reduced for a person who is on continuous tube feedings. Although opinions of the best way to handle this problem differ, clinicians often suggest that for most clients on either intermittent or continuous feedings, the feeding should be stopped for 2 hours before and 2 hours after giving phenytoin.[13] For clients requiring continuous feedings, the rate of delivery is increased during the times the feeding is given to ensure that nutrient needs are met.

Some clients have a specific type of feeding jejunostomy called a *needle catheter jejunostomy* through which phenytoin cannot be delivered. In such cases, phenytoin is given intravenously.

To sum up, enteral formulas may be used whenever a client can digest and absorb nutrients via the GI tract, but cannot eat enough food to meet nutrient needs. Among the choices are standard formulas, which contain complete proteins, and hydrolyzed formulas, which contain free amino acids, dipeptides, and tripeptides. Complete formulas may be used to supply all the nutrients a person needs; alternatively, modular formulas, which supply individual nutrients, may be used to construct or supplement formulas as needed. Each type of formula has distinguishing characteristics that influence the formula selection (see Figure 23–2). When giving formulas by mouth, clinicians can improve palatability by adding flavors and serving them cold and attractively. When giving formulas by tube, attention must be given to the appropriate preparation of the formula, selection of the tube, delivery schedule, and administration of medications.

Addressing Tube-Feeding Complications

When formulas are correctly selected, prepared, and administered, and problems are promptly identified and corrected, chances are good that the formulas will successfully support nutritional health. Table 23–4 on p. 772 provides a monitoring schedule that helps detect problems before they become serious.

Mechanical problems, such as a clogged feeding tube, a malfunctioning feeding pump, or a tube that has become dislodged from its appropriate location, can interrupt the feeding schedule and prevent the delivery of nutrients. Complications related to the formula or its administration can result in such GI complaints as nausea, vomiting, diarrhea, cramps, constipation, delayed gastric emptying, and abdominal distention. Metabolic complications such as dehydration, electrolyte imbalance, and elevated blood glucose can also occur. Table 23–5 on p. 773 summarizes problems associated with tube feedings, their causes, and ways to prevent them. These complications have been discussed in appropriate sections throughout this chapter, but two of them deserve further attention here: failure to achieve or maintain adequate nutrition status and diarrhea.

FAILURE TO ACHIEVE OR MAINTAIN ADEQUATE NUTRITION STATUS

Sometimes a client does not respond to a tube feeding as expected. If the client continues to lose weight, for example, health care professionals must find out why. Perhaps they have underestimated energy and nutrient requirements.

Table 23–4

Checklist for Monitoring Clients Recently Placed on Tube Feedings

Before starting a new feeding:	Complete a nutrition assessment.
	Check tube placement.
Before each intermittent feeding:	Check gastric residual.
Every half hour:	Check gravity drip rate, when applicable.
Every hour:	Check pump drip rate, when applicable.
Every 4 hours:	Check vital signs, including blood pressure, temperature, pulse, and respiration.
Every 6 hours:	Check blood glucose; monitoring blood glucose can be discontinued after 48 hours if test results are consistently negative in a nondiabetic client.
Every 4 to 6 hours of continuous feeding:	Check gastric residual.
Every 8 hours:	Check intake and output.
	Check specific gravity of urine.
	Check tube placement.
	Chart client's total intake of, acceptance of, and tolerance to tube feeding.
Every day:	Weigh client.
	Check electrolytes and blood urea nitrogen until stabilized.
	Clean feeding equipment.
Every 7 to 10 days	Check all laboratory findings.
	Reassess nutrition status.
As needed:	Observe client for any undesirable responses to tube feeding; for example, delayed gastric emptying, nausea, vomiting, or diarrhea
	Check nitrogen balance.
	Check laboratory data.
	Chart significant details.

Remember that even the best calculations for determining energy and protein needs are only estimates. One study of people in a nursing home who were being tube fed found that those who developed pressure sores were malnourished, even though they were receiving formulas that were high in energy and protein.[14]

Inappropriate formula selection may explain failure to reach nutrition goals. If a formula is prescribed without calculating its nutrient composition, the formula may not be meeting all of the client's nutrient needs. The selected formula may need to be changed; a client with fat malabsorption, for example, may need a lower-fat formula, additional calcium, or extra fat-soluble vitamins.

Table 23–5

Causes and Prevention or Correction of Tube-Feeding Complications

Complications	Possible Causes	Preventive/Corrective Measures
Aspiration pneumonia	Compromised gastroesophageal sphincter, delayed gastric emptying, gastric obstruction	Use nasoenteric, gastrostomy, or jejunostomy feedings in high-risk clients; use small-diameter transnasal tube; elevate head of bed during and 30 minutes after feeding; use continuous drip method of delivery; check gastric residual.
Clogged feeding tube	Formula too thick for tube	Select appropriate tube size; dilute formula with water; flush tubing with water before and after giving formula.
	Medications	Use oral, liquid, or injectable drugs whenever possible; dilute thick or sticky liquid drugs with water before administering; crush tablets to a fine powder and mix with water; flush tubing with water before and after drugs are given; give drugs individually; do not mix drugs with formula.
Constipation	Low-fiber formula	Provide additional fluids; use high-fiber formula.
	Lack of exercise	Encourage walking and other activities, if appropriate.
	Drug therapy	Change drug therapy if possible; give laxatives or enemas if indicated.
Dehydration and electrolyte imbalance[a]	Excessive diarrhea	See items under *Diarrhea*.
	Inadequate fluid intake	Provide additional fluid.
	Carbohydrate intolerance	Use continuous drip administration of formula; monitor blood glucose; consider administering insulin; change amount or type of carbohydrate.
	Excessive protein intake	Monitor blood electrolyte levels; reduce protein intake.
Diarrhea, cramps, distention	Bacterial contamination	Use fresh formula every 24 hours; store opened or mixed formula in a refrigerator; rinse feeding bag and tubing before adding fresh formula; change feeding bag every 24 hours; prepare formula with clean hands using clean equipment in a clean environment.
	Lactose intolerance	Use lactose-free formula in lactose-intolerant and high-risk clients.
	Hypertonic formula	Use a small volume of formula and increase volume gradually; dilute formula; use isotonic formula.
	Rapid formula administration	Slow administration rate or use continuous drip feedings.
	Malnutrition/low serum albumin	Use a small volume of dilute formula and increase volume and concentration gradually.
	Drug therapy	Use antidiarrheal agents; change drug, drug form, or dosage; if possible.
Hyperglycemia	Primary medical condition	Treat disorder.
	Diabetes, hypermetabolism, drug therapy	Check blood glucose; slow administration rate; provide adequate fluids; limit type or amount of carbohydrate; consider administering insulin.
Nausea and vomiting	Obstruction	Discontinue tube feeding.
	Delayed gastric emptying	Check gastric residual; slow administration rate, use continuous drip feedings, or discontinue tube feeding.
	Intolerance to concentration or volume of formula	Use small volume of dilute formula and increase volume and concentration gradually; use continuous drip feedings.
	Drug therapy	Change drug, drug form, or dosage if possible; use antinausea and antiemetic drugs.
	Psychological reaction to tube feeding	Address client's concerns.
Skin irritation at enterostomy site	Leakage of GI secretions and friction caused by the tube	Keep site clean; inspect area for redness, tenderness, and drainage; use protective skin cream.

Note: Many of the complications presented here can be caused by the client's primary disorder rather than the tube feeding itself. In such a case, the corrective measure would include treatment of the disorder. Additionally, many of the corrective measures require a physician's order.

[a]This cluster of symptoms is sometimes called the tube-feeding syndrome. Imbalances of any electrolytes are possible, and corrective measures would vary.

It is also possible that the formula is not being delivered as intended. Sometimes feedings are withheld to perform medical procedures or to deal with complications; gastric retention of formula, inadvertent removal of the feeding tube, GI intolerances, or difficulty in positioning or retaining the tube in the appropriate feeding site (duodenum, jejunum) can all necessitate stopping the feeding. Whenever a client fails to achieve or maintain adequate nutrition status while on a tube feeding, the health care team should investigate the causes. Some questions to answer include:

- Is the client receiving the prescribed formula?
- Is the client receiving the amount of formula that has been ordered? If not, why not? When changing the feeding bag or adding fresh formula to a bag that has been rinsed with water, check and record the amount of formula left from the previous feeding.
- Is the formula being delivered at the correct flow rate? If a pump is being used, is it working correctly?
- If the formula is being delivered as prescribed, has the nutrient content of the formula been calculated to ensure that it meets the client's needs?
- Have the client's nutrient needs changed, or have they been incorrectly estimated?

Be alert to signs that the tube feeding is not being delivered as ordered so that problems can be corrected early and nutrient needs met.

DIARRHEA

Diarrhea is a commonly cited and troublesome complication associated with tube feedings. Its actual incidence and significance are difficult to determine, because diarrhea in tube-fed clients has not been clearly defined.[15] Traditionally, the enteral formula was blamed for diarrhea. It now seems clear, however, that diarrhea may often be related to the client's illness or its treatments.[16] Drug therapy is frequently the culprit. Liquid drugs (frequently used to deliver medications through feeding tubes) often contain sorbitol, a sugar alcohol that causes diarrhea when given in large doses. This scenario is particularly likely when an adult receives a liquid pediatric preparation in high doses. When drugs cause diarrhea, the client's medications must be carefully reviewed, and corrective steps taken, if possible. In some cases, a substitute drug with similar pharmaceutical action, but without the side effects, can be used to reduce GI problems. In other cases, giving the drug more frequently in smaller doses may be effective. Oftentimes, antidiarrheal agents are prescribed.

For more information about lactose intolerance, see Chapter 4.

Other reasons for diarrhea include bacterial contamination of the formula, lactose intolerance, rapid delivery of the formula, use of nutrient- or kcalorie-dense formulas, or use of high-fat formulas. Following the suggestions provided earlier (see p. 767) can reduce the risk of formula contamination. Carefully selecting formula suitable to the client's needs and delivering it appropriately can minimize diarrhea as well.

WHAT TO CHART

Chapter 17 emphasized the importance of the medical record as a communication tool. The health care team should document tube-feeding information in each client's medical record, including:

- Education of the client regarding the tube-feeding procedures.
- Type of feeding tube.
- Tube placement.
- Client's response to tube insertion.
- Administration schedule (concentration and rate).
- Method of delivery (intermittent or continuous, gravity drip or infusion pump).
- Client's tolerance to tube feeding (note any complications and any corrective actions taken).
- Client's emotional and physical responses to tube feeding.
- Reasons that a tube feeding was interrupted or could not be delivered as ordered, if necessary.
- Drugs, drug form, and problems noted when drugs are delivered through feeding tubes.

The dietitian records the client's estimated nutrient needs, the selected formula's name, and its nutrient composition. If a person on a tube feeding does not seem to be responding adequately, investigate to see if the feeding has been delivered as intended. Be sure to correct any problems early.

To review, problems with tube feedings can usually be detected and alleviated by monitoring clients regularly and taking corrective measures promptly (see Tables 23–4 and 23–5). Careful charting also helps to identify and correct problems early. The checklist on p. 776 reviews key points for assessing nutrition status in people receiving tube feedings.

From Tube Feedings to Table Foods

Once the problem causing the need for a tube feeding resolves, the client can gradually shift to an oral diet as the volume of formula is tapered off. The client should be eating adequate amounts of foods by mouth before the tube feeding is discontinued. In many cases, the person can drink the same formula that was earlier given by tube. Some people cannot make the transition to oral intake for medical reasons and go home on tube feedings. Chapter 24 discusses specialized nutrition support at home. The case study on p. 777 reviews the many factors involved in tube feedings.

Tube feeding is a practical solution to feeding the person who is unable to consume adequate nutrients by mouth. A person without a functional GI tract cannot benefit from a tube feeding, however. In such a case, intravenous nutrition (the subject of the next chapter) can be a life-saving treatment option.

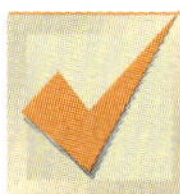

Nutrition Assessment Checklist

For People Receiving Tube Feedings

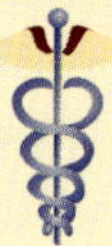

Medical Review the client's medical record for the information necessary to select the appropriate feeding site (gastric versus intestinal), insertion procedure (transnasal or enterostomy), and formula. The development of undesirable symptoms associated with the client's medical condition, therapy (especially drug), or formula selection requires prompt intervention.

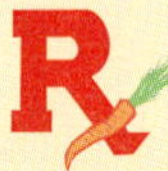

Drug Review the client's drug therapy for possible drug-nutrient interactions and GI side effects that may affect the client's tolerance for the tube feeding. If the feeding tube is used to deliver drugs, follow the precautions on pp. 769–771.

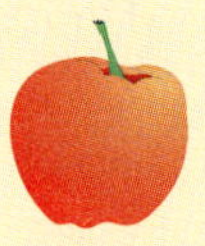

Nutrient Intake Ensure that formula is being delivered as prescribed, and take corrective actions as needed (see p. 774). For clients beginning to eat, determine the degree to which nutrient needs are being met by table foods or formula taken orally, and reduce the volume of the tube feeding accordingly.

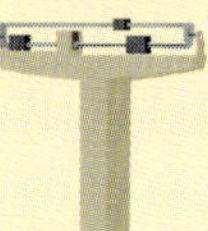

Anthropometric Assess the client's weight daily to make sure that the client is meeting nutrition goals.

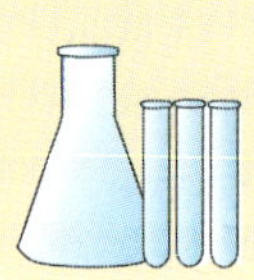

Laboratory Monitor serum and urine lab values for signs of fluid and electrolyte imbalances and glucose intolerance. Check serum protein levels to ensure that they are improving or being maintained. When available, assess nitrogen balance to determine if the tube feeding is meeting the client's protein needs.

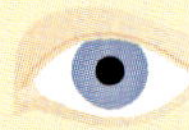

Physical Check gastric residual for signs of delayed gastric emptying to prevent GI complications and reduce the risk of aspiration. Check tube placement and gravity drip rate or infusion pump drip rate as needed (see Table 23-4). Assess blood pressure, temperature, pulse, and respiration every 4 hours. Look for physical signs of malnutrition or dehydration.

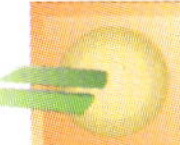

Case Study Graphics Designer Requiring Enteral Nutrition

Mrs. Innis is a 24-year-old graphics designer who suffered multiple fractures when she fell from a cliff while hiking. She has been in the hospital for seven days and has no appetite. Mrs. Innis has lost 8 pounds over the course of her hospitalization. Due to the nature of her injuries, Mrs. Innis is in traction and is immobile, although the head of her bed can be elevated to 30 degrees. From the history, the dietitian determined that Mrs. Innis's nutrition status was adequate prior to hospitalization. The health care team agrees that a nasoduodenal tube feeding should be instituted before nutrition status deteriorates further. The standard formula selected for the feeding is lactose-free, and Mrs. Innis's nutrient requirements can be met with 2200 milliliters of the formula per day.

What steps can the health care team take to prepare Mrs. Innis for tube feeding? Why might nasoduodenal placement of the feeding tube be preferred to nasogastric placement for Mrs. Innis? Based on the limited information available, is the choice of formula appropriate?

The physician's orders specified that the feeding should be given continuously over 18 hours. Develop a tube-feeding schedule for Mrs. Innis.

What parameters should be monitored to ensure that Mrs. Innis's fluid needs are being met? How can additional fluids be given? Describe precautions that should be taken if Mrs. Innis is to receive medications through the feeding tube.

After three days of feeding, Mrs. Innis develops diarrhea. Look at Table 23–5 on p. 773 to determine the possible causes. What measures can be taken to correct the various causes of diarrhea?

What tube-feeding information should be charted in Mrs. Innis's medical record? When Mrs. Innis is ready to eat table foods again, what steps will the health care team take?

Study Questions

1. Describe standard formulas, hydrolyzed formulas, complete formulas, and modular formulas, explaining the characteristics of each and how they differ.
2. What factors are considered in selecting an appropriate formula for an oral or tube feeding? Explain how each of the following narrows the formula choice: medical and nutrient needs; digestive and absorptive function; feeding route; and individual tolerances.
3. Suggest ways for improving acceptance of enteral formulas by mouth.
4. What are tube feedings? In what ways and in what locations can feeding tubes be placed?
5. Discuss the ways in which tube feedings can be administered to clients. Why are feeding tubes usually removed after each feeding when an infant is tube fed?
6. Describe the problems that can occur when drugs are delivered through feeding tubes. What guidelines can be used to help prevent these problems?
7. What complications are associated with tube feedings? What steps help to identify and prevent complications before they become serious?

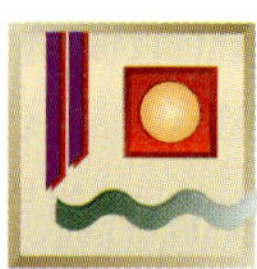

Clinical Applications

1. Complex procedures, such as those necessary to deliver enteral nutrition, require attention to many technical details, making it easy to focus on the procedure and forget about the client. Imagine that you need a transnasal tube feeding. How might you react to news that you need the feeding and to the insertion procedure? What would you miss most about eating table foods? Think of ways health care professionals might help you deal with these feelings.
2. Take a look at the checklist for monitoring clients on tube feedings (Table 23–4). You can see that the person on a tube feeding requires a great deal of care. Discuss the advantages of a nutrition support team in monitoring clients on tube feedings. What contributions might various members of the health care team make in working with tube-fed clients (see Highlight 17)?
3. Review Chapters 21 and 22 and note the symptoms and disorders that may require the use of tube feedings. For each symptom or disorder, consider when and why a tube feeding might be appropriate and which conditions might require a hydrolyzed formula. Also note those conditions associated with a risk for gastric reflux that might preclude the use of a nasogastric feeding. What alternatives are possible in these cases?

Notes

1. D. K. Bernard, J. Mandt, and E. P. Shronts, Creation of a unique modular enteral feeding system, *Support Line*, April 1993, pp. 10–14.
2. H. M. Storm and P. Lin, Forms of carbohydrate in enteral formulas, *Support Line*, June 1996, pp. 7–9.
3. D. C. Frankenfield and P. L. Beyer, Dietary fiber and bowel function in tube-fed patients, *Journal of the American Dietetic Association* 91 (1991): 590–596; J. Slavin, Commercially available enteral formulas with fiber and bowel function measures, *Nutrition in Clinical Practice* 5 (1990): 247–250.
4. J. C. Palacios and J. L. Rombeau, Dietary fiber: A brief review and potential application to enteral nutrition, *Nutrition in Clinical Practice* 5 (1990): 99–106; K. Shankardass and coauthors, Bowel function of long-term tube-fed patients consuming formulae with or without dietary fiber, *Journal of Parenteral and Enteral Nutrition* 14 (1990): 508–512.
5. D. F. Bowers, The logistics of enteral nutrition support: Current practices for the initiation and progression of tube feeding, A summary, in *Enteral Nutrition Support for the 1990s: Innovations in Nutrition, Technology, and Techniques*, Report of the Twelfth Ross Roundtable on Medical Issues, Ross Laboratories, 1992.
6. K. Teahon and coauthors, Practical aspects of enteral nutrition in the management of Crohn's disease, *Journal of Parenteral and Enteral Nutrition* 19 (1995): 365–368.
7. W. W. Souba, Nutritional support, *New England Journal of Medicine*, 336 (1997): 41–48: E. P. Shronts, Enteral vs. parenteral nutrition: A clinical review, *Support Line*, June 1996, pp. 10–13.
8. Shronts, 1996.
9. F. W. Clevenger and D. J. Rodriguez, Decision-making for enteral feeding administration: The why behind where and how, *Nutrition in Clinical Practice* 10 (1995): 104–113; Q. Duh, Decision tree for route of enteral nutrition support: Placement techniques, A summary, in *Enteral Nutrition Support*, Report of the First Ross Conference on Enteral Devices, Ross Laboratories, 1996.
10. S. P. Marcuard, K. L. Stegall, and S. Trogdon, Clearing obstructed feeding tubes, *Journal of Parenteral and Enteral Nutrition* 13 (1989): 81–83.
11. G. Moe, Enteral feeding and infection in the immunocompromised patient, *Nutrition in Clinical Practice* 6 (1991): 55–64.
12. G. P. Zaloga, Enteral nutrition in hospitalized patients: A summary, in *Enteral Nutrition Support for the 1990s: Innovations in Nutrition, Technology, and Techniques*, Report of the Twelfth Ross Roundtable on Medical Issues, Ross Laboratories, 1992.
13. J. Hatton and B. Magnuson, How to minimize interaction between phenytoin and enteral nutrition: Two approaches, *Nutrition in Clinical Practice* 11 (1996): 28–31.
14. R. A. Breslow, J. Hallfrisch, and A. P. Goldberg, Malnutrition in tubefed nursing home patients with pressure sores, *Journal of Parenteral and Enteral Nutrition* 15 (1991): 663–668.
15. S. Mobarhan and M. DeMeo, Diarrhea induced by enteral feeding, *Nutrition Reviews* 53 (1995): 67–70.
16. P. G. Eisenberg, Causes of diarrhea in tube-fed patients: A comprehensive approach to diagnosis and management, *Nutrition in Clinical Practice* 8 (1993): 119–123.

Enteral Formulas: Who's Minding the Market?

The medical marketplace offers an astounding array of enteral formulas. New products appear regularly, paralleling the trend that favors the use of enteral over parenteral nutrition to feed people who cannot meet their nutrient needs with conventional foods. Enteral formulas were originally manufactured simply to provide the nutrients of table foods in a liquid form. Gradually, formulas with specific nutrition profiles were developed for specific uses; lactose was eliminated from some formulas to improve GI tolerance, for example, and free amino acids replaced whole proteins in other formulas to improve absorption. Even more recently, formulas have been designed not only to meet nutrient needs, but also to directly affect the disease process.[1] Some of these formulas contain nutrients or other dietary constituents in types or amounts that differ considerably from those found in standard diets. Are such formulas foods or drugs? This highlight addresses the concerns of health care professionals about the expanding enteral formula market and its regulation.

CURRENT PRACTICE

In the United States, enteral formulas are exempt from the testing for safety and effectiveness that drugs must go through before they can be marketed. Enteral formulas are currently regulated as medical foods.[2] The Food and Drug Administration (FDA) notes that to qualify as medical foods, products must meet the following criteria:

- They must be specifically formulated and processed, as opposed to a naturally occurring food used in a natural state.
- They must be designed for oral or tube feeding.
- They must be labeled for the dietary management of a disorder that has distinctive nutritional requirements.
- They must be intended for use with medical supervision.[3]

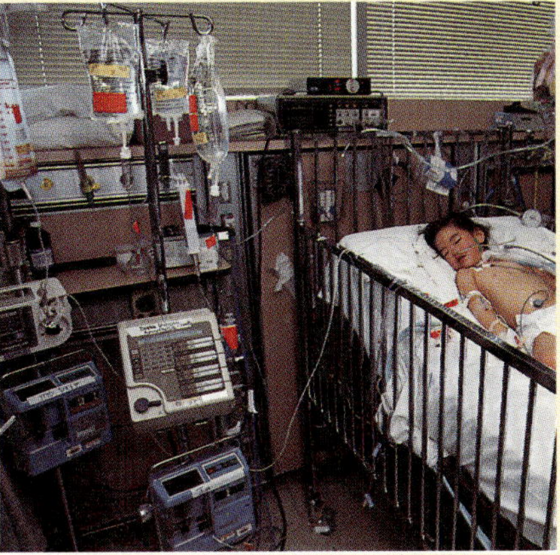

Enteral formulas, which serve as the primary source of nutrients for some people who are ill, are exempted from regulations that govern labeling, nutrient content claims, and health claims.

Products that do not qualify as medical foods include parenteral nutrients, single-nutrient preparations, weight-loss products, and foods recommended by a physician or other health care professional as part of an overall diet to reduce the risk of a medical disease.

As medical foods, enteral formulas must conform to the manufacturing standards applied to all foods. These standards ensure that products are prepared in a sanitary environment and are free of contamination. Manufacturers, motivated to protect their reputations and limit their legal liabilities, generally conduct clinical trials before marketing their products and maintain high quality control standards.[4]

Potential Problems

Medical foods are exempt from regulations that govern nutrition labeling, nutrient content claims, and health claims.[5] A medical food can technically be sold without any nutrition information on its label. The product may reach the market before the formulation's suitability for its intended purpose has been evaluated. Furthermore, a label on a medical food may make unsubstantiated health claims.

These exemptions would probably not be a cause for concern if enteral formula use was always supervised by a physician (as the definition of medical foods asserts), but such is not always the case. Many formulas are marketed directly to the public on television and in print and are widely available without a prescription in pharmacies and grocery stores.

In effect, medical foods, which are intended for use with people who are ill, receive less scrutiny than table foods, which are intended for the general population. Thus the public is currently not protected from potential safety hazards or inappropriate treatment claims for these products.

Standard and Special Formulas

Standard enteral formulas mimic regular diets in their sources of nutrients and proportions of protein, carbohydrate, and fat. Thus these formulas are nutritionally similar to traditional foods, and they are generally considered safe.

Other formulas, designed for use in specific medical situations, differ from standard formulas in either the types or the amounts of nutrients they supply. Hydrolyzed formulas, for example, are special because they supply free amino acids rather than intact proteins; they are also much lower in fat than standard formulas. Other special formulas may go a step further—for example, they may provide high levels of certain amino acids and low levels of others. Still other formulas may contain added amounts of dietary constituents that are not known to be essential. Formulas designed to stimulate immune function, for example, have added nucleotides, omega-3 fatty acids, and the nonessential amino acid arginine.

Special formulas pose a greater potential risk to client health than standard formulas, primarily because far less is known about nutrient requirements in specific medical conditions and because such products are often the sole source of nutrients. Manufacturers can develop formulas for a specific medical condition and market them before their safety and effectiveness have been fully documented. For example, preliminary studies suggest that glutamine, a nonessential amino acid, may help protect the integrity of the GI tract during severe stress (see Chapter 25). Because the body may not be able to make enough glutamine to meet its needs, researchers are examining whether supplemental glutamine might be a safe and effective therapy. Spurred by these potentially important studies, formulas with added glutamine have been quickly developed and marketed. The potential benefits and risks of these products, however, have not been satisfactorily documented. Consider some of these unanswered questions:

- Is glutamine a conditionally essential amino acid during stress?
- How are glutamine needs during stress affected by the degree of stress or by the person's age, gender, or other medical conditions?
- At what level should glutamine be supplemented?
- Is there a measurable benefit from using a glutamine-enriched formula over a standard formula provided in appropriate amounts?
- Are any risks associated with providing too much glutamine?

These questions remain to be answered. An example of a potential risk associated with glutamine-enriched formulas involves their use in people with compromised liver and kidney function. End products of glutamine metabolism include ammonia and urea, substances that can be toxic to people with inadequate liver and kidney function, respectively.

As mentioned, an enteral formula often represents the sole source of nutrients for the person who needs it. In addition, the person may be quite ill, and there may be little leeway for errors that could hinder recovery. Clinical trials could help to refine the art of selecting and administering enteral formulas, but conducting truly adequate clinical trials in human beings is extremely difficult, particularly in people with metabolic stresses. The type and degree of stress, individual responses to stress, prior nutrition status, age, preexisting medical conditions, and varying techniques for providing care are but a few of many factors that complicate clinical studies and limit their application to other clinical situations.

Finally, highly modified formulas are often considerably more expensive than standard formulas. In today's cost-conscious health care environment, it is important to know whether such a formula provides benefits that justify its cost.

PROPOSED REGULATIONS

Since the 1970s, the FDA has considered proposals for medical food regulations, although none have been approved to date. The FDA's most recent notice of proposed rulemaking for medical foods appeared late in 1996.[6] With the formula market expanding and new manufacturers entering the field, the FDA is aware of the increased potential for injury to consumers and fraudulent claims. For these reasons, the FDA is seeking comments from medical professionals, industry, and consumers to help it determine the most effective ways to regulate the medical food industry.

The FDA's proposed rules note that labeling regulations for medical foods might include:

- Labeling of nutrient content and inclusion of adequate directions for use.
- Assurances of product composition and quality.
- Substantiation of suitability for intended purpose and for health claims.

As of this writing, the enteral formulas are still governed as medical foods, and no further action has been taken.

PROFESSIONAL RESPONSIBILITY

In the meantime, how can health care professionals ensure the safe and effective use of enteral formulas? First of all, most clients on tube feedings are on standard formulas that have been used safely for many years. The benefits of these formulas outweigh the risks of starving or subsisting on nutrient-deficient intakes.

Special formulas should be thoroughly investigated by the nutrition support team or by a skilled dietitian or physician. The investigation should include evaluating clinical studies, reviewing product literature, and determining the values of different formulas for their intended uses. Sound medical judgment that weighs the expected benefits against the potential risks of different formulas will factor heavily in the final selection of new products.

Both individuals and organizations with extensive experiences with enteral formulas should submit their recommendations to the FDA to ensure that the final regulations will be adequate and feasible. The comments of the American Society for Parenteral and Enteral Nutrition (A.S.P.E.N.) have recently been published.[7]

Conscientious professionals know that availability of an enteral formula does not ensure safety and effectiveness. These professionals will keep abreast of new regulations and consider how these regulations will affect formula development and selection.

NOTES

1. S. B. Heymsfield, Enteral solutions: Is there a solution? *Nutrition in Clinical Practice* 10 (1995): 4–7.
2. C. Mueller and M. Nestle, Regulation of medical foods: Toward a rational policy, *Nutrition in Clinical Practice* 10 (1995): 8–15.
3. Regulation of Medical Foods, *Federal Register,* November 29, 1996, pp. 60661–60671.
4. I. S. Bass, A legal overview of the status of medical foods in the United States, *Food Drug Cosmetic Law Journal* 44 (1989): 467–477.
5. Regulation of Medical Foods, 1996.
6. Regulation of Medical Foods, 1996.
7. A.S.P.E.N. Medical Foods Task Force, A.S.P.E.N.'s response to FDA notice of proposed rulemaking, *Nutrition in Clinical Practice* 12 (1997): 131–136.

Chapter 24

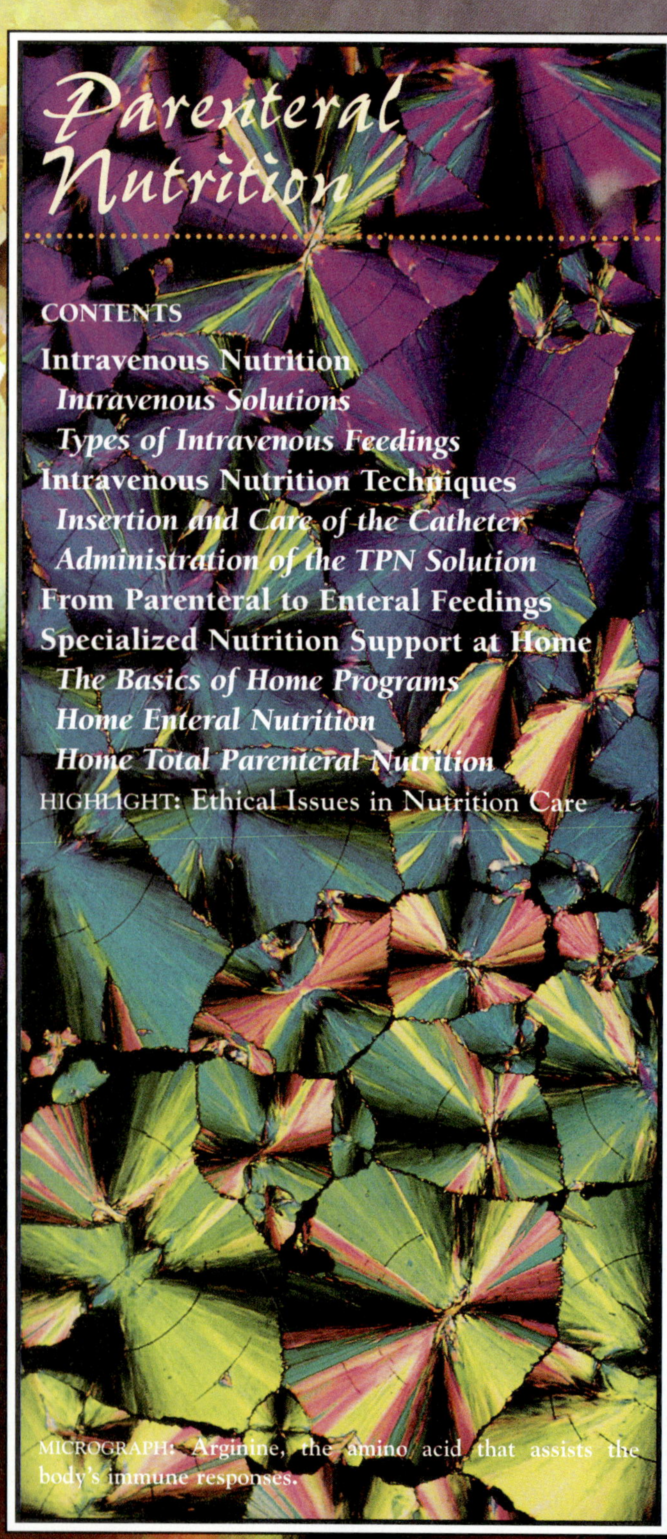

Parenteral Nutrition

CONTENTS

MICROGRAPH: Arginine, the amino acid that assists the body's immune responses.

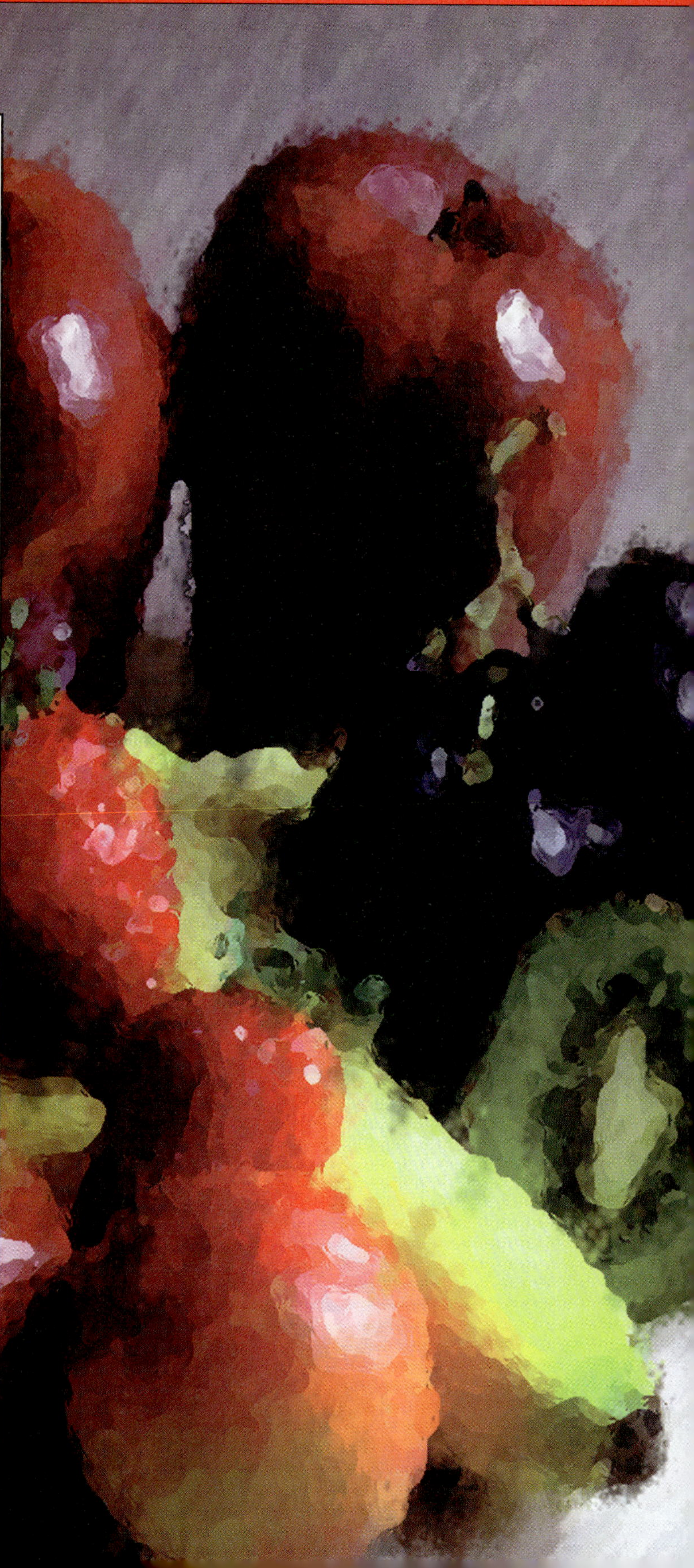

The science of medical nutrition as we know it today was shaped tremendously by the demonstration in 1968 that all nutrient needs could be met by vein.[1] Practitioners now had a way to feed people who otherwise might have died from malnutrition before their primary medical disorders could be corrected. With time, clinicians learned which solutions and which delivery methods served their clients best. They also discovered that while intravenous nutrition is a life-saving treatment, it is very costly and is associated with serious complications including liver dysfunction, progressive kidney problems, bone disorders, and many nutrient deficiencies. These findings prompted a renewed appreciation for the GI tract and for the value of using it to deliver nutrients whenever possible. Health care professionals first make every effort to feed clients an oral diet of conventional foods, supplements (including enteral formulas), or a combination of foods and supplements. When a person with a functional GI tract cannot, will not, or should not eat an oral diet, tube feedings provide an alternative. Only when people cannot meet their nutrient requirements using the enteral route should they receive parenteral or intravenous (IV) nutrition.

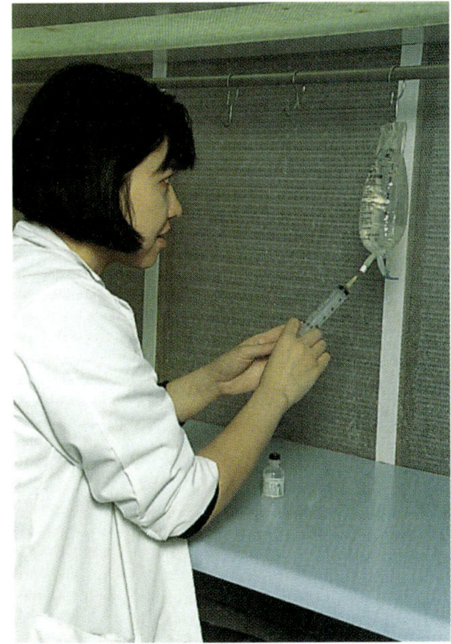

Skilled pharmacists carefully compound IV solutions under sterile conditions to ensure safety and stability.

Intravenous Nutrition

As is true of all medical nutrition therapy, the decision to use intravenous solutions, the method of delivery, and the type and amount of nutrients to provide are based on a thorough assessment of the client's medical condition and nutrient needs. Infusion of intravenous nutrients immediately changes blood levels of fluids, electrolytes, and other nutrients and, therefore, requires vigilant attention to the individual's responses.

parenteral nutrition: delivery of nutrient solutions directly into a vein, bypassing the intestines.
para = outside
enteron = intestine

intravenous (IV): through a vein.
intra = within
vena = vein

INTRAVENOUS SOLUTIONS

A variety of nutrient solutions can be administered by vein. These IV solutions may contain any or all of the essential nutrients: water, amino acids, carbohydrate, fat, vitamins, and minerals. Skilled pharmacists can compound individualized IV solutions to meet a client's specific needs.

Amino Acids Intravenous amino acid solutions usually contain both essential and nonessential amino acids to meet the body's need for protein. Special products that contain only essential amino acids or large amounts of certain amino acids and small amounts of others are available for specific medical conditions. Products designed for liver failure, for example, may contain more branched-chain amino acids and fewer aromatic amino acids (see Chapter 26).

A nonessential amino acid may be omitted from standard solutions because it does not mix well or is not stable. For example, glutamine, which may be a conditionally essential amino acid for some clients, is not stable in IV solutions. Providing glutamine as a dipeptide solves the instability problem, and studies suggest that short-chain peptides can be digested to free amino acids by enzymes bound to cell membranes.[2]

Glutamine may be a conditionally essential amino acid following intestinal resections (see Highlight 22) and during recovery from stress (see Chapter 25).

Carbohydrate Standard IV solutions provide carbohydrate as dextrose (glucose). Because the form of dextrose in IV solutions contains some water, dextrose solutions provide only 3.4 kcalories per gram, whereas glucose provides 4.

dextrose monohydrate: a form of glucose that contains water and is stable in IV solutions. Dextrose solutions provide 3.4 kcal/g, whereas glucose provides 4 kcal/g.

IV lipid emulsions are made from egg phospholipids (see p. 151) and plant-derived oils.

A 10% IV fat emulsion provides 1.1 kcal/ml, so a 500 ml bottle delivers 550 kcal.

A 20% IV fat emulsion provides 2 kcal/ml, so a 500 ml bottle delivers 1000 kcal.

bilirubin: a pigment in the bile whose concentration in the blood may rise as a result of some disorders.

Hyperlipidemia and atherosclerosis are discussed in Chapter 28. Liver disorders are the subject of Chapter 26.

Lipid Intravenous lipid emulsions are the vehicle for fat in IV solutions. Intravenous fats are provided either daily or periodically (two or three times a week). If provided daily, IV fat serves as a concentrated source of energy; if offered less often, it serves primarily as a source of essential fatty acids.

Intravenous fat emulsions are contraindicated for newborns with markedly elevated bilirubin levels, people with some types of hyperlipidemia, people with severe liver disease, and those with severe egg allergies. Cautious use of IV lipids is recommended for people with atherosclerosis, moderate liver disease, blood coagulation disorders, pancreatitis, and some types of lung problems. After long-term administration, brown pigments may accumulate in certain liver cells, but these pigments disappear after parenteral therapy is discontinued; their effects on liver function are unknown. Prolonged IV lipid use may also enlarge the liver and spleen and reduce the number of blood platelets and white blood cells.

Micronutrients Vitamins, electrolytes (minerals), and trace elements may be used in IV solutions. Currently available IV multivitamin solutions for adults meet the recommendations of the Nutrition Advisory Group of the American Medical Association, which do not include a recommendation for vitamin K.[3] Vitamin K must be added separately or given by injection. Pediatric multivitamin solutions contain vitamin K.

Some electrolytes (particularly calcium and phosphorus) can precipitate with other IV solution components, posing life-threatening problems. As an indication of the seriousness of this problem, the Food and Drug Administration recently alerted health care professionals that a precipitate of calcium phosphate might have been responsible for at least two deaths and two cases of respiratory distress.[4] A skilled pharmacist knows how to mix solutions to minimize the risk of precipitation.

Other Additives Intravenous medications are sometimes added directly to the solution or infused into it through a separate port. Common examples include heparin, insulin, cimetidine, ranitidine, and famotidine. Providing medications along with the IV solution saves time and avoids the need for a separate infusion site. Interactions between medications and IV solutions, however, can and do occur. Deliver medications along with the IV solution only if they have been proven physically compatible with, and biochemically stable in, the solution. When drugs are added directly to the IV solution, the health care team must remember that if the total volume of solution is not infused, then the client may not receive the full dose of medication. Conversely, if the medication is not noted on the drug record, the physician may inadvertently reorder the drug, and the client may suffer potentially severe consequences.

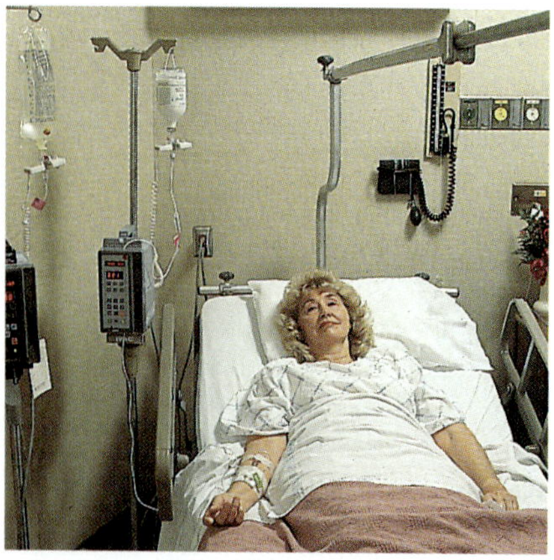

Intravenous fat emulsions provide energy and essential fatty acids and can be easily identified by their milky white color.

TYPES OF INTRAVENOUS FEEDINGS

Intravenous solutions can be provided in different ways. The method used depends on the person's immediate medical and nutrient needs, nutrition status, and anticipated length of time on IV nutrition support.

Simple IV Solutions Simple IV solutions are used routinely in hospitals to provide water, dextrose, and electrolytes to maintain the body's fluid and electrolyte and acid-base balances. Most people are expected to be able to eat within

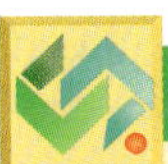

How to Calculate the Nutrient Content of IV Solutions

You can have confidence in IV solutions if you know what they contain. The basic thing to remember is that the percentage of a substance in solution tells you how many grams of that substance are present in 100 milliliters. For example, a 5 percent dextrose solution contains 5 grams of dextrose per 100 milliliters. A 3.5 percent amino acid solution contains 3.5 grams of amino acids per 100 milliliters. A 0.9 percent normal saline solution contains 0.9 grams of sodium chloride per 100 milliliters.

Suppose a person is receiving 3 liters of an intravenous solution containing 1500 milliliters of 50 percent dextrose and 1500 milliliters of 7 percent amino acids. For dextrose, the person would get:

$$\frac{50 \text{ g dextrose}}{100 \text{ ml}} = \frac{x \text{ g dextrose}}{1500 \text{ ml}}.$$

$$\frac{50 \text{ g} \times 1500 \text{ ml}}{100 \text{ ml}} = 750 \text{ g dextrose}.$$

And for amino acids:

$$\frac{7 \text{ g amino acids}}{100 \text{ ml}} = \frac{x \text{ g amino acids}}{1500 \text{ ml}}.$$

$$\frac{7 \text{ g} \times 1500 \text{ ml}}{100 \text{ ml}} = 150 \text{ g amino acids}.$$

To calculate the total kcalories in 3000 milliliters of the solution, simply multiply by kcalories per gram:

$$\begin{aligned} 750 \text{ g dextrose} \times 3.4 \text{ kcal/g} &= 2550 \text{ kcal} \\ 105 \text{ g amino acids} \times 4.0 \text{ kcal/g} &= 420 \text{ kcal} \\ \text{Total} &= 2970 \text{ kcal} \end{aligned}$$

a few days following surgery, trauma, or illness, and simple IV solutions usually meet their needs satisfactorily.

Total Parenteral Nutrition Simple IV solutions fall short of meeting total nutrient needs. People who cannot use their GI tracts for a long time, those who are malnourished, and those who have high nutrient requirements need complete parenteral nutrition support. The box above explains how to calculate the nutrient content of IV solutions.

Highly concentrated dextrose and amino acid solutions cannot be infused into the small-diameter peripheral veins, such as those in the forearm and on the back of the hand, because they become irritated and eventually collapse. To deliver all the nutrients needed using less-concentrated solutions would typically require more than 12 liters of solution a day, a volume far greater than the body could safely handle. Two options remain: peripheral parenteral nutrition or central parenteral nutrition.

Simple IV solutions typically contain 5% dextrose and normal saline. Other electrolytes or salts may be added as needed. Often 3 liters of the solution are provided daily and deliver about 150 g glucose, or about 510 kcal per day.

peripheral veins: the small-diameter veins that bring blood to the extremities (arms and legs).

Peripheral Parenteral Nutrition (PPN) For some people, nutrient needs can be met using the peripheral veins to deliver IV solutions that provide dextrose, amino acids, IV fat, vitamins, minerals, and trace elements—*peripheral parenteral nutrition (PPN)*. A typical PPN solution delivers about 2500 kcalories per day and provides about 150 grams of amino acids; IV lipid emulsions contribute more than half of the total kcalories. Intravenous lipid emulsions make it possible to deliver needed nutrients by peripheral vein because they provide a concentrated source of kcalories in a form that is isotonic to blood and less irritating to the blood vessels than highly concentrated dextrose solutions.

peripheral parenteral nutrition (PPN): the use of the peripheral veins to provide a solution that meets nutrient needs.

A typical PPN solution contains 10% dextrose and 5% amino acids. Often 3 liters of the solution are provided daily along with one 500 ml bottle of a 20% fat emulsion.

Peripheral parenteral solutions best suit people with normal renal function who need only short-term nutrition support (about 7 to 14 days), people who need additional nutrients temporarily to supplement an oral diet or tube feeding, or those in whom inserting an IV catheter into a central vein might be difficult.[5] People with very high energy requirements, people with weak peripheral veins that collapse easily, and those with fluid restrictions are not candidates for PPN.

IV catheter: a thin tube inserted into a vein through which nutrient solutions or medications can be given directly.

Total Parental Nutrition (TPN) by Central Vein Another method for meeting all nutrient needs by vein is central total parenteral nutrition, or TPN for short. In TPN, the tip of the IV catheter is either placed directly in a large-diameter central vein (see Figure 24–1) or threaded into a central vein through a peripheral vein. Almost a gallon of blood rushes through one such central vein, the superior vena cava, each minute, so highly concentrated solutions quickly become diluted. By the time these solutions reach the peripheral veins, they are no longer concentrated enough to irritate the blood vessels.

central total parenteral nutrition (TPN): a method for meeting all nutrient needs by infusing formula into a large-diameter central vein.

central veins: the large-diameter veins located close to the heart (see Figure 24–1).

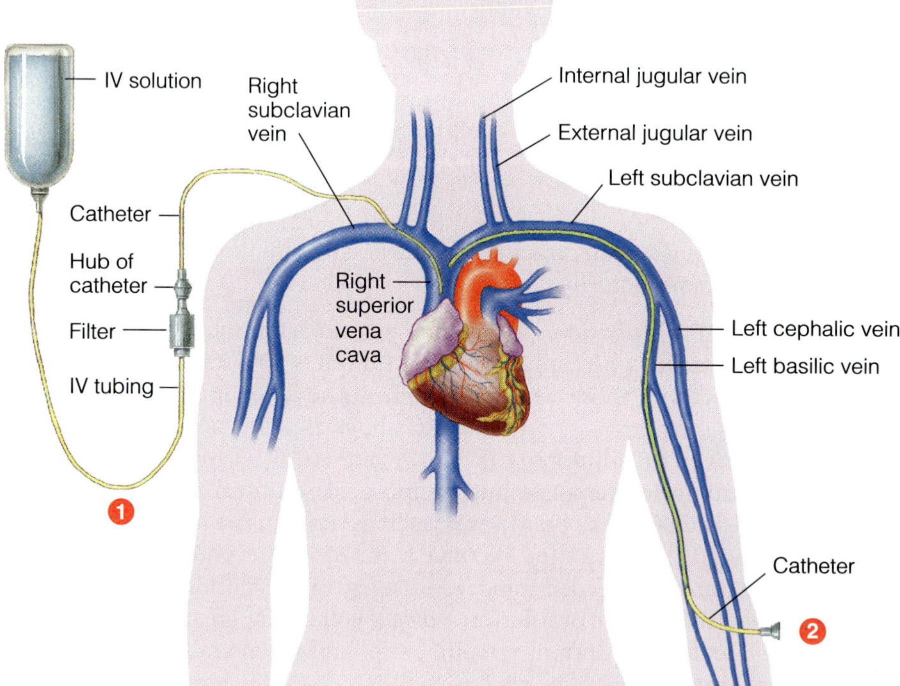

Figure 24–1

The Veins Used for TPN

1 Traditionally, TPN catheters enter the circulation at the right subclavian vein and are threaded into the superior vena cava with the tip of the catheter lying close to the heart. Sometimes catheters are threaded into the superior vena cava from the left subclavian vein, the internal jugular veins, or the external jugular veins.

2 Peripherally-inserted central catheters usually enter the circulation at the basilic or cephalic vein and are guided up toward the heart so that the catheter tip rests in a central vein, often the superior vena cava.

Table 24–1

Possible Indications for TPN by Central Vein

Acquired immune deficiency syndrome (AIDS)
Extensive small bowel resections
Radiation enteritis (inflammation of intestine caused by radiation)
Intractable diarrhea
Intractable vomiting
Severe GI tract obstructions
Bone marrow transplants
Severe acute pancreatitis
Severe malnutrition if surgical or intensive medical intervention is necessary
Hypermetabolic disorders, or major surgery, when it is anticipated that the GI tract will be unusable for more than 2 weeks
High-output enterocutaneous fistulas
Severe nausea and vomiting associated with pregnancy (hyperemesis gravidarum) when they last for more than 14 days
Low birthweight with necrotizing enterocolitis (severe GI inflammatory disease) or bronchopulmonary dysplasia (chronic lung disease)
When it is anticipated that adequate enteral nutrition cannot be established within 14 days of hospitalization

Note: If short-term parenteral nutrition support is anticipated (less than 14 days), PPN is preferred.

Source: Adapted from A.S.P.E.N. Board of Directors, Guidelines for the use of parenteral and enteral nutrition in adult and pediatric patients, *Journal of Parenteral and Enteral Nutrition* (supplement) 17 (1993): 1–49.

TPN is indicated whenever long-term parenteral nutrition will be required, when nutrient requirements are high, or when people are severely malnourished (see Table 24–1). People who need TPN for weeks or months, but risk serious complications if a catheter is inserted directly into a central vein, may be candidates for peripherally inserted central catheters.[6]

peripherally inserted central catheter (PICC): a catheter inserted into a peripheral vein and advanced into a central vein.

Regardless of how the catheter is placed, TPN should be initiated before nutrition status is severely compromised. It is much easier to maintain nutrition status than to try to replenish lost nutrient stores.

Composition of TPN Solutions The actual concentrations of amino acids, dextrose, and lipids that compose the final TPN solution are determined by each person's unique nutrient needs. TPN solutions meet energy needs primarily from dextrose. Providing too much dextrose, however, can result in hyperglycemia, a common metabolic complication associated with TPN. Clinicians recommend that the solution provide not more than 4 to 5 milligrams of dextrose per minute per kilogram of body weight.[7]

To prevent hyperglycemia, provide no more than 4 to 5 mg dextrose/min/kg body weight.

One liter of a typical central TPN solution contains 25% dextrose and 3.5% amino acids. Often 3 liters of the solution are given daily and provide about 3000 kcal and 105 g protein.

If additional energy is needed, IV lipids can be used. Intravenous fat can provide about 50 to 60 percent of the total daily energy requirement for an adult who is not severely stressed.[8] During stress, clinicians frequently restrict fat to 30 percent of the total daily energy requirement (see Chapter 25).[9]

respiratory acidosis: a condition of too much acid in the blood caused by failure of the lungs to expel carbon dioxide properly. Excess carbon dioxide is normally released from the lungs during exhalation; diseased lungs, however, are unable to perform this function rapidly enough.

Providing energy from fat helps to minimize hyperglycemia in people who are sensitive to high glucose loads. Providing more energy from fat may also help prevent respiratory acidosis in people with respiratory failure, because they are unable to expel carbon dioxide efficiently, and fat oxidation produces less carbon dioxide than glucose oxidation does. If lipids are not used as an energy source, essential fatty acid requirements may be met by giving IV lipid periodically (two to three times per week).

Researchers are actively working to identify the best types and amounts of amino acids, carbohydrates, and lipid for TPN solutions, as well as the factors affecting the bioavailability of vitamins, minerals, trace minerals, and drugs. Many of these studies are particularly relevant for clients with severe stresses and will be described in Chapter 25.

Nutrient solutions delivered by vein are called intravenous or parenteral solutions and typically contain all or a combination of the essential nutrients. Sometimes drugs are added to the solution as well. Simple IV solutions provide water, dextrose, and electrolytes; they support well-nourished people with average nutrient needs for a short time. Other people need complete parenteral nutrition, delivered either by peripheral vein (PPN) or central vein (TPN).

Intravenous Nutrition Techniques

Intravenous solutions are like tube feedings in that careful attention to selection, preparation, and delivery helps support nutrition status while minimizing the risks of complications. To prevent bacterial contamination and ensure the stability of IV solutions, they should be shielded from light and refrigerated until used. As Table 24–2 shows, many of the risks associated with IV nutrition are more serious than those associated with enteral nutrition.

INSERTION AND CARE OF THE CATHETER

Insertion of a catheter for PPN is the same as for simple IV solutions. Skilled nurses can place peripherally inserted central catheters for TPN, but a catheter for direct central access is inserted surgically by a qualified physician either at bedside or in an operating room. The client is often awake for the procedure, but is given a local anesthetic. Unnecessary apprehension can be avoided by explaining the procedure to the client.

Maintaining the integrity of peripheral veins is often a problem with PPN. Veins may become inflamed and sometimes infected. Often the infusion catheter must be removed and reinserted at a new site; consequently, long-term feedings are difficult and rarely indicated. Peripherally inserted central catheters are less irritating to the veins and can be in place longer than catheters for PPN.

The presence of disease-causing bacteria in the blood is called **sepsis**—a major complication of TPN.

Infections can develop at the catheter site in both PPN and central TPN. Compared with peripherally inserted catheters (for either PPN or TPN), though, central TPN presents a greater risk of introducing disease-causing microorganisms into the bloodstream, because the catheter is inserted so near the heart. Health care workers must inspect the catheter site regularly and change the dressing frequently to keep the site clean.

Table 24–2

Complications Associated with TPN

Catheter- or Care-Related Complications
Fluid in the chest (hydrothorax)
Air or gas in the chest (pneumothorax)
Blood in the chest (hemothorax)
Catheter tip broken off, obstructing blood flow (catheter embolism)
Air leaking into catheter, obstructing blood flow (air embolism)
Hole or tear in heart made by catheter tip (myocardial perforation)
Catheter inadvertently placed in subclavian artery (arterial puncture)
Improperly positioned catheter tip
Sepsis
Blood clot (thrombosis)
Infusion pump malfunctions
Metabolic or Nutrition-Related Complications
Elevated blood glucose (hyperglycemia)
Low blood glucose (hypoglycemia)
Dehydration
Fluid overload
Coma from excessive glucose load (hyperosmolar, hyperglycemic, nonketotic coma)
Electrolyte imbalances
Essential fatty acid deficiency
Vitamin and mineral deficiencies
Trace element deficiencies
High blood ammonia levels (hyperammonemia)
Acid-base imbalances
Elevated liver enzymes
Fatty liver
Bone demineralization

ADMINISTRATION OF THE TPN SOLUTION

Just as a tube feeding is started slowly to allow the GI tract time to adapt to the formula, a central TPN feeding is started slowly to allow the blood time to adapt to the high glucose concentration and osmolality of the TPN solution. Typically, 1 liter of TPN solution is infused at a constant rate (about 40 milliliters per hour) during the first 24 hours. An infusion pump ensures an accurate and steady delivery rate. Electrolytes and blood glucose are monitored periodically. If tests indicate electrolyte imbalances or unacceptably high blood glucose, the causes are investigated and treated. After the first 24 hours, the infusion rate is increased by 1 liter a day until the desired volume of solution is being given every 24 hours.

Recall from Chapter 23 that infusion pumps may seem like toys to young children and must be kept at a safe distance from the bed so that the child will not change the flow rate or topple the pump or IV pole.

Rapid changes in the infusion rate can cause severe hyperglycemia and hypoglycemia, which can lead to coma, convulsions, or even death, so all changes must be made gradually and cautiously. Problems are more likely to occur in people with organ dysfunction or in infants with immature organ systems. When the administration of solution gets behind or ahead of schedule, the drip rate should be adjusted to the correct hourly infusion rate, but no attempt should be made to speed up or slow down the drip rate to meet the originally ordered volume. When a person is being taken off TPN, the infusion rate of the solution must be tapered off gradually to prevent hypoglycemia. Table 24–3 provides guidelines for monitoring clients on TPN.

Peripheral TPN Infusion Unlike central TPN solutions, peripheral TPN does not have to be increased gradually when feedings are initiated or tapered off gradually when feedings are discontinued. Peripheral TPN solutions do not have the high concentrations of glucose or the high osmolality of central TPN solutions and do not present the associated problems.

IV Lipid Infusion Traditionally, IV lipid emulsions are infused separately from the TPN solution containing dextrose, amino acids, and micronutrients (see the photo on p. 784). Occasionally, people experience adverse reactions to IV lipid emulsions, particularly when the IV lipids are given in large amounts or administered too rapidly. Immediate reactions may include fever, warmth, chills, backache, chest pain, allergic reactions, palpitations, rapid breathing, wheezing, cyanosis, nausea, and an unpleasant taste in the mouth. To guard against adverse reactions, the client receives only small amounts of lipid emulsion over the first 15 to 30 minutes. After that time, the rate can be increased.

TPN solutions that contain all nutrients, including fat, are called **total nutrient admixtures, 3-in-1 admixtures,** or **all-in-one admixtures.**

When IV lipid emulsions are used as an energy source, they are often added directly to the base solution and infused along with it. The use of total nutrient admixtures for clients in the hospital as well as at home has grown dramati-

Table 24–3

Guidelines for Monitoring People on TPN

Before starting TPN:	Complete nutrition assessment.
	Confirm placement of catheter tip by X ray.
	Check blood glucose, electrolytes, chemical profile, and complete blood count.
Every 4 to 6 hours:	Check blood glucose.
	Monitor vital signs.
	Check pump infusion rate.
Daily:	Monitor weight changes.
	Record intake and output.
	Check urine specific gravity.
Daily until stable, and then 2 to 3 times weekly:	Monitor serum electrolytes, calcium, magnesium, phosphorus, and blood urea nitrogen.
Weekly:	Reassess nutrition status.
	Monitor serum proteins, ammonia, and triglycerides.
	Check the complete blood count.

cally.[10] Total nutrient admixtures must be compounded carefully, refrigerated prior to use, and mixed gently before they are infused.

Cyclic Infusion A person on cyclic parenteral nutrition receives the TPN solution at a constant rate for 8 to 12 hours a day. Because the infusion can be given during the night to allow freedom for routine daytime activities, cyclic parenteral nutrition is often used for long-term TPN. When a person receives a TPN solution continuously, insulin levels stay high. As a result, the person cannot mobilize fat stores for energy or for essential fatty acids; eventually, fat may be deposited in the liver. Cyclic TPN reverses these problems.[11] Additionally, fewer kcalories seem to be necessary to maintain nitrogen balance, probably because the person uses body fat for energy. Some people, however, cannot tolerate the delivery of a day's volume of solution over a short period of time.

cyclic parenteral nutrition: the continuous administration of TPN solutions for 8 to 12 hours with time periods when no nutrients are infused.

Careful attention to the selection, preparation, and delivery of parenteral solutions minimizes the risks of complications (review Table 24–2). Table 24–3 presents a schedule for monitoring people on TPN.

From Parenteral to Enteral Feedings

Once the problem causing the need for IV nutrition resolves, the client can gradually shift to an enteral diet while the volume of the IV solution is tapered off. The transition requires careful planning. During long periods of disuse, the intestinal villi shrink and lose some of their function. Reintroducing nutrients to the GI tract at the appropriate rate and volume will stimulate the progressive restoration of the villi's normal structure and function and prevent malabsorption and other GI discomforts.

Transitional Feedings The transition from IV feeding to an enteral diet can be accomplished in different ways and often involves a combination of feeding methods. One way is to start an oral diet while the person is still on IV nutrition. The diet is often progressive, beginning with liquids provided in small amounts. If the person cannot eat enough food to meet at least 50 percent of daily nutrient needs within a few days, and intake does not seem to be improving, tube feedings should be considered.[12]

Whether a person is given a tube feeding initially or provided an oral diet and then switched to a tube feeding, the volume of the IV solution is reduced as the volume of tube feeding is increased. The person who cannot tolerate large volumes of tube feeding can still rely on TPN to meet nutrient needs. Parenteral nutrition can be discontinued when at least 60 percent of estimated energy needs are being met by oral intake, tube feeding, or a combination of the two.[13] Chapter 23 described the transition from tube feedings to table foods.

Psychological Effects Returning to oral intake after having been fed either intravenously or by tube can have a variety of psychological effects. Some people may be extremely eager to eat again, and food can be an important morale booster. Others may be apprehensive about eating, particularly if they have had extensive GI problems. Appetite may be slow to return for some. In such circumstances, all members of the health care team can support the successful

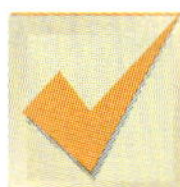

Nutrition Assessment Checklist

For People on Parenteral Nutrition Support

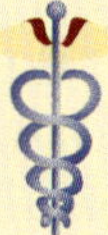

Medical Review the client's medical record for information necessary to select the appropriate feeding site (peripheral versus central), insertion method (PPN, peripherally inserted central catheter, or central TPN catheter), and IV solution. The development of undesirable symptoms related to IV fluids requires prompt treatment.

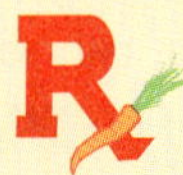

Drug Assure that drugs delivered along with IV solutions are physically compatible with the solution and that drug activity will not be adversely affected. Remember that all of the drug dosage will not be delivered if the drug has been added to the solution and the infusion is stopped for any reason.

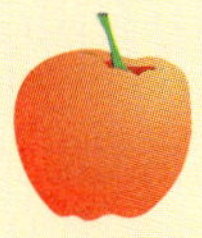

Nutrient Intake Ensure that IV solutions are being delivered as prescribed. For clients beginning enteral nutrition, determine the degree to which nutrient needs are being met by enteral formulas (orally or by tube) or by table foods, and reduce the volume of nutrient IV solutions accordingly.

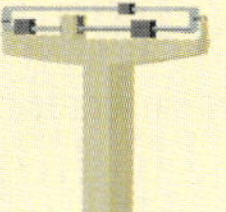

Anthropometric Assess the client's weight daily to make sure that nutrient goals are being met.

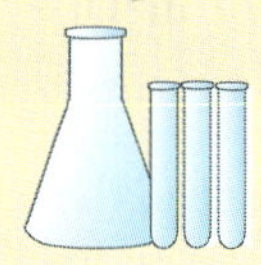

Laboratory Monitor serum and urine lab values for signs of glucose intolerance and fluid and electrolyte imbalances. Check serum protein levels to ensure that they are rising or being maintained. When available, assess nitrogen balance to determine if the IV solution is meeting the client's protein needs.

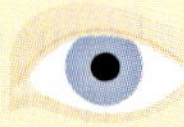

Physical Inspect catheter insertion sites for signs of infection or inflammation. Check the infusion pump drip rate as needed. Assess blood pressure, temperature, pulse, and respiration about every 4 hours. Look for physical signs of malnutrition and dehydration.

reintroduction of food. Recognize the person's concerns, and provide reassurances that you will be there to help throughout the process.

A gradual transition from an IV feeding to an oral diet helps to prevent GI problems. During the transition, the client may experience various psychological effects ranging from apprehension to eagerness.

The many decisions surrounding the provision of TPN require careful consideration. The nutrition assessment checklist reviews the areas of nutrition assessment that require attention in people on IV nutrition support, and the case study presents an example for your review.

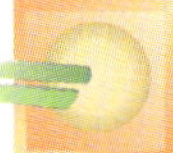

Case Study Mail Carrier Requiring Parenteral Nutrition

Mr. Rossi, a 37-year-old mail carrier has been admitted to the hospital for Crohn's disease (see Chapter 22). He has been steadily losing weight and appears emaciated. A thorough examination indicates that Mr. Rossi needs surgery as soon as possible to remove a portion of his small intestine. In the meantime, he cannot be placed on enteral feedings. The nutrition assessment reveals severe protein-energy malnutrition.

Mr. Rossi is placed on central TPN before surgery. He progresses well, gains weight, and undergoes surgery one week after admission.

What factors in Mr. Rossi's history indicate the need for central TPN? How would you explain the need for TPN to Mr. Rossi?

Describe the components of a typical TPN solution. Calculate the energy and protein that 1 liter of this solution provides.

Consider some of the physiological and psychological problems Mr. Rossi might face when enteral nutrition is reintroduced. How will the health care team know when it will be safe to take Mr. Rossi off central TPN? Describe the different ways the transition from TPN to enteral feedings can be accomplished.

Specialized Nutrition Support at Home

Occasionally, a client must continue to receive specialized nutrition support (tube feedings or parenteral nutrition) after the primary medical condition has stabilized. In such a case, continuing nutrition support at home may be an option.

Since the first report of a person sent home successfully on TPN in 1969,[14] the use of nutrition support at home has expanded rapidly. Since 1992, the number of people on home parenteral nutrition has grown from 17,000 to 40,000, while the number of people on home enteral nutrition has grown from 48,000 to 150,000.[15] As the number of people on home nutrition programs continues to grow, health care professionals who work with these programs are gaining valuable experience and improving the quality of home nutrition support. Medical supply companies provide the equipment, formulas, and services necessary to support home nutrition care.

THE BASICS OF HOME PROGRAMS

As with tube feedings and TPN in the hospital, the main objective of home enteral and parenteral nutrition is to maintain or achieve adequate nutrition status. Nutrition support at home, however, has an added dimension: it permits the person to receive nutrition care in familiar surroundings. If you have ever been in the hospital, or taken a long trip for that matter, you probably remember the comfort you experienced when you returned to your own bed, knew where things were, and could get things when you needed them. Certainly, a home nutrition support program has a big impact on the person's lifestyle, but clients report that they feel their lives have improved with home nutrition therapy.[16] Many people who require nutrition support at home can also eat some foods by mouth, and some resume activities, such as going to work, driving, and playing sports.

Cost Savings When the responsibilities formerly performed by hospital staff are assumed by the client or caregiver, the costs of nutrition support decline dramatically. One institution reports a cost savings of $1.5 million a year for ten clients maintained on home TPN versus TPN in the hospital.[17] Costs for home care are rising, however, because of the increasingly complex care available for home clients and the strict regulation of the home care industry.[18] As a result, more skilled professionals and additional time are required, and both increase costs.

Candidates for Home Nutrition Support The nutrition support team most frequently decides whether a client is a candidate for home enteral or parenteral nutrition. In addition to medical considerations, the candidate for home nutrition support and those who care for that person must have rational, stable personalities so they can successfully handle any problems that may arise. They must be capable of learning the necessary techniques and of dealing with complications. They must have adequate financial resources and access to the equipment, supplies, and professional support that are integral components of a successful home program.

Roles of Health Care Professionals Once a home nutrition program is initiated, a nurse visits the client at home, and the person also sees a physician at regular intervals. In some programs, dietitians also make home visits. A qualified nurse, dietitian, or physician must be available to answer questions and handle problems as they arise.

HOME ENTERAL NUTRITION

People on home enteral nutrition programs most commonly have cancer or swallowing disorders. Gastrostomies, and sometimes jejunostomies, usually provide access to the GI tract for long-term tube feedings (see Chapter 23). Some people learn to use transnasal tubes, which they insert at each feeding. Others have a transnasal tube inserted by a health care professional. When possible, intermittent feeding schedules are arranged so that clients are free to move around between meals. Clients on continuous feedings who must use pumps can obtain small pumps that are easily concealed and allow more freedom of movement.

The person on a home program usually purchases commercially prepared, premixed formulas. Most clients prefer these, and such formulas should certainly be used whenever a person's ability to mix the formula safely and appropriately is questionable.

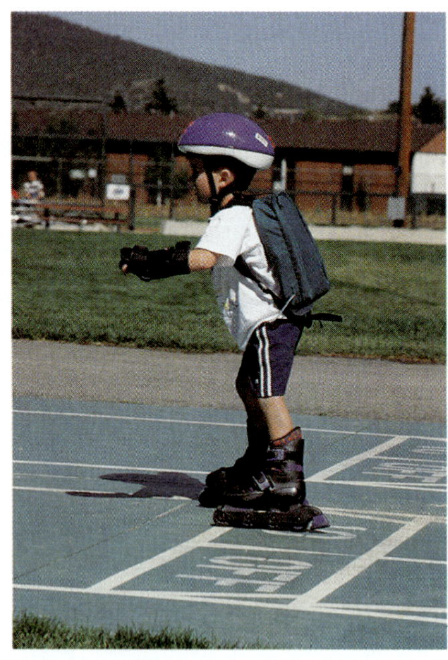

Portable pumps and convenient carrying cases allow clients who require nutrition support at home to move about freely.

HOME PARENTERAL NUTRITION

People on home TPN often have acquired immune deficiency syndrome (AIDS), cancer, Crohn's disease, or other intestinal disorders. Different types of home TPN programs are currently in use. Ideally, clients assume as much responsibility for their own care as they can handle. For example, a client who is capable of changing the catheter dressing is trained to do so. Typically, caregivers also learn the procedures so that they can assist as needed.

Special catheters, designed for long-term use, often are inserted for home TPN. The day's volume of TPN solution is frequently delivered within 8 to 12 hours using an infusion pump. Many clients prefer to infuse the solution while sleeping, so they can move about unencumbered during the rest of the day.

For people who cannot tolerate an 8- to 12-hour infusion rate, nutrients are infused over 24 hours. Those who are ambulatory may use a lightweight carrying case that holds a small pump and IV bags. This system allows the client to move around freely with little inconvenience.

Unquestionably, specialized nutrition support provides life-saving alternatives for nourishing people who cannot eat traditional diets either in the hospital or at home. Such support can be adapted for use in virtually any medical disorder, including those of the GI tract described in Chapters 21 and 22, and in severe stress, described in the next chapter.

Study Questions

1. What are the components of a typical TPN solution? What other additives may be present?
2. Describe the differences between simple IV solutions, PPN solutions, and central TPN solutions. When would each type be used?
3. How have IV lipid emulsions made it possible to meet energy requirements by peripheral vein? When are IV lipids preferable to IV dextrose for meeting energy needs?
4. How are PPN and TPN catheters inserted? Describe how PPN and TPN solutions are started and discontinued, and discuss the reasons for any differences.
5. Describe two ways that lipid emulsions can be delivered. What precautions should be taken when giving IV lipid emulsions?
6. Why is cyclic feeding of TPN solutions preferable to continuous feeding?
7. Describe some ways in which a person on parenteral nutrition can be weaned to ordinary table foods.
8. What are the advantages of home enteral and parenteral nutrition programs over hospital-administered programs?
9. Discuss how a home enteral nutrition program works. Describe some features of TPN that are unique to home programs.

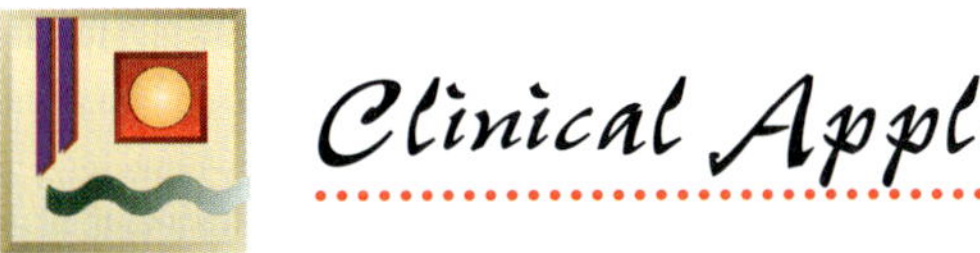

Clinical Applications

1. The development of technology for feeding people by vein has expanded our knowledge in many areas and has raised important issues as well. Specifically, the ability to meet all nutrient needs by vein has:
   - Spurred appreciation of the role of nutrition in recovery from illness and fostered identification of specific nutrients and other therapies that may aid recovery (Highlight 22 and Chapter 25).
   - Enlightened health care professionals about the importance of the GI tract during stress (see Chapter 25), thus spurring a greater understanding of both parenteral and enteral nutrition.
   - Expanded the home health care industry.

   Important issues raised as a result of the increased use of nutrition support techniques include:
   - Formula safety and efficacy. How should formulas be regulated so that their safe use can be assured (Highlight 23)?
   - Cost containment. Do the benefits of specialized nutrition support techniques justify their costs (Highlight 30)?
   - Ethics. When are special feedings appropriate (Highlight 24)?

   As you read about these developments and issues in the remaining chapters of this book, reflect on the contributions special nutrition support has made to medical care.

2. One liter of a TPN solution contains 500 milliliters of 50 percent dextrose and 500 milliliters of 8.5 percent amino acids. Determine the daily kcalorie and protein intakes of a person who receives 2 liters of this TPN solution. Calculate the average daily energy intake if the person also receives 500 milliliters of a 10 percent fat emulsion three times a week.
3. Consider what it must be like to be on a home TPN program with no foods allowed by mouth. What advantages would there be to being at home instead of in the hospital? Think of how you would manage feedings. How would you feel about the time, costs, and commitment required to maintain this therapy? How would you feel about not being able to eat after a long time? How would you handle holidays and special occasions that often center around food?

Notes

1. D. W. Wilmore and S. J. Dudrick, Growth and development of an infant receiving all nutrients exclusively by way of the vein, *Journal of the American Medical Association* 203 (1968): 860–864.
2. M. S. Dahn, Intravenous peptides, *Nutrition in Clinical Practice* 8 (1993): 93–94; J. A. Vazquez, H. Daniel, and S. A. Adibi, Dipeptides in parenteral nutrition: From basic science to clinical applications, *Nutrition in Clinical Practice* 8 (1993): 95–105; P. Fürst and P. Stehle, The potential use of parenteral dipeptides in clinical nutrition, *Nutrition in Clinical Practice* 8 (1993): 106–114.
3. J. D. Anderson, Components and compounding of total parenteral nutrition, *Support Line*, February 1993, pp. 12–15.
4. B. T. McKinnon, FDA safety alert: Hazards of precipitation associated with parenteral nutrition, *Nutrition in Clinical Practice* 11 (1996): 59–65.
5. M. A. Stokes and G. L. Hill, Peripheral parenteral nutrition: A preliminary report on its efficacy and safety, *Journal of Parenteral and Enteral Nutrition* 17 (1993): 145–147.
6. J. Z. Rogers, K. McKee, and E. McDermott, Peripherally inserted central venous catheters, *Support Line*, October 1995, pp. 6–9; S. C. Loughran and M. Borzatta, Peripherally inserted central catheters: A report of 2506 catheter days, *Journal of Parenteral and Enteral Nutrition* 19 (1995): 133–136.
7. D. K. Rosmarin, G. M. Wardlaw, and J. Mirtallo, Hyperglycemia associated with high, continuous infusion rates of total parenteral nutrition dextrose, *Nutrition in Clinical Practice* 11 (1996): 151–156: A.S.P.E.N. Board of Directors, Guidelines for the use of total parenteral nutrition in adult and pediatric patients, *Journal of Parenteral and Enteral Nutrition* (supplement) 17 (1993): 21.
8. A. M. Karch, *Lippincott's Nursing Drug Guide* (Philadelphia: Lippincott-Raven Publishers, 1997), p. 468.
9. R. G. Barton, Nutrition support in critical illness, *Nutrition in Clinical Practice* 9 (1994): 127–139.
10. D. F. Driscoll, Total nutrient admixtures: Theory and practice, *Nutrition in Clinical Practice* 10 (1995): 114–119.
11. L. M. Gramlich and B. Bistrian, Cyclic parenteral nutrition: Considerations of carbohydrates and lipid metabolism, *Nutrition in Clinical Practice* 9 (1994): 49–50.
12. R. S. DeChicco and L. E. Matarese, Selection of nutrition support regimens, *Nutrition in Clinical Practice* 7 (1992): 239–245.
13. M. F. Winkler and coauthors, Transitional feeding: The relationship between nutritional intake and plasma protein components, *Journal of the American Dietetic Association* 89 (1989): 969–970.
14. M. E. Shils and coauthors, Long-term parenteral nutrition through an external arteriovenous shunt, *New England Journal of Medicine* 283 (1970): 341–344.
15. As cited in M. Evans, Home nutrition support materials, *Nutrition in Clinical Practice* 10 (1995): 37–39.
16. M. Malone, Effect of home nutrition support on patient's lifestyle (abstract), *Journal of Parenteral and Enteral Nutrition* (supplement) 19 (1995): 23.
17. E. T. Herfinal and coauthors, Survey of home nutritional support patients, *Journal of Parenteral and Enteral Nutrition* 13 (1989): 255–261.
18. K. S. Crocker, Current status of home infusion therapy, *Nutrition in Clinical Practices* 7 (1992): 256–263.

Ethical Issues in Nutrition Care

Chapters 23 and 24 described how enteral and parenteral feedings can meet nutrient needs and support recovery in many cases. Only in the past few decades have we had the capability of providing nourishment to clients unable to eat by mouth. The technical advances made in the areas of enteral and parenteral nutrition have been life-saving for many people. Like other medical technologies, however, the availability of special nutrition support forces health care professionals and society to face ethical issues. Such treatments can prolong life by merely delaying death; the remaining life may be of low quality. Is it ever morally and legally appropriate to withhold or withdraw nutrition support?

In answering such a question, ethics experts are guided by the following principles:

- *Autonomy*—the client's right to make decisions concerning his or her own well-being.
- *Beneficence* and *maleficence*—the treatment or its withdrawal will do more good than harm, and the caregivers will promote well-being and act without selfish intent.
- *Justice*—the actions are based on fairness, honesty, and loyalty to agreements.

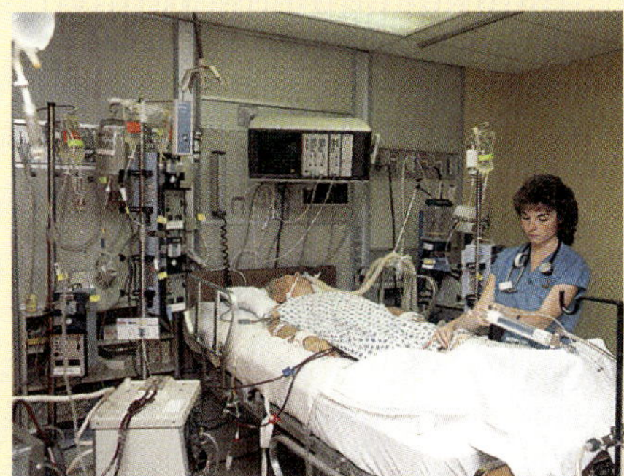

When is it morally and legally appropriate to use special nutrition support?

Glossary

advance directive: the means by which competent adults record their preferences for future medical interventions. The living will and durable power of attorney are types of advance directives.

artificial feeding: parenteral and enteral nutrition; feeding by a route other than the normal ingestion of food.

comatose: in a state of deep unconsciousness from which the person cannot be aroused.

competent: having sufficient mental ability to understand a treatment, weigh its risks and benefits, and comprehend the consequences of refusing or accepting the treatment.

death: permanent cessation of vital functions.

durable power of attorney: a legal document in which one competent adult authorizes another competent adult to make decisions for her or him in the event of incapacitation. The phrase "durable power" means that the agent's authority survives the client's incompetence; "attorney" refers to an attorney-in-fact (not an attorney-at-law).

ethical: in accordance with moral principles or professional standards. Socrates described *ethics* as "how we ought to live."

legal: established by law.

living will: a document signed by a competent adult that specifically states whether the person wishes any heroic measures to be taken in the event of terminal illness or irreversible coma from which the person is not expected to recover.

persistent vegetative state: exhibiting motor reflexes but without the ability to regain cognitive behavior, communicate, or interact purposefully with the environment.

terminal illness: a progressive, irreversible disease that will lead to death in the near future.

Ideally, these principles help people find the answers to ethical questions. In reality, though, the answers often lie entangled in personal values, charged emotions, and legal conflict. Answers rarely come easily. This highlight explores some of the ethical questions that surround the use of special nutrition support; the accompanying glossary defines related terms.

A LOOK AT THE PROBLEMS

To put the problems into perspective, consider the circumstances under which health care professionals make their decisions to feed clients. Most often, they readily provide whatever form of nutrition is necessary to support all clients who have any chance of recovering from a disease. Clearly, health care professionals cannot rightfully withhold nutrition support because of poor judgment or negligence. If a client were to die because nourishment was withheld, the staff and facility would be held responsible, and in all likelihood, a malpractice lawsuit would result. A discipline known as "medical ethics" has developed out of the need to discuss and solve problems of this nature.

The decision of whether to feed a client becomes less clear, however, when the client is not expected to recover. How aggressively do we support the person who is terminally ill or in a persistent vegetative state? How do we respond to elderly or physically disabled people who refuse special nutrition support because they feel the quality of their lives is so poor that they do not wish to be sustained? Do we (as a society) allow them such choices? Are health care professionals morally and legally obligated to comply with, or to deny, requests to discontinue feedings? Furthermore, when clients are incompetent and unable to speak for themselves, who, if anyone, should be allowed to make such life-and-death decisions?

These unanswered questions are but a few that have evolved along with the technology of special nutrition support. Occasionally, they spark intense controversy and give rise to court cases. Then the courts define the questions more clearly and lay down rules to answer them. Much more often, though, families and physicians work out their own answers to these questions. This highlight reviews the court decisions that have resolved some of the legal issues raised by these questions and also reports on how people are resolving the same questions in daily life.

NANCY CRUZAN AND THE COURTS' DECISIONS

Nancy Cruzan was a young woman who suffered permanent and irreversible brain damage after a car crash in 1983. For eight years, she was in a persistent vegetative state—awake but unaware. Her physicians and parents held no hope for recovery. They knew that few people who have had traumatic injuries recover consciousness after a year; those who do remain severely disabled.[1] Yet given food and water, Cruzan might have lived for another 30 years. Her parents requested permission to discontinue tube feeding, but their request was rejected by the Missouri Supreme Court in 1987. The court held that Cruzan never definitively stated her "right to die" wishes and that Cruzan's parents had no legal right to make such a request for her. The court said that preserving life, no matter its quality, takes precedence over all other considerations.

Unsatisfied with the Missouri Supreme Court decision, the Cruzans took further legal action. In 1989 the U.S. Supreme Court agreed to hear the *Cruzan* case. Several professional organizations—including the American Medical Association, American Academy of Family Physicians, American Association of Neurological Surgeons, American College of Surgeons, American College of Physicians, and American Society for Parenteral and Enteral Nutrition—filed briefs with the Supreme Court in support of the Cruzans.

The Cruzans tried to convince the Supreme Court that their once independent and vivacious daughter would not want to live in a vegetative state. Their lawyer argued that Cruzan had a right to be free from medical intervention. No one questioned that Cruzan's parents knew their daughter's wishes better than anyone and had the highest and most loving motives. The question for the Court was whether families (or anyone) can make life-and-death decisions on behalf of incompetent persons.

The Supreme Court recognized that competent adults have the right to stop life-sustaining treatments. But, in a 5-to-4 decision, the Court held that life-sustaining treatment could not be withdrawn without "clear and convincing" evidence that the incompetent person would refuse treatment.[2] Cruzan's statements to her roommate and family about her desire to live or die under certain conditions were insufficient to convince the Court. In making its decision, the Supreme Court entrusted state legislatures with the task of enacting laws that address the issue of whether families (or other third parties) can authorize the withdrawal of life-sustaining treatment on behalf of incompetent persons in the absence of exacting evidence.

After another round of court battles in which additional evidence did convince the Missouri trial court of Nancy Cruzan's wishes, her feeding tube was removed. She died from dehydration two weeks later. The financial and emotional costs of supporting Cruzan were enormous. In terms of money, health care costs to support her ran about $130,000 per year (paid by the state). The emotional costs are more difficult to calculate, of course. Cruzan's parents first faced the initial shock of their daughter's accident. Then, for several years, they maintained hope that with continued care she would survive and regain consciousness. Finally, they endured court battles over their child's fate—a fate that meant grief whichever way the courts decided.

Some 30,000 other families of people who live in a persistent vegetative state face similar struggles. No doubt, the Supreme Court's decision had widespread implications for these people and the health professionals who care for them. In fact, this decision touches all of us, because it influences the extent to which our society views life-sustaining treatment as optional not only for our clients, but for ourselves and our families.[3] It decides how we may be allowed to die.[4]

INDIVIDUAL RIGHTS

The emerging ethical, medical, and legal consensus seems to support the view that individual rights outweigh those of the state. Competent individuals have a legal right to refuse medical treatment—including nourishment and hydration—even when medical experts consider that treatment necessary to sustain life. In other words, even when treatment is life-saving and its refusal may bring an earlier death, clients' rights remain paramount.

Many people will agree that competent adults have the right to accept or refuse medical treatment.[5] The controversy heightens, however, when the adult is comatose, incompetent, or otherwise unable to refuse or accept medical treatment—especially when the person's wishes are not known. Without clear and convincing evidence of an incompetent person's wishes, a court must decide in favor of protecting and preserving the client's life. For many families such as the Cruzans, it becomes their burden to provide such evidence; the Supreme Court rejected the argument that families have a constitutional right to speak on behalf of their incompetent relatives.

Several court cases over the years have raised the question of whether there is a distinction between providing "extraordinary" medical care such as ventilators and providing "ordinary" care such as nourishment and hydration.[6] Some people have suggested that "pulling the plug" on a life-support machine is acceptable, but that denying food and water—the basics of life—is inhumane. The courts have defined special nutrition support as a medical procedure, and in reviewing the Cruzan case, the Supreme Court did not distinguish between nutrition and other life-saving treatments. Nor did the Court recognize a moral or legal difference between not starting life support and discontinuing it.

INFORMED CONSENT

How can people protect their rights to retain or refuse treatment in the event of incompetency? How can health care professionals provide treatment in accordance with their clients' wishes? The answers rest with the attending health care professionals, the clients, and the clients' families.

Health care professionals should initiate discussions about advance directives as part of their routine care.[7] They should encourage their competent clients to express ahead of time their preferences for medical treatments, including artificial feedings, should terminal illness or coma develop. These professionals can be a valuable source of information, but they must be careful not to project their personal views onto their clients. Each client's preferences should be noted in the medical records.

The rights and personal beliefs of both the client and health care professionals must be respected. Any health care professional who is uncomfortable or unwilling to abide by the client's stated preferences should arrange for continuing care by an equally qualified professional and then withdraw from that client's care.[8] The law does not force health care professionals to withdraw or provide treatment that is contrary to their personal beliefs or professional standards. Clients should expect that health care professionals and facilities will comply with their preferences and not merely tolerate them grudgingly.

In addition to informing their physicians, clients can state their preferences in legal documents known as living wills (see Form H24–1). A living will allows a competent adult to express clear directions regarding medical treatment in the event that the person is unable to make the necessary decisions at that time. The living will may specify that no extraordinary treatments should be administered, or alternatively it may declare that every effort should be made to maintain life. Some people regard the providing of nourishment and hydration as ordinary care, and they consider withholding or withdrawing nutrition support for any reason to be unjustified. Others consider artificial nutrition support intrusive and believe the refusal of nutrition support is justified for people who want no heroic measures taken to sustain life.[9] People who prefer that nourishment and hydration be continued or discontinued need to write this specification into their living wills to ensure that their wishes will be carried out. Physicians seem more likely to comply with a *specific* living will than with a standard one.[10]

Most states have statutes regarding the use of living wills; health care professionals should be aware of these regulations. Some states'

Form H24–1
An Example of a Living Will

DECLARATION TO MY FAMILY, MY PHYSICIAN, MY LAWYER, AND MY SPIRITUAL ADVISER

If the time arrives when I can no longer take part in decisions for my own future, this statement and Declaration shall stand as the expression of my wishes.

I recognize that death is as much a reality as birth, growth, maturity, and old age. It is but one phase in the cycle of life and is the only certainty. I do not fear death as much as I fear there is no reasonable expectation of my recovery from physical or mental disability, I wish to be allowed to die and not to be kept alive by artificial means or heroic measures, but wish only that drugs be mercifully administered to me for terminal suffering, even if they hasten the moment of my death.

I recognize that my wishes place a heavy burden of responsibility upon you, and I therefore make the following declaration with the intention of sharing this responsibility and this decision with you and of mitigating any feelings of guilt that you may have:

THIS DECLARATION is made this _____ day of __________, 19____.

I, ______________________________, willfully and voluntarily make known my desire that my dying not be artificially prolonged under the circumstances set forth below, and I do hereby declare:

If at any time I should have a terminal condition and if my attending physician has determined that there can be no recovery from such condition and that my death is imminent, I direct that life-prolonging procedures be withheld or withdrawn when the application of such procedures would serve only to prolong artificially the process of dying, and that I be permitted to die naturally with only the administration of medication or the performance of any medical procedures deemed necessary to provide me with comfort care or to alleviate pain. I desire that nutrition and hydration (food and water) be withheld or withdrawn when the application of such procedures would serve only to prolong artificially the process of dying.

In the absence of my ability to give directions regarding the use of such life-prolonging procedures, it is my intention that this declaration be honored by my family and physician as the final expression of my legal right to refuse medical or surgical treatment and to accept the consequences for such refusal.

I understand the full import of this declaration, and I am emotionally and mentally competent to make this declaration.

____
(signature)

The declarant is known to me, and I believe him/her to be of sound mind.

____
Witness

____
Witness

The foregoing instrument was acknowledged before me this _____ day of __________, 19____, by __________.

____
Notary Public

laws allow withdrawal of nutrition support; others specifically prohibit it; and still others do not mention it.[11] Form H24–1 shows how a living will might begin, and Appendix F provides an address for obtaining additional information. People should make their wishes known in writing to their attending physicians and family. Unfortunately, only one out of five adults has taken such steps.

Although most health care professionals advocate the use of living wills and agree that clients' wishes

Form H24-2
Durable Power of Attorney

I, ______________________ now residing at ______________________________ hereby constitute and appoint ______________________ as my true and lawful attorney-in-fact for me and in my name, place and stead, giving and granting unto my said attorney full power and authority to do and perform every act as fully as I might do if personally present, with full power of substitution and revocation. I hereby ratify and confirm all that my attorney shall lawfully do or cause to be done pursuant to this power.

This Power includes, but is not limited to, the right to encumber, assign or convey realty, including homestead realty. In addition, my attorney-in-fact is authorized to arrange for and consent to medical, therapeutical and surgical procedures for me as principal, including the administration of drugs.

I have executed this Power while in command of my faculties and with knowledge of the consequences, both legal and practical.

This Durable Power of Attorney shall not be affected by my disability as principal except as provided by statute.

IN WITNESS WHEREOF, I have hereunto set my hand and seal this _____ day of __________, 19___.

WITNESSES:

______________________________ ______________________________ (SEAL)

____

STATE OF ________________
COUNTY OF ________________

I HEREBY CERTIFY that on this day, before me, a Notary Public duly authorized in the State and County named above to take acknowledgments, personally appeared ______________________ to me known to be the person described in and who executed the foregoing DURABLE POWER OF ATTORNEY, and said individual acknowledged before me that execution of this instrument was for the uses and purposes herein expressed.

WITNESS my hand and official seal in the State and County named above this _____ day of __________, 19___.

(SEAL)

____
NOTARY PUBLIC

should be honored, actual medical care may not always reflect these beliefs. In practice, physicians are more likely to follow family directives concerning tube feedings and other life support than the instructions in a living will.[12] If people wish to ensure that they receive medical care consistent with their individual wishes, they need to discuss their living wills and hypothetical scenarios with family members before medical conditions arise that will necessitate others making decisions for them.

In many states, the durable power of attorney offers clients a way to ensure that their wishes will be carried out (see Form H24–2). Some states have enacted statutes authorizing the use of durable powers of attorney specifically for health care.[13] A durable power of attorney allows a competent adult to designate another competent adult (usually a relative or close friend) as an agent to make health care decisions in the event of incapacitation. In essence, it says, "I give this person the right to make health care decisions on my behalf should I become unable to make them."

Ideally, the person representing the client will make decisions that reflect the client's health care preferences. In reality, though, when faced with hypothetical situations, clients and those who would have to decide for them agree on treatment only 70 percent of the time.[14] Such discrepancy is natural because each views the other's experience as most important when making decisions. Clients want to avoid burdening their families, and families want to provide any treatment that offers a possible cure or relief from pain.

The person who plans ahead for future care in the case of a terminal illness or irreversible state of unconsciousness relieves others of the guilt and some of the anxiety of having to make decisions. Imagine the anguish a family member goes through in directing the health care team to stop nutrition support, knowing its cessation will hasten death. That decision is a little easier if the family member knows that it is what the individual would want or, better yet, if a legal document takes the decision out of the family's hands altogether.

When the person's wishes regarding life-sustaining measures are unknown, life support can be discontinued only if the burden of providing it clearly and markedly outweighs the benefits to the individual. Providers must also consider the pain caused by withdrawing the treatment in weighing the benefits against the negative aspects of treatment.

The questions raised in this highlight have no easy answers, yet decisions must be made. Each case must be carefully decided individually. Most hospitals have established ethics committees to deal with problems such as those presented here. Health care professionals should ensure that their disciplines are represented on such committees and become familiar with their profession's ethics policies and guidelines.[15] In addition, education programs designed to help professionals develop the analytical skills needed to resolve ethical dilemmas can be most beneficial.[16] Education enables professionals to make informed decisions and promote greater public awareness of these issues.[17]

NOTES

1. The Multi-Society Task Force on PVS, Medical aspects of the persistent vegetative state, *New England Journal of Medicine* 330 (1994): 1572–1579.
2. *Cruzan v. Director, Missouri Department of Health*, __ U.S. __, 110 S.Ct. 2841, 111 L.Ed.2d 224 (1990).
3. M. Angell, Prisoners of technology: The case of Nancy Cruzan, *New England Journal of Medicine* 322 (1990): 1226–1228; B. Lo, F. Rouse, and L. Dornbrand, Family decision making on trial—Who decides for incompetent patients? *New England Journal of Medicine* 322 (1990): 1228–1232.
4. The Court and Nancy Cruzan, *Hastings Center Report*, January/February 1990, pp. 38–50.
5. R. Burck, Feeding, withdrawing, and withholding: Ethical perspectives, *Nutrition in Clinical Practice* 11 (1996): 243–253.
6. T. W. Mayo, Forgoing artificial nutrition and hydration: Legal and ethical considerations, *Nutrition in Clinical Practice* 11 (1996): 254–264.
7. *Advance Directives: The Role of Health Care Professionals* (Columbus, Ohio: Ross Products Division, Abbott Laboratories, 1996).
8. C. R. Gallagher-Allred, Managing ethical issues in nutrition support of terminally ill patients, *Nutrition in Clinical Practice* 6 (1991): 113–116.
9. G. Chapman, An oncology patient's choice to forgo novolitional nutrition support: Ethical considerations, *Nutrition in Clinical Practice* 11 (1996): 265–268.
10. J. W. Ely and coauthors, The physician's decision to use tube feedings: The role of the family, the living will, and the *Cruzan* decision, *Journal of the American Geriatrics Society* 40 (1992): 471–475.
11. H. Brody and M. B. Noel, Dietitians' role in decisions to withhold nutrition and hydration, *Journal of the American Dietetic Association* 91 (1991): 580–585.
12. Ely and coauthors, 1992.
13. A. M. Capron, The implications of the *Cruzan* decision for clinical nutrition teams, *Nutrition in Clinical Practice* 6 (1991): 89–94.
14. J. Hare, C. Pratt, and C. Nelson, Agreement between patients and their self-selected surrogates on difficult medical decisions, *Archives of Internal Medicine* 152 (1992): 1049–1054.
15. American Dietetic Association, Position of The American Dietetic Association: Legal and ethical issues in feeding permanently unconscious patients, *Journal of the American Dietetic Association* 95 (1995): 231–234; American Academy of Pediatrics Committee on Bioethics, Guidelines on forgoing life-sustaining medical treatment, *Pediatrics* 93 (1994): 532–536; A.S.P.E.N. Board of Directors, Ethical and legal issues in specialized nutrition support, *Journal of Parenteral and Enteral Nutrition* (supplement) 17 (1993): 50–52; American Dietetic Association, Position of The American Dietetic Association: Issues in feeding the terminally ill adult, *Journal of the American Dietetic Association* 92 (1992): 996–1005.
16. S. Edelstein and S. Anderson, Bioethics and dietetics: Education and attitudes, *Journal of the American Dietetic Association* 91 (1991): 546–548.
17. M. G. Wall and coauthors, Feeding the terminally ill: Dietitians' attitudes and beliefs, *Journal of the American Dietetic Association* 91 (1991): 549–552.

Nutrition and Severe Stress

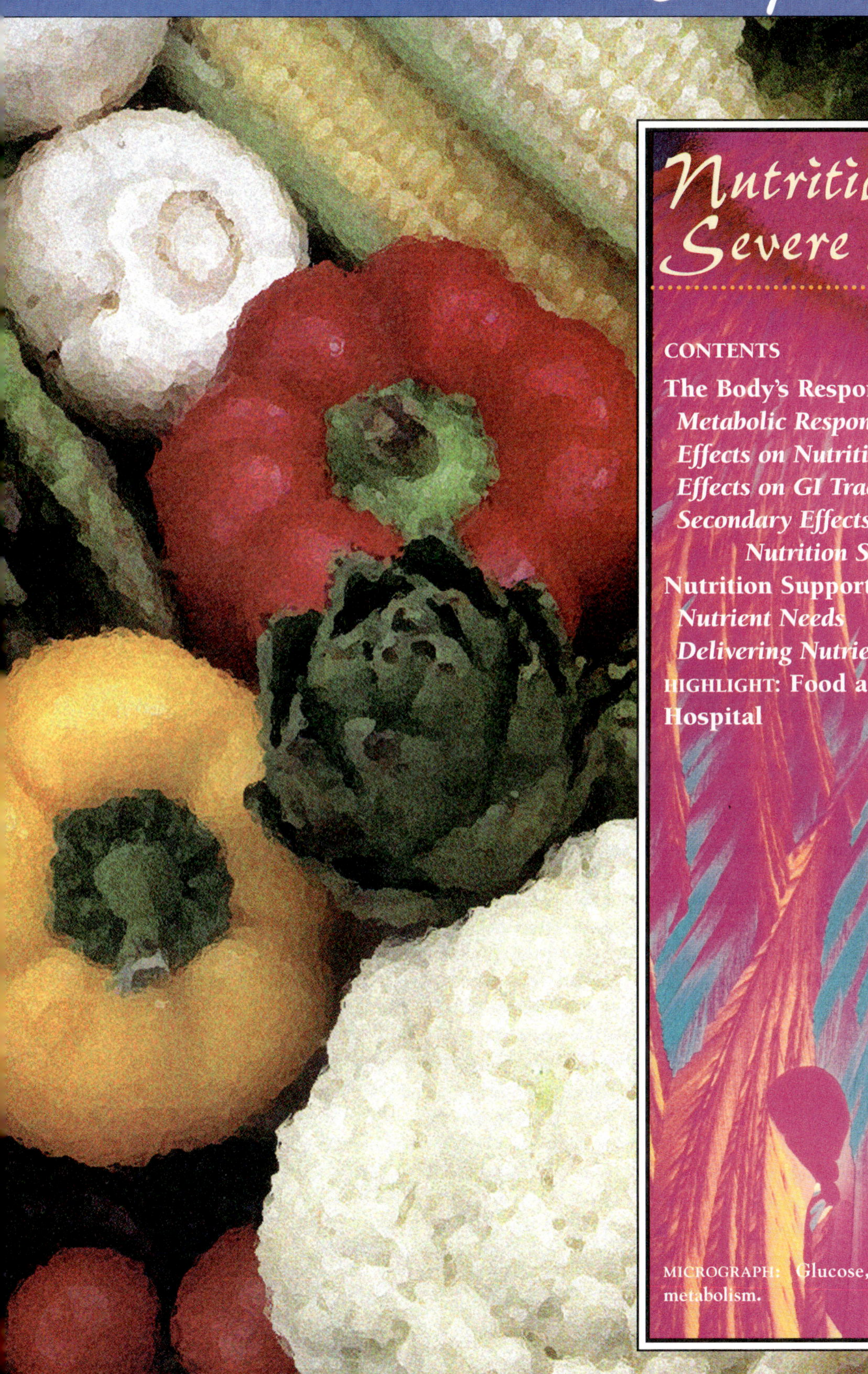

CONTENTS

MICROGRAPH: Glucose, the central player in energy metabolism.

Reminder: Any threat to a person's well-being is a *stress*. Some stresses fall within the body's normal and healthy functioning and are known **physiological stresses**. Outside these limits, additional stresses imposed by disease or trauma are **pathological stresses**. The term **severe stresses** is used here to refer to pathological stresses that rapidly and markedly raise the body's metabolic rate and significantly upset its normal internal balance.

trauma: physical insult to the body that causes tissue damage including fractures, wounds, burns, or surgery.

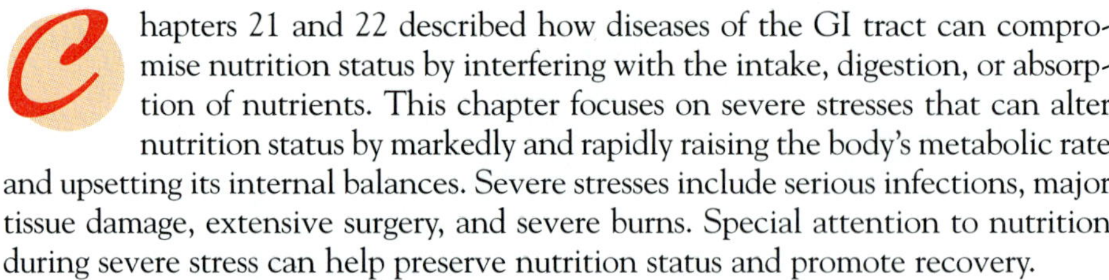

Chapters 21 and 22 described how diseases of the GI tract can compromise nutrition status by interfering with the intake, digestion, or absorption of nutrients. This chapter focuses on severe stresses that can alter nutrition status by markedly and rapidly raising the body's metabolic rate and upsetting its internal balances. Severe stresses include serious infections, major tissue damage, extensive surgery, and severe burns. Special attention to nutrition during severe stress can help preserve nutrition status and promote recovery.

The Body's Response to Stress

All illnesses can threaten the body and impair nutrition status to some extent, but the burden of severe stresses is exceptionally great. Such stresses require that the body employ complicated mechanisms to reestablish its balance. These mechanisms, which are collectively called the stress response, constitute an adaptation that is sustained for as long as is necessary or until the body can no longer sustain them and exhaustion leads to death.

Reminder: The *stress response* is an elaborate series of metabolic events orchestrated by the body in response to *stressors* such as severe infections, extensive surgery, major burns, serious or multiple fractures, and deep, penetrating wounds such as gunshot wounds, fistulas, and surgical incisions. These stressors lead to tissue injury or necrosis (death), inflammation, or shock.

METABOLIC RESPONSES TO SEVERE STRESS

In response to severe stresses, the body speeds up its metabolic rate (hypermetabolism) and mobilizes nutrients into glucose and amino acid pools, so that it can synthesize the special factors it needs to limit and repair damage and to regain homeostasis. These metabolic responses are mediated by immune, inflammatory, and hormonal factors.

The exact factors the body makes depends on the type of stress. Mending a broken bone requires different factors than does healing a wound or fighting an infection. Researchers are working to elucidate the complex and interrelated mechanisms of the stress response in order to find new approaches to promote recovery.

inflammatory response: the changes that occur in tissues when they are injured by such forces as blows, wounds, foreign bodies (chemicals, microorganisms), heat, cold, electricity, or radiation.

The fluid containing plasma proteins, electrolytes, and immune factors that leaks out through the capillaries is called the **exudate**.

exudare = to sweat out

During an infection, the body is invaded by disease-causing microorganisms or viruses. An infection may remain localized in one area and form an abscess or granuloma, or it may enter the bloodstream and, thereby, the whole body. The presence of microorganisms or their poisonous products in the bloodstream is known as **sepsis** or **septicemia** (sep-tih-SEE-me-ah).

Immune System and Inflammatory Responses The body's natural defense against pathogens—the immune system—enables the body to fight off infectious agents. The immune system defends the body so alertly and silently that most healthy people are unaware that thousands of microbes mount attacks against them every day. Occasionally, though, an infection succeeds in making a person ill, and the immune system must then mount a counterattack. Of all severe stresses, serious infections most intensely tax the immune system, and if the system fails, death may follow.

In other severe stresses, the immune system plays a key, although less obvious, role. Tissue damage renders the body vulnerable to invading organisms. The body's inflammatory response to tissue injury inactivates invaders, removes foreign particles, and repairs tissue damage. At the site of injury, the capillaries dilate and become more permeable, allowing blood, blood proteins, and immune system factors to flow into the injured area. The accumulation of fluid in the interstial space causes edema. Eventually, blood flow to the injured tissue slows, and clots form around the injured area, sealing it off from the rest of the body and limiting the spread of invaders. Meanwhile, immune system factors at the injury site begin to attack and neutralize the foreign substances. If the immune factors fail, the infection may remain localized and form an abscess or granuloma, or it may spread throughout the body. When infectious microorganisms or their poisonous by-products invade the bloodstream, sepsis develops. Critically ill people who develop sepsis may experience progressive failure of multiple organ systems. Such a combination is the most common cause of serious complications and death in critically ill people.

The immune and inflammatory responses to stressors result in redness, swelling, heat, and pain at the injury site. Body temperature, heart rate, and respiratory rate increase; blood concentrations of iron and zinc fall; and anorexia develops. All of these changes are believed to assist the immune system in fighting infection. In some responses, particularly if a bacterial infection is involved, white blood cell production increases. Among the hundreds of factors that mediate the body's complex response to inflammation are the *cytokines,* factors believed to contribute to the hypermetabolism, GI tract changes, anorexia, fever, and malaise that accompany the inflammatory response.[1]

Hormonal Factors Hormonal changes characteristic of the immediate stress response drive catabolism by shifting the balance between insulin, which promotes the storage of carbohydrate and lipid and the synthesis of protein, and the counterregulatory hormones, which promote the breakdown of glycogen, the mobilization of fatty acids from lipids, and the synthesis of glucose from protein (see Table 25–1). As a result, the metabolic rate rises, and the body mobilizes energy stores and elevates blood glucose at the expense of protein tissue. Other

Reminder: An abscess is an accumulation of pus and may contain immune system cells and foreign bodies. Treatment involves draining the abscess.

Reminder: A granuloma is a granular growth that contains foreign bodies surrounded by immune system cells and covered with a fibrous coat; the body may retain live bacteria in the form of a granuloma for years without exhibiting symptoms of infection.

The changes that result from the activation of immune and inflammatory factors during stress are sometimes called the **systemic inflammatory response syndrome (SIRS)**

cytokines (SIGH-toe-kynes): immune system factors that help regulate the inflammatory response. During infections, the cytokine *interleukin-1* (in-ter-LOO-kin) causes fever-induced anorexia, the cytokine *cachetin* (ka-KEK-tin) also induces anorexia, and the cytokine *gamma-interferon* (in-ter-FEAR-on) induces fever and malaise.

Reminder: The metabolic breakdown of large molecules into smaller ones is *catabolism*. Catabolic reactions usually release energy.

counterregulatory hormones: hormones such as glucagon, cortisol, and catecholamines that oppose insulin's actions and promote catabolism.

Table 25–1

Hormonal Changes That Occur during Severe Stress

Hormone	Alteration	Metabolic Effect
Catecholamines	Increase	Glucagon release increases. Insulin-to-glucagon ratio decreases.[a] Glycogen breakdown increases. Glucose production from amino acids increases. Mobilization of free fatty acids increases.
Cortisol	Increases	Mobilization of free fatty acids increases. Glucose production from amino acids increases.
Glucagon	Increases	Insulin-to-glucagon ratio decreases.[a] Glucose production from amino acids increases. Glycogen breakdown increases. Storage of glucose, amino acids, and fatty acids decreases.
Antidiuretic hormone	Increases	Retention of water increases.
Aldosterone	Increases	Retention of sodium increases.

Note: These changes are part of the immediate stress response. As adaptation occurs and recovery is in progress, hormone levels gradually return to normal.
[a]The net effect of a decrease in the ratio of insulin to glucagon is that catabolism predominates.

The acute, or flow, phase of the stress response is the catabolic period immediately following the onset of stress. During the adaptive phase, the body adjusts to the stress to minimize losses. If adaptation succeeds, recovery follows. If adaptation fails, exhaustion follows.

Not all amino acids can be used to make glucose. The most important amino acids in glucose production are alanine and glutamine; they are synthesized in the body from the branched-chain amino acids.

Reminder: *Ketone bodies* are compounds formed during the incomplete oxidation of fatty acids.

hormones promote the retention of water and sodium and the excretion of potassium. With recovery, hormones gradually return to normal. To understand the impact of severe stress on nutrient stores, it is helpful to compare the body's response to simple fasting and severe stress.

Response to Simple Fasting Fasting (see pp. 239–244) and severe stresses both require the body to use its stored carbohydrate and fat for energy and to mobilize amino acids to make glucose. The body adapts to simple starvation by reducing its use of glucose, thus conserving its vital proteins. The liver begins to produce an alternate energy source from fat—ketone bodies. At the same time, the metabolic rate and body temperature fall, reducing the body's need for energy from any source. The person feels fatigued and uses less energy.

Response to Severe Stress In contrast to simple fasting, severe stress raises the metabolic rate for an extended time. Carbohydrate continues to be oxidized for energy, but despite high blood glucose levels, amino acids continue to be used for glucose synthesis. Fat metabolism increases as well, but the high insulin levels suppress the mobilization of fat from body stores. Plasma levels of essential fatty acids fall dramatically, and clinical signs of deficiency may develop in as few as 10 days.[2] Figure 25–1 illustrates the metabolic differences between simple fasting and severe stress.

Figure 25–1

Metabolic Responses to Fasting and Stress

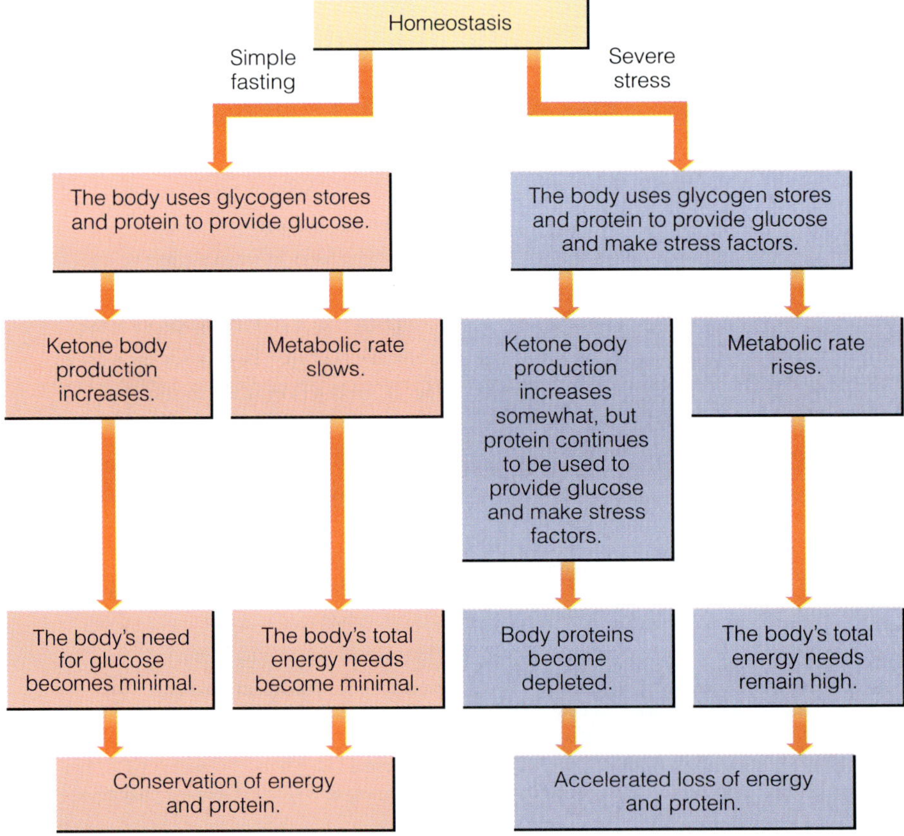

Generally, hypermetabolism peaks at about 3 to 4 days and subsides in about 7 to 10 days.[3] Clinical findings typical of the stress response—elevated blood glucose (hyperglycemia), negative nitrogen balance, elevated blood urea nitrogen (from protein catabolism), increased retention of fluid and sodium, and increased excretion of potassium—gradually return to normal as the stress resolves.

EFFECTS ON NUTRITION STATUS

The effects of hypermetabolic illnesses and protein-energy malnutrition (PEM) show astonishing similarities. Both deplete energy reserves, cause the breakdown of protein tissue, impair nutrient absorption, and tax the immune system.

Unlike glucose and fat, protein is not held in reserve in case the body needs it. All of the body's proteins are already in use as skeletal muscle, cell structures, enzymes, hormones, immune system factors, and other blood proteins and body components. During stress, the body needs extra protein to synthesize additional hormones to orchestrate metabolism, immune factors to fight infection, collagen to rebuild damaged tissue and bone, muscle cells to maintain the physical work of taxed organ systems, and many more vital tissue constituents. Without adequate protein, the body loses its ability to adapt, and it becomes vulnerable and defenseless.

Acute Malnutrition In a previously healthy person, extreme or prolonged stress can trigger a dramatic and immediate form of acute malnutrition. The rerouting of nutrients to make stress response factors leaves the body unable to meet its regular protein and energy needs. The body is effectively "starved" for these nutrients. In addition, the body's organs and cells have not had time to adapt to conserving protein by using fat (ketone bodies) for energy. That adaptation is also made more difficult by stress. Providing adequate nutrition support to the client with acute malnutrition precipitated by stress is extremely difficult.

Chronic Malnutrition People with chronic PEM do not have the nutrient reserves to successfully mount a stress response. They require immediate nutrition support and generally respond well when the stress is not too severe. The person's body has adapted to limited energy and protein intake over a prolonged period by conserving lean body mass to the greatest extent possible and depending on fat stores for energy.

Mixed Malnutrition When the person with chronic malnutrition is faced with an extreme or prolonged stress, or when adequate nutrients are not provided, the person experiences the deficits of both conditions. Likewise, the person with acute malnutrition may progress to mixed malnutrition. Table 25–2 shows the clinical findings that distinguish the different forms of malnutrition.

Nutrient Absorption Organs that undergo rapid cell replacement—such as the GI tract—are among the first to suffer the consequences of protein losses, whether they occur due to stress or to malnutrition. The intestinal microvilli gradually shrink and become nonfunctional; up to 90 percent of them can be lost.

Gastric Motility Severe stress reduces blood flow to the GI tract and slows gastric motility, prohibiting the use of oral diets in the early poststress period. But

Figure 25–2

Stress, Malnutrition, and Immunity

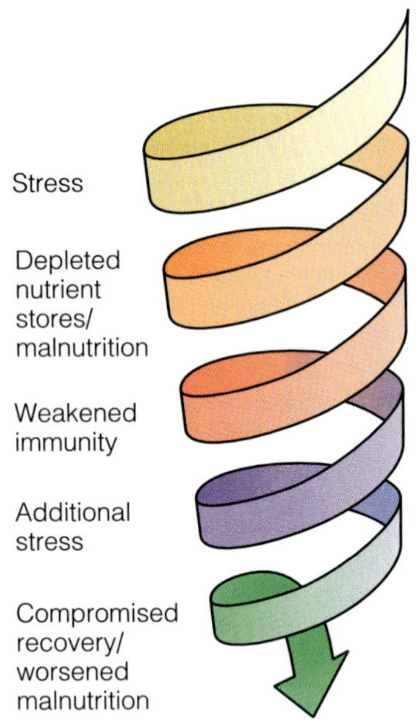

Regardless of where a person enters the spiral, the effects of stress, malnutrition, and impaired immunity can interact to worsen malnutrition and compromise recovery.

Table 25–2

Clinical Findings Used to Distinguish Different Types of PEM

	Weight and Fat Stores	Blood Protein, Internal Organs, and Immune Function
Acute Malnutrition (Kwashiorkor)	Excessive or adequate	Depleted/compromised
Chronic Malnutrition (Marasmus)	Low/depleted	Adequate
Mixed Malnutrition	Low/depleted	Depleted/compromised

when people—even healthy people— are fed entirely by vein, their intestinal tracts undergo structural and functional changes.[4] Lack of enteral nutrients in the GI tract further contributes to reduced GI blood flow and reduced motility. Thus stress interferes with the person's ability to handle oral nutrients, and even though adequate nutrients are provided, the GI tract will have a compromised ability to absorb them. Consequently, PEM may develop or worsen, and the body may have difficulty providing the extra energy and protein it needs to fight the stress.

Appetite and Eating As described earlier, immune factors involved in the stress response cause fever, malaise, and pain and interfere with appetite and eating, even when oral diets are possible. The location of an injury may also interfere with eating. A person with burned hands, for example, may be unable to hold eating utensils. A person with a surgical incision near the waist may find sitting up to eat uncomfortable.

Other GI Effects Some severe stresses further impair GI tract function. Wounds or trauma to the GI tract, including surgical resections, can interfere with nutrient intake and aggravate malabsorption and nutrient losses.

To understand the relationship of PEM to severe stress, think of energy stores and protein status as money in the bank. Severe stress can be compared to a major expense that arises unexpectedly. The person who has saved enough money can pay off the expense without too much difficulty. If more and more expenses arise, however, the money may run out. The person with little or no savings is unable to pay even a small expense.

Left unattended, PEM can interact with stress in a deadly cycle: stress worsens malnutrition, and malnutrition hinders the stress response (see Figure 25–2). Malnutrition renders the body vulnerable to infections and markedly interferes with the ability to recover.

EFFECTS ON GI TRACT IMMUNE FUNCTION

The significant role of the GI tract in preventing foreign invaders from entering the body has only recently received the attention it deserves. A protective coating of mucus lines the entire GI tract. The mucus contains antimicrobial chemicals and enzymes to destroy foreign bodies and forms a slippery coat that prevents invaders from attaching to the lining of the GI tract. To reach the intestine, invaders must also avoid destruction by the highly acidic contents of the stomach. Invaders that enter the intestine directly (through breaks in tissue) or avoid destruction by mucus or gastric acidity encounter other formidable obstacles in the intestinal tract.

Recall from Chapter 22 that disorders or drug therapies that significantly raise gastric pH may result in bacterial overgrowth and malabsorption.

Intestinal Barrier Function Healthy intestinal villi are crowded close together, forming a physical barrier that prevents anything from passing between them. Damaged cells allow substances to cross the intestinal cells' membranes and enter the body.

Immune System Cells Interspersed among the villi are mucus-secreting cells and lymph tissue that houses immune cells to fend off invaders. To appreciate the vast importance of the intestinal lymph tissue in fighting foreign invaders, consider that of all the body's immunologic-secreting cells, 70 to 80 percent of them are located in the intestine.[5]

Bacterial Flora The large intestine also supports a bacterial population that inhibits the growth of harmful bacteria by competing with them for nutrients and space. The normal bacterial flora also produce short-chain fatty acids (see Highlight 22) that prevent harmful bacteria from sticking to the intestinal surface.

Bacterial Translocation Conditions that compromise the GI tract's barrier, alter the normal bacterial flora, or compromise the function of the immune system may allow infectious agents to cross the intestinal barrier and enter the body—a process called translocation.[6] Table 25–3 lists conditions that may increase the likelihood of translocation; many of these conditions exist during severe stress or malnutrition. In small amounts, the translocation of infectious

translocation: the passage of infectious agents into the body through the intestinal tract.

Table 25–3

Conditions That Increase the Likelihood of Translocation

Conditions
Altered structure and function of GI tract barrier
Prolonged fasting or lack of enteral nutrients
Injury to the GI tract
Inflammatory responses
Malnutrition
Changes in bacterial flora
Lack of enteral nutrients
Decreased GI tract motility
Use of broad-spectrum antibiotics
Compromised function of immune factors
Malnutrition
Hypermetabolism

Source: Adapted from M. T. DeMeo, The role of enteral nutrition in maintaining the structural and functional integrity of the GI tract, in *Enteral Nutrition Support,* Report of the First Ross Conference on Enteral Devices, Ross Laboratories 1996, pp. 4–8.

agents may stimulate the immune system, but extensive translocation may cause serious infection and even death.

Research suggests that translocation may be a major factor in the development of sepsis and multiple organ failure.[7] Frequently, multiple organ failure does not occur until days or weeks after the initial stress. Regardless of the type of stress, the typical course of multiple organ failure is remarkably similar in all people, suggesting that common factors may be involved. People with multiple organ failure develop sepsis, and the first organs to fail are the lungs, followed by the liver and kidneys. Some of the infectious agents associated with multiple organ failure arise from the intestinal tract.[8] Clinical evidence to support a role for intestinal translocation as a primary factor, or even one of the factors, leading to sepsis and multiple organ failure following severe stress is lacking, and the theory remains unproven.[9] In practice, however, measures to support intestinal integrity including early enteral nutrition (described later) are widely accepted and utilized by clinicians.

SECONDARY EFFECTS OF STRESS AND ILLNESS ON NUTRITION STATUS

Some effects of stress or illness on nutrition status arise not from the stress itself, but rather from its consequences or treatment. A person suffering from anxiety and psychological stress associated with an injury, for example, may lose all interest in eating.

Immobility and Pressure Sores Stresses often necessitate bed rest and immobility. Immobility further compromises nutritional health. Without the muscle tension and weight load incurred by normal activity, the muscles and bones are not stimulated to maintain themselves and begin to lose nitrogen and calcium, respectively. In prolonged immobilization, blood and urinary calcium may rise so high that calcium stones form in the bladder and kidneys.

Immobility, severe stress, and poor food intake are all associated with the development of pressure sores.[10] Pressure sores can form whenever there is constant pressure on the skin. The elderly and people who are unable to respond to pain or change body positions are at great risk for developing pressure sores. These sores can be extremely painful and are an open invitation to infections, which can further contribute to stress and tax nutrient stores.

pressure sores: the breakdown of skin and underlying tissues due to constant pressure and lack of oxygen to the affected area; often called decubitus (dee-CUE-bih-tis) ulcers or bedsores.

Diagnostic Tests and Medical Procedures Diagnostic tests and medical procedures may require special diets or no food by mouth in order to obtain accurate test results or to protect health. Such restrictions further interfere with a person's ability to receive adequate nourishment.

Nutrient-Drug Interactions Drug therapy, critical in the treatment of many stresses and illnesses, may further tax nutrition status. When people who are severely stressed or malnourished are given multiple drugs, the likelihood of drug-nutrient interactions increases, and serious deficiencies may result. Furthermore, the intestinal changes associated with both stress and malnutrition can hinder the absorption of both drugs and nutrients.

Severe stresses and malnutrition can also interfere with the metabolism and excretion of drugs. Many drugs are transported in the blood bound to serum pro-

Rx PRESCRIPTION PAD

Drugs used in the treatment of severe stresses may include:

- Analgesics
- Antidiarrheals
- Anti-infective agents
- Anti-inflammatory agents
- Antiulcer agents
- Immunosuppressants

See Appendix E for timing with meals and nutrition-related side effects.

teins such as albumin, and low serum albumin is a symptom of both stress and PEM. Without sufficient carriers, drugs may be slow to reach their sites of action. Once drugs do arrive at their target cells, the lack of carriers may delay the drugs' transport to the liver and kidneys, where many drugs are detoxified and excreted. Thus drugs may take a long time to work and then may remain active for a longer time, making side effects more likely.

In summary, severe stresses spark a series of hormonal and metabolic responses to reestablish balance. These changes demand energy and drain nutrient stores, which can lead a well-nourished body rapidly into PEM and send a malnourished body perilously close to death.

Nutrition Support during Stress

Following stress, the immediate concerns are to restore blood flow and maintain oxygen transport and to prevent or treat infection. Possible measures include giving transfusions, providing IV solutions to correct fluid and electrolyte imbalances, removing dead tissues, draining abscesses, and administering antibiotics. Nutrition support following stress helps to prevent acute malnutrition, preserve organ function, maintain immune defenses, and minimize nutrient losses—all of which aid the client's recovery. Restoring nutrient deficits before the hypermetabolism that initially accompanies stress subsides is difficult, however. Once hypermetabolism does subside, nutrition support can promote positive nitrogen balance and weight gain.

Nourishment must be introduced cautiously to the stressed person with PEM. If nutrients are introduced too rapidly, severe complications, including malabsorption, cardiac insufficiency, respiratory distress, congestive heart failure, convulsions, coma, and even death, can result. Collectively, these complications are called the refeeding syndrome.

When a sudden drop in the blood volume disrupts the supply of oxygen to the tissues and the return of blood to the heart, **shock** results. Shock is a critical event that must be corrected immediately. Many severe stresses can lead to shock through massive bleeding or severe dehydration.

The removal of dead tissue resulting from burns and other wounds, called **debridement** (dee-BREED-ment), speeds healing and helps prevent infection.

Chapter 22 described dietary modifications beneficial in treating malabsorption. Dietary therapy for other organ system failures is described in later chapters: liver failure (Chapter 26), heart failure (Chapter 28), respiratory failure (Chapter 28), and kidney failure (Chapter 29).

refeeding syndrome: a set of physiologic and metabolic complications associated with reintroducing adequate nutrition too rapidly for a person with severe PEM. These complications can include malabsorption, cardiac insufficiency, respiratory distress, congestive heart failure, convulsions, coma, and possibly death.

NUTRIENT NEEDS

Health professionals caring for severely stressed individuals face a challenge. Providing enough nourishment, but not too much, is critical to recovery.

Fluids and Electrolytes People experiencing severe stress often lose fluids and electrolytes through bleeding, wounds, vomiting, diarrhea, and fever. To restore blood volume and prevent dehydration and electrolyte imbalances, the medical team must act quickly to stabilize the body's fluid and electrolyte balances.

The physician determines the person's fluid needs based on clinical measures such as blood pressure, heart rate, respiratory rate, urinary output, level of consciousness, and body temperature. Serum electrolytes are closely monitored and adjustments are made as necessary.

With catabolism, electrolytes normally concentrated in the intracellular fluids (potassium, phosphorus, magnesium, and calcium) rise and disrupt the body's chemical balances. Once hypermetabolism subsides, these intracellular electrolytes move into the cells along with glucose and amino acids to begin rebuilding tissue. Without careful attention to replacement, circulating levels of these electrolytes can plummet, resulting in life-threatening complications.

Table 25–4

The Harris-Benedict Equation for Estimating Energy Needs

Harris-Benedict equation for estimating basal energy expenditure (BEE):[a]

Women:

BEE = 655 + (9.6 × wt[b] in kg[c]) + (1.7 × ht in cm[c]) − (4.7 × age in yr)

Men:

BEE = 66 + (13.7 × wt[b] in kg[c]) + (5 × ht in cm[c]) − (6.8 × age in yr)

Add to BEE for activity:

20% Sedentary

35% Moderately active

50% Active

Add to BEE for stress:

10–15% Uncomplicated elective surgery

20–40% Complicated surgery or fractures

50–100% Major burn

Add to BEE for fever (if present):

13% per degree centigrade over normal body temperature (37°C)[c]

Add to BEE to promote weight gain (if necessary):

5% if weight loss is moderate

10–15% if weight loss is severe

For people with a %IBW greater than 125, adjust the weight used in the BEE equation by following this equation:[d]

(Actual body weight − IBW) × 25%[e] + IBW = Adjusted body weight

[a]Basal metabolic rate (BMR, described on p. 262) and BEE express the same thing: basal energy need. The equation for BMR is traditionally used in physiology and fitness laboratories; that for BEE, in hospitals. The two equations yield slightly different results, each suitable for the purposes intended. Adjustments for activity used in the hospital differ from those on p. 264 for similar reasons. All are approximations; all require judgment in their application.

[b]Use actual body weight, not ideal body weight.

[c]See Appendix D for equations to convert pounds to kilograms, inches to centimeters, and degrees Fahrenheit to degrees centigrade.

[d]From J. M. Karkeck, Adjustment for obesity, *American Dietetic Association Renal Practice Group Newsletter*, Winter, 1984.

[e]Approximately 25 percent of body fat tissue is metabolically active.

Reminder: Indirect calorimetry is the estimation of energy output from measures of the amount of oxygen used and carbon dioxide eliminated.

Energy Energy needs during severe stress depend on both the type and severity of the stress, organ function, and the individual's metabolic state and nutrition status. Energy requirements may double for clients with severe burns, for example.[12] When measurements are carefully taken and cautiously interpreted, indirect calorimetry provides an accurate assessment of energy needs during severe stress.[11] Many facilities lack the equipment necessary to perform this measurement, however, so clinicians often rely on various other estimates of energy needs. The Harris-Benedict equation shown in Table 25–4 is frequently used.* Alternatively, some clinicians simply provide minimally stressed clients

*Several studies suggest that the Harris-Benedict equation overestimates energy needs during severe stress.

with 25 to 30 nonprotein kcalories per kilogram of body weight per day. (Note: kcalories from protein are not counted as meeting part of the energy needs when this formula is used.) The box on p. 814 shows how to estimate energy and protein needs during severe stress. Clinical judgment and continual monitoring of nutrition status are always necessary to confirm that energy needs are being met without overfeeding.

Supplying too much energy contributes to an elevated metabolic rate, which increases the use of oxygen and the production of carbon dioxide. Then the heart and lung muscles, already working hard as a consequence of stress, must work even harder to keep the body's gases in balance. If these vital organs are weakened by malnutrition, they may not be able to respond to the additional insult. Supplying too little energy compromises recovery.

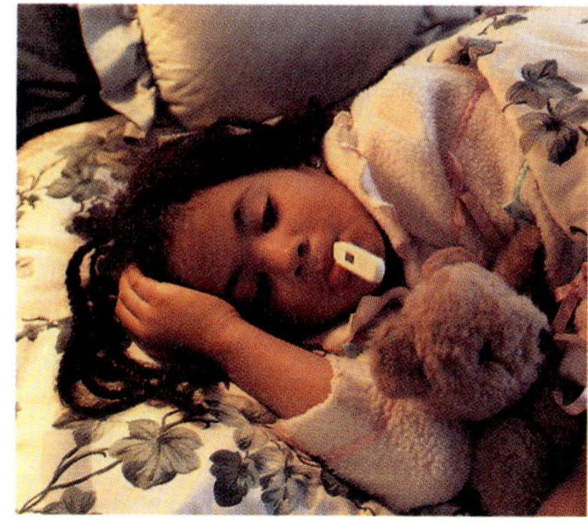

The energy needs of a child with a fever (a mild stress) are elevated, but not nearly as high as those of a person with extensive burns (a severe stress).

Fever, a frequent consequence of stress, is associated with an elevated basal metabolic rate (BMR) of approximately 13 percent for each degree centigrade (7 percent for each degree Fahrenheit) that the temperature rises above normal (98.6° Fahrenheit; 37° centigrade). Thus a person with a fever of 4 degrees (Fahrenheit)—that is, a temperature of 102.6°F—will have a BMR that is running about a fourth faster than normal (4 degrees × 7 percent = 28 percent). Since the BMR requires some 1000 to 2000 kcalories a day (recall from Chapter 8), this person may need an additional 300 to 600 kcalories a day.

A **fever** is an elevation of body temperature above normal. A person who is **febrile** (FEE-brile) has a fever; **afebrile** (AY-fee-brile) means "without fever."

Reports suggest that people who are obese and mildly to moderately stressed may be able to attain positive nitrogen balance and recover while receiving about half of their estimated energy needs, provided that protein needs are met.[13] Obese people who are severely stressed, however, need no less energy during the hypermetabolic phase than people of normal weight.[14] Energy restriction is not appropriate, and weight-loss efforts should wait until recovery is well under way.

Protein The greater the stress, the more body protein is broken down (up to the limit of the body's capabilities), the more nitrogen is excreted in the urine, and the greater the need for protein. Only after the hypermetabolic stage of stress subsides can negative nitrogen balance be fully corrected. Clinicians can use nitrogen balance studies to determine how much dietary protein the stressed person needs. Alternatively, they can estimate protein needs by providing 1 to 2 grams of protein per kilogram of body weight per day. People with severe burns may require up to 3 grams of protein per kilogram of body weight per day.[15] As always, adequate energy from nonprotein kcalories is necessary to spare protein use for energy.

Amino Acids In recent years, increasing attention has been placed on supplying higher amounts of specific amino acids during stress, rather than simply supplying protein. Research has been far from conclusive, but some studies suggest that supplementing branched-chain amino acids (leucine, isoleucine, and valine) may minimize negative nitrogen balance.

Reminder: Branched-chain amino acids and glutamine participate in gluconeogenesis. Glutamine and arginine may help augment the immune system.

Another amino acid receiving wide attention in relation to stress is glutamine. As Highlight 22 described, glutamine provides fuel for intestinal cells and helps maintain their structure and function. During stress, glutamine may become a conditionally essential amino acid. Most enteral and parenteral formulas lack glutamine because it is unstable in solution. Studies to determine whether supplemental glutamine helps to minimize negative nitrogen balance,

How to Estimate Energy and Protein Needs Following Severe Stress

Bernadette is a 39-year-old female, who is 5 feet 3 inches tall and weighs 130 pounds. She recently underwent extensive surgery and currently has a temperature of 101°F. Her energy needs can be estimated using the Harris-Benedict equation as follows:

$$\text{Weight in kilograms} = 130 \text{ lb} \div 2.2 \text{ kg} = 59 \text{ kg}.$$

$$\text{Height in centimeters} = 63 \text{ in} \times 2.54 \text{ cm} = 160 \text{ cm}.$$

$$\text{BEE} = 655 + (9.6 \times \text{wt in kg}) + (1.7 \times \text{ht in cm}) - (4.7 \times \text{age in yr}).$$

$$655 + (9.6 \times 59 \text{ kg}) + (1.7 \times 160 \text{ cm}) - (4.7 \times 39) = 655 + 566 + 272 - 183 = 1310 \text{ kcal}.$$

Next add 20–40% × BEE for surgery (see Table 25–4 on p. 812):

$$1310 \text{ kcal} \times 20\% = 262 \text{ kcal}.$$

$$1310 \text{ kcal} \times 40\% = 524 \text{ kcal}.$$

$$1310 + 262 = 1572 \text{ kcal}.$$

$$1310 + 524 = 1834 \text{ kcal}.$$

Bernadette needs between 1572 and 1834 kcalories to meet her BEE and additional energy needs due to surgery.

To determine additional energy needs for fever, you must first convert degrees Fahrenheit to degrees centigrade (see Appendix D):

$$°\text{C} = \tfrac{5}{9}(°\text{F} - 32°).$$

$$°\text{C} = \tfrac{5}{9}(101° - 32°) = \tfrac{5}{9}(69°) = 38°\text{C}.$$

Normal body temperature is 37°C, so Bernadette has a body temperature elevation of 1°C.

To determine the percentage of the BEE needed due to fever:

$$1° \times 13\% = 13\%.$$

Add 13% BEE for fever:

$$1310 \times 13\% = 170 \text{ kcal}.$$

Add fever needs to energy needs:

$$1572 \text{ kcal} + 170 \text{ kcal} = 1742 \text{ kcal}.$$

$$1834 \text{ kcal} + 170 \text{ kcal} = 2004 \text{ kcal}.$$

Bernadette's estimated energy needs range from about 1750 to 2000 kcalories; clinicians monitor weight changes to determine if actual needs are higher or lower. Her energy needs will change as stress resolves.

Protein needs for Bernadette can be estimated at 1 to 2 grams of protein per kilogram of body weight per day. Use her weight of 59 kilograms to make the calculation:

$$59 \text{ kg} \times 1 \text{ g/kg} = 59 \text{ g protein}.$$

$$59 \text{ kg} \times 2 \text{ g/kg} = 118 \text{ g protein}.$$

Bernadette needs an estimated 59 to 118 grams of protein daily. Clinicians can monitor serum proteins (see Chapter 16) or use nitrogen balance studies to determine if the estimate is meeting actual protein needs.

protect the structure and function of the intestinal tract, and enhance the immune system have produced promising, yet inconclusive results.[16] Whether these effects can prevent translocation also remains to be proven.

Other nitrogen-containing substances, including arginine and nucleotides, may be important following severe stress. Studies suggest that supplemental arginine may help minimize negative nitrogen balance, improve wound healing, and stimulate the immune system. Nucleotides may help improve the function of certain immune cells. Studies are sparse, however, and their results have been variable.

nucleotides: nitrogen-containing components of RNA and DNA. Nucleotides can be synthesized in the body and therefore are not essential in the diets of healthy individuals. In severely stressed individuals, however, a dietary source may be beneficial.

Carbohydrate and Fat Nonprotein energy sources spare protein, so the amount of carbohydrate and fat to recommend has ramifications for stressed people. Carbohydrate provides a readily usable source of energy, but the body can only metabolize a fixed amount (about 500 grams per day) of glucose during stress. Excess glucose may contribute to hyperglycemia and its consequences.[17] Fat provides essential fatty acids and energy, but given in excess, it can also tax metabolic functions and hamper immune responses. Clinicians often supply nonprotein kcalories through a mixture of 70 to 75 percent glucose and 25 to 30 percent lipids.[18] For clients with burns, restricting fat further (15 to 20 percent of the nonprotein kcalories) appears to be beneficial.

Fatty Acids Intravenous lipid emulsions and enteral formulas are rich sources of omega-6 fatty acids. When given in excess of essential fatty acid requirements, however, omega-6 fatty acids may impair immune function and, therefore, may be inappropriate for severely stressed clients.[19] Alternate lipid sources such as fish oils (a rich source of omega-3 fatty acids) are currently under investigation. Triglycerides chemically modified to contain both long- and medium-chain fatty acids may also be advantageous during stress.[20] Highlight 22 described short-chain fatty acids and their potential benefits.

Micronutrients Vitamin and mineral needs during stress are highly variable, and specific requirements are unknown. The need for many B vitamins increases when energy and protein intakes increase. Some micronutrients act as cofactors in the many metabolic reactions that are occurring, so their levels dwindle quickly. Other micronutrients play specific roles in healing wounds and mending broken bones. Levels of antioxidant nutrients fall, and although research is lacking, supplementing these nutrients is believed to be of value.[21] Other vitamins and minerals are frequently supplemented at levels above the RDA as well.

Stress Formulas Clinicians eager to improve a client's outcome often rely on enteral formulas designed to meet nutrient needs during stress. Many such formulas are high in kcalories and protein. Some contain extra vitamins A and C, zinc, and other nutrients designed to promote wound healing. Formulas designed to preserve immune function often contain added glutamine, arginine, nucleotides, and omega-3 fatty acids. Although such formulas appear to be beneficial for specific situations, further research is necessary to determine their impact on recovery.[22]

Growth Hormone and Insulinlike Growth Factor Researchers have begun to study nondietary factors that might improve nitrogen balance and lessen the

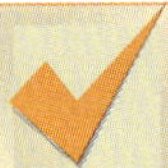

Nutrition Assessment Checklist
For People with Swallowing Disorders

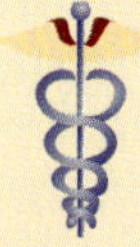

Medical Use the medical record to determine the degree and type of stress and to help estimate prestress nutrition status.

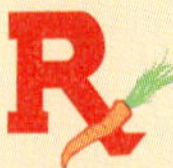

Drug Assess the client's drug history for drug-nutrient interactions that might alter nutrient needs.

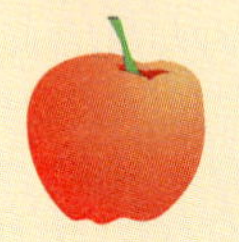

Nutrient Intake Calculate nutrient intake from parenteral and enteral formulas and oral diets to determine if intake is meeting calculated needs. If not, investigate the cause and take corrective actions, when possible. For severely stressed clients, indirect calorimetry may provide a more accurate assessment of energy needs. For clients on oral diets, a careful history of food preferences will be invaluable in encouraging adequate oral intake.

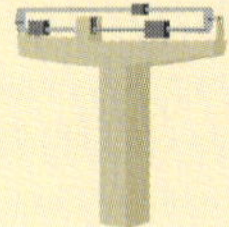

Anthropometric Interpret anthropometrics cautiously in the immediate poststress period. Weights may reflect the infusion of fluids or edema and can be deceptively high. The location of injuries may make anthropometric measurements impossible.

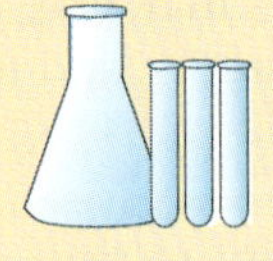

Laboratory Anticipate low serum protein in stressed clients, especially those with burns or severe wounds. (Remember that plasma proteins leak through the capillaries to the injury site.) Use nitrogen balance studies for a more accurate assessment of protein needs for severely stressed clients when necessary. Check blood glucose at regular intervals and treat hyperglycemia according to the hospital's protocol or physician's orders. Monitor electrolytes to replace losses immediately after stress and to prevent metabolic complications once hypermetabolism subsides.

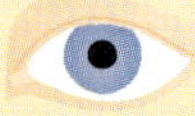

Physical Check for physical signs of nutrient deficiencies, energy level, and emotional state. Regular assessment of blood pressure, pulse, and intake and output records can help prevent dehydration or overhydration.

impact of severe stress on the host. Highlight 22 described two such factors, growth hormone and insulinlike growth factor-1 (IGF-1), which stimulate the growth of intestinal cells. Although research is limited, growth hormone has been shown to improve nitrogen balance in both animals and people.[23] Similarly, IGF-1 improves nitrogen balance in animals.[24]

DELIVERING NUTRIENTS DURING STRESS

Selecting the appropriate amounts and types of nutrients to help people recover from stress is only part of diet therapy. Just as important is supplying nutrients in a form that best serves the body's ability to recover.

Oral Diets Well-nourished clients who are expected to eat within a few days following a mild-to-moderate stress receive simple IV solutions to maintain fluid and electrolyte balances and provide minimal kcalories. Once GI motility returns, they begin an oral diet that often progresses from clear liquids to full liquids and on to soft and then regular foods as tolerated (see Chapter 22). Highlight 25 describes how foods are prepared and delivered to meet clients' needs while hospitalized.

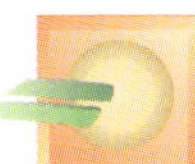

Case Study Journalist with a Third-Degree Burn

Mr. Sampson, a 48-year-old journalist, has been admitted to the emergency room. He suffered a severe burn covering over 40 percent of his body when he was trapped in a building fire. His height on admission was 6 feet, and he weighed 175 pounds. The physician ordered lab work, including serum proteins; the results are not back yet.

Identify Mr. Sampson's immediate postinjury needs. How can these needs be met?

Do you have enough information to determine Mr. Sampson's preinjury, preburn nutrition status? If not, what information would be useful? Is information about preburn nutrition status important in this case? Why or why not?

Considering Mr. Sampson's condition, what problems might the dietitian encounter in getting information from him about his preburn nutrition status?

Calculate Mr. Sampson's energy and protein needs to support burn healing (use 2 × the BEE for energy and 2 to 3 grams of protein per kilogram of body weight). What other nutrients must be considered?

Describe the possible benefits of early enteral nutrition to Mr. Sampson. How might these benefits be particularly important following a severe burn injury?

Specialized Nutrition Support People with severe malnutrition, those who undergo severe stresses, and those who are not expected to be able to eat within 10 days benefit from parenteral nutrition or tube feedings. Oral or gastric feedings have to wait until gastric motility is restored to prevent abdominal distention, nausea, vomiting, and the possible aspiration of foods or formula into the lungs. Peristalsis returns more quickly to the small intestine than to the stomach, however, and feeding formula directly into the small intestine through a tube is not only possible, but provides advantages over parenteral nutrition.[25] Early feeding (initiated within about 36 hours following stress) stimulates intestinal blood flow, function, and adaptation and may minimize hypermetabolism and help prevent translocation. Most significantly, however, early enteral feeding improves recovery following stress by reducing septic complications.[26] Early enteral feeding following major trauma, head injuries, extensive burns, and surgery improves clinical outcomes. Early enteral feedings are not possible in cases where blood flow to the intestine is severely disrupted, however. Additionally, some clients may need both enteral feedings and parenteral nutrition until they are able to meet all nutrient needs orally.

Once hypermetabolism subsides and oral feeding is possible, clients can begin to receive enteral formulas or table foods. Chapters 23 and 24 described the different ways that clients can be weaned from tube feedings or parenteral nutrition. The box on p. 757 described ways to encourage oral intake. The nutrition assessment checklist summarizes the important information necessary to monitor the nutrition care of stressed clients. The accompanying case study of a client with burns tests your knowledge of nutrition and severe stress.

The stresses of surgery, infections, and burns can place tremendous demands on the body. The body uses all of its resources to fight the battle to survive and regain health. Recovery depends, in part, on the body's receiving the energy and nutrients required to mount a defense, repair damaged tissues, and replenish nutrient reserves. The next chapter describes the ways liver diseases affect nutrition status.

Study Questions

1. What is the stress response, and what does it achieve?
2. How do immune system factors and hormones mediate the stress response?
3. How do acute and chronic PEM relate to stress? Describe the effect of nutrition status on the body's ability to respond to stress. How can stress rapidly lead to PEM?
4. How do stress and PEM affect vital organ systems, gastric motility, and GI tract absorptive and immune functions?
5. Describe how nutrient needs change during severe stress. Describe precautions that must be taken when feeding the acutely or chronically malnourished person with stress.
6. Why might enteral nutrition be preferable to parenteral nutrition after a severe stress? Why can enteral nutrients be delivered by tube into the small intestine but not be taken by mouth in the early poststress period? When are enteral feedings inappropriate?

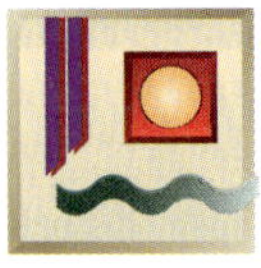

Clinical Applications

1. Returning to Bernadette from the box on p. 814, recalculate her energy needs using the estimate of 25 to 30 nonprotein kcalories per kilogram of body weight per day. Now add the kcalories to meet protein needs. Compare these results with those obtained using the Harris-Benedict equation. Are the estimates similar?
2. Assuming that Bernadette can tolerate an intact enteral formula, find at least three formulas in Appendix K that meet her energy and protein needs and supply at least 100 percent of the RDA for vitamins and minerals.
3. Susan Griff is a 28-year-old woman admitted to the hospital following a car accident in which she broke several bones, ruptured a portion of her small intestine, and suffered a severe burn. Aside from the nutrient demands imposed by these stresses, describe how the following factors can impair her nutrition status:

   - Susan's injuries are painful.
   - Susan's medications cause extreme drowsiness.
   - Susan is depressed.
   - Susan is often out of her room for X rays and other diagnostic tests when her food trays arrive.
   - Susan's food intake is often restricted for diagnostic tests she will be receiving.

   How might these problems be resolved to improve Susan's ability to eat?

Notes

1. R. G. Barton, Nutrition support in critical illness, *Nutrition in Clinical Practice* 9 (1994): 127–139.
2. Barton, 1994.
3. J. D. Anderson, F. A. Moore, and E. E. Moore, Enteral feeding in the critically injured patient, *Nutrition in Clinical Practice* 7 (1992): 117–122.
4. A. L. Buchman and coauthors, Parenteral nutrition is associated with intestinal morphologic and functional changes in humans, *Journal of Parenteral and Enteral Nutrition* 19 (1995): 453–460.
5. P. Brandtzaeg and coauthors, Immunobiology and immunopathology of human gut mucosa: Humoral immunity and intraepithelial lymphocytes, *Gastroenterology* 97 (1989): 1562–1584.
6. M. T. DeMeo, The role of enteral nutrition in maintaining the structural and functional integrity of the gastrointestinal tract, in *Enteral Nutrition Support*, Report of the First Ross Conference on Enteral Devices, Ross Laboratories, 1996, pp. 4–8.
7. DeMeo, 1996; E. V. Shronts, Enteral versus parenteral nutrition: A clinical review, *Support Line*, June 1996, pp. 10–13; K. A. Kudsk, Clinical applications of enteral nutrition, *Nutrition in Clinical Practice* 9 (1994): 165–171.
8. Shronts, 1996.

9. T. O. Lipman, Bacterial translocation and enteral nutrition in humans: An outsider looks in, *Journal of Parenteral and Enteral Nutrition* 19 (1995): 156–165.
10. B. J. Braden, Using the Braden Scale for predicting pressure sore risk, *Support Line,* August 1996, pp. 14–17.
11. C. Porter and N. H. Cohen, Indirect calorimetry in critically ill patients: Role of the clinical dietitian in interpreting results, *Journal of the American Dietetic Association* 96 (1996): 49–54.
12. W. W. Souba, Nutritional support, *New England Journal of Medicine* 336 (1997): 41–48.
13. J. C. Burge and coauthors, Efficacy of hypocaloric total parenteral nutrition in hospitalized obese patients: A prospective, double-blind randomized trial, *Journal of Parenteral and Enteral Nutrition* 18 (1994): 203–207.
14. P. Amato and coauthors, Formulaic methods of estimating calorie requirements in mechanically ventilated obese patients: A reappraisal, *Nutrition in Clinical Practice* 10 (1995): 229–232.
15. D. J. Rodriguez, Nutrition in major burn patients: State of the art, *Support Line,* August 1995, pp. 1–8.
16. T. R. Ziegler, Glutamine supplementation in catabolic illness, *American Journal of Clinical Nutrition* 64 (1996): 645–647.
17. D. K. Rosmarin, G. M. Wardlaw, and J. Mirtallo, Hyperglycemia associated with high, continuous infusion rates of total parenteral nutrition dextrose, *Nutrition in Clinical Practice* 11 (1996): 151–156, A.S.P.E.N. Board of Directors, Guidelines for the use of total parenteral nutrition in adult and pediatric patients, *Journal of Parenteral and Enteral Nutrition* (supplement) 17 (1993): 21.
18. M. M. Gottschlich, Selection of optimal lipid sources in enteral and parenteral nutrition, *Nutrition in Clinical Practice* 7 (1992): 152–165; R. H. Bower, Nutritional and metabolic support of critically ill patients, *Journal of Parenteral and Enteral Nutrition* (supplement) 14 (1990): 257–259; G. L. Blackburn, In search of the "preferred fuel," *Nutrition in Clinical Practice* 4 (1989): 3–5; F. Negro and F. Cerra, Nutritional monitoring in the ICU: Rational and practical application, *Critical Care Clinics* 4 (1988): 34–47.
19. A. Hyltander, R. Sandström, and K. Lundholm, Metabolic effects of structured triglycerides in humans, *Nutrition in Clinical Practice* 10 (1995): 91–97.
20. Hyltander, Sandström, and Lundholm, 1995; E. Pscheidi and coauthors, Effects of chemically defined structured lipid emulsions on reticuloendothelial system function and morphology of liver and lung in a continuous low-dose endotoxin rat model, *Journal of Parenteral and Enteral Nutrition* 19 (1994): 33–40.
21. V. Sardesai, Role of antioxidants in health maintenance, *Nutrition in Clinical Practice* 10 (1995): 19–25.
22. R. G. Barton, Immune-enhancing enternal formulas: Are they beneficial in critically ill patients? *Nutrition in Clinical Practice* 12 (1997): 51–62.
23. K. Takagi and coauthors, Recombinant human growth hormone and protein metabolism of burned rats and esophagectomized patients, *Nutrition* 11 (1995): 22–26.
24. T. Inaba and coauthors, Effects of growth hormone and insulin-like growth factor-1 (IGF-1) treatments on the nitrogen metabolism and hepatic IGF-1–messenger RNA expression in postoperative parenterally fed rats, *Journal of Parenteral and Enteral Nutrition* 20 (1996): 325–331.
25. Souba, 1997; Shronts, 1996; Kudsk, 1994.
26. K. A. Kudsk, Immunologic support: Enteral vs parenteral feeding, in *Enteral Nutrition Support,* Report of the First Ross Conference on Enteral Devices, Ross Laboratories 1996, pp. 70–74.

Highlight 25

Food and Foodservice in the Hospital

People who suffer severe stresses, as well as many others, require a level of care that necessitates hospitalization. These people often have illnesses that interfere with appetite either directly or through the psychological stress of the illness or the hospitalization itself. The hospital's dietary department, under the direction of management dietitians and foodservice managers, faces a challenge in planning, producing, and delivering meals designed to accommodate dozens of special diets and food preferences. This highlight explores the problems health care professionals must resolve when feeding clients in the hospital and describes how hospital foodservice systems work. Although this discussion focuses on hospitals, much of the discussion applies to any health care facility that serves meals to large groups of people, including nursing homes, assisted living centers, and residential mental health care facilities. While people in hospitals may eat poorly, they can make up for nutrient deficits by eating well when they return home. The resident of a long-term care facility does not have this option. For this reason, dietary departments in long-term care facilities must make even greater efforts to ensure that their clients receive nutritious and appealing foods.

THE CLIENT'S PERSPECTIVE

What comes to mind when you see or hear the words "hospital food"? What are your own experiences with hospital food or the experiences of someone close to you? Viewing hospital food from a client's perspective will add to your understanding of nutrition care.

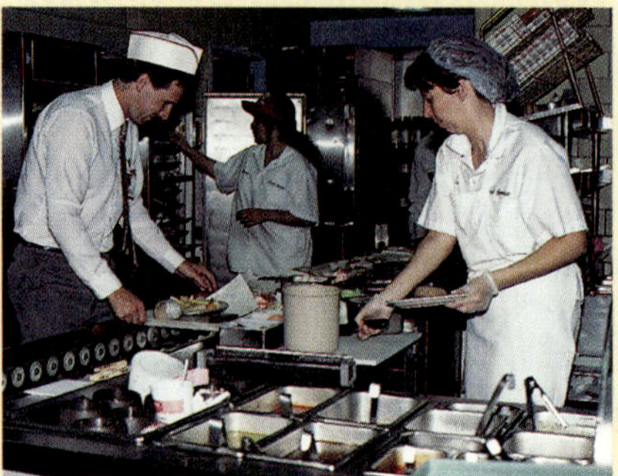

Dietary departments prepare foods to accommodate dozens of special diets and hundreds of food preferences.

Most people generally look forward to eating, and in the hospital, eating may become even more enjoyable than usual, for it offers clients familiarity in an otherwise strange environment. It is also one of the few experiences in the hospital where clients have a choice. Consider that clients usually cannot choose when they will receive tests, how much blood will be drawn, what nurse will care for them, or what time they will have surgery. But they usually can select their meals, and they can also exercise some control: they can eat or refuse to eat!

Clients may complain about hospital food. Complaining may have little to do with the food itself, but serves instead as a way to vent fear, frustration, anger, and physical pain. Clients need opportunities to express their feelings, and often you may find that a problem can be resolved simply by listening and providing emotional support.[1] Actual food problems need to be corrected by the dietary department as soon as possible.

Problems with foodservice unrelated to a client's physical or mental state can interfere with appetite. For one, the hospital does not cook food the same way a client does at home—a considerable problem when the client must eat three meals a day for many days in the hospital. Unfortunately, hot foods may not be hot and cold foods may not be cold by the time they arrive in the client's room. In addition, the client receives meals at specified times regardless of hunger and often must eat without companionship in bed, which can be more of a chore than a pleasurable experience. Meals may be unwelcome if they follow painful treatments. Food is so important to most people that a bad experience with it in the hospital can make both the client and those who work with the client agitated and angry.

All of this is not to say that every person in the hospital has a problem with meals. The majority of clients will eat adequate amounts of food, even though they complain about it. If their intakes decrease somewhat, the deficit will be easy to correct once they are at home eating familiar foods.

Suggestions for helping people to eat were provided in the box on p. 757. In some cases, the solution to a problem can be handled directly by the person caring for the client. In other cases, the dietary department must be contacted to solve a food-related problem. Understanding how the foodservice system works will help you deal with problems more efficiently.

HOW FOODSERVICE SYSTEMS WORK

The responsibility of budgeting, planning, preparing, and serving food in

Figure H25–1

Sample Lunch Menus

Lunch

REGULAR **SUNDAY**

Meats

Baked chicken❤ Fried fish
Hamburger on bun with chips (with lettuce and tomato)

Starchy Vegetables

Cornbread dressing Parsleyed potatoes❤

Vegetables

Baby carrots❤ Stewed tomatoes

Soup/Salad/Juice
Coleslaw
Clam chowder
Gelatin
Tossed salad❤

Dressings
French
Thousand Island
Italian
Diet Thousand Island❤

Desserts

Apple pie
Fresh fruit❤
Butterscotch pudding

Breads

Dinner roll
White bread
Wheat bread
Bran bread❤
Crackers

Beverages & Condiments

Coffee
Decaf. coffee
Hot tea
Decaf. hot tea
Iced tea
Whole milk
Buttermilk
2% milk
Skim milk❤
Chocolate milk

Sugar
Sugar substitute
Herb seasoning
Creamer
Lemon
Mustard
Mayonnaise
Catsup
Margarine

PLEASE DO NOT LEAVE MENU ON THE TRAY

NAME ____________ **ROOM** ______

People on regular diets select the foods of their choice. The regular menu may also be used for high-kcalorie, high-protein diets. The menu items marked with a heart guide people in selecting foods that are lower in fat, cholesterol, sodium, and caffeine or higher in fiber than other menu choices.

Lunch

SOFT/BLAND/LOW RESIDUE **SUNDAY**

Meats

Baked chicken
Hamburger on bun
Baked fish (cod)

Starchy Vegetables

Rice Boiled potatoes

Vegetables

Baby carrots Green beans

Soup/Salad/Juice
Gelatin
Lemonade
Tomato soup

Dressings
Mayonnaise
Catsup

Desserts

Apple pie Pears

Breads

Dinner roll
White bread
Crackers

Beverages & Condiments

Decaf. coffee
Decaf. hot tea
Decaf. iced tea
Hot chocolate
Whole milk
2% milk
Buttermilk
Skim milk

Sugar
Sugar substitute
Creamer
Lemon
Margarine

NO PEPPER
PLEASE DO NOT LEAVE MENU ON TRAY

NAME ____________ **ROOM** ______

Foods for soft/bland/low-residue diets are similar to those for regular diets. Foods from the regular menu that are not appropriate have been eliminated from the menu, and substitutes have been made. For clients on bland diets, decaffeinated coffee and tea would be crossed off the menu.

Lunch

KCALORIE RESTRICTED, DIABETIC
1200 **CALORIES** **SUNDAY**

LF = Low Fat LSLF = Low Sodium, Low Fat

Meat Exchange (Select 1)
LSLF Baked chicken (2 oz) LSLF Baked fish (2 oz)
LSLF Hamburger on bun (with lettuce and tomato, 2 oz meat) omit 2 starches

Starch Exchange (Select 1)
Clam chowder (1 c)
LSLF Rice (1/3 c)
LSLF Boiled potatoes (1/2 c)
Angel food cake (1" slice)
LF Dinner roll (1)
White bread (1 slice)
Wheat bread (1 slice)
Bran bread (1 slice)
Crackers (6)

Vegetable Exchange (Select 2)
LSLF Baby carrots (1/2 c) LSLF Green beans (1/2 c)

Fruit Exchange (Select 1)
Diet pears (1/2 c) Fresh fruit

Milk Exchange (Select 1)
Whole milk (1 c) omit 2 fats
2% milk (1 c) omit 1 fat
Buttermilk (1 c)
Skim milk (1 c)

Fat Exchange (Select 1)
Margarine (1 tsp)
Diet mayonnaise (1/2 oz)
Creamer (1 = 1/2 fat)

Calorie-free Foods
Coffee
Decaf. coffee
Hot tea
Decaf. hot tea
Iced tea
Sugar substitute
Lemon
Herb seasoning

LSLF Coleslaw (1/2 c)
Tossed salad (1 c)
Diet gelatin (1/2 c)
Diet French
Diet Thousand Island
Diet Italian
Mustard
Diet catsup

PLEASE DO NOT LEAVE MENU ON THE TRAY

NAME ____________ **ROOM** ______

For kcalorie-restricted and diabetic diets, the number of exchanges allowed is written on the menu beforehand. (This example uses a 1200-kcalorie diet.) Note that the meat exchange is written in 2-ounce portions so that 1 serving = 2 exchanges. (Chapter 17 describes the exchange system.)

the hospital rests with either a chief administrative dietitian or a foodservice manager. In some hospitals, foodservice companies from outside the hospital perform these duties.

Clinical dietitians work directly with clients to assess their nutrition status, plan appropriate diets, and provide nutrition education. In some hospitals, dietetic technicians assist dietitians in both administrative and clinical responsibilities. Other dietary employees include clerks, aides, cooks, porters, and other assistants. Keep in mind that only dietitians have extensive formal training in nutrition. Other dietary employees do not have such training, and their ability to interpret diet orders or provide accurate information may be limited.

Menu Procedures

Most hospitals provide menus from which clients can select their meals. A client who must follow a special diet receives menus that list only foods specified in the hospital's diet

Figure H25–1

(continued)

Lunch

LOW-FAT/LOW CHOLESTEROL/CARDIAC **SUNDAY**

LF = Low Fat LSLF = Low Sodium, Low Fat

Meats

LSLF Baked chicken LSLF Baked fish (cod)
LSLF Hamburger on bun (with lettuce and tomato)

Starchy Vegetables

LSLF Rice LSLF Boiled potatoes

Vegetables

LSLF Baby carrots LSLF Green beans

Soup/Salad/Juice

LSLF Coleslaw
Gelatin
Tomato soup
LS Chicken broth
Tossed salad

Dressings

Diet French
Diet Thousand Island
Diet Italian

Desserts

Pears Angel food cake
Fresh fruit

Breads

LF Dinner roll Bran bread
White bread Crackers
Wheat bread LS Crackers

Beverages & Condiments

Coffee Creamer
Decaf. coffee Sugar
Hot tea Sugar substitute
Decaf. hot tea Herb seasoning
Iced tea Lemon
Buttermilk Margarine
Skim milk Mustard
Diet mayonnaise
Catsup

PLEASE DO NOT LEAVE MENU ON THE TRAY

NAME ____________ **ROOM** ______

People on low-fat, low-cholesterol diets who also need kcalorie restriction receive a kcalorie-restricted menu to control portion sizes and number of servings. Both menus provide low-fat, low-cholesterol foods. Foods not appropriate for a low-fat, low-cholesterol diet, such as whole milk, would be crossed off the menu beforehand.

Lunch

LOW SODIUM **SUNDAY**

LF = Low Fat LSLF = Low Sodium, Low Fat

Meats

LSLF Baked chicken LSLF Baked fish (cod)
LSLF Hamburger on bun (with lettuce and tomato)

Starchy Vegetables

LSLF Rice LSLF Boiled potatoes

Vegetables

LSLF Baby carrots LSLF Green beans

Soup/Salad/Juice

LSLF Coleslaw
LS Chicken broth
Apple juice
Tossed salad

Dressings

Diet French
Diet Thousand Island
Diet Italian

Desserts

Angel food cake Pears
Fresh fruit

Breads

Dinner roll Bran bread
White bread LS Crackers
Wheat bread

Beverages & Condiments

Coffee Sugar
Decaf. coffee Sugar substitute
Hot tea Creamer
Decaf. hot tea Lemon
Iced tea Herb seasoning
Whole milk Margarine
2% milk Diet mustard
Skim milk Diet mayonnaise
Diet catsup

NO SALT

PLEASE DO NOT LEAVE MENU ON THE TRAY

NAME ____________ **ROOM** ______

Low-sodium menus are similar to those provided for low-fat, low-cholesterol diets, but they eliminate high-sodium foods, such as tomato soup. The person on a low-sodium, low-fat, low-cholesterol diet selects foods from a low-fat menu with high-sodium foods crossed off beforehand. If the person is also on a low-kcalorie diet, foods would be selected from a low-kcalorie menu with high-sodium foods crossed off the menu beforehand.

Lunch

RENAL **SUNDAY**

LF = Low Fat LSLF = Low Sodium, Low Fat

Meats (2 oz)

LSLF Baked chicken LSLF Baked fish
LSLF Hamburger on bun (with lettuce)

Starchy Vegetables

LSLF Rice LSLF Dialyzed potatoes

Vegetables

LSLF Baby carrots LSLF Green beans

Soup/Salad/Juice

Lemonade
LSLF Coleslaw
Tossed salad (no tomato)

Dressings

Diet French
Diet Thousand Island
Diet Italian

Desserts

Pears Apple pie

Breads

Dinner roll Bran bread
White bread LS Crackers
Wheat bread

Beverages & Condiments

Coffee Sugar
Decaf. coffee Sugar substitute
Hot tea Creamer
Decaf. hot tea Lemon
Iced tea Margarine
Diet mustard
Mayonnaise

NO SALT

PLEASE DO NOT LEAVE MENU ON THE TRAY

NAME ____________ **ROOM** ______

Renal diets must be highly individualized and the person checking the menu has to carefully consider the client's selections and make appropriate changes when necessary.

manual for that diet. By allowing a choice, this system helps to ensure that clients receive foods they enjoy and will eat. An added advantage for people on special diets is that they become familiar with their diets by marking the appropriate menus.

Although procedures vary somewhat between hospitals, generally dietary employees deliver menus to each client's room early in the day and pick them up again later in the day. Each menu shows the client's name and room number as well as the name of the meal, the type of diet, and the day the menu will be served. Generally, the client makes selections for the next day or for the next few days to give the dietary department time to collect the menus and estimate the amount of food to prepare. Menus are usually color coded by diet. Color coding helps ensure that foodservice employees put the right foods on a client's tray and helps the person delivering the tray to quickly determine whether the client has received the right diet. Figure H25–1 shows lunch menus from several different diet menus and explains how each menu might be used.

Clients typically select one or more items from each food category on the menu. Clients may not receive foods they enjoy if they fail to mark the appropriate selections. If menus are not marked or if a menu is lost, the client receives meals preselected by the dietary department. Menus may not be marked for several reasons:

- Clients may have trouble seeing, reading, understanding, or physically marking the menus.
- Clients may not understand that their selections will be for the *next* (or another) day.
- Clients may be out of their rooms (for tests, procedures, or exercise) or asleep when the menus arrive; when the clients return or wake up, they may not see the menus or may have missed the menu pickup time.
- Clients may be too ill or too disinterested in food to make menu selections.

Occasional problems with menu selections can usually be corrected simply by explaining the menu system to clients or taking extra time to help them mark the menus. If clients continue to complain about food selections, the dietitian should be contacted.

Once food selections have been made, menus are often checked by a member of the dietary staff (often a registered dietetic technician) to make sure selections are appropriate. Completed menus can provide valuable clues about a client's food habits or understanding of a modified diet. In checking menus, the technician may notice that one person on a regular diet is selecting very little or that another is selecting too much. In another case, the technician may see that a person on a low-kcalorie diet is not selecting the appropriate number of servings from each exchange list. Such problems suggest the need for intervention by a dietitian.

Some hospitals do not offer selective menus. Instead, they serve a standard house diet, adjusting the menu for individual food preferences or special diets when necessary. For example, clients can request simple changes, such as the substitution of one vegetable for another. Similarly, if the regular menu offers fried fish, a person on a low-fat or low-kcalorie diet would receive baked fish.

Food Preparation and Delivery

The logistics of preparing foods tailored to each modified diet can be overwhelming. For this reason, foodservice departments use special systems designed to limit costs and keep errors to a minimum. Foods prepared for regular and soft/bland/low-residue diets are prepared with some fat and salt, because these dietary components are not restricted on such diets. Note that the other diet menus in Figure H25–1 provide a number of low-fat (LF) or low-sodium, low-fat (LSLF) foods.

If the dietary department were to prepare a food (baked chicken, for example) for each different diet, it would have to prepare regular baked chicken, low-fat baked chicken, low-sodium baked chicken, and low-sodium, low-fat baked chicken, Using the system illustrated in the menus of Figure H25–1, only two types of baked chicken need to be prepared, one with some fat and salt, the other without fat or salt.

Keep in mind that baked chicken is only one of many menu items in a day, and you can see why preparing individual foods for each diet is not feasible. Instead, clients can add allowed items to their foods. For example, the person on a low-salt diet could add margarine to a serving of vegetables; the person on a low-fat diet could add salt to a serving of rice.

Sometimes foods are prepared in a main kitchen, assembled on trays, and heated in areas close to the clients' rooms. In other cases, foods are delivered directly to the floor from the main kitchen. In either case, dietary personnel deliver the food carts directly to the nursing unit. Once at the unit, nursing or dietary personnel take a tray to each client. Efficient delivery of foods to the nursing unit and then to the clients' rooms helps ensure that clients receive foods at the appropriate temperature.

Once a client has finished eating, the tray is returned to the food cart. Dietary personnel pick up the carts and return them to the dietary department.

Working with the System

You can help your clients greatly—and save yourself needless aggravation and time—by learning about the foodservice system in the health care facility where you work. Better yet, ask to spend a few hours or a day working with a dietary employee to see firsthand how the department operates. If that is not possible, learn the facility's procedure for ordering diets, making diet changes, reporting problems with a client's tray, or making special requests. Remember that requests are not simply made by one individual to another. Often many people are involved in processing even a simple request, and the number of requests made during a short period can be considerable. Translating requests (for example, requesting a diet change or another tray) takes time, and delays are often unavoidable.

One of the most important things to know about your facility's foodservice system is the time when meals are actually assembled, so that you can call in any requests before that time. Once tray assembly begins, dietary employees are extremely busy, and requests will be difficult to process.

With so many people and steps involved in the delivery of food and so many clients with individual dietary needs and food preferences, it is easy to see many opportunities for problems to arise regarding food in the hospital. Once you understand how the dietary department operates, you can use the system to tackle problems efficiently and avoid needless frustration for your client and yourself.

NOTES

1. M. Bélanger and L. Dubé, The emotional experience of hospitalization: Its moderators and its role in patient satisfaction with foodservices, *Journal of the American Dietetic Association* 96 (1996): 354–360.

Chapter 26

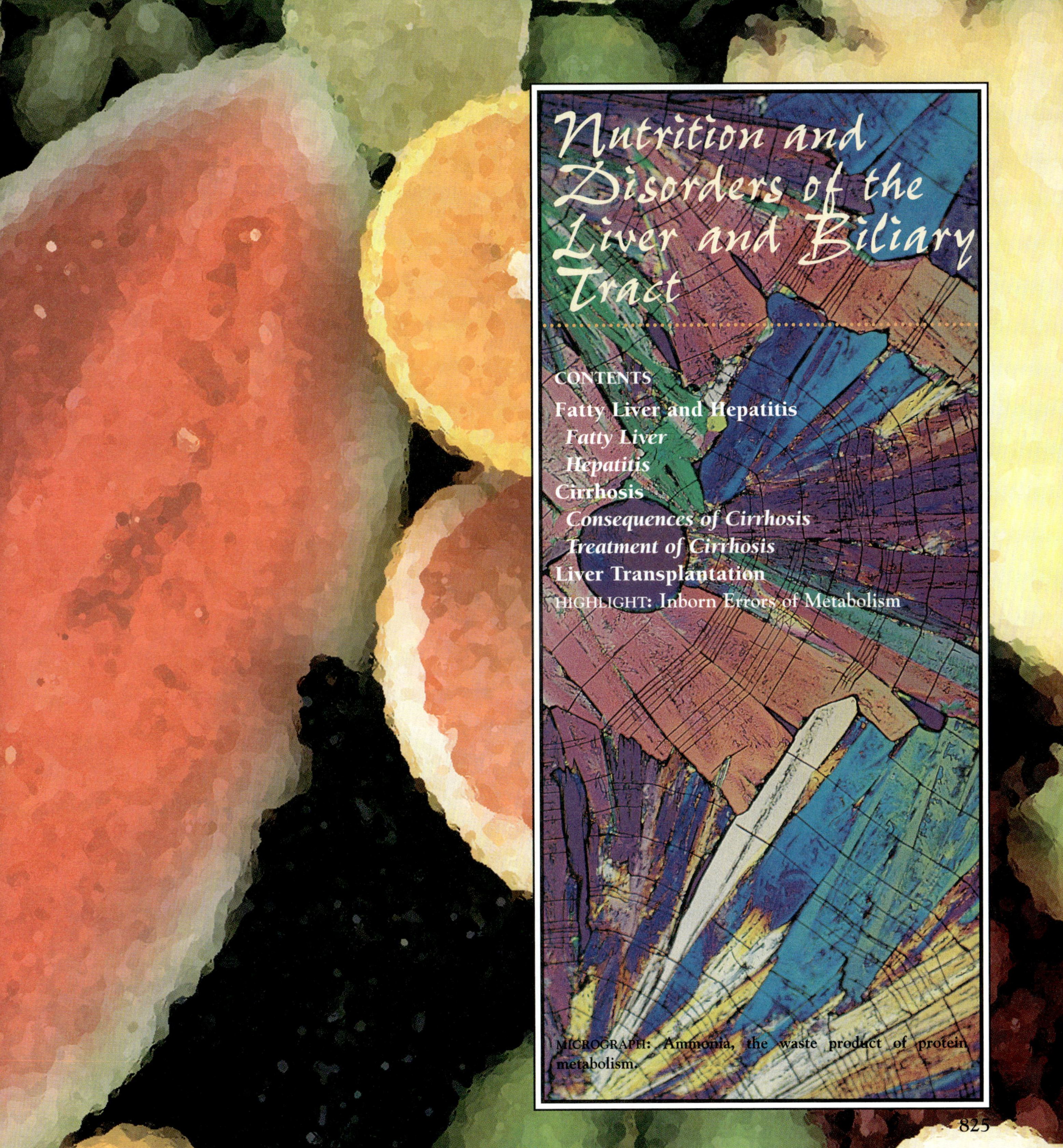

Nutrition and Disorders of the Liver and Biliary Tract

CONTENTS

MICROGRAPH: Ammonia, the waste product of protein metabolism.

During severe stress, hypermetabolism necessitates that the liver work diligently to synthesize stress factors and provide glucose. Indeed, the liver is the metabolic crossroad of the body, and its health is crucial to every body function. The liver receives nutrients and metabolizes, packages, stores, or ships them out for use by the other organs. It manufactures bile, which the body uses to emulsify fat in preparation for digestion and absorption. The liver also detoxifies drugs, prepares waste products for excretion, and participates in iron recycling and the manufacture of red blood cells. No wonder hepatic disorders can profoundly affect both nutrition and general health status. Figure 26–1 shows the liver, its circulatory system, and the biliary tract.

hepatic (he-PAT-ik): of, like, or pertaining to the liver.

Liver disease can be caused by a variety of conditions, including alcohol abuse, congenital disorders, poisoning by toxins, infections, biliary tract obstructions, and heart disease. This chapter describes several types of liver disorders for which dietary management is appropriate.

Figure 26–1

The Liver, Biliary Tract, and Associated Blood Vessels

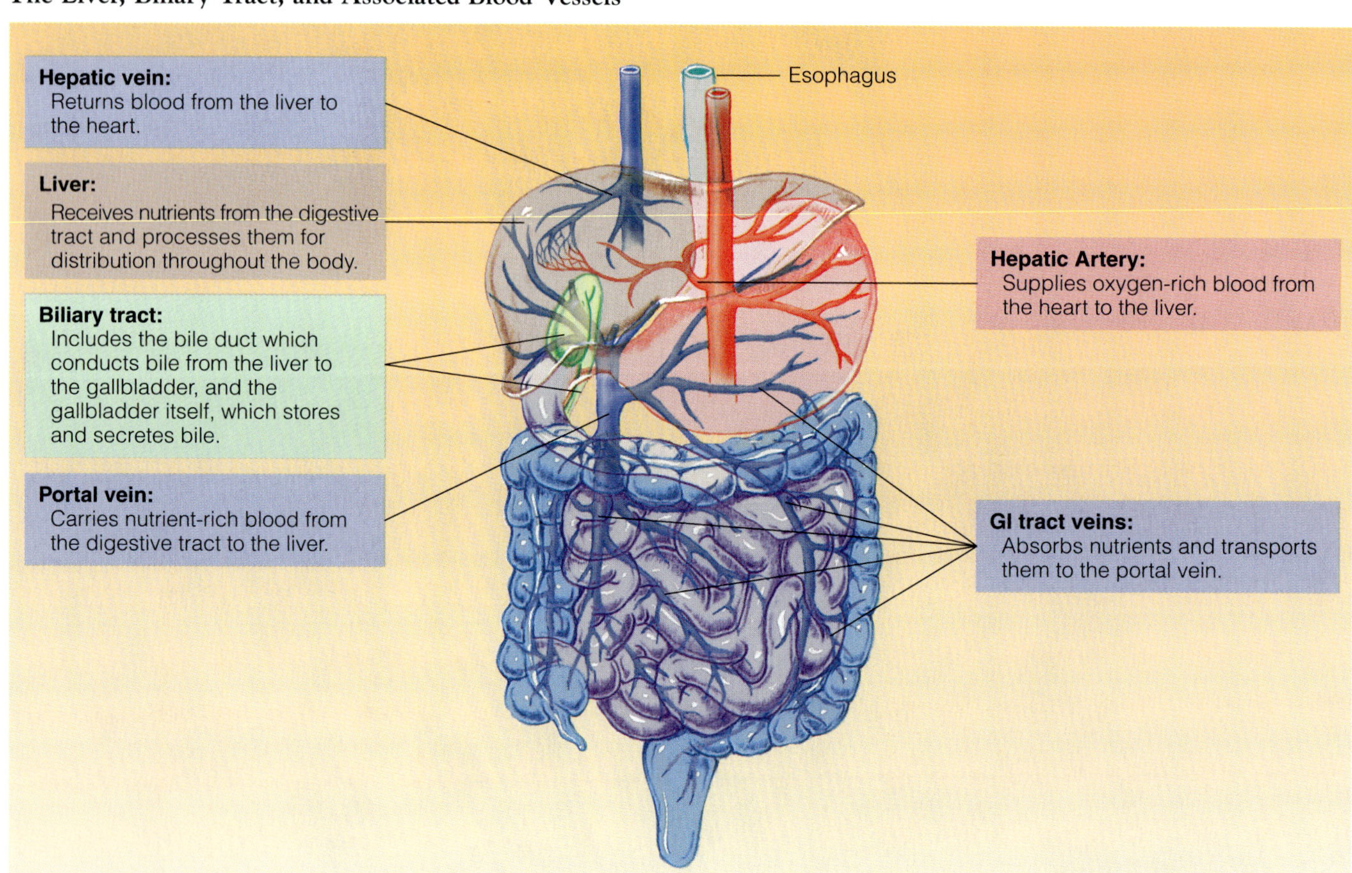

Fatty Liver and Hepatitis

Two of the more common disorders of the liver are fatty liver and hepatitis. Dietary factors can play a role in the development of both disorders, although both may also arise from other causes. Similarly, diet management may play a role in the treatment of both disorders.

FATTY LIVER

Fatty liver is not a disease, but rather a clinical finding common to many conditions. Fatty liver may develop from damage to liver cells or from altered nutrient availability to the liver. Most commonly, fatty liver develops from the liver's exposure to toxic substances such as alcohol (see Highlight 7), from an inadequate intake of protein (as in PEM), or as the result of infection or malignant disease. Fatty liver can also develop as a complication of drug therapy (such as therapy with corticosteroids or tetracycline), obesity, long-term TPN, or small bowel bypass surgery.

Reminder: *Fatty liver* is an early sign of liver deterioration seen in several diseases, including acute malnutrition and alcoholic liver disease. Fatty liver is characterized by an accumulation of fat in the liver cells and liver enlargement. Fatty liver is also called **hepatic steatosis** (STEE-ah-TOE-sis).

Fatty liver occurs when the liver either synthesizes too much fat, oxidizes too little, takes up too much from the blood, releases too little back into the blood, or any combination of these errors. Whatever the reason, triglycerides accumulate in the liver and cause it to enlarge. In severe cases, liver weight may increase from a normal weight of about 3½ pounds to as much as 11 pounds, with triglycerides making up approximately 40 percent of the weight (normally, triglycerides account for only about 5 percent of liver weight). Other clinical findings associated with fatty liver may include elevated serum transaminases (ALT and AST), alkaline phosphatase, and bilirubin.[1]

Two transaminase enzymes—alanine transaminase (ALT) and aspartate transaminase (AST)—increase in liver disease.

Excessive bilirubin in the blood is **hyperbilirubinemia**.

Consequences of Fatty Liver Fatty liver alone usually causes no harm. Fatty liver associated with TPN, for example, may resolve as the feeding continues, when the feeding is changed to a cyclic infusion, or when TPN is discontinued. In other cases, however, the liver's accumulation of fat suggests the presence of an underlying primary disorder that can progress to permanent liver damage, metabolic and blood coagulation disturbances, renal failure, and death, if left unattended.

Treatment of Fatty Liver The appropriate therapy for fatty liver focuses on eliminating the cause and reversing its effects. Fatty liver due to alcohol abuse requires abstinence from alcohol and an adequate diet to replenish nutrient stores. Fatty liver caused by malnutrition requires the gradual introduction of a diet adequate in protein, energy, and all other nutrients. Fatty liver caused by drug therapy requires alternative drugs or other therapies.

HEPATITIS

In hepatitis, the destruction of liver cells causes inflammation and liver enlargement. Most often hepatitis results from a viral infection, although it can also occur as a consequence of excessive or chronic ingestion of alcohol, certain drugs, or toxins. Among the five types of viruses known to cause hepatitis (types A, B, C, D, and E), type A is the highly contagious form that is often spread

hepatitis: inflammation of the liver caused by a virus, alcohol, drug, or other toxin.
hepat = liver
itis = inflammation

through contaminated foods and water. Recent hepatitis A outbreaks have been traced to contaminated berries, although most often, seafood harvested from polluted water is to blame.

Reminder: *Jaundice* is the yellowing of the skin caused by bile pigments (bilirubin) from the liver spilling into the bloodstream.

Symptoms of Hepatitis During the early states of hepatitis, the person may develop fatigue, joint and muscle pain, anorexia, nausea, vomiting, diarrhea or constipation, and fever. In some cases, the symptoms are mild and may go unnoticed. In other cases, hepatitis progresses, and yellow bile pigments accumulate in the inflamed liver and spill into the blood, causing jaundice and producing a dark urine. Serum transaminase levels (AST and ALT) are elevated. The liver enlarges and becomes tender.

Consequences of Hepatitis The origin and type of hepatitis, the extent of liver damage, and the person's response to treatment all determine how seriously the disease will affect health. In many cases, liver cells gradually regenerate and liver function recovers. Hepatitis A is often mild, although relapses may occur after apparent recovery. Sometimes chronic hepatitis develops, particularly as a late consequence of hepatitis B. Liver cancer may develop after infection with hepatitis B or C. Much less commonly, severe hepatitis can rapidly lead to liver failure, hepatic coma (described in later sections), and death.

Treatment of Hepatitis Liver cells need nutrients to help them recover from hepatitis. Recovery also aims to reduce further insult to the liver cells; thus the person must abstain from alcohol. The person with hepatitis who is in good nutrition status receives a regular, well-balanced diet. The malnourished person with hepatitis receives a high-kcalorie, high-protein diet to replenish nutrient stores. For the person with mild anorexia, suggest small, frequent meals, enteral formula supplements, or both. Persistent anorexia and nausea may make tube feedings necessary. For the person who experiences persistent vomiting, parenteral nutrition is an alternative.

Fatty liver develops when liver cells are damaged, as commonly occurs in alcohol abuse, PEM, infection, and long-term TPN. Treatment focuses on correcting the cause. Further destruction of liver cells leads to hepatitis. When fatty liver or hepatitis goes unresolved, chronic hepatitis or cirrhosis can develop. Not only is cirrhosis the most serious type of liver injury, but it is also irreversible.

cirrhosis (seer-OH-sis): an advanced form of liver disease in which scar tissue replaces liver cells that have permanently lost their function.

The type of cirrhosis associated with alcohol abuse and malnutrition is called **Laennec's** (lay-eh-NECK'S) **cirrhosis**. **Postnecrotic cirrhosis** develops as a complication of hepatitis. **Biliary cirrhosis** can develop when the biliary tract is obstructed or inflamed, usually as a result of a gallstone that blocks the flow of bile from the liver to the gallbladder. **Cardiac cirrhosis** is associated with failure of the heart's right ventricle, which disrupts blood flow to the liver. In still other cases, cirrhosis may be **idiopathic**, having no identifiable cause.

Cirrhosis

In cirrhosis, a serious and chronic form of liver failure, liver cells destroyed by chronic inflammation do not regenerate. Instead, scar tissue (fibrosis) forms within the liver, altering the structure of the liver and the blood flow through it. (Recall that fibrosis associated with chronic pancreatitis leads to the loss of pancreatic function and the fibrosis associated with inflammatory bowel diseases alters the function of the intestine.)

Chronic alcohol abuse is the most common cause of cirrhosis in the United States, although not all people with cirrhosis are alcohol abusers, and not all alcohol abusers develop cirrhosis. Other causes of cirrhosis include infections, biliary tract obstructions, heart disease, and exposure to some drugs and toxic chemicals.

CONSEQUENCES OF CIRRHOSIS

Unlike healthy liver tissue, which is soft and flexible, scar tissue is unyielding. This difference leads to major consequences, as shown in Figure 26–2 and described in the following paragraphs.

Portal Hypertension The portal vein (see Figure 26–1) and the hepatic artery carry 1½ quarts of blood every minute to the miles of intermeshed capillaries within the liver. This huge volume of blood cannot pulse easily through the scarred tissue of a cirrhotic liver. Consequently, blood backs up and pressure in the portal vein rises sharply, causing portal hypertension.

Reminder: The *portal vein* is the blood vessel that carries nutrients from the GI tract to the liver. The *hepatic vein* returns blood from the liver to the heart. The *hepatic artery* delivers oxygen-rich blood from the heart back to the liver.

portal hypertension: elevated blood pressure in the portal vein caused by obstructed blood flow through the liver.

Esophageal Varices With normal blood flow through the liver blocked, pressure forces some of the blood to take a detour through smaller vessels around the liver. These collaterals, or shunts, often develop in the area around the esophagus. Frequently, high pressure enlarges the collaterals so that they bulge into the lumen of the esophagus much as varicose veins in the legs do, creating

Figure 26–2

The Consequences of Cirrhosis

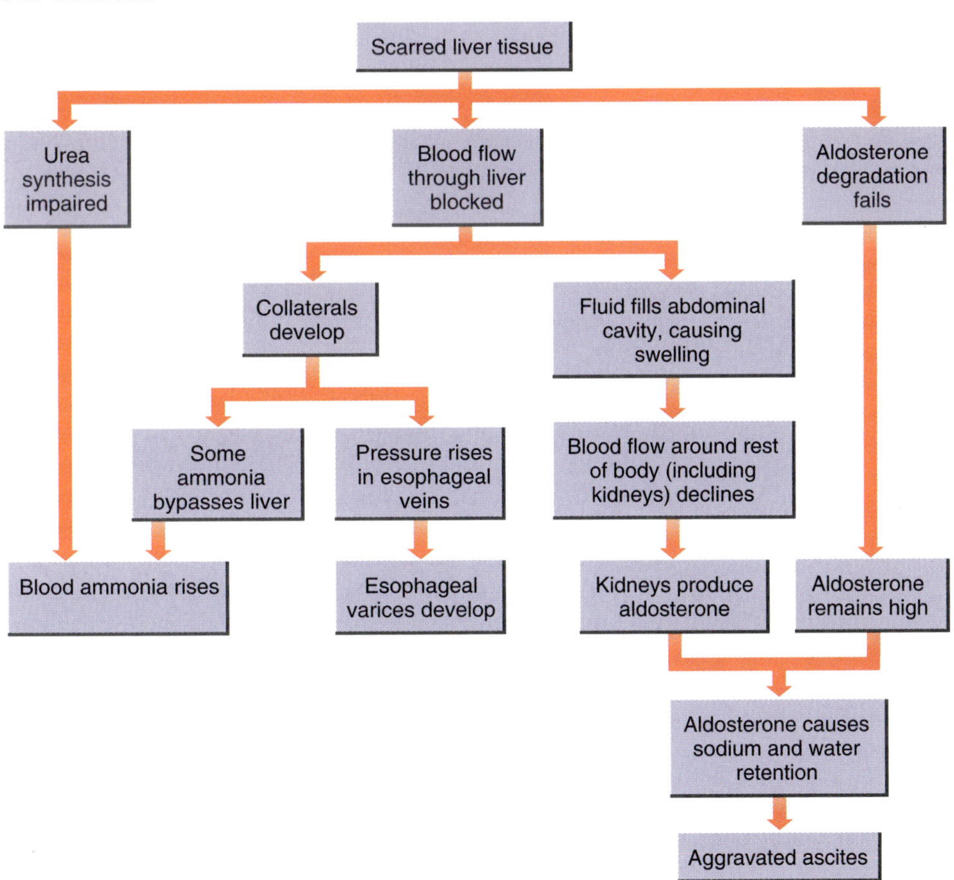

collaterals: small blood vessels that develop to divert blood flow away from an obstructed organ; also called **shunts**.
shunt = to avoid

esophageal varices (ee-SOFF-ah-GEE-al VAIR-ih-seez): tangles of distended blood vessels that protrude into the esophagus.

ascites (ah-SIGH-teez): a type of edema characterized by the accumulation of fluid in the abdominal cavity.

esophageal varices. Eventually, the thin esophageal lining that covers the varices may wear away, and massive bleeding follows. Bleeding esophageal varices tend to recur, and people can bleed to death.

Ascites The rising pressure in the portal vein forces plasma out of the liver's blood vessels into the abdominal cavity, causing the abdomen to swell. This accumulation of fluid in the abdominal cavity is called ascites. Ascites tends to be a self-aggravating condition. Because less blood reaches the kidneys, the body responds by making more aldosterone, the hormone that expands the body's blood volume by triggering the retention of sodium and water. As a result of the sodium and water retention, ascites worsens and edema spreads to all body compartments. To make matters worse, the diseased liver cannot dispose of aldosterone as it normally does, so aldosterone levels remain high.

An elevated blood ammonia level is called **hyperammonemia**. Normal blood ammonia levels are less than 50 µg/100 ml.

Elevated Blood Ammonia Levels Normally, the healthy liver removes ammonia from circulation and converts it to urea, but a severely diseased liver fails at this task, and blood ammonia rises. Even if the liver does handle the ammonia it receives, some ammonia-laden blood bypasses the liver by way of the collaterals. Elevated blood ammonia levels disrupt central nervous system function, compounding the risk of hepatic coma. Thus therapy aims to control ammonia production.

hepatic coma: a state of unconsciousness that results from severe liver disease; also called **hepatic encephalopathy** or **portal systemic encephalopathy**.

Hepatic Coma Hepatic coma is a dangerous complication of liver failure. Its exact cause remains elusive; high blood ammonia plays an important role, but the degree of elevation does not correlate with the severity of coma. A possible explanation for this poor correlation is that *blood* ammonia levels do not parallel *brain* ammonia concentration. When brain ammonia is elevated, the body produces greater quantities of two substances (glutamine and ketoglutarate), and the degree of their elevation tends to correlate with the degree of coma. Other nitrogen-containing compounds may also be involved.

Phenylalanine and tyrosine are the aromatic amino acids; they are characterized by a ringlike structure.

Leucine, isoleucine, and valine are the branched-chain amino acids, so named because their side chains have a branched structure.

Blood amino acid patterns also change in hepatic coma. The liver fails to break down aromatic amino acids, so their blood concentrations rise. Hormonal changes that accompany liver disease (specifically, elevated insulin levels) promote the uptake of branched-chain amino acids by muscle cells, so the blood concentrations of these amino acids fall. The resulting high ratio of aromatic to branched-chain amino acids interferes with the formation of certain neurotransmitters (dopamine and norepinephrine) and causes the production of substances that may contribute to hepatic coma.[2] Altered amino acid metabolism also adds ammonia to the blood.

The odor that may develop in people with impending hepatic coma is called **fetor hepaticus**.

flapping tremor: uncontrolled movement of the muscle group that causes the outstretched arm and hand to flap like a wing; occurs in hepatic coma and other diseases that cause encephalopathy; also called **asterixis** (AS-ter-ICK-sis).

Typically, the person with impending hepatic coma exhibits mental disturbances such as changes in judgment, personality, or mood. The person may be unable to draw even a simple shape, such as a star. A sweet, musty, or pungent odor may develop on the breath. Flapping tremor may also develop in the precoma state. Just before passing into coma, the person becomes very difficult to arouse.

TREATMENT OF CIRRHOSIS

Treatment of cirrhosis includes diet and drugs to preserve remaining organ function to the greatest extent possible, to control clinical manifestations of the disorder, and to prevent hepatic coma. When liver failure has progressed to a severe stage, liver transplantation becomes an option.

How to Adjust Diets for Liver Disease

Health care professionals adjust diets in liver disease to meet each client's medical needs. The following guidelines help to determine nutrient needs for liver failure:

Energy: 35 to 45 kcalories per kilogram of actual body weight.

Protein in cirrhosis: 1.0 to 1.5 grams of protein per kilogram of body weight.

Protein in impending coma: 40 to 60 grams per day from foods; additional protein to meet needs can be supplied from special formulas.

Protein in hepatic coma: Protein from all sources may need to be restricted. Tolerances are determined individually; protein intake is gradually increased as the condition improves.

Sodium and fluids: 1000 to 2000 milligrams of sodium per day and 1500 to 2000 milliliters of fluid per day if ascites has developed; intake is increased as liver function improves.

As noted earlier, therapy seeks to limit blood ammonia levels. The GI tract produces about two-thirds of the body's ammonia. Intestinal bacteria make ammonia from undigested proteins (including dietary proteins, proteins from shed mucosal cells, and protein from GI tract bleeding). Digestive enzymes also produce ammonia as they dismantle proteins. Thus diet and drug therapy also aim to control intestinal ammonia production.

Drug Therapy Drug therapy for cirrhosis often includes broad-spectrum antibiotics to limit the growth of intestinal bacteria and laxatives to speed intestinal transit time, thus limiting the time available for bacteria to produce ammonia. In addition, diuretics are frequently given to reduce fluid retention and prevent ascites.

Energy and Protein In providing diet therapy for cirrhosis, health care professionals must pay attention to clients' intakes of energy, protein, sodium, and fluid. Adequate carbohydrate and fat prevent the catabolism of protein for energy, which would further raise blood ammonia. Dietary protein should be sufficient to regenerate liver cells and prevent infections, but not so excessive as to aggravate ammonia buildup and induce hepatic coma. A diet adequate in energy and restricted, but not low, in protein is the cornerstone of cirrhosis treatment. The accompanying box shows how diets are adjusted to meet nutrient needs for different stages of liver failure. (Note that protein needs actually exceed the RDA of 0.8 grams of protein per kilogram of body weight per day.)

A person who shows signs of impending coma requires additional dietary modifications. Protein intake must be restricted to 40 to 60 grams of high-quality protein per day. Restricting protein reduces the risk of coma, but may threaten protein status. Although research is limited and controversial, many clinicians recommend special enteral or parenteral formulas that are low in aromatic amino acids and high in branched-chain amino acids to meet the demand for additional protein.[3] If coma ensues, some people may be able to tolerate these special formulas, but for others, both dietary protein and special formulas may be restricted.[4] As the client's neurological status improves, protein can gradually be increased.

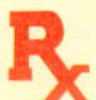

PRESCRIPTION PAD

Drugs used in the treatment of liver failure may include:

- Antibiotics
- Diuretics
- Laxatives (lactulose)

See Appendix E for timing with meals and nutrition-related side effects.

Avoiding hypermetabolism is critical for a person with compromised liver function. The impaired liver is already taxed in maintaining homeostasis. The added demands of stress factor synthesis and gluconeogenesis can easily overwhelm the liver and lead to death.

Appendix K includes enteral formulas for hepatic insufficiency.

People with liver disease may tolerate vegetable and dairy proteins better than meat proteins, perhaps because vegetables contain fewer ammonia-forming constituents and aromatic amino acids and more branched-chain amino acids than meats. In addition, diets high in plant foods contain more fiber, which speeds up intestinal transit time and reduces the time available for ammonia absorption from the gut.

Fat Because fat helps make foods more appetizing and delivers energy efficiently, it serves an important role in the diet of a person with cirrhosis. Fat needs to be restricted only if the cirrhotic person develops steatorrhea, a clear sign of fat malabsorption. Even then, the body can usually handle MCT fat (see Chapter 22, p. 729).

Fluid and Sodium For people with ascites, the diet often restricts fluid and sodium (see the box on p. 831 for details). To assess changes in fluid balance, health care professionals monitor weight changes and measure abdominal girth. Rapid weight gain indicates fluid retention; sudden weight loss indicates successful fluid excretion. To measure abdominal girth, the assessor places a tape measure around the back and over the person's abdomen directly over the umbilicus. A decreasing abdominal girth indicates fluid mobilization; an increasing abdominal girth signifies worsening ascites. Table 26–1 shows diet patterns for two levels of sodium restriction. The menu on p. 834 provides sample protein- and sodium-restricted meals.

Alcohol To protect the liver from further injury, clients with cirrhosis must completely abstain from alcohol use. A cirrhotic liver exposed to the toxic effects of alcohol cannot function.

Vitamins The liver's central role in the metabolism and storage of vitamins and minerals, combined with coexisting conditions (such as malabsorption, alcoholism, and malnutrition), explains why nutrient deficiencies commonly occur in people with liver disorders. Virtually all people with advanced liver disease require supplementation of some vitamins, minerals, and trace elements. Physicians determine which nutrients to supplement by monitoring serum levels and by checking for clinical signs of deficiencies.

The B vitamins serve as coenzymes for the liver's many metabolic reactions and repair work; deficiencies of thiamin, vitamin B_6, riboflavin, and folate are common. Fat-soluble vitamins may be malabsorbed if steatorrhea develops. If the diseased liver fails to synthesize adequate amounts of retinol-binding protein, body tissues may not receive the vitamin A they need. Vitamin D nutrition status may suffer if the impaired liver fails to activate vitamin D for the body's use. Vitamin K deficiencies can prolong the time blood takes to clot, a dangerous complication that increases the risk of massive bleeding from esophageal varices or other areas of the GI tract.

One laboratory test that evaluates the time it takes for blood to clot is called the **prothrombin time.** Both vitamin K deficiency and liver disease can prolong prothrombin time.

Minerals Calcium deficiencies can develop from three causes: steatorrhea, low serum albumin (albumin, which carries calcium in the blood, is manufactured in the liver), and impaired vitamin D metabolism. Fluid and electrolyte imbalances and ascites may necessitate that diuretics be used, and these may lead to deficiencies of potassium, magnesium, and zinc.

Table 26–1

One- and Two-Gram Sodium-Restricted Diets

Foods Restricted	Number of Servings[a]		Serving Size	Sodium per Serving (mg)
	1 gram (1000 mg) sodium	2 grams (2000 mg) sodium		
Regular breads and cooked cereals	3	4	1 slice	125
Fresh, frozen, or canned vegetables without salt: artichokes; beets; carrots; celery; beet, collard, dandelion, mustard, and turnip greens; kale; swiss chard; white turnips; low-sodium vegetable juice	3 per week	Avoid excessive use	½ cup	50
Canned or frozen vegetables with salt; frozen corn, lima beans, mixed vegetables, and peas	0	2	½ cup	250
Regular nonfat, whole, and evaporated milk and milk products	2	2	8 oz	120
Fresh and fresh frozen meats, poultry, and freshwater fish; low-sodium canned meats and fish, peanut butter, cheese; unsalted soybeans, textured vegetable protein, and cottage cheese	8	8	1 oz	25
Eggs	1	1	1	70
Regular butter and margarine	0	6	1 tsp	50

Foods Allowed

1. Low-sodium breads, bread products, and cereals; bread products made without salt and with low-sodium baking powder; puffed rice and wheat and shredded wheat cereals; rice; pasta.
2. Fresh, unsalted frozen, and low-sodium canned vegetables (except those listed above); low-sodium tomato juice.
3. All fruits and fruit juices.
4. Unsalted butter, margarine, nuts, and gravy; low-sodium salad dressings and mayonnaise; shortening.
5. Low-sodium catsup, mustard, and tabasco sauce.
6. Soups, casseroles, and recipes made with allowed foods and food ingredients.

Foods Not Allowed (Unless Calculated Into the Diet)

1. Table, celery, garlic, and onion salts; reduced-sodium salts; regular catsup, mustard, and tabasco sauce; monosodium glutamate; Worcestershire, barbeque, and soy sauces; baking powder and soda.
2. Instant and quick-cooking hot cereals; commercial bread products made from self-rising flour or cornmeal, salt, baking powder, or baking soda; salted snack foods such as potato chips, corn chips, tortilla chips, popcorn, and pretzels.
3. Sauerkraut, pickles, and salted vegetable juices.
4. Maraschino cherries; crystallized or glazed fruits, and dried fruits with sodium sulfite added.
5. Buttermilk, chocolate milk, instant milk mixes, regular cheeses, and prepared pudding mixes; commercial ice cream, sherbet, and frozen desserts.
6. Cured, canned, salted, or smoked meats, poultry and fish such as bacon, luncheon meats, corned beef, kosher meats, and canned tuna and salmon; imitation fish products; salted textured vegetable protein; regular peanut butter; salted nuts.
7. Salt pork and bacon fat; commercial salad dressings and mayonnaise; olives; regular gravy.
8. Regular canned soups and bouillon.

[a]Number of servings daily, except as noted.

Sample Protein-Restricted (60 g), Sodium-Restricted (1000 mg) Diet Menu

Foods on this low-sodium menu are cooked without salt. To raise sodium intake, add salt to foods. To reduce sodium, use unsalted margarine and low-sodium milk. The kcalories provided by this menu depend on how much fat is used in cooking. To raise energy intake, encourage the liberal use of fats and sugars from foods that do not contain protein (for example, margarine and table sugar).

Menu

Breakfast	Lunch	Supper
Orange juice	Sandwich with	2 oz baked chicken
½ c oatmeal	2 oz roast beef,	½ c mashed potatoes
½ c milk	2 slices bread, lettuce,	Broccoli
1 egg	and mayonnaise	1 low-sodium dinner roll
Margarine	Cole slaw	Margarine
Coffee	Cinnamon applesauce	Fruit cocktail
Cream	½ c milk	½ c milk
Sugar		

Diet Planning Dietitians face a challenge in devising a diet plan that is low in sodium, supplies adequate energy and nutrients, and also stimulates the appetite. Many high-quality protein foods (for example, eggs, meat, and milk) also contain significant amounts of sodium. To circumvent this problem, planners recommend special supplements and milk products that are low in sodium. Diet offers critical support in the care of liver failure, and health professionals should make every effort to solve food-related problems.

Offer encouragement and work closely with clients and their caregivers to individualize the diet and serve foods attractively. Try the tactics suggested in Chapter 23 to encourage clients to eat.

Enteral and Parenteral Nutrition If the person with cirrhosis cannot take enough food or formula by mouth, health care professionals should promptly begin tube feedings or TPN. As mentioned earlier, enteral and parenteral formulas designed for liver failure provide fewer aromatic and more branched-chain amino acids than standard formulas. Both types of special nutrition support have been used successfully in people with cirrhosis.

People with bleeding esophageal varices will be unable to consume food by mouth and are often given simple IV solutions to maintain fluid and electrolyte balances. Parenteral nutrition should be considered if the person is malnourished or unable to resume oral intake for an extended period of time. The accompanying box presents a case study on cirrhosis. Use your clinical knowledge and judgment in answering the questions presented.

Liver Transplantation

When liver failure progresses to a severe and irreversible stage, liver transplantation may become an option. Surgeons remove the diseased liver, replace it with

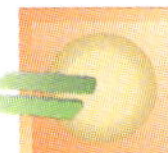

Case Study Carpenter with Cirrhosis

Mr. Sloan, a 48-year-old carpenter, has been hospitalized many times. He recognizes his problem with alcohol abuse and has entered alcohol rehabilitation programs several times over the last few years. Nevertheless, he is still drinking. Mr. Sloan was recently admitted to the hospital, and a diagnosis of alcoholic cirrhosis has been confirmed. At 5 feet 7 inches tall, Mr. Sloan, who once weighed 150 pounds, now weighs 120 pounds. He looks thin, although his abdomen is distended with ascites, and his skin is yellow. He has advanced liver disease and is showing signs of impending hepatic coma. Laboratory findings include elevated AST, ALT, alkaline phosphatase, and blood ammonia. Compare these findings with Table 26–2 to determine if they are consistent with liver disease.

Can you explain to Mr. Sloan what cirrhosis is and what its consequences are? From the limited information available, what can you determine about Mr. Sloan's nutrition status? What medical problem makes it difficult to interpret Mr. Sloan's actual weight? How can his weight measurements help determine if his condition is improving?

What dietary changes do clients with cirrhosis generally receive? How will Mr. Sloan's diet be altered now that he is in a precoma state? What signs suggest that a person is in a precoma state?

Why is Mr. Sloan's abdomen distended? Explain the development of ascites in liver disease and how diet is adjusted.

Would you expect Mr. Sloan's blood ammonia levels to be high? Why or why not?

Describe portal hypertension, jaundice, and esophageal varices. How would Mr. Sloan's diet be changed if he were found to have esophageal varices?

a donor liver, and reconnect the blood vessels and the biliary tract. In some liver transplant cases, the graft fails to function, and retransplantation forestalls an otherwise inevitable death.

Nutrition before Transplantation In severe liver failure, malnutrition has often progressed for some time. Clinicians report malnutrition in over 70 percent of liver transplant recipients and note that malnutrition increases the risk of

Table 26–2

Standards for Tests Used to Diagnose and Monitor Liver Disease

Test	Normal Values	Values in Liver Disease
Albumin	3.5–5.0 g/100 ml	Decreased
Alkaline phosphatase	Varies[a]	Normal or elevated
ALT (formerly SGPT)[b]	Varies[a]	Elevated
Ammonia	<50 μg/100 ml	Elevated
AST (formerly SGOT)[b]	Varies[a]	Elevated
Bilirubin (direct)	0.1–0.3 mg/100 ml	Elevated
Prothrombin time		Prolonged

Note: To convert albumin (g/100 ml) to standard international (SI) units, multiply by 10; to convert ammonia (μg/100 ml) to SI units, multiply by 0.5872; to convert bilirubin (mg/100 ml) to SI units (μmol/L) multiply by 17.10

[a]Reference ranges vary depending on the test used. Consult laboratory report for normal ranges.

[b]ALT = alanine transaminase; SGPT = serum glutamic pyruvic transaminase; AST = aspartate transaminase; SGOT = serum glutamic oxaloacetic transaminase.

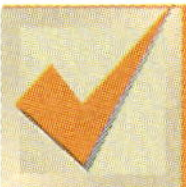

Nutrition Assessment Checklist
For People with Liver Disorders

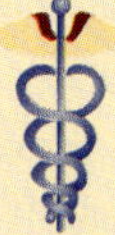

Medical Review the medical record to determine the type and cause of liver disease, as well as any history of alcohol abuse, hepatitis, or biliary tract obstruction. Recognize that the effects of advanced liver disease and malnutrition are often difficult to distinguish.

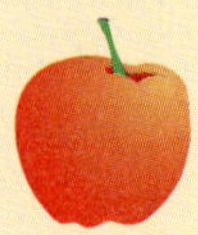

Nutrient Intake Obtain an accurate diet history to determine nutrition status, calculate nutrient requirements, and identify inadequate nutrient intake. Assess current intake to help pinpoint tolerance for protein in people with advanced liver disease. People who abuse alcohol normally derive much of their daily energy intake from alcohol. Without that energy source, as occurs during hospitalization, special care must be taken to ensure that the diet supplies sufficient energy.

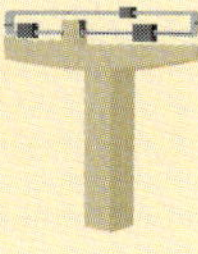

Anthropometric Interpret anthropometric data cautiously in people with edema and ascites. In advanced liver disease, weight is measured daily to assess changes in fluid status. Abdominal girth measurements are also useful for assessing fluid status.

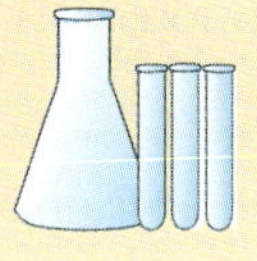

Laboratory Anticipate low serum protein levels in people with advanced liver diseases. Many laboratory tests, including serum albumin, reflect liver function as well as nutrition status. Supplying adequate protein may fail to raise serum proteins if the liver is unable to synthesize them. AST, ALT, ammonia, and bilirubin levels increase with deteriorating liver function.

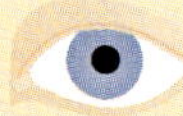

Physical Note physical signs of altered liver function including ascites, edema, and jaundice. Gynecomastia (abnormally large mammary tissue) and testicular atrophy may be present in men with liver failure. Other physical signs of liver dysfunction include angiomas (masses of dilated capillaries and arterioles) and distended abdominal blood vessels. Flapping tremor suggests impending hepatic coma.

complications and death following a liver transplant.[5] A liver transplant candidate must often wait for a liver donor before surgery is possible. Wise health care professionals use this time to identify and correct nutrient imbalances whenever possible. Often TPN is used to provide nutrients prior to a transplant. The person equipped with adequate nutrient stores faces the transplant better prepared to fight infections, heal wounds, and mount a stress response.

Difficulties arise in assessing nutrition status in liver transplant candidates because the metabolic effects of liver disease and those of malnutrition are difficult to distinguish. Edema may mask weight loss and alter other anthropometric measurements. Low serum protein may reflect liver disease itself, rather than nutrition status.

Nutrition following Transplantation Following liver transplantation, liver function determines nutrient needs. All people are hypermetabolic after surgery, and energy needs must be met. Immunosuppressant drugs given to prevent tissue rejection can contribute to nutrient imbalances by causing nausea, vomiting, diarrhea, and mouth sores. The client has an increased susceptibility to infection, and if an infection does occur, nutrient stores are further taxed. The nutrition support team often uses indirect calorimetry to estimate energy needs and carefully monitors clinical and laboratory data to make specific nutrient recommendations.

Although TPN has been the traditional source of nutrients in the posttransplant period, researchers report equal success with intestinal tube feedings.[6] Early enteral nutrition support may reduce the incidence of infection, a particularly important consideration for people with suppressed immune systems.[7]

The complications of cirrhosis outlined in Figure 26–2 all result from the scar tissue that forms within the liver. Dietary and drug treatment aims to preserve liver function and prevent hepatic coma. Perhaps the greatest dietary challenge is providing enough protein to heal, but not so much as to generate ammonia.

The recovery of people with disorders of the liver depends in large part on attention to nutrition and nutrition assessment parameters. The accompanying nutrition assessment checklist reviews important points to keep in mind when assessing the nutrition status of people with liver diseases.

Without a doubt, liver disorders wreak havoc on the body's metabolic work. Equally disturbing to the body's homeostasis are disorders that alter blood glucose concentrations, the topic of the next chapter.

Study Questions

1. What is fatty liver, and what are its causes? What diet modifications, if any, are useful for the treatment of fatty liver?
2. What is hepatitis, and what nutrition concerns arise in the person suffering from hepatitis?
3. Discuss cirrhosis, and describe how it leads to portal hypertension, esophageal varices, ascites, formation of collaterals, and elevated blood ammonia levels.
4. Describe the dietary treatment of the person with cirrhosis and hepatic coma. Consider special dietary concerns of the person with ascites and esophageal varices.
5. How does nutrition status influence recovery from a liver transplant?

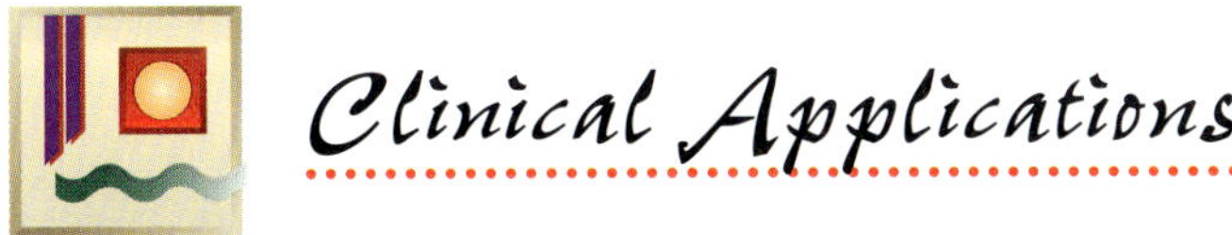

Clinical Applications

1. Think about the problems a person might have in receiving adequate energy from a diet restricted to 40 grams of protein. On such a diet, the total protein allowance could be used up on just one scrambled egg, 3 ounces of meat, a cup of milk, and two slices of bread. Using Figure 17–1 on pp. 572–573

for reference, write down the exchange lists that contain no protein, and add enough of these foods to the diet to meet energy needs (assume an energy need of 2000 kcalories).

Now compare the results with the Daily Food Guide on pp. 42–43. Which food groups have you offered in the recommended quantities? Which food groups are in short supply? Which nutrients might be low? How might fats and sugars be useful in such a diet?

2. The more restrictive a diet is, the harder it usually is to comply with it. The person given the diet in question 1, for example, may miss eating large amounts of meat or meat alternates, breads and grains, or milk and milk products. What effect might additional restrictions, such as fluid and sodium restrictions, have on dietary compliance? Consider, in addition, how much more difficult compliance might be for an alcohol abuser, who must also abstain from alcohol.

Notes

1. Springhouse Corporation, *Diseases*, 2nd ed. (Springhouse, Pa.: Springhouse Corporation, 1997), p. 933.
2. J. E. Fischer, Branched-chain-enriched amino acid solutions in patients with liver failure: An early example of nutritional pharmacology, *Journal of Parenteral and Enteral Nutrition* (supplement) 14 (1990): 249–256.
3. A. Fabri and coauthors, Overview of randomized clinical trials of oral branched-chain amino acid treatment in chronic hepatic encephalopathy, *Journal of Parenteral and Enteral Nutrition* 20 (1996): 159–164.
4. A.S.P.E.N. Board of Directors, Practice guidelines: Liver failure, *Journal of Parenteral and Enteral Nutrition* (supplement) 17 (1993): 14–15; E. P. Shronts and coauthors, Nutrition support of the adult liver transplant candidate, *Journal of the American Dietetic Association* 87 (1987): 441–451.
5. J. Hasse, Nutrition and transplantation, *Nutrition in Clinical Practice* 8 (1993): 3–4; J. Pikul and coauthors, Degree of preoperative malnutrition is predictive of postoperative morbidity and mortality in liver transplant recipients, *Transplantation* 57 (1994): 469–472.
6. C. Wicks and coauthors, Comparison of enteral feeding and total parenteral nutrition after liver transplantation, *Lancet* 344 (1994): 837–840; J. M. Hasse, Early enteral nutrition support in patients undergoing liver transplantation, *Journal of Parenteral and Enteral Nutrition* 19 (1995): 437–443.
7. Hasse, 1995.

Inborn Errors of Metabolism

The discussion in Chapter 26 of the metabolic consequences of liver disorders sets the stage for a closer look at metabolic disorders caused by genetic errors in protein synthesis. When the body makes certain proteins in an insufficient quantity or with an abnormal structure, body functions that depend on those proteins, such as metabolic reactions and transports, cannot proceed. If an enzyme that converts compound A to compound B is missing or malfunctioning in the metabolic pathway, then compound A accumulates and compound B becomes deficient. Both the excess of compound A and the lack of compound B can lead to a variety of problems and, in many cases, to death. Furthermore, this imbalance creates excesses and deficiencies in other metabolic pathways that present another array of problems. The diseases that result from inherited biochemical blocks in normal metabolic pathways are known as inborn errors of metabolism. The accompanying glossary defines related terms.

In some instances, the accumulated compound is not toxic and the deficient compound is not essential, so individuals experience no problem. In all likelihood, they will never know about the error. In other cases, however, inborn errors have severe consequences, including possible mental retardation. Without proper diagnosis and treatment, they can be lethal. As is true of most medical disorders, the earlier the diagnosis and treatment, the better the prognosis.

The primary treatment for many inborn errors of metabolism is nutrition intervention. With an understanding of the biochemical pathway involved, a clinician can often manipulate the diet to compensate for excesses and inadequacies. Management involves restricting dietary precursors that occur prior to the error in the metabolic pathway, replacing needed products that fail to be produced, or both. The goal of therapy is to:

- Prevent the accumulation of toxic metabolites.
- Replace essential nutrients that are deficient as a result of the defective metabolic pathway.
- Provide a diet that supports normal growth, development, and maintenance.

Meeting these three objectives is a major challenge that was previously unattainable. New knowledge about the body's many biochemical pathways, coupled with current technol-

A simple blood test screens newborns for PKU—the most common inborn error of metabolism.

Glossary

carrier: an individual who possesses one dominant and one recessive gene for a recessive trait, such as an inborn error of metabolism. Such a person may show no signs of the trait but can pass it on.

dominant gene: a gene that has an observable effect on an organism even when it is paired with a normal gene; see also *recessive gene*.

galactosemia (ga-LAK-toe-SEE-me-ah): an inborn error of metabolism in which galactose cannot be metabolized normally to compounds the body can handle and an alternative metabolite accumulates in the tissues, causing damage.

genes: the basic units of hereditary information, made of DNA, that are passed from parent to offspring in the chromosomes. Each gene codes for a protein.

inborn error of metabolism: an inherited flaw evident as a metabolic disorder or disease present from birth.

mutation: an alteration in a gene such that an altered protein is produced.
muta = change

PKU, phenylketonuria (FEN-el-KEY-toe-NEW-ree-ah): an inborn error of metabolism in which phenylalanine, an essential amino acid, cannot be converted to tyrosine. Alternative metabolites of phenylalanine (phenylketones) accumulate in the tissues, causing damage, and overflow into the urine.

recessive gene: a gene that has no observable effect on an organism as long as it is paired with a normal gene that can produce a normal product. In this case, the normal gene is said to be *dominant*.

ogy for synthesizing formulas of specific nutrient compositions, has greatly enhanced the treatment of inborn errors.

CLASSIC PHENYLKETONURIA

This discussion focuses primarily on the most common inborn error of metabolism—phenylketonuria (PKU). PKU is only one of several inborn errors that affect amino acid metabolism. Other disorders affect not only amino acid metabolism but also carbohydrate, lipid, and vitamin metabolism. The number of possible inborn errors is limited only by the number of possible gene mutations, for genes carry the codes to make the enzymes in the body.

PKU affects approximately 1 out of every 10,000 newborns in the United States each year. The ability to detect and treat PKU has saved and significantly improved the lives of many people. The achievements in this area offer hope to those suffering from other inborn errors.

Classic PKU results from a deficiency of the enzyme phenylalanine hydroxylase, which converts the essential amino acid phenylalanine to tyrosine (see Figure H26–1). Without the enzyme, abnormally high concentrations of phenylalanine and other related compounds accumulate and damage the developing nervous system. Simultaneously, the body cannot make tyrosine or other compounds (such as the neurotransmitter epinephrine) that normally derive from tyrosine. Under these conditions, tyrosine becomes an essential amino acid; that is, the body cannot make it, and therefore the diet must supply it.

PKU is a hidden disease that cannot be seen at birth, yet diagnosis and treatment beginning in

Figure H26–1

The Biochemical Pathway in PKU

Normal:

Normally, the amino acid phenylalanine follows two pathways, one in the liver, the other in the kidneys. In the liver, the enzyme phenylalanine hydroxylase adds a hydroxyl group (OH) to produce the amino acid tyrosine. Tyrosine, in turn, produces melanin, the pigmented compound found in skin and brain cells; the neurotransmitters epinephrine and norepinephrine; and the hormone thyroxin. In the kidneys, enzymes convert phenylalanine to by-products that are excreted.

In the liver:

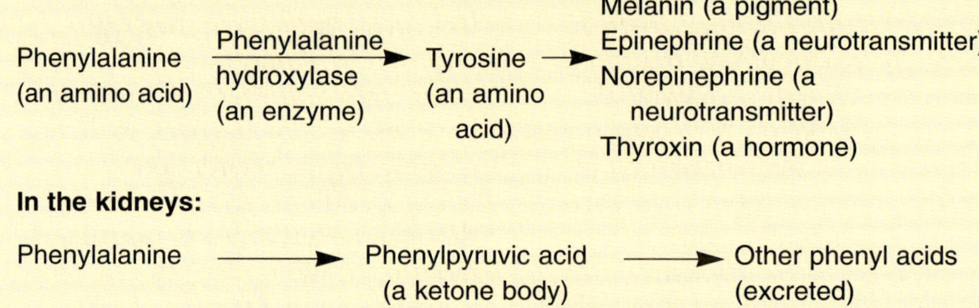

In PKU:

Individuals with PKU lack the liver enzyme phenylalanine hydroxylase, impairing conversion of phenylalanine to tyrosine. Phenylalanine accumulates in the liver and blood, reaching the kidneys in abnormally high concentrations. In the kidneys, an aminotransferase enzyme converts phenylalanine to the ketone body phenylpyruvic acid, which spills into the urine—thus the name phenylketonuria.

In the liver:

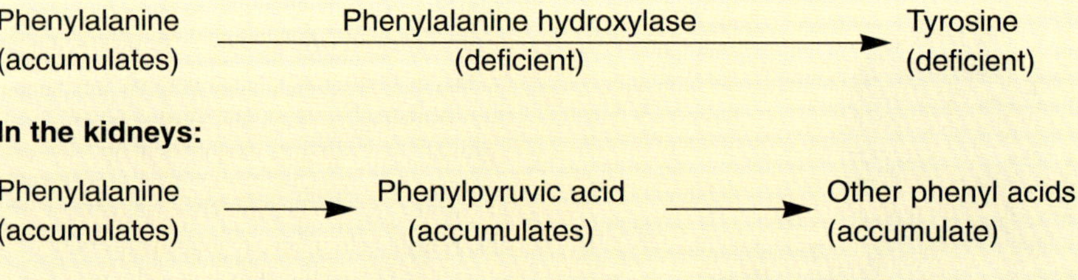

the first few days of life can prevent its devastating effects. For these reasons, and because PKU is the most common inborn error of metabolism, all newborns in the United States receive a screening test for PKU.[1] The test must be conducted after the infant has consumed several meals containing protein (usually after 24 hours and before seven days). Before screening became routine, an infant with PKU would suffer the dire consequences of uncorrected high phenylalanine concentrations. At first, the only signs are a skin rash and light skin pigmentation. Between three and six months, signs of developmental delay begin to appear. The infant becomes irritable and frantic and is unable to sleep restfully. By one year, irreversible brain damage is clearly evident, and the child will score poorly on developmental and intellectual tests.

Sample Phenylalanine-Restricted Menu for a Child with PKU

Note: Lofenalac is a special low-phenylalanine formula that is commercially available.

Menu

Breakfast	Lunch	Supper
2 tbs raisins 5 tbs cream of rice 2 tsp sugar 8 oz Lofenalac	½ small banana 2 tbs tomato soup (without milk) 3 tbs rice 1½ tsp margarine 8 oz Lofenalac	2 tbs instant potatoes (without milk) 3 tbs green beans 4 tbs vegetable and beef broth 1½ tsp margarine ¾ c sliced peaches 8 oz Lofenalac
Midmorning Snack	**Afternoon Snack**	**Bedtime Snack**
4 oz orange juice	4 oz Lofenalac 5 round butter crackers	2 tbs raisins 4 oz Lofenalac

Nutrition Therapy

The effect of nutrition intervention in PKU is remarkable. In almost every case, dietary management can prevent the devastating array of symptoms described. Essentially, the diet restricts phenylalanine and supplements tyrosine to maintain blood concentrations within a safe range. As most dietitians can attest, the diet is more easily described than designed.

Because phenylalanine is an essential amino acid, the diet cannot exclude it completely. If phenylalanine intake is too low, children suffer bone, skin, and blood disorders; growth and mental retardation; and death. Therefore, the diet must strike a balance, providing enough phenylalanine to support normal growth and health but not enough to cause harm. The problem is not that children with PKU require less phenylalanine than other children, but that they cannot handle excesses without detrimental effects. To ensure that blood phenylalanine and tyrosine concentrations remain within an acceptable range, children with PKU receive blood tests periodically and alterations in their diets when necessary. With a controlled phenylalanine intake, children with PKU can lead normal, healthy lives.

To control phenylalanine intake requires strict dietary management that was impossible prior to 1958, when a special low-phenylalanine formula became commercially available. Low-phenylalanine formulas are now the primary source of energy and protein for children with PKU. Their diets exclude high-protein foods such as meat, fish, poultry, cheese, eggs, milk, nuts, and dried beans and peas. Also excluded are commercial breads and pastries made from regular flour, which has a high phenylalanine content. Basically, the diet allows foods that contain some phenylalanine, such as fruits, vegetables, and cereals, and those that contain none, such as fats, sugars, jellies, and some candies. Clearly, it is impossible to create such a diet using only whole, natural foods, but children who depend primarily on a formula for their nourishment risk multiple trace mineral deficiencies.[2] Health care professionals monitor trace mineral status and supplement as needed. The accompanying menu provides a sample phenylalanine-restricted diet for a child with PKU.

Infants receive a special casein hydrolysate formula with a low-phenylalanine content. It does not contain all the phenylalanine an infant requires, so parents supplement it with measured quantities of milk, rice cereal, and baby foods as the infant develops. Other formulas and products are available that provide a synthetic mixture of amino acids without phenylalanine. This enables older children to receive their entire phenylalanine quota from foods.

People with PKU must also be aware of the phenylalanine in products containing the sweetener aspartame (see Table H4–1 on p. 134) and use these products only with guidance from their physicians or dietitians. For adolescents on phenylalanine-restricted diets, occasional diet beverages appear to cause no harm.[3]

Perhaps one of the hardest aspects of this diet is the children's sense of social isolation. From birth, children with PKU are on a "special diet" and cannot eat the foods that other children are eating. Some low-protein cookies and other products containing very little, if any, phenylalanine are commercially available and allow children to share treats with others. Teachers, friends, and family members must understand that they cannot offer foods to children with PKU without permission from the children's parents. Until the children are old enough to know their dietary restrictions, parents must teach them to ask before eating any food. Parents who have learned positive and creative problem-solving skills can effectively resolve situations involving dietary decisions. Consequently, their children are more likely to eat appropriate foods and maintain phenylalanine levels within normal ranges than children of parents without such skills.[4] Routine blood tests and the threat of possible brain damage motivate children and their parents to adhere to the diet.

During the early years of central nervous system development, prompt nutrition intervention is clearly critical to preventing irreversible mental retardation in the young PKU child. Less clear is the length of time the nervous system is vulnerable to the PKU defect. Until the late 1970s, researchers assumed that the child with PKU could abandon the special diet after the first few years of life when the central nervous system had completed its development. They realized that with a regular diet, phenylalanine and associated metabolite concentrations would rise, but thought perhaps these high levels would not be damaging. Unfortunately, elevated phenylalanine concentrations in the older child do cause problems such as short attention span, poor short-term memory, and poor eye-to-hand coordination, although the damage is less severe than at an earlier age. In general, children with PKU who have discontinued their controlled diet experience problems in school performance, mood, and behavior. For these reasons, clinicians now encourage children to continue the low-phenylalanine diet indefinitely. Convincing adolescents to return to the phenylalanine-restricted diet after several years of an unrestricted diet requires intense education and reinforcement. Even then the effort is quite often unsuccessful. Reinstitution of a controlled diet, however, does improve blood phenylalanine concentrations, behavior, and IQ scores.

Therapy for inborn errors goes beyond nutrition to include psychological counseling for the people who are affected and their families. A genetic disorder is a lifelong problem that affects the entire family. All family members are at high risk for being carriers, and they inevitably become involved in the care and management of the person with the inborn error. Therefore, families must learn how to handle the impact such a diagnosis has on their relationships.

Maternal PKU

PKU, like all inborn errors, is a recessive disorder; that is, it appears only when a person inherits two defective genes—one from each parent. This can occur even if neither parent has PKU, because both may be carriers (see Figure H26–2). A carrier is a person who inherits one defective gene and one normal gene. The carrier may be unaware of having a defective gene, for the symptoms are usually mild or absent.

Before the development of routine metabolic screenings, special formulas, and restricted diets, children with PKU died young. Now that people with PKU are living longer and reaching reproductive age, the chances of women with PKU conceiving children have increased significantly. The chance that a mother with PKU will have a child with PKU is about 1 out of 120.[5]

The risks for a PKU mother primarily affect her baby. When a woman is off the diet as an adult, her blood phenylalanine concentrations are high. When she becomes pregnant, her fetus's blood concentrations rise even higher than hers, and fetal development is impaired. The mother may experience a spontaneous abortion; or her infant is likely to suffer mental retardation, microcephaly, congenital heart disease, and low birthweight.[6]

Dietary control of maternal PKU may protect the fetus, at least in part, if implemented early enough.[7] Dietary control does not ensure a successful outcome of pregnancy, but the children of women who follow a low-phenylalanine diet from at least one to two months prior to conception and continue it throughout pregnancy are more likely to have higher birthweights, larger head circumferences, fewer malformations, and higher scores on intelligence tests than the children of women who begin diet therapy during their pregnancy or not at all.[8]

As mentioned, many physicians recommend adherence to a restricted diet throughout life. Resuming a low-phenylalanine diet is not easy. Special formulas that meet the energy, protein, vitamin, and mineral needs of pregnant PKU women are now available. These special formulas are costly and may be inconvenient and unpalatable to an adult who has been eating foods freely. Many women have forgotten that they were ever on a special diet as a child or may never have understood why.

Given the genetic risks and fetal abnormalities associated with a poorly controlled PKU pregnancy, a woman with PKU needs genetic and medical counseling. She must consider the possible consequences of pregnancy, her ability to follow the special diet, and the options of contraception to prevent pregnancy and adoption if she wants children.

Before closing this discussion, it is appropriate to briefly describe another inborn error of metabolism to illustrate the similarities and differences between these types of disorders. To this point, the discussion has focused on PKU, an example of a defect in amino acid metabolism. The following paragraphs describe a defect in carbohydrate metabolism—galactosemia.

Figure H26–2

The Inheritance of PKU

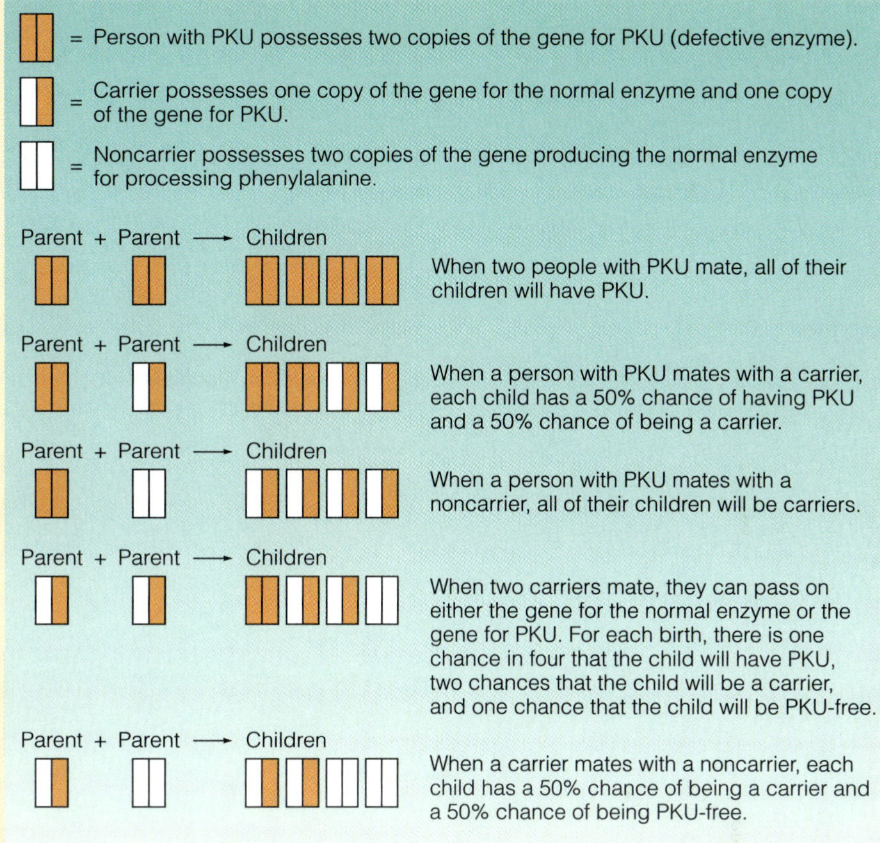

GALACTOSEMIA

Galactosemia is an inborn error of carbohydrate metabolism in which the body cannot use the monosaccharide galactose. Three enzymes are required for the conversion of galactose to glucose; in galactosemia, at least one of those enzymes is missing or defective. When infants with galactosemia are given standard infant formula or breast milk (which contains a galactose unit in each molecule of lactose), they vomit and have diarrhea. The unmetabolized product accumulates and follows an alternative metabolic pathway to form an abnormal product that causes growth failure, liver enlargement, and other neurological abnormalities that lead to coma and death. Early introduction of a galactose-restricted diet prevents or minimizes most of these symptoms. However, it may not prevent ovarian damage, some visual and speech problems, and other neurological abnormalities.

Dietary adjustment in galactosemia is simpler than in PKU for a couple of reasons. First, unlike phenylalanine, galactose is not an essential nutrient. The PKU diet is a balancing act between providing enough phenylalanine for normal growth and development on the one hand and assuring that not enough is left over to be toxic on the other. The galactosemia diet needs only to exclude galactose. Second, galactose occurs primarily in lactose (the sugar in milk), so treatment depends chiefly on the careful restriction of milk and all milk products. This is not to say that the diet is easy to follow; many commercially prepared products contain milk. Still, milk is less widespread in the diet than the amino acid phenylalanine, which appears in all proteins.

As scientific understanding of human genetics and biochemistry increases, more and more inborn errors affecting enzyme function are being recognized. Understanding the roles of enzymes in metabolism makes it possible to compensate for these defects of metabolism that otherwise would destroy the quality of life. Diet cannot always be tailored to prevent the defects of inborn errors, but in many such diseases diet can make a dramatic difference in people's lives.

NOTES

1. Committee on Genetics, Newborn screening fact sheet, *Pediatrics* 98 (1996): 473–501.
2. C. Reilly and coauthors, Trace element nutrition status and dietary intake of children with phenylketonuria, *American Journal of Clinical Nutrition* 52 (1990): 159–165.
3. L. C. Wolf-Novak and coauthors, Aspartame ingestion with and without carbohydrate in phenylketonuric and normal subjects: Effect on plasma concentrations of amino acids, glucose, and insulin, *Metabolism* 39 (1990): 391–396.
4. A. M. B. Fehrenbach and L. Peterson, Parental problem-solving skills, stress, and dietary compliance in phenylketonuria, *Journal of Consulting and Clinical Psychology* 57 (1989): 237–241.
5. Committee on Genetics, Maternal phenylketonuria, *Pediatrics* 88 (1991): 1284–1285.
6. P. B. Acosta, Phenylketonuria—Impact of nutrition support on reproductive outcomes, *Nutrition Today*, January/February 1991, pp. 43–47.
7. The Maternal Phenylketonuria Collaborative Study: A status report, *Nutrition Reviews* 52 (1994): 390–393.
8. Committee on Genetics, 1991; Acosta, 1991.

Chapter 27

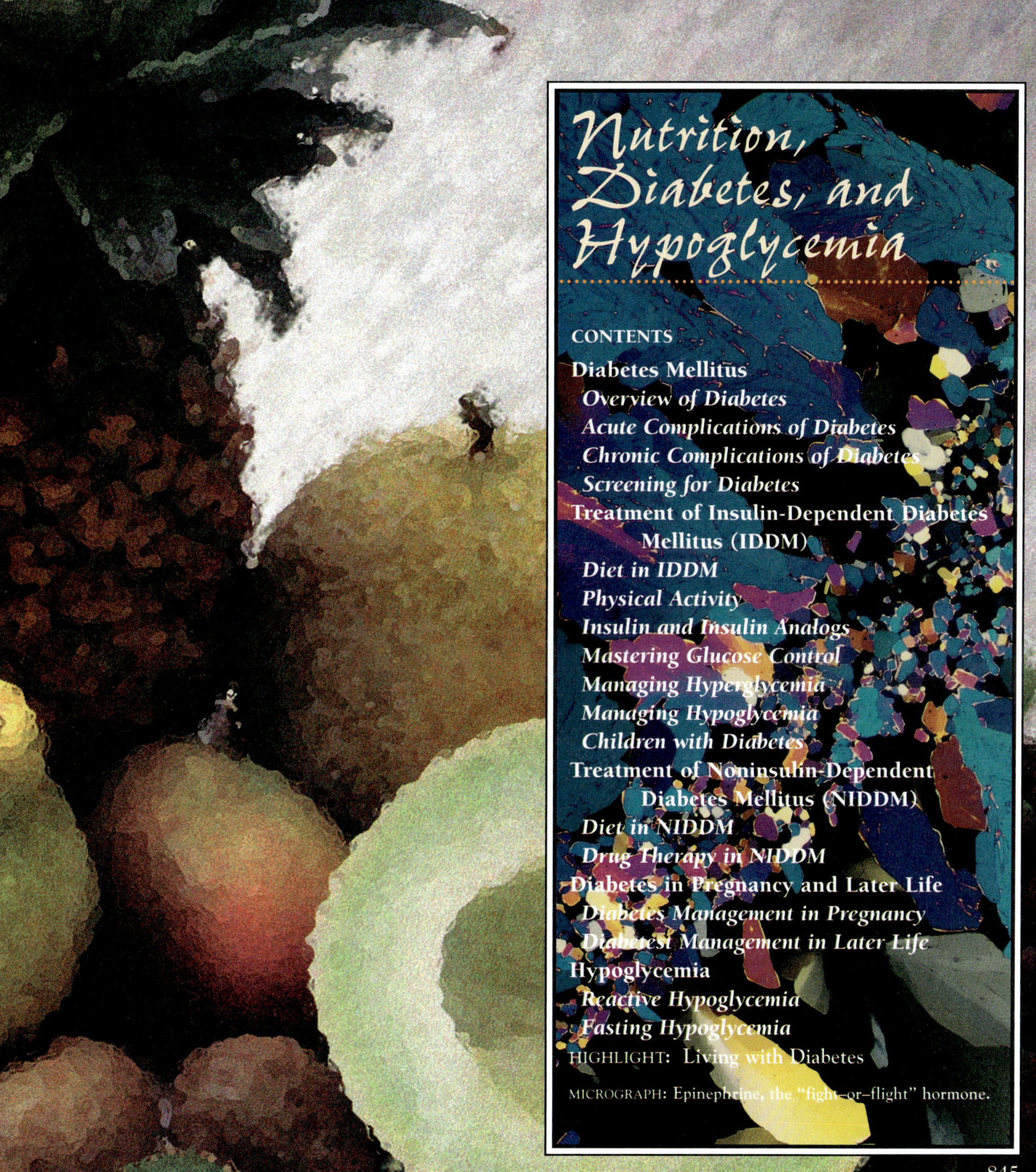

Nutrition, Diabetes, and Hypoglycemia

CONTENTS

MICROGRAPH: Epinephrine, the "fight-or-flight" hormone.

The body's metabolic work is so vital to survival that metabolic disturbances, such as those imposed by severe stresses and liver dysfunction, are often severe and even fatal. Likewise, diabetes mellitus, a disorder of energy metabolism, and hypoglycemia, a symptom of altered glucose metabolism, can lead to serious consequences. Medical nutrition therapy for both conditions serves not only to maintain nutrition status, but also to control symptoms and prevent complications associated with each disorder.

Diabetes Mellitus

diabetes (DYE-uh-BEET-eez) **mellitus** (MELL-ih-tus or mell-EYE-tus): a metabolic disorder characterized by altered blood glucose regulation and utilization, usually caused by insufficient or relatively ineffective insulin.
diabetes = passing through (the body)
mellitus = honey-sweet (sugar)

Diabetes mellitus is a chronic disorder characterized by elevated blood glucose and altered energy metabolism caused by an absolute deficiency of insulin or ineffective insulin. About 8 million people in the United States have been diagnosed with diabetes, and estimates suggest that another 8 million people have the disorder but remain undiagnosed.[1] Still others have the first signs that they may develop diabetes later; the prevalence increases with age.

OVERVIEW OF DIABETES

Diabetes ranks among the leading causes of death in the United States. It is a major cause of blindness, kidney failure, infections necessitating leg amputations, and birth defects. In addition, people with diabetes are twice as likely to develop cardiovascular problems as those without diabetes. Table 27–1 shows the distinguishing features of the two main forms of diabetes, which are described next. Both forms appear to develop as a consequence of both hereditary and environmental factors.

Insulin-Dependent Diabetes Mellitus Insulin, which signals the body to store energy fuels following meals, is produced by the islets of Langerhans—the

Table 27–1

Features of IDDM and NIDDM

	IDDM	NIDDM
Other names	Type I diabetes Juvenile-onset diabetes Ketosis-prone diabetes Brittle diabetes	Type II diabetes Adult-onset diabetes Ketosis-resistant diabetes Lipoplethoric diabetes Stable diabetes
Age of onset	<20 (mean age, 12)	>40
Associated conditions	Viral infection	Obesity
Insulin required?	Yes	Sometimes
Cell response to insulin	Normal	Resistant
Symptoms	Relatively severe	Relatively moderate
Prevalence in diabetic population	5 to 10%	90 to 95%

endocrine cells of the pancreas. The pancreatic islets consist of several cell types including the beta cells, which produce insulin, and the alpha cells, which produce glucagon. In insulin-dependent diabetes (IDDM), the less common type of diabetes (about 5 to 10 percent of all diagnosed cases), the pancreas cannot synthesize insulin. Without insulin, the body's energy metabolism is dramatically altered with such serious consequences that people with IDDM cannot survive unless they obtain insulin from another source.

insulin-dependent diabetes mellitus (IDDM): the less common type of diabetes in which the person produces no insulin at all.

IDDM most frequently develops in people younger than 20, although the incidence peaks again in individuals over 40 who initially develop noninsulin-dependent diabetes and later become insulin dependent. Researchers believe that the individual with IDDM may have inherited a defect in which immune cells mistakenly attack and destroy insulin-producing pancreatic cells. IDDM frequently develops following exposure to certain viruses, further suggesting an immune system connection. Indeed, the detection of antibodies to the insulin-producing pancreatic cells indicates the destruction of such cells and predicts the subsequent development of IDDM.[2] Diabetes can develop secondary to other disorders, such as pancreatitis and cystic fibrosis (discussed in Chapter 22), or as a result of exposure to certain drugs or chemicals.

The immune system disorders in which the body destroys its own tissues are called **autoimmune disorders**.

Noninsulin-Dependent Diabetes Mellitus The predominant type of diabetes mellitus (90 to 95 percent of all cases), and the type likely to go undiagnosed, is called noninsulin-dependent diabetes mellitus (NIDDM). Although the exact cause of NIDDM remains unknown, high blood glucose and insulin resistance are the hallmarks of the disorder. In the initial stages, the pancreas produces insulin, but the cells become less and less sensitive to its effects. As blood glucose rises, the pancreas makes more insulin, and blood insulin rises to abnormally high levels (hyperinsulinemia). The chronic demand for insulin exhausts the beta cells, and finally insulin production falters as the disease progresses. NIDDM develops most often in people over 40 and appears to be associated with obesity (often of long duration), abdominal fat, and physical inactivity.[3] As body fat increases, body tissues become less able to respond to insulin. Thus NIDDM appears to be a self-aggravating condition.

noninsulin-dependent diabetes mellitus (NIDDM): the more common type of diabetes that develops gradually and is associated with insulin resistance. A type of NIDDM that develops during the teen years has been termed maturity-onset diabetes in the young (MODY).

insulin resistance: the condition in which a set amount of insulin produces a subnormal effect.

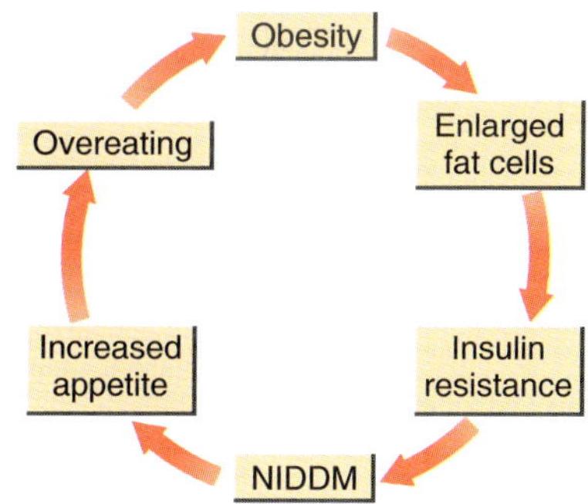

Diabetes-Related Risk Disorders A nationwide multicenter study (the Diabetes Prevention Program) is currently under way to determine whether early interventions for people with impaired glucose metabolism can prevent NIDDM.[4] People with impaired glucose tolerance have mild hyperglycemia without the symptoms of diabetes. Those most likely to develop impaired glucose tolerance include people from certain ethnic groups (Native Americans, Hispanic Americans, and African Americans); people who are obese, are over age 45 (especially those over 65), and have close relatives with diabetes; and women who have given birth to babies weighing more than 9 pounds or have developed hyperglycemia while pregnant—gestational diabetes (described in a later section).

Consequences of Diabetes To appreciate the problems caused by either insufficient or ineffective insulin, recall that insulin enhances cellular uptake of glucose and fatty acids and stimulates protein synthesis, glycogen synthesis, and fat synthesis. Disruption of energy metabolism and exposure of the tissues to high glucose concentrations result in both acute and chronic complications. The accompanying glossary defines diabetes-related symptoms and complications.

glucose tolerance: the ability of the body to regulate its blood glucose concentration to either the intake of dietary carbohydrate or the release of glucose from cells during fasting or metabolic stress.

Glossary of Diabetes-Related Symptoms and Complications

acetone breath: a distinctive fruity odor that can be detected on the breath of a person who is experiencing ketosis.

diabetic coma: unconsciousness precipitated by hyperglycemia, dehydration, ketosis, and acidosis in uncontrolled IDDM.

gangrene: death of tissue due to a deficient blood supply and/or infection.

gastroparesis: delayed gastric emptying.

glycosuria (GLY-ko-SUE-ree-ah) or **glucosuria** (GLUE-ko-SUE-ree-ah): glucose in the urine, which generally occurs when blood glucose exceeds 180 mg/100 ml.

hyperglycemia: elevated blood glucose.

hyperosmolar hyperglycemia nonketotic coma: coma that occurs in uncontrolled NIDDM precipitated by the presence of hypertonic blood and dehydration.

hypoglycemia: low blood glucose.

ketonemia: ketones in the blood.

ketonuria: ketones in the urine.

macroangiopathies: disorders of the large blood vessels.

microangiopathies: disorders of the capillaries.

nephropathy: a disorder of the kidneys.

neuropathy: a disorder of the nerves.

polydipsia (POLL-ee-DIP-see-ah): excessive thirst.

polyphagia (POLL-ee-FAY-gee-ah): excessive eating.

polyuria (POLL-ee-YOU-ree-ah): excessive urine production.

retinopathy: a disorder of the retina.

ACUTE COMPLICATIONS OF DIABETES

Figure 27–1 presents an overview of the metabolic changes and acute complications that occur in uncontrolled diabetes. The metabolic consequences of IDDM are more immediate and severe than those of NIDDM because in IDDM no glucose enters the cells.

Symptoms of hyperglycemia:

- Intense thirst and hunger.
- Increased urination.
- Weight loss.
- Blurred vision.
- Fatigue.
- Acetone breath.
- Glycosuria.
- Labored breathing.

renal threshold: the point at which blood glucose rises so high that the kidneys cannot reabsorb it.

Hyperglycemia, Dehydration, and Glycosuria With insufficient or ineffective insulin, blood glucose rises and hyperglycemia results. High blood glucose creates an osmotic effect, drawing water from tissues into the blood. Then the high blood concentration of glucose overwhelms the kidneys' ability to reabsorb glucose (the renal threshold). The excess glucose "spills" into the urine along with fluid and electrolytes. Glycosuria generally occurs when blood glucose exceeds 180 milligrams per 100 milliliters. As a result of hyperglycemia, both the intracellular and the extracellular fluid compartments become depleted, leading to severe dehydration. This series of events explains why the person with uncontrolled diabetes produces excessive urine (polyuria) and exhibits excessive thirst (polydipsia).

Ketosis and Coma in IDDM IDDM continuously deprives cells of the energy fuels they need. Amino acids and glucose may abound in the body fluids, but the cells have limited access to them. Consequently, the body mobilizes fat for energy. The liver responds to the mobilization of fatty acids by producing ketone bodies, which accumulate in the blood (ketonemia). A fruity odor on the

Figure 27–1

Metabolic Consequences and Acute Clinical Manifestations of Untreated IDDM and NIDDM

As you can see, when glucose cannot enter the cells, a cascade of metabolic changes follows. In NIDDM, some glucose enters the cells. Because the cells are not "starved" for glucose, the body does not shift into the metabolism of fasting (losing weight and producing ketones).

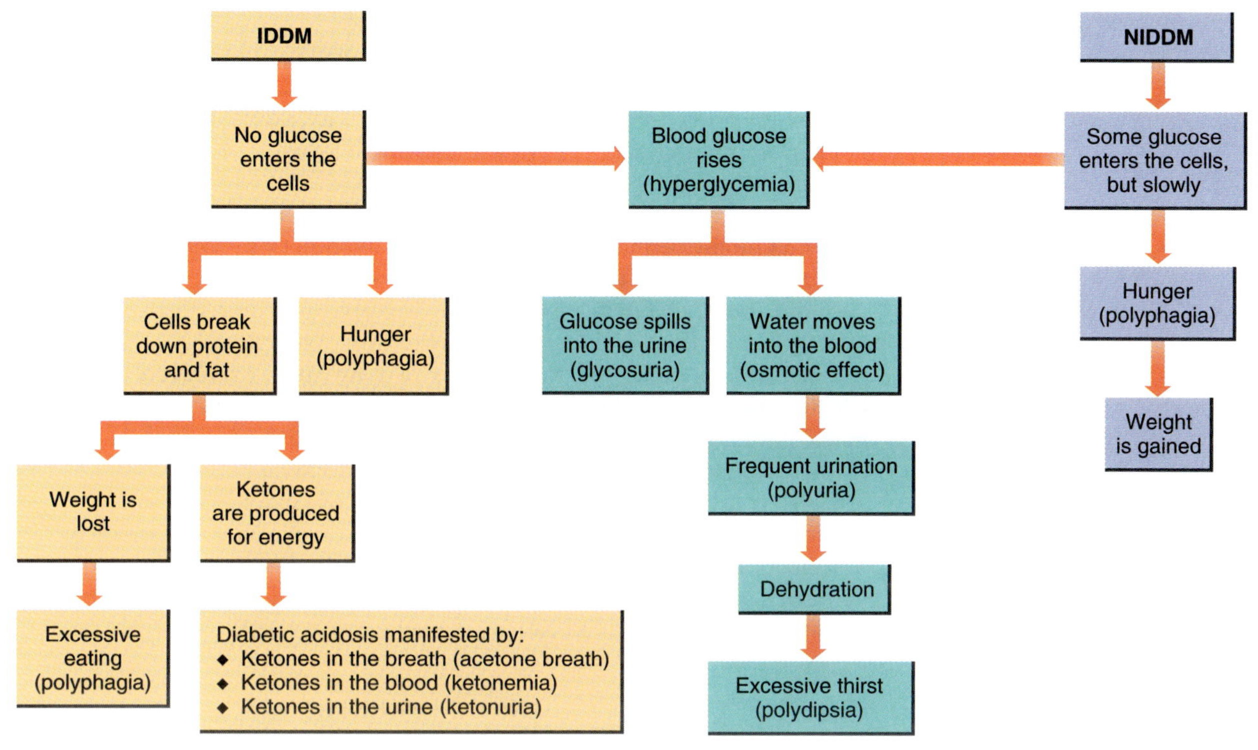

breath of a person with uncontrolled IDDM reflects the presence of the ketone acetone. Ketone bodies in the blood lower its pH (acidosis) because they contain acid groups. Ketone bodies also begin to appear in the urine (ketonuria). In addition, the kidneys excrete sodium and potassium along with the ketone bodies in a way that worsens acidosis. When acidosis becomes severe enough, a potentially fatal coma may follow.

Reminder: *Ketone bodies* are produced by the incomplete breakdown of fat when glucose is not available in the cells.

Nonketotic Coma in NIDDM People with NIDDM generally are not prone to ketosis and acidosis, but they can develop another kind of coma caused by extremely high blood glucose. This problem is common in the elderly because they may not recognize thirst and drink enough water to compensate for high blood glucose levels. Logically, this kind of coma is termed hyperosmolar hyperglycemic nonketotic coma.

Weight Loss in IDDM With the loss of glucose and ketone bodies (both energy sources) in the urine, combined with protein breakdown, serious weight loss follows. The person with poorly controlled IDDM is likely to be thin despite eating excessively (polyphagia).

Weight Gain in NIDDM NIDDM also deprives cells of the energy fuels they need, not continuously, but enough to make the cells hungry. As a result, people with NIDDM often overeat. Then the insulin they do have slowly takes effect, and the body ends up storing fat from the excess energy consumed. This explains why the person with NIDDM is likely to remain overweight and also why ketone bodies do not accumulate in the blood and urine.

Hypoglycemia Hypoglycemia is a consequence, not of untreated diabetes, but rather of inappropriate management. It can result from too much insulin or glucose-lowering drugs, strenuous physical activity, skipped meals, delayed meals, inadequate food intake, vomiting, or severe diarrhea.

Left untreated, severe hypoglycemia can lead to loss of consciousness, brain damage, and even death. Some research suggests that repeated episodes of hypoglycemia might permanently impair cognitive function.[5] Mental confusion and shakiness may make it difficult for the person to recognize symptoms of hypoglycemia (see the margin) and to take corrective measures. Recovery from severe hypoglycemia requires the assistance of another person.

Symptoms of hypoglycemia:
- Hunger.
- Headache.
- Sweating.
- Shakiness.
- Nervousness.
- Confusion.
- Disorientation.
- Slurred speech.

Adults who have had diabetes for a long time risk severe hypoglycemia because the warning signs become less noticeable over time. People who tightly manage their blood glucose levels (intensive therapy) are more likely to develop hypoglycemia than others with diabetes. Symptoms can also occur while the person is sleeping, making hypoglycemia difficult to detect.

Notice that many of the symptoms of hypoglycemia are those of alcohol intoxication. If the true problem goes unrecognized, the person may die. To prevent such a tragic mistake, advise every person with IDDM to wear medical identification in the form of a bracelet or necklace.

CHRONIC COMPLICATIONS OF DIABETES

Chronic hyperglycemia damages the structures of the blood vessels and nerves. Circulation becomes poor and nerve function falters. Infections are more likely to occur due to poor circulation coupled with glucose-rich blood and urine. People with diabetes must pay special attention to hygiene and keep alert for early signs of infection.

Cardiovascular Diseases Atherosclerosis (see Chapter 28) tends to develop early, progress rapidly, and be more severe in people with diabetes. More than 80 percent of people with diabetes die as a consequence of cardiovascular diseases, especially heart attacks. If nerve function is also impaired, the person may have a heart attack and not even realize it.

Disorders of the large blood vessels, including atherosclerosis, are called **macroangiopathies**.
macro = large
angio = blood vessel
pathy = disease

A heart attack that goes unnoticed is called a **silent heart attack**.

Microangiopathies Disorders of the small blood vessels (capillaries) may also develop and lead to loss of kidney function and retinal degeneration with accompanying loss of vision. About 85 percent of people with diabetes have nephropathy, retinopathy, or both (see the glossary on p. 848). Consequently, as mentioned earlier, diabetes is a leading cause of both kidney failure and blindness.

Disorders of the small blood vessels are called **microangiopathies**.
micro = small

Neuropathy Nerve tissues may also deteriorate, resulting in neuropathy. Neuropathy may express itself at first as a painful prickling sensation, often in the arms and legs. Later, the person loses sensation in the hands and feet. Injuries to these areas may go unnoticed, and infections can progress rapidly. With loss of both circulation and nerve function, undetected injury and infection may lead to death of tissue (gangrene), necessitating amputation of the limbs (most often the legs or feet). People with neuropathy are advised to take conscientious care of their feet and visit a podiatrist regularly.

Neuropathy can also delay gastric emptying. When the stomach empties slowly after a meal, the person may experience a premature feeling of fullness, bloating, nausea, vomiting, weight loss, and poor blood glucose control due to irregular nutrient absorption.

SCREENING FOR DIABETES

A major multicenter clinical trial, the Diabetes Control and Complications Trial (DCCT), showed that carefully controlling blood glucose in a near-normal range can reduce the risks of chronic complications in IDDM by 50 to 80 percent.[6] Evidence that similar results might be possible in NIDDM is mounting. Recognizing that many people may have diabetes and not know it, and that early treatment might reduce the risk of serious complications, efforts are under way to screen for diabetes.

Because the lifetime risk of developing NIDDM is one in five, screening all people over age 30 for the early detection of diabetes would be ideal.[7] The American Diabetes Association recommends that all people over the age of 45 be tested for diabetes every three years.[8] Those at high risk for diabetes (see p. 847) need screening at earlier ages or more frequently.

Major risk factors for NIDDM:

- Obesity.
- Family history.
- High-risk ethnic background.
- Gestational diabetes or mother giving birth to a baby weighing over 9 lb.

Blood tests help identify people with diabetes or impaired glucose tolerance. Most commonly, high fasting blood glucose on two occasions suggests diabetes. Fasting blood glucose higher than normal, but not high enough to confirm diabetes, indicates impaired glucose tolerance. Health care professionals often advise people with impaired glucose tolerance to begin diet therapy for diabetes. Some physicians prefer to test a person's fasting blood glucose and then retest several times more after glucose is given orally—a procedure called a glucose tolerance test.

Interpretation of fasting blood glucose:
Normal: <110 mg/100 ml.
Impaired glucose tolerance: 110–126 mg/100 ml.
Diabetes: >126 mg/100 ml.

Impaired glucose tolerance is sometimes called **borderline diabetes**

Diabetes mellitus is characterized by elevated blood glucose caused by either an absolute deficiency of insulin (IDDM) or ineffective insulin (NIDDM). Table 27–1 summarizes the distinguishing features of IDDM and NIDDM, and Figure 27–1 shows their metabolic consequences and symptoms. Long-term complications of diabetes include cardiovascular diseases, kidney failure, blindness, and nerve damage. Screening for diabetes through blood and urine tests allows for early detection and early treatment, which helps to minimize complications.

Treatment of Insulin-Dependent Diabetes Mellitus (IDDM)

A diagnosis of IDDM can be devastating. The parents of a young child with IDDM may feel overwhelmed, angry, anxious, and even guilty. A teenager may feel that it is the end of the world. A person of any age may fear the prospect of daily insulin injections, possible complications, and the new diet. To control blood glucose successfully, the person must master the complex task of

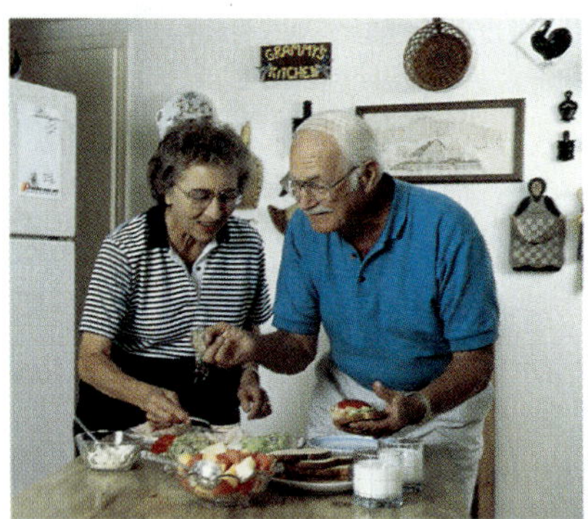

The diet for diabetes emphasizes a consistent intake of carbohydrate spaced evenly throughout the day.

coordinating diet, physical activity, and insulin. On the bright side, however, is that with such mastery the person can live a full and active life and significantly reduce the risk of chronic complications. Highlight 27 describes how health care professionals can assist in this process.

The goals of medical and nutrition therapy for diabetes are to maintain blood glucose within a fairly normal range, achieve optimal blood lipid levels, control blood pressure, support health and well-being, and treat complications. The most important of these goals is to maintain blood glucose control.

To the student reading about diabetes today, such a goal may seem obvious: of course, blood glucose should be maintained at or near levels observed in people without diabetes. Only recently, however, have improvements in the technology for monitoring blood levels at home made such tight control possible. Only recently, too, have the benefits of tight control been clearly demonstrated. (A later section describes blood glucose monitoring in more detail.)

Assessment is important in diabetes: an accurate history enables the health care team to work out acceptable goals for a diet, physical activity, and insulin program. To promote success, the health care team plans and adjusts therapy for the client's medical needs, motivational level, educational ability, and lifestyle. Successful diabetes education takes time and must be flexible to accommodate changing needs.

DIET IN IDDM

The diet for diabetes parallels a healthy diet for all people in both amounts and types of nutrients. It differs from a regular diet in that carbohydrate intake must be consistent from day to day and at each meal and snack, or adjustments must be made in insulin administration. The actual distribution of nutrients for each client depends on medical needs and current food habits.

Energy The diet for IDDM first focuses on providing adequate food energy to achieve or maintain a healthy and realistic body weight and to support growth in children and pregnant women. To determine whether energy intake is appropriate, the planner uses the RDA for energy as a guide, takes height and weight measures periodically, and adjusts the diet as necessary.

Carbohydrate Carbohydrate-containing foods provide energy and directly affect blood glucose. The more carbohydrate a person eats in a meal, the higher blood glucose rises, but the diet for IDDM does not restrict carbohydrate intake. Carbohydrate is necessary to maintain a steady supply of glucose. Typically, diet plans provide from 45 to 60 percent of the total kcalories from carbohydrate. Eating about the same amount of carbohydrate at about the same time each day helps the person avoid hyperglycemia and hypoglycemia and eases the task of coordinating insulin doses and food intake.

Recall that authorities recommend 20 to 35 g of dietary fiber a day.

Encourage clients to select foods rich in complex carbohydrates: whole-grain breads and cereals, legumes, fruits, and vegetables. In addition to carbohydrates, these foods provide vitamins and minerals and offer many health benefits (see Chapter 4).

Traditionally, concentrated sweets were strictly excluded from the diet for diabetes, but now they are restricted only to the same extent as they are for all people. Health care professionals recognize that the *total* carbohydrate is of greater concern in diabetes than the *type* of carbohydrate.[9] The person with diabetes can use concentrated sweets as a limited part of a healthy diet, as long as they are counted as part of the carbohydrate allowance. Artificial sweeteners that contain minimal kcalories, and products made from them, can be used in place of sugar.

Carbohydrate Replacement for Missed Meals A person with IDDM who misses a meal needs to eat about 15 to 30 grams of complex carbohydrate to forestall hypoglycemia. If appetite is poor, people can use juice, flavored gelatin, soft drinks, or frozen juice bars to meet their carbohydrate needs. In the hospital, if a person with IDDM misses a meal, different procedures may be employed. One procedure provides at least half the prescribed carbohydrate and kcalories within three hours of the missed meal. If this cannot be done, the physician may change the insulin schedule, give IV dextrose, or change the diet prescription to include more simple carbohydrates.

Carbohydrate from Enteral and Parenteral Formulas When people with diabetes require enteral or parenteral formulas, adjustments may need to be made for the large amount of carbohydrates the formulas contain. Often health care professionals adjust insulin doses to meet the higher carbohydrate load.[10] If additional insulin fails to control hyperglycemia, people on parenteral nutrition may need to receive less energy from dextrose and more from IV fat emulsions (see Chapter 24). People who cannot tolerate the carbohydrate in standard enteral formulas may benefit from specially designed formulas that contain less total carbohydrate (see Appendix K).

Protein Protein provides about 10 to 20 percent of the total kcalories in the diet for diabetes. Providing adequate, but not excessive, protein may help delay the onset or progression of kidney disease (see Chapter 29). At the first sign of kidney disease, people with diabetes may need to restrict protein to 0.8 grams per kilogram of body weight per day (same as the RDA).[11]

An early sign of impending kidney disease is elevated albumin in the urine or microalbuminuria (see Chapter 29).

Fat People with diabetes who have normal blood lipids benefit from a fat intake consistent with the *Dietary Guidelines for Americans* (30 percent or less of total kcalories from fat and less than 10 percent from saturated fat). Those who need to lose weight may need to restrict fat further. People with diabetes and elevated LDL may need to restrict saturated fat to 7 percent or less of total kcalories and cholesterol to less than 200 milligrams daily (see Chapter 28). To lower fat and cholesterol intakes, clients can use low-fat and nonfat milk and lean meats, among other strategies (see p. 168).

Sodium People with diabetes frequently develop hypertension and are likely to be salt sensitive. Practitioners generally advise all clients with diabetes to limit sodium to less than 3000 milligrams per day.[12] People with diabetes and hypertension may need to restrict sodium to 2400 milligrams or less per day. Chapter 12 (p. 421) describes strategies to lower sodium intake.

Alcohol The person whose blood glucose is well controlled can usually include some alcoholic beverages with the consent of the physician. Because alcohol can cause hypoglycemia in any person, however, people with IDDM are advised to take only moderate amounts (no more than two drinks a day), with

One drink is defined as 1½ oz liquor or 5 oz wine or 12 oz beer. Note: light beer contains the same amount of alcohol as regular beer, with half the carbohydrate. When counting kcalories, 1 drink = 2 fat exchanges.

meals, and in addition to the usual meal plan. Remember, too, that the person with hypoglycemia may appear to be intoxicated, and alcohol use can add confusion to a potentially dangerous situation.

Alcohol intake is discouraged for people with a history of alcohol abuse; those with pancreatitis, abnormal blood lipids, or neuropathy; and pregnant women. Alcohol use is also discouraged for people who are overweight; if it is used, alcohol should be substituted for fat exchanges. Drinks that contain simple sugars (mixers, sweet wines, and liqueurs) are best avoided. If they are used, the person must count their carbohydrate contents as part of the daily carbohydrate allowance.

Timing and Composition of Meals In diabetes, consistent timing and composition of meals and snacks from day to day improve glucose control. An evening snack is especially important because it helps sustain the person's blood glucose through the night. A person with a regular physical activity program who takes a prescribed dose of insulin at a set time and then eats about the same amount of carbohydrate at about the same time each day knows that glucose and insulin will be available to the body when they are needed. Meal patterns and physical activity programs that change dramatically from day to day require careful blood glucose monitoring and insulin adjustments to help maintain control. People who find a set schedule difficult to maintain need to work with skilled health care professionals to learn how to adjust their insulin doses to fit their food intakes and physical activity schedules.

Diet-related behaviors that may improve blood glucose control include:

- Adherence to the meal plan.
- Appropriate treatment of hypoglycemia.
- Prompt treatment of hyperglycemia.
- Consistent and appropriate bedtime snacking.[13]

Dietitians teach the diet in stages, starting first with simple concepts and progressing to more difficult ones as the client's abilities and needs dictate.

Meal-Planning Strategies No single approach to diet therapy meets everyone's needs, and diet planners use several approaches to help clients achieve blood glucose control. Some diet strategies teach clients to use food guides or simple menus to plan diets. Traditionally, however, diet planners use the exchange patterns described in Chapter 17 (see pp. 570–575). Recall that the foods within each list of the exchange system are similar in food energy and in carbohydrate, protein, and fat per serving. The person using this system learns that the food portions on any one list can be exchanged freely for one another. For example, a person who needs a starch exchange might select one slice of bread or ½ cup of bran cereal or one small (3 ounce) baked potato. The accompanying box shows how to plan a diet for diabetes using exchange lists.

Appendix G includes the U.S. Exchange System, and Appendix I shows the Canadian Exchange System.

A strategy gaining wide use, called *carbohydrate counting,* teaches clients to focus mainly on the carbohydrate contents of foods. Clients can use food composition tables, food labels, and exchange lists to determine the carbohydrate contents of the foods they eat. Clients using this system learn to eat consistent amounts of carbohydrates at meals and snacks. They must have the motivation to weigh or measure portion sizes and the ability to perform the mathematical operations necessary to calculate their carbohydrate intakes. Regardless of the

How to Plan a Diet for Diabetes Using Exchange Lists

The dietitian most often plans the diet for a client with diabetes. In doing so, the dietitian carefully considers the client's lifestyle and medical needs. Planning a diet using exchange lists takes time, but with practice, a dietitian can learn to plan diets quickly. This box describes a simplified diet plan.

Dietitians begin by assessing each individual to determine what weight is reasonable and how many kcalories are necessary to achieve or maintain that body weight. Chapter 16 described ways of estimating desirable body weights, and the box on p. 265 in Chapter 8 showed how to estimate energy needs based on body weight and physical activity levels. Chapter 9 described kcalorie needs for safe weight loss (see p. 302) and weight gain (see p. 310). The growth charts in Appendix E can be used to estimate desirable weights for children, and Chapter 19 (see p. 638) described their energy needs. Remember, though, that desirable weights and calculated energy needs are estimates only.

For this example, we will use a man who is 6 feet tall and is comfortable with the weight of 178 pounds that he has maintained throughout his adult life. From an assessment of food intake, the dietitian estimates that the man has maintained his weight on about 2900 kcalories per day with 25 percent of kcalories from protein, 45 percent from carbohydrate, and 30 percent from fat.

1. The first step is to determine the grams of protein, carbohydrate, and fat recommended for a diet for diabetes.
   - 10 to 20% of the kcalories from protein.
   - 45 to 60% of the kcalories from carbohydrate.
   - 30% or less of the kcalories from fat.

   For 2900 kcalories, this division of nutrients translates into grams as follows:

   - Protein:

$$10\% \times 2900 \text{ kcal} = 290 \text{ kcal.} \qquad 290 \text{ kcal} \div 4 \text{ kcal/g} = 73 \text{ g.}$$
$$20\% \times 2900 \text{ kcal} = 580 \text{ kcal.} \qquad 580 \text{ kcal} \div 4 \text{ kcal/g} = 145 \text{ g.}$$

Thus the man needs between 73 and 145 g protein.

   - Carbohydrate:

$$45\% \times 2900 \text{ kcal} = 1305 \text{ kcal.} \qquad 1305 \text{ kcal} \div 4 \text{ kcal/g} = 326 \text{ g.}$$
$$60\% \times 2900 \text{ kcal} = 1740 \text{ kcal.} \qquad 1740 \text{ kcal} \div 4 \text{ kcal/g} = 435 \text{ g.}$$

Thus the man needs between 326 and 435 g carbohydrate.

   - Fat:

$$30\% \times 2900 \text{ kcal} = 870 \text{ kcal.} \qquad 870 \text{ kcal} \div 9 \text{ kcal/g} = 97 \text{ g.}$$

Thus the man needs about 97 g fat or less.

2. The dietitian recognizes that the client will need to make dietary changes to conform to a healthy eating plan. To minimize the changes the client must make, the dietitian decides to plan the diet to include 20 percent protein or 580 kcalories. Thus 80 percent or 2320 kcalories remain for carbohydrate and fat. After reviewing information about the man's blood lipids, which are within acceptable limits, the dietitian plans the diet to keep fat at the current level of 30 percent (870 kcalories). This means that 50 percent of the kcalories (1450 kcalories) remain for carbohydrate.

$$2900 \text{ total kcal} - 580 \text{ protein kcal} - 870 \text{ fat kcal} = 1450 \text{ carbohydrate kcal.}$$

3. To translate the kcalories from fat and carbohydrate to grams:

$$870 \text{ fat kcal} \div 9 \text{ kcal/g} = 96.6 \text{ g (round down to 96 to limit fat).}$$

How to Plan a Diet for Diabetes Using Exchange Lists (continued)

$$1450 \text{ carbohydrate kcal} \div 4 \text{ kcal/g} = 362.5 \text{ g (round up to 363).}$$

Thus the diet will provide 2900 kcalories with a distribution of 20 percent protein (145 grams or 580 kcalories), 50 percent carbohydrate (363 grams or 1450 kcalories), and 30 percent fat (96 grams or 870 kcalories).

4. Now it is time to translate the diet prescription into a meal plan. Table 17–2 on p. 571 shows the grams of carbohydrate, protein, and fat and the energy value in each serving on an exchange list. Using this table and the client's food intake record as a guide, the dietitian first plans servings of foods that contain carbohydrate, then protein, and finally fat, trying to match foods as closely as possible to the client's usual food intake. This process takes practice and requires some adjusting based on trial and error. Most often, the final result does not fit the meal plan exactly, but comes close. Table 27–2 shows how the dietitian might plan a day's exchanges for the man in this example. Note that the plan falls within the guidelines of the Daily Food Guide on p. 42. The plan uses nonfat milk and lean meat exchanges for calculations. Lower-fat foods are encouraged. If the client occasionally chooses to use another type of milk or meat, the number of fat servings must be adjusted accordingly. For example, if the client eats 4 ounces of a high-fat meat (32 grams of fat) instead of lean meat (12 grams of fat), he must then use four fewer fat exchanges during the day (20 grams of fat). The plan shown in Table 27–2 does not include the "other carbohydrates" list; starches and other foods (described later) can be substituted for foods on this list.
5. Distribute foods into meals that fit the client's usual eating patterns. Table 27–3 shows how the day's exchanges might be divided for the man in this example. With this information in hand, the dietitian and client can begin to fill in the plan with real foods to create a sample menu such as the one shown on p. 858. The client is reminded to eat about the same amount of carbohydrate at about the same time each day.
6. Teach clients how to tailor the diet to meet their own preferences. For example, foods from the starch, fruit, milk, and other carbohydrate lists contain similar amounts of energy and carbohydrate and can be substituted for one another from time to time. Regular substitution is discouraged, however, because each list makes unique contributions to other nutrient needs. A client who regularly substitutes fruit for milk, for example, may not be getting enough calcium. The client who regularly substitutes milk for a starch or fruit may not be getting enough fiber.[a]

   Several servings of free foods can be used as long as their use is spread throughout the day. Free foods contain up to 20 kcalories and 5 grams of carbohydrate per serving.

[a]M. Wheeler, M. J. Franz, and P. Barrier, Helpful hints: Using the 1995 exchange lists for meal planning, *Diabetes Spectrum* 8 (1995): 325–326.

diet strategy, all clients receive instructions on planning well-balanced and healthy meals, eating consistent amounts of foods at regular times, and maintaining a desirable weight.

PHYSICAL ACTIVITY

Fitness programs confer benefits on the cardiovascular system that people with diabetes especially need. People with IDDM must take certain precautions when engaging in physical activity, however.

Physical Activity and Blood Glucose in IDDM For the person without diabetes, blood glucose generally varies little during physical activity unless the activity is intense and of very long duration, such as marathon running. This is

Table 27–2

A Day's Exchanges for a Sample 2900-kCalorie Diet

Exchange Group/List	Number of Exchanges	Carbohydrate (g)	Protein (g)	Fat[a] (g)
Carbohydrate Group[b]				
Starch	13	195	39	0
Fruit	7	105	—	—
Milk	3	36	24	0
Vegetable	6	30	12	—
Meat and Meat Substitutes Group				
Lean	10	—	70	30
Fat Group	13	—	—	65
Total grams		366	145	95
Total kcalories		1464	580	855
% kcalories		50.5	20	29.5

[a]To ease calculation, exchanges from the carbohydrate groups are assumed to have 0 grams fat. If the client uses a fat-containing exchange, the fat can be deducted from the daily fat allowance.
[b]Foods from the "other carbohydrates" list can be substituted for a starch, fruit, or milk list exchange. Any fat in the selected food is then deducted from the daily fat allowance.

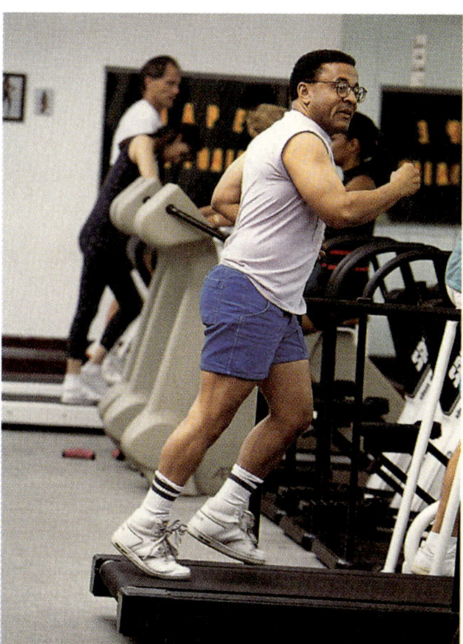

Physical activity plays an important role in the management of diabetes.

not the case in IDDM, where blood glucose can vary markedly with exercise. People with IDDM who have mild hyperglycemia may experience a *fall* in blood glucose during physical activity, whereas those with marked hyperglycemia may experience a still greater *rise* in blood glucose. For this reason, people with IDDM check their blood glucose prior to exercise and refrain from vigorous physical activity if their blood glucose levels are too high (greater than 300 milligrams per 100 milliliters).

Table 27–3

Translating a Day's Exchanges into Meals

Exchange Group/List	Number of Exchanges[a]	Breakfast	Lunch	Midafternoon Snack	Supper	Bedtime Snack
Carbohydrate Group						
Starch	13	3	3	2	3	2
Fruit	7	2	1	1	1	2
Milk	3	1	1		1	
Vegetable	6		3		3	
Meat and Meat Substitutes Group						
Lean	10		3	1	4	2
Fat Group	13	3	3	2	3	2

[a]From Table 27–2.

Sample 2900-kCalorie Diet Menu

Menu
Breakfast
½ c bran cereal
1 c nonfat milk
1 bagel (2 oz)
3 tsp margarine
1 banana
Coffee
Lunch
1 c pasta made with:
½ c spaghetti sauce
2 oz meatballs
(medium fat)
2 tbs grated
parmesan cheese
1½ c broccoli
2 tsp margarine
17 small grapes
1 c nonfat milk
Midafternoon Snack
1 fat-free granola bar
2 tbs peanut butter spread
over slices of 1 small apple
Supper
4 oz grilled salmon
⅔ c rice
1 whole-wheat roll
1 c cooked carrots
1 tsp margarine
1 c mixed green salad
Salad dressing made
with 2 tsp olive oil
and wine vinegar
1 c diced cantaloupe
1 c nonfat milk
Bedtime Snack
¼ c lowfat cottage cheese
1 c fruit cocktail
1 small frosted cupcake
1 c nonfat milk
MILK MILK

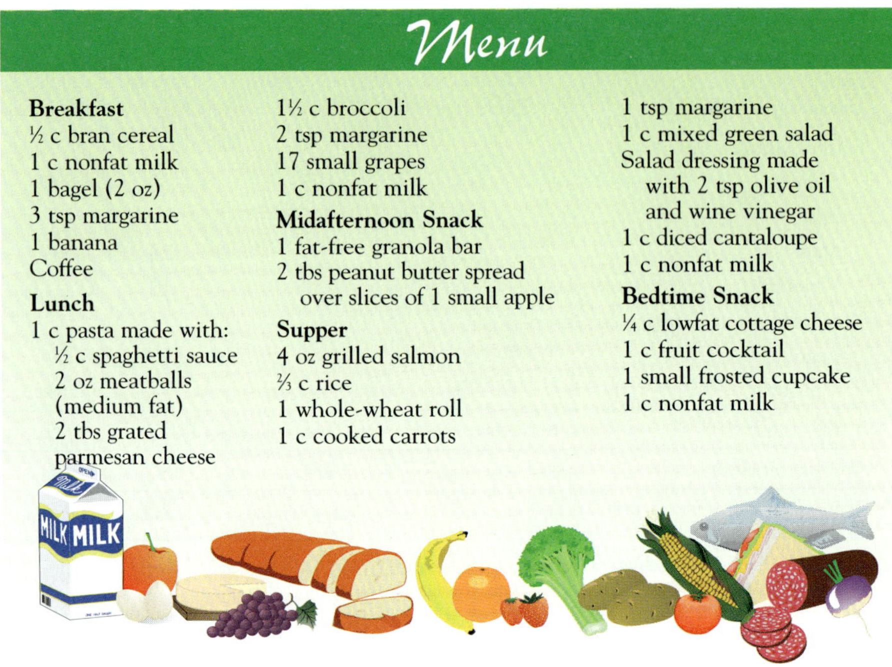

Physical Activity and Food Intake The person with IDDM may need to eat before, during, and after vigorous physical activity. Especially important is carbohydrate, which is readily available from fruits, fruit juices, yogurt, crackers, and other starches. As a general guideline, the exerciser should have about 10 to 15 grams of additional carbohydrate before moderate activity or about 20 to 30 grams of carbohydrate before vigorous activity. Clients are advised to check blood glucose 30 minutes before and 1 hour after physical activity and adjust carbohydrate accordingly. Table 27–4 lists general guidelines for providing additional carbohydrate for various activity intensities and blood glucose concentrations.

INSULIN AND INSULIN ANALOGS

Because people with IDDM cannot make their own insulin, they must receive it from another source. Human insulin, the most widely used insulin, is synthesized from pork insulin (by modifying the amino acid patterns) or from bacteria using recombinant DNA.* Insulins extracted from animal sources that have a slightly different amino acid pattern than human insulin are also available. Insulins are either rapid acting (regular), intermediate acting (NPH and lente), or long acting (ultralente) depending on how quickly they begin to work and how long they are effective (see Figure 27–2). Insulin analogs act as rapid-acting forms.

Although the availability of insulin has been life-saving, insulin therapy cannot achieve the same degree of blood glucose control as a body that produces its own insulin.

Some people develop an **insulin allergy** to a particular type of insulin or an additive in the insulin. A person experiencing such a reaction must switch to a different type of insulin.

Insulin Analogs Insulin analogs (lispro) are rapid-acting human insulins whose amino acid composition has been slightly modified to make them work

*Insulin was first used successfully in diabetic dogs by F. G. Banting and C. H. Best in 1922. The first does of human insulin was given to a person in the United Kingdom in 1980. Since then, it has become the most commonly used insulin type.

Table 27–4

Guidelines for Providing Additional Carbohydrate for Activity in IDDM

Exercise Intensity	Blood Glucose (mg/100 ml)	Additional Carbohydrate to Provide (g)	Examples of Snacks to Provide Carbohydrate
Low	<100	10–15	½ English muffin
	>100	none	—
Moderate	<100	15–20	½ English muffin with jelly
	100–180	10–15	Large pretzel
	180–300	none	—
Strenuous	<100	35–40	1 c yogurt with a banana
	100–180	25–50	Sandwich with 1 c milk
	180–300	10–15	½ c apple juice

Note: These values are estimates only. The individual should monitor blood glucose to determine specific needs more accurately.

Source: Adapted from M. J. Franz, Exercise and the management of diabetes mellitus, *Journal of the American Dietetic Association* 87 (1987): 872–880.

faster.[14] Unlike regular insulin, which must be administered 30 to 45 minutes before meals, lispro is taken 5 to 10 minutes before meals. Lispro reduces after-meal hyperglycemia to a greater extent than regular insulin, and its duration of action is about 3 hours rather than 5 to 6 hours. Thus lispro reduces the risk of hypoglycemia between meals and during the night.

The Honeymoon Phase Some clients experience a temporary remission of diabetes after their initial treatment with insulin—a time referred to as the "honeymoon phase." Why this honeymoon occurs remains a bit of a mystery. Perhaps

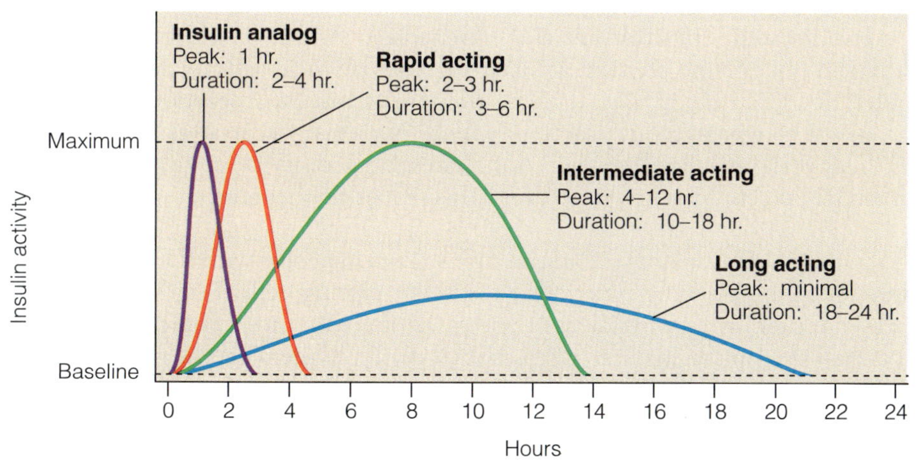

Figure 27–2

Actions of Insulin Types

with insulin treatment and relief from the constant hyperglycemia of uncontrolled diabetes, the insulin-producing cells of the pancreas become able to function normally again—but only temporarily. Tight control of blood glucose—whether by diet, insulin, or hypoglycemic agents—helps prolong the "honeymoon."

multiple daily injections (MDI): delivery of different types of insulin by injection three or more times daily.

Insulin Delivery People with IDDM inject insulin or use pumps to deliver the insulin they need. The person with IDDM who chooses injections often receives a mixture of two or more types of insulin, three or more times daily; single injections are seldom effective.

External pumps, about the size of a pager, hold enough insulin to meet needs for two to three days. From the pump, the insulin enters the body through tubing and a needle that has been inserted into the abdominal area. Personal preferences, motivational level, and financial considerations guide clients in deciding which delivery system works best for them.

Researchers continue to search for better and more comfortable methods of delivering insulin. Although not yet commercially available, researchers report promising results using implantable pumps that automatically deliver scheduled doses of insulin.[15] Each pump is approximately the size of a hockey puck and holds a three-month supply of insulin. Once the pump is surgically implanted in the abdomen, the client can release extra doses of insulin as needed by sending signals to the pump with a transmitter. The pump can be refilled as needed at the physician's office. Researchers are also working to develop glucose sensors that will continuously monitor blood glucose and adjust insulin delivery as needed.

Insulin and Food Intake Insulin delivery is timed to mimic the body's normal insulin action as closely as possible. Normally, the body secretes a constant, baseline amount of insulin at all times and secretes more as blood glucose rises following meals. The person with IDDM often receives NPH (intermediate-acting) insulin to meet baseline needs and regular (rapid-acting) insulin or insulin analogs to process energy nutrients following meals. The physician initially prescribes the types and dosages of insulin based on individual needs. Although these needs vary greatly, as a rule of thumb, a total of about 0.5 to 1.0 unit of insulin is given per kilogram of body weight per day. The health care team teaches people with IDDM to adjust their insulin doses to accommodate changes in eating patterns, physical activity, or health status.

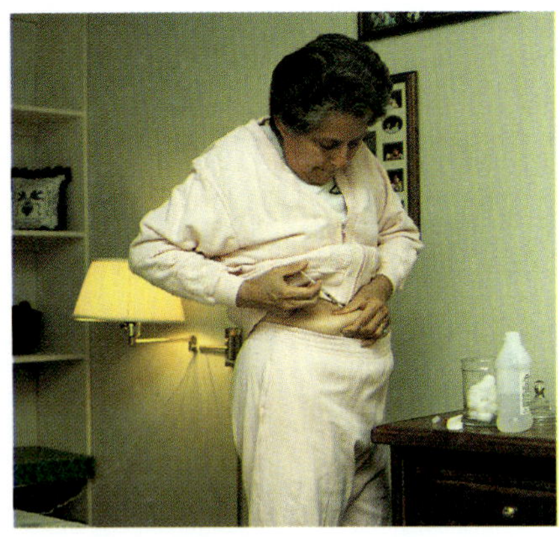

Injections are one option for delivering insulin for people with diabetes.

Insulin and Physical Activity Generally, insulin should be taken more than an hour before physical activity. Vigorous physical activity and warm temperatures speed blood flow, increase the rate of insulin absorption, and set the stage for a hypoglycemic reaction, which may even occur after several hours. Reducing the insulin doses before and after the activity by up to 30 percent, or even 50 percent, can help to prevent this sequence of events.

Pancreas Transplants Pancreas transplants in people with IDDM have been successful in providing functional, insulin-producing cells. People with IDDM who are candidates for pancreas transplants often are those who encounter serious problems managing their diseases with insulin. Otherwise, the risks associated with the surgery and the need for immunosuppressant drugs would outweigh the benefits of the transplant. Most often, however, a pancreas transplant is combined with a kidney transplant. For the person with IDDM who needs a kidney transplant, the addition of a pancreas transplant can enhance the quality of life.[16] One year after surgery, 75 percent of people who received a simultaneous pancreas-kidney transplant do not need insulin.[17] For people undergoing a pancreas transplant only, 50 percent do not need insulin after one year.

MASTERING GLUCOSE CONTROL

Motivated clients who keep accurate records of food intake, physical activity, blood glucose measurements, and insulin doses learn how to control their blood glucose even when they change their usual eating habits or activity schedule. The health care team determines acceptable fasting and after-meal blood glucose goals for each client. People with IDDM on intensive therapy receive insulin three or four times a day, either through injections or from an external pump. They test their blood glucose levels about four times daily and have monthly medical checkups that include measurement of hemoglobin A_{1c} (described below). People on standard therapy receive insulin one or two times a day, monitor blood glucose once a day, and have medical checkups that include measurement of hemoglobin A_{1c} three or four times a year. The team uses the client's records to make sure goals are being met; if not, the team investigates the reasons and suggests solutions.

The Diabetes Control and Complications Trial sought to maintain fasting and premeal glucose between 80 and 120 mg/100 ml. In this study, groups receiving intensive treatment achieved an average fasting blood glucose of 155 mg/100 ml.

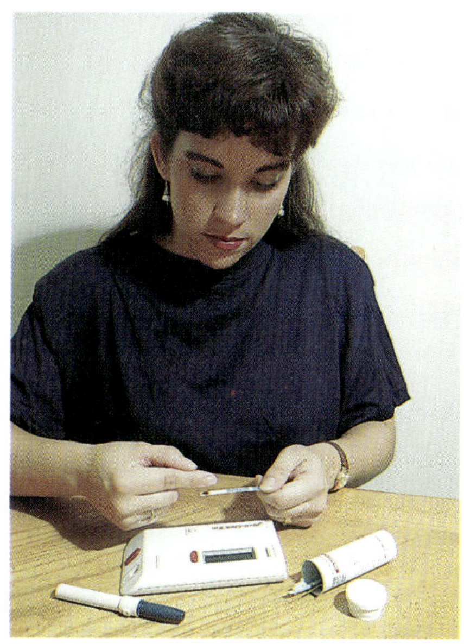

Blood glucose monitoring helps people with diabetes maintain blood glucose in a safe range.

Blood Glucose Monitoring To test blood glucose at home, the client pricks a finger to get a blood sample (the same method used to determine hematocrit) and transfers the blood to a strip. Most clients today rely on computerized meters that measure the blood glucose concentration from the blood sample. Less accurate and less costly are paper strips that change to different colors, depending on the blood glucose concentration.

At first, the person performs blood tests at least seven times during the day: before each meal, two hours after each meal, and at bedtime. During this time, clients who conscientiously adhere to a consistent diet and physical activity program learn how their blood glucose levels respond to diet, physical activity, and insulin. Once people learn to control their blood glucose levels, they can test blood glucose less often.

Glycated Hemoglobin In addition to blood glucose records, physicians monitor blood glucose control by evaluating hemoglobin A_{1c}. As blood glucose rises, small glucose molecules spontaneously attach to an amino acid on each hemoglobin. The glucose molecules remain attached to the hemoglobin molecules until the cells die (about 120 days). Therefore, hemoglobin A_{1c} reflects diabetes control over the past two to three months, whereas a single blood glucose test reflects diabetes control just prior to the test.

Glycated hemoglobin is also called **glycosylated hemoglobin**. The type of glycated hemoglobin most commonly measured to screen for diabetes or monitor control of diabetes is **hemoglobin A_{1c}**, which normally averages <6%.

In the Diabetes Control and Complications Trial, groups receiving intensive treatment achieved an average hemoglobin A_{1c} of 7.2%.

Urinary Ketones Health care professionals often recommend that clients with consistently high blood glucose also monitor ketones in the urine, especially during illness. As described earlier, the individual with diabetes can develop a type of coma associated with high ketone levels.

Other Measures The health care team also monitors the client's weight, blood lipid levels, blood pressure, and reflexes and checks for early signs of complications. As described earlier, urine tests can help detect the early signs of kidney disease. Eye exams help identify the early signs of retinopathy, and foot exams detect early signs of infection.

At medical appointments, the health care team reviews the client's records to monitor the client's progress and look for patterns that suggest the need for adjustments in the treatment plan. In making recommendations, the team keeps in mind the four factors that influence blood glucose regulation: diet, physical activity, insulin dose, and the level of counterregulatory hormones.

The counterregulatory hormones (including glucagon, cortisol, and catecholamines) oppose insulin's actions.

MANAGING HYPERGLYCEMIA

Table 27–5 on p. 863 summarizes strategies for adjusting treatment plans to correct problems with hyperglycemia and hypoglycemia. Regular detection of hyperglycemia before lunch or dinner in a person with a consistent carbohydrate intake signals the health care professional to look back to the previous meal to make corrections. (Recall that it takes time for food to be digested and absorbed before blood glucose rises.) Treatment may involve adjusting the dose of regular insulin, adding physical activity to the plan, reducing the amount of carbohydrate at the previous meal, or spacing the meals so that the available insulin has time to work. The client's medical needs, lifestyle, and preferences dictate which course is best.

dawn phenomenon: early morning hyperglycemia that develops in response to counterregulatory hormones that act to raise glucose levels during an overnight fast.

Dawn Phenomenon Early morning (before breakfast) hyperglycemia can occur in people with diabetes as a natural response to an overnight fast. During the night, levels of counterregulatory hormones increase and act to raise blood glucose. Without adequate insulin, glucose fails to enter the cells and hyperglycemia results. Treatment of this form of hyperglycemia may require adjustment of the intermediate-acting insulin given at bedtime. Many clients need more regular insulin to cover their needs in the morning, until counterregulatory hormone levels fall.

rebound hyperglycemia: hyperglycemia resulting from excessive secretion of counterregulatory hormones in response to excessive insulin; also called the **Somogyi** (so-MOHG-yee) **effect**.

Rebound Hyperglycemia A similar but more dramatic and severe form of hyperglycemia can occur when a person uses too much insulin to meet needs. People who take high insulin doses or engage in strenuous physical activity (which reduces insulin needs) are more likely than others with diabetes to experience this form of hyperglycemia. At first, the insulin drives glucose into the cells, and hypoglycemia results. Then, the body reacts by markedly raising the level of counterregulatory hormones, which causes blood glucose levels to rise rapidly. Giving more insulin at this point makes the problem worse, so treatment includes reducing the insulin dose.

Illness Even a minor illness such as a cold or flu may cause blood glucose to rise dramatically, and the client may require higher insulin doses. Thus a record of illness helps evaluators interpret blood glucose test results. During this precarious time, clients with diabetes should vigilantly monitor blood glucose and urinary ketones and carefully follow insulin and dietary instructions. Physicians may advise clients to reduce total energy and carbohydrate intakes slightly to limit the need for extra insulin. A major concern is the prevention of starvation, dehydration, and vomiting.

Table 27–5

Strategies for Managing Hyperglycemia and Hypoglycemia

Problem	Possible Solutions[a]
HYPERGLYCEMIA	
Before breakfast	• Adjust dose of intermediate-acting insulin at bedtime.[b]
Before lunch	• Adjust morning dose of rapid-acting insulin.[b] • Reduce amount of carbohydrate at breakfast. • Reduce or omit midmorning snack. • Change time of breakfast or midmorning snack. • Add physical activity after breakfast.
Before dinner	• Adjust afternoon dose of rapid-acting insulin.[b] • Reduce carbohydrate at lunch. • Reduce or omit midafternoon snack. • Change time of lunch or midafternoon snack. • Add physical activity between lunch and dinner.
At bedtime	• Adjust insulin dose before dinner.[b] • Reduce amount of carbohydrate at dinner. • Reduce or omit evening snack. • Add physical activity after dinner.
HYPOGLYCEMIA	
Before breakfast	• Adjust dose of intermediate- or long-acting insulin at bedtime.[b] • Add carbohydrate at evening snack. • Avoid strenuous activity late in the day.
Before lunch	• Adjust morning dose of rapid-acting insulin.[b] • Add carbohydrate at breakfast. • Add a morning snack. • Change time of breakfast, lunch, or morning snack. • Adjust physical activity schedule.
Before dinner	• Adjust afternoon dose of rapid-acting insulin.[b] • Add carbohydrate at lunch. • Add an afternoon snack. • Change time of lunch, dinner, or afternoon snack. • Adjust physical activity schedule.
At bedtime	• Adjust insulin dose before dinner.[b] • Add carbohydrate at dinner. • Add an evening snack. • Change time of dinner or evening snack.

[a]Skilled health care professionals gather additional data to find the best solution for problems with blood glucose control. Is the problem an isolated occurrence or a pattern? Has food intake changed? If yes, why? Has the activity level changed? Has illness been a problem? Whenever diet changes might be difficult for the client, insulin is adjusted to correct problems, if possible.
[b]Insulin doses can be adjusted in amount or timing or both.

Severe Hyperglycemia and Ketoacidosis Severe hyperglycemia and ketoacidosis can occur in untreated IDDM or when the person with IDDM omits an insulin dose, makes an error in the type of insulin taken, overeats without taking additional insulin, experiences rebound hyperglycemia, or suffers a stress (infection, trauma) that causes blood glucose to rise. Severe hyperglycemia and ketoacidosis is a medical emergency that can lead to coma and death. Prevention is the best treatment. Educating the client to follow the treatment plan (including regular blood glucose monitoring) is critical. When prevention fails, a physician treats hyperglycemia and ketoacidosis by carefully administering insulin and correcting fluid and electrolyte and acid-base balances using IV fluids.

MANAGING HYPOGLYCEMIA

insulin reaction: hypoglycemia that results from an overdose of insulin, strenuous physical activity, skipped meals, or inadequate intake of food; also called **insulin shock**.

Tightly controlling blood glucose reduces the risk of chronic complications, but increases the risk of hypoglycemia. Hypoglycemia in the person with IDDM is also known as an *insulin reaction* or *insulin shock*. An insulin reaction can result from an overdose of insulin, strenuous physical activity, skipped meals, or inadequate food intake. People with IDDM and those who spend time with them need to learn to recognize the symptoms of hypoglycemia (see margin note on p. 850).

Easy-to-eat sources of carbohydrate (10 to 15 g per serving):

- 2 to 3 tsp honey.
- 4 to 5 hard candies (such as Lifesavers).
- 5 to 6 large jelly beans.
- 4 to 6 oz regular soft drink.
- 4 oz orange juice.
- 1 tbs icing from a tube.
- Glucose tablets (check label for amount).

Judicious treatment of hypoglycemia prevents overtreatment and thus avoids subsequent hyperglycemia. As soon as the symptoms are observed, the person needs to receive 10 to 15 grams of carbohydrate. Any carbohydrate source that is readily available and easy to eat is a good choice.[18] It is best to avoid carbohydrate sources that also contain fat (such as a candy bar), because fat slows the absorption of carbohydrate. Blood glucose is then checked within 15 to 20 minutes to see if it has risen to an acceptable level. If not, an additional 10 to 15 grams of carbohydrate are given, and blood glucose is rechecked. The procedure continues until blood glucose returns to an acceptable range. Advise clients to carry some convenient source of carbohydrate with them at all times, so that they can act immediately when hypoglycemic symptoms occur.

If the person frequently experiences hypoglycemia, treatment can lead to excessive weight gain. Therefore, repeated episodes of hypoglycemia require investigation, so their causes can be corrected.

Hypoglycemia before Meals Consistent hypoglycemia before meals suggests the need to reduce the prior insulin dose, increase the prior carbohydrate intake, or eat the next meal earlier. The best solution depends on the person's medical needs and preferences.

nocturnal hypoglycemia: hypoglycemia that occurs while a person is sleeping.

Nocturnal Hypoglycemia Hypoglycemia that occurs during sleep makes symptoms difficult to detect. People prone to nocturnal hypoglycemia may be advised to wake up during the night and test their blood glucose. Nocturnal hypoglycemia may occur more readily in people who engage in strenuous physical activity late in the day. For this reason, strenuous activity should be undertaken earlier in the day, if possible. Other strategies that may help eliminate the problem are to snack consistently at bedtime or reduce the insulin dose following evening activity.

Severe Hypoglycemia In severe cases, the person may be disoriented, unable to recognize a hypoglycemic reaction, and unable to swallow safely. In such cases, the person needs to receive intravenous glucose, the hormone glucagon, or both to counteract the insulin reaction. Without treatment, the person may lapse into shock and die.

CHILDREN WITH DIABETES

The overall approach to diabetes remains the same throughout life, but special problems may become apparent at different stages. Consider some of the problems of children with diabetes. Like those of all children, the energy and nutrient needs of children with diabetes keep changing throughout the growing years. Children's appetites and activities vary widely from day to day. A child may eat like a horse one day and like a mouse the next. A teen may spend hours walking around the mall one day and spend the next day watching TV. Growth and activity influence the needs for food and insulin, and management must adjust to meet those needs.

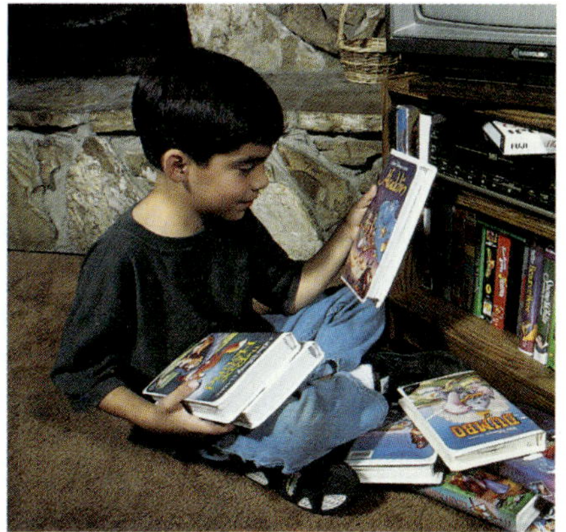

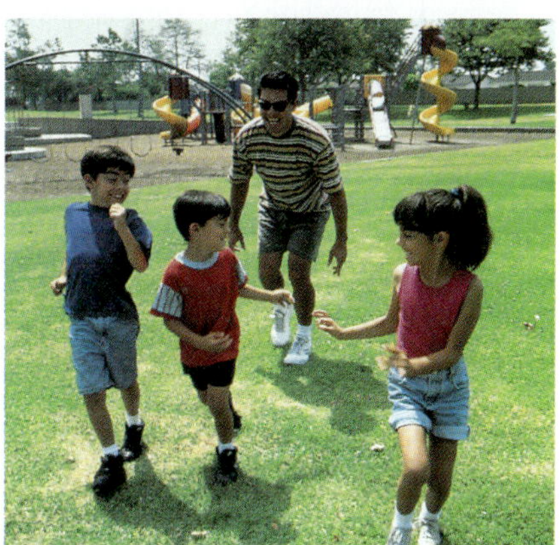

Because a child's activities vary from day to day, food and insulin needs may also change.

Meal Plans To support growth and development, children with IDDM need flexible, balanced meals and snacks that offer wide varieties of foods from each of the food groups. Dietitians often teach children and caregivers carbohydrate counting to provide flexibility from day to day. Concentrated sweets are allowed within the context of a healthy diet. Caregivers need not force children to finish meals, but should encourage them not to skip meals either, because hypoglycemia can result. Meals are best taken at about the same times each day, and children with diabetes can eat the same foods as the rest of the family.

Family Lifestyles Successful diet management incorporates prescribed meals into existing family lifestyles and eating patterns. Depending on insulin administration and personal preferences, children generally receive three meals with two to three snacks a day. Snacks before bedtime help prevent nocturnal hypoglycemia, especially if the child engages in strenuous activity late in the day. Caregivers should vary snacks to prevent boredom, provide enough to share with friends, and avoid identifying foods as "good" or "bad." Such connotations create unrealistic expectations or fears and invite the development of manipulative eating behaviors. The case study presents a child with IDDM.

The goals of IDDM therapy are to control blood glucose, blood lipids, and blood pressure; support health; and treat complications. To maintain blood glucose within a fairly normal range, people with IDDM need to be consistent in their carbohydrate intake each day. They also need to coordinate their food intake, physical activity, and insulin. Regular glucose monitoring allows clients to make the adjustments necessary to avoid hypoglycemia and hyperglycemia (review Table 27–5).

Treatment of Noninsulin-Dependent Diabetes Mellitus (NIDDM)

The striking results of the Diabetes Control and Complications Trial clearly show the value of tight blood glucose control for preventing long-term complications in IDDM and suggest that similar benefits might be possible for the vast

Case Study Child with IDDM

One year ago, Yusuf, a 12-year-old boy, was diagnosed with IDDM. The initial diagnosis was made after Yusuf's parents became concerned when he began to lose weight, urinate excessively, and complain of thirst. Aware of a family history of diabetes, the parents quickly sought medical help. Since that time, Yusuf's diabetes has been well controlled. Recently, however, Yusuf was admitted to the emergency room, complaining of nausea, vomiting, and intense thirst. He had a fever, and his blood glucose records from the previous day showed that his blood glucose was high throughout the day. The physician observed that Yusuf was confused and breathing with difficulty and also noted the smell of acetone on his breath. Urine tests were positive for glycosuria and ketonuria, and Yusuf's blood glucose was 400 milligrams per 100 milliliters. The diagnosis was diabetic ketoacidosis.

Describe the metabolic events that led to the symptoms associated with diabetes (before diagnosis), as well as those associated with diabetic ketoacidosis. Were Yusuf's physical symptoms and laboratory tests consistent with this diagnosis? How can you distinguish between diabetic ketoacidosis and hypoglycemia?

When Yusuf recovers, what advice can you offer him to prevent future incidents of ketoacidosis? Assume that Yusuf had instructions for a diet for diabetes. What dietary modifications would you advise him to make?

Think about and discuss the influence of Yusuf's age on his outlook and ability to cope with diabetes. What problems does his age pose? Consider some ways you might help him deal with these problems. Regarding his future, describe the possible role of diet in preventing the chronic complications of diabetes.

majority of people with diabetes—those with NIDDM.[19] The goals of therapy for NIDDM mimic those for IDDM, namely:

- To achieve and maintain acceptable blood glucose levels, blood lipid concentrations, and blood pressure.
- To prevent the acute and chronic complications associated with diabetes.
- To support quality of life by enabling people to continue the activities they enjoy with the best possible health.

DIET IN NIDDM

The benefits of medical nutrition therapy in NIDDM are receiving increasing attention.[20] The diet for NIDDM is designed to maintain near-normal blood glucose by delivering a balanced nutrient intake with carbohydrates spaced evenly throughout the day. As in IDDM, many approaches can be used to plan diets in NIDDM. The diet's balance typifies healthy eating for all people and is the same as for people with IDDM.

Timing and Distribution of Meals Providing a consistent carbohydrate intake spaced throughout the day helps people with NIDDM maintain appropriate blood glucose levels and maximizes the effectiveness of drug therapy. Giving too much carbohydrate at one time can raise blood glucose too high, stressing the already-compromised insulin-producing cells. Giving too little carbohydrate can lead to hypoglycemia, especially for people on drug therapy (some oral drugs or insulin).

Altering the distribution of kcalories from carbohydrate and fat may be especially important for controlling blood glucose and lipids for people with NIDDM. Although a low-fat diet might be appropriate in some cases, studies suggest that diets providing 40 percent of kcalories from carbohydrate and 45 percent of kcalories from fat (25 percent monounsaturated, 10 percent polyunsaturated, and 10 percent saturated) result in lower blood glucose and insulin levels following meals and lower day-long blood levels of triglycerides. Results such as these remind practitioners to individualize diet prescriptions.[21]

Chapter 28 provides more information on the associations of different blood lipids to cardiovascular disease.

Weight Control Weight loss is often prescribed for people with NIDDM. Even moderate weight loss (10 to 20 pounds) can help reverse insulin resistance, improve the blood lipid profile, and reduce blood pressure. Weight-reduction diets that provide at least 10 kcalories per pound of body weight allow a safe and gradual weight loss. In some cases, very-low-kcalorie diets (less than 800 kcalories per day) may help establish blood glucose control, but the value of such diets remains controversial.[22] The person at a healthy weight may not need to limit energy intake, but still needs to follow the principles of the diet for diabetes.

Alcohol The guidelines for alcohol use in NIDDM are the same as for IDDM (see p. 853). Alcohol use is discouraged for people who are overweight—a kcalorie-restricted diet has little room for high-kcalorie foods of limited nutritional value. Furthermore, the combination of alcohol and some oral antidiabetic agents may cause flushing of the skin and a rapid heartbeat.

oral antidiabetic agents: drugs taken by mouth to lower blood glucose levels. They include sulfonylureas, metformin, acarbose, and troglitazone. Sulfonylureas (sull-FAH-nal-you-RE-ahs) are also called **hypoglycemic agents** because they stimulate insulin secretion.

Physical Activity A regular program of moderate physical activity improves blood glucose control, contributes to weight loss, improves blood lipid levels, and lowers blood pressure in people with NIDDM. Authorities recommend a program of 20 to 30 minutes of low-impact aerobic activity (such as walking) at least three days a week.[23] Many clinicians believe that 80 to 90 percent of overweight people with NIDDM can achieve metabolic control by following a kcalorie-restricted diet combined with a moderately intense physical activity program. The Diabetes Prevention Program (see p. 847) is studying the effects of diet and physical activity in delaying or preventing the development of NIDDM.[24]

DRUG THERAPY IN NIDDM

People with NIDDM may also monitor their blood glucose to maintain it within an acceptable range. When diet and physical activity fail to control blood glucose adequately, oral drugs called antidiabetic agents may be prescribed to lower blood glucose. Drugs do not replace diet and physical activity; advise clients to continue these therapies as instructed. Physicians select drug therapy based on the client's fasting and after-meal blood glucose, body weight, and response to the current therapy.

Oral Antidiabetic Agents Sulfonylureas are antidiabetic agents that have been in wide use for many years. Sulfonylureas stimulate the release of insulin from the pancreas, sensitize the insulin-producing cells of the pancreas to glucose, and reduce insulin resistance.[25] Because sulfonylureas raise insulin levels, people taking them may experience hypoglycemia and weight gain.

Caution: People taking sulfonylureas who also consume alcohol may experience hypoglycemia, flushing of the skin, and a rapid heartbeat.

A more recently approved antidiabetic agent is metformin. Metformin suppresses the liver's production of glucose and may reduce insulin resistance; it does not stimulate insulin secretion, however, and therefore does not cause hypoglycemia. Metformin is not associated with weight gain, and it has a further advantage of reducing serum triglycerides and cholesterol and raising HDL.

Because acarbose inhibits sucrose absorption, people taking it who develop hypoglycemia need to use glucose for treatment.

Another recently approved antidiabetic agent is acarbose, an enzyme inhibitor that reduces the rate of complex carbohydrate and sucrose digestion and the subsequent absorption of glucose from the intestine. Acarbose may be used alone for people with mild NIDDM or in combination with sulfonylureas or metformin in other cases.

Finally, troglitazone, the newest class of oral antidiabetic agents, works primarily by lessening peripheral insulin resistance without stimulating insulin secretion.[26] In addition to lowering blood glucose, troglitazone reduces triglyceride levels and raises HDL. Troglitazone has also been shown to improve insulin resistance and reduce blood pressure in people with impaired glucose tolerance. For these reasons, troglitazone may prove valuable in preventing or delaying the development of NIDDM or complications associated with insulin resistance, and it is being included as an intervention in the Diabetes Prevention Program.[27]

Insulin and Insulin Analogs Oral antidiabetic agents have a maximum dose; if blood glucose cannot be adequately controlled at the maximum dose, physicians prescribe insulin or insulin analogs, alone or in combination with oral drugs. Diabetes management for a person with NIDDM who is on insulin therapy is the same as for a person with IDDM. The accompanying case study provides practice in working with clients with NIDDM.

The goals of NIDDM therapy are similar to those of IDDM, but the approach differs slightly. Weight loss receives a high priority because of its beneficial effect in reversing insulin resistance, improving blood lipids, and reducing blood pressure. If diet and physical activity cannot control blood glucose, physicians may prescribe oral antidiabetic agents, insulin, insulin analogs, or a combination of these.

Diabetes in Pregnancy and Later Life

All stages of growth and development have unique characteristics that influence nutrient needs and affect nutrition education. An earlier section mentioned some special considerations for children and teenagers who most often have IDDM. Special considerations also apply to pregnant women and to elderly people with diabetes.

DIABETES MANAGEMENT IN PREGNANCY

As Chapter 18 noted, pregnancy elevates blood insulin and alters insulin resistance in all women. Blood insulin begins to rise soon after conception, and the cells respond by storing energy nutrients to provide for the developing fetus. Later in pregnancy, insulin remains high, but the cells become insulin resistant. Hormones that act antagonistically to insulin rise. This hormonal shift signals the body to stop storing energy fuels and allows the fetus to rapidly take up

The hormones that oppose the action of insulin during late pregnancy are placental lactogen, cortisol, prolactin, and progesterone.

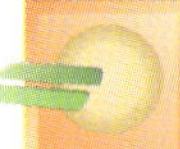

Case Study Truck Driver with NIDDM

Mr. Evans, a truck driver, was 52 years old when he was first diagnosed with NIDDM. He visited his physician after experiencing excessive thirst, excessive urination, and excessive appetite. Mr. Evans, who stands 5 feet 11 inches tall and currently weighs 200 pounds, experienced a 30-pound weight gain over the past two years. His fasting blood glucose is 235 milligrams per 100 milliliters. His fasting triglycerides and cholesterol are also elevated.

The diabetes health care team members have evaluated Mr. Evans's case. They are eager to help him achieve the first goal of diabetes management—to bring his blood glucose under control. The team has helped Mr. Evans plan a diet and physical activity program that considers the nature of his job and life on the road.

Mr. Evans is concerned about his health. He is worried that he may need insulin injections and overwhelmed by all the information presented to him over the past few days.

What are the differences between NIDDM and IDDM? Describe the factors in Mr. Evans's history that might have predisposed him to NIDDM. Can you explain to Mr. Evans why he will not need insulin injections at this time?

What will be the primary objective of the diet therapy for Mr. Evans? Determine Mr. Evans's desirable body weight, and describe two diet plans that might help him control both his blood glucose and his lipids. Select one of these diet plans and plan Mr. Evans's diet using the information in the box on pp. 855–856. Suggest some types of physical activities that might be appropriate for Mr. Evans. Remember that he travels frequently and needs a plan he can follow regularly. In what ways do diet and physical activity plans benefit clients with NIDDM?

What alternative treatments might Mr. Evans's physician consider if diet and physical activity fail to control his blood glucose?

Consider Mr. Evans's emotional health. How can the health care team help him during this difficult period?

energy nutrients. Because pregnancy stresses the glucose regulatory system in these ways, women with diabetes should expect control to become more difficult during pregnancy.

Risks of Diabetes during Pregnancy Women with diabetes who are contemplating pregnancy should know that poorly controlled diabetes before and during pregnancy presents risks for both mother and infant.[28] Women face a high infertility rate, and those who do conceive may experience episodes of severe hypoglycemia or hyperglycemia, spontaneous abortion, and pregnancy-induced hypertension. Infants also have increased mortality and morbidity, including macrosomia, congenital abnormalities, and other complications such as severe hypoglycemia or respiratory distress, both of which can be fatal. The greatest risk of fetal malformations from poorly controlled diabetes occurs during the first trimester, a time when the woman with diabetes may not realize she is pregnant. Therefore, women with diabetes should receive preconceptual care, which aims to achieve excellent blood glucose control before conception, and continued prenatal care to maintain blood glucose control during pregnancy.

Reminder: High blood pressure that develops in pregnancy is known as *pregnancy-induced hypertension* and may signal the onset of other complications (see p. 599).

respiratory distress: a disorder of the lung membranes that results in delayed onset of respiration at birth and difficulty in breathing after birth.

Gestational Diabetes Women who never had diabetes or never knew they had it may be diagnosed with diabetes for the first time during pregnancy (see Chapter 18). Gestational diabetes is relatively common, and the American

Diabetes Association recommends that health care professionals screen all women for diabetes between 24 and 28 weeks gestation.

Blood Glucose Monitoring Obstetricians recommend blood glucose monitoring for all pregnant women with any type of diabetes. Establishing blood glucose control is important to the health of both mother and infant. Pregnant women with diabetes may also monitor their urine for ketones, either daily or periodically, because ketosis in early pregnancy can lead to congenital malformations, central nervous system disorders, and low measures of intelligence in infants.

Diet Therapy For the pregnant woman with diabetes, a diet tailored to meet the increased demands of pregnancy and carefully coordinated with insulin therapy (when necessary) is central to therapy. The diet plan aims to provide adequate but not excessive kcalories to support weight gain (see the weight-gain recommendations in the margin on p. 589). Carbohydrate is often provided at lower amounts (40 to 45 percent of kcalories) than in the usual diet for diabetes to keep blood glucose levels from rising too high after meals.[29] Limiting carbohydrate to about 15 to 30 grams at breakfast helps maintain morning blood glucose levels in an acceptable range until counterregulatory hormone levels have diminished (see p. 862). Frequent small meals and snacks help assure an ongoing supply of glucose without inducing hyperglycemia. A bedtime snack is recommended to prevent nocturnal hypoglycemia in the mother and to provide fuel and prevent ketosis in the developing fetus.

Preventive Measures after Gestational Diabetes For most women with gestational diabetes, glucose tolerance returns to normal after pregnancy. Nevertheless, those with gestational diabetes are likely to develop NIDDM later in life, especially if they are overweight. In women with previous gestational diabetes, being 20 percent or more overweight doubles the risk of NIDDM. For this reason, health care professionals encourage clients with gestational diabetes to avoid excessive weight gain during pregnancy and to achieve or maintain a healthy weight thereafter. Yearly screenings for diabetes are recommended so that treatment can begin promptly and complications avoided.

DIABETES MANAGEMENT IN LATER LIFE

The elderly face special problems in dealing with diabetes. They have greater risks of hyperglycemia and hypoglycemia because of reduced appetite, altered thirst regulation, altered kidney and liver functions, depression or mental deterioration, multiple medications, and other medical conditions.

Many elderly people have NIDDM, and with aging their insulin resistance may progress until they can no longer maintain glucose levels within acceptable ranges with diet and oral drugs. The prospect of daily insulin injections and the need for additional blood glucose monitoring may be overwhelming to the elderly client. Those who have also suffered a loss of vision as a consequence of aging or diabetes may be unable to draw correct insulin doses, give self-injections, or use glucose strips or meters. The inability to perform these necessary tasks may make it impossible for the person to live independently.

The elderly may also lack the financial resources or social support necessary to help them cope with their diabetes. Caring health care professionals address these problems and help elderly clients find solutions.

Poorly controlled diabetes during pregnancy is associated with infertility, spontaneous abortion, and congenital abnormalities. Some women first develop diabetes during pregnancy—gestational diabetes. To minimize complications, women need to control blood glucose levels by carefully coordinating a diet that meets the nutrient needs of pregnancy with insulin therapy (when necessary). Changes that occur with aging present special problems for the management of diabetes.

Hypoglycemia

Strictly speaking, the term *hypoglycemia* simply means "low blood glucose," and it refers not to a disease, but to a symptom of an alteration in carbohydrate metabolism. Ordinarily, blood glucose initially rises and then falls after eating; in healthy people the decline is gradual, blood glucose remains in the normal range, and the transition occurs without notice. In some people, however, blood glucose falls too low as the body shifts from the fed to the fasting state. Hypoglycemia may or may not be accompanied by other symptoms, and the symptoms may or may not be uncomfortable. There are two major types of hypoglycemia, reactive and fasting.

REACTIVE HYPOGLYCEMIA

Reactive hypoglycemia occurs within an hour or two after eating and is triggered by the release of the hormone epinephrine in response to rapidly falling blood glucose. Hypoglycemia may occur, for example, after gastric surgery (see Chapter 21), when central parenteral solutions are discontinued too quickly (see Chapter 24), or early in NIDDM when insulin levels are elevated. In most cases, however, the reason for the rapid decline in blood glucose is unknown. This section describes reactive hypoglycemia of unknown origin.

reactive hypoglycemia: hypoglycemia experienced simultaneously with epinephrine-release symptoms one to three hours after a meal; also called **postprandial hypoglycemia**.

Symptoms of Reactive Hypoglycemia The symptoms of reactive hypoglycemia are similar to those of an anxiety attack: weakness, rapid heartbeat, sweating, anxiety, hunger, and trembling. These symptoms are not surprising, as they are caused by the "emergency hormone," epinephrine.

Diagnosis of Reactive Hypoglycemia True reactive hypoglycemia can be identified by directly testing blood glucose at intervals after a meal. Low blood glucose and the simultaneous presence of symptoms confirm a diagnosis of reactive hypoglycemia. True reactive hypoglycemia is rare, although it is often misdiagnosed and has been the subject of much misguided advice. Many dishonest or ill-informed practitioners "diagnose" hypoglycemia on the basis of their clients' verbal reports alone and prescribe all sorts of "remedies" for it with transparently thin rationale. People also "diagnose" themselves so commonly that physicians have identified a special category for their condition: *non*hypoglycemia.

Carbohydrate-Modified Diet for Reactive Hypoglycemia For people who experience true reactive hypoglycemia, a judicious carbohydrate-modified diet may bring relief. Avoiding both low-carbohydrate dieting (see p. 243) and sudden large carbohydrate doses may be all that is required. The remedy, then, is similar to the diet for diabetes: eat a consistent amount of carbohydrate from balanced meals at regular times. If average-sized meals fail to relieve symptoms, smaller meals eaten more frequently may help. A registered dietitian, if consulted, develops a diet plan that is appropriate to achieve or maintain a healthy body weight.

FASTING HYPOGLYCEMIA

fasting hypoglycemia: hypoglycemia that develops gradually and primarily affects the brain and central nervous system.

A person who has symptoms while well advanced into the fasting state (for example, overnight) is experiencing a different kind of hypoglycemia. So is the person whose symptoms occur because insulin has driven too much glucose into the cells. Fasting hypoglycemia arises from medically diverse disorders, such as diabetes or tumors of the pancreas or liver, that interfere with normal blood glucose regulation. Table 27–6 lists the major distinguishing characteristics of fasting and reactive hypoglycemia.

Symptoms of Fasting Hypoglycemia The symptoms of fasting hypoglycemia differ from those of reactive hypoglycemia because they are not related to epinephrine release. Instead, blood glucose falls slowly, and the major effect is on the brain and central nervous system. The symptoms include headache, blurred vision, mental dullness, fatigue, confusion, amnesia, and even seizures and unconsciousness.

Carbohydrate-Modified Diets for Fasting Hypoglycemia Earlier sections of this chapter described how an evenly spaced, consistent carbohydrate intake can help prevent fasting hypoglycemia in people with diabetes and also discussed how

Table 27–6

Characteristics of Reactive and Fasting Hypoglycemia

	Reactive Type	Fasting Type
Onset of symptoms	Sudden; occurs 1 to 3 hours after meals	Gradual
Type of symptoms	Anxiety, weakness, sweating, rapid heartbeat, hunger, trembling	Headache, mental dullness, fatigue, confusion, amnesia, seizures, unconsciousness
Duration of symptoms	Transient	Persistent
Possible causes	Early NIDDM, gastric surgery, TPN	Hormonal imbalance, diabetes, drugs, tumors
Clinical course	Less serious; treat with diet	Can be serious; treat underlying problems

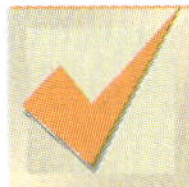

Nutrition Assessment Checklist
For People with Diabetes and Hypoglycemia

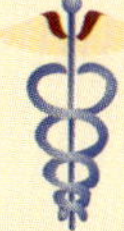

Medical For people with diabetes, use the medical record to determine the person's type of diabetes, its duration, acute and chronic complications, and other medical conditions that may affect nutrient needs. For people with hypoglycemia, check the medical record for the cause, if known, and for a confirmation of the diagnosis.

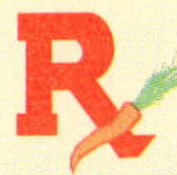

Drug For clients with preexisting diabetes who use insulin, note the types of insulin and schedule of administration. Note drug therapy, if any, for clients with NIDDM. Check for other drug therapy including antilipemics (to lower blood lipids) and antihypertensives (to reduce blood pressure). Note possible nutrient-drug interactions.

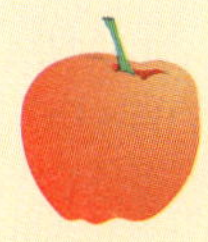

Food Intake Obtain an accurate diet and physical activity record from the person with diabetes to plan an acceptable plan and to coordinate drug therapy. During reassessment, use food intake and physical activity records along with records of blood glucose monitoring to evaluate the effectiveness of the treatment plan and to help make acceptable adjustments, when necessary. An assessment of food intake for the person with hypoglycemia helps pinpoint foods or amounts of foods that cause undesirable symptoms.

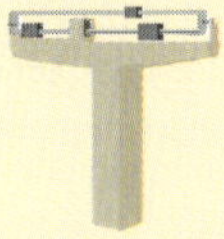

Anthropometric Take accurate height and weight measurements and determine desirable weight. Initial doses of insulin and calculated energy needs rely on body weight. Food energy intakes may need to be adjusted regularly to account for weight changes, particularly for growing children.

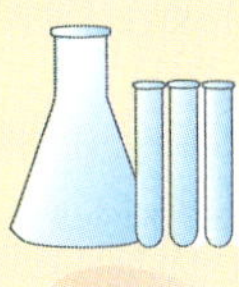

Laboratory Monitor blood glucose, hemoglobin A_{1c}, and blood lipids regularly for people with diabetes. Check results of urine tests for microalbuminuria when available.

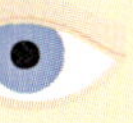

Physical Check results of eye and foot exams and monitor blood pressure. Look for physical signs of dehydration in elderly people with diabetes.

carbohydrates are used to treat hypoglycemia. Surgery is the primary treatment of fasting hypoglycemia caused by tumors, although carbohydrate-controlled diets (as described for reactive hypoglycemia) may be used temporarily.

Hypoglycemia means low blood glucose and is a symptom of disturbed carbohydrate metabolism. Table 27–6 summarizes the distinguishing features of the two major types of hypoglycemia—reactive and fasting.

Diet therapy has proved to be an essential component of an intensive treatment plan to prevent the complications of diabetes. Although such a plan may be difficult to master, the reward to clients and health care professionals appear to be well worth the effort. The nutrition assessment checklist highlights areas of concern for people with diabetes and hypoglycemia.

Study Questions

1. Name the two major types of diabetes. Which type is more common? Design a table to show the differences between the two types.
2. Give the physiological reasons for the following: hyperglycemia, glycosuria, weight loss, weight gain, dehydration, polyuria, polydipsia, polyphagia, acetone breath, ketosis, diabetic coma, and hyperosmolar hyperglycemic nonketotic coma.
3. List the types of chronic complications that can arise as a result of diabetes.
4. What biochemical tests are used to diagnose diabetes? Why is screening for diabetes important? What risk factors indicate the need for additional screening?
5. What are the goals of therapy for all people with diabetes? Name three aspects of lifestyle that must be coordinated for the person with IDDM.
6. What is the usual distribution of nutrients in the diet in the treatment of IDDM? How does this distribution compare with the healthy diet recommended to all people? What determines the actual distribution of nutrients?
7. Why are the timing and composition of meals important considerations in planning a diet for a person with IDDM?
8. How does physical activity affect blood glucose levels in IDDM? Give general guidelines for adjusting food intake for physical activity (both moderate and vigorous).
9. In what ways does the body normally secrete insulin, and how is commercially available insulin given to simulate these actions? What are the advantages of insulin analogs?
10. How are blood glucose monitoring results used to coordinate insulin, diet, and physical activity plans for people with diabetes? Describe ways that diet, physical activity, and insulin can be adjusted for people with diabetes who experience hyperglycemia or hypoglycemia.
11. How is the diet adjusted to meet the special needs of children with IDDM?
12. What is the primary goal of diet therapy in the person with NIDDM? How does diet therapy for NIDDM differ from that for IDDM? Describe the advantages and disadvantages of different oral antidiabetic drugs.
13. What are the risks of poorly controlled diabetes during pregnancy? How are pregnant women with diabetes managed to control blood glucose?
14. Define gestational diabetes. What preventive measures are important following gestational diabetes?
15. What special concerns arise in elderly people with diabetes?
16. Besides diabetes, what are some other causes of hypoglycemia? What diet is recommended for the treatment of reactive hypoglycemia?

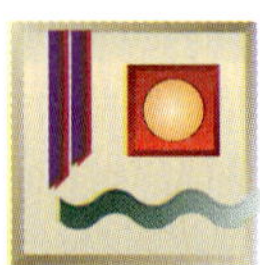

Clinical Applications

1. Using the box on pp. 855–856, plan a diet using the exchange lists for a sedentary woman with IDDM who is 5 feet 9 inches tall and weighs 160 pounds. Assume that the distribution of kcalories will be 55 percent from carbohydrate, 20 percent from protein, and 25 percent from fat. Round off kcalories to develop a sample diet pattern.
2. An important part of learning is being able to apply

knowledge and guidelines to real-life situations. Using Table 27–5 as a guide, think about the possible remedies for either hyper- or hypoglycemia. Describe at least one situation when it might be preferable to alter the insulin dose and one situation when it might be preferable to alter the carbohydrate intake.

3. Take a trip to a pharmacy and price these items: blood glucose meter, test strips for the meter selected, glucose test strips for use without a meter, lancets, insulin, and syringes. Determine the approximate cost of insulin injections for a person who uses 14 units of regular insulin and 26 units of NPH insulin daily (don't forget to include the cost of the syringes). Then estimate the cost of testing blood glucose four times daily. How does the cost of using a blood glucose meter compare to the cost of regular blood glucose test strips? How much do lancets add to the total daily cost? Consider how an external pump might affect the total cost of managing diabetes. How does the need for a balanced diet influence the cost of diabetes care? If intensive therapy requires more expenditures for insulin injections, blood glucose testing, and medical checkups than does traditional therapy, how might the added costs be justified?

Notes

1. M. I. Harris, NIDDM: Epidemiology and scope of the problem, *Diabetes Spectrum* 9 (1996): 26–29.
2. R. B. Lyon and D. M. Vinci, Nutrition management of insulin-dependent diabetes mellitus in adults: Review by the Diabetes Care and Education dietetic practice group, *Journal of the American Dietetic Association* 93 (1993): 309–314, 317.
3. Harris, 1996.
4. W. Y. Fujimoto, A national multicenter study to learn whether type II diabetes can be prevented: The Diabetes Prevention Program, *Clinical Diabetes* 15 (1997): 13–15.
5. I. J. Deary, Hypoglycemia-induced cognitive decrements in adults with Type I: A case to answer? *Diabetes Spectrum* 10 (1997): 42–47.
6. The Diabetes Control and Complications Trial Research Group, The effect of intensive treatment of diabetes on the development and progression of long-term complications in insulin-dependent diabetes mellitus, *New England Journal of Medicine* 329 (1993): 977–987.
7. M. C. Riddle and D. M. Karl, Screening for diabetes, *Clinical Diabetes* 14 (1996): 38–40.
8. The Expert Committee on the Diagnosis and Classification of Diabetes Mellitus, Report of the Expert Committee on the diagnosis and classification of diabetes mellitus, *Diabetes Care* 20 (1997): 1183–1197.
9. American Diabetes Association, Nutrition recommendations and principles for people with diabetes mellitus, *Diabetes Care* 17 (1994): 519–522.
10. P. J. Charney, Nutrition support in patients with diabetes mellitus, *Support Line*, April 1993, pp. 1–4.
11. American Diabetes Association, 1994.
12. M. Karlsen, D. Khakpour, and L. L. Thomson, Efficacy of medical nutrition therapy: Are your patients getting what they need? *Clinical Diabetes* 14 (1996): 54–60.
13. American Diabetes Association, 1994.
14. American Diabetes Association, Lispro: A new fast-acting insulin option, *Diabetes Spectrum* 9 (1996): 253.
15. M. Scavini and D. S. Schade, Implantable insulin pumps, *Clinical Diabetes* 14 (1996): 30–35.
16. D. E. Sutherland, The case for pancreas transplantation, *Diabetes Metabolism* 22 (1996): 132–138.
17. J. D. Pirsch and coauthors, Pancreas transplant for diabetes mellitus, *American Journal of Kidney Diseases* 27 (1996): 444–450.
18. M. Franz and coauthors, Who, what, and where—questions from "Maximizing the role of nutrition in diabetes management" contininug education program, *Diabetes Spectrum* 8 (1995): 369–374.
19. American Diabetes Association, Postition statement: Implications of the Diabetes Control and Complications Trial, *Diabetes Care* (supplement) 19 (1996): 50–52.
20. M. J. Franz and coauthors, Outcomes and cost-effectiveness of medical nutrition therapy for non-insulin-dependent diabetes, *Diabetes Spectrum* 9 (1996): 122–127; E. Q. Johnson and S. Valera, Medical nutrition therapy in non-insulin-dependent diabetes improves clinical outcome, *Diabetes Spectrum* 9 (1996): 131–133; M. J. Franz and coauthors, Effectiveness of medical nutrition therapy provided by dietitians in management of non-insulin-dependent diabetes mellitus: A randomized, controlled clinical trial, *Diabetes Spectrum* 9 (1996): 133–135.
21. A. Garg and coauthors, Effects of varying carbohydrate content of diet in patients with non-insulin-dependent diabetes mellitus, *Journal of the American Medical Association* 271 (1994): 1421–1428; L. V. Campbell and coauthors, The high-monounsaturated fat diet as a practical alternative for NIDDM, *Diabetes Care* 17 (1994): 177–182.
22. R. R. Wing, Use of very-low-calorie diets in the treatment of persons with non-insulin-dependent diabetes mellitus, *Journal of the American Dietetic Association* 95 (1995): 569–572.
23. American Diabetes Association, Position statement: Dia-

betes mellitus and exercise, *Diabetes Care* (supplement) 19 (1996): 30.
24. Fujimoto, 1997.
25. J. R. White, The pharmacologic management of patients with type II diabetes in the era of new oral agents and insulin analogs, *Diabetes Spectrum* 9 (1996): 227–234.
26. S. V. Edelman, Troglitazone: A new and unique oral antidiabetic agent for the treatment of Type II diabetes and the insulin resistance syndrome, *Clinical Diabetes* 15 (1997): 60–65.
27. T. Antonucci and coauthors, Impaired glucose tolerance is normalized by treatment with the thiozolidinedone troglitazone, *Diabetes Care* 20 (1997): 188–193.
28. A. Elixhauser and coauthors, Cost-benefit analysis of preconception care for women with established diabetes mellitus, *Diabetes Care* 16 (1993): 1146–1157.
29. C. Fagen, J. D. King, and M. Erick, Nutrition management in women with gestational diabetes mellitus: A review by ADA's Diabetes Care and Education dietetic practice group, *Journal of the American Dietetic Association* 95 (1995): 460–467.

Living with Diabetes

A healthy person goes about daily activities with little thought to how the body will react to everyday routines or disruptions to those routines. If you usually eat breakfast at 8:00 A.M. you may sleep in and choose not to eat breakfast on weekends without a second thought. If your friend asks you to play tennis and the match interferes with dinner, you simply eat later. If you get hungry during the day, you eat a snack. If you're not hungry at your usual dinner hour, you wait and eat later. For people with diabetes, even such simple variations in a daily schedule require thought and adjustment. They need to learn facts, master techniques, and develop new attitudes and behaviors that will provide for a healthy life.

Health care professionals who simply "prescribe" remedies and then expect their clients to comply with those remedies fail to consider the impact that lifestyle changes impose on a person's quality of life. Clients can easily be overwhelmed, and their motivation and compliance may be poor. This highlight describes a different educational approach—client empowerment—that is directed by the client. To use this approach, health care professionals provide clients with the information and skills they need to make decisions about their treatment plans and manage their diseases.

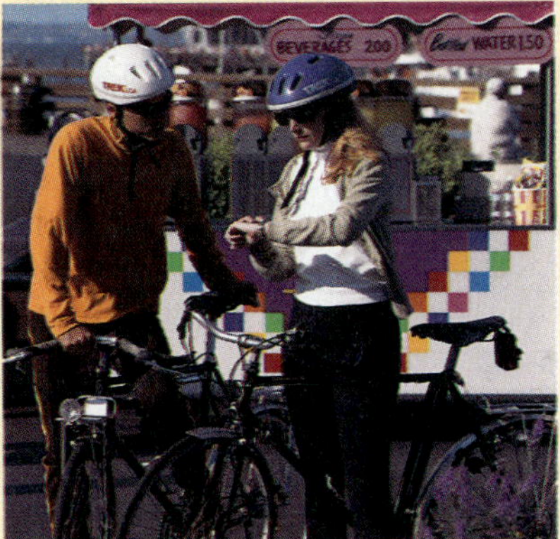

For a person with diabetes, even simple changes in routine require planning and adjustments.

BALANCING MEDICAL NEEDS WITH PERSONAL NEEDS

Some aspects of disease management are critical for survival. Other aspects may be beneficial but less critical. Still other aspects may be ideal but less pressing when considered in the total context of a treatment plan. The health care team must use clinical judgment in assigning priorities to various treatments. A person with IDDM, for example, must take insulin or face death. The person's goals, motivation, finances, and ability help determine if intensive therapy or traditional therapy is more appropriate. A 30-year-old client with IDDM may be eager to learn intensive therapy, while an 80-year-old client with NIDDM may refuse insulin therapy, even if it means poor blood glucose control. Health care professionals who practice client empowerment explain the ramifications of treatment choices, but respect the individual's right to make health care decisions without judgment.

The health care team uses a similar approach to balancing medical needs and personal needs in planning diet changes. For example, the health care team may agree on a diet plan that encourages a consistent carbohydrate intake at each meal and snack. Once the client has mastered that goal, the next step may be to work on diet behaviors that improve blood lipid levels or encourage a greater variety of foods. At each step, the health care team balances clinical needs with the individual's goals and motivation.

Health care professionals cannot knowingly encourage clients to practice behaviors that are medically harmful. Nor can they "force" clients to follow advice. With that in mind, the next section describes some of the basic concepts clients with diabetes should ideally learn about their treatment plan.

LEARNING ABOUT DIABETES

Health care professionals encourage their clients to learn about many aspects of diabetes so they can manage their disease and prevent complications:

- *Medication*. Clients need to learn the appropriate type, dose, and schedule. Clients on insulin need to learn how to draw insulin, give themselves an injection, and rotate injection sites. Clients who use external pumps need to know how to operate and maintain them and have them refilled.
- *Blood testing*. Clients need to learn how to administer the tests, record and interpret results, and bring glucose levels within a desirable range.
- *Diet*. Clients need to know how to schedule their meals, distribute carbohydrate throughout the day, and control portion sizes.
- *Changes to accommodate physical activity, missed meals, or illness*. Clients need to know how to meet these demands.
- *Complications associated with diabetes*. Clients need to learn how

to prevent complications and how to recognize and treat them when they occur.

- *Record keeping*. Clients need to learn how to keep accurate food, activity, and insulin administration records so that they can learn how their bodies respond to diabetes and how they can gain control over their disease.

For clients with diabetes and their families, all this new information and simply the time required to manage the disease can be overwhelming. They may find the diagnosis of diabetes and all it entails difficult to grasp and accept. Clients need a great deal of support to cope with their fears, stay motivated when they feel overwhelmed, gain confidence in their abilities to manage the disorder, and live a high-quality life.

Health care professionals facilitate the learning process by working out a highly individualized plan that carefully considers the client's motivation, goals, and ability to grasp new concepts and make lifestyle changes. The plan must be flexible to accommodate changing needs; a person who is highly motivated at one point, for example, may become totally discouraged at another time and need to restructure goals temporarily. The combined expertise of many health care professionals including physicians, nurses, dietitians, counselors, and physical therapists or exercise physiologists enhances diabetes management. Along with the client, these professionals form the health care team. Throughout this discussion, keep in mind that the client is the central member of the team.

PROMOTING DIABETES MANAGEMENT

Health care professionals recognize that all newly diagnosed clients and their families need intensive diabetes care training and counseling and that the learning process takes time. Even highly motivated clients who listen attentively need several counseling sessions to learn the basics of diabetes management. Inevitably, efforts at in-depth, short-term counseling will meet with failure. Diabetes education is a continuous process that is a routine part of diabetes management.

Health care professionals can help clients make lifestyle changes by using a stepwise process that includes assessment, goal setting, intervention, and evaluation.[1] As Chapter 27 describes, a complete assessment serves as the first step in formulating a treatment plan.[2] The more detailed the assessment, the more closely the plan can be tailored to meet the individual's needs and the better the chances for success. Using assessment data, the health care team sets long-term medical goals to provide the health care team and the client with a tool to measure the success of therapy; therefore, they are stated in terms of measurable outcomes such as target ranges for blood glucose, blood lipids, and body weight.

Health care professionals also work with the client to negotiate short-term goals geared toward making lifestyle adjustments. To be successful, short-term goals consider clients' personal views of their health goals and the steps they are willing and ready to take to reach these goals. Let's look at an example. After a complete nutrition assessment of a 55-year-old woman newly diagnosed with NIDDM, the dietitian may find that in addition to the elevated blood glucose, blood lipids are also elevated; the client is 30 pounds overweight, does not have a regular physical activity plan, skips breakfast, has a large dinner, eats many fried and high-fat foods and snacks, and seldom eats vegetables. The dietitian recognizes that several dietary changes are warranted, but works with the client to find an acceptable treatment goal. The client tells the dietitian that she wants to lose weight, but she feels very stressed and doesn't know how to get started. With the guidance of the dietitian, the woman sets these goals: she will eat a consistent amount of carbohydrate three times a day, with careful attention to portion sizes, and begin a physical activity program. By involving the client in goal setting, the dietitian improves the chances for success and encourages the client to take responsibility for her health.

Once goals have been set, the next step is intervention. What specific activities can help the client meet goals? Returning to our example, the dietitian and client might discuss a diet plan that includes appropriate portion sizes for breakfast, lunch, and dinner; review several menu options; practice weighing and measuring foods; and develop a physical activity plan in which the client agrees to walk after dinner for 20 minutes three times a week. The dietitian would like records of food, activity, and blood glucose, but the client feels she cannot handle that task right now. Instead, she will monitor blood glucose as instructed by the nurse.

Once the client tries the plan, the next step is evaluation.[3] Which strategies were successful and which were not? Suppose the client in our example returns for her next appointment. She has been successful at eating breakfast, inconsistent about reducing her portion sizes at lunch and dinner, and has managed to walk for 20 minutes only once or twice a week. From the client's records, the dietitian sees that her blood glucose levels have improved somewhat and that she has lost half a pound. The dietitian reinforces the value of the positive changes the client has made and praises her efforts. At this point, the dietitian, keeping in mind the client's medical goals, must reassess the client's motivation and decide what steps to take next. The client may want to continue the plan and agree to renew her commitment to control portion sizes and to walk more frequently. Alternatively, she may be so pleased with how she is feeling that she is ready to do more. She may then agree to keep up with her original plan, but also keep food and activity records and limit servings of fried foods to two a week, for example.

To help people adjust to the physiological demands imposed by diabetes, health care professionals guide clients through management plans with measurable goals set by the client. Clients' responses to the interventions and level of motivation dictate future actions. Health care professionals who are aware of the psychological burdens associated with diabetes are better equipped to support their clients' emotional health—an important factor in diabetes management.

COPING WITH DIABETES

Consider that in the example just discussed, the plan focused only on the nutrition component of diabetes education. Clients have many other diabetes-related tasks to master. In addition, they have responsibilities related to work, family, and community. It should come as little surprise that even when clients know what to do and why they should do it, they may be unable to carry out the plan at times.[4] Many people with diabetes report feeling overwhelmed and frustrated by the multitude of self-care demands.[5] In the words of one diabetes educator: "No one but another person who has diabetes can fully appreciate the demands of diabetes. It is 24 hours a day, 365 days a year (except on Leap Year when you get an extra day of diabetes). It involves all manner of imposition and deprivation. And even when you do everything right, there are no guarantees."[6]

People with diabetes often feel that health care professionals, family, and friends "blame" them for diabetes-related problems and complications.[7] They may feel guilt and remorse because their efforts at diabetes control were not good enough.[8] Health care professionals are wise to remain nonjudgmental when working with clients with diabetes and to recognize that diabetes control must be balanced with quality of life. Clients also need to know that they may experience complications even when they are doing everything possible. Expecting perfection can only meet with failure.

Teenagers often have intense difficulty accepting the initial diagnosis of diabetes. At a time when they are striving to develop their identity with a group and to be as similar to their peers as possible, they are faced with an unwelcome diagnosis and new rules they are expected to follow; their response may be denial and refusal to cooperate. Yet their refusal to cooperate might result in serious consequences. The person who appreciates a teen's special views on life is best prepared to help with the adjustment. Adolescents especially need to know that they can manage the disease themselves—that it won't turn them back into dependent children.

Parents and other family members also face the challenge of living with diabetes. The intensity of the situation can either reinforce or disrupt family unity. Parents may resent the demands of caring for a child with a chronic illness and also may experience guilt for having those feelings. They may feel anxious and be reluctant to allow their child to follow the diabetes care plan without their constant assistance. Especially in the case of an older child, they may press their care and control on a child who needs to develop autonomy and self-care. Parents may also become emotionally upset when they see their child feeling anxious, depressed, or withdrawn. Parents need time to work through these feelings. They might want to attend meetings for parents of children with diabetes.* Such meetings offer opportunities to share feelings, ideas, and frustrations with others in similar situations. Sometimes just knowing that you're not alone helps.

OTHER RESOURCES

After an initial introduction to the world of diabetes, clients may benefit from educational programs designed to expand their knowledge and promote independence.[9] Some programs encourage clients to bring friends, which makes the experience more comfortable and fun. Some programs are designed specifically for parents, grandparents, and other caregivers.

*The American Diabetes Association provides information about the disease and referrals to local support groups. See Appendix F for the address and phone numbers.

Children can combine education and summer vacation at camps designed especially for children with diabetes. These camps offer the chance to learn more about diabetes while "living" the lifestyle with companions under supervision. Children trade snack ideas, try new recipes, and help prepare meals. Older children assist younger ones, and all benefit.

The results of the Diabetes Control and Complications Trial clearly show that tightly managing diabetes can dramatically reduce the complications associated with it. Helping clients with diabetes make the necessary adjustments in a continuous process that balances medical and individual needs.

Many chronic diseases require diet and other lifestyle changes to ensure health. Even relatively minor diet changes can be important to the individual. A person with a hiatal hernia, for example, may be unwilling to give up coffee, even though the consequences include the pain of heartburn and worsening esophagitis. The biggest change the person may be willing to make may be to reduce coffee intake from 6 cups to 2 cups a day or to agree to drink coffee only along with foods. Clients with extremely serious disorders who lack motivation to change their lifestyles may benefit from professional counseling along with the encouragement of health care professionals, family, and friends, but in the end, only the client can determine the course that he or she can accept.

NOTES

1. American Diabetes Association and the American Dietetic Association, *Facilitating Lifestyle Change: A Resource Manual* (Alexandria, Va.: American Diabetes Association, 1996).
2. J. G. Pastors, Nutrition assessment for diabetes medical nutrition therapy, *Diabetes Spectrum* 9 (1996): 99–103.
3. M. Peyrot, Evaluation of patient education programs: How to do it and how to use it, *Diabetes Spectrum* 9 (1996): 86–93.
4. M. M. Funnell and R. M. Anderson, Judge not: Lessons learned from simulated diabetes regimens, *Diabetes Spectrum* 8 (1995): 328–329.
5. W. H. Polonsky, Listening to our patients' concerns: Understanding and addressing diabetes-specific emotional distress, *Diabetes Spectrum* 9 (1996): 8–11.
6. R. R. Rubin, Life's work they have *not* chosen, *Diabetes Spectrum* 8 (1995): 308.
7. K. F. McFarland, The power of words, *Diabetes Spectrum* 8 (1995): 308.
8. J. Betschart, Neither good nor bad, *Diabetes Spectrum* 8 (1995): 309.
9. G. L. Grossan and M. L. Uster, Islet pilots—An educational program for children with diabetes, *Journal of the American Dietetic Association* 88 (1988): 471.

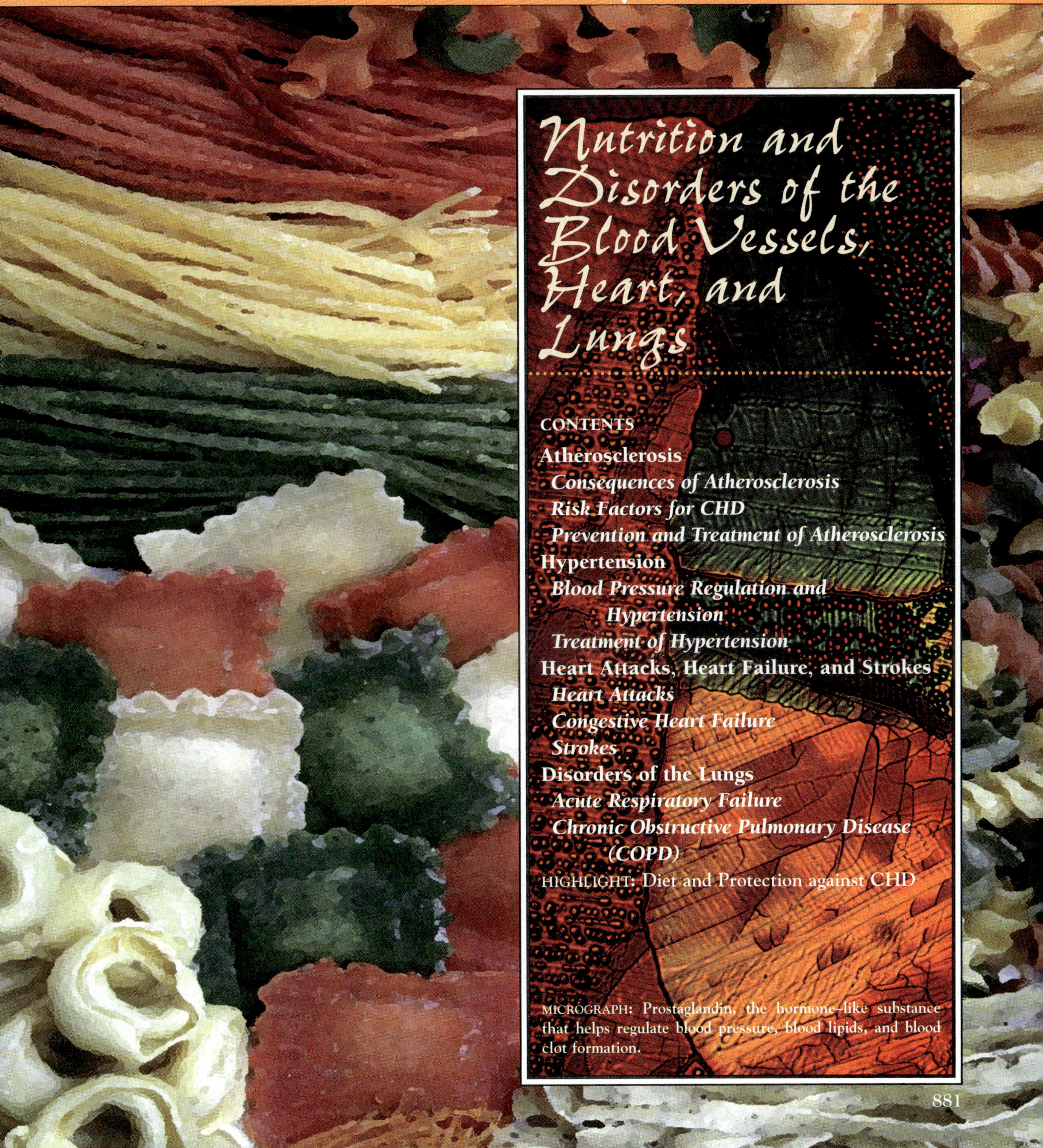

Nutrition and Disorders of the Blood Vessels, Heart, and Lungs

CONTENTS

MICROGRAPH: Prostaglandin, the hormone-like substance that helps regulate blood pressure, blood lipids, and blood clot formation.

For decades, the major causes of death in many developed countries have been diseases of the heart and blood vessels, collectively known as cardiovascular disease (CVD). Cardiovascular disease is the leading cause of death around the world today.[1] In the United States, death rates from cardiovascular disease in men (ages 35 to 50) are three times greater than in women of the same age, but in later years (65 to 74), the incidence is similar. The consequences of cardiovascular disease are usually heart disease and strokes, the first and third leading causes of death for adults, respectively.[2]

Reminder: *Atherosclerosis*, the most common cause of CVD, is characterized by plaques along the inner walls of the arteries, which occlude the affected artery and restrict blood flow. (The related term *arteriosclerosis* refers to all conditions in which the arteries lose elasticity, including some rare diseases.)

Coronary heart disease (CHD), the most common form of cardiovascular disease, usually involves atherosclerosis and hypertension. This chapter first examines atherosclerosis and hypertension, then describes the major consequences of ignoring these conditions—heart attacks, congestive heart failure, and strokes. It concludes with discussions of disorders of the lungs. Figure 28–1 shows the heart, major blood vessels, and lungs.

Figure 28–1

The Heart, Blood Vessels, and Lungs

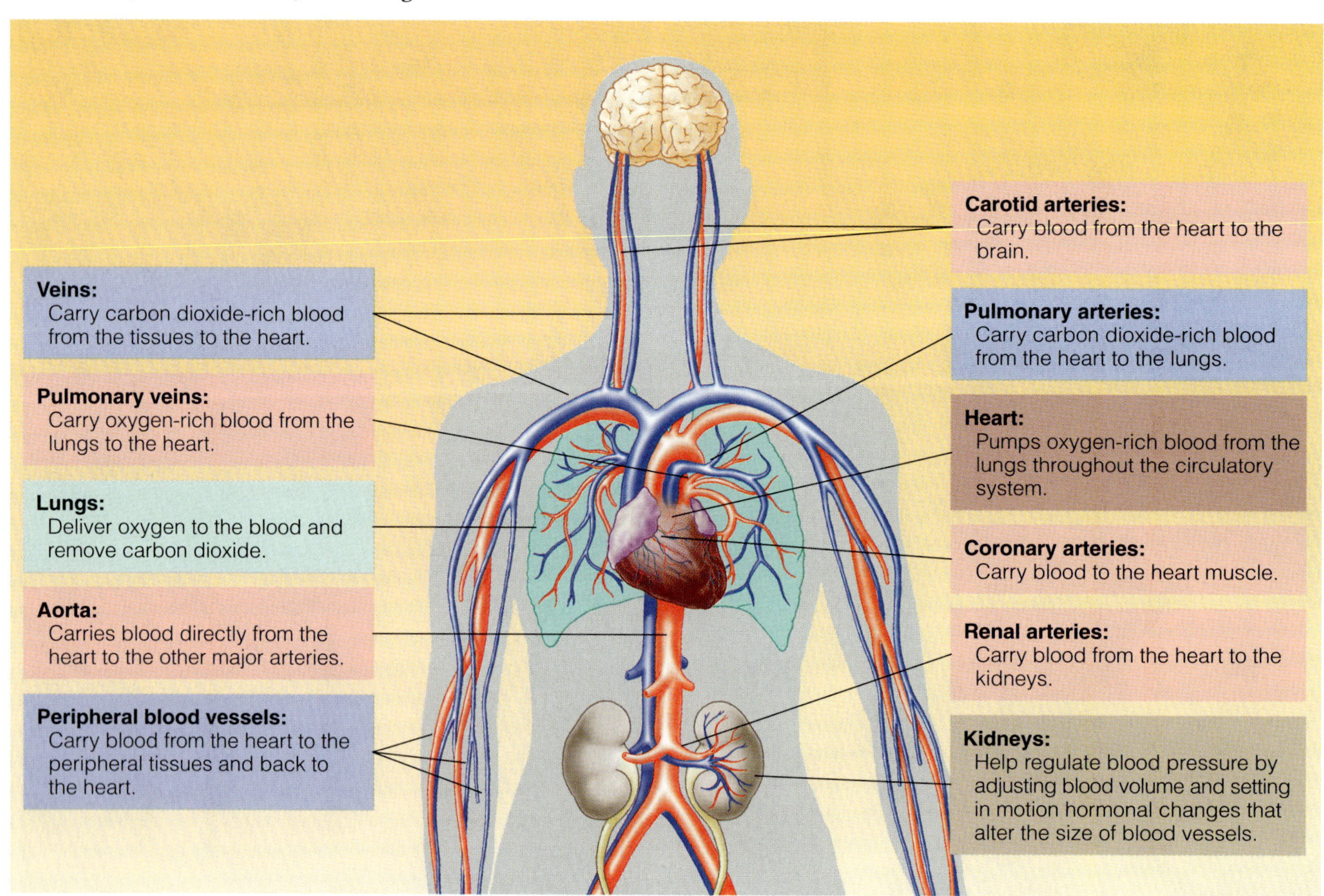

Atherosclerosis

Atherosclerosis usually begins with the accumulation of soft fatty streaks along the inner arterial walls, especially at branch points. These fatty streaks gradually enlarge and become hardened with minerals, forming plaques. Figure H19–1 on p. 659 illustrates the formation of plaques in atherosclerosis. Plaques stiffen the arteries and narrow the passages through them. Most people have well-developed plaques by the age of 30. Preventive efforts focus on preventing plaque development from an early age or delaying or reversing the progression of existing plaques.

plaques (PLACKS): mounds of lipid material, mixed with smooth muscle cells and calcium, which develop in the artery walls in atherosclerosis. This type of plaque is known as **atheromatous** plaque.
placken = patch or plate

CONSEQUENCES OF ATHEROSCLEROSIS

Atherosclerosis directly and indirectly obstructs blood flow through the arteries, damages tissues, and raises blood pressure. When blood flow in the arteries feeding the heart is obstructed, coronary artery disease results. When coronary artery disease damages the heart muscle (coronary heart disease), the person may experience pain and pressure in and around the area of the heart (angina). If the blood flow to the heart muscle is cut off, that area of heart muscle dies, and a heart attack results. When blood flow to the brain is obstructed, a transient ischemic attack (TIA) or stroke results.

angina: a painful feeling of tightness or pressure, felt in the area in and around the heart, often radiating to the back, neck, and arms; caused by a lack of oxygen to an area of heart muscle.

Blood Clots Form Small, cell-like bodies in the blood, known as platelets, cause clots to form whenever they encounter injuries in blood vessels. Clots normally form and dissolve in the blood all the time, but in atherosclerosis, clots form faster than they dissolve, because the platelets respond to plaques as they normally do to injuries.

platelets: tiny, disc-shaped bodies in the blood, important in blood clot formation.

A blood clot may stick to a plaque and gradually grow large enough to restrict or close off a blood vessel (thrombosis). A coronary thrombosis blocks blood flow through an artery that feeds the heart muscle. A cerebral thrombosis blocks blood flow through an artery that feeds the brain. A clot may also break free from the artery wall and travel through the circulatory system until it lodges in a small artery and suddenly shuts off blood flow to that area (embolism). The gradual or sudden loss of blood flow to the portion of the tissue supplied by the clotted artery robs the tissue of oxygen and nutrients, and the tissue may eventually die.

thrombosis: the formation of a **thrombus**, a blood clot that may obstruct a blood vessel, causing gradual tissue death.
thrombo = clot

embolism: the obstruction of a blood vessel by an **embolus** (EM-boh-luss), or traveling clot, causing sudden tissue death.
embol = to insert, plug

Blood Pressure Rises The heart must create enough pressure to push blood through the circulatory system. When arteries are narrowed by plaques, clots, or both, blood flow is restricted, and the heart must then generate more pressure to deliver blood to the tissues. This higher blood pressure further damages the artery walls, and plaques and clots are especially likely to form at damage points. Thus the development of atherosclerosis is a self-accelerating process. (A later section describes additional consequences of hypertension.)

RISK FACTORS FOR CHD

Although atherosclerosis can invade any blood vessel, the coronary arteries are most often affected. The margin lists the risk factors for CHD identified by health authorities.[3] Obesity and lack of physical activity significantly affect several of the major risk factors. Obesity, for example, especially central obesity (see p. 272), is associated with high blood lipids, hypertension, and diabetes. Researchers continue to look for modifiable risk factors for CHD, and many diet-

Major risk factors for CHD:

- High LDL cholesterol.
- Male, 45 years or older.
- Female, 55 years or older, or with premature menopause and not on estrogen replacement therapy.
- Low HDL cholesterol. (Subtract 1 risk factor if HDL cholesterol ≥60 mg/dL.)
- Hypertension.
- Smoking.
- Diabetes mellitus.
- Family history of heart attacks or sudden death prior to age 55 in a male parent or sibling or prior to age 65 in a female parent or sibling.

related factors are under investigation. Highlight 28 examines some of the most widely publicized and promising areas of investigation.

Highlight 19 describes the development of atherosclerosis in childhood and shows cholesterol standards for children and adolescents.

Screening for Risk Factors To determine an individual's risk of CHD, health care professionals consider the person's health history and lifestyle (see the box on p. 886) and measure several blood lipids including total cholesterol, LDL cholesterol, HDL cholesterol, and triglycerides. Ideally, at least two measurements are taken at least one week apart and then compared to standards (shown in Table 28–1). Single measurements may fail to identify those at risk

Reminder: Cholesterol is carried in several lipoproteins, chief among them LDL and HDL (see Chapter 5 for details). Remember them this way:

- **H**DL = **H**igh-density lipoproteins = **H**ealthy.
- **L**DL = **L**ow-density lipoproteins = **L**ess healthy.

Table 28–1

Standards for CHD Risk Factors

LDL Cholesterol	Total Cholesterol[b]
<130 mg/dL = desirable[a]	<200 mg/dL = desirable
130–159 mg/dL = borderline high	200–239 mg/dL = borderline high
≥160 mg/dL = high	≥240 mg/dL = high
HDL Cholesterol	**Triglycerides (Fasting)[d]**
HDL ≤35 mg/dL indicates risk[c]	<200 mg/dL = desirable
LDL-to-HDL ratio:	200–400 mg/dL = borderline high
Men: >5.0 indicates risk	400–1000 mg/dL = high
Women: >4.5 indicates risk	>1000 mg/dL = very high
Hypertension	**Obesity**
Diastolic pressure:[e]	Body mass index:
<85 = normal	Men: >27.8
80–89 = high-normal	Women: >27.3
90–99 = mild	
100–109 = moderate	
110–119 = severe	
>120 = very severe	

[a]For people with existing CHD, desirable LDL cholesterol values are lower (≤100 mg/dL).

[b]To convert cholesterol (mg/dL) to standard international units (mmol/L), multiply by 0.02586. For cholesterol values for children and adolescents, see Table H19–1.

[c]This HDL value may be too low for women; no alternative value has yet been proposed. NIH Consensus Development Panel on Triglyceride, High-Density Lipoprotein, and Coronary Heart Disease, Triglyceride, high-density lipoprotein, and coronary heart disease, *Journal of the American Medical Association* 269 (1993): 505–510.

[d]High triglycerides alone normally do not indicate *direct* risk, but may reflect lipoprotein abnormalities associated with CHD. The risk of CHD increases as triglyceride levels increase in people with other risk factors. High triglycerides also occur in conditions such as kidney disease and diabetes, which suggest a high CHD risk.

[e]Diastolic pressure is the lower of the numbers in the blood pressure reading—for example, the 70 in 105/70. Blood pressure is measured in millimeters of mercury (mm Hg), a standard unit for the measurement of pressure.

Sources: Blood lipid standards adapted from The Expert Panel, Summary of the second report of the National Cholesterol Education Program (NCEP) Expert Panel on Detection, Evaluation, and Treatment of High Blood Cholesterol in Adults (Adult Treatment Panel II), *Journal of the American Medical Association* 269 (1993): 3015–3023; hypertension standards adapted from the Fifth Report of the Joint National Committee on Detection, Evaluation, and Treatment of High Blood Pressure, National High Blood Pressure Education Program, National Heart, Lung, and Blood Institute, National Institutes of Health, October 30, 1992, p. 5.

or may misclassify them because blood cholesterol and other lipid concentrations vary significantly from day to day.

Recommendations for Screening Population studies have found most middle-aged and older adults have at least one risk factor and many have more than one. Both the United States and Canada recommend screening to identify individuals at high risk so as to offer preventive advice and treatment. Such programs are proving successful: since 1960, both blood cholesterol levels and deaths from cardiovascular disease among U.S. adults have shown a continuous and substantial downward trend.[4]

Diet-Related Risk Factors It befits a nutrition book to focus on diet and physical activity strategies to reduce CHD risk. Several of the major risk factors can be modified by diet and activity: high LDL cholesterol, low HDL cholesterol, hypertension (the subject of a later section in this chapter), and diabetes mellitus (discussed in Chapter 27).

LDL Cholesterol and Other Lipids The blood cholesterol linked to atherosclerosis risk is LDL cholesterol (see Figure 28–2). HDL also carry cholesterol, but raised HDL represent cholesterol returning from the cells to the liver, so HDL indicate a *reduced* risk. In general, the higher the LDL cholesterol, the greater the risk of CHD (review Table 28–1).

The exact reasons why high LDL increase the risk of CHD remain unclear. Mounting evidence suggests, however, that the process is promoted by the oxidation of LDL by free radicals. (Highlight 11 describes free-radical formation and its consequences.)

Most often, men have higher LDL cholesterol and a greater risk of CHD at an earlier age than women. Men's blood cholesterol early in adulthood strongly correlates with their risk of developing heart disease later in life.[5] Until menopause, estrogen protects women from cardiovascular disease. Cardiovascular disease occurs about 10 to 12 years later in women than in men.[6] About one-third of women in the United States have LDL cholesterol high enough to pose a serious risk of heart disease.[7]

To a lesser extent, other blood lipids have also been linked to CHD. Triglycerides, mostly concentrated in VLDL, are elevated in some people with CHD, especially those with diabetes and those who are overweight. Yet others with high triglycerides and VLDL do not appear to have a high risk of heart disease. Elevated triglycerides are also associated with a high fasting blood glucose and low HDL.[8] Further studies are needed to determine whether triglycerides directly increase heart disease risk.[9]

Hypertension Chronic high blood pressure frequently accompanies atherosclerosis, diabetes, and obesity. The higher the blood pressure above normal, the greater the risk of heart disease.

Diabetes Mellitus More than 80 percent of people with diabetes die from cardiovascular disease, often a heart attack. People with diabetes have two to five times the incidence of coronary artery disease than those without diabetes.[10] Women with diabetes have the same rate of cardiovascular disease as men; thus diabetes increases the risk of cardiovascular disease more in women than in men.[11] Diabetes, like CHD, is associated with high LDL, high triglycerides, low HDL, hypertension, and obesity, particularly central obesity.

Figure 28–2

HDL and LDL Compared

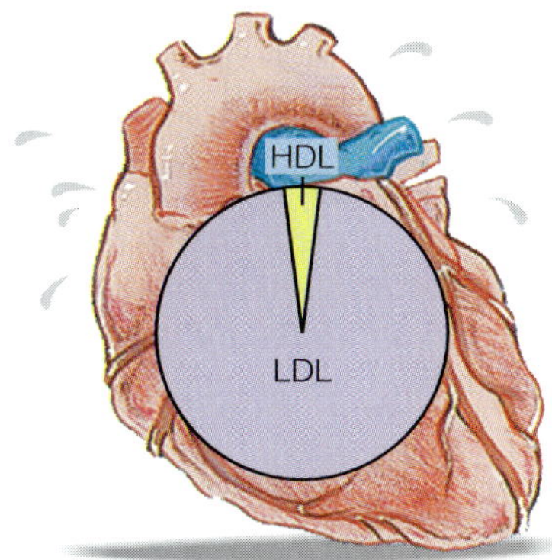

Low HDL relative to **LDL**
Increased risk of heart attack

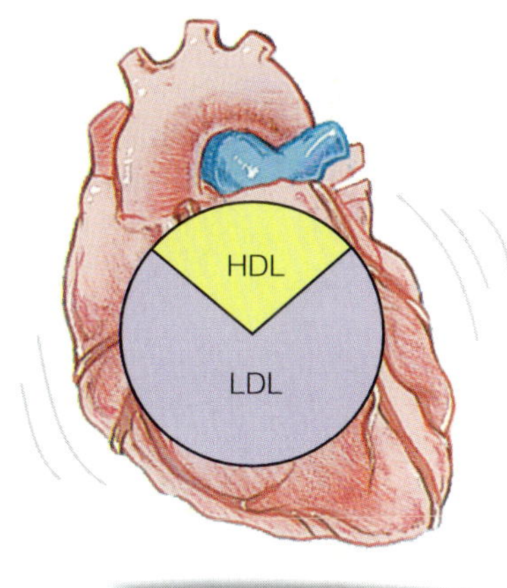

High HDL relative to **LDL**
Decreased risk of heart attack

The technical term for abnormal blood lipids is **dyslipidemia**; elevated LDL and low HDL are examples. Elevated blood lipids may also be called **hyperlipidemia**.

The combination of insulin resistance, glucose intolerance, hypertension, elevated blood lipids, and obesity frequently observed in people with cardiovascular disease is sometimes called **Syndrome X**.

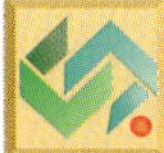

How to Assess Your Heart Disease Risk

Do you know your heart disease risk score? Respond to the statements below, and score yourself as directed. Be aware that a high risk score does not mean you *will* develop heart disease, but it should warn you of the possibility. Consult your physician if you have questions about your score results.

Heart Disease Risk Scorecard

	If you:	**Add:**	
Age	Are 56 or over	1	______
Sex	Are male	1	______
Family history	Have blood relatives who have had a heart attack or stroke before age 60	12	______
	Have blood relatives who have had a history of heart disease at or before age 60	10	______
	Have blood relatives who have had a heart attack or stroke after age 60	6	______
Personal history	Are 50 or under and have had a heart attack, stroke, or cardiovascular surgery	20	______
	Are 51 or over and have had any of the above	10	______
Diabetes	Have diabetes that appeared before age 40 and you take insulin	10	______
	Have diabetes that appeared at or after 40 and you take insulin or pills	5	______
	Have diabetes that appeared after age 55 and you control it with diet	3	______
Smoking	Smoke 2 or more packs/day	10	______
	Smoke 1 to 2 packs/day or quit within past year	6	______
	Smoke 6 or more cigars/day or use a pipe regularly	6	______
	Smoke less than 1 pack/day or quit over a year ago	3	______
Cholesterol[a]	Have a cholesterol level of 240 or higher	10	______
	Have a cholesterol level of 200 to 239	5	______
Diet[a]	Normally eat		
	Red meat daily; more than 7 eggs weekly; and butter, whole milk, and cheese daily	8	______
	Red meat 4 to 6 times weekly; margarine, low-fat dairy products, and some cheese	4	______
	Poultry, fish, little or no red meat; 3 or fewer eggs weekly; some margarine, nonfat milk and milk products	0	______
Blood pressure	Have a blood pressure higher than 160/100 (either number)	10	______
	Have a blood pressure higher than 140/90 but less than 160/100 (either number)	5	______
Weight[b]	Are 25 lb overweight	4	______
	Are 10 to 24 lb overweight	2	______
	Are less than 10 lb overweight	0	______
Exercise	Engage in aerobic exercise more than 20 minutes less than once a week	4	______
	Engage in aerobic exercise more than 20 minutes 1 to 2 times a week	2	______
	Engage in aerobic exercise more than 20 minutes 3 or more times a week	0	______
Stress	Are frustrated and easily angered when waiting	4	______
	Are impatient and occasionally moody when waiting	2	______
		TOTAL POINTS	______

[a]Answer the diet question only if you do not know your cholesterol level.

[b]Use the formula 106 lb + 6 lb per inch over 5 feet for men, or 100 lb + 5 lb per inch over 5 feet for women.

If you answered the blood pressure question:

High risk	36 and above
Medium risk	19 to 35
Low risk	18 and below

If you did not answer the blood pressure question:

High risk	40 and above
Medium risk	20 to 30
Low risk	19 and below

Source: Adapted from Arizona Heart Institute, Cardiovascular Risk Factor Analysis.

PREVENTION AND TREATMENT OF ATHEROSCLEROSIS

Strategies for preventing and treating atherosclerosis aim to normalize blood lipids, alter modifiable risk factors, and prevent complications. Treatment plans may include major changes in lifestyle involving diet, physical activity, and smoking cessation. Drugs and surgery may also be necessary. Dietary changes can be especially effective when combined with other strategies, such as quitting smoking and being physically active. These three strategies—quitting smoking, dietary changes, and physical activity—are always recommended before drug therapy.

For people with advanced atherosclerosis, therapy may also include surgery to restore blood flow to the affected organ. When elevated LDL or related abnormalities develop as a consequence of another disorder such as diabetes, treatment of the disorder may help normalize blood lipid levels.

Surgery to restore blood flow to the heart muscle to prevent a heart attack is called a **coronary artery bypass graft (CABG)**. Alternative, less invasive procedures to restore coronary blood flow include **laser** or **balloon angioplasty**. Surgery to restore blood flow through the carotid artery to the brain is called a **carotid endartectomy**.

Diet Therapy As Table 28–2 shows, the goals of diet therapy for preventing and treating CHD focus on reducing LDL cholesterol. To that end, people are advised to control their body weights and their intakes of total fat, saturated fat, and dietary cholesterol. A panel of experts recommends a two-step plan, shown in Table 28–3.[12] The Step 1 diet was originally designed for people with borderline-high or high LDL cholesterol, but because atherosclerotic disease is so common, many experts advocate its use for everyone. If blood lipids do not improve, therapy moves on to Step 2. People with existing CHD are immediately placed on the Step 2 diet.

Although the goal of diet therapy for CHD is to reduce blood levels of LDL cholesterol, the primary diet strategy to achieve that end is to reduce fat, especially saturated fat. A low-fat diet is likely to be lower in total kcalories and dietary cholesterol.

Highlight 19 on pp. 658–664 discusses dietary recommendations for preventing atherosclerosis in children.

Control Weight Both steps of the diet to reduce LDL cholesterol recommend energy intakes to achieve or maintain desirable weights. With weight loss, heart disease risk factors improve: blood pressure, blood cholesterol, and blood triglycerides decline.[13] For people with NIDDM, weight loss diminishes insulin resistance.

People with elevated triglycerides are advised to restrict alcohol because alcohol raises triglyceride levels.

Table 28–2

Dietary Treatment Guidelines Based on LDL Cholesterol

Risk Factor Status	Cholesterol Values When Diet Therapy Should Begin	Goals for Cholesterol Values with Diet Therapy
• Without existing CHD and with one other risk factor	≥160 mg/dL[a]	<160 mg/dL
• Without existing CHD and with two or more risk factors	≥130 mg/dL[b]	<130 mg/dL
• With existing CHD	>100 mg/dL	≤100 mg/dL

[a]Note that ≥160 mg/dL indicates high risk.
[b]Note that ≥130 mg/dL indicates borderline-high risk.

Source: Adapted from The Expert Panel, Summary of the second report of the National Cholesterol Education Program (NCEP) Expert Panel on Detection, Evaluation, and Treatment of High Blood Cholesterol in Adults (Adult Treatment Panel II), *Journal of the American Medical Association* 269 (1993): 3015–3023.

Table 28–3

Diet Strategies to Reduce LDL Cholesterol

	Step 1	Step 2
Energy	Adequate to achieve or maintain desirable weight	Adequate to achieve or maintain desirable weight
Total fat[a]	≤30%	≤30%
Saturated fat[a]	<10%	<7%
Polyunsaturated fat[a]	<10%	<10%
Monounsaturated fat[a]	5–15%	5–15%
Cholesterol	<300 mg/day	<200 mg/day

[a]All fats except cholesterol are expressed as percentages of total food energy.

Source: Adapted from E. J. Schaefer, New recommendations for the diagnosis and treatment of plasma lipid abnormalities, *Nutrition Reviews* 51 (1993): 246–252.

Notice that the low-fat diet described here restricts both the amount and the types of fat. By comparison, the low-fat diet described in Chapter 22's discussion of malabsorption syndromes concentrates on simply limiting the total amount of fat.

Reduce Fat, Especially Saturated Fat The Step 1 diet recommends a total fat intake of less than 30 percent of daily kcalories, with saturated fat no more than one-third of that and dietary cholesterol less than 300 milligrams a day. Such a diet restricts obvious sources of fat, saturated fat, and cholesterol and can be accomplished by following the practical suggestions for reducing fat outlined in Chapter 5 on p. 168.

The Step 2 diet further reduces saturated fat to 7 percent of the daily fat kcalories and cholesterol to less than 200 milligrams per day. For persons requiring the Step 2 diet, the help of a registered dietitian can ensure that saturated fat and cholesterol are reduced as needed without sacrificing nutritional quality.

Interestingly, men may benefit more from such a dietary regimen than women.[14] Even though total blood cholesterol levels decrease similarly, the decline in LDL is greater and the decline in HDL is smaller in men than in women.

Other Dietary Measures In addition to the dietary recommendations of the expert panel, many other diet-related strategies for reducing CHD risk are under investigation. Some researchers have shown, for example, that a diet that provides up to 45 percent of total kcalories from fat can effectively lower LDL and triglyceride levels, provided that the additional fat comes from monounsaturated sources.[15] As an added benefit, the diet does not appear to lower HDL. As Chapter 27 described, such a diet may be particularly useful for improving blood lipid levels in people with NIDDM. Highlight 28 describes other diet-related strategies that may help to lower LDL or otherwise reduce the risk of CHD, including antioxidant nutrients, fiber, homocysteine and folate, fish oils, and alcohol.

Physical Activity Physical activity deserves attention in any program to reduce CHD risk. Some evidence suggests that weight training can raise HDL somewhat if undertaken regularly, but frequent and sustained *aerobic* activity may be most effective in lowering LDL and raising HDL. Furthermore, aerobic, endurance-type activities, such as brisk walking, undertaken faithfully for 30 minutes or more as a daily or every-other-day routine can strengthen the heart and blood vessels; alter body composition in favor of lean over fat tissue; expand the volume of oxygen the heart can deliver to the tissues at each beat and so reduce the heart's workload; change the hormonal climate in which the body does its work in such a way as to lower blood pressure; and bring about a redistribution of body water that eases the transit of blood through the peripheral arteries. These changes are so beneficial that some experts believe that physical activity should be the primary focus of cardiovascular disease prevention efforts.[16]

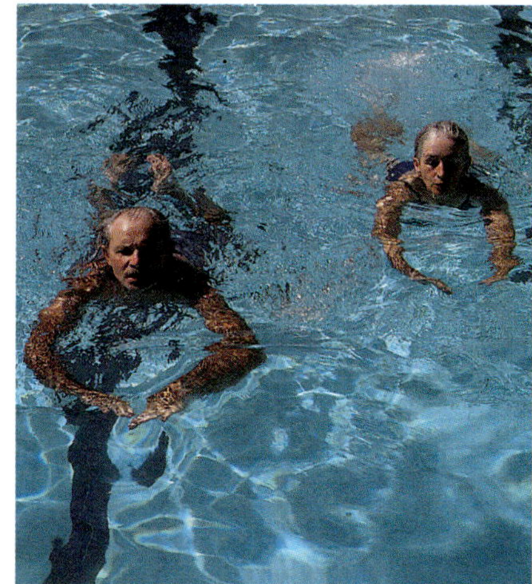

Regular aerobic exercise can help to defend against heart disease by strengthening the heart muscle, promoting weight loss, reducing blood pressure, and improving blood lipid and blood glucose levels.

If heart and artery disease has already set in, a monitored program of physical activity may actually help to reverse it.[17] Activity may stimulate development of new arteries to feed the heart muscle. These arteries may help account for the excellent recovery seen in some heart attack victims who exercise.

Some researchers wonder if physical activity itself raises blood HDL or if the weight loss that often accompanies exercise is the real factor. For women, diet alone appears to *lower* HDL, but when diet is combined with moderate aerobic activity, HDL do not decline.[18] In men, diet raises HDL, and activity in conjunction with diet results in a significantly greater rise in HDL than diet alone.

Diet helps a little, physical activity helps a little, and the combination is better still. People with CHD have been able to reduce plaque buildup in their arteries by following a comprehensive plan combining a low-fat vegetarian diet, no cigarette smoking, stress management training, and moderate physical activity.[19] Without such a program, atherosclerosis would most likely have progressed; instead, it regressed and did so without lipid-lowering drugs.

Drug Therapy When used together with diet therapy and a physical activity program, drug therapy can effectively lower blood lipids. Lipid-lowering drugs carry potential risks, however, and are costly. Therefore, physicians as a rule do not prescribe drugs to treat hyperlipidemia until after a six-month trial of intensive diet therapy and physical activity alone has proved unsuccessful in lowering blood lipid concentrations. For people with very high LDL cholesterol (greater than 220 milligrams per deciliter), a shorter diet trial may be considered. Besides lipid-lowering drugs, the treatment of atherosclerosis may include aspirin and anticoagulants to prevent clot formation and antihypertensives to reduce blood pressure. All of these drugs are associated with significant risks and nutrition-related side effects, a problem compounded by the fact that drug therapy often includes multiple drugs and continues for many years or even for life.

℞ **PRESCRIPTION PAD**

Drugs used in the treatment of cardiovascular disease may include:

- Anticoagulants (including aspirin)
- Antihypertensives
- Antilipemics
- Diuretics (isosorbide nitrate)
- Nitroglycerin (to ease angina)

See Appendix E for timing with meals and nutrition-related side effects.

Plaques in atherosclerosis raise blood pressure and trigger abnormal blood clotting, which can cause heart attacks and strokes. Dietary recommendations to lower the risks of these cardiovascular diseases focus on reducing saturated fat and cholesterol intake. Smoking cessation and engaging in regular physical activity are also important. Anyone concerned about atherosclerosis and the risk it presents must also be concerned about hypertension. The two together are a life-threatening combination.

Hypertension

Chronic elevated blood pressure, or hypertension, is a major CHD risk factor; it is believed to affect some 60 million people in the United States, more than a

hypertension: higher-than-normal blood pressure. Hypertension that develops without an identifiable cause is known as **essential** or **primary hypertension**; hypertension that is caused by a specific disorder such as kidney disease is known as **secondary hypertension**.

Normal resting blood pressure for adults averages about 120 over 80 millimeters of mercury (mm Hg). At readings of 140 over 90 mm Hg or higher, the risks of heart attacks and strokes increase in direct proportion to increasing blood pressure, especially diastolic pressure (review Table 28–1).

peripheral resistance: resistance to the flow of blood caused by the reduced diameter of the vessels at the periphery of the body—the smallest arteries and capillaries.

third of the entire adult population.[20] Hypertension contributes to half a million strokes and over a million heart attacks each year. The higher the blood pressure is above normal, the greater the risk of heart disease. (Low blood pressure, on the other hand, is generally a sign of long life expectancy and low heart disease risk.) People cannot feel the physical effects of high blood pressure, but it can impair life's quality and end life prematurely.

BLOOD PRESSURE REGULATION AND HYPERTENSION

The body's ability to maintain its blood pressure is vital to life. The heart's pumping action must create enough force to push blood through the major arteries into the smaller arteries and finally into the tiny capillaries, whose thin, porous walls permit fluid exchange between the blood and the tissues (see Figure 28–3). The nervous system helps maintain blood pressure by adjusting the size of the

Figure 28–3

How Normal Blood Pressure Supports Fluid Exchange

At the same time the heart pushes blood into an artery, the small-diameter arteries and capillaries at its other end resist the blood's flow (peripheral resistance). Both actions contribute to the pressure inside the artery. Another determining factor is the volume of fluid in the circulatory system, which depends in turn on the number of dissolved particles in that fluid.

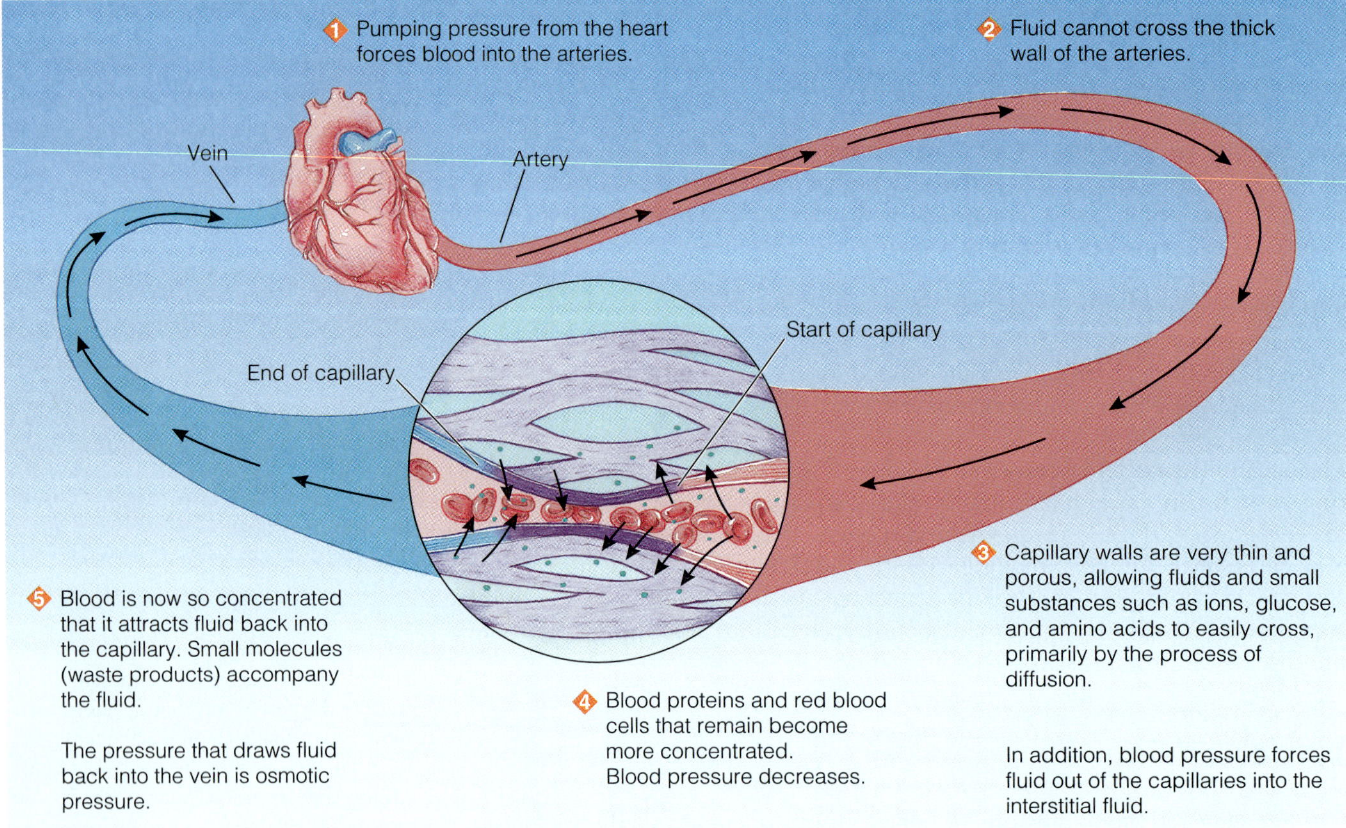

blood vessels and by influencing the heart's pumping action. The kidneys help regulate blood pressure by setting in motion mechanisms that change the blood volume. The narrower the blood vessels or the greater the volume of blood in the circulatory system, the harder the heart must pump (and the more pressure the heart must create) to feed the tissues.

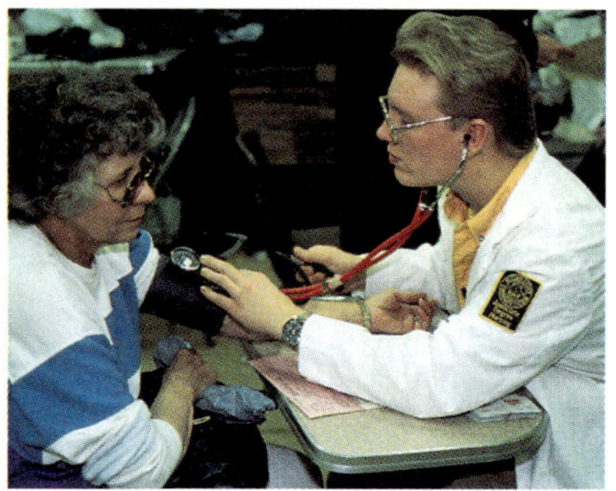

Screening people for high blood pressure is a first step in reducing CHD risk from hypertension.

The Kidneys and Hypertension What triggers chronic hypertension remains for the most part unknown, although one of the mechanisms involving the kidneys has been defined. The kidneys are highly sensitive to changes in blood pressure because their ability to filter the blood and form urine depends on it. When blood flow to the kidneys is reduced (as occurs in atherosclerosis), the kidneys respond by setting in motion actions that raise blood pressure by expanding blood volume and constricting peripheral blood vessels. Unfortunately, the pressure increases not only in the kidneys, but all over the body. High blood pressure stresses the heart, which has to pump extra hard to push the expanded blood volume against resistant arteries.

Obesity and Hypertension Obesity can contribute to the development of hypertension or make it worse. The added adipose tissue that obesity incurs means miles of extra capillaries through which the blood must be pumped. The combination of hypertension, atherosclerosis, and obesity puts a severe strain on the heart and arteries, which intensifies cardiovascular complications.

Insulin Resistance and Hypertension Insulin resistance, most commonly associated with obesity, triggers the pancreas to produce more insulin to move glucose into the cells. High blood insulin signals the kidneys to retain sodium and may precipitate the development of hypertension.[21] Hypertension is two to three times more common in people with NIDDM (characterized by insulin resistance) than in the general population.[22] The interrelationships among NIDDM, obesity, hypertension, and atherosclerosis may explain why 80 percent of people with diabetes die from cardiovascular diseases.

Consequences of Hypertension Strain on the heart's pump, the left ventricle, can enlarge and weaken it, until it gradually fails (heart failure). Constant elevated pressure in an artery may cause it to gradually balloon out and eventually burst (aneurysm). Aneurysms that go undetected can lead to massive bleeding and death, particularly if a large vessel such as the aorta is affected. In the small arteries of the brain, an aneurysm may lead to stroke, and in the eye, it may lead to blindness. Likewise, the kidneys can be damaged (kidney disease) when the heart is unable to adequately pump blood through them. Hypertension injures the artery linings and accelerates plaque formation, thus setting the stage for atherosclerosis or worsening existing atherosclerosis. Then the plaques and reduced blood flow induce a further rise in blood pressure, and hypertension and atherosclerosis become mutually aggravating conditions.

Major risk factors for hypertension:

- *Age*. Arteries lose their elasticity and blood pressure increases with age; most people who develop hypertension do so in their 50s and 60s.
- *Heredity*. A family history of hypertension and heart disease raises the risk of developing hypertension two to five times.
- *Obesity*. Obese people are more likely to develop hypertension.
- *Race*. Hypertension is twice as common among African Americans as among whites; it tends to develop earlier and become more severe.

Prevention Significant risk factors for the development of hypertension are listed in the margin. Among the risk factors listed, obesity is the only one that might be modified; it is discussed in a later section. The single most effective step people can take against hypertension is to find out whether they have it. A major national effort to identify and treat hypertension is currently under way. Even mild hypertension can be serious.[23] Early treatment promotes health and a higher-quality, longer life.

TREATMENT OF HYPERTENSION

The treatment of hypertension often focuses on weight loss, physical activity, and drugs. Treatment of underlying disorders such as atherosclerosis and diabetes is also important. The next sections describe the diet-related strategies to reduce blood pressure, which often include weight control and salt-restricted, potassium-rich, fat-controlled diets.

Weight Control Excess body fat, especially central fat, can precipitate hypertension, thus increasing the risks of heart attacks and strokes. Weight loss is one of the most effective and long-lasting treatments for hypertension.[24] Those who are using drugs to control their blood pressure can often reduce the dose or discontinue the drugs if they lose weight. Even a modest weight loss of 10 pounds may significantly lower blood pressure.[25] Many professionals recommend a fat-controlled diet, such as the Step 1 diet shown in Table 28–3 on p. 888, both for weight loss and to control blood lipids and blood pressure.

Physical Activity Not only does physical activity help with weight control, but moderate aerobic activity also helps to lower blood pressure directly. Those who engage in regular, aerobic activity may not need medication for mild hypertension.[26]

People with chronic renal disease or diabetes, people with one or two parents who have hypertension, African Americans, and people over 50 years of age are most likely to be salt sensitive.

Reminder:
- 5 g salt = 2 g sodium = 1 tsp table salt.

Sodium/Salt Sodium in combination with chloride (table salt) may aggravate hypertension in some people who are genetically sensitive, but sodium combined with other ions does not have this effect.[27] Most studies show that weight loss lowers blood pressure more effectively than salt restriction.[28] Salt-sensitive individuals, however, may be able to lower their blood pressure somewhat with a no-added-salt diet that limits salt to about 5 grams a day. Clients can adjust their diets by following the suggestions on p. 421.

The person who normally uses salt liberally may find unsalted foods unpalatable. Clients may be able to adjust to the flavor of unsalted foods if they make changes gradually. A registered dietitian can help a client identify the behaviors associated with salt intake. As the client's motivation and needs dictate, each of these behaviors can be modified using the techniques described in Highlight 27.

Caution: People with renal disease and those on potassium-sparing diuretics should not use salt substitutes.

Salt substitutes and low-sodium products may be helpful for some people, but palatable diets can be planned without them. Caution clients that some of these products contain considerable amounts of salt and cannot be used freely. Furthermore, tell clients not to heat salt substitutes because they turn bitter.

Many health care agencies have advocated a no-added-salt diet for everyone, reasoning that at best it may help to prevent hypertension and at worst it will do no harm. Such wisdom has been called into question by a recent study that found that people with mild-to-moderate hypertension who consumed the lowest sodium intakes had a greater likelihood of suffering a heart attack than those with the highest sodium intakes.[29] The lack of evidence that lowering salt intakes provides a consistent benefit by preventing or reducing hypertension, coupled with evidence that low-sodium diets may be harmful, may prompt many agencies to rethink their recommendations regarding salt restriction.

Potassium, Calcium, and Magnesium Mounting evidence suggests a link between salt sensitivity and the adequacy of potassium, calcium, and magnesium in the diet. For people who regularly consume adequate intakes of these minerals, high-salt diets may not be associated with elevated blood pressure. Some authorities suggest that educating clients to consume diets adequate in potassium, calcium, and magnesium on a daily basis may be a useful intervention for preventing and treating hypertension.[30]

Potassium may be of special concern for people taking diuretics to treat hypertension. A later section describes how these diuretics can lead to potassium imbalances.

Tables 12–5, 12–6, and 12–9 in Chapter 12 list significant sources of potassium, calcium, and magnesium, respectively. Diets rich in fresh fruits and vegetables, whole grains, and legumes and adequate in milk and milk products can help ensure an adequate intake of these minerals.

Alcohol Alcohol, especially if consumed in large amounts, is associated with hypertension. An expert committee recommends that if people with hypertension drink, they should do so in moderation.[31] People who need to lose weight must consider the kcalories contributed by alcohol as well.

A moderate alcohol intake has previously been defined as no more than 1 to 2 drinks per day, but recent studies suggest that men should drink no more than 2 to 6 drinks per week and women no more than 1 to 3 drinks per week. See Highlight 28 for more information.

Other Dietary Modifications Because people with hypertension already have at least one risk factor for CHD, and because fat restriction helps with weight loss, a fat-restricted diet is appropriate (see Table 28–3). People with diabetes are advised to follow a fat-restricted diet as part of their overall meal plan. The sample menu illustrates a day's meals for a fat-restricted, no-added-salt, high-potassium diet—a typical diet for people with hypertension.

Drug Therapy Nondrug treatments such as diet changes, physical activity, and smoking cessation can sometimes control hypertension, especially in mild cases. If nondrug therapies are ineffective, drug therapy may include one or a

Menu

Breakfast	Lunch	Supper
¾ c cantaloupe	Broiled chicken breast	Baked flounder
½ c all-bran cereal	Baked potato	Brown rice
Nonfat milk	Tossed salad	Broccoli
1 slice toast	Hard roll	Hard roll
Margarine	Margarine	Margarine
Coffee or tea	Low-fat dressing	1 medium orange
Sugar (optional)	Nonfat milk	Coffee or tea
	1 small banana	

Sample Fat-Controlled, No-Added-Salt, High-Potassium Diet Menu
Foods for this menu are prepared with little or no salt and a minimal amount of fat. The fats used for cooking or for flavor would be monounsaturated and polyunsaturated.

PRESCRIPTION PAD

Drugs used in the treatment of hypertension may include:

- Antihypertensives
- Diuretics
- Potassium supplements

See Appendix E for timing with meals and nutrition-related side effects.

combination of several types of antihypertensive agents and diuretics. Many clients may also be receiving drugs to treat CHD as described earlier. The risk of side effects, including drug-drug and drug-nutrient interactions, is heightened because several drugs may be necessary, and the drugs must be used for long time periods.

Diuretics can cause potassium imbalances and lead to muscle weakness, unexplained numbness and tingling sensations, irregular heartbeats (arrhythmias), and cardiac arrest. Thiazide and loop diuretics increase the urinary excretion of potassium, and clients on these diuretics need to include rich sources of potassium or potassium supplements daily. Clinicians should regularly monitor blood potassium in clients on these drugs and advise clients to watch for the signs of potassium imbalances just mentioned. Potassium-sparing diuretics, on the other hand, lead to potassium retention. Clients taking potassium-sparing diuretics should be cautioned to avoid excessive potassium intakes, potassium supplements, and salt substitutes.

Of the risk factors that contribute to hypertension, obesity is the only one with a dietary relationship; weight control is the most effective treatment. Researchers continue to study how the minerals sodium, potassium, and calcium influence blood pressure.

Heart Attacks, Heart Failure, and Strokes

When atherosclerosis and hypertension run their courses without treatment, the consequences can be fatal. Most often, these conditions lead to heart attacks and strokes.

HEART ATTACKS

heart attacks: sudden tissue death caused by blockages of vessels that feed the heart muscle; also called **myocardial infarction** or **cardiac arrest**.
myo = muscle
cardial = heart
infarct = tissue death

rheumatic (roo-MAT-ik) **heart disease:** heart damage (often affecting the heart valves) that follows rheumatic fever (caused by a systemic bacterial infection).

The enzymes that increase in the blood after a heart attack include aspartate transaminase (AST), lactate dehydrogenase (LDH), and creatine phosphokinase (CPK).

The heart receives nutrients and oxygen not from inside its chambers, but from arteries on its surface (see Figure 28–1). As mentioned earlier, a heart attack, or myocardial infarction (MI), occurs when the supply of blood to the heart muscle is suddenly cut off. Most commonly, atherosclerosis and hypertension contribute to heart attacks; other contributors include abnormal blood clotting, electrical disturbances that alter the heart rate (arrhythmias), spasms of the coronary arteries, infection of the membrane covering the heart, and rheumatic heart disease.

As an area of heart tissue dies, enzymes specific to heart tissue leak out into the general circulation, much as digestive enzymes leak out of the pancreas in people with pancreatitis. Physicians use blood tests for elevated concentrations of these enzymes to help diagnose heart attacks.

Immediate Care Treatment aims to relieve pain, stabilize the heart rhythm, and reduce the heart's workload. The client is confined to bed rest at first. Like an accident victim, a heart attack victim is initially in shock, and diet therapy cannot begin until shock resolves. After several hours of observation, the person can usually begin to eat again, as outlined in the accompanying box.

The diet aims to reduce the work of the heart and therefore restricts energy, the amount of food or drink provided at each feeding, sodium, and caffeine. Because nausea is a common problem following an MI, liquids are provided first. Low-sodium foods prevent fluid retention, and soft foods prevent abdominal dis-

How to Manage Diets after a Myocardial Infarction (MI)

- Offer nothing by mouth until shock resolves.
- After several hours, give a 1000- to 1200-kcalorie diet that progresses from low-sodium liquids to low-sodium soft foods of moderate temperature in frequent, small feedings.
- After five to ten days, adjust the diet to meet individual needs, generally in three meals a day.
- Although controversial, many practitioners restrict caffeine completely during the first few days after an MI and generally recommend a moderate restriction (no more than 3 cups of a caffeine-containing beverage per day) thereafter.

tention, which would push the diaphragm up toward the heart and stress the heart muscle. Temperature extremes can stimulate nerves that slow the heart rate, so foods should be neither too hot nor too cold. Caffeine stimulates the metabolic rate, increasing the workload of the heart, and therefore is usually restricted.

Long-Term Diet Therapy After the person is out of immediate danger (in about five to ten days), the diet is tailored to meet individual needs and to deal with conditions such as hyperlipidemia, hypertension, obesity, diabetes, and the like. Whatever else may be necessary, a fat-restricted diet to prevent further heart disease or hypertension is appropriate. Such a diet can be planned to provide three meals a day, but people who continue to have chest pain after an MI may benefit from eating frequent, small meals. Advise them to eat slowly and to avoid strenuous physical activity immediately before and after meals.

Encourage Lifestyle Changes The overweight, hard-driving person with elevated LDL cholesterol and hypertension who jokes about smoking cigarettes, being a "couch potato," and eating "junk food" may experience a dramatic change in attitude after a heart attack. Almost overnight, the person places a new value on life and eagerly seeks the advice of health care professionals. Such clients listen carefully and are highly motivated to follow advice. This is an opportune time to recommend changing lifestyle habits and improving the chances for survival. With time, clients may return to old habits as symptoms disappear. To make permanent lifestyle changes, clients need continuing evaluation, support, and encouragement and can benefit from the techniques described in Highlight 27.

CONGESTIVE HEART FAILURE

While heart attacks represent acute heart failure, heart failure can also be gradual. Many disorders—CHD, hypertension, and kidney disease—can lead to congestive heart failure (CHF). In CHF, heart muscle gradually weakens as it strains to supply adequate blood to the tissues despite its own reduced blood supply. The

congestive heart failure (CHF): a syndrome in which the heart can no longer adequately pump blood through the circulatory system.

weakened muscle stretches as it fills with blood it cannot adequately push through the circulatory system. Most often, the left ventricle of the heart is affected first. When this occurs, blood begins to pool in the pulmonary veins and capillaries, and pulmonary edema may eventually result. As heart failure progresses, reduced blood flow impairs the function of all organs. Reduced blood flow to the kidney triggers the retention of fluid (see p. 891), further stressing the heart and compounding the stagnation of fluid in the organs. The heart enlarges and begins to beat more rapidly to try to compensate for its inability to pump. Peripheral, pulmonary, and hepatic edema may develop as the person becomes increasingly "congested" with excess fluids. CHF threatens life, particularly when accompanied by pulmonary edema. Pulmonary congestion increases the likelihood of pneumonia and other respiratory infections, which can further stress the heart and lungs.

pulmonary: of or pertaining to the lungs.

Enlargement of the heart is **cardiomegaly** (CAR-dee-oh-MEG-ah-lee). A rapid heart rate is **tachycardia** (TACK-ee-CAR-dee-ah).

cardio = heart
mega = large
tachys = rapid

Malnutrition in CHF The person with CHF has high energy needs because organ systems, particularly the heart and lungs, must work extra hard to maintain their functions. At the same time, the disrupted blood flow that occurs in CHF limits the supply of nutrients and oxygen to the organs and tissues. Repeated respiratory infections further tax nutrition status. People with CHF are often unable to eat enough to meet energy demands; oral intake may be limited due to anorexia, altered taste sensitivity, intolerance to food odors, physical exhaustion, the diet used for treatment (described later), and medications. Studies suggest that cytokines contribute to malnutrition in people with CHF.[32] Undernutrition in people with CHF may go unnoticed until it has progressed considerably, because edema masks their underweight condition. Thus severe protein-energy malnutrition is a frequent consequence, particularly as the disorder progresses. Malnutrition can further contribute to the weakness of heart muscle and lungs and the development of respiratory infections.

Chronic PEM that develops as a consequence of heart disease is called **cardiac cachexia** (ka-KEKS-ee-ah).

Treatment of CHF Drug therapy for CHF includes diuretics to reduce the fluid volume and cardiac glycosides to increase the strength of heart muscle contractions. People taking thiazide or loop diuretics and cardiac glycosides are at high risk for potassium deficiency and may be prescribed a potassium supplement as well. Stool softeners may be prescribed, particularly for elderly clients who frequently experience constipation, because straining to empty the bowels can stress the heart. Initially, bed rest helps reduce the heart's workload. Once recovery is under way, the person must rest frequently and avoid overexertion.

Rx PRESCRIPTION PAD

Drugs used in the treatment of CHF may include:

- Antihypertensives (vasodilators)
- Cardiac glycosides
- Diuretics
- Potassium supplements

See Appendix E for timing with meals and nutrition-related side effects.

Diet Therapy Diet therapy for CHF is similar to that for acute heart failure (MI), because it aims to reduce the work of the heart (see the accompanying box). Providing adequate nutrients is vital, but overfeeding the severely malnourished person may cause serious problems. Giving too much energy increases the body's metabolic rate; giving too much fluid and sodium expands the body's fluid volume; both consequences tax the heart. For the person who is overweight, judicious weight loss will help relieve strain on the heart.

The extent of sodium restriction depends on the degree of heart failure. Generally, a person with a moderate degree of heart failure benefits from restricting sodium to 2 grams a day. In many cases, a fat-restricted diet is indicated. Dietary fiber is carefully adjusted. The goal is to provide some fiber to prevent constipation, but to avoid amounts and types of fibers that produce gas and abdominal distension.

How to Manage Diets for Congestive Heart Failure (CHF)

- Restrict sodium, caffeine, and fat.
- Encourage gradual weight loss, if necessary. Replace nutrients gradually if the person is malnourished.
- Provide frequent, small meals; use foods that are least likely to produce gas (see Chapter 22).
- Adjust dietary fiber carefully to prevent constipation.
- Use liquid formulas of high nutrient density as an oral supplement or tube feeding to prevent or reverse malnutrition. In some cases, TPN may be required.
- Whether enteral or parenteral, select all formulas carefully and give cautiously to ensure that energy, fluid, and sodium intake will not overload the body.

STROKES

Temporary interference with blood flow to the brain may result in a transient ischemic attack (TIA), a condition that causes changes in mental status that may last for a few moments or a few hours. People who experience a TIA may or may not develop a total blockage of blood flow to a portion of the brain that results in a stroke, or cerebrovascular accident (CVA). Most strokes occur as a consequence of atherosclerosis, hypertension, or a combination of the two.

transient ischemic attack (TIA): a temporary reduction in blood flow to the brain that causes temporary symptoms that depend on the part of the brain that is affected. Some common symptoms include light-headedness, visual disturbances, paralysis, staggering, numbness, or dysphagia.

stroke: an event in which the blood flow to a part of the brain is cut off; also called a **cerebrovascular accident (CVA)**.
cerebro = brain
vascular = blood vessels

Complications Affecting Food Intake For some stroke victims, recovery is unremarkable. For others, recovery requires many months of rehabilitative therapy. Victims may suffer from temporary or permanent problems that interfere with the ability to communicate. This inability to communicate effectively makes it difficult for them to tell health care professionals about foods they can or would like to eat or about problems they may be having with swallowing foods.

Dysphagia Dysphagia (see p. 697 in Chapter 21) affects many stroke victims. The stroke victim may fail to respond to the presence of food in the trachea with a coughing response, and food may enter the lungs. "Silent" aspiration has been documented in a number of people who develop dysphagia following a stroke.[33] Tube feedings may be indicated initially until clients are able to work with a speech therapist and dietitian to determine what foods they can safely chew and swallow. (Chapter 21 described cautions for tube feeding clients with dysphagia.)

Reminder: *Dysphagia* refers to an inability to coordinate swallowing appropriately.

Physical Problems Some stroke victims have problems with the physical process of eating. They may be unable to grasp utensils or coordinate movements that bring foods or liquids from the table to the mouth. Highlight 21 describes ways to handle such problems.

Long-Term Diet Therapy Long-term diet therapy for stroke victims depends on the underlying medical condition. A diet that restricts kcalories, fat, and sodium is often appropriate. Food energy may need to be limited due to inactivity. A client who must relearn how to walk or use other muscle groups will be better able to do so if not overweight. Underweight can also hinder physical

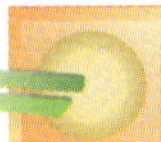

Case Study History Professor with Cardiovascular Disease

Mr. Jablonski, a 48-year-old history professor, has a blood lipid profile that includes elevated LDL cholesterol. He is 5 feet 7 inches tall and weighs 200 pounds. Mr. Jablonski has a family history of CHD. His diet history shows excessive intakes of food energy, cholesterol, total fat, saturated fat, and salt. He smokes a pack of cigarettes a day, and his lifestyle leaves him little time for physical activity. Mr. Jablonski also has hypertension, for which diuretics have been prescribed. He frequently forgets to take his pills, though, and his blood pressure is often quite high.

Name the risk factors for CHD in Mr. Jablonski's history. Which of them can he control? Which can be helped by diet? What complications might you expect if his condition goes untreated?

What type of diet, if any, would you recommend to treat Mr. Jablonski's high LDL cholesterol? Explain the rationale for each diet change. How will his current diet change? Prepare a day's menus for Mr. Jablonski.

What type of diet, if any, would you recommend for Mr. Jablonski's hypertension? What suggestions might you offer to help him make the necessary diet changes? Are these diet changes consistent with those you would recommend for high LDL cholesterol?

What laboratory and clinical tests would you expect to see monitored regularly? Why?

Name at least three ways in which Mr. Jablonski could benefit from losing weight. How does physical activity fit into a weight-loss plan? Describe other ways Mr. Jablonski might benefit from a physical activity program.

Discuss nutrition considerations if Mr. Jablonski should suffer a heart attack, develop congestive heart failure, or have a stroke. Describe the relationships of these disorders to elevated blood lipids and hypertension.

rehabilitation, another reason to ensure that the person does not become malnourished.

The accompanying case study presents a client with CHD. Carefully consider the questions posed to review the information presented thus far in the chapter.

Disorders of the Lungs

The heart and lungs work together to ensure the delivery of oxygen to the cells of the body and to remove wastes generated by metabolic processes in these cells. Thus lung disorders can affect nutrition status. This section describes the nutrition implications of two types of lung disorders, acute respiratory failure and chronic obstructive pulmonary disease.

ACUTE RESPIRATORY FAILURE

respiratory failure: failure of the lungs to exchange gases; also known as **adult respiratory distress syndrome (ARDS)**.

Recall from Chapter 25 that the lungs are often the first organ to fail in people who develop multiple organ failure as a consequence of severe stress. In today's intensive care units, respiratory failure is a frequent and sudden cause of serious illness and death.

Causes of Acute Respiratory Failure Severe stress is the most frequent cause of acute respiratory failure, but other possible causes include emboli lodged in the lungs, severe allergic reactions, aspiration pneumonia, inhalation of toxic gases, and some drug overdoses. In respiratory failure, the inflammatory responses described in Chapter 25 increase the permeability of the capillaries of the lungs' alveoli, fluids accumulate in the lungs' interstitial spaces, and pulmonary edema develops. The lungs stiffen and are unable to exchange gases.

alveoli (al-VEE-oh-lie): air sacs in the lungs; one sac is an *alveolus*.

Consequences of Acute Respiratory Failure To compensate for altered gas exchange, the person breathes faster, the heart rate increases, breathing becomes labored, and the person becomes restless. Lack of oxygen causes the person to look pale and cyanotic. If respiratory failure progresses to a severe stage, mental status diminishes. The person may eventually lapse into a coma, and heart failure may ensue. Clients who recover from respiratory failure, however, often regain normal lung function.

Lack of oxygen in the blood is called hypoxemia.

cyanosis: a bluish discoloration of the skin caused by a lack of oxygen.

Treatment of Acute Respiratory Failure Treatment focuses on correcting the underlying disorder and preventing the progression of respiratory failure. The person often requires mechanical ventilation. Intravenous fluids are used to correct fluid and electrolyte and acid-base imbalances. Diuretics help mobilize fluids.

mechanical ventilator: a machine that "breathes" for the person who can't.

Diet Therapy Diet therapy for respiratory failure aims to provide enough energy and protein to support lung function and prevent infections without overtaxing the respiratory system. Actual energy needs depend on the underlying stress and can be highly variable. Adequate protein and energy help prevent infections and weakening of the lung muscle, which is working hard to produce forceful respirations. Weak muscles, in turn, fail to push blood along through the veins, worsening circulatory problems and contributing to poor nutrition. The combination of poor respiration, poor circulation, and poor local nutrition makes pulmonary infections likely.

The person being weaned from mechanical ventilation also has high energy and protein needs. The switch from mechanical ventilation to normal breathing is a stressful and energy-consuming process. The person's lungs were weak before mechanical ventilation was offered, and they have become weaker with disuse. Now they must do more work as the ventilator does less of the breathing.

Energy Sources With respect to energy needs, the ratio of carbohydrate to fat affects the lungs' workload; so does the total energy delivered. During metabolism, glucose generates more carbon dioxide per kcalorie delivered than does fat. Overfeeding also generates excess carbon dioxide. Therefore, carbohydrate or energy in excess of the body's needs taxes the lungs. For these reasons, authorities recommend that total kcalories and carbohydrate be carefully controlled for people in respiratory failure.[34] Early reports suggested that fat should supply as much as 50 to 60 percent of the total kcalories, but as Chapter 25 described, high fat intakes may impair immune function. Many authorities recommend indirect calorimetry to determine the ratio of carbon dioxide produced to oxygen consumed and use the results to develop an individualized diet plan.

The ratio of carbon dioxide produced to oxygen consumed is the respiratory quotient (RQ). Clinicians use the RQ to estimate total energy needs and the appropriate mix of carbohydrate and fat to meet those needs.

Fluids and Electrolytes Fluid and sodium restrictions may be necessary to ease pulmonary edema. Maintaining appropriate levels of other electrolytes, particularly phosphorus, potassium, calcium, and magnesium, is also important. These electrolytes play important roles in maintaining the structure and function of muscle tissue.[35]

Enteral and Parenteral Nutrition People in acute respiratory failure are generally ventilator-dependent and unable to meet their nutrient needs with an oral diet. Tube feedings are preferred to IV feedings: they are safer and help to maintain GI tract integrity. Possibly, they support immune function better, too. Intestinal feedings are preferred over gastric feedings because they minimize the risk of aspiration—a consideration of particular importance to the person in respiratory failure. Special enteral formulas, designed for respiratory failure, are available (see Appendix K). When enteral nutrition is contraindicated, TPN should be started without delay. Both enteral and parenteral formulas can be tailored to meet specific nutrient needs.

CHRONIC OBSTRUCTIVE PULMONARY DISEASE (COPD)

chronic obstructive pulmonary disease (COPD): one of several disorders, including emphysema and bronchitis, that interfere with respiration.

emphysema (EM-fe-SEE-ma): a type of COPD in which the lungs lose their elasticity and the victim has difficulty breathing; often occurs along with bronchitis.

bronchitis (bron-KYE-tis): inflammation of the lungs' air passages.
bronchos = windpipe
itis = inflammation

Chronic obstructive pulmonary disease (COPD) is a term that describes several conditions characterized by persistent obstruction of airflow through the lungs. The two major types of COPD are emphysema and chronic bronchitis. COPD ranks as the fourth leading cause of death in the United States.[36] Smoking is a primary risk factor for COPD, and most people with COPD are smokers. Other risk factors include exposure to environmental pollution (including exposure of nonsmokers to cigarette smoke) and, possibly, repeated respiratory tract infections.

Experts believe that COPD may be largely preventable by encouraging people not to smoke and by controlling environmental pollutants.[37] Early identification of people with COPD is important; quitting smoking before the disorder has progressed can help preserve lung function.

Consequences of COPD Regardless of the type of COPD, the lungs gradually lose their functional surface area and strength, making it difficult for them to deliver oxygen to the blood and to remove carbon dioxide from it. As lung function becomes increasingly compromised, pulmonary infections, respiratory failure, and heart failure can follow.

COPD and Nutrition Status People with advanced COPD frequently experience PEM and infection, and they account for many cases of malnutrition in hospitals. The extent of malnutrition appears to correlate with the severity of pulmonary disease.

Weight loss in people with COPD may be rapid and dramatic. The weight loss may occur for many reasons, including the following:

- Anorexia and poor food intake.
- High energy expenditures associated with labored breathing.
- Steroid drug therapy, which raises nutrient requirements and compromises nutrition status.
- Use of mechanical ventilators, because people who require them are in a hypermetabolic state. Furthermore, people in the end stages of COPD who need long-term mechanical ventilation often experience weakness and discomfort that make it extremely difficult to meet nutrient needs orally.
- Repeated infections, which raise nutrient needs and deplete nutrient stores. Nutrient deficiencies, in turn, open the way for infection, a vicious cycle.

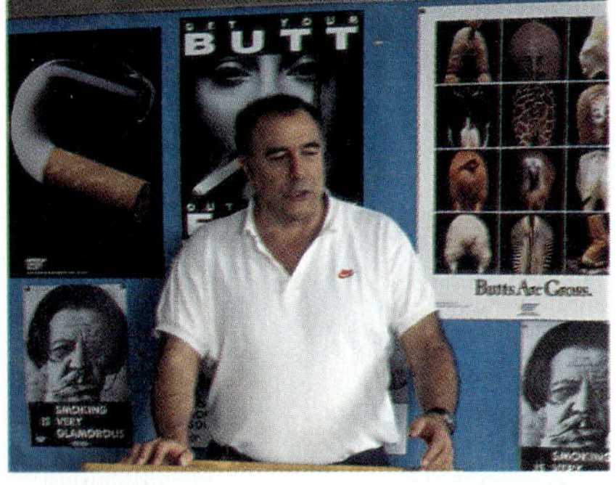

Health care professionals urge clients not to smoke to reduce the incidence of both COPD and heart disease.

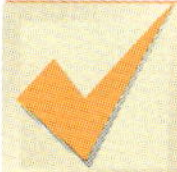

Nutrition Assessment Checklist

For People with Disorders of the Heart, Blood Vessels, and Lungs

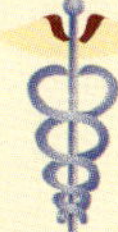

Medical Use the health history to note risk factors or existing cardiovascular disease or COPD, complications associated with those disorders, and other medical conditions that might affect nutrition status.

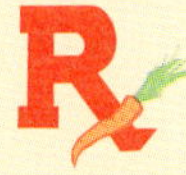

Drug Assess the client's drug history for drug-nutrient interactions. Note that the likelihood of adverse affects on nutrition status is heightened when cardiovascular disease and COPD occur in the elderly who frequently take multiple medications over long periods of time. People in respiratory failure are hypermetabolic, and they, too, are at high risk for drug-nutrient interactions. Keep in mind the special potassium needs of those taking diuretics and/or cardiac glycosides.

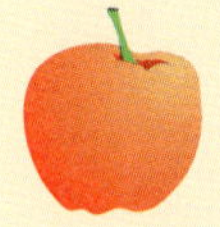

Food Intake For clients with cardiovascular disease, assess nutrient intake for total energy; saturated, monounsaturated, and polyunsaturated fats; and cholesterol. In addition, check intakes for salt, sodium, potassium, and alcohol. For clients with COPD, assess intakes for total energy and protein. For clients in respiratory failure, respiratory quotients can provide estimates of total energy needs as well as an acceptable ratio of carbohydrate and fat.

Anthropometric Assess weight, body fat, and central fat for people with cardiovascular and lung diseases. Weight measurements must be interpreted cautiously in people with CHF and pulmonary edema because fluid retention may mask significant undernutrition. For people with heart and lung disorders, achieving or maintaining a healthy body weight prevents the additional stress of either obesity or undernutrition on the cardiovascular and respiratory systems.

Laboratory Anticipate low serum albumin levels in people who are retaining fluids or experiencing respiratory failure. Monitor serum lipids in people at risk for CHD and in those with hyperlipidemia. Monitor serum potassium in people taking thiazide or loop diuretics and cardiac glycosides.

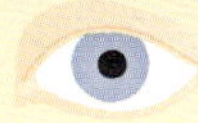

Physical Check for physical signs of nutrient deficiencies, energy level, and fluid status. Monitor blood pressure, heart rate, and respiratory rate. Watch for physical signs of potassium imbalances (muscle weakness, numbness and tingling sensations, and irregular heartbeats). Clients with heart and lung disorders may experience shortness of breath and chest pain, especially when they are physically active.

Diet Therapy For the person with COPD, repleting and maintaining nutrient stores can help to maintain lung function and prevent lung infections. Overfeeding people with COPD, however, can be as harmful as underfeeding them. Overfeeding produces high carbon dioxide levels, which tax the already stressed lungs. Clients replete nutrient stores best when refed gradually. They benefit from a high-kcalorie, high-protein diet of easy-to-eat foods. A severely depleted person may require tube feedings or parenteral nutrition.

Chronic diseases of the heart and lungs gradually lead to loss of organ function and can eventually progress to acute events that are fatal. Health care professionals seek to identify people at high risk for heart and lung disorders and encourage clients to modify behaviors known to increase that risk. Early detection and treatment can help prevent the development or progression of the heart and lung diseases and reduce mortality. The nutrition assessment checklist helps to identify diet-related practices that may help prevent or treat heart and lung disorders.

Study Questions

1. What is atherosclerosis? How can atherosclerosis lead to hypertension, thrombosis, heart attacks, and strokes?
2. What risk factors for CHD can be helped by diet? What dietary and physical activity measures are recommended to reduce CHD risk?
3. What is hypertension? Discuss the role of diet in hypertension. Describe some steps that people with hypertension can take to lower their blood pressure.
4. What is a myocardial infarction, and what events trigger an attack? Describe the diet therapy for a heart attack victim immediately after the attack, after several hours, and after a week. State the rationale for each diet modification you list.
5. What is congestive heart failure? Why is malnutrition common in the person with CHF?
6. Describe the diet recommended for the person with CHF. What is the rationale for each recommendation? Discuss some special concerns that must be considered when feeding the person with CHF by tube feeding or TPN.
7. Consider some of the ways in which a person's nutrition needs are affected by a stroke. How can nutrition affect the way a person responds to physical therapy?
8. What is respiratory failure? How can malnutrition affect the course of respiratory failure? Describe how the nutrient needs of the person with respiratory failure should be met.
9. What is COPD? What circumstances alter nutrition status in people with COPD?

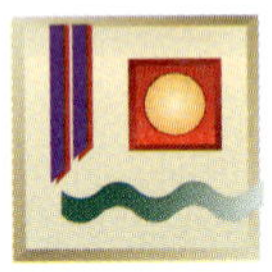

Clinical Applications

1. Consider the list of risk factors for CHD and include obesity and lack of physical activity, as well. Describe possible interrelationships among the factors. For example, an overweight woman over age 55 is at high risk of diabetes; a person with diabetes is likely to have hypertension.
2. Pull together what you know about stress from Chapter 25, tube feedings from Chapter 23, parenteral nutrition from Chapter 24, and respiratory failure from this chapter. If a person suffers a major stress (a severe burn, for example) and later develops an infection and respiratory failure, many factors are influencing nutrient needs. List these factors and consider how nutrient needs might be met by tube feedings or parenteral nutrition. What would be the advantages of a tube feeding for this person? The possible disadvantages? What would be the advantages of parenteral nutrition? The possible disadvantages? Describe some special problems that both tube feedings and parenteral nutrition might pose for a severely stressed, infected person in respiratory failure.

Notes

1. A Leaf and H. A. Hallaq, The role of nutrition in the functioning of the cardiovascular system, *Nutrition Reviews* 50 (1992): 402–406.
2. National Institutes of Health, National Heart, Lung, and Blood Institute, *The Healthy Heart Handbook for Women* (Washington, D.C.: NIH Publication No. 92-2720, 1992).
3. The Expert Panel, Summary of the second report of the National Cholesterol Education Program (NCEP) Expert Panel on Detection, Evaluation, and Treatment of High Blood Cholesterol in Adults (Adult Treatment Panel II), *Journal of the American Medical Association* 269 (1993): 3015–3023.
4. C. L. Johnson and coauthors, Declining serum total cholesterol levels among US adults—The National Health and

Nutrition Examination Surveys, *Journal of the American Medical Association* 269 (1993): 3002–3008.

5. M. J. Klag and coauthors, Serum cholesterol in young men and subsequent cardiovascular disease, *New England Journal of Medicine* 328 (1993): 313–318.
6. P. M. Kris-Etherton and D. Krummel, Role of nutrition in the prevention and treatment of coronary heart disease in women, *Journal of the American Dietetic Association* 93 (1993): 987–993.
7. National Institutes of Health, 1992.
8. M. H. Criqui and coauthors, Plasma triglyceride level and mortality from coronary heart disease, *New England Journal of Medicine* 328 (1993): 1220–1225.
9. NIH Consensus Development Panel on Triglyceride, High-Density Lipoprotein, and Coronary Heart Disease, Triglyceride, high-density lipoprotein, and coronary heart disease, *Journal of the American Medical Association* 269 (1993): 505–510; Criqui and coauthors, 1993.
10. F. O. Karlsson and A. J. Garber, Lipoprotein disorders in diabetes mellitus, *Clinical Diabetes* 14 (1996): 124–127.
11. A. J. Garber, The complication most often overlooked, *Clinical Diabetes* 15 (1997): 46–48.
12. The Expert Panel, 1993.
13. R. E. Andersen and coauthors, Relation of weight loss to changes in serum lipids and lipoproteins in obese women, *American Journal of Clinical Nutrition* 62 (1995): 350–357; A. M. Dattilo and P. M. Kris-Etherton, Effects of weight reduction on blood lipids and lipoproteins: A meta-analysis, *American Journal of Clinical Nutrition* 56 (1992): 320–328; R. R. Wing and coauthors, Change in waist-hip ratio with weight loss and its association with change in cardiovascular risk factors, *American Journal of Clinical Nutrition* 55 (1992): 1086–1092.
14. P. M. Clifton and P. J. Nestel, Influence of gender, body mass index, and age on response of plasma lipids to dietary fat plus cholesterol, *Atherosclerosis and Thrombosis* 12 (1992): 955–962.
15. A. Garg and coauthors, Effects of varying carbohydrate content of diet in patients with non-insulin-dependent diabetes mellitus, *Journal of the American Medical Association* 271 (1994): 1421–1428.
16. A. L. Macnair, Physical activity, not diet, should be the focus of measures for the primary prevention of cardiovascular disease, *Nutrition Reviews* 51 (1993): 151–152.
17. P. D. Wood and coauthors, The effects of plasma lipoproteins of a prudent weight-reducing diet, with or without exercise in overweight men and women, *New England Journal of Medicine* 325 (1991): 461–466.
18. Wood and coauthors, 1991.
19. D. Ornish and coauthors, Can lifestyle changes reverse coronary heart disease? The Lifestyle Heart Trial, *Lancet* 336 (1990): 129–133.
20. D. Farley, High blood pressure: Controlling the silent killer, *FDA Consumer*, December 1991, pp. 28–33.
21. K. M. Finta and coauthors, Urine sodium excretion in response to an oral glucose tolerance test in obese and nonobese adolescents, *Pediatrics* 90 (1992): 442–446.
22. C. F. Steil, J. Otwell, and K. Pennington, Diabetes and hypertension, *Diabetes Spectrum* 8 (1992): 364–365.
23. M. J. Klag and coauthors, Blood pressure and end-stage renal disease in men, *New England Journal of Medicine* 334 (1996): 13–18; P. R. Liebson and coauthors, Echocardiographic correlates of left ventricular structure among 844 mildly hypertensive men and women in the Treatment of Mild Hypertension Study (TOMHS), *Circulation* 87 (1993): 476.
24. Joint National Committee on Detection, Evaluation, and Treatment of High Blood Pressure, The fifth report of the Joint National Committee on Detection, Evaluation, and Treatment of High Blood Pressure (JNCV), *Archives of Internal Medicine* 153 (1993): 154–183.
25. S. A. Corrigan and coauthors, Weight reduction in the prevention and treatment of hypertension: A review of representative clinical trials, *American Journal of Health Promotion* 5 (1991): 208–214.
26. M. H. Keleman and coauthors, Exercise training combined with antihypertensive drug therapy: Effects on blood lipids, blood pressure, and left ventricular mass, *Journal of the American Medical Association* 263 (1990): 2766–2771.
27. T. A. Kotchen and J. M. Kotchen, Dietary sodium and blood pressure: Interactions with other nutrients, *American Journal of Clinical Nutrition* (supplement) 65 (1997): 708–711.
28. Hypertension Prevention Collaborative Research Group, The effects of nonpharmacologic interventions on blood pressure of persons with high normal levels, *Journal of the American Medical Association* 267 (1992): 1213–1220; J. Wylie-Rosett and coauthors, Trial of Antihypertensive Intervention and Management: Greater efficacy with weight reduction than with a sodium-potassium intervention, *Journal of the American Dietetic Association* 93 (1993): 408–415.
29. M. Alderman and coauthors, Low urinary sodium excretion is associated with greater risk of myocardial infarction among treated hypertensive men, *Hypertension* 25 (1995): 1144–1152; M. Alderman and coauthors, Urinary sodium excretion and myocardial infarction in hypertensive patients: A prospective cohort study, *American Journal of Clinical Nutrition* (supplement) 65 (1997): 682–686.
30. Kotchen and Kotchen, 1997; P. K. Whelton and coauthors, Effects of oral potassium on blood pressure, *Journal of the American Medical Association* 277 (1997): 1624–1632; D. A. McCarron, Role of dietary calcium intake in the prevention and management of salt-sensitive hypertension, *American Journal of Clinical Nutrition* (supplement) 65 (1997): 712–716.
31. National Institutes of Health, Fifth report of the Joint Committee on Detection, Evaluation, and Treatment of High Blood Pressure (Washington, D.C.: NIH Publication No. 93-1088, October 1992).
32. S. D. Katz and coauthors, Pathophysiological correlates of increased serum tumor necrosis factor in patients with congestive heart failure, *Circulation* 90 (1994): 12–16.

33. J. Horner and E. W. Massey, Silent aspiration following stroke, *Neurology* 38 (1988): 317–319.
34. A.S.P.E.N. Board of Directors, Practice guidelines: Respiratory failure, *Journal of Parenteral and Enteral Nutrition* (supplement) 17 (1993): 16–17; C. S. Ireton-Jones, K. R. Borman, and W. W. Turner, Nutrition considerations in the management of ventilator-dependent patients, *Nutrition in Clinical Practice* 8 (1993): 60–64.
35. Ireton-Jones, Borman, and Turner, 1993; R. A. Landon and E. A. Young, Role of magnesium in regulation of lung function, *Journal of American Dietetic Association* 93 (1993): 674–677.
36. T. Petty, Building a national strategy for the prevention and management of and research in chronic obstructive pulmonary disease, *Journal of the American Medical Association* 277 (1997): 246–253.
37. Petty, 1997.

Diet and Protection against CHD

In general, experts agree that lowering LDL cholesterol reduces complications and mortality from CHD, but the value of lowering LDL to *prevent* CHD is less clear.[1] What is obvious is that there is much to learn about how cardiovascular diseases develop and what yet-to-be-defined factors might be protective. Furthermore, as Chapter 28 noted, the current dietary recommendations to reduce CHD risk, which include reducing total fat and saturated fat and maintaining a healthy weight, may not be as effective as other measures at lowering LDL. Such findings have led researchers to explore other avenues for pieces of the puzzle. A good deal of that research continues to focus on dietary factors; those that appear most promising are featured in this highlight.

THE ANTIOXIDANT NUTRIENTS

A discussion of dietary factors to reduce CHD risk must include the antioxidant nutrients—a hot topic in both the popular press and scientific journals today. Highlight 11 describes the antioxidant nutrients in detail and explains how they attack free radicals and protect against heart disease. Evidence continues to mount that antioxidant nutrients, particularly vitamin E, may be protective against CHD by preventing the toxic effects of free radicals. Vitamin E may also slow the progression of plaques that have already formed in the arteries or may lower the risk of developing a heart attack in people with existing CHD.[2]

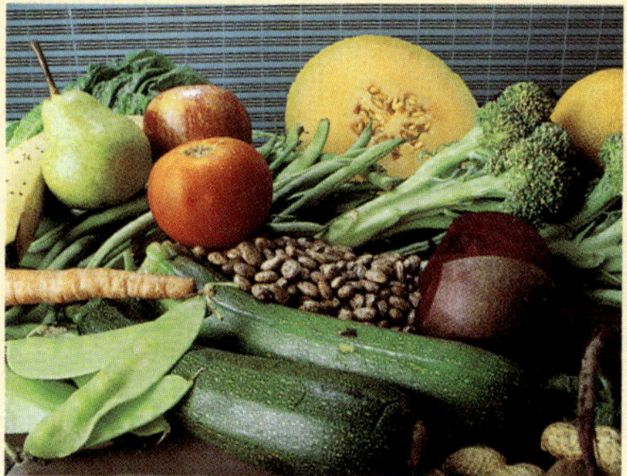
Eating a variety of fruits and vegetables may confer special protection against CHD.

The amount of vitamin E that appears to be protective against CHD exceeds the RDA and is difficult to consume from a standard diet, particularly from a diet that obtains less than 30 percent of its energy from fat. (The most frequently consumed dietary sources of vitamin E are vegetable oils, polyunsaturated margarines, some nuts, and wheat germ.) Therefore, vitamin E supplements may be necessary to maximize its effects. When provided in large amounts, vitamin E may have pharmacological, rather than nutritional, effects. Before such supplements can be recommended, large-scale studies (and several are under way) are needed to rule out whether other dietary factors or lifestyle behaviors are actually responsible for the protective effects attributed to vitamin E.[3] The safety of the long-term use of high doses of vitamin E also requires further investigation.

DIETARY FIBER

Soluble fiber lowers blood cholesterol, especially in those with high blood cholesterol.[4] A recent study of more than 43,000 male health care professionals found that men who had the highest fiber intakes (about 29 grams per day) had the lowest rate of heart attacks.[5] Similarly, a Finnish study of more than 21,000 male smokers found that those with high-fiber intakes (over 25 grams per day) had fewer heart attacks than those with lower-fiber intakes (about 16 grams a day). People with diabetes (NIDDM) showed improved blood glucose control and an improved ratio of LDL to HDL with a diet that provided 18 grams of fiber from breads made from oat bran concentrates.[6]

As Chapter 4 noted (see pp. 126–128), the reasons why high-fiber diets may be protective are difficult to determine. High-fiber diets tend to be lower in fat and cholesterol and higher in vitamins (including folate, discussed later) and other nonnutrient compounds (phytochemicals). These properties may actually account for some of the findings. Regardless, consuming from 20 to 35 grams of fiber daily seems a prudent health measure with few risks and possible protection from CHD.

HOMOCYSTEINE AND FOLATE

As Chapter 6 noted (see p. 202), elevated blood levels of the amino acid homocysteine may be a risk factor for cardiovascular disease.[7] For many years researchers have recognized that people with homocysteinuria, a genetic disorder characterized by markedly elevated blood and urine levels of homocysteine, show characteristic patterns of accelerated atherosclerosis, blood clots, and emboli.

Researchers have also suspected a link between moderately elevated homocysteine and cardiovascular disease, but early studies failed to show whether cardiovascular disease itself was the cause of elevated homocysteine or elevated homocysteine was the cause of cardiovascular disease.[8] More recently, several prospective studies of people who entered the study without preexisting heart disease have shown a positive association between elevated blood homocysteine and risk of cardiovascular disease.[9] How elevated homocysteine contributes to heart disease remains unclear, but researchers speculate that it may structurally change the blood vessels to promote plaque formation, increase the likelihood of clot formation, and interfere with the metabolism of cholesterol in the liver.[10]

What causes elevated homocysteine in people without homocysteinuria? Again, the answer is not always clear. In many cases, elevated homocysteine is associated with suboptimal concentrations of the B vitamins involved in the metabolism of homocysteine. Most commonly, a suboptimal dietary intake of folate is to blame, but an optimal intake has yet to be defined. Some research suggests that folate intakes that meet the current RDA may be insufficient to prevent elevated homocysteine.[11] In people with low folate intakes, supplementation brings homocysteine back to desirable levels.[12] Supplementation may not be necessary, though, if rich sources of folate are selected daily.[13]

The question that remains to be answered is whether providing adequate dietary folate to reduce homocysteine also reduces the risk of cardiovascular disease.[14] One study followed more than 5000 men and women for 15 years and found that those with the lowest serum folate had a significantly higher risk of dying from cardiovascular disease.[15] As noted earlier, foods high in folate (fruits, vegetables, and legumes) also tend to be high in other nutrients, nonnutrients, and fiber; further research may help to define exactly which factors provide protective effects.

For most people, selecting at least five servings of folate-rich fruits and vegetables daily should be sufficient to normalize homocysteine concentrations. The Food and Drug Administration's recent decision to require folate fortification of grain products in an effort to reduce the incidence of birth defects will also increase folate intakes.[16] Whether folate fortification confers an added benefit of reducing CHD risks remains to be seen.

FISH OIL

From the dietary factors described up to now and the information presented in Chapter 28, it seems logical to assume that diets low in saturated fats and cholesterol that include abundant fruits and vegetables would be protective against heart disease. Yet the Inuit peoples of Alaska and Greenland, who eat a diet consisting almost entirely of meat (rich in saturated fat) and fish (rich in cholesterol and relatively rich in saturated fat), have a remarkably low incidence of heart disease. In searching for factors that might account for the low incidence of CHD, researchers discovered that compared to other populations, the Inuit had lower blood triglycerides, their platelets contained higher amounts of omega-3 fatty acids, and their blood took longer to clot.

Early research regarding fish oil suggested that its protective effects were related to blood clotting, which is under the control of certain hormonelike substances (eicosanoids), the prostaglandins and thromboxanes. Thromboxanes, which the body makes from the omega-6 fatty acids abundant in vegetable oils, *promote* platelet aggregation (sticking together). Prostaglandins, which the body makes from the omega-3 fatty acids abundant in fish oil, *inhibit* platelet aggregation. Although a diet rich in omega-3 fatty acids can limit clot formation by changing the balance between the prostaglandins and thromboxanes, researchers have found that only large amounts of fish oils are effective. Yet the protective effects of fish oils have been seen even in cases where people consume only one or two fish meals per week, suggesting that a different mechanism is involved.[17] Furthermore, the effects of fish oils on platelet function are modest when compared to even tiny doses of aspirin, which is known to significantly reduce clot formation.[18]

A recent, large, carefully conducted study failed to show a correlation between fish oil and CHD risk.[19] The authors noted, however, that very few men in the study group ate no fish at all, and eating one or two fish meals per week may confer the same benefits as eating five to six fish meals per week.

Fish oils may help prevent cardiac arrhythmias (irregular heartbeats that can lead to a sudden and fatal heart attack) and sudden death in people with CHD.[20] When men with no known heart disease who suffered a heart attack were compared to a matched control group, researchers found that men who ate about one fish meal per week had a 50 percent lower incidence of heart attacks and a 29 percent reduction in two-year mortality from all causes.[21]

Eating one or two fish meals per week may be beneficial and is certainly safe. Fish oil supplements are unnecessary and may be toxic; people who dislike fish may want to review the warnings on p. 169 before choosing a fish oil supplement.

ALCOHOL

Research suggests that a *moderate* consumption of alcohol may reduce the risk of heart disease by raising HDL cholesterol and preventing blood clot formation.[22] These benefits are more apparent in people over age 50, in those with other risk factors, and in those with high LDL.[23] Researchers speculate that when LDL levels are high, alcohol may cause changes that reduce the likelihood of clot formation.[24] Early studies suggested that red wine was more effective than other alcoholic beverages in reducing CHD risk, indicating that perhaps something other than alcohol was responsible for the protective effect. A review of studies to date, however, found that alcohol from any source—red or white wine, beer, or liquor—appears to be equally effective, and that alcohol itself may be the protective factor.[25]

These findings pose a dilemma for health care professionals who are well aware of the potentially damaging effects of alcohol on many body systems (see Highlight 7). Any benefits that alcohol may confer on cardiovascular health must be weighed against the risks of raising complications and mortality from other causes.[26] The question to answer is how much alcohol is protective, and how much is harmful? Early studies suggested that total mortality was reduced in people who drank 1 to 2 drinks per day as compared to abstainers, but in larger amounts (more than 3 drinks per day), alcohol was associated with increased mortality.[27] More recent studies suggest that the beneficial effects of alcohol occur at lower intakes. In one study, researchers examined alcohol intake and mortality over a ten-year period in more than 22,000 male physicians with no history of heart attacks, strokes, transient ischemic attacks, or cancer.[28] Men who consumed 2 to 6 drinks per *week* had the lowest mortality risk, and those who consumed 2 or more drinks per *day* had the highest mortality risk. The lower mortality risks found in men who consumed some alcohol were largely the result of a reduced risk of death from cardiovascular causes. Studies of Danish adults found the lowest mortality risk in people who drank 1 to 6 drinks per week.[29] Among British male physicians, researchers found that 5 to 9 drinks per week were protective.[30] The amount of alcohol that exerts a positive effect on CHD risk for women may be lower still. A study of more than 85,000 women found the most beneficial alcohol consumption level to be no more than 1 to 3 drinks per week.[31]

The advice clinicians offer clients regarding the use of alcohol to lower CHD risks rests largely on clinical judgment.[32] The number of deaths attributed to alcohol is greatest for people between the ages of 15 and 44—and their risk of heart disease is relatively minor. Clearly, for these people, the benefits do not outweigh the risks. Additionally, people with a personal or family history of alcohol abuse and those with medical conditions complicated by alcohol use (liver and pancreatic disorders, for example) should not use alcohol. Clients who do use alcohol should be cautioned to avoid alcohol use during times when clear judgment is important, such as when they are driving, working, or operating potentially dangerous equipment. These clients should also be evaluated periodically to assure that alcohol intake has not become excessive or problematic.

CONFOUNDING FACTORS

As this discussion has pointed out, diets are complex and foods that contain one protective factor for CHD may contain several. Is one factor responsible or is it the combination of factors?

Furthermore, groups of people with low risks of CHD may have lifestyle habits or genetic characteristics that explain the low risks. The native people of Alaska (described early) may have a low incidence of CHD, but their lifestyles differ significantly from other populations, and many do not live to a very old age.[33] Certainly, major lifestyle factors and other characteristics account for some differences in CHD risks.

In making decisions regarding the value of dietary changes to protect against CHD, one must weigh the potential benefits against the potential risks. Certainly, including plenty of fruits, vegetables, and legumes would be safe and may offer the beneficial effects of antioxidant nutrients, phytochemicals, fiber, and folate. With respect to vitamin E supplements, the issues become somewhat complicated. Research regarding vitamin E's protective effects is inconclusive, and because vitamin E must be taken in large doses, it may prove to have some adverse effects. The issues surrounding alcohol's protective effects are clearly the most complex. While alcohol may have a protective effect against CHD, its potential for abuse and its damaging effects on many body systems limit its usefulness as a protective factor. Clinicians must use clinical judgment in helping clients decide if alcohol consumption is warranted.

NOTES

1. J. B. Ubbink, Homocysteine—An atherogenic and a thromogenic factor? *Nutrition Reviews* 53 (1995): 323–326.
2. H. N. Hodis and coauthors, Serial coronary angiographic evidence that antioxidant vitamin intake reduces progression of coronary artery atherosclerosis, *Journal of the American Medical Association* 273 (1995): 1849–1854; N. G. Stephens and coauthors, Randomised controlled trial of vitamin E in patients with coronary disease: Cambridge Heart Antioxidant Study (CHAOS), *Lancet* 347 (1996): 781–786.
3. J. M. Gaziano, Antioxidants in cardiovascular disease: Randomized trials, *Nutrition Reviews* 54 (1996): 175–184.
4. C. Dubois and coauthors, Chronic oat bran intake alters post-prandial lipemia and lipoproteins in healthy adults, *American Journal of Clinical Nutrition* 61 (1995): 325–333; S. R. Glore and coauthors, Soluble fiber and serum lipids: A literature review, *Journal of the American Dietetic Association* 94 (1994): 425–436; C. M. Ripsin and coauthors, Oat products and lipid lowering, *Journal of the American Medical Association* 267 (1992): 3317–3325.
5. E. B. Rimm and coauthors, Vegetable, fruit, and cereal fiber intake and risk of coronary heart disease among men, *Journal of the American Medical Association* 275 (1996): 447–451.
6. M. E. Pick and coauthors, Oat bran concentrate bread products improve long-term control of diabetes: A pilot study, *Journal of the American Dietetic Association* 96 (1996): 1254–1261.
7. J. Selhub and coauthors, Association between plasma homocysteine concentrations and extracranial carotid-artery stenosis, *New England Journal of Medicine* 332 (1995): 286–289; E. Arnesen and coauthors, Serum total homocysteine and coronary heart disease, *International Journal of Epidemiology* 24 (1995): 704–709; K. Robinson and coauthors, Hyperhomocysteinemia and low pyridoxal phosphate: Common and independent reversible risk factors for coronary artery disease, *Circulation* 92 (1995): 2825–2830.
8. P. Verhoef and M. J. Stampfer, Prospective studies of homocysteine and cardiovascular disease, *Nutrition Reviews* 53 (1995): 283–288.
9. M. J. Stampfer and coauthors, A prospective study of plasma homocyst(e)ine and risk of myocardial infarction in US physicians, *Journal of the American Medical Association* 268 (1992): 877–880; Arnesen and coauthors, 1995; P. Verhoef and coauthors, A prospective study of plasma homocyst(e)ine and risk of ischemic stroke, *Stroke* 25 (1994): 1924–1930.
10. J. S. Stamler and A. Slivka, Biological chemistry of thiols in the vasculature and in vascular-related disease, *Nutrition Reviews* 54 (1996): 1–30.
11. J. Selhub and coauthors, Vitamin status and intake as primary determinants of homocysteinemia in an elderly population, *Journal of the American Medical Association* 270 (1993): 2693–2698.
12. J. B. Ubbink, P. J. Becker, and W. J. H. Vermaak, Will an increased dietary folate intake reduce the incidence of cardiovascular disease? *Nutrition Reviews* 54 (1996): 213–216.
13. J. B. Ubbink, Vitamin nutrition status and homocysteine: An atherogenic risk factor, *Nutrition Reviews* 52 (1994): 383–393; Ubbink, Becker, and Vermaak, 1996.
14. M. J. Stampfer and E. B. Rimm, Folate and cardiovascular disease, *Journal of the American Medical Association* 276 (1996): 1929–1930.
15. H. I. Morrison and coauthors, Serum folate and risk of fatal coronary heart disease, *Journal of the American Medical Association* 275 (1996): 1893–1896.
16. J. Foulke, Folic acid to fortify U.S. food products to prevent birth defects, Food and Drug Administration press release, February 29, 1996.
17. M. B. Katan, Fish and heart disease: What is the real story? *Nutrition Reviews* 53 (1995): 228–229.
18. N. W. Schoene and G. A. Fitzgerald, Thromogenic potential of dietary long-chain polyunsaturated fatty acids: Session summary, *American Journal of Clinical Nutrition* (supplement) 56 (1992): 977–982.
19. A. Ascherio and coauthors, Marine *n*-3 fatty acids, fish intake, and the risk of coronary disease among men, *New England Journal of Medicine* 332 (1995): 977–982.
20. A. Sellmayer and coauthors, Effects of dietary fish oil on VPC's, *American Journal of Cardiology* 76 (1995): 974–977; D. S. Siscovick and coauthors, Fish intake and risk of primary cardiac arrest, *Journal of the American Medical Association* 274 (1995): 1363–1367.
21. Siscovick and coauthors, 1995.
22. J. M. Gaziano and coauthors, Moderate alcohol intake, increased levels of high-density lipoprotein and its subfractions, and decreased risk of myocardial infarction, *New England Journal of Medicine* 329 (1993): 1829–1834; P. R. Ridker and coauthors, Association of moderate alcohol consumption and plasma concentration of endogenous tissue-type plasminogen activator, *Journal of the American Medical Association* 272 (1994): 929–933.
23. C. S. Fuchs and coauthors, Alcohol consumption and mortality among women, *New England Journal of Medicine* 332 (1995): 1245–1250; H. O. Hein, P. Suadicani, and F. Gyntelberg, Alcohol consumption, serum low density lipoprotein cholesterol concentration, and risk of ischaemic heart disease: Six year follow up in the Copenhagen male study, *British Medical Journal* 312 (1996): 736–741.
24. Hein, Suadicani, and Gyntelberg, 1996.
25. E. B. Rimm and coauthors, Review of moderate alcohol consumption and reduced risk of coronary heart disease: Is the effect due to beer, wine, or spirits? *British Medical Journal* 312 (1996): 731–736.
26. G. D. Friedman and A. L. Klatsky, Is alcohol good for your health? *New England Journal of Medicine* 329 (1993): 1882–1883.
27. T. A. Pearson and P. Terry, What to advise patients about drinking alcohol, *Journal of the American Medical Association* 272 (1994): 967–968.
28. C. A. Camargo and coauthors, Prospective study of moderate alcohol consumption and mortality in US male physicians, *Archives of Internal Medicine* 137 (1997): 79–85.
29. N. Grønbaek and coauthors, Influence of sex, age, body mass index, and smoking on alcohol intake and mortality, *British Medical Journal* 308 (1994): 302–306.
30. R. Doll and coauthors, Mortality in relation to consumption of alcohol, *British Medical Journal* 309 (1994): 911–918.
31. Fuchs and coauthors, 1995.
32. Pearson and Terry, 1994.
33. Katan, 1995.

Chapter 29

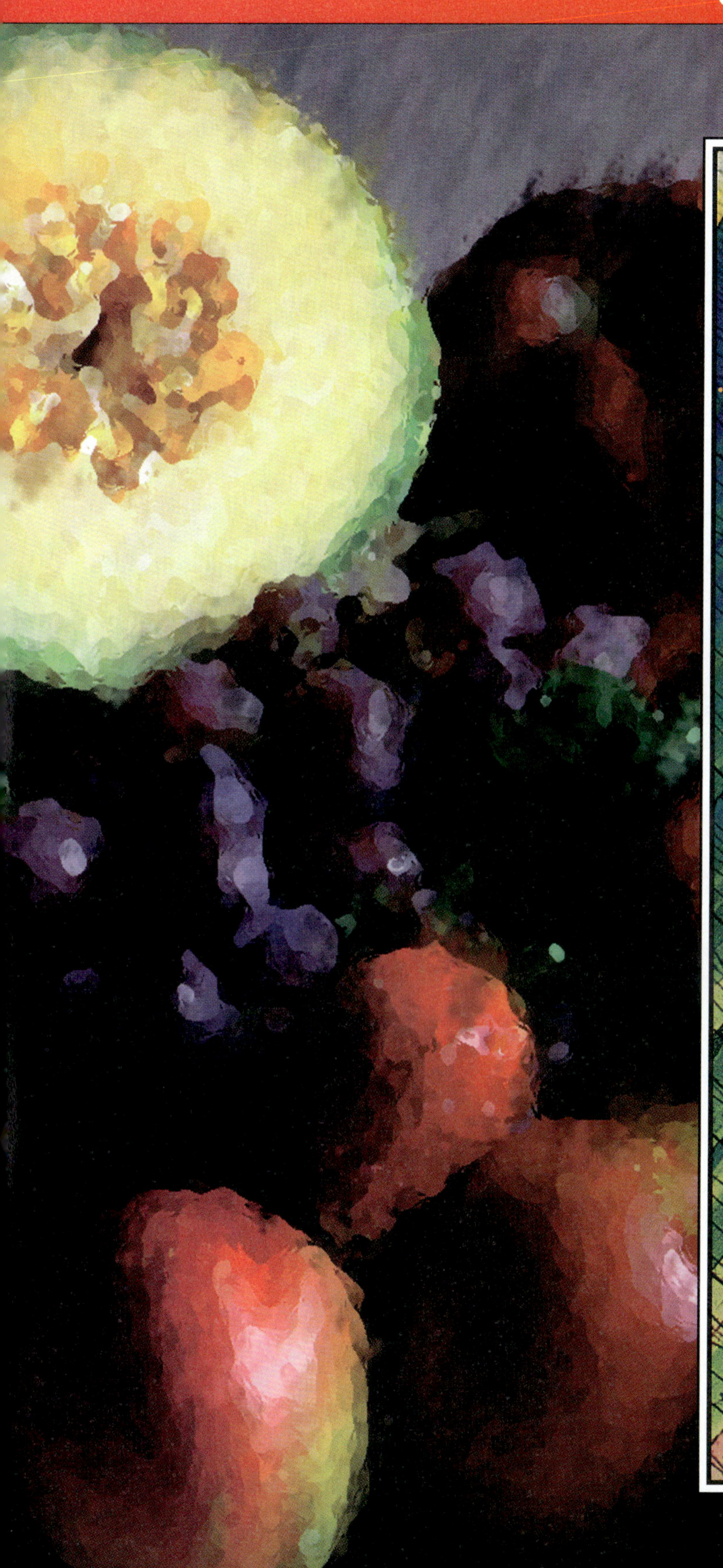

Nutrition and Disorders of the Kidneys

CONTENTS

MICROGRAPH: Urea, the body's vehicle for eliminating excess nitrogen.

The kidneys:

- Help maintain fluid, electrolyte, and acid-base balances.
- Eliminate metabolic waste products.
- Help regulate blood pressure.
- Produce a hormone that stimulates red blood cell production.
- Activate vitamin D.

nephrotic syndrome: the complex of symptoms that occur when glomerular function fails; it includes proteinuria and albuminuria.

The loss of protein in the urine is called **proteinuria**, and the loss of the protein albumin in the urine is called **albuminuria**. Sensitive laboratory tests allow clinicians to detect **microalbuminuria**, the loss of albumin in the urine in quantities that are greater than normal but not enough to precipitate symptoms. Tests for microalbuminuria are routinely performed in people are high risk for renal disease.

renal failure: failure of the kidneys to maintain normal function.

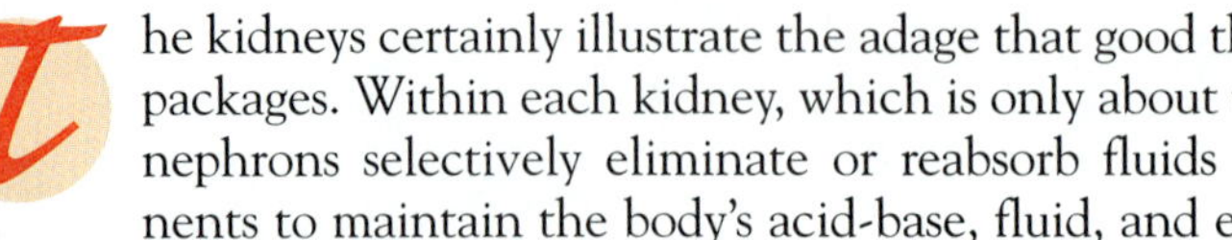

The kidneys certainly illustrate the adage that good things come in small packages. Within each kidney, which is only about the size of a fist, the nephrons selectively eliminate or reabsorb fluids and blood components to maintain the body's acid-base, fluid, and electrolyte balances. The kidneys also help to regulate blood pressure, stimulate red blood cell production, and maintain bone structure. The accompanying glossary reviews terms related to the kidneys and their functions. Figure 29–1 illustrates the kidneys and the urinary tract, and Figure 3–8 (on page 88) shows how the nephrons filter wastes from the blood. This chapter describes disorders that disrupt renal function, including nephrotic syndrome and kidney failure. Highlight 29 discusses kidney stones, which can lead to complications that affect the kidneys.

The Nephrotic Syndrome

The nephrotic syndrome is not a disease, but rather a distinct cluster of symptoms including proteinuria, low serum albumin, edema, and elevated blood lipids. Causes of nephrotic syndrome include damage to the kidneys from infections, blood clots in the renal veins, metabolic disorders (including diabetes mellitus), and some drugs and toxins. As a consequence, the permeability of the glomerular capillaries increases, and plasma proteins, which are normally retained in the blood, escape into the urine instead. Nephrotic syndrome is sometimes an early sign of renal failure, especially in people with diabetes (see page 853). In other cases, treatment of the underlying condition can correct the disorder before renal failure develops.

Figure 29–1

The Kidneys and Urinary Tract

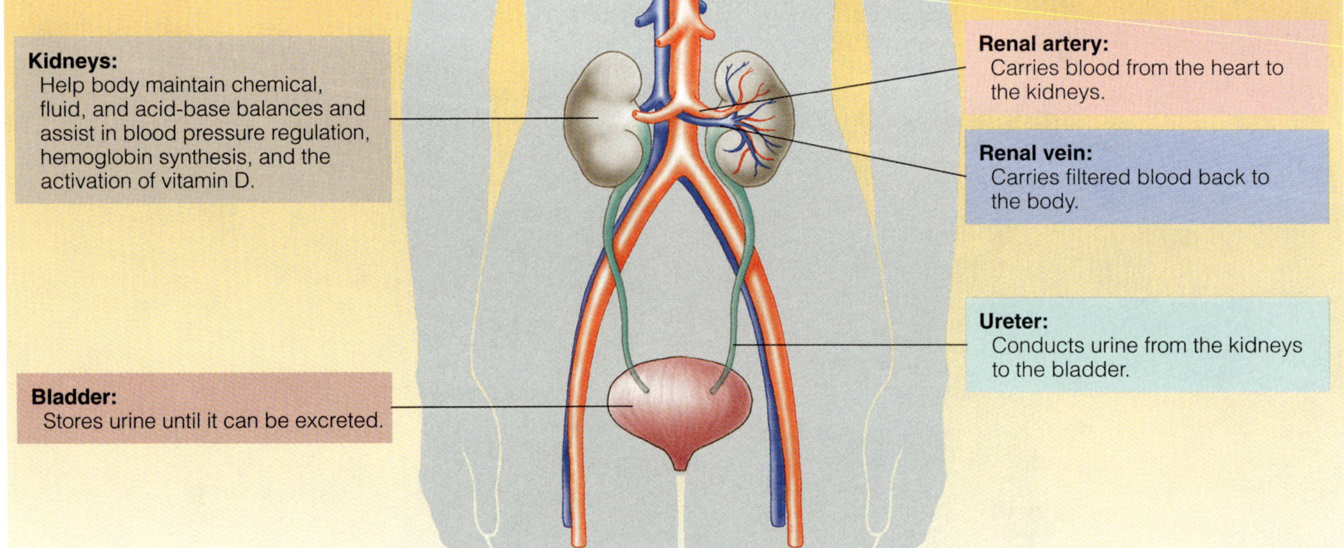

Glossary of Kidney-Related Terms

active vitamin D: the 1,25-dihydroxy form of vitamin D that promotes calcium balance and bone mineralization. Figure 11–8 (on p. 387) shows how the kidneys participate in the final conversion of vitamin D to its most active form.

erythropoietin (eh-REE-throw-POY-eh-tin): a hormone secreted by the kidneys in response to oxygen depletion or anemia that stimulates the bone marrow to produce red blood cells.
- *erythro* = red (blood cell)
- *poiesis* = creating (like poetry)

filtrate: in the kidneys, the fluid that passes from the blood through the capillary walls of the glomeruli, eventually forming urine.

glomerular filtration rate (GFR): the rate at which the kidneys form filtrate. Normally, the GFR is between 90 and 120 ml/min.

glomerulus (glow-MARE-you-lus): a cup-shaped membrane enclosing a tuft of capillaries within a nephron. (The plural is *glomeruli.*)

nephrons (NEF-rons): the working units of the kidneys; each consists of a glomerulus and a tubule.

renal: pertaining to the kidneys.

renin: an enzyme secreted by the kidneys in response to a reduced blood flow that triggers the release of the hormone aldosterone from the adrenal glands. Aldosterone, in turn, signals the kidneys to retain sodium and water.

tubule: a tube like structure that surrounds the glomerulus and descends through the nephron. A pressure gradient between the glomerular capillaries and the tubule returns needed materials to the blood and moves wastes into the tubule to be sent to the bladder.

CONSEQUENCES OF NEPHROTIC SYNDROME

The major consequences of nephrotic syndrome include protein-energy malnutrition (PEM), infection, blood coagulation disorders, occlusion of blood vessels from clots in the lungs and legs, and accelerated atherosclerosis. Many of the consequences of the disorder are the same as those of malnutrition, which is not surprising because both alter protein status (see Figure 29–2). If nephrotic syndrome progresses to renal failure, the person develops other complications, as a later section describes.

Blood Proteins Fall and Malnutrition Develops As plasma proteins are lost in the urine, blood proteins fall sharply. Albumin, the major plasma protein, is also the major protein lost in the urine, and its blood level is markedly reduced. Among the other blood proteins lost are immunoglobulins, transferrin, and the vitamin D–binding protein. Losses of immunoglobulins render the person prone to infections, which can further compromise health and nutrition status. Loss of transferrin, the iron-carrying protein, may lead to anemia. When the vitamin D–binding protein is lost in the urine, vitamin D deficiency may develop, which impairs calcium absorption. Some calcium is also lost directly along with the albumin that carries it. Consequently, rickets may develop as a result of the nephrotic syndrome, particularly in children. If protein loss continues without replacement, lean body tissues break down, and PEM and general malnutrition follow.

Figure 29–2

Consequences of Urinary Protein Losses in the Nephrotic Syndrome

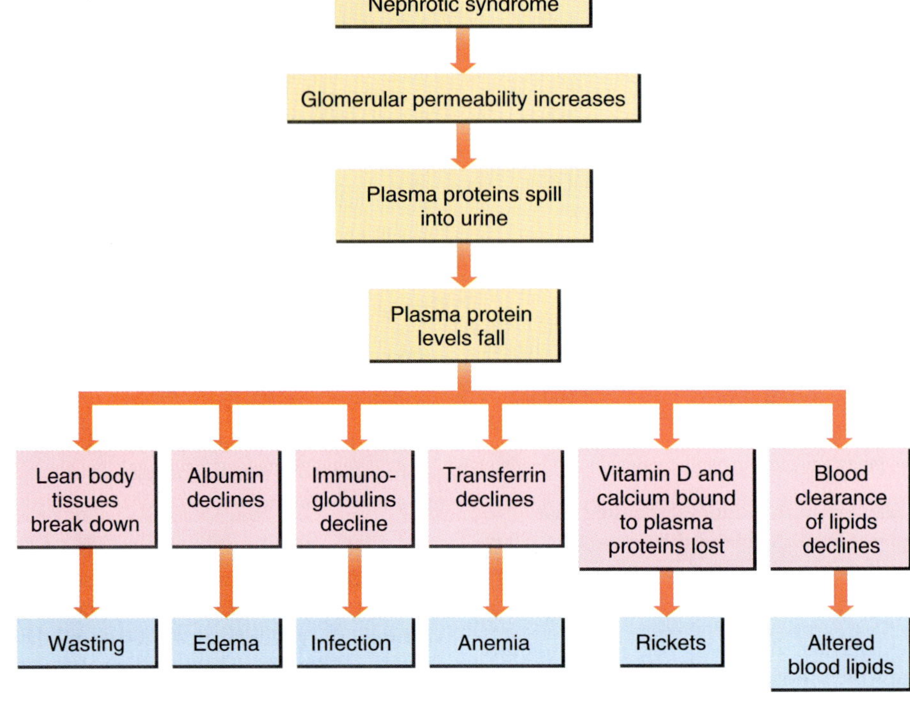

Edema Develops Low blood protein contributes to edema by failing to exert enough pressure to keep fluids from moving into the interstitial spaces. As fluids enter the interstitial spaces, blood volume diminishes, and the kidneys respond by retaining sodium and fluid, further aggravating edema.

Blood Lipids Change Elevated cholesterol, triglycerides, LDL, and VLDL and low HDL are characteristics of nephrotic syndrome. This lipid pattern increases the risk of cardiovascular disease and stroke and may damage the kidneys further.[1]

Exactly why blood lipids increase in nephrotic syndrome remains unknown, but the defective clearance of lipids by the kidneys may be partially to blame. Animal studies suggest that these lipid changes occur as a consequence of urinary protein loss.[2]

PRESCRIPTION PAD

Drugs used in the treatment of nephrotic syndrome may include:

- Antibiotics
- Anti-inflammatory agents
- Antilipemics
- Diuretics
- Immunosuppressants

See Appendix E for timing with meals and nutrition-related side effects.

TREATMENT OF NEPHROTIC SYNDROME

Medical treatment first requires treatment of the underlying disorder and then drug and diet therapy to resolve the nephrotic syndrome. Corticosteroids are sometimes used in the treatment of nephrotic syndrome, but they must be used judiciously because they can contribute to nutrient imbalances (see Appendix E). Diet is central to preventing protein malnutrition and alleviating edema.

Energy A diet adequate in energy sustains desirable weight and spares protein. Additional kcalories may be appropriate if the person loses weight or develops an infection or fever. Obese people with nephrotic syndrome may be advised to reduce their energy intakes to help control blood lipid levels.

Protein In the past, high-protein diets (about 120 grams per day) were often prescribed for people with nephrotic syndrome, stemming from the belief that protein intakes would compensate for protein losses. High-protein diets do accelerate albumin synthesis, but they also produce greater urinary losses of albumin as well.[3] Furthermore, extra dietary protein may accelerate deterioration of renal function.[4] For these reasons, protein is provided in amounts consistent with the RDA.

Fat A low-fat diet such as the plan shown in Chapter 28 (see p. 893) can help control the elevated blood lipids associated with nephrotic syndrome. Such a diet limits total fat, saturated fat, and cholesterol. Often, however, people with nephrotic syndrome are unable to control blood lipids adequately using diet alone, and physicians must prescribe drugs.

Sodium Because the body avidly retains sodium in nephrotic syndrome, sodium must be restricted. Early treatment combines a diet very low in sodium (250 milligrams) with diuretics to help mobilize the accumulated fluid from the interstitial spaces.

Hidden sources of sodium can undermine severely restricted diets. If the local water has a high-sodium concentration and is used for preparing and cooking foods, it can significantly contribute to sodium intake. (Health departments can supply information on the sodium content of local water supplies.) Medications such as antacids, antibiotics, cough medicines, laxatives, pain relievers, and sedatives may also contain sodium. Some toothpaste and mouthwashes also contain large amounts of sodium; people should not swallow these compounds and should rinse thoroughly after brushing their teeth or using a mouthwash.

Once edema is resolved and sodium balance is achieved, sodium restriction relaxes, but is still fairly stringent. Chapter 26 provides more information on sodium-restricted diets. Clients on thiazide or loop diuretics should be encouraged to select foods rich in potassium.

The kidneys maintain the body's acid-base, fluid, and electrolyte balances, eliminate waste products, regulate blood pressure, stimulate red blood cell production, and activate vitamin D. Damage to the kidneys can lead to nephrotic syndrome, a disorder characterized by protein losses, fluid imbalances (edema), and elevated blood lipids. Because nephrotic syndrome alters protein status in the same way malnutrition does , the consequences are similar (review Figure 29–2). Treatment includes a diet adequate in energy and protein, with less than 30 percent of the total kcalories from fat, and low in saturated fat, cholesterol, and sodium (see the box on p. 914).

Acute Renal Failure

In acute renal failure, the nephrons suddenly lose function and are unable to maintain homeostasis. The degree of renal dysfunction varies among individuals and can range from mild to severe. With prompt treatment, acute renal failure may be reversible, but in some cases, the damage is permanent.

Chronic renal failure [is like] a downhill course for your patient; acute renal failure is like seeing him go over a cliff no one quite knew was there.

—J. L. Stark

How to Modify the Diet for Nephrotic Syndrome

- Energy: Adequate to maintain a healthy body weight (about 35 kcalories per kilogram of body weight per day).
- Protein: 0.8 to 1.0 gram per kilogram of body weight per day.
- Fat: Less than 30 percent of the total kcalories, low in saturated fat and cholesterol.
- Sodium: 250 to 1500 milligrams per day.

Reduced blood flow to the kidneys is a **prerenal** cause of acute renal failure.

A urinary tract obstruction is a **postrenal** cause of acute renal failure. The kidneys can make urine, but the urine cannot be excreted.

Damage to the kidneys' cells is an **intrarenal** cause of acute renal failure.

Acute renal failure frequently develops when blood flow to the kidneys suddenly drops, often as a result of a severe stress such as heart failure, shock, or severe blood loss following surgery or trauma. Less than normal amounts of blood reach the kidneys, less blood is filtered, and less urine is produced. Urinary tract obstructions can also precipitate acute renal failure. In this case, the kidneys can make urine initially, but the urine cannot be excreted. In still other cases, infections, toxins, and some drugs directly damage the kidney's cells.

CONSEQUENCES OF ACUTE RENAL FAILURE

Acute renal failure is characterized by a sudden and precipitous drop in the glomerular filtration rate (GFR) and urine output. As the nephrons fail, the composition of the blood and urine changes.

Abnormal accumulation of nitrogen-containing substances in the blood is called **uremia** (you-REE-me-ah) or **azotemia** (AZE-oh-TEE-me-ah). Normal BUN levels are 10 to 20 mg/dL. A BUN of 50 to 150 mg/dL indicates serious impairment of renal function. BUN may rise as high as 150 to 250 mg/dL in end-stage renal disease.

hyperkalemia: an excessive amount of potassium in the blood.

The early phase of acute renal failure, when urine volume is reduced, is the **oliguric phase**; the phase characterized by large fluid and electrolyte losses in the urine is the **diuretic phase**; the gradual return of renal function marks the **recovery phase**.

Waste Products Accumulate When the kidneys fail to function, the body's principal nitrogen-containing metabolic waste products—blood urea nitrogen (BUN), creatinine, and uric acid—accumulate in the blood. Clinicians evaluate renal function by performing laboratory tests to measure blood levels of these waste products and urinary clearance tests to measure the GFR.

Potassium Rises Blood potassium rises as renal function deteriorates because the kidneys can no longer excrete it. A severe stress taxes the kidneys further as the body's cells break down and intracellular fluids release potassium. Blood potassium rises sharply (hyperkalemia) and can result in sudden heart failure.

Blood Volume Changes In the early stages of acute renal failure, the kidneys fail to excrete fluids, and blood pressure may rise to dangerously high levels. During this stage, clients, particularly elderly clients, may develop fluid overload, which may lead to pulmonary edema.

Later in the course of acute renal failure, the kidneys cannot conserve water, and the person begins to excrete large amounts of fluids and electrolytes. If recovery occurs, kidney function gradually normalizes.

Clinical Symptoms Develop As toxic waste products build up, the person may experience uremic syndrome—a wide array of symptoms in virtually every body system. Hemorrhages may be visible on the skin, and GI bleeding sometimes occurs. In advanced stages, seizures and coma may ensue.

uremic (you-REE-mic) **syndrome:** the many symptoms that accompany the buildup of toxic waste products in the blood. Symptoms include:
- Fatigue.
- Weakness.
- Diminished mental alertness.
- Agitation.
- Muscular twitches.
- Muscle cramps.
- Anorexia.
- Nausea.
- Vomiting.
- Stomatitis.
- Unpleasant taste in the mouth.
- Diarrhea.

TREATMENT OF ACUTE RENAL FAILURE

The primary goal in acute renal failure is to treat the underlying disorder in order to prevent permanent or further damage to the kidneys. For example, a blood transfusion may be given to restore blood volume in the case of severe blood loss. Diet therapy, drug therapy, and dialysis may be undertaken to restore fluid and electrolyte balance and minimize blood concentrations of toxic waste products. Health care professionals diligently monitor indices of renal function to determine the best treatment plan.

Energy The person in acute renal failure is often unable to obtain enough energy to meet needs. Without sufficient energy to fuel hypermetabolism, proteins break down and blood urea and potassium concentrations rise even higher—all taxing the kidneys further. Thus wasting and malnutrition complicate recovery. The person's energy needs depend on the rate of catabolism; usually 30 to 50 kcalories per kilogram of body weight will meet these needs.

Take a moment to consider the high energy needs of an 80 kg (176 lb) person: 2400 to 4000 kcal/day.

Protein The protein needs of people with acute renal failure depend on the degree of renal function, the metabolic rate, and nutrition status. People who are not on dialysis (described later in this section) receive about 0.6 to 1.0 gram of protein per kilogram of body weight per day.[5] Complicating factors must also be considered, however. Impaired wound healing, infections, muscle wasting, and negative nitrogen balance are commonly seen in individuals with acute renal failure, and these complications may prove to be fatal. Accordingly, some practitioners consider it most important to prevent negative nitrogen balance and its possible consequences; they prefer to provide a higher protein intake, even if it necessitates dialysis. If dialysis is instituted, a more liberal protein intake is indicated because some amino acids are lost during the procedure. Depending on the type of dialysis, people receive from 1.1 to 2.5 grams of protein per kilogram of body weight per day.[6]

Fluids Fluid balances are carefully restored in clients who are either overhydrated or dehydrated. Thereafter, health care professionals determine fluid needs by measuring urine output and then adding about 500 milliliters to account for water lost through the skin, lungs, and perspiration. The person who is vomiting, has diarrhea, has a high fever, or otherwise loses fluids has greater fluid needs. In the oliguric stage, the person needs small amounts of fluids. In the diuretic stage, urine volume may increase significantly, and large amounts of fluids may have to be provided.

Electrolytes Sodium may be restricted (to 500 to 1000 milligrams) in the oliguric phase, but this may change as the person enters the diuretic phase. Likewise, potassium is often restricted to less than 2 grams per day in the oliguric phase, but may need to be supplemented in the diuretic phase.

Enteral and Parenteral Nutrition Because clients with acute renal failure are often severely stressed, they frequently receive their nutrients from tube feedings or TPN. Special enteral and parenteral formulas meet nutrient needs in small volumes. Compared with standard enteral formulas, renal formulas have less protein, fewer electrolytes, and more kcalories per milliliter (see Appendix K). TPN formulas are compounded with mixtures of both nonessential and essential amino acids at lower concentrations and dextrose at higher concentrations than in standard TPN solutions. Electrolytes are added in appropriate amounts.

The carbohydrate-dense enteral and parenteral formulas used for acute renal failure may exacerbate the hyperglycemia that frequently accompanies both hypermetabolic disorders and renal failure. Fat can be used to add kcalories, reduce the need for carbohydrate, and limit the glucose load. Insulin may be provided to lower blood glucose.

Rx PRESCRIPTION PAD

Drugs used to treat acute renal failure may include:

- Diuretics
- Exchange resins (sodium polystyrene)
- Insulin

See Appendix E for timing with meals and nutrition-related side effects.

Drug Therapy In the oliguric phase of acute renal failure, diuretics may be used to mobilize fluids. Drugs called exchange resins may be used to treat hyperkalemia. These drugs, provided by mouth or through an enema, cause sodium to be exchanged for potassium in the colon, and the potassium is then excreted in the stool.

As mentioned, insulin may be provided to help lower blood glucose. Insulin also temporarily lowers blood potassium in two ways. First, as insulin moves glucose into the cells, potassium follows. Second, as an anabolic hormone, insulin minimizes tissue breakdown and, consequently, retains potassium in the cells.

dialysis (dye-AL-ih-sis): removal of waste from the blood using the principles of simple diffusion and osmosis through a semipermeable membrane.

In **hemodialysis** (HE-mo-dye-AL-ih-sis), a blood vessel is tapped, and the blood is routed through a dialysis machine where excess fluids and wastes are removed. Blood is then returned from the machine to the body.

In **peritoneal** (PERR-ee-toe-NEE-al) **dialysis**, excess fluids and wastes are removed from the blood using the peritoneum as a semipermeable membrane.

nephritis (nef-RYE-tis): inflammation of the kidneys.

Impairment of renal blood flow because of renal artery damage is called **nephrosclerosis** (NEF-ro-skle-ROH-sis). It can be caused by hypertension or atherosclerosis.

Common nephropathies include **pyelonephritis** (PIE-eh-loh-neh-FRY-tis), an inflammation of the kidneys and bladder, and **glomerulonephritis** (glo-MARE-you-loh-neh-FRY-tis), an inflammation of the glomerular capillaries.

Dialysis Dialysis removes excess fluids and wastes from the blood by employing the principles of simple diffusion and osmosis across a semipermeable membrane. In so doing, dialysis reduces the symptoms of uremia, but the hormonal functions of the kidneys are not restored. The two major types of dialysis are hemodialysis and peritoneal dialysis.

In acute renal failure, the nephrons suddenly fail to maintain homeostasis, most often because of an abrupt decline in blood flow to the kidneys. Waste products accumulate, blood potassium rises, blood volume changes, and the clinical symptoms of uremic syndrome develop. Energy and protein needs are high, but those not on dialysis may need to restrict their protein intake. In the early oliguric stage, treatment includes small amounts of fluids, a diet restricted in sodium and potassium, and diuretics to mobilize fluids. In the later diuretic phase, treatment provides large amounts of fluids and may supplement potassium. The accompanying box provides a case study of a client with acute renal failure. Take a moment to review the many parameters health care professionals must consider when treating such clients.

Chronic Renal Failure

Most often chronic renal failure develops gradually from disorders that progressively and permanently damage the kidneys. Some of these disorders include nephritis, renal artery obstruction, kidney stones (see Highlight 29), renal tubular disorders, diabetic nephropathy (Chapter 27), hypertension (Chapter 28), and atherosclerosis (Chapter 28). Recall that nephrotic syndrome sometimes

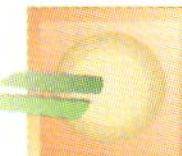

Case Study Store Manager with Acute Renal Failure

Mrs. Calley is a 35-year-old woman admitted to the hospital's intensive care unit. She was first seen in the emergency room after she sustained multiple and severe injuries in an auto accident. She had lost so much blood she almost died before reaching the hospital. Her injuries include a fractured leg, broken ribs, a collapsed lung, and internal bleeding. Following emergency surgery to stop the internal bleeding and repair injuries, she developed acute renal failure. Mrs. Calley is 5 feet 3 inches tall and weighs 125 pounds.

Mrs. Calley has a urine volume of less than 50 ml/day and a BUN of 75 mg/dL. A test of GFR could not be performed due to the low volume of urine she was excreting.

Describe the most probable reason why Mrs. Calley developed acute renal failure. What other problems can cause acute renal failure? Describe the phases of acute renal failure.

What are Mrs. Calley's dietary needs in the early phase? What waste products and electrolytes are of greatest concern? Why? What factors do you have to keep in mind in determining Mrs. Calley's energy and protein needs during acute renal failure? How will these needs change if dialysis is begun?

How will Mrs. Calley's nutrient needs change as she progresses to the second stage of acute renal failure? Why?

progresses to chronic renal failure. In a few cases, chronic renal failure develops from a disorder that rapidly causes irreversible kidney damage, as may occur following acute renal failure.

CONSEQUENCES OF CHRONIC RENAL FAILURE

Chronic renal failure progresses in stages. In the early stages, the body compensates for the loss of some nephron function by enlarging the remaining functional nephrons. The hypertrophied nephrons work so efficiently that the GFR may fall to 75 percent of its normal rate before symptoms appear. This efficiency explains why renal failure is often advanced before its presence is detected.

The capacity of the kidneys to function despite loss of some nephrons is referred to as **renal reserve**.

The body eventually exhausts the overworked nephrons, and renal function deteriorates further. (This effort is similar to the pancreatic cells in NIDDM, which at first produce more and more insulin in response to high blood glucose and later become exhausted and unable to produce adequate insulin.) In end-stage renal disease, the GFR drops below 20 percent of normal.

end-stage renal disease: the severe stage of renal failure in which dialysis or a kidney transplant is necessary to sustain life.

Blood Chemistry Alterations As renal function deteriorates, nitrogen-containing waste products accumulate in the blood, and the uremic syndrome (described on p. 915) develops. The skin becomes dry and scaly, and the person may itch uncomfortably. Skin hemorrhages may be visible. In later stages, urea (which can be excreted through sweat) may crystallize on the skin, a symptom known as uremic frost.

Reminder: The nitrogen-containing waste products that accumulate in renal failure include blood urea nitrogen (BUN), creatinine, and uric acid.

uremic frost: the appearance of urea crystals on the skin.

Normal metabolic processes generate more acid than base, and in healthy people, the kidneys excrete this excess acid. Lacking this ability, the person with chronic renal failure easily develops acidosis.

Reminder: The condition of having above-normal acidity in the blood and body fluids is *acidosis*.

In addition to nitrogen-containing compounds, the body retains excess fluids and electrolytes that are normally excreted in the urine. The retention of fluids and sodium causes edema and stresses the cardiovascular and pulmonary systems. Elevated blood potassium can trigger arrhythmias (irregular heartbeats) that further stress the heart and lead to heart failure. Elevated phosphorus alters bone metabolism (described later).

Uremia, together with altered hormonal activity, upsets the body's homeostasis and frequently leads to hypertension, hyperglycemia, elevated blood lipids (especially triglycerides), low serum albumin levels, and altered bone metabolism. All of these conditions further impair health.

Cardiovascular Complications Accelerated atherosclerosis and cardiovascular disease frequently accompany renal failure. Retention of fluid, sodium, and potassium, together with elevated blood lipids, hormonal changes, and hyperglycemia, can lead to hypertension, congestive heart failure, heart attacks, and pulmonary edema (see Chapter 28). In addition, some people with renal failure have elevated homocysteine levels, which may be an independent risk factor for cardiovascular disease (see Highlight 28).[7] Whether lowering homocysteine levels in people with renal disease can reduce their risk of cardiovascular disease remains to be determined. Cardiovascular disease is the cause of death in about a third of people with end-stage renal failure.[8]

Bone Disease The blood's normal balance between calcium and phosphorus prevents the two minerals from precipitating and forming calcium phosphate salts. When blood phosphorus rises too high because the kidneys are unable to excrete it, however, the excess phosphorus forms salts with calcium, which are then deposited in soft tissues such as eyes, skin, lungs, heart, and blood vessels. As calcium phosphate salts precipitate, serum levels of both phosphorus and calcium fall. As serum calcium, which were not elevated to begin with, falls, low calcium levels trigger the release of parathormone (PTH), which promotes excretion of phosphorus from the kidneys.

The deposition of phosphorus and calcium salts in soft tissue is called **metastatic** (MET-ah-STAT-ik) **calcification**.

Reminder: **Parathormone** (PTH) is a hormone secreted by the parathyroid glands that regulates calcium and phosphorus metabolism; also known as **parathyroid hormone**.

For a while, PTH effectively restores calcium and phosphorus balance, but as the GFR progressively declines, more PTH is needed to promote phosphorus excretion. Eventually, serum phosphorus remains high and calcium remains low despite markedly elevated levels of PTH (hyperparathyroidism).

To compound these problems, the diseased kidneys are unable to effectively activate vitamin D, which normally responds to low blood calcium by increasing calcium absorption from the GI tract. With lower levels of active vitamin D available, less calcium is absorbed. Besides all this, renal diets tend to be low in calcium as well. Hence the body is forced to draw calcium from bone tissue to raise blood calcium.

For all these reasons, bone disorders are common in chronic renal failure as evidenced by bone pain, diminished bone mass, soft (demineralized) bones, and fractures. Figure 29–3 summarizes the events leading to renal osteodystrophy.

renal osteodystrophy (OS-tee-oh-DIS-tro-fee): bone disorders resulting from calcium and phosphorus imbalances in renal disease. In **osteopenia**, bone mass is reduced; in **osteomalacia** (see p. 388), bones soften and fracture easily.

A type of renal osteodystrophy that results from hyperparathyroidism and is characterized by kidney stones, decalcification and softening of bones, and, sometimes, formation of cysts and tumors is called **osteitis** (os-tee-EYE-tis) **fibrosis**.

Gastrointestinal Disturbances Nausea, vomiting, diarrhea, and constipation commonly accompany the uremic syndrome. Gastritis and GI bleeding are also prevalent. All of these conditions can reduce food intake and increase nutrient losses.

Growth Failure and Wasting Syndrome Both children and adults with chronic renal disease frequently develop wasting and PEM. Nutrition status becomes more difficult to maintain as renal failure progresses. Taking multiple drugs over long periods of time further compromises nutrition status. Table 29–1

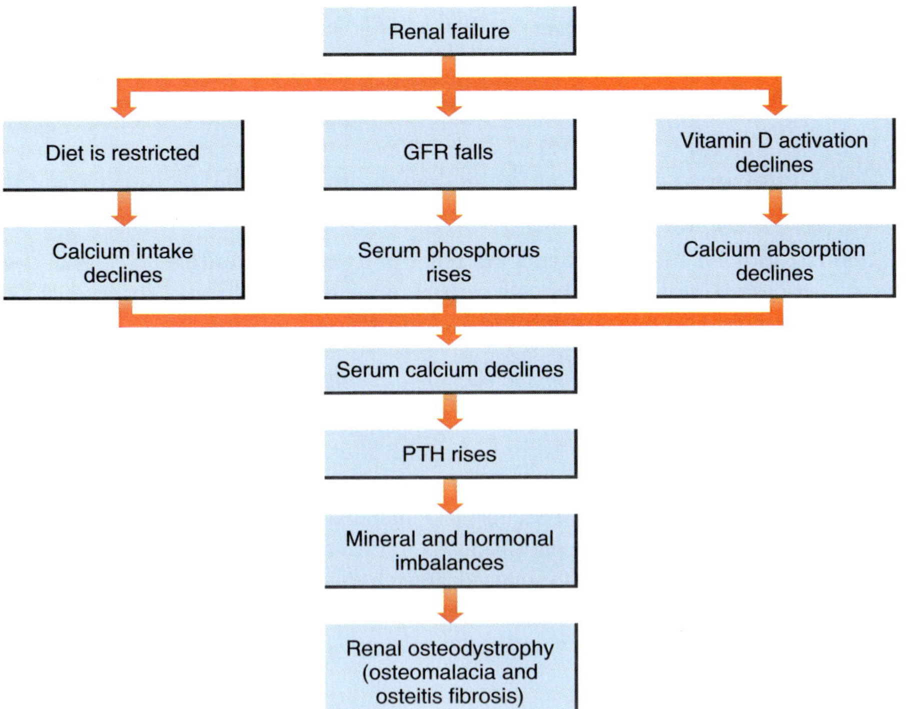

Figure 29–3

Events Leading to Renal Osteodystrophy

summarizes the causes of wasting associated with renal failure. Children with renal disease need nutrition intervention before the end of puberty if they are to make up growth deficits. Adults with renal disease can maintain or restore nutrition status, avoid complications, and improve quality of life by conscientiously attending to their diets as well.

Anemia People with functional kidneys respond to any type of anemia by increasing their production of erythropoietin, a hormone that stimulates hemoglobin and red blood cell synthesis. Depressed erythropoietin synthesis by the

Table 29–1

Possible Causes of Wasting in Renal Failure

Reduced Nutrient Intake	Excessive Nutrient Losses	Raised Nutrient Needs
Anorexia	Dialysis	Drugs
Drugs	Diarrhea	Hormonal alterations
Fatigue	Drugs	Infection
Nausea	GI bleeding	
Pain	Numerous blood tests	
Restrictive diet	Poor absorption	
Taste alterations	Vomiting	

damaged kidneys often results in anemia. Other factors that contribute to iron-deficiency anemia in renal failure include:

- Limited iron intake from the restrictive diet.
- Impaired intestinal absorption of iron.
- Blood (and iron) losses from hemodialysis, frequent blood tests, and GI bleeding.

When the kidneys fail, the effects are felt throughout the entire body, and the consequences are severe. Although renal failure is fatal without intervention, proper treatment can help sustain life and improve its quality.

TREATMENT OF CHRONIC RENAL FAILURE

Treatment for chronic renal failure includes diet, drugs, dialysis, and kidney transplants. Treatments aim to delay the progression of renal failure, prevent the buildup of toxic metabolic products and associated complications, maintain nutrition status, and alleviate symptoms to improve the client's well-being.

renal insufficiency: reduced renal function but not to the degree that requires dialysis or a kidney transplant.

Diet therapy is highly individualized and changes as renal disease progresses from renal insufficiency to end-stage renal disease. Table 29–2 summarizes nutrient needs for renal insufficiency and shows how these needs change for hemodial-

Table 29–2

Nutrient Needs in Chronic Renal Failure

Nutrients	Renal Insufficiency (Predialysis)	Hemodialysis	Peritoneal Dialysis
Energy (kcal/kg)	35–40	30–35	25–35
Protein (g/kg)	0.6–0.8	1.2–1.4	1.2–1.5
Fluid (ml)	Typically not restricted	500–750 plus daily urine output, or 1000 if anuric	≥2000
Sodium (g)	2–4	2–3	2–4
Potassium (g/kg)	Typically not restricted	3–4	Typically not restricted
Phosphorus (mg/g protein)	10–12[a]	12–15[a]	12–15[a]
Supplements			
Calcium (mg)	1000–1500	1000–1500	1000–1500
Folate (mg)	1	1	1
Vitamin B_6 (mg)	5	10	10
Other water-soluble vitamins	RDA	RDA	RDA
Vitamin D	As appropriate	As appropriate	As appropriate

Note: The actual amounts of these nutrients in the diet must be highly individualized based on each person's responses. For example, calcium supplementation may be as high as 3000 milligrams per day.

[a]The extent of phosphorus restriction depends on serum phosphorus. The goal is to maintain serum phosphorus between 4.5 and 6.0 milligrams per deciliter. Often, phosphate binders are useful for this purpose.

Sources: Adapted from Meeting the challenge of the renal diet: A preview of the 'National Renal Diet' educational series, *Journal of the American Dietetic Association* 93 (1993): 637–639; J. A. Beto, Which diet for which renal failure: Making sense of the options, *Journal of the American Dietetic Association* 95 (1995): 898–903.

ysis and peritoneal dialysis. The complexity of the renal diet, as well as its crucial role in the treatment of renal disease, underscores the need for a specialist, a renal dietitian, to educate clients and provide diet plans. Other health care professionals need not know the specifics of diet therapy, but they must understand the general concepts in order to communicate effectively with clients.

To evaluate dialysis and guide diet therapy, renal teams often use a mathematical model that takes into account the kidneys' ability to clear urea and the person's protein catabolic rate. The technique is called **urea kinetic modeling**.

Energy All people with renal failure need adequate food energy to achieve or maintain a desirable body weight and to prevent protein catabolism. Diet restrictions and the nausea associated with uremia may make it difficult for people with renal insufficiency to eat enough food. Most adults need at least 35 kcalories per kilogram of body weight per day. People on peritoneal dialysis, however, may need to restrict food intake because they absorb a significant amount of energy as glucose from the dialysate. For children, 100 or even more kcalories per kilogram of body weight per day is desirable, but 80 kcalories per kilogram of body weight per day is considered a reasonable intake. At the minimum, energy intake should meet the RDA.[9]

Protein Providing the right amount of protein in renal failure is like walking a tightrope. Too little protein, and the person develops malnutrition. Too much protein, and blood urea (the toxic waste product of protein metabolism) rises. For people with renal insufficiency, restricting protein may help protect the remaining nephrons, but human studies have not clearly demonstrated a beneficial effect.[10] Because dietary protein is limited, the diet emphasizes high-quality protein sources such as eggs, milk, meat, poultry, and fish.

People at high risk for developing chronic renal failure (such as those with diabetes) are often advised to limit protein intake to about the RDA.

A diet that includes protein from both animal and plant sources may be best because it combines the high quality of animal proteins with the low saturated fat and low cholesterol of plant proteins. As renal failure progresses, some clinicians prescribe very-low-protein diets supplemented with essential amino acids or their precursors (keto acids). Once the client begins dialysis, protein restrictions can be relaxed somewhat because dialysis incurs protein losses, peritoneal dialysis more so than hemodialysis.

Lipid The ideal renal diet restricts total fat, saturated fat, and cholesterol to help control elevated blood lipids and reduce the risk of cardiovascular disease. A later section describes the difficulties of meeting this dietary goal.

Carbohydrate A diet rich in complex carbohydrate helps to minimize the elevated blood glucose and triglycerides commonly seen in people with chronic renal failure. People on peritoneal dialysis may need to further restrict the intake of total carbohydrate, and especially simple carbohydrates, because they absorb a considerable amount of glucose from the dialysate.

Sodium and Fluids As renal failure progresses, the person excretes less urine and cannot handle even normal amounts of sodium and fluids. At this point, limiting sodium and fluids helps to prevent hypertension, edema, and heart failure. Individual needs for sodium and fluids are determined by carefully monitoring each person's weight, blood pressure, urine output, and blood electrolyte levels. A rise in body weight and blood pressure suggests that the person is retaining sodium and fluid; conversely, a decline in body weight and blood pressure (a desirable outcome of dialysis) represents fluid loss.

Minimal urine volume is **oliguria**; no urine excretion is **anuria**.

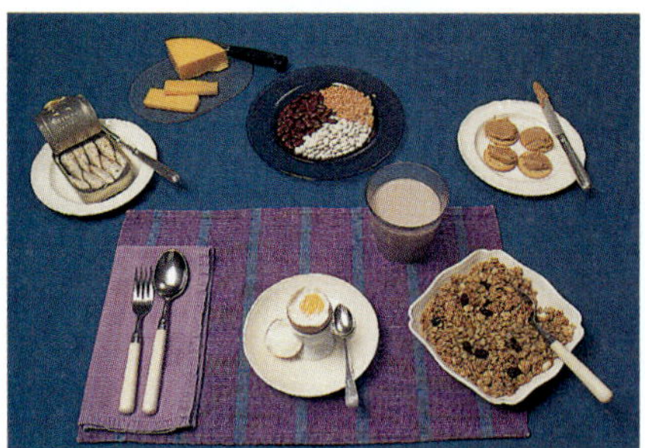

Foods such as milk and milk products, cheese, peanut butter, bran cereal, sardines, and legumes are high in phosphorus and so must be restricted in a renal diet. See Appendix H for other foods high in phosphorus.

Fluids are not restricted in renal insufficiency until urine output decreases. For the person who is neither dehydrated nor overhydrated, daily fluid needs amount to the daily urine output plus about 500 to 750 milliliters to provide for insensible water losses.

Once a person is on dialysis, sodium and fluid intake is controlled to allow a weight gain of about 2 pounds (of fluid) between dialysis treatments, although larger weight gains are common.[11] Typical renal diets provide from 2 to 4 grams of sodium and 500 to 3000 milliliters (about ½ to 3 quarts) of fluids daily. Table 29–3 lists foods considered part of the fluid allowance.

Potassium Most people with renal insufficiency and those on peritoneal dialysis can handle typical intakes of potassium.[12] People on hemodialysis, however, may experience elevated potassium levels between dialysis treatments. When hyperkalemia is a problem, potassium may be moderately restricted to about 2 to 3 grams per day. Figure 12–7 on p. 425 lists the potassium contents of commonly eaten foods; the person who must restrict potassium limits potassium-rich foods. Remember, however, that individual needs vary. People with renal disease who are taking potassium-wasting diuretics may need to adjust their potassium intakes accordingly.

Phosphorus Dietary phosphorus restrictions help control rising phosphorus levels and may help slow the progression of renal failure. Fortunately, when a client follows a protein-restricted diet, phosphorus is restricted as well. In addition, the person must limit foods high in phosphorus, such as those shown in the margin photo.

Physicians may also prescribe drugs that bind phosphorus in the GI tract, thus making it unavailable for absorption. These phosphate binders must be taken with meals. Calcium salts—calcium carbonate and calcium acetate—are the preferred phosphate binders for people with end-stage renal disease. Aluminum and magnesium salts also bind phosphate, but they carry a risk of toxicity and are therefore avoided.

Caution: People with renal failure who must restrict potassium must avoid using low-sodium products and salt substitutes that contain potassium.

People with renal failure should avoid aluminum- and magnesium-containing antacids and laxatives or enemas containing magnesium; aluminum toxicity or serious hypermagnesemia can result.

Calcium Supplements As mentioned, impaired calcium absorption due to the lack of active vitamin D and limited calcium intake may contribute to bone disease in people with renal failure. Most people with renal disease need calcium supplements; some, however, develop hypercalcemia. The renal team monitors serum calcium closely to prevent both low and high blood calcium. Calcium-containing phosphate binders provide some calcium, but the absorption of calcium from these products varies widely.

Water-Soluble Vitamins People with renal failure frequently develop vitamin B_6 and folate deficiencies because of the restrictive diet, loss of vitamins during dialysis, drug therapy, and altered metabolism. For these reasons, clients receive generous amounts of vitamin B_6 and folate, along with RDA amounts of the other water-soluble vitamins. Intakes of vitamin C from both the diet and supplements should be limited to less than 100 milligrams per day to prevent the formation of oxalate stones (see Chapter 22 p. 728).[13]

The active form of supplemental vitamin D, or calcitriol, can be given orally or intravenously. A new, experimental form of active vitamin D called 22 oxa calcitriol is associated with a less marked rise in serum calcium than calcitriol.

Fat-Soluble Vitamins Supplemental vitamin D in its active form can help maintain blood calcium and prevent bone disease. The dosages and methods of administering vitamin D supplements must be carefully adjusted for each client to maintain serum calcium levels within the normal range. Supplementation of the other fat-soluble vitamins is usually not necessary.

Trace Minerals The administration of human erythropoietin along with the iron needed to synthesize hemoglobin is effective in treating iron-deficiency anemia, once a common and persistent problem in people with chronic renal disease. Poor iron absorption and the GI side effects of iron supplements may make it difficult for clients to fully meet their iron needs. Clients should be cautioned to avoid iron supplements that also contain vitamin C.

People on dialysis frequently complain of anorexia and altered taste perceptions (dysgeusia), symptoms typical of zinc deficiency. Clients with these symptoms may need supplements if their serum zinc levels are inadequate.

Enteral and Parenteral Nutrition Enteral and parenteral nutrition can provide nutrients to people with chronic renal failure who are unable to eat adequate amounts of foods. If the GI tract is functional, health care professionals first try to supplement the diet with enteral formulas orally. Glucose polymer powders may be used to add food energy without requiring clients to eat extra food or use their fluid allowances. In addition, formulas designed for use with renal failure (as described earlier on p. 916) can be given by tube (see Appendix K). Parenteral formulas are also available.

Diet Planning The ideal renal diet presents a challenge: provide adequate energy, but restrict protein, fat, and, sometimes, simple carbohydrate. Complex carbohydrates, which might appear to be the ideal energy source, are rich sources of electrolytes, which are also restricted on the renal diet. Complex carbohydrates are also rich sources of fiber; and because fibers absorb fluids, which are often restricted, they must be used cautiously. Diet planners must accept that under such circumstances, no diet is truly ideal. They must recognize that the need to meet protein and electrolyte requirements outweighs the need to restrict fats and simple carbohydrates.

To help meet energy needs, clients include as many complex carbohydrate foods as their diet plans allow. They supplement their meals with formulas high in kcalories but restricted in protein and electrolytes (see Appendix K) and use foods such as sugars (glucose polymers, hard candy, and jelly) and fats (margarine, oil) freely. The person with elevated blood lipids may be advised to restrict fat and modify the type of fat if possible. The person with diabetes or hyperglycemia is advised to maintain a consistent carbohydrate intake at regular intervals and to adjust insulin to cover carbohydrate intake.

To help individuals on renal diets find foods they will accept and enjoy, food lists similar to the exchange system are available. Whereas the exchange system for diabetes groups foods by their energy, carbohydrate, protein, and fat contents, renal food lists group foods by their energy, protein, sodium, potassium, and phosphorus contents. The box on p. 924 provides suggestions to ease the task of complying with a renal diet. A sample renal diet menu is shown on p. 925.

Diet Compliance The challenges dietitians face in designing renal diets pale in comparison to those encountered by clients and caregivers who must follow a complicated medical care plan of which diet is only one part. Successful

Table 29–3

Substances Controlled on Fluid-Restricted Diets

Foods
Cream
Frozen yogurt
Fruit ice
Gelatin
Ice cream
Ice milk
Popsicles
Sherbet
Soup
Other
Ice
Liquid medications

Note: All foods contain some water, but these foods contain considerable amounts of water and, therefore, must be considered part of the fluid allowance on a fluid-restricted diet.

How to Help Clients Comply with a Renal Diet

The following suggestions can assist clients in complying with the renal diet:

1. To keep track of fluid intake:
   - Fill a container with an amount of water equal to your total fluid allowance. Each time you use a liquid food or beverage, discard an equivalent amount of water from the container. The amount remaining in the container will show you how much fluid you have left for the day.
   - Be sure to save enough fluid to take medications.
2. To help control thirst:
   - Chew gum or suck hard candy.
   - Freeze fluids so they take longer to consume.
   - Add lemon juice to water to make it more refreshing.
   - Gargle with refrigerated mouthwash.
3. To prevent the diet from becoming monotonous:
   - Experiment with new combinations of allowed foods.
   - Use favorite foods whenever possible.
   - Substitute nondairy products for regular dairy products. Nondairy products are lower in protein, phosphorus, and potassium than regular dairy foods, and they can substitute for milk and add energy to the diet.
   - Add zest to foods by seasoning with garlic, onion, chili, curry powder, oregano, pepper, or lemon juice.
   - Consult a dietitian when you want to eat restricted foods. Many restricted foods can be used occasionally and in small amounts if the diet is carefully adjusted.

treatment hinges on compliance with the medical plan. To help clients understand medical plans and support their efforts, the health care team must effectively communicate with their clients and, just as important, listen to them. Within a tangled web of abnormal metabolic processes, dialysis lines, and toxic waste products is a person, often a frightened or discouraged one. All of the members of the health care team need to understand the plan if they are to offer the most effective support.

A nutrition education approach that emphasizes self-management appears to be a useful strategy for helping clients comply with a renal diet.[14] This approach (described in Highlight 27) guides clients in identifying goals, selecting strategies to meet their goals, and evaluating their progress. Both psychosocial and behavioral factors play key roles in helping clients adhere to protein-restricted diets.[15]

Psychosocial factors include:
- Knowledge.
- Attitude.
- Support.
- Satisfaction.
- Self-perception of success.

Behavioral factors include:
- Self-monitoring of protein intake.
- Provision of feedback by a dietitian.

Menu

Breakfast
1 egg, fried with
1 tbs margarine
1 slice toast
2 tsp margarine
Jelly
½ c grape juice
Coffee
Nondairy creamer
Sugar

Snacks
Hard candy, gum drops, marshmallows
Carbonated beverages

Lunch
Sandwich with
2 oz turkey
2 slices bread
1 tbs mayonnaise
Lettuce leaf
1 c green beans
2 tsp margarine
½ c strawberries
2 tbs whipping cream
Sugar
½ c milk

Supper
3 oz roast beef
½ c rice
2 tsp margarine
½ c mushrooms sautéed in 2 tsp olive oil and seasonings
½ c applesauce
Iced tea
2 tsp sugar

Sample Renal Diet Menu

This diet menu provides 60 grams of protein and controls phosphorus, potassium, and sodium intake. To increase the kcalories in this diet, prepare food with oil or unsalted margarine (regular margarine, if allowed) and use additional fat, sugar, or syrup whenever possible. For example, canned fruit packed in heavy syrup, rather than juice, adds kcalories.

KIDNEY TRANSPLANTS AND DIET

A preferable alternative to dialysis in end-stage renal disease is a kidney transplant. Kidney transplants can successfully restore kidney function and normal growth. For this reason, transplants are particularly desirable in children. Given a choice, many would prefer transplants, but suitable kidney donors cannot always be found.

Immunosuppressant Drug Therapy After receiving a new kidney, the person must take very large doses of immunosuppressants to prevent rejection (see Table E–1 in Appendix E for nutrient-drug interactions). Muscular weakness, GI bleeding, protein catabolism, carbohydrate intolerance, sodium retention, fluid retention, hypertension, weight gain, and a characteristic puffy-faced appearance commonly accompany immunosuppressant therapy. Infections and increased susceptibility to malignant tumors are also common. Diuretics are frequently prescribed to promote the excretion of sodium and fluid and prevent hypertension. The kidney may be rejected or fail to function, in which case dialysis must be reinstituted either temporarily until another kidney can be found or permanently.

Dietary Interventions Immediately following a kidney transplant, enough energy and protein are provided to limit catabolism and preserve organ function and nutrition status. Once recovery is underway, the degree of renal function guides diet therapy. Typical post-transplant diet modifications appear in Table 29–4. Dietary protein is provided in amounts adequate to prevent the protein catabolism that immunosuppressants may incur, but not too much to tax renal function. Because blood lipids are frequently elevated, clients are advised to follow a low-fat diet. Sodium restrictions help prevent fluid

Table 29–4

Dietary Guidelines Following Kidney Transplant

Energy: Adequate to achieve or maintain desirable body weight.

Protein: 1g per kg body wt. (Adjust based on renal function tests.)

Fat: ≤30 percent of total kcal; ≤300 mg cholesterol.

Sodium: 3 to 4 g per day.

Potassium: Adjust according to diuretic therapy.

Source: Adapted from J. A. Beto, Which diet for which renal failure: Making sense of the options, *Journal of the American Dietetic Association* 95 (1995): 898–903.

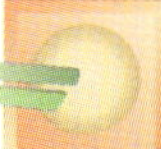

Case Study Child with Chronic Renal Failure

Jason is a nine-year-old child who developed chronic glomerulonephritis several months after suffering from a streptococcal infection (strep throat). Jason's renal function has declined steadily over the last three years. His mother consulted his pediatrician because the boy had been very tired, unable to eat, and complaining of stomach cramps and unpleasant taste sensations. Laboratory tests revealed the following information:

- GFR: 4 ml/min (below normal).
- BUN: 102 mg/dL (above normal).

Jason was admitted to the hospital, and after further testing, dialysis was instituted, and a search for a suitable kidney donor was begun. Jason is 4 feet 3 inches tall and weighs 55 pounds. Before coming to the hospital, he was following a fluid-, sodium-, potassium-, and phosphorus-restricted diet that allowed 30 grams of protein. His typical energy intake is 1100 kcalories per day.

Describe chronic renal failure. Are the symptoms Jason complained of typical of renal failure? Why did his GFR fall, and why did his BUN levels rise?

Look closely at Jason's height and weight. How do they compare with the height and weight of other children of the same age? (Use the growth charts in Appendix E.) Discuss reasons why growth may be compromised in the child with renal failure.

Think about Jason's diet before he came to the hospital. Describe the reasons why protein, fluid, sodium, potassium, and phosphorus were restricted. Calculate Jason's energy range, and compare this estimate with his actual energy intake. Consider the effect of Jason's energy intake on his growth.

Describe ways Jason's nutrient needs will change when he begins hemodialysis. How will his needs change if he receives a kidney transplant?

Discuss some diet strategies you can suggest to Jason and his parents to help him comply with his diet. Consider the impact of renal disease on Jason, his family, and his interactions with friends. How can all members of the health team help support Jason and his family during this difficult time?

retention and hypertension. Depending on the type of diuretic prescribed, potassium intakes may have to be adjusted as well.

As mentioned, people with kidney transplants may reject their new kidneys either temporarily or permanently. During these times, they must return to the prescribed diet for renal failure. Clients may find this regression difficult to accept and need to be prepared for the possibility before it occurs. The accompanying case study helps direct your thoughts toward the special needs of a client with chronic renal failure.

Chronic renal failure develops gradually from any disorder that progressively and permanently damages the kidneys. At first, the nephrons compensate for the loss of function, making detection in the early stages difficult. Eventually, end-stage renal disease will dramatically affect every body system and compromise nutrition status. Diet plans control fluid, energy, protein, sodium, potassium, and phosphorus intakes; plans differ depending on the degree of renal insufficiency, the type of dialysis, and the success of a transplant. Use the nutrition assessment checklist to review assessment findings of concern in renal failure.

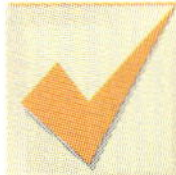

Nutrition Assessment Checklist

For People with Renal Diseases

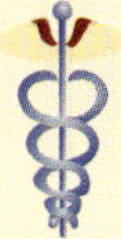

Medical Use the medical record to evaluate the cause of renal insufficiency or renal failure and the treatment plan. Determine what other conditions such as severe stress, hyperlipidemia, hypertension, congestive heart disease, or diabetes may alter nutrient needs.

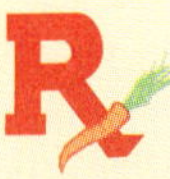

Drug Review the client's drug therapy for possible drug-nutrient interactions, particularly for clients with chronic renal diseases that will require long-term use of various drugs including antilipemics, antihypertensives, diuretics, and immunosuppressants. Assess the client's over-the-counter drug use for sources of electrolytes.

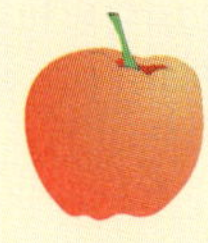

Food Intake Assess food intake to evaluate usual intake of energy, protein, fluids, sodium, potassium, phosphorus, calcium, vitamins, and minerals. Use food records to assess the client's compliance with diet therapy and to make additional suggestions.

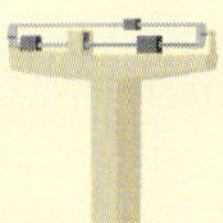

Anthropometric Monitor changes in height and weight in children and weight in adults. Interpret anthropometric measurements cautiously in people with oliguria, anuria, or edema because anthropometrics may be deceptively normal or high due to fluid retention. For people on dialysis, the weight measured immediately after a treatment most accurately reflects the person's true weight and is sometimes called the "dry weight." Rapid weight gain between dialysis treatments often reflects fluid retention. Weight loss should be expected following dialysis treatment.

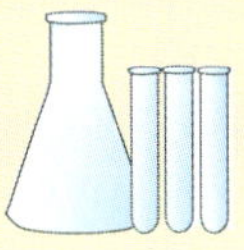

Laboratory Check serum protein levels, which are often low in people with nephrotic syndrome and renal failure and may be even lower if malnutrition complicates renal disease. Review laboratory measurements of GFR, electrolytes, BUN, and creatinine, which are commonly used to determine dietary and medical treatments. Note whether serum lipids are elevated, as frequently occurs in people with nephrotic syndrome, renal failure, and kidney transplants.

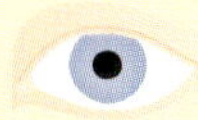

Physical Check for physical signs of fluid retention or dehydration, iron deficiency (pale skin and conjunctiva), uremia (fatigue, mental confusion, dry itchy skin, skin hemorrhages, nausea, vomiting, altered taste perceptions), osteodystrophy (bone pain, fractures, and bowed legs in children), hyperkalemia (arrhythmias and muscle weakness), and zinc deficiencies (altered taste perceptions). Record blood pressure and vital signs.

Study Questions

1. What functions do the kidneys perform? What roles do they play in maintaining chemical homeostasis?
2. What is nephrotic syndrome? What are its consequences? What are the energy and protein needs of the person with nephrotic syndrome? Why is a low-fat, low-cholesterol diet important in nephrotic syndrome? What are the fluid and electrolyte needs of these individuals?
3. Describe acute renal failure and list some of its causes. What symptoms are associated with the buildup of toxic metabolic products in the blood? What are the consequences of acute renal failure?
4. What are the nutrient needs of the person in the oliguric phase of acute renal failure? How do these needs change as the person progresses to the diuretic phase?
5. Can tube feedings and TPN be used safely for the person with renal failure? What special considerations are involved in selecting an enteral or parenteral formula for the person with acute renal failure?
6. What are the causes of chronic renal failure? Why is it often difficult to detect in the early stages? What happens in the end stage of renal failure?
7. What are the objectives of dietary treatment of chronic renal failure? When is a special diet instituted in the course of renal failure? When is dialysis or a kidney transplant considered for the person with renal failure?
8. What are the energy needs of adults with chronic renal failure? Of children? What are the consequences of providing too little energy in the diet of the person with chronic renal failure?
9. Why is the protein (nitrogen) intake of the person with chronic renal failure a particular concern? How does dialysis affect protein needs?
10. What fluid and electrolyte modifications are made to the diet of the person with chronic renal failure? What modifications are made concerning phosphorus, calcium, and vitamin D? Why?
11. What other vitamins and minerals need special consideration in the diet of the person with chronic renal failure? Describe why each of the nutrients you list may be a problem.
12. Discuss the nutrient needs of the person with a kidney transplant.

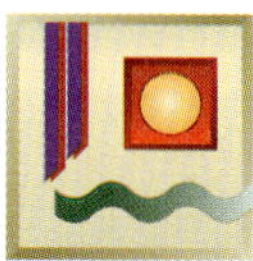

Clinical Applications

1. Chapter 25 described severe stresses and discussed how the combination of severe stress, hypermetabolism, and malnutrition can lead to multiple organ failure. The sequence of multiple organ failure often begins with respiratory failure (Chapter 28), followed by liver failure (Chapter 26), and then renal failure. Design a table with four columns: severe stress, respiratory failure, liver failure, and renal failure. Make the following rows: energy, protein, fat, fluid, and other nutrients. Fill the appropriate block with a brief description if there is a need for consideration: Which nutrient modifications are common to all four disorders? Do some of the necessary modifications for one disorder conflict with those for another? If yes, describe how the final decision might be made for the most appropriate diet.
2. Using the box on p. 924 as a guide, suggest ways to help people adjust to different aspects of their renal diets.

Notes

1. J. D. Dwyer, Vegetarian diets for treating nephrotic syndrome, *Nutrition Reviews* 51 (1993): 44–56; G. A. Kaysen, Nutritional management of nephrotic syndrome, *Journal of Renal Nutrition* 2 (1992): 50–58.
2. R. W. Davies and coauthors, Proteinuria, not altered albumin metabolism, affects hyperlipidemia in the nephrotic rat, *Journal of Clinical Investigations* 86 (1990): 600–605.
3. R. Rodrigo and M. Pino, Proteinuria and albumin homeostasis in the nephrotic syndrome: Effect of dietary protein intake, *Nutrition Reviews* 54 (1996): 337–347.
4. Kaysen, 1992.
5. J. D. Kopple, Nutrition management of the patient with acute renal failure, *Journal of Parenteral and Enteral Nutrition* 20 (1996): 3–12.
6. Kopple, 1996.
7. J. A. Friedman and J. T. Dwyer, Hyperhomocysteinemia as a risk factor for cardiovascular disease in patients undergoing hemodialysis, *Nutrition Reviews* 53 (1995): 197–201.
8. K. W. Ma, G. L. Greene, and L. Raij, Cardiovascular risk factors in chronic renal failure and hemodialysis populations, *American Journal of Kidney Diseases* 19 (1992): 505–513.
9. A.S.P.E.N. Board of Directors, Practice guidelines: Kidney failure—Pediatric, *Journal of Parenteral and Enteral Nutrition* (supplement) 17 (1993): 43.
10. The Modification of Diet in Renal Disease Study Group, The effects of dietary protein restriction and blood pressure control on the progression of chronic renal disease, *New England Journal of Medicine* 330 (1994): 877–884.
11. J. A. Beto, Which diet for which renal failure: Making sense of the options, *Journal of the American Dietetic Association* 95 (1995): 898–903.
12. Beto, 1996.
13. Beto, 1996.
14. B. P. Gillis and coauthors, Nutrition intervention program of the Modification of Diet in Renal Disease Study: A self-management approach, *Journal of the American Dietetic Association* 95 (1995): 1288–1294.
15. N. C. Milas and coauthors, Factors associated with adherence to the dietary protein intervention in the Modification of Diet in Renal Disease Study, *Journal of the American Dietetic Association* 95 (1995): 1295–1300; T. Coyne and coauthors, Dietary satisfaction correlated with adherence in the Modification of Diet in Renal Disease Study, *Journal of the American Dietetic Association* 95 (1995): 1301–1306.

Highlight 29

Kidney Stones—Treatments and Prevention

Kidney stones affect 10 to 20 percent of the U.S. population, with about one in a thousand people requiring hospitalization for this painful, although rarely fatal, condition. Most people with kidney stones are men over age 25, and although they may have recurrences, many report only a single episode. Kidney stones are prevalent in certain geographical locations, particularly in the southeastern United States. These findings suggest that kidney stones may be preventable. The glossary on p. 931 defines terms related to kidney stones.

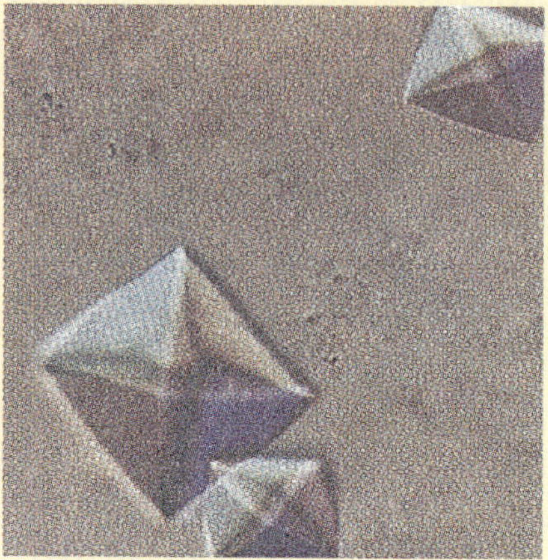

Most kidney stones are formed from calcium oxalate crystals, shown here.

KIDNEY STONES

Kidney stones may form anywhere in the urinary tract, but most often they form in the area just above the ureter called the renal pelvis (review Figure 29–1 on p. 910). Kidney stones vary in size, and a person may form a single stone or multiple stones. Kidney stones form when stone constituents become concentrated in the urine and form crystals that grow. Stone constituents vary, but most stones are composed of calcium oxalate. The incidence of calcium oxalate kidney stones has climbed steadily in affluent countries.[1] Less commonly, stones are composed of calcium phosphate, uric acid, the amino acid cystine, or magnesium ammonium phosphate (known as struvite). Table H29–1 on p. 931 lists some conditions associated with stone formation.

Consequences of Kidney Stones

In most cases, kidney stones pose no problems, especially when they are few and small. Small stones (less than one-fifth of an inch in diameter) may pass readily through the ureters and out of the body via the urine with minimal treatment. Large stones, on the other hand, cannot pass easily through the ureter. When a large stone or a large piece of a stone enters a ureter, it produces a sharp, stabbing pain, called *renal colic*. Typically, the pain starts suddenly in the back and intensifies as the stone follows the course down the abdomen toward the groin. The intense pain is often accompanied by nausea and vomiting. When the stone reaches the bladder, the pain subsides abruptly. Large stones that fail to pass through the ureter may cause a urinary tract obstruction or infection and serious bleeding. Symptoms may include frequent urination, urgency of urination, painful urination (dysuria), and bloody urine (hematuria).

Treatment of Kidney Stones

Clinicians analyze the chemical composition of urine, blood, and stones (when available) to determine the composition of the stone and its cause. Whenever the cause can be determined, treatment depends on resolving the underlying condition.[2]

Clients with small kidney stones may more readily pass the stone if

Glossary

cystinuria (SIS-te-NEW-ree-ah): the presence of cystine in the urine; the symptom of an inherited metabolic disorder in which large amounts of the amino acids cystine, lysine, arginine, and ornithine are excreted in the urine. Cystinuria commonly results in kidney stone formation.

dysuria (dis-YOU-ree-ah): painful or difficult urination.

gout: a metabolic disorder that results in excess uric acid in the blood and sometimes in the urine; characterized by acute arthritis and inflammation of the joints.

hematuria (HEME-at-YOU-ree-ah): blood in the urine.

hypercalciuria (HIGH-per-kal-see-YOU-ree-ah): excessive urinary excretion of calcium. When not related to a known underlying medical condition, it is known as **idiopathic hypercalciuria**.

renal colic: the severe pain that accompanies the movement of a kidney stone from the kidney through the ureter to the bladder.

struvite: crystals of magnesium ammonium phosphate.

Table H29–1

Conditions Associated with Kidney Stones

Cystinuria
Fat malabsorption
Glucocorticoid excess
Gout
Hyperparathyroidism
Hyperthyroidism
Immobilization
Malignancies (some types)
Osteoporosis
Paget's disease
Recurrent urinary tract infections
Renal tubular acidosis
Vitamin D toxicity

they drink plenty of fluids (more than 3 liters a day). They may also need antimicrobials if an infection is present and may sometimes need diuretics to help maintain urine output so that stones do not have a chance to form or enlarge. Large stones that block the flow of urine or cause an infection require removal either surgically or, more commonly, by using shock waves to break the stone into pieces small enough to pass readily through the urinary tract.

PREVENTION OF KIDNEY STONES

Treatment of the underlying medical condition is necessary to help prevent recurrences of kidney stones. Dietary measures vary according to the composition of the stone, but prevention of all stones includes this advice: increase fluid intake to dilute the urine. People who have had kidney stones need to drink enough fluid (mostly water) to maintain a urine volume of at least 2 liters a day. This level of output requires an intake of 3 or 4 liters of fluids throughout the day. People who are physically active or who live in warm climates may need additional fluids. People with fevers, diarrhea, or vomiting also need additional fluids until these conditions resolve.

Dietary therapies for specific types of stones are described next. Phosphate stones are not responsive to diet and are treated with drugs or surgery.

Calcium Stones

About half of all people with calcium stones excrete normal amounts of calcium in the urine, and the other half excrete excess calcium (hypercalciuria). People with hypercalciuria are either more efficient at absorbing calcium from the intestine or more wasteful in their excretion of calcium than most people. Diet therapy for people with hypercalciuria limits calcium intake to the RDA appropriate for age and sex. It is important that the diet not fall below the RDA, however. Those with hypercalciuria who follow a low-calcium diet generally excrete more calcium than they ingest, indicating that they are losing calcium from their bones.

Oxalate-Restricted Diets Calcium restriction increases urinary oxalate excretion (see p. 728), which poses a problem for people with calcium oxalate stones. Hyperoxaluria increases the likelihood of calcium oxalate stone formation even more than hypercalciuria does.

People with calcium oxalate stones, including people with fat malabsorption, are advised to limit their intakes of foods high in oxalate—spinach, rhubarb, beets, nuts, chocolate, tea, wheat bran, and strawberries.[3] Some clinicians report that for most people, only nuts (and peanut butter) need to be restricted.[4]

Most of the oxalate in the urine, however, comes from the body's synthesis of oxalate. One of the pathways of oxalate synthesis in the body begins with vitamin C. Consequently, megadoses of vitamin C can raise urinary oxalate concentrations. People at risk for oxalate stones are therefore advised to avoid vitamin C supplements.

Sodium-Restricted Diets In addition to calcium and oxalate, attention to salt intake may be important in preventing calcium oxalate stones. Studies suggest that excess salt increases urinary calcium excretion in all people, but causes a proportionately greater amount of calcium to be excreted in people with hypercalciuria.[5] Thus people who form calcium oxalate stones and who have hypercalciuria may benefit by moderately restricting salt. Further research is necessary to determine if such a restriction can prevent calcium stones from forming.[6]

People with calcium stones may be treated with thiazide diuretics, which effectively reduce the excretion of calcium and increase the excretion of fluids, thus reducing the likelihood of stone formation. A high salt intake can offset the beneficial effects of thiazide diuretics and can cause excessive potassium excretion. Thus people taking thiazide diuretics have an additional reason to lower their salt intake. Potassium-rich foods are recommended. Potassium supplements may also be prescribed.

Uric Acid Stones

Uric acid stones are frequently associated with gout, a metabolic disorder characterized by elevated levels of uric acid in the blood and urine. Uric acid stones form when the urine becomes persistently acid, contains excessive uric acid, or both. Purine-restricted diets are commonly prescribed to prevent uric acid stones. A purine-restricted diet limits red meats, particularly organ meats, anchovies, sardines, and meat extracts. The benefits of such a diet are unproven, but avoiding excessive protein may be useful; health care professionals recommend a diet limited to 100 grams of protein per day. Alcohol intake is also limited. Drug therapy (allopurinol) is often prescribed to inhibit uric acid production, reducing both uric acid levels and urinary acidity.

Cystine Stones

Cystine stones form when an inherited disorder of amino acid metabolism (cystinuria) causes an abnormally high urinary excretion of cystine. For cystine stones, health care professionals recommend a diet restricted in the amino acid methionine, because the body makes cystine from methionine. Drug therapy to reduce urinary acidity may also be beneficial.

Struvite Stones

Struvite stones, sometimes called "infection stones," form when the urinary tract becomes infected with a specific type of microorganism that hydrolyzes urea, creating an ammonia-rich, alkaline urine. (You may want to review the discussion of how the body disposes of excess nitrogen on p. 234.) Unlike most stones, struvite stones are about twice as prevalent in women as in men. Effective treatment includes removal of the stones and antimicrobial drugs.

Many people experience kidney stones during the course of their lives, and the incidence of kidney stones is increasing. Modifying dietary and other risk factors for kidney stones has the potential to save many people from the pain and possible complications of kidney stones.

NOTES

1. L. K. Massey, Dietary salt, urinary calcium, and kidney stone risk, *Nutrition Reviews* 53 (1995): 131–139.
2. F. L. Coe, J. H. Parks, and J. R. Asplin, The pathogenesis and treatment of kidney stones, *New England Journal of Medicine* 327 (1992): 1141–1152.
3. L. K. Massey, H. Roman-Smith, and R. A. L. Sutton, Effect of dietary oxalate and calcium on urinary oxalate and risk of formation of calcium oxalate kidney stones, *Journal of the American Dietetic Association* 93 (1993): 901–906.
4. C. L. Smith, M. Davis, and R. O. Berkseth, Dietary factors in calcium nephrolithiasis, *Journal of Renal Nutrition* 2 (1992): 146–153.
5. W. J. Burtis and coauthors, Dietary hypercalciuria in patients with calcium oxalate kidney stones, *American Journal of Clinical Nutrition* 60 (1994): 424–429.
6. Massey, 1995.

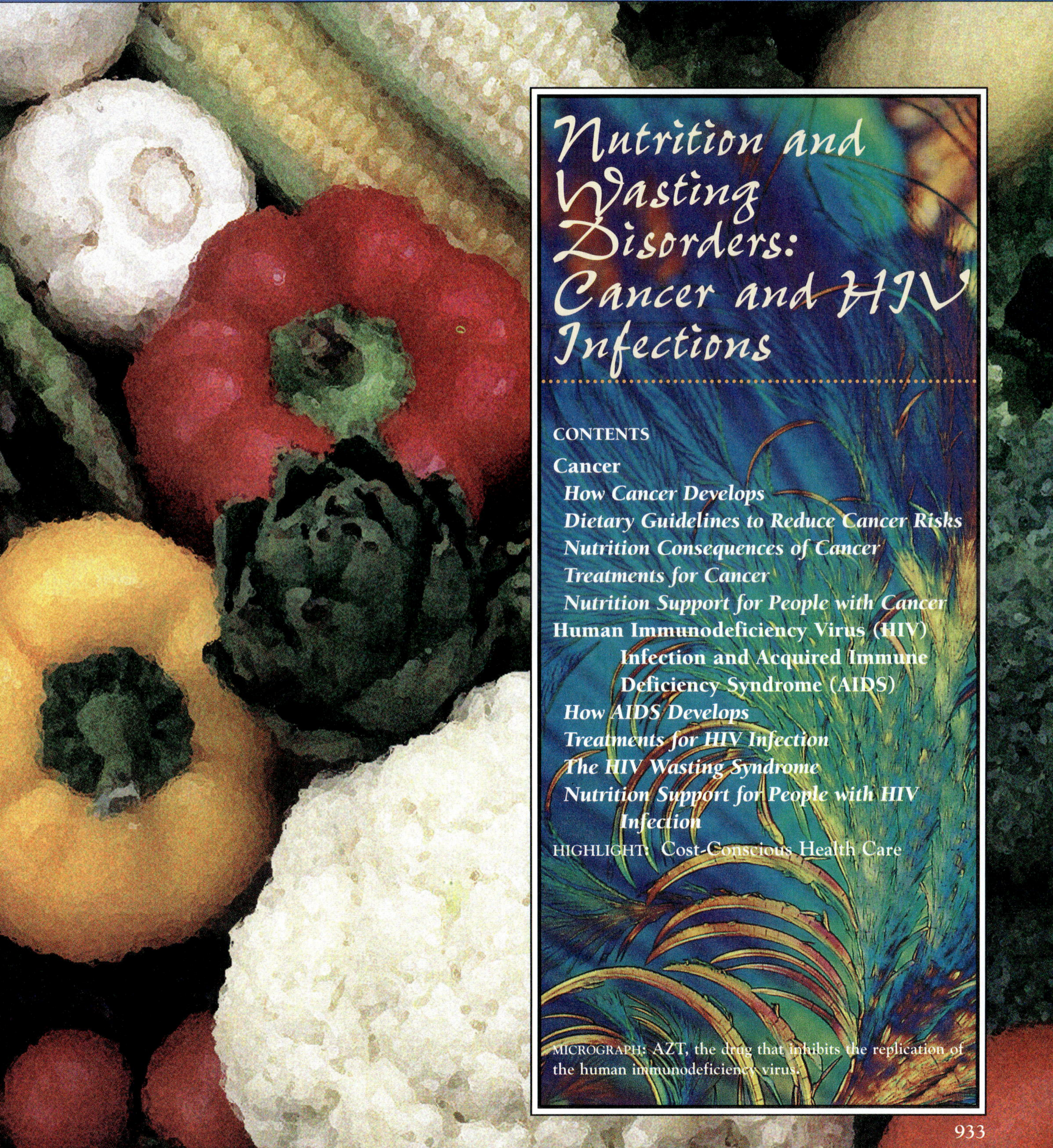

Chapter 30

Nutrition and Wasting Disorders: Cancer and HIV Infections

CONTENTS

MICROGRAPH: AZT, the drug that inhibits the replication of the human immunodeficiency virus.

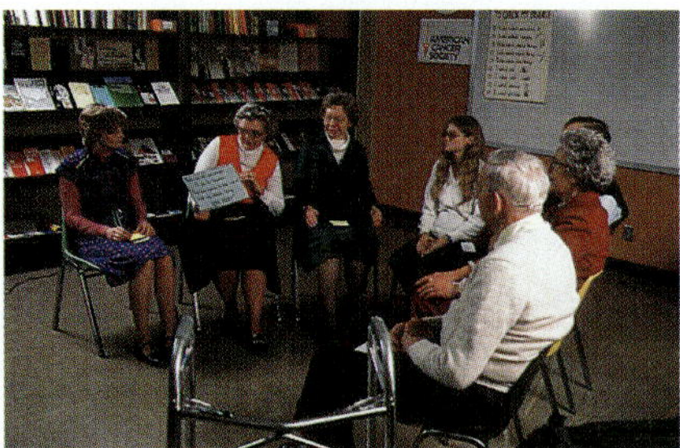

People with cancer take comfort from the support of others and from the knowledge that medical science is waging an unrelenting battle in their defense.

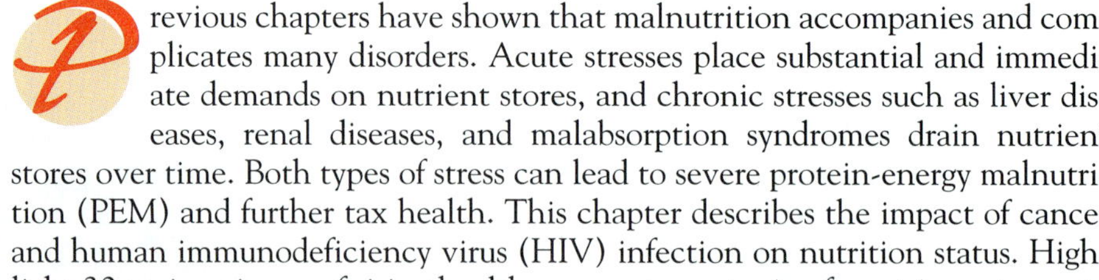

Previous chapters have shown that malnutrition accompanies and complicates many disorders. Acute stresses place substantial and immediate demands on nutrient stores, and chronic stresses such as liver diseases, renal diseases, and malabsorption syndromes drain nutrient stores over time. Both types of stress can lead to severe protein-energy malnutrition (PEM) and further tax health. This chapter describes the impact of cancer and human immunodeficiency virus (HIV) infection on nutrition status. Highlight 30 reviews issues of rising health care costs—a topic of great importance in the treatment of prolonged diseases like cancer and HIV infections that incur considerable costs.

From a nutrition standpoint, cancer and HIV infection present many similarities. Both affect many organ systems. Both involve symptoms that limit nutrient intake. Both are associated with wasting, and in both, the wasting is caused not only by the diseases themselves but also by their treatments. In both cases, malnutrition aggravates the symptoms, impairs the quality of life, and shortens life expectancy. A diagnosis of cancer or HIV infection alerts health care professionals to potential nutrition problems so that remedial steps can be taken to improve the quality of life and prevent early death.

Cancer

The thought of cancer often strikes fear in people. Indeed, cancer ranks just below cardiovascular disease as a cause of death, and thus many people have personal experiences with cancer. As with cardiovascular diseases, however, the prognosis for cancer today is far brighter than in the past. Identification of risk factors, new detection techniques, and innovative therapies offer hope and encouragement.

Cancer is not a single disorder. There are many *cancers*, that is, many different kinds of malignancies. They have different characteristics, occur in different locations in the body, take different courses, and require different treatments.

cancers: diseases that result from the unchecked growth of malignant tumors.

tumor: a new growth of tissue forming an abnormal mass with no function; also called a **neoplasm** (NEE-oh-plazm). Tumors that multiply out of control, threaten health, and require treatment are **malignant** (ma-LIG-nant). Tumors that stop growing without intervention or can be removed surgically and pose no threat to health are **benign** (bee-NINE).

malignus = of bad kind
benign = mild

Cancers are classified by the tissues or cells from which they develop:

- **Adenomas** (ADD-eh-NO-mahz) arise from glandular tissues.
- **Carcinomas** (KAR-see-NO-mahz) arise from epithelial tissues.
- **Gliomas** (gly-OH-mahz) arise from glial cells of the central nervous system.
- **Leukemias** (loo-KEY-mee-ahz) arise from the white blood cells.
- **Lymphomas** (lim-FOE-mahz) arise from lymph tissue.
- **Melanomas** (MEL-ah-NO-mahz) arise from pigmented skin cells.
- **Sarcomas** (sar-KO-mahz) arise from muscle, bone, or connective tissues.

A cancer that spreads from one part of the body to another is said to **metastasize** (me-TAS-tah-size).

HOW CANCER DEVELOPS

The genes in a healthy body work together regulating cell division to ensure that each new cell is a replica of the parent cell. In this way, the healthy body grows, replacing dead cells and repairing damaged ones. Cancers develop from mutations in the genes that regulate cell division. The mutations silence the genes that ordinarily monitor replicating DNA for chemical errors. The affected cells seemingly have no built-in brakes to halt cell division. As the abnormal mass of cells, called a malignant *tumor* or *neoplasm*, grows, blood vessels form to supply the tumor with the nutrients it needs to support its growth. Eventually, the tumor invades healthy tissue and may spread. Clinicians describe cancers by their size and extent, specifically noting if the tumor has spread to surrounding lymph nodes or to distant sites in the body. Figure 30–1 illustrates tumor formation.

Genetic Factors Some cancers appear to have a genetic component. A person with a family history of breast cancer, for example, has a greater risk of developing breast cancer than a person without such a genetic predisposition. This does not mean, however, that the person *will* develop cancer, only that the risk is greater.

Figure 30–1

Tumor Formation

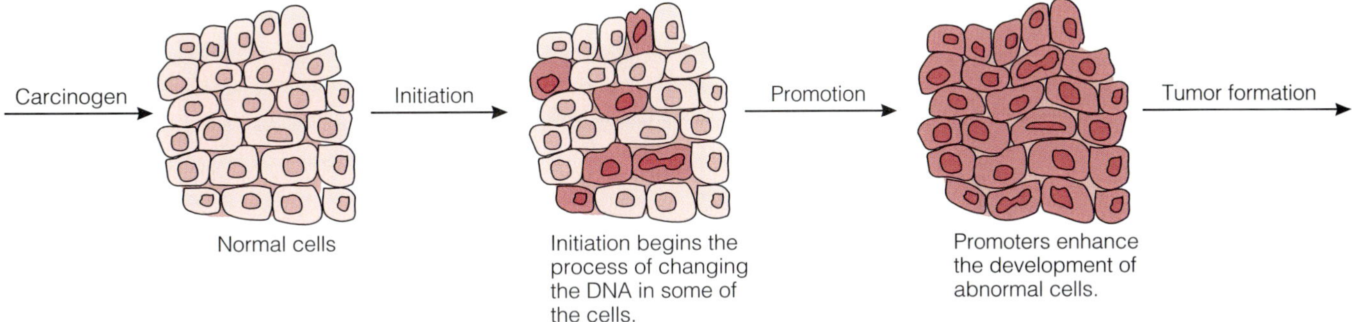

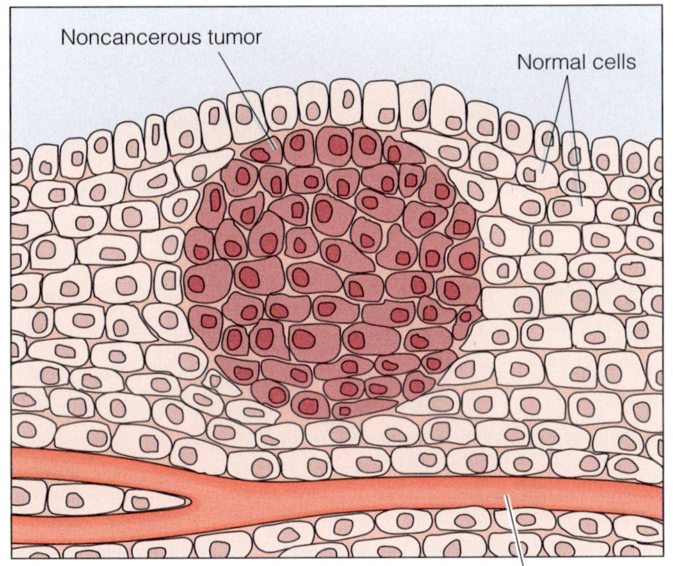

A noncancerous (benign) tumor usually grows within a self-contained capsule. It does not invade nearby tissue, nor does it spread.

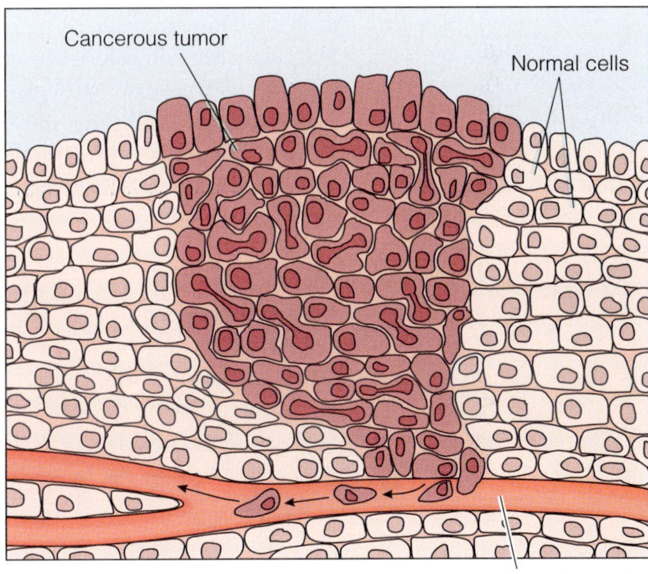

A cancerous (malignant) tumor usually grows out of control and may spread to other parts of the body through the blood or lymph systems.

Immune Factors A healthy immune system recognizes foreign cells and destroys them. Researchers theorize that an ineffective immune system may interfere with the recognition of tumor cells as foreign, thus allowing tumor growth. Aging affects immune function, and the incidence of cancer increases with age. Medications that suppress the immune system and viral infections (including HIV infection) and other disorders that severely tax the immune system may increase the risk of cancer.

Environmental Factors Among environmental factors exposure to radiation and sun, water and air pollution, and smoking are known to cause cancer. As Table 30–1 shows, dietary constituents are also associated with an increased

Table 30–1

Factors Associated with Cancer at Specific Sites

Cancer Sites	High Incidence Associated with:	Protective Effect Associated with:
Esophageal cancer	High alcohol use, tobacco use, and especially combined use; use of preserved foods (such as pickles); low intakes of vitamins and minerals; high intakes of vitamin A supplements	
Stomach cancer	High intakes of salt-preserved foods (such as dried, salted fish); low intakes of fresh fruits and vegetables	Fresh fruit and vegetables
Colorectal cancer	High intakes of fat (particularly saturated fat), meat, and alcohol (especially beer); low intakes of fiber, folate, and vegetables; inactivity	High intake of vegetables
Liver cancer	Infection with hepatitis B or aflatoxins; high intakes of alcohol; iron overload	
Pancreatic and lung cancer	No dietary risk factors have been established; correlated primarily with cigarette smoking	Fruits and vegetables, especially green and yellow ones
Breast cancer	High intakes of food energy and alcohol; little or no association with dietary fat specifically	Fruits and vegetables, especially green and yellow ones
Ovarian cancer	No dietary risk factors have been established; inversely correlated with oral contraceptive use	Fruits and vegetables, especially green and yellow ones
Cervical cancer	Folate deficiency	
Endometrial cancer	No dietary risk factors have been established; associated with estrogen therapy, obesity, hypertension, and diabetes (NIDDM)	
Bladder cancer	*Possible* associations with coffee, artificial sweeteners, and alcohol; associated with cigarette smoking	Fruits and vegetables, especially green and yellow ones
Prostate cancer	High fat intake, especially saturated fats from meats	Fruits and vegetables, especially green and yellow ones

Note: Findings based on epidemiological studies.

Sources: Committee on Diet and Health, *Diet and Health: Implications for Reducing Chronic Disease Risk* (Washington, D.C.: National Academy Press, 1989), pp. 594–600; J. H. Weisburger, Nutritional approach to cancer prevention with emphasis on vitamins, antioxidants, and carotenoids, *American Journal of Clinical Nutrition* (supplement) 53 (1991): 226–237; R. G. Ziegler, Vegetables, fruits, and carotenoids and the risk of cancer, *American Journal of Clinical Nutrition* (supplement) 53 (1991): 251–259; Potential mechanisms for food-related carcinogens and anticarcinogens: A scientific status summary by the Institute of Food Technologists' Expert Panel on Food Safety and Nutrition, *Food Technology* 47 (1993): 105–118.

Factors such as radiation and carcinogens (car-SIN-oh-jenz) which cause mutations that give rise to cancer are called **initiators**.

Factors that favor the development of cancer once it has begun are called **promoters**.

Factors that oppose the development of cancer are called **antipromoters**.

risk of certain cancers. Some dietary factors may initiate cancer development, others may promote cancer development once it has started, and still others may protect against the development of cancer.

Dietary Factors—Cancer Initiators We do not know to what extent diet contributes to cancer development, although some experts estimate that diet may be responsible for a third or more of all cases. Many people think that certain foods are carcinogenic, especially those that contain additives or pesticides. As Chapter 14 explained, however, our food supply is one of the safest in the world. Additives that have been approved for use in foods are not carcinogenic. Some pesticides are carcinogenic at high doses, but not at the concentrations allowed on fruits and vegetables.[1]

The incidence of cancers, especially stomach cancers, is high in parts of the world where people eat a lot of heavily smoked, pickled, or salt-cured foods that produce carcinogenic nitrosamines. Most commercial manufacturers in the United States use different preservative methods, and all are carefully controlled to minimize carcinogenic contamination.

Alcohol has also been associated with a high incidence of some cancers, especially of the mouth and throat. Beverages such as beer and scotch may contain damaging nitrosamines as well as alcohol.[2] The amounts of these compounds found in alcoholic beverages currently on the market are not considered harmful—assuming consumption in moderate amounts. These findings illustrate clearly why any potential benefit of moderate alcohol consumption on cardiovascular disease (see Highlight 28) must be weighed against potential dangers.

Dietary Factors—Cancer Promoters Unlike carcinogens, which initiate cancers, some dietary components may accelerate cancers that have already begun to develop. Studies suggest that certain dietary fats eaten in excess may promote cancer, in part by contributing to obesity. More specifically, linoleic acid, the omega-6 fatty acid of vegetable oils, has been implicated in enhancing cancer development in rats.[3] (In contrast, omega-3 fatty acids from fish oils appear to delay cancer development.)

Dietary Factors—Antipromoters It seems apparent that, besides promoters, foods may contain antipromoters. Almost without exception, epidemiological studies find a link between eating plenty of fruits and vegetables and a low incidence of cancers.[4] The fiber in fruits and vegetables helps to protect against some cancers by speeding up the transit time of all materials through the colon so that the colon walls are not exposed to cancer-causing substances for long. In addition to fiber, fruits and vegetables contain both nutrients and nonnutrients that protect against cancer. By acting as scavengers of oxygen-derived free radicals, the antioxidant nutrients beta-carotene, vitamin C, and vitamin E may help to prevent cell and tissue damage that can give rise to cancer. Phytochemicals common to many vegetables, especially those of the cabbage family, can activate enzymes that are capable of destroying carcinogens. (Highlight 11 describes the cancer preventive properties of antioxidants and phytochemicals in more detail.)

DIETARY GUIDELINES TO REDUCE CANCER RISKS

On the basis of current knowledge and available evidence, the following dietary guidelines are recommended for cancer prevention:

- Control weight and prevent obesity.
- Reduce consumption of total fat to 30 percent or less of total food energy.
- Increase fiber intake to 20 to 30 grams per day.
- Include a variety of vegetables and fruits in the daily diet.
- Minimize consumption of salt-cured, salt-pickled, and smoked foods.
- Consume alcoholic beverages in moderation, if at all.

One additional recommendation is in order: *vary food choices*. This last suggestion is based on an important concept—dilution. Switching from food to food dilutes the negative qualities of a food. For example, it is safe to eat *some* salt-cured or smoked meats, but not all the time. Combine such foods with a variety of others so that any carcinogens that may be present will be diluted in the total diet.

Some dietary factors, such as alcohol and heavily smoked or salted foods, may initiate cancer development; others, such as dietary fat, may promote cancer once it has gotten started; and still others, such as fiber and antioxidant nutrients and nonnutrients, may serve as antipromoters that protect against the development of cancer. Eating many green, yellow, and orange vegetables, including high-fiber foods, and reducing fat intake offer the best possible nutrition at the lowest possible risk.

NUTRITION CONSEQUENCES OF CANCER

Once cancer has developed, its consequences depend on its severity, location, and treatment. An isolated, nonspreading type of skin cancer may be removed in a physician's office with no observable effect on nutrition status, but a pancreatic cancer may seriously impair the person's ability to digest and absorb nutrients. Similarly, cancers of the gastrointestinal tract can severely affect nutrition status. The following sections describe the kinds of nutrition problems that often occur in certain types of cancers.

cancer cachexia (ka-KEKS-ee-ah) **syndrome:** a syndrome that frequently accompanies many types of cancer; characterized by anorexia, inadequate intake of food, malnutrition, accelerated metabolism and wasting, and general ill health.

Cancer Cachexia Just as cardiac cachexia describes the PEM associated with heart failure, cancer cachexia describes the PEM associated with cancer. Loss of appetite, weight loss, and depletion of lean body mass and serum proteins typify the cancer cachexia syndrome, which affects about two-thirds of people with cancer. It is often evident at the time of diagnosis. The combination of poor appetite, accelerated and abnormal metabolism, and the diversion of nutrients to support tumor growth simultaneously reduces the supply of energy and nutrients and increases the demand for them.

People who develop cachexia swiftly fall into a downward spiral. Poor food intake paired with heightened nutrient demands leads to muscle wasting and general poor health, which diminishes intake further. The body is unable to respond to this reduced nutrient supply as it does during uncomplicated fasting, so it continues to deplete its nutrient stores at an accelerated rate. The resulting malnutrition compromises the quality of life and may lead to complications and early death. Figure 30–2 summarizes some of the many known causes of the cancer cachexia syndrome.

Reminder: *Cytokines* are proteins secreted as part of the immune response (see Chapter 25). Some of the cytokines identified as mediators of cancer cachexia include tumor necrosis factor (cachectin), interleukin-1 alpha and beta, interleukin-6, interferon-τ, and differentiation factor.

Mechanisms of Cachexia Altered metabolism begins early in tumor development, even before weight loss occurs. Cachexia appears to be tumor derived; that is, the tumor itself causes the changes that lead to cachexia, and removal of the tumor can reverse the cachexia. Cytokines, secreted by the host's immune system in response to tumors, appear to be important mediators of the cancer cachexia syndrome.[5] They induce anorexia and alter metabolism. Current research into the roles of various cytokines and possible ways to block their actions holds promise for treating cachexia.

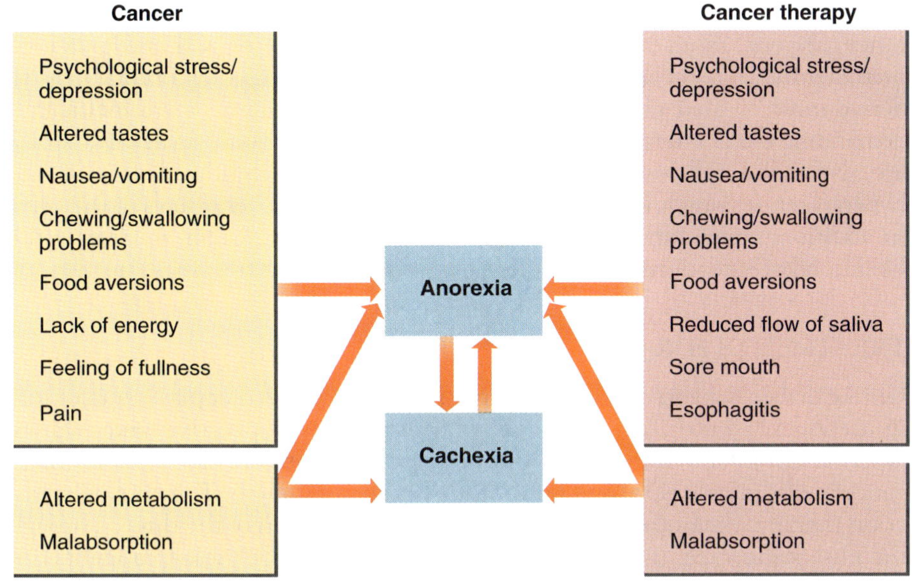

Figure 30–2

Causes of the Cancer Cachexia Syndrome

Anorexia and cachexia contribute to each other. Cancer itself and the available treatments for it make both problems worse.

Anorexia and Inadequate Nutrient Intake Anorexia is widely recognized as the major precipitating event in cancer cachexia. Factors contributing to anorexia in the person with cancer include:

- *Early satiety and nausea*. A premature feeling of fullness after eating small amounts of food or nausea may interfere with the appetite.
- *Fatigue*. People with cancer often tire easily and lack energy to prepare meals and eat.
- *Pain*. People in pain may have little interest in food, particularly if eating aggravates the pain.
- *Psychological stress*. The very diagnosis of cancer as well as its treatment can cause so much anxiety that eating becomes unimportant.
- *Obstructions*. A tumor may partially or completely obstruct any portion of the GI tract and interfere with chewing and swallowing; cause delayed gastric emptying, nausea, or vomiting; or make oral diets impossible.

Nutrient Losses Excessive nutrient losses in the person with cancer can contribute to deteriorating nutrition status. Depending on the location and type of cancer as well as its treatments, the person may experience nutrient losses due to inadequate digestion, malabsorption, vomiting, and diarrhea.

Maldigestion and malabsorption frequently accompany cancer of the pancreas (which depletes digestive enzymes) or liver (which depletes bile salts). Tumors of the small intestine can cause malabsorption, as does a tumor that obstructs the upper small intestine, creating a blind loop (see Chapter 22). Some tumors directly cause severe vomiting, diarrhea, or both, and electrolyte imbalances and dehydration may result. (Later sections describe the nutrient losses associated with various cancer treatments.)

Cancer-induced causes of nutrient losses include:
- Inadequate digestion.
- Malabsorption.
- Vomiting.
- Diarrhea.

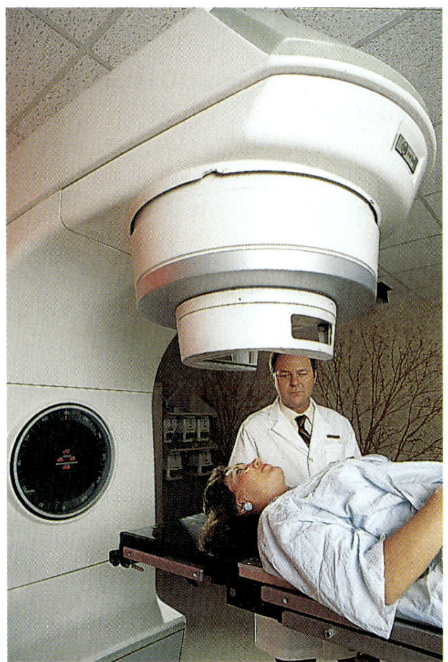
Radiation therapy is one of several weapons in the fight against cancer.

Metabolic Alterations Some people with cancer are hypermetabolic while others are not. In all cases, metabolic pathways are altered and nutrients used inefficiently. In comparison to the metabolic pathways used by normal cells to derive most of their energy, the pathways used by tumor cells are inefficient, demanding extra energy nutrients and wasting vital protein tissues. Fat stores are also mobilized. Many people with cancer develop insulin resistance and hyperglycemia, which interferes with the availability of energy fuels to the cells. In addition, cancer and its treatments tax the immune system, increasing the likelihood of infections, which raise energy and nutrient needs still further.

TREATMENTS FOR CANCER

Unlike diabetes, heart disease, and renal failure, in which diet plays a major role in treatment, nutrition therapy in cancer is only supportive and will be described in a later section. The primary cancer treatments aim to annihilate cancer cells, relieve pain, and prevent further tumor growth. They include radiation therapy, chemotherapy, surgery, or any combination of the three. Through their use, cancer can sometimes be arrested, but ironically, these treatments can also threaten health and nutrition status. Table 30–2 summarizes the nutrition-related side effects of radiation and chemotherapy, and Table 30–3 shows how various cancer surgeries can affect nutrition status.

Table 30–2

Possible Causes of Wasting Associated with Radiation and Chemotherapy

	Reduced Nutrient Intake	Accelerated Nutrient Losses	Altered Metabolism
Radiation	Anorexia Damage to teeth and jaws Esophagitis Mouth ulcers Nausea Reduced salivary secretions Taste alterations Thick salivary secretions Vomiting	Chronic blood loss from intestine and bladder Diarrhea Fistula formation Intestinal obstructions Malabsorption Vomiting	Secondary effects of malnutrition or infection
Chemotherapy	Abdominal pain Anorexia Mouth ulcers Nausea Taste alterations Vomiting	Diarrhea Intestinal ulcers Malabsorption Vomiting	Fluid and electrolyte imbalances Hyperglycemia Interference with vitamins or other metabolites Negative nitrogen and calcium balance Secondary effects of malnutrition or infection

Table 30–3

Possible Effects of Surgery for Cancer on Nutrition Status

Head and Neck Resection	
Difficulty in chewing/swallowing	Inability to chew/swallow
Esophageal Resection	
Diarrhea	Reduced gastric motility
Fistula formation	Steatorrhea (fat malabsorption)
Reduced gastric acid secretion	Stenosis (constriction)
Gastric Resection	
Dumping syndrome	Lack of gastric acid
General malabsorption	Vitamin B_{12} malabsorption
Hypoglycemia	
Intestinal Resection	
Blind loop syndrome	General malabsorption
Diarrhea	Hyperoxaluria
Fluid and electrolyte imbalance	Steatorrhea
Pancreatic Resection	
Diabetes mellitus	General malabsorption

Radiation Therapy Radiation therapy disrupts DNA replication and, consequently, cell division. In doing so, radiation damages all actively dividing cells—normal body cells as well as tumor cells. Treatment is often effective because cancer cells divide more rapidly than normal cells, they are damaged more severely by radiation, and they are slower to recover from its effects. Therapists must carefully administer radiation treatments in doses that target tumor cells and minimize damage to normal cells.

radiation therapy: the use of radiation to arrest or destroy cancer cells.

The cells of the GI tract, bone marrow, hair, and skin are actively dividing and are often affected by cancer treatments.

Radiation therapy can cause fatigue, anorexia, nausea, vomiting, and diarrhea. Radiation may inflame tissues in the mouth and esophagus, lead to the development of mouth ulcers, interfere with the flow of saliva, and damage teeth and the bones of the jaws—all of which can make chewing and swallowing painful and difficult. The person may develop food aversions if certain foods are associated with the radiation therapy. Radiation therapy to the small intestine can alter the structure of the intestinal cells (radiation enteritis) and result in malabsorption, chronic blood loss, and fluid and electrolyte imbalances. The intestinal wall may become thick and fibrotic, narrowing the intestinal lumen and increasing the likelihood that an intestinal obstruction or a fistula will develop. Small blood vessels may become so inflamed that blood flow to some sections of the bowel may be blocked. Any of these events can be fatal. Intestinal function may return after radiation therapy ends, but for some, the changes are permanent.

radiation enteritis: radiation damage to intestine.

chemotherapy: the use of drugs to arrest or destroy cancer cells. Drugs used for chemotherapy are called **chemotherapeutic** or **antineoplastic agents**.
chemo = chemical

Chemotherapy Medications can also be used to interrupt cell division, but like radiation, they have undesirable side effects. Chemotherapeutic agents include some antibiotics, alkaloids, alkylating agents, antimetabolites, steroids, and others. The current trend in chemotherapy is to use high doses of several chemotherapeutic agents together in cycles. This method helps ensure that malignant cells will be destroyed. Although these treatments are often effective, they frequently intensity undesirable side effects.

Chemotherapy can dramatically reduce food intake by causing nausea, vomiting, altered taste perceptions, mouth ulcers, reduced flow of saliva, and food aversions. Additionally, chemotherapy may cause diarrhea, malabsorption, and peptic ulcers that aggravate nutrient losses. Chemotherapy using vitamin antagonists interferes with normal metabolic pathways, further compromising nutrition status.

Rx PRESCRIPTION PAD

Drugs used in the treatment of cancer may include:

- Analgesics
- Antidiarrheals
- Anti-inflammatory agents
- Antinauseants
- Antineoplastics
- Appetite stimulants
- Sedatives

See Appendix E for timing with meals and nutrition-related side effects.

Other Drug Therapy Depending on which organ systems are affected by cancer and by the side effects of treatment, many other medications may also be used in treatment. Medications commonly used to treat symptoms of cancers include antinausea agents, antidiarrheals, analgesics, and sedatives.

Several medications may be useful in the treatment of wasting.[6] The most promising medication, megestrol acetate, stimulates the appetite and promotes weight gain (primarily as body fat). Preliminary studies suggest that growth hormone and insulin-like growth factor can promote weight gain, particularly a gain in lean body mass. Dronabinol (a medication containing the principal psychoactive ingredient in marijuana) works as both an appetite stimulant and an antiemetic and may be useful in some cases.

Surgery Often surgery is necessary to remove the tumor. The side effects of surgery depend on the location of the tumor and its size (see Table 30–3). Surgery is often followed by radiation or chemotherapy to prevent new tumor growth.

Surgery can also cause anorexia, nausea, and vomiting. Some surgeries, such as a partial or total removal of the tongue, resection of the muscles of the mouth, esophagus, or salivary glands, and removal of the jaw, invariably create extensive problems with chewing and swallowing. Surgeries may also aggravate nutrient losses through diarrhea, malabsorption, and blood loss. Surgery also accelerates metabolism because it initiates the stress response.

bone marrow transplant: the replacement of diseased bone marrow in a recipient with healthy bone marrow from a donor; used as a treatment for breast cancer, leukemia, and other blood disorders.

Bone marrow transplants may be a treatment for leukemia, lymphomas, and certain blood disorders.

graft-versus-host disease (GVHD): destruction of healthy donor cells by the recipient's immune system, which recognizes the donor cells as foreign.

Bone Marrow Transplants The use of bone marrow transplants to treat certain cancers and blood disorders has grown markedly.[7] During a bone marrow transplant, the individual's diseased bone marrow is replaced with healthy bone marrow from a donor, usually a close relative. Before the bone marrow transplant is performed, the recipient is treated with high doses of chemotherapy and sometimes whole-body radiation therapy. In addition, immunosuppressants are given before and after the procedure. Although these procedures effectively kill abnormal cells and help prevent tissue rejection, they also render the individual defenseless against infections. Antibiotics are frequently prescribed.

Graft-versus-host disease (GVHD), a serious complication of bone marrow transplants, develops when the recipient's body mounts an immune system attack against healthy donor cells, which it recognizes as foreign. Most often, the skin, liver, and GI tract are affected. Acute GVHD develops within a few months of transplantation; chronic GVHD may develop later.

The preparatory procedures for a bone marrow transplant frequently result in anorexia, taste alterations, nausea, vomiting, and inflammation of mucous membranes of the GI tract. Following transplantation, severe diarrhea and malabsorption, with fluid losses often exceeding 10 liters per day, signal acute GVHD.[8] Immunosuppressive drugs used to help treat or prevent GVHD can lead to negative nitrogen and calcium balances, sodium and fluid retention, muscular weakness, osteoporosis, and glucose intolerance.

Other Treatments Researchers continue to search for more effective ways of treating people with cancer. One such treatment, immunotherapy, provides antigens to bolster the immune system so that it can recognize and attack cancer cells. Another treatment being investigated uses highly specific antibodies to deliver chemotherapy directly to the cancer site, thus leaving healthy cells unaffected. The overall effectiveness of these therapies remains undetermined at present.

Alternative Therapies People who feel they are making little progress in their fight against cancer or think conventional medicine offers little hope of recovery may try alternative therapies. (Highlight 20 provides a perspective on alternative therapy.) Fortunately, most people with cancer rely on traditional medical treatments, although they may supplement them with alternative therapies.[9]

Health care professionals should be alert to alternative therapies that include nutrition components. Potentially harmful practices include:

- Discontinuing prescribed therapy to adhere to an unproven remedy.
- Following a diet that eliminates or severely restricts specific food groups.
- Taking vitamins or minerals that can be toxic in large doses.
- Using herbal preparations that may be contaminated.

Cancer and its treatments lead to cachexia—a combination of anorexia, accelerated nutrient losses, and altered metabolism. In fact, many people with cancer die from cachexia rather than the cancer itself.[10] Providing optimal nutrition care supports recovery and improves quality of life.

NUTRITION SUPPORT FOR PEOPLE WITH CANCER

Prior to the widespread use of tube feedings and TPN, the deteriorating nutrition status that accompanies cancer was largely accepted. Without a way to feed people who simply could not eat, many practitioners believed that emaciation and physical debilitation were inevitable. Others believed that if you fed the client, you also fed the tumor, so to "starve the tumor," they would almost starve the client.

The Scope of Nutrition Support for Cancer Nutrition cannot cure cancer, nor is it a primary treatment. Whether nutrition support directly prolongs survival or improves tolerance for chemotherapy or radiation therapy has not been proven.[11] The wide variety of cancers and their various stages of development make proving a beneficial effect difficult. In some malnourished people with cancer, nutrition support has proven to be beneficial.[12] Attention to diet can help prevent or reverse poor nutrition status and its associated complications, and in this way, nutrition plays a supportive role in cancer therapy. Compared with the malnourished person, the person in good nutrition status:

- Feels better.
- Functions better.
- Is more active.
- Is stronger.
- Eats more.
- Resists infections better.
- Enjoys a better quality of life.

Although it is sometimes hard to quantify these benefits, they are of great importance to the person with cancer.[13]

Dietary Interventions Considering the many adverse effects that threaten the appetite of a person with cancer, health care professionals face an enormous challenge in helping these individuals maintain nutrition status. Every bit of nutrition knowledge and interpersonal skill helps, beginning with the professional's awareness of the client's predicament. Oral food intake can often be improved once the individual's specific problems are addressed. The box on pp. 946–947 is long and detailed, reflecting both the complexity and the importance of offering specific suggestions to deal with specific problems.

Energy and Protein Needs Actual nutrient needs vary depending on the type and severity of the cancer, its treatment, and the person's nutrition status. Table 30–4 shows diet modifications that may be necessary for different types of cancer. Often clinicians aim to provide about 1.5 times the basal energy expenditure and 1.5 to 2.0 grams of protein per kilogram of body weight per day.

To review calculations of basal energy expenditure, see Table 25–3 on p. 809.

Women diagnosed with breast cancer often gain, rather than lose, weight, and this weight gain can be distressing.[14] Health care professionals serve these clients best by helping them avoid unnecessary weight gain.

Vitamins and Minerals Vitamin and mineral needs are highly variable depending on the specific treatment and the presence and severity of complications such as vomiting and malabsorption. The individual must be carefully monitored for early signs of nutrient deficiencies to prevent the development of serious deficiencies.

Tube Feedings and TPN Because studies have failed to confirm that aggressive nutrition support directly benefits survival and response to cancer treatment, tube feedings or TPN are not routinely recommended for adequately nourished or mildly malnourished people with cancer who must undergo surgery, chemotherapy, or radiation therapy.[15] Special nutrition support may be indicated, however, when anorexia persists or when a person is severely malnourished, particularly during and immediately after other cancer treatments. As is true whenever special nutrition support is indicated, tube feedings are preferred to TPN when the GI tract is functional. People requiring head and neck resections may need long-term tube feedings and may need to continue tube feedings at home. People with severe radiation enteritis may require home TPN.

Table 30–4

Dietary Considerations for Various Cancers

Cancer Sites	Dietary Considerations
Brain	Physical feeding disabilities (see Highlight 21); chewing and swallowing problems see (Chapter 21).
Head/neck	Chewing and swallowing problems.
Mouth/esophagus	Chewing and swallowing problems; if obstructed, tube feeding below the obstruction may be necessary.
Stomach	Nausea, vomiting; if obstructed, tube feeding below the obstruction or TPN may be necessary; if resection is performed, a postgastrectomy diet (see Chapter 21) may be needed; nutrient deficiencies due to bacterial overgrowth (Chapter 22) may occur.
Intestine	If obstructed, tube feeding or TPN may be necessary; resections or inflammation may cause multiple nutrition problems (see Chapter 22); fat- and lactose-restricted diet may be useful.
Liver	Protein-, sodium-, and fluid-restricted diet may be necessary (see Chapter 26).
Pancreas	Fat-restricted diet and enzyme replacements may be necessary (see Chapter 22); diabetic diet may be necessary if insulin production is affected (see Chapter 27).
Kidneys	Protein-, electrolyte-, and fluid-controlled diet may be necessary (see Chapter 29).

Note: The considerations listed here are specific to the type of cancer; they do not include other nutrition-related concerns, such as anorexia, nausea, and vomiting.

Ethical Issues Every malnourished person with cancer who cannot consume an adequate diet orally is a potential candidate for aggressive nutrition support. Before tube feeding or parenteral nutrition is undertaken, some important questions should be considered. What is the prognosis if the cachexia can be reversed and progressive wasting can be arrested? Will the person survive longer? Will the quality of life improve? Will therapy be more successful? Does the client want aggressive nutrition support? Special nutrition support should be undertaken only if it can provide direct benefits and the client is in agreement. For the person with little hope of recovery, the as yet unproven benefits of specialized nutrition support may not be worth the cost and discomfort involved. Making this decision requires good clinical judgment from the health care team as well as consideration of the client's feelings about the goals of nutrition therapy. (Highlight 24 describes these and other ethical issues that must be considered when people receive tube feedings or TPN.)

Nutrition Support before Bone Marrow Transplants Because the GI tract is severely compromised by the preparatory procedure for a bone marrow transplant, TPN is routinely provided. Although not extensively studied, tube

How to Help Clients Handle Food-Related Problems

For each problem, find a solution using these suggestions.

1. *To improve nutrient intake:*
   - Explain why eating is important.
   - Encourage clients to eat the most when they feel the best.
   - Encourage people to eat extra food between chemotherapy or radiation treatments.
   - Suggest that clients eat nutrient-dense foods first.
   - Recommend indulging in favorite foods throughout the day.
   - Encourage clients to eat with family and friends.
   - Recommend smaller, more frequent meals.
   - Advise clients to avoid drinking large amounts of liquids with meals.
   - Work out a medication schedule that allows the client to take pain or antinausea medications at times when they will be effective during meals.
   - Provide a pleasant and relaxed environment.
   - Serve foods attractively.
   - Reassess clients regularly to solve problems as they arise.
2. *To save energy for eating:*
   - Recommend that others prepare foods.
   - Suggest foods that are easy to prepare and eat.
   - Encourage the use of time-saving appliances for food preparation.
3. *To combat bitter or metallic taste perceptions:*
   - Advise clients to brush their teeth or use a mouthwash before eating.
   - Recommend adding sauces and seasonings to meats.
   - Suggest that meats be served cold or at room temperature.
   - Encourage clients to try using eggs, fish, poultry, and dairy products instead of meats.
   - Encourage clients to try new foods and experiment with herbs and spices.
4. *To control nausea and vomiting:*
   - Give antinausea drugs at times when they will be effective during meals.
   - Recommend small, frequent meals.
   - Advise clients to avoid spicy and high-fat foods.
   - Suggest that clients avoid food odors that cause nausea. It may help to have others prepare meals, if possible.
   - Encourage clients to save most liquids for after meals. Clear liquids or popsicles after meals help prevent dehydration.
   - Suggest that clients get fresh air, loosen tight clothing, or rest after meals.

5. *To prevent food aversions:*
   - Suggest that clients save favorite foods for time when they are feeling relatively good.
   - Advise clients not to eat their favorite foods during the times of day when they usually experience nausea or vomiting.
   - Suggest that clients maintain a food-free "window" of an hour or so before and after treatment times, if the treatments cause nausea or vomiting.
6. *To alleviate problems with chewing and swallowing:*
   - Work with clients to find the consistency of food that will be easiest to handle. Thin liquids, true solids, and sticky foods are often difficult to swallow.
   - Recommend that clients add sauces and gravies to dry foods.
   - Provide fluids with meals to ease chewing and swallowing.
   - Advise clients with mouth sores to try foods at cooler temperatures. They are often soothing.
   - Recommend that clients with mouth ulcers avoid foods that are spicy, acidic, or coarse; foods that contain seeds that can be trapped in an ulcer; or sticky foods such as peanut butter that may be difficult to swallow.
   - Recommend that clients experiment with tilting the head forward and backward to see if swallowing is easier with the head positioned differently.
   - Suggest a straw for drinking.
   - Encourage clients who suffer from a reduced flow of saliva to rinse the mouth frequently. Artificial saliva from the pharmacy can also help. Sour candy or gum can stimulate the flow of saliva.
   - Encourage good oral and dental hygiene to prevent cavities and oral infections.
7. *To add kcalories and protein:*
   - Add milk powder to liquid milk, meat loafs, casseroles, soups, puddings, and cereals.
   - Add ground meats, chicken, fish, or grated cheeses to sauces, soups, casseroles, or vegetables.
   - Eat peanut butter on fruit, celery, or crackers.
   - Use plenty of butter, margarine, mayonnaise, cream cheese, oil, and salad dressings on breads, sandwiches, potatoes, vegetables, salads, pasta, and rice.
   - Use yogurt, sour cream, or a sour cream dip with vegetables.
   - Add whipping cream to deserts and hot chocolate, or use it to lighten coffee.
   - Have snacks available at all times.
   - Add nuts and dried fruits such as raisins to desserts, cereals, or salads.
   - Use cream instead of milk with cereal.
   - Try commercially available liquid supplements or instant breakfast mixes for milk shakes, meals, or between-meal snacks.
   - Use whole milk instead of low-fat or nonfat milks.

feedings have also proven effective in providing nutrition support for bone marrow transplant recipients.[16] Appropriate nutrition support helps to heal the GI tract and support the immune system. Glutamine added to the TPN solution may be particularly beneficial for people undergoing bone marrow transplants (see Highlight 22). Researchers have found that adding glutamine to TPN solutions results in fewer infections and shorter hospital stays for bone marrow transplant recipients.[17]

Nutrition Support after Bone Marrow Transplants After a bone marrow transplant, the person usually continues TPN until GI function returns. As the person begins to receive food orally, parenteral nutrition is gradually tapered off (see Chapter 24). The nutrition-related side effects of the bone marrow transplant procedure make oral intake difficult, and the individual needs encouragement from all members of the health care team. Early oral feedings often start with lactose-free, low-residue, low-fat liquids to maximize absorption and minimize nausea, vomiting, and steatorrhea. Gradually, solid foods are introduced. For about three months after a transplant, the diet excludes most fresh fruits and vegetables, undercooked meats, poultry and eggs, and ground meats to minimize the risk of food-borne bacterial infections. Fiber and lactose are gradually added to the diet as individual tolerances allow. Additional fat is given if steatorrhea is not evident.

After a bone marrow transplant, nutrition complications can be severe and debilitating, especially for people with gastrointestinal GVHD. Because the bone marrow recipient must take immunosuppressants following the procedure, recommendations include a high-protein, high-calcium diet. In addition, physicians often prescribe calcium and vitamin D supplements. Individuals with persistent diarrhea are encouraged to eat high-potassium foods (see Figure 12–7 on p. 425). The accompanying box provides a case study for cancer.

human immunodeficiency virus (HIV): the virus that causes AIDS. The infection progresses to become an immune system disorder that leaves its victims defenseless against numerous infections.

acquired immune deficiency syndrome (AIDS): the end stage of HIV infection, in which severe complications are manifested.

Human Immunodeficiency Virus (HIV) Infection and Acquired Immune Deficiency Syndrome (AIDS)

For many years, the devastating effects of infection by the human immunodeficiency virus (HIV), the infection that eventually causes acquired immune deficiency syndrome (AIDS), seemed unstoppable. And although the disease still has no cure, remarkable progress has been made in understanding and treating HIV infections, giving rise to a renewed hope that a cure may be possible. Without a cure, however, the best course is prevention. Transmission of the virus requires sexual activity, direct blood contact, or passage of the infection from a mother to her infant during pregnancy, birth, or breastfeeding. Table 30–5 on p. 950 presents strategies for preventing HIV transmission.

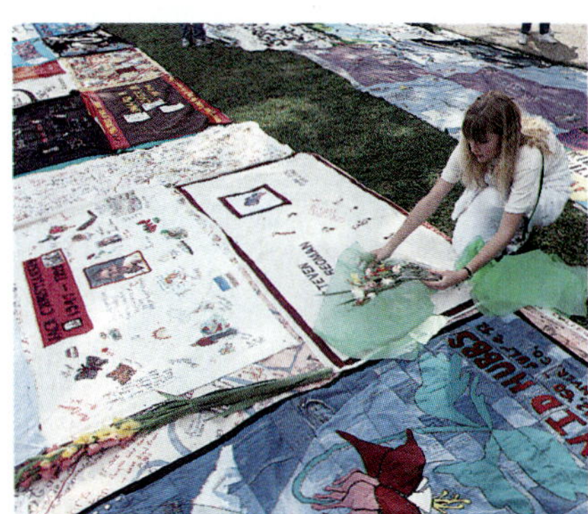

The countless lives touched by AIDS serve as a potent reminder of the need to continue the search for a cure.

Once a person has been infected with HIV, it takes about 6 to 12 weeks before laboratory tests can confirm a diagnosis. Because people remain symptom-free in the early stages of infection, however, they may not even be tested for HIV for several years following infection. Thus early detection to prevent the spread of HIV infection and to ensure early treatment for the person infected is an important health goal.

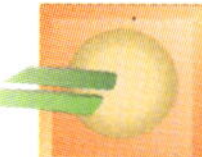

Case Study Retired Newscaster with Cancer

Mr. Bustamante is a retired newscaster who first visited his doctor when he noticed that he was losing weight rapidly and was easily fatigued. He also had a lesion in his mouth that wouldn't heal. Mr. Bustamante smokes a pack of cigarettes a day and has a history of alcohol abuse. After he was admitted to the hospital, tests confirmed a diagnosis of cancer of the mouth. The doctor would like to prepare Mr. Bustamante nutritionally before proceeding with radiation therapy. Radical surgery is a possibility. A thorough nutrition assessment reveals that Mr. Bustamante is suffering from severe mixed PEM. His height is 5 feet 10 inches, and he weighs 125 pounds.

What is Mr. Bustamante's ideal weight? His %IBW? What other anthropometric measurements would you expect to see affected?

Given his PEM status, what lab test results would you expect to find? How might Mr. Bustamante's past history have affected his nutrition status before he developed cancer?

In what ways can cancer affect his nutrition status? How can radiation therapy affect his nutrition status? Discuss the possible impact of radical head and neck surgery on his nutrition status.

Describe cancer cachexia. What are some of its causes? What are the benefits of preventing or correcting it?

If Mr. Bustamante is able to take food by mouth, what suggestions will you give him for dealing with poor appetite, nausea and vomiting, dry and sore mouth, and chewing and swallowing problems?

If Mr. Bustamante is unable to eat an oral diet, is aggressive nutrition support indicated? Why or why not?

HOW AIDS DEVELOPS

HIV infection attacks the immune system and leaves its victims defenseless against opportunistic infections and disorders from which most people are protected. The disorder begins with infection by the virus and progresses in stages. The virus gradually destroys cells with a specific protein called CD4+ on their surfaces. Among the cells most affected are CD4+ T-lymphocytes, essential components of the immune system. At first, CD4+ lymphocytes decline gradually, and the HIV-infected individual remains symptom-free. As the infection progresses, though, depletion of CD4+ lymphocytes greatly impairs immune function. Early symptoms may include fatigue, skin rashes, fevers, diarrhea, muscle pain, night sweats, weight loss, oral lesions and infections, and other opportunistic infections that are not life-threatening. In the final stages, frequent and often fatal complications arise, such as severe weight loss; tuberculosis; recurrent bacterial pneumonia; serious infections of the central nervous system, GI tract, and skin; cancers; and severe diarrhea. On average, it takes about 10 years for an HIV infection to progress to AIDS. Clinicians monitor the progress of HIV infection by measuring the concentrations of CD4+ lymphocytes and the circulating virus (viral load).

opportunistic infections: infections from microorganisms that normally do not cause disease in the general population but can cause great harm in people once their immune systems are compromised (as in HIV infection).

CD4+ T-lymphocyte: a type of circulating white blood cell that has the CD4+ protein on its surface and is a necessary component of the immune system.

The cluster of mild symptoms that sometimes occur early in the course of AIDS is called **AIDS-related complex (ARC)**.

People with AIDS frequently experience severe PEM and wasting. The wasting often begins early in the progression of the disease and becomes worse. People with AIDS may lose up to 34 percent of their ideal body weight in the four to five months before death, a degree of wasting similar to that seen in people who die from starvation.[18] Such findings prompt clinicians to speculate that severe wasting alone causes the death of some individuals with AIDS.[19] Even

Table 30–5

Strategies to Prevent HIV Transmission

HIV is transmitted from one person to another by direct contact with contaminated body fluids, most often through sexual intercourse, through contaminated needles or blood products, or from mother to infant during pregnancy or lactation. To prevent the transmission of HIV infection:

- Avoid sexual contact with anyone with an HIV infection.
- Use a latex condom and a spermicidal agent during sexual contact unless you are in a monogamous relationship with a person who is free from AIDS and whose sexual history you know.
- Do not share toothbrushes, razors, or other implements that could be contaminated with blood.
- Exercise caution when undergoing procedures such as acupuncture, tattooing, or ear piercing, in which needles might be contaminated.
- If you are an IV drug user, seek help for your addiction. Meanwhile, use only sterile, unused needles and dispose of them so that others will not use them. Avoid unprotected sexual contact with others.

when other complications ultimately cause death, malnutrition appears to be an important cofactor. Studies suggest that for people with AIDS, malnutrition contributes to disease-related complications and morbidity.[20] Finally, although direct evidence is lacking, the effects of PEM on the immune system, combined with those of HIV infection, may hasten the course of the disease. A later section describes the wasting associated with HIV infection.

TREATMENTS FOR HIV INFECTION

The antiviral drugs used in the treatment of HIV infection include zidovudine (AZT), didanosine (ddl), zalcitabine (ddC), stavudine (d4T), lamivudine (3TC), nevirapine, indinavir, ritonavir, and saquinavir.

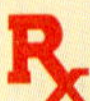

PRESCRIPTION PAD

Drugs used in the treatment of HIV infection may include:

- Analgesics
- Antidiarrheals
- Anti-infectives
- Antinauseants
- Antineoplastics
- Appetite stimulants

See Appendix E for timing with meals and nutrition-related side effects.

Treatments for HIV infection focus on improving the individual's comfort and quality of life by slowing the course of the infection and controlling its symptoms. Clinical trials of new drug treatments for HIV infection have yielded encouraging results and have expanded the array of medications available for treatment.

Drug therapy often includes a combination of AZT (zidovudine) and other medications called protease inhibitors that prevent the virus from replicating. Studies are underway to determine if providing combinations of medications in the earliest stages of infection might destroy the virus. In addition to drugs targeted to destroy the HIV virus, other medications are used to treat the symptoms and complications of HIV infection. The medications described on p. 942 can also be used to prevent wasting due to HIV infection. Diet therapy, which plays a supportive role in the treatment of HIV infection, is described in a later section.

THE HIV WASTING SYNDROME

The wasting associated with HIV infection occurs in the later stages and shares many similarities with the wasting associated with cancer. In both, the causes of malnutrition are related to the disease, its complications, and its treatments. Both result in inadequate nutrient intake, excessive nutrient losses, and hypermetabolism. As is true for cancer cachexia, the cytokines appear to play an important role in HIV wasting. Slow, progressive weight loss is usually associated with reduced food intake and gastrointestinal complications, whereas rapid weight loss is most often associated with infections.[21] The strongest predictors of weight loss and depletion of lean body mass and fat in people with HIV infection include anorexia, diarrhea, and other infections.[22] Table 30–6 lists the many factors that lead to progressive wasting from HIV infection.

Anorexia and Inadequate Nutrient Intake People with AIDS have inadequate nutrient intakes for reasons similar to those of people with cancer. Clinicians report that the oral intakes of hospitalized people with AIDS meet only 70 percent of their *basal* energy needs and 65 percent of their protein needs.[23] These percentages would be even lower if the extra energy and protein needs imposed by hypermetabolism and activity were taken into account. Indeed, another group of investigators found that HIV-infected people with additional infections did not consume adequate energy to meet their high metabolic needs.[24]

HIV-related causes of anorexia include:

- *Psychological stress and pain*. Depression over the HIV diagnosis, progression, and prognosis and the medical, personal, and financial problems that lie ahead, as well as the pain associated with the disorder, can destroy the appetite.
- *Oral infections*. Infections and fever cause anorexia. In addition, oral infections associated with HIV cause further problems. Thrush, a common oral infection associated with HIV infection, can alter taste sensitivity, reduce the flow of

HIV-related causes of anorexia include:
- Depression.
- Fever.
- Pain.
- Mouth blindness.
- Dry mouth.
- Difficulty swallowing.
- Mouth ulcers.
- Esophageal lesions and obstructions.
- Use of oxygen masks.
- Drug therapy.
- Lethargy.
- Dementia.

Table 30–6

Possible Causes of Wasting in HIV Infection

Reduced Food Intake	
Altered taste perceptions	Infections
Cancer/cancer therapy	Lack of energy to eat
Difficulty chewing/swallowing	Mouth blindness
Drug therapy	Nausea/vomiting
Dry mouth	Oral lesions
Esophageal lesions/obstructions	Pain
Fear, depression, and dementia	Use of oxygen masks
Fever	
Accelerated Nutrient Losses	**Altered Metabolism**
Cancer/cancer therapy	Cancer
Diarrhea	Drug therapy
Drug or other therapy	Infections
Infections	
Malabsorption	
PEM	

thrush: a fungal infection of the mouth and esophagus caused by *Candida albicans*; the technical term for this infection is candidiasis. Thrush is characterized by a thick white coating of the tongue that alters taste sensations and causes pain on chewing and swallowing.

herpes virus: a virus that can lead to mouth lesions and may also affect the lower GI tract, causing diarrhea.

Kaposi's (cap-OH-seez) **sarcoma:** a type of cancer rare in the general population but common in people with HIV infection.

saliva, and cause pain on swallowing. Oral infections caused by the herpes virus can cause painful mouth ulcers that interfere with chewing and swallowing.

- *Respiratory infections*. Pneumonia and tuberculosis cause fever and pain that contribute to anorexia. The person who uses an oxygen mask may find eating difficult.
- *GI tract complications and altered organ function*. In addition to the problems associated with oral infections, people with HIV may experience belching, gastric reflux, and heartburn that may interfere with eating. Intestinal complications and altered organ function contribute to anorexia, early satiety, and food aversions.[25]
- *Cancer*. As previously described, cancer leads to anorexia. Kaposi's sarcoma, a cancer associated with HIV infection, can cause lesions and obstructions in the esophagus that make eating very painful.
- *Medical treatments*. Drugs used to treat HIV infection, associated infections, and cancer often cause anorexia, nausea, and vomiting that reduce food intake. Food aversions associated with medical treatments can also arise.
- *Lethargy and dementia*. In the later stages of AIDS, lethargy and dementia become common problems that interfere with food intake. The individual may be chronically exhausted and may not care or even remember to eat.

AIDS-induced causes of nutrient losses include:

- HIV infection.
- GI tract infections.
- Cancer.
- Cancer therapy.
- Anti-infective drugs.
- Megadoses of vitamins.
- Home remedies for AIDS.
- Reduced gastric acid secretion.
- Bacterial overgrowth.
- Malnutrition.

The diarrhea and malabsorption associated with AIDS for which no known cause has been identified are called **AIDS enteropathies**.

Nutrient Losses In addition to anorexia, AIDS and its complications and treatments accelerate nutrient losses and contribute to wasting. From 50 to 90 percent of people with AIDS experience chronic or recurrent diarrhea and malabsorption, often associated with GI tract infections (see Table 30–7). Foods may serve as a source of infectious agents, and people with advanced HIV infection are highly susceptible to food-borne illness. Diarrhea may be severe and unresponsive to drug therapy—the person may lose from 10 to 15 liters of diarrheal fluids daily.

Nutrient losses may also arise when advanced HIV infection suppresses gastric acid secretion. A high gastric pH limits the absorption of iron and calcium

Table 30–7

Causes of GI Infections in AIDS

Bacterial	**Protozoan**
Clostridium dificile	*Cryptosporidium* species
Mycobacterium avium-intracellulare	*Giardia lamblia*
Mycobacterium tuberculosis	*Isosporia belli*
Salmonella species	*Microsporidium* species
Fungal	*Pneumocystitis carinii*
Candida albicans	*Toxoplasma gondii*
Cryptococcus neoformans	**Viral**
Parasitic	AIDS enteropathy
Nonpathogenic amoeba	*Cytomegalovirus* species
Entamoeba histolytica	Epstein-Barr
	Herpes simplex

and allows bacteria to grow in the upper GI tract. Bacterial overgrowth can lead to fat malabsorption and vitamin B_{12} and folate deficiencies (see Chapter 22).

Treatments common among HIV-infected individuals, especially anti-infective agents, chemotherapy, and radiation therapy, can accelerate nutrient losses due to vomiting, diarrhea, and malabsorption. Megadoses of vitamin C and other home remedies that some people with HIV infection use may also cause diarrhea. Once malnutrition is underway, it, too, contributes to malabsorption.

Metabolic Alterations The accelerated metabolism associated with repeated infections significantly taxes nutrition status in people with HIV infection (see Chapter 25). Metabolic alterations associated with cancer also affect people with HIV infection who have cancer.

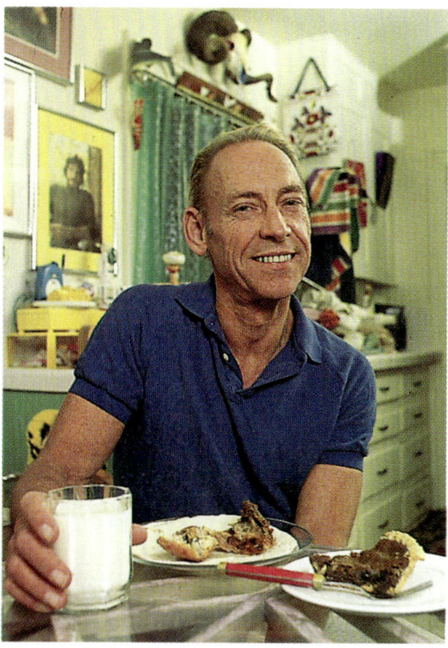

Nutrition provides an edge in maintaining quality of life and encouraging independence.

NUTRITION SUPPORT FOR PEOPLE WITH HIV INFECTION

In an era of improved treatments and prolonged survival for people with HIV infection, measures that improve the quality of life assume great importance. Attention to nutrition cannot change the ultimate outcome of an HIV infection, but it can offer an improved quality of life and possibly slow disease progression. Good nutrition status may also improve a person's response to drug therapy, reduce duration of hospital stays, and promote physical independence.[26] At a minimum, meeting nutrient needs eliminates the additional stresses imposed by malnutrition.

Benefits of Early Nutrition Support Nutrition intervention takes a high priority from the moment an individual receives a positive diagnosis for HIV infection. The initial nutrition assessment evaluates the individual's current nutrition status and establishes baseline parameters from which to monitor changes. Nutrition therapy may be most effective in the early stages of HIV infection when reduced food intake is more likely to lead to malnutrition than in the later stages when repeated infections and hypermetabolism quickly deplete nutrient stores.[27] Clinicians can begin to encourage gradual improvements in eating habits before the person becomes debilitated and the task becomes monumental.

Oral Diets Nutrition counseling for clients with HIV infection often includes recommendations for high-energy, high-protein diets; strategies for avoiding food-borne illnesses; and suggestions for alleviating anorexia, altered taste sensations, nausea and vomiting, and difficulty with chewing and swallowing (see the box on pp. 946–947). Often clinicians recommend that clients take daily vitamin and mineral supplements that provide at least 100 percent of the RDA. Health care professionals remind clients that supplements are intended to augment dietary sources, not to replace them.

Energy and protein needs for people with HIV infection depend on the stage of the infection and the complications associated with each case. Typical diets provide 1.5 times the basal energy expenditure (see Chapter 25) and at least 1.5 g of protein per kilogram of body weight per day.

Provided early in the course of HIV infection, nutrition counseling, a standard high-energy, high-protein diet, and oral supplements have been successful in halting weight loss and restoring weight in people without secondary infections.[28] Limited research suggests that immune-enhancing formulas that include omega-3 fatty acids, arginine, and nucleotides (see p. 815) may improve nutrition status early in the course of HIV infection, possibly by modulating the effects of tumor necrosis factor, a cytokine associated with wasting.[29] Other researchers report that supplementing the diet with hydrolyzed protein and fish oil (rich in omega-3 fatty acids) may help prevent weight loss and reduce the frequency of hospitalizations in the early stages of HIV infection.[30] Whether special formulas confer benefits over regular high-energy, high-protein foods and formulas in the early stages of HIV infection remains to be proven. Because special formulas are quite expensive and people with HIV infection face an enormous financial burden in treating their disorders, standard formulas (see Chapter 23) may be appropriate for people with weight loss related to poor food intake. Special formulas, however, may be beneficial for people who develop malabsorption or secondary infections.[31]

Treatment of Diarrhea Treatment of HIV-associated diarrhea depends on its cause and the extent to which the intestine is affected. Although diarrhea is sometimes unresponsive to therapy, often a pathogen can be identified. Appropriate drug therapy along with the provision of adequate fluids and electrolytes is at the core of treatment. Drinking plenty of fluids is essential. The liberal use of table salt, salty broths, and high-potassium foods and juices can help replace electrolytes. Oral rehydration formulas (see Chapter 22) may be useful for severe cases of diarrhea. Other dietary modifications may include lactose and fat restrictions.

Susceptibility to food-borne illnesses requires that the individual with HIV infection be given written and oral instructions on the safe handling of foods. Table 14–1 on p. 488 summarizes food-borne illnesses and describes ways to prevent them.

Tube Feedings and Parenteral Nutrition Individuals unable to consume adequate oral diets to prevent nutrition complications and unintentional weight loss need aggressive nutrition support. Both enteral and parenteral nutrition support have been shown to be effective in repleting lean body mass and promoting weight gain in some people with AIDS.[32] As a guideline, aggressive nutrition support should be considered when:

- The individual loses 5 percent of body weight within one month.
- The individual loses more than 10 percent of body weight over the past six months.[33]
- It can provide direct benefits and the client is in agreement.

As always, tube feedings are preferred to parenteral feeding. Tube feedings given at night can supplement oral diets during the day. If pain or obstructions in the upper GI tract make nasogastric passage of the feeding tube difficult or painful, gastrostomy or jejunostomy feedings are indicated. Preventing bacterial contamination of the formula is particularly important because of the susceptibility of HIV-infected individuals to GI infections.

TPN is generally reserved for people with HIV infection who are unable to tolerate enteral nutrition, but need to maintain their nutrition status while undergoing a therapy that is expected to improve their condition. TPN may be more useful in repleting the body mass of people whose primary problems are reduced food intake or malabsorption than in supporting those who have other

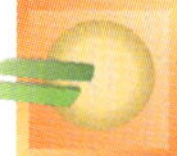

Case Study Travel Agent with HIV Infection

Mr. Sands, a travel agent, sought medical help at age 34 when he began feeling run-down and developed a painful white coating over his mouth and tongue. The presence of thrush and anemia alerted Mr. Sands's physician to the possibility of an HIV infection. When Mr. Sands tested positive for an HIV infection, he and his family and friends were devastated by the news. Fortunately, those closest to him have been supportive during this difficult time, and he has a strong desire to live out his life as independently as possible.

Four months after the diagnosis of HIV infection, Mr. Sands developed a serious, continuous diarrhea that required hospitalization to classify and control. Since the diagnosis of HIV infection was made, Mr. Sands has lost 10 pounds. At 6 feet tall, he currently weighs 158 pounds.

Describe how HIV infection can lead to reduced food intake, nutrient losses, and hypermetabolism.

From the limited information given here, what factors could have contributed to Mr. Sands's weight loss? Is his weight loss significant? What is Mr. Sands's %IBW? What steps could prevent further weight loss?

Discuss nutrition strategies for dealing with thrush and diarrhea.

What additional nutrition consequences might be anticipated if Mr. Sands develops cancer?

systemic diseases.[34] People with GI tract obstructions, severe vomiting, or GI infections affecting the entire small bowel may benefit from TPN.

systemic: affecting the whole body rather than one part or organ system.

The concern for infection when receiving TPN is magnified in people with AIDS because their immune systems are already compromised. Data are scarce, but seem to indicate that TPN can be used safely and effectively in AIDS treatment.[35] The accompanying box presents a case study on HIV infection.

Wasting and severe malnutrition are commonly associated with both cancer and HIV infection. Health care professionals who work with people with these disorders serve their clients best by identifying nutrition problems early (see the nutrition assessment checklist) and offering solutions before nutrition status seriously deteriorates.

This chapter brings to a close your introduction to normal and clinical nutrition. Congratulations! You have received an abundance of information since you first turned to page 1. The normal nutrition chapters of this text provided you with current recommendations to promote optimal health. You learned how the body transforms food into nutrients and how those nutrients support the body's growth and well-being. The clinical chapters of the text addressed you as a future health care professional, concerned not only with your own health, but also with the well-being of others throughout the life cycle and during times of illness. They provided guidelines on diet for a variety of disorders. Along the way, you learned about tube feedings, parenteral nutrition, and a variety of modified diets.

We hope that this text has served you well and that when selecting food for yourself or making recommendations for others, you will remember to honor the body. It is a prized possession. Nourish it well.

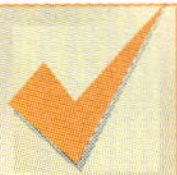

Nutrition Assessment Checklist

For People with Cancer and HIV Infection

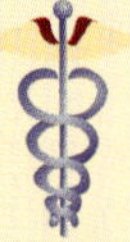

Medical Check the client's medical history for the type of cancer or stage of HIV infection, associated complications, medical therapy, and symptoms. A diagnosis of cancer or HIV infection alerts health care professionals to the need for a thorough nutrition assessment.

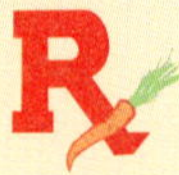

Drug Record the client's drug therapy for possible drug-nutrient interactions and nutrient-related complications. Antineoplastic agents, antiviral agents, anti-inflammatory agents, and antimicrobical agents can significantly and adversely affect nutrition status. Medications used to treat wasting can promote weight gain. Ask clients if they are using alternative therapies, including megadoses of vitamins and herbal preparations.

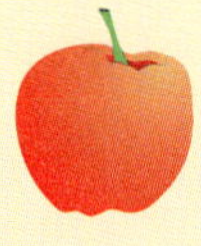

Food Intake Determine if anorexia or nutrition-related complications are interfering with the client's ability to eat. Aggressively work with clients to improve nutrient intake and preserve nutrition status in the early stages of cancer or HIV infection. For clients with pain or nausea, check the timing of the administration of analgesics and antinausea agents to be sure they are given at times when they will improve appetite.

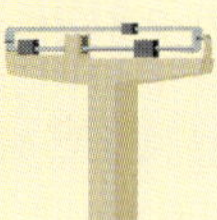

Anthropometric Measure height and weight at regular intervals to detect wasting early.

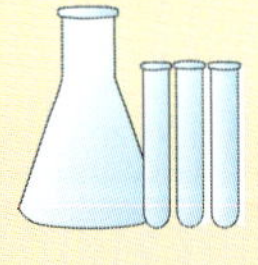

Laboratory Assess laboratory data for changes in nutrition status, fluid and electrolyte balance, organ function, and response to therapy. Low serum protein levels are common in both cancer and advanced HIV infection.

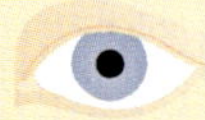

Physical Check for physical signs of nutrient deficiencies, dehydration (especially for those with fever, diarrhea, or vomiting), and mouth ulcers.

Study Questions

1. What is cancer? What events are believed to lead to its development?
2. What roles may dietary factors play in cancer development or cancer prevention? What dietary advice might be most effective in reducing the risk of cancer?
3. What is cancer cachexia? What factors contribute to its development?
4. Describe the anorexia that is associated with cancer. How does it differ from anorexia in other disease states? Discuss how cancer and its therapies contribute to anorexia.

5. How can cancer result in excessive nutrient losses, and how do these losses contribute to the cancer cachexia syndrome?
6. Describe the metabolic changes that occur in the person with cancer, and discuss their role in the cancer cachexia syndrome.
7. What are some of the treatments for cancer, and how do they work? In what ways can each treatment for cancer contribute to malnutrition?
8. Discuss strategies for combating anorexia, bitter or metallic tastes in the mouth, nausea and vomiting, problems with mouth ulcers, reduced flow of saliva, or other problems with chewing or swallowing.
9. What are the recommended uses for tube feedings and parenteral nutrition for people with cancer?
10. What is HIV infection? What are the consequences of HIV infection? What is the HIV wasting syndrome?
11. Describe factors that can lead to reduced nutrient intake, excessive nutrient losses, and altered metabolism in people with HIV infection.
12. In what ways might good nutrition status possibly alter the course of HIV infection?
13. Why are people with HIV infection highly susceptible to food-borne illness?

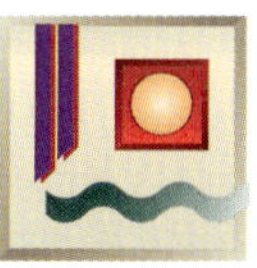

Clinical Applications

1. Many disorders can lead to wasting. For some of these, such as renal disease, diet is a cornerstone of treatment. For others, such as cancer and HIV infection, nutrition plays a supportive role. What determines whether nutrition plays a major or supportive role in the treatment of a disorder? Review the effects of PEM on pp. 199–202 and p. 551. Carefully consider how severe malnutrition can further debilitate people with cancer and advanced HIV infection.
2. Consider problems associated with nutrition in a 36-year-old woman with a malignant brain tumor affecting her ability to move the right side of her body (including the tongue) and to speak coherently. She has an expected length of survival of six months and is taking a pain medication that makes her nauseated and sleepy. What would be a realistic goal of nutrition support? If she is right-handed, how can her impairment interfere with eating? What suggestions might you have for overcoming this problem? How might nutrition be affected by her speech problems? Describe ways that the medications she is taking can affect her nutrition status. Would tube feedings or TPN be appropriate for this woman? Why or why not?

Notes

1. Council on Scientific Affairs, American Medical Association, Report of the Council on Scientific Affairs, Diet and cancer: Where do matters stand? *Archives of Internal Medicine* 153 (1993): 50–56.
2. H. Hwang, J. Dwyer, and R. M. Russel, Diet *Heliobacter pylori* infection, food preservation and gastric cancer risk: Are there new roles for preventative factors? *Nutrition Reviews* 52 (1994): 75–83.
3. R. A. Karmali, Fatty acid metabolism and biochemical mechanisms in cancer, in *Health Effects of Dietary Fatty Acids*, ed. G. J. Nelson (Champaign, Ill.: American Oil Chemists Society, 1991), pp. 150–156.
4. Y. Kim and J. B. Mason, Nutrition chemoprevention of gastrointestinal cancers: A critical review, *Nutrition Reviews* 54 (1996): 259–279.
5. T. C. Hardin, Cytokine mediators of malnutrition: Clinical implications, *Nutrition in Clinical Practice* 8 (1993): 55–59.
6. A. M. Herrington, J. D. Herrington, and C. A. Church, Pharmacologic options for the treatment of cachexia, *Nutrition in Clinical Practice* 12 (1997): 101–113.

7. T. Duell and coauthors, Health and functional status of long-term survivors of bone marrow transplantation. EBMT Working Party on Late Effects and EULEP Study Group on Late Effects. European Group for Blood and Marrow Transplantation, *Annals of Internal Medicine* 126 (1997): 184–192.
8. K. Ringwald-Smith, R. Krance, and L. Stricklin, Enteral nutrition support in a child after bone marrow transplantation, *Nutrition in Clinical Practice* 10 (1995): 140–143.
9. B. R. Cassileth and C. C. Chapman, Alternative and complementary cancer therapies, *Cancer* 77 (1996): 1026–1034.
10. C. Grunfeld, Therapy for treatment of the wasting syndrome in cancer and AIDS: What can we do and what should we do? *Nutrition in Clinical Practice* 12 (1997): 99–100.
11. W. W. Souba, Nutritional support, *New England Journal of Medicine* 336 (1997): 41–48.
12. A. M. B. Hunter, Nutrition management of patients with neoplastic disease of the head and neck treated with radiation therapy, *Nutrition in Clinical Practice* 11 (1996): 157–169.
13. D. F. Cella, Overcoming difficulties in demonstrating health outcome benefits, *Journal of Parenteral and Enteral Nutrition* (supplement) 16 (1992): 106–111.
14. W. Demark-Wahnefried, B. K. Rimer, and E. Winer, Weight gain in women diagnosed with breast cancer, *Journal of the American Dietetic Association* 97 (1997): 519–526, 529.
15. A.S.P.E.N. Board of Directors, Practice guidelines: Cancer, *Journal of Parenteral and Enteral Nutrition* (supplement) 17 (1993): 12–13.
16. Ringwald-Smith, Krance, and Stricklin, 1995.
17. T. R. Ziegler and coauthors, Clinical and metabolic efficacy of glutamine-supplemented parenteral nutrition after bone marrow transplantation, *Annals of Internal Medicine* 116 (1992): 821–828; P. R. Schloerb and M. Amare, Total parenteral nutrition with glutamine in bone marrow transplantation and other clinical applications (randomized, double-blind study), *Journal of Parenteral and Enteral Nutrition* 17 (1993): 407–413.
18. D. P. Kotler and coauthors, Magnitude of body-cell-mass depletion and the timing of death from wasting in AIDS, *American Journal of Clinical Nutrition* 50 (1989): 444–447.
19. D. O. Jacobs, Bioelectrical impedance analysis: A way to assess changes in body cell mass in patients with acquired immunodeficiency syndrome? *Journal of Parenteral and Enteral Nutrition* 17 (1993): 401–402.
20. U. Süttmann and coauthors, Incidence and prognostic value of malnutrition and wasting in human immunodeficiency virus–infected outpatients, *Journal of Acquired Immune Deficiency Syndromes and Human Retrovirology* 8 (1995): 239–246.
21. D. C. Macallan and coauthors, Prospective analysis of patterns of weight change in stage IV human immunodeficiency virus infection, *American Journal of Clinical Nutrition* 58 (1993): 417–424.
22. A. Schwenk and coauthors, Clinical risk factors for malnutrition in HIV-1-infected patients, *AIDS* 7 (1993): 1213–1219.
23. E. B. Trujillo and coauthors, Assessment of nutritional status, nutrient intake, and nutrition support in AIDS patients, *Journal of the American Dietetic Association* 93 (1993): 477–478.
24. C. Grunefeld, M. Pange, and L. Shimizu, Resting energy expenditure, caloric intake, and short-term change in HIV infection and AIDS, *American Journal of Clinical Nutrition* 55 (1992): 455–460.
25. C. Fields-Gardner, A review of mechanisms of wasting in HIV disease, *Nutrition in Clinical Practice* 10 (1995): 167–176.
26. Federation of American Societies for Experimental Biology, Nutrition and HIV infection: A review and evaluation of the extant knowledge of the relationship between nutrition and HIV infection, *Nutrition in Clinical Practice* (supplement) 6 (1991): 46–48.
27. J. A. Stack and coauthors, High-energy, high-protein, oral, liquid, nutrition supplementation in patients with HIV infection: Effect on weight status in relation to incidence of secondary infection, *Journal of the American Dietetic Association* 96 (1996): 337–341.
28. Stack and coauthors, 1996.
29. Süttmann and coauthors, 1995.
30. R. T. Chelowski and coauthors, Long-term effects of early nutrition support with new enterotropic peptide-based formula vs. standard enteral formula in HIV-infected patients: Randomized prospective study, *Nutrition* 9 (1993): 507–512.
31. Stack and coauthors, 1996.
32. A.S.P.E.N. Board of Directors, Acquired immune deficiency syndrome, *Journal of Parenteral and Enteral Nutrition* (supplement) 17 (1993): 13–14; P. Singer and coauthors, Risks and benefits of home parenteral nutrition in the acquired immunodeficiency syndrome, *Journal of Parenteral and Enteral Nutrition* 15 (1991): 75–79.
33. Department of Continuing Education in Health Sciences, UCLA Extension, 1989.
34. D. P. Kotler and coauthors, Effect of home total parenteral nutrition on body composition in patients with acquired immunodeficiency syndrome, *Journal of Parenteral and Enteral Nutrition* 14 (1990): 454–458.
35. Singer and coauthors, 1991.

Cost-Conscious Health Care

Decades of medical research have resulted in an explosion of knowledge and technologies to diagnose and treat diseases. This astounding progress, however, has come at a tremendous financial cost. Anyone who has paid an insurance premium or needed medical attention recently has felt the effects of skyrocketing health care costs. The United States spends more money on health care than any other nation, yet some citizens go without needed care. Without attention to cost containment, the health status of the nation is threatened; sophisticated medical services do little good if people cannot use them.

To address this problem, government officials, health care professionals, and insurance executives look for ways to cut costs without sacrificing quality and to make health care affordable to all people in the United States. Thus the medical community, which once embodied the idealistic approach of sparing no cost when it came to health care, has embraced the reality that cost is an element of quality.[1]

The full implications of cost containment and its impact on the nation's health remain to be seen. In the words of one clinician, "Our American society is in the midst of the most far reaching and profoundly disturbing uncontrolled study in the history of health care. We are experiencing major changes in the way we practice and pay for health care with very little evidence that these changes will achieve the desired outcome."[2] To address all of the ramifications of cost containment for health care delivery and payment systems is beyond the scope of this highlight. Instead, this highlight focuses on how cost containment affects nutrition services and how attention to nutrition might help reduce health care costs. As you read, keep in mind that as new strategies are implemented and studied, some will prove successful and others will not.

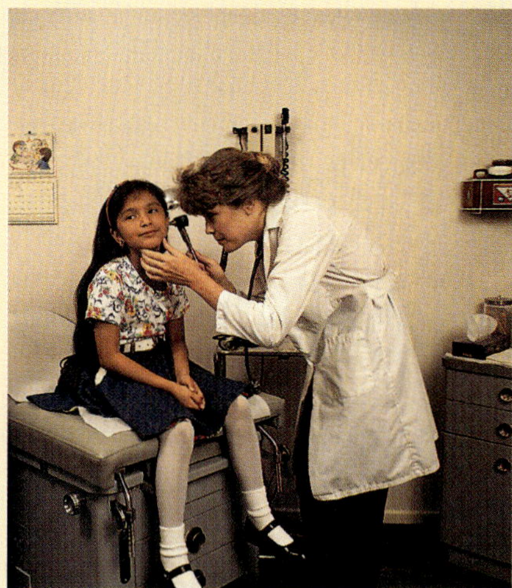

Health care professionals work diligently to deliver high-quality health care while controlling costs.

OUTCOME-ORIENTED CARE

Among other things, efforts to control health care costs aim at eliminating duplication of services, limiting access to unnecessary services, and reducing the number of hours or professionals involved in client care. Spurred by changes in the government insurance program (Medicare), which successfully lowered health costs by limiting reimbursement for services, traditional fee-for-service medical insurance is increasingly being replaced by managed care systems. (The glossary defines insurance-related and other terms.) Managed care organizations, which were rare just 15 years ago, now account for over 40 percent of the insurance provided by employers, and that percentage appears to be rising.[3] Managed care, which includes health maintenance organizations (HMOs) and preferred provider organizations (PPOs), is a health care delivery system that strives to control the use of resources to achieve the best health outcomes at tolerable costs.[4]

Glossary

health maintenance organization (HMO): a form of managed care that limits the subscriber's choice of health care professionals and controls access to services by directing care through a primary care physician.

indemnity insurance: traditional insurance that pays a fee for service.

managed care: a health care delivery system that is directed at providing quality health care at tolerable costs by coordinating services.

preferred provider organization (PPO): a form of managed care that encourages subscribers to select health care providers from a group that has contracted with the organization to provide services at lower costs.

Implicit in managed care and any effort to reduce medical costs is the need to identify which services provide the best outcomes at the lowest costs. The more expensive the procedure or test, the more critical justifying its costs becomes. For example, the clinical benefits of highly technical, costly, and potentially hazardous nutrition services, such as tube feedings and parenteral nutrition, are justified only when they have a reasonable chance of improving the client's outcome. Examples of desirable outcomes include the person's ability to function independently (the more care a person needs, the more expenses incurred), reduced hospital stays, prevention of complications, and extended survival time. For a person with cancer, the costs of tube feedings or parenteral nutrition might be justified if the person's inability to eat, rather than the cancer itself, is interfering with treatment or quality of life.[5] In other cases, the ability of tube feedings or parenteral nutrition to improve outcomes remain unproven; thus their associated costs are difficult to justify.

In representing nutrition professionals, the American Dietetic Association takes the position that managed care organizations and integrated health delivery systems should provide medical nutrition therapy as an essential component of health care and that it should be provided by qualified nutrition professionals.[6] Nutrition professionals must keep abreast of changing health care delivery systems and document how their unique knowledge and skills provide cost-effective care.[7]

Nutrition advocates continue to respond to the challenge of cost containment by documenting the proper use of nutrition services, improved outcomes associated with medical nutrition therapy, and innovative ways to reduce costs associated with nutrition therapy.[8] In one analysis of data from several sources, researchers report that early attention to malnutrition in hospitalized clients may result in cost savings of approximately $8300 per hospital bed per year.[9]

The speed at which cost containment measures are sweeping through the medical community suggests that there is little time to hesitate. Without data to support the costs of valuable health services such as nutrition, third-party payers (insurers) may opt to exclude services that might ultimately improve the quality of health care. Trying to implement changes later will be far more difficult. The rest of this highlight describes specific strategies nutrition professionals have begun to use to control costs and ensure the inclusion of their services.

CLINICAL PATHWAYS

To ensure that people's nutrition needs are addressed in the changing health care environment, nutrition professionals must be actively involved in the development of outcome measures and standards of care that guide health care. One such example, clinical pathways, is described here. Clinical pathways, also called *critical pathways* or *care maps*, are used to provide coordinated, outcome-oriented, cost-effective care. Clinical pathways are charts or tables that map out a plan of care for a specific diagnosis, procedure, or treatment. The plan defines a time frame for each intervention with a goal of providing the best outcome at the lowest cost. The development of a clinical pathway requires a multidisciplinary approach that focuses on the goal of the pathway, rather than on individual professional interests.[10]

The health care team develops each clinical pathway after careful study of their unique client population. Once in place, each pathway must be reassessed by studying unexpected outcomes or variances from the expected plan. When necessary, the pathway is improved.

To ensure that clients' nutrition needs are addressed in clinical pathways, nutrition professionals must actively participate in the multidisciplinary teams that develop the pathways and monitor their effectiveness. To be successful, nutrition professionals must educate themselves in areas beyond nutrition; they need to understand how to manage data, resources, programs, finances, and people.[11] They must develop skill in balancing nutrition needs with other medical needs and in making compromises that will not jeopardize the overall quality of care.[12]

HOME CARE

Another change in health care delivery, spurred by rising health care costs, is a shift from hospital care to home care. Early discharges lower hospital costs. Because clients may be discharged before they have regained health, however, they may require additional medical care at home. By teaching clients and caregivers to perform many of the procedures formerly performed by hospital staff, health care costs can be reduced. Some home care clients receive therapeutic diets as part of their treatment plans; others continue tube feedings and parenteral nutrition programs at home (see Chapter 24).

Nutrition professionals seek to ensure that nutrition services are included in home health care delivery systems. With their specialized knowledge and skills, nutrition professionals are uniquely qualified to assess nutrition status and to implement measures to prevent or correct malnutrition. They are also uniquely qualified to resolve eating problems (such as anorexia or nausea) and to evaluate the best feeding method (such as oral diet, tube feedings, or TPN) and composition of the diet (such as high protein or low sodium). The task for nutrition professionals is to document how these nutrition services improve outcomes and save money.[13] Dietitians in home health care need business and marketing skills to ensure that their nutrition services will be available to clients and that their position in the market will be secure.[14]

Clearly, health care professionals need to work within the health care system to provide cost-effective nutrition care without sacrificing quality. Suggestions for providing cost-saving, yet appropriate, nutrition care include:

- Use a qualified professional (registered dietitian) to complete a nutrition assessment and determine the most appropriate nutrition care plan for each person.
- Identify nutrition interventions that can prevent or treat disease and document the positive effects and cost savings of these services.
- Recommend the most cost-effective method of feeding people (oral, enteral, or parenteral).

Whatever the final direction of health care delivery, one thing is certain. Health care professionals must continue to provide high-quality nutrition care in a cost-effective manner. In doing so, they help to ensure that quality, affordable health care will be available to all.

NOTES

1. A. Bothe, Consensus: We should not lower quality to cut costs, *Nutrition in Clinical Practice* (supplement) 10 (1995): 1–7.
2. J. R. Wesley, Managing the future of nutrition support, *Journal of Parenteral and Enteral Nutrition* 20 (1996): 383–384.
3. J. K. Iglehart, The American health care system: Introduction, *New England Journal of Medicine* 326 (1992): 962–967; D. A. August, Creation of a specialized nutrition support outcomes research consortium: If not now, when? *Journal of Parenteral and Enteral Nutrition* 20 (1996): 394–400.
4. A. W. Wojner and A. Hedberg, Incorporating nutrition care into critical pathways for improved outcomes, in *Integrating Nutrition Care into Critical Pathways*, Report of the Fifteenth Ross Roundtable on Medical Issues (Columbus, Ohio: Ross Laboratories, 1995), pp. 1–8.
5. W. W. Souba, Nutritional support, *New England Journal of Medicine* 336 (1997): 41–48.
6. American Dietetic Association, Position of The American Dietetic Association: Nutrition services in managed care, *Journal of the American Dietetic Association* 96 (1996): 391–395.
7. August, 1996; R. Chernoff, Managing managed care—A mission impossible? *Journal of the American Dietetic Association* 96 (1996): 715.
8. E. L. Johnson and S. Valera, Medical nutrition therapy in non-insulin-dependent diabetes mellitus improves clinical outcomes, *Journal of the American Dietetic Association* 95 (1995): 700–701; B. R. Dahl and M. H. Read, Effect of a nutrition education program on the reduction of serum cholesterol level in Veterans Administration outpatients, *Journal of the American Dietetic Association* 95 (1995): 702–703; M. R. Gallagher-Allred and coauthors, Malnutrition and clinical outcomes: The case for medical nutrition therapy, *Journal of the American Dietetic Association* 96 (1996): 361–369; D. B. Schwartz, Enhanced enteral and parenteral nutrition practice and outcomes in an intensive care unit with a hospital-wide performance improvement process, *Journal of the American Dietetic Association* 96 (1996): 484–489; M. A. Puangco, H. L. Nguyen, and M. J. Sheridan, Computerized PN ordering optimizes timely nutrition therapy in a neonatal intensive care unit, *Journal of the American Dietetic Association* 97 (1997): 258–261; J. Maurer and coauthors, Reducing the inappropriate use of parenteral nutrition in an acute care teaching hospital, *Journal of Parenteral and Enteral Nutrition* 20 (1996): 272–274.
9. H. N. Tucker and S. G. Miguel, Cost containment through nutrition intervention, *Nutrition Reviews* 54 (1996): 111–121.
10. L. Wolf, Integrating nutrition care into critical pathways: An example, in *Integrating Nutrition Care into Critical Pathways*, Report of the Fifteenth Ross Roundtable on Medical Issues (Columbus, Ohio: Ross Laboratories, 1995) pp. 28–31.
11. Chernoff, 1996.
12. Wolf, 1995.
13. T. Byars, Dietetics professionals are paving new paths in home care, *Support Line*, December 1996, pp. 1–4.
14. A. Arkin, Marketing nutrition services to home health care: A client-focused, three-step marketing strategy, *Support Line*, December 1996, pp. 11–13.

Appendixes

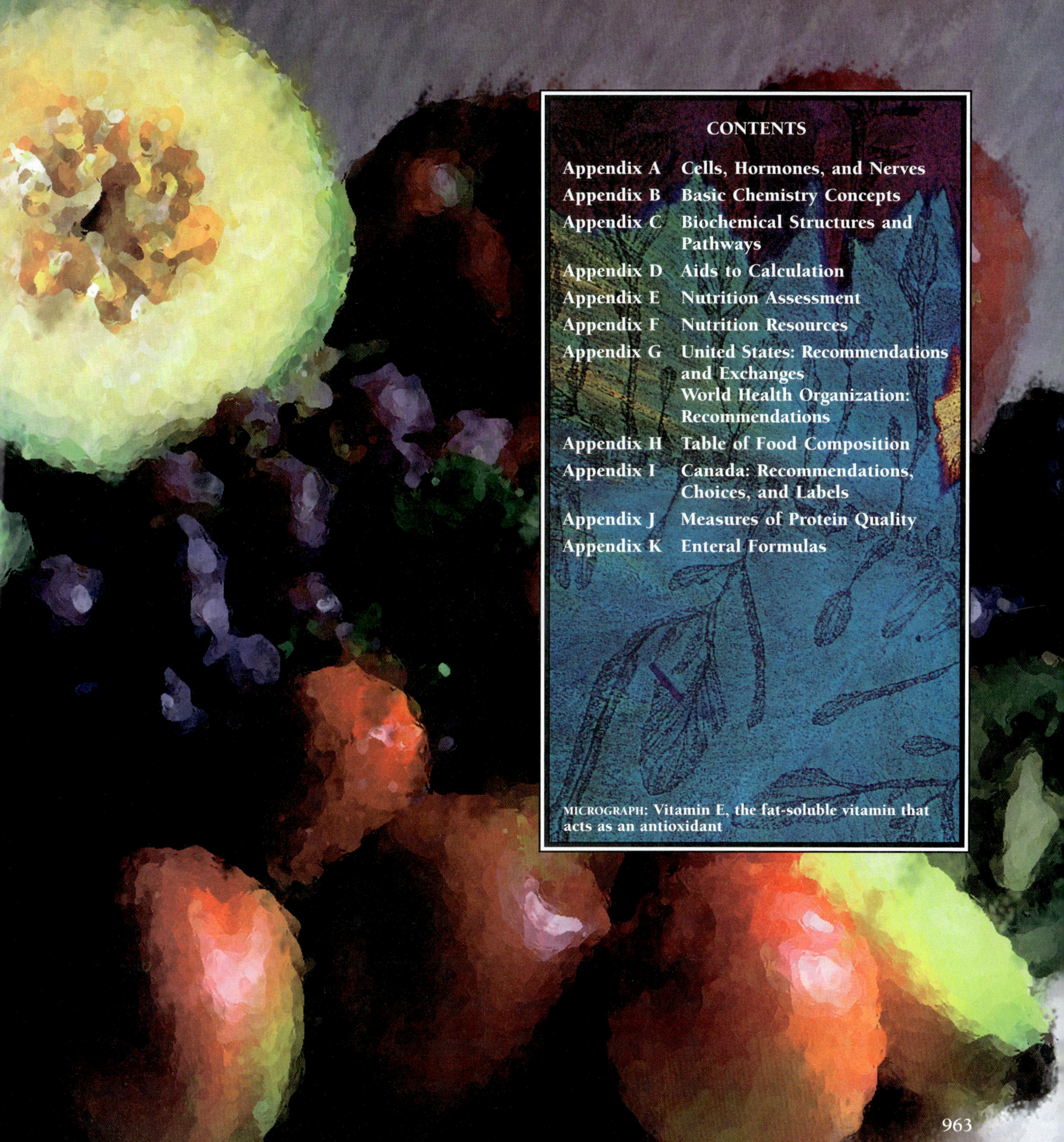

CONTENTS

MICROGRAPH: Vitamin E, the fat-soluble vitamin that acts as an antioxidant

APPENDIX A

Contents

CELLS, HORMONES, AND NERVES

This appendix is offered as an optional chapter for readers who want to enhance their understanding of the body's ways of coordinating its activities. The text presents a brief summary of the structure and function of the body's basic working unit (the cell) and of the body's two major regulatory systems (the hormonal system and the nervous system).

THE CELL

The body's organs are made up of millions of cells and of materials produced by them. Each cell is specialized to perform its organ's functions, but all cells have common structures (see Figure A–1). Every cell is contained within a cell membrane. The cell membrane assists in moving materials into and out of the cell, and some of its special proteins act as "pumps" (described in Chapter 6). Some features of cell membranes, such as microvilli (Chapter 3), permit cells to interact with other cells and with their environments in highly specific ways.

Inside the membrane lies the cytoplasm, or cell "fluid." The cytoplasm contains much more than just fluid, though. It is a highly organized system of fibers, tubes, membranes, particles, and subcellular organelles as complex as a city. These parts intercommunicate, manufacture and exchange materials, package and prepare materials for export, and maintain and repair themselves.

Within each cell is another membrane-enclosed body, the nucleus. Inside the nucleus are the chromosomes, which contain the genetic material, DNA. The DNA encodes all the instructions for carrying out the cell's activities. The role of DNA in coding for cell proteins is summarized in Chapter 6, Figure 6–6. Chapter 6 also describes the variety of proteins produced by cells and the ways they perform the body's work.

Among the organelles within a cell are ribosomes, mitochondria, and lysosomes. Figure 6–6 briefly refers to the ribosomes; they assemble amino acids into proteins, following directions conveyed to them by RNA copies from the DNA in the chromosomes.

The mitochondria are made of intricately folded membranes that bear thousands of highly organized sets of enzymes on their inner and outer surfaces. Although mentioned only briefly in this book's chapters, their presence is implied whenever the enzymes of the TCA cycle and electron transport chain are mentioned because

cell: the basic unit of life, of which all living things are composed. Every cell is surrounded by a membrane and contains cytoplasm, within which are organelles and a nucleus; the cell nucleus contains chromosomes.

cell membrane: the membrane that surrounds the cell and encloses its contents; made primarily of lipid and protein.

cytoplasm (SIGH-toe-plazm): the cell contents, except for the nucleus.
cyto = cell
plasm = a form

nucleus: a major membrane-enclosed body within every cell, which contains the cell's genetic material, DNA, embedded in chromosomes.
nucleus = a kernel

chromosomes: a set of structures within the nucleus of every cell that contain the cell's genetic material, DNA, associated with other materials (primarily proteins).

organelles: subcellular structures such as ribosomes, mitochondria, and lysosomes.
organelle = little organ

ribosomes: protein-making organelles in cells; composed of RNA and protein.
ribo = containing the sugar ribose (in RNA)
some = body

mitochondria (my-toe-KON-dree-uh); singular **mitochondrion**: the cellular organelles responsible for producing ATP aerobically; made of membranes (lipid and protein) with enzymes mounted on them.
mitos = thread (referring to their slender shape)
chondros = cartilage (referring to their external appearance)

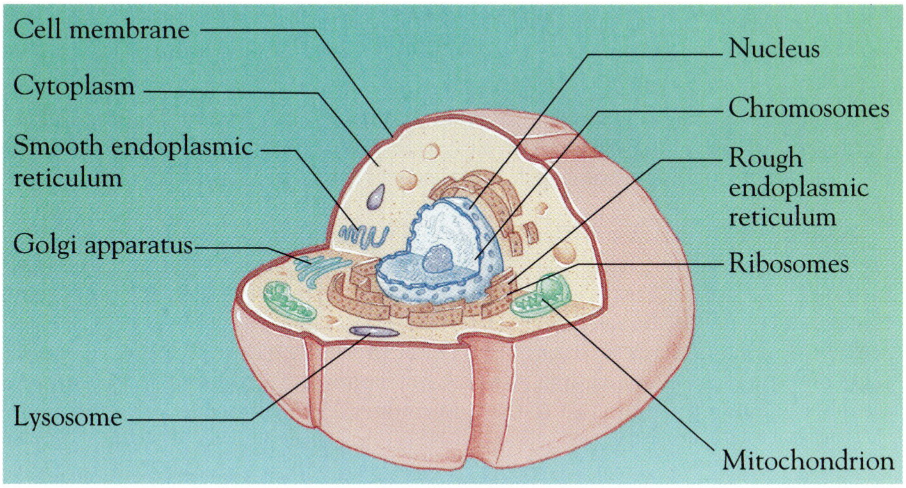

Figure A–1
The Structure of a Typical Cell

The cell shown might be one in a gland (such as the pancreas) that produces secretory products (enzymes) for export (to the intestine). The rough endoplasmic reticulum with its ribosomes produces the enzymes; the smooth reticulum conducts them to the Golgi region; the Golgi membranes merge with the cell membrane, where the enzymes can be released into the extracellular fluid.

the mitochondria house all these enzymes.* Mitochondria are therefore crucial to aerobic metabolism, described in Chapter 7, and muscles conditioned to work aerobically are packed with them.

The lysosomes are membranes that enclose degradative enzymes. When a cell needs to self-destruct or to digest materials in its surroundings, its lysosomes free their enzymes. Lysosomes are active when tissue repair or remodeling is taking place—for example, in cleaning up infections, healing wounds, shaping embryonic organs, and remodeling bones.

lysosomes: cellular organelles; membrane-enclosed sacs of degradative enzymes.
lysis = dissolution

Besides these and other cellular organelles, the cell's cytoplasm contains a highly organized system of membranes, the endoplasmic reticulum. The ribosomes may either float free in the cytoplasm or be mounted on these membranes. A membranous surface dotted with ribosomes looks speckled under the microscope and is called "rough" endoplasmic reticulum; such a surface without ribosomes is called "smooth." Some intracellular membranes are organized into tubules that collect cellular materials, merge with the cell membrane, and discharge their contents to the outside of the cell; these membrane systems are named the Golgi apparatus, after the scientist who first described them. The rough and smooth endoplasmic reticula and the Golgi apparatus are continuous with one another, so secretions produced deep in the interior of the cell can be efficiently transported to the outside and released. These and other cell structures enable cells to perform the multitudes of functions for which they are specialized.

rough endoplasmic reticulum (en-doh-PLAZ-mic reh-TIC-you-lum): intracellular membrane dotted with ribosomes, where protein synthesis takes place.
endo = inside
plasm = the cytoplasm

smooth endoplasmic reticulum: smooth intracellular membrane bearing no ribosomes.

Golgi (GOAL-gee) **apparatus:** a set of membranes within the cell where secretory materials are packaged for export.

The actions of cells are coordinated by both hormones and nerves, as the next sections show. Among the types of cellular organelles are receptors for the hormones delivering instructions that originate elsewhere in the body. Some hormones penetrate the cell and its nucleus and attach to receptors on chromosomes, where they activate certain genes to initiate, stop, speed up, or slow down synthesis of certain proteins as needed. Other hormones attach to receptors on the cell surface and transmit their messages from there. The hormones are described in the next section; the nerves, in the one following.

The study of hormones and their effects is **endocrinology**.

*For the reactions of glycolysis, the TCA cycle, and the electron transport chain, see Chapter 7 and Appendix C. The reactions of glycolysis take place in the cytoplasm; the end product acetyl CoA moves into the mitochondria; and the TCA and electron transport reactions take place there. The mitochondria then release carbon dioxide, water, and ATP as their end products.

THE HORMONES

hormone: a chemical messenger. Hormones are secreted in response to altered conditions by a variety of endocrine glands in the body. Each hormone travels to one or more specific target tissues or organs, where it elicits a specific response.

A hormonal message originates in a gland and travels as a chemical compound—a hormone—in the bloodstream. The hormone flows everywhere in the body, but only its target organs respond to it, because only they possess the receptors to receive it.

The hormones, the glands they originate in, and their target organs and effects are described in this section. Many of the hormones you might be interested in are included, but only a few are discussed in detail. Figure A–2 identifies the glands that produce the hormones discussed in this section.

The hormonal system is a complex system in which many of the parts interact with one another. For example, several hormones are produced in the anterior pituitary gland in the brain. All of these hormones are regulated by other hormones

Figure A–2
The Endocrine System

These organs and glands release hormones that regulate body processes.

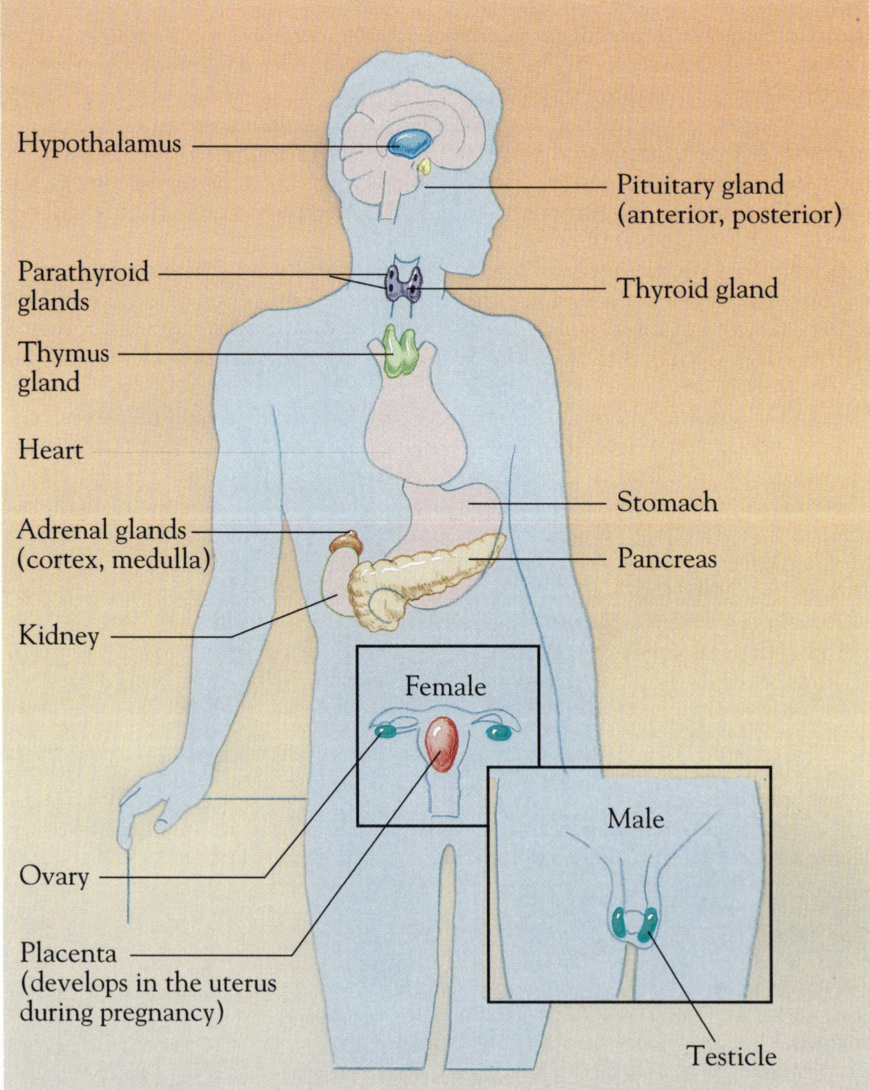

endocrine: with reference to a gland, one that secretes its product directly into (*endo*) the blood; for example, the pancreas cells that produce insulin. An **exocrine** gland secretes its product(s) out (*exo*) of the gland through a duct into a cavity; the sweat glands of the skin and the enzyme-producing glands of the pancreas are both examples. The pancreas is therefore both an endocrine and an exocrine gland.

produced in another part of the brain, the hypothalamus. Furthermore, each of the pituitary gland hormones has effects on the production of compounds elsewhere in the body. Some of these compounds are also hormones that will affect still other body parts. A hormone may travel far from its point of origin and ultimately have profound, even unexpected, effects.

hypothalamus: a brain region (see Figure A–2) that is connected by a channel to the pituitary and can produce many hormones in response to signals from it or from other body conditions.
hypo = below
thalamus = another brain region

A

HORMONES OF THE PITUITARY GLAND AND HYPOTHALAMUS

The anterior pituitary gland produces the following hormones, each of which acts on one or more target organs and elicits a characteristic response:

- Adrenocorticotropin (ACTH) acts on the adrenal cortex, promoting the making and release of its hormones.
- Thyroid-stimulating hormone (TSH) acts on the thyroid gland, promoting the making and release of thyroid hormone.
- Growth hormone (GH) works on all tissues, promoting growth, fat breakdown, and the formation of antibodies.
- Follicle-stimulating hormone (FSH) works on the ovaries in the female, promoting their maturation, and on the testicles in the male, promoting sperm formation.
- Luteinizing hormone (LH) also acts on the ovaries, advancing their maturation, the making of progesterone and estrogens, and ovulation; and on the testicles, promoting the making and release of androgens (male hormones).
- Prolactin, secreted in the female during pregnancy and after she has borne a baby, acts on the mammary glands to stimulate their growth and the making of milk.
- Melanocyte-stimulating hormone (MSH) acts on the pigment cells, promoting the making and dispersal of pigment.

The **pituitary** gland in the brain has two parts—the **anterior** (front) and the **posterior** (hind) parts.

adrenocorticotropin: so named because it stimulates (*trope*) the adrenal cortex. The adrenal gland, like the pituitary, has two parts, in this case an outer portion (*cortex*) and an inner core (*medulla*).

follicle (ovarian): that part of the female reproductive system where the ovary lies and eggs are produced.

luteinizing: so called because the follicle turns orange as it matures.
lutein = an orange pigment

prolactin: so named because it promotes *(pro)* the production of milk *(lacto)*.

melanocyte (MEL-an-oh-cite)**:** a cell containing the pigment melanin.
cyte = cell

The controls over this array of actions are sensitive and specific. Each of these seven hormones has one or more signals that turn it on and another (or others) that turns it off. Among the controlling signals are several hormones from the hypothalamus:

- Corticotropin-releasing hormone (CRH), which promotes release of ACTH, is turned on by stress and turned off by ACTH when enough has been released.
- TSH-releasing hormone (TRH), which promotes release of TSH, is turned on by large meals or low body temperature.
- GH-releasing hormone (GRH), which stimulates the release of GH, is turned on by insulin.
- GH-inhibiting hormone (GIH or somatostatin), which inhibits the release of GH and interferes with the release of TSH, is turned on by hypoglycemia and/or exercise and is rapidly destroyed by body tissues so that it does not accumulate.
- FSH/LH–releasing hormone (FSH/LH–RH) is turned on in the female by nerve messages or low estrogen and in the male by low testosterone.
- Prolactin-inhibiting hormone (PIH) is turned on by high prolactin levels and off by estrogen, testosterone, and suckling (by way of nerve messages).
- MSH-inhibiting hormone (MIH) is turned on by the hormone melatonin.

Hormones that are turned off by their own effects are said to be regulated by **negative feedback.** For example, when a pituitary gland hormone has caused the release of a substance from a target organ, that substance itself switches off the original hormone signal (that is, it feeds back negatively).

somatostatin (GIH): a hormone that inhibits the release of growth hormone; the opposite of **somatotropin (GH)**.
somato = body
stat = keep the same
tropin = make more

Let's examine some of these controls. PIH, for example, responds to high prolactin levels (remember, prolactin promotes the making of milk). High prolactin levels ensure that milk is made and—by calling forth PIH—ensure that prolactin levels don't get too high. But when the infant is suckling—and creating a demand for milk—PIH is not allowed to work (suckling turns off PIH). The consequence: prolactin remains high, and milk manufacture continues. Demand from the infant thus directly adjusts the infant's supply of milk. This example not only shows how the need is met but also illustrates the cooperation between nerves and hormones that achieves this effect.

As another example, consider CRH. Stress, perceived in the brain and relayed to the hypothalamus, switches on CRH. On arriving at the pituitary, CRH switches on ACTH. Then ACTH acts on its target organ, the adrenal cortex, which responds by producing and releasing stress hormones, and the stress response is under way. Events cascading from there involve every body cell and many other hormones.

The numerous steps required to set the stress response in motion make it possible for the body to fine-tune the response; control can be exerted at each step. These two examples illustrate what the body can do in response to two different stimuli—producing milk in response to an infant's need and gearing up for action in an emergency.

Two hormones produced by the posterior pituitary gland are:

- Antidiuretic hormone (ADH), or vasopressin.
- Oxytocin.

antidiuretic hormone (ADH): the hormone that prevents water loss in urine (also **vasopressin**).
anti = against
di = through
ure = urine
vaso = blood vessels
pressin = pressure

oxytocin: the hormone of childbirth.
oxy = quick
tocin = childbirth

cervix: the circular muscle that guards the opening of the uterus. When a baby is about to be born, the cervix begins to stretch.
cervic = neck

ADH promotes contraction of arteries and acts on the kidney to prevent water from being excreted. It is turned on whenever the blood volume is depleted, the blood pressure is low, or the salt concentration of the blood is too high (see Chapter 12). It is turned off by the return of these conditions to normal. Oxytocin is produced in response to reduced progesterone levels, suckling, or the stretching of the cervix and acts on two target organs. One, the uterus, contracts, thus inducing labor; the other, the mammary glands, release milk.

HORMONES THAT REGULATE ENERGY METABOLISM

Hormones produced by a number of different glands have effects on energy metabolism:

- Insulin from the pancreas beta cells.
- Glucagon from the pancreas alpha cells.
- Thyroxin from the thyroid gland.
- Norepinephrine and epinephrine from the adrenal medulla.
- Growth hormone (GH) from the anterior pituitary (already mentioned).
- Glucocorticoids from the adrenal cortex.

Norepinephrine and epinephrine were formerly called noradrenalin and adrenalin.

glucocorticoid: a hormone from the adrenal cortex that affects the body's management of glucose.
gluco = glucose
corticoid = from the cortex

Insulin is turned on by many stimuli, including raised blood glucose. It acts on cells to increase glucose and amino acid uptake into them and to promote the secretion of GRH. Glucagon responds to low blood glucose and acts on the liver to promote the breakdown of glycogen to glucose, the conversion of amino acids to glucose, and the release of glucose. Thyroxin responds to TSH and acts on many cells to increase their metabolic rate, growth, and heat production. The hormones norepinephrine and epinephrine respond to stimulation by sympathetic nerves and produce reactions in many cells that facilitate the body's readiness for fight or flight: increased heart activity, blood vessel constriction, breakdown of glycogen and glucose, raised blood glucose levels, and fat breakdown. Norepinephrine and epinephrine also influence the secretion of the many hormones from the hypothalamus that exert control on the body's other systems. The glucocorticoid hormones become active during times of stress and carbohydrate metabolism.

Every body part is affected by these hormones. Each different hormone has unique effects; and hormones that oppose each other are produced in carefully regulated amounts, so each can respond to the exact degree that is appropriate to the condition.

A

HORMONES THAT ADJUST OTHER BODY BALANCES

Hormones are involved in moving calcium into and out of the body's storage deposits in the bones:

- Calcitonin (CT) from the thyroid gland.
- Parathormone (parathyroid hormone or PTH) from the parathyroid gland.
- Vitamin D from the kidneys.

calcitonin: so called because it regulates (tones) the calcium level.

parathyroid: named for their location, the four parathyroid glands nestle in the surface layers of the two thyroid lobes in the neck.
para = beside, next to

One of calcitonin's target tissues is the bones, which respond by storing calcium from the bloodstream whenever blood calcium rises above the normal range. Calcitonin also acts on the kidneys to increase excretion of both calcium and phosphorus in the urine. Parathormone responds to the opposite condition—lowered blood calcium—and acts on three targets: the bones, which release stored calcium into the blood; the kidneys, which slow the excretion of calcium; and the intestine, which increases calcium absorption. Vitamin D acts with parathormone and is essential for the absorption of calcium in the intestine. Figure 12–9 in Chapter 12 diagrams the ways vitamin D, and the hormones calcitonin and parathormone, regulate calcium homeostasis.

Vitamin D is sometimes viewed as a hormone because it is produced in one body organ and regulates others.

Another hormone has effects on blood-making activity:

- Erythropoietin from the kidneys.

erythropoietin (eh-REE-throw-POY-eh-tin)**:** named for its red blood cell–making function.
erythro = red (blood cell)
poiesis = creating (like poetry)

Erythropoietin is responsive to oxygen depletion of the blood and to anemia. It acts on the bone marrow to stimulate the making of red blood cells.

Another hormone, special for pregnancy, is:

- Relaxin from the ovary.

relaxin: the hormone of late pregnancy.

This hormone, which is secreted in response to the raised progesterone and estrogen levels of late pregnancy, acts on the cervix and pelvic ligaments to allow them to stretch so that they can accommodate the birth process without strain.

Other agents help regulate blood pressure:

- Renin (an enzyme), from the kidneys, in cooperation with angiotensin in the blood.
- Aldosterone, a hormone from the adrenal cortex.

renin (REN-in)**:** an enzyme from the kidneys, which works by activating angiotensin.
ren = kidney

angiotensin: a hormone involved in blood pressure regulation.
angio = blood vessels
tensin = pressure

aldosterone: a hormone from the adrenal gland involved in blood pressure regulation.
aldo = aldehyde

Renin responds to a reduced blood supply experienced by the kidneys and acts in several ways. Encountering the inactive form of angiotensin in the bloodstream, renin converts this molecule to active angiotensin I and then to the very active angiotensin II. The angiotensins constrict the blood vessels, thus raising the blood pressure. They also stimulate thirst, leading to increased water intake, another way of raising the blood pressure. The angiotensins also cause the kidneys to retain water and salt. Thus the angiotensins increase blood pressure by several means at once.

Renin and angiotensin also stimulate the adrenal cortex to secrete the hormone aldosterone. This hormone's target is also the kidneys, which respond by excreting less sodium and with it, less water. The effect is to retain more water in the bloodstream—thus, again, raising the blood pressure. Figure 12–1 in Chapter 12 provides more details.

THE GASTROINTESTINAL HORMONES

Several hormones are produced in the stomach and intestines in response to the presence of food or the components of food:

- Gastrin from the stomach and duodenum.
- Cholecystokinin from the duodenum.
- Secretin from the duodenum.
- Gastric-inhibitory peptide from the duodenum and jejunum.

Gastrin stimulates the stomach to make and release its acid and digestive juices and to move and churn its contents actively. Cholecystokinin signals the gallbladder and pancreas to release their contents into the intestine to aid in digestion. Secretin calls forth acid-neutralizing bicarbonate from the pancreas into the intestine and slows the action of the stomach and its secretion of acid and digestive juices. Gastric-inhibitory peptide inhibits the secretion of gastric acid and slows the process of digestion. These hormones are presented in more detail in Chapter 3.

THE SEX HORMONES

The three major sex hormones are:

- Testosterone from the testicles.
- Estrogens from the ovary.
- Progesterone from the ovary's corpus luteum in preparation for, and during, pregnancy.

testosterone: a steroid hormone from the testicles, or testes. The steroids, as explained in Chapter 5, are chemically related to, and some are derived from, the lipid cholesterol.
sterone = a steroid hormone

estrogens: hormones responsible for the menstrual cycle and other female characteristics.
oestrus = the egg-making cycle
gen = gives rise to

progesterone: the hormone of gestation (pregnancy).
pro = promoting
gest = gestation (pregnancy)
sterone = a steroid hormone

In the male, testosterone is released in response to LH (described earlier). It acts on all the tissues that are involved in male sexuality and promotes their development and maintenance. Estrogens, released in response to both FSH and LH, act similarly in females. Progesterone, released in response to raised LH and prolactin, acts on the uterus and mammary glands, stimulating them to grow and develop.

THE PROSTAGLANDINS

Reminder: A *prostaglandin* is a hormonelike compound, derived from the polyunsaturated fatty acids.

The prostaglandins are a group of hormonelike substances produced by many different body organs. They perform a multitude of diverse functions including the regulation of blood vessel contractions, nerve impulses, and hormone responses. They don't have descriptive names but are designated by letters and numbers: E_1, E_2, and so forth. The prostaglandins are all derived from the polyunsaturated fatty acids and account in part for the necessity for these fatty acids in the diet.

This brief description of the hormones and their functions should suffice to provide an awareness of the enormous impact these compounds have on body processes. The other overall regulating agency is the nervous system.

THE NERVOUS SYSTEM

central nervous system: the central part of the nervous system, the brain and spinal cord.

peripheral (puh-RIFF-er-ul) **nervous system:** the peripheral (outermost) part of the nervous system, the vast complex of wiring that extends from the central nervous system to the body's outermost areas. It contains both somatic and autonomic components (defined next).

The nervous system has a central control system—a sort of computer—that can evaluate information about conditions within and outside the body, and a vast system of wiring that receives information and sends instructions. The control unit is the brain and spinal cord, called the central nervous system; and the vast complex of wiring between the center and the parts is the peripheral nervous system. The smooth functioning that results from the system's adjustments to changing conditions is homeostasis.

The nervous system has two general functions: it controls voluntary muscles in response to sensory stimuli from them, and it controls involuntary, internal muscles and glands in response to nerve-borne and chemical signals about their status. In fact, the nervous system is best understood as two systems that use the same or similar pathways to receive and transmit their messages. The somatic nervous system controls the voluntary muscles; the autonomic nervous system controls the internal organs.

When scientists were first studying the autonomic nervous system, they noticed that when something hurt one organ of the body, some of the other organs reacted as if in sympathy for the afflicted one. They therefore named the nerve network they were studying the sympathetic nervous system. The term is still used today to refer to that branch of the autonomic nervous system that responds to pain and stress. The other branch is called the parasympathetic nervous system. (Think of the sympathetic branch as the responder when homeostasis needs restoring and the parasympathetic branch as the commander of function during normal times.) Both systems transmit their messages through the brain and spinal cord. Nerves of the two branches travel side by side along the same pathways to transmit their messages, but they oppose each other's actions (see Figure A–3).

An example will show how the sympathetic and parasympathetic nervous systems work to maintain homeostasis. When you go outside in cold weather, your skin's temperature receptors send "cold" messages to the spinal cord and brain. Your conscious mind may intervene at this point to tell you to zip your jacket, but let's say

somatic (so-MAT-ick) **nervous system:** the division of the nervous system that controls the voluntary muscles, as distinguished from the autonomic nervous system, which controls involuntary functions.
soma = body

autonomic nervous system: the division of the nervous system that controls the body's automatic responses. Its two branches are the **sympathetic** branch, which helps the body respond to stressors from the outside environment, and the **parasympathetic** branch, which regulates normal body activities between stressful times.
autonomos = self-governing

A

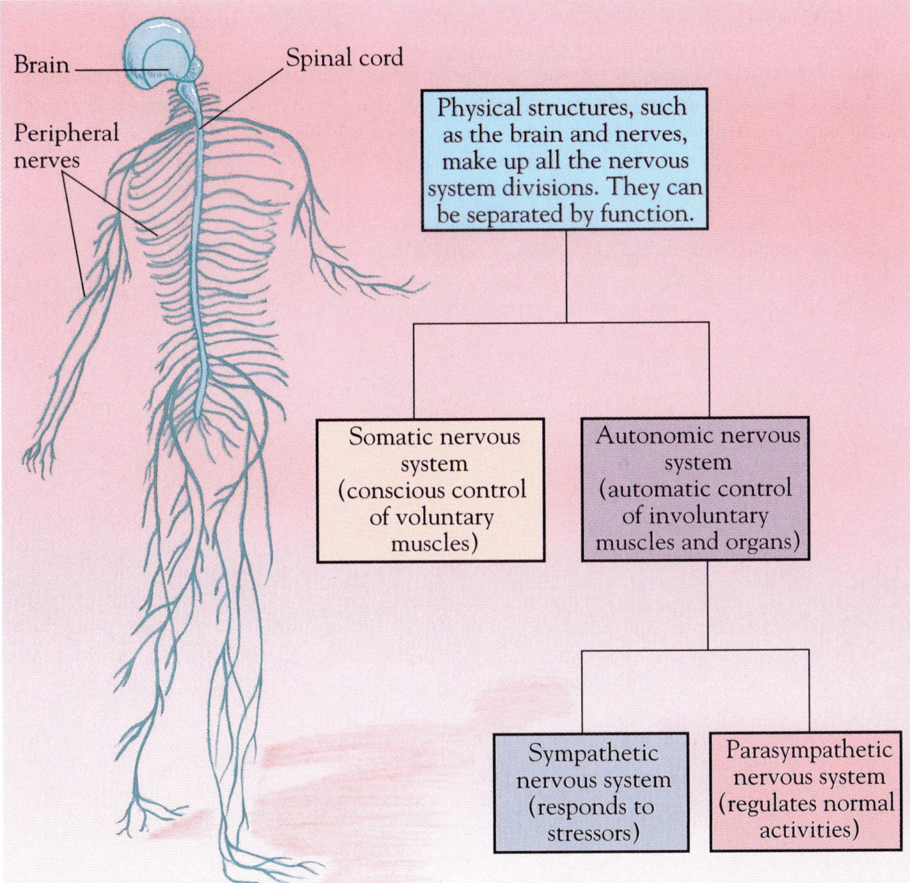

Figure A–3
The Organization of the Nervous System
The brain and spinal cord evaluate information about conditions within and outside the body, and the peripheral nerves receive information and send instructions.

you have no jacket. Your sympathetic nervous system reacts to the external stressor, the cold. It signals your skin-surface capillaries to shut down so your blood will circulate deeper in your tissues, where it will conserve heat. Your sympathetic nervous system also signals involuntary contractions of the small muscles just under the skin surface. The product of these muscle contractions is heat, and the visible result is goose bumps. If these measures do not raise your body temperature enough, then the sympathetic nerves signal your large muscle groups to shiver; the contractions of these large muscles produce still more heat. All of this activity adds up to a set of adjustments that maintain your homeostasis (with respect to temperature) under conditions of external extremes (cold) that would throw it off balance. The cold was a stressor; the body's response was resistance.

Now let's say you come in and sit by a fire and drink hot cocoa. You are warm and no longer need all that sympathetic activity. At this point, your parasympathetic nerves take over; they signal your skin-surface capillaries to dilate again, your goose bumps to subside, and your muscles to relax. Your body is back to normal. This is recovery.

PUTTING IT TOGETHER

The hormonal and nervous systems coordinate body functions by transmitting and receiving messages. The point-to-point messages of the nervous system travel through a central switchboard (the spinal cord and brain), whereas the messages of the hormonal system are broadcast over the airways (the bloodstream), and any organ with the appropriate receptors can pick them up. Nerve impulses travel faster than hormonal messages do—although both are remarkably swift. Whereas your brain's command to wiggle your toes reaches the toes within a fraction of a second and stops as quickly, a gland's message to alter a body condition may take several seconds or minutes to get started and may fade away equally slowly.

Together, the two systems possess every characteristic a superb communication network needs: varied speeds of transmission, along with private communication lines or public broadcasting systems, depending on the needs of the moment. The hormonal system, together with the nervous system, integrates the whole body's functioning so that all parts act smoothly together.

BASIC CHEMISTRY CONCEPTS

Contents

This appendix is intended to provide the background in basic chemistry that you need to understand the nutrition concepts presented in this book. Chemistry is the branch of natural science that is concerned with the description and classification of matter, the changes that matter undergoes, and the energy associated with these changes. Matter is anything that takes up space and has mass. Energy is the ability to do work.

MATTER: THE PROPERTIES OF ATOMS

Every substance has characteristics or properties that distinguish it from all other substances and thus give it a unique identity. These properties are both physical and chemical. The physical properties include such characteristics as color, taste, texture, and odor, as well as the temperatures at which a substance changes its state (from a solid to a liquid or from a liquid to a gas) and the weight of a unit volume (its density). The chemical properties of a substance have to do with how it reacts with other substances or responds to a change in its environment so that new substances with different sets of properties are produced.

A physical change does not change a substance's chemical composition. For example, the three states ice, water, and steam all consist of two hydrogen atoms and one oxygen atom bound together. However, a chemical change occurs if an electric current passes through water. The water disappears and two different substances are formed: hydrogen gas, which is flammable, and oxygen gas, which supports life. Chemical changes are also referred to as chemical reactions.

SUBSTANCES: ELEMENTS AND COMPOUNDS

Molecules are one or more atoms of the same element or two or more atoms of different elements joined by chemical bonds. They constitute the smallest part of a substance that can exist separately without losing its physical and chemical properties. If a molecule is composed of atoms that are alike, the substance is an element (for example, O_2). If a molecule is composed of two or more different kinds of atoms, the substance is a compound (for example, H_2O).

Just over 100 elements are known, and these are listed in Table B–1. A familiar example is hydrogen, whose molecules are composed only of hydrogen atoms linked together in pairs (H_2). On the other hand, over a million compounds are known. An example is the sugar glucose. Each of its molecules is composed of 6 carbon, 6 oxygen, and 12 hydrogen atoms linked together in a specific arrangement (as described in Chapter 4).

THE NATURE OF ATOMS

Atoms themselves are made of smaller particles. Within the atomic nucleus are protons (positively charged particles), and surrounding the nucleus are electrons (negatively charged particles). The number of protons (+) in the nucleus of an atom determines the number of electrons (−) around it. The positive charge on a proton is equal to the negative charge on an electron, so the charges cancel each other out and leave the atom neutral to its surroundings.

The nucleus may also include neutrons, subatomic particles that have no charge. Protons and neutrons are of equal mass, and together they give an atom its weight. Electrons bond atoms together to make molecules, and they are involved in chemical reactions.

B

Table B–1
Chemical Symbols for the Elements

Number of Protons (Atomic Number)	Element	Number of Electrons in Outer Shell	Number of Protons (Atomic Number)	Element	Number of Electrons in Outer Shell
1	Hydrogen (H)	1	52	Tellurium (Te)	6
2	Helium (He)	2	53	Iodine (I)	7
3	Lithium (Li)	1	54	Xenon (Xe)	8
4	Beryllium (Be)	2	55	Cesium (Cs)	1
5	Boron (B)	3	56	Barium (Ba)	2
6	Carbon (C)	4	57	Lanthanum (La)	2
7	Nitrogen (N)	5	58	Cerium (Ce)	2
8	Oxygen (O)	6	59	Praseodymium (Pr)	2
9	Fluorine (F)	7	60	Neodymium (Nd)	2
10	Neon (Ne)	8	61	Promethium (Pm)	2
11	Sodium (Na)	1	62	Samarium (Sm)	2
12	Magnesium (Mg)	2	63	Europium (Eu)	2
13	Aluminum (Al)	3	64	Gadolinium (Gd)	2
14	Silicon (Si)	4	65	Terbium (Tb)	2
15	Phosphorus (P)	5	66	Dysprosium (Dy)	2
16	Sulfur (S)	6	67	Holmium (Ho)	2
17	Chlorine (Cl)	7	68	Erbium (Er)	2
18	Argon (Ar)	8	69	Thulium (Tm)	2
19	Potassium (K)	1	70	Ytterbium (Yb)	2
20	Calcium (Ca)	2	71	Lutetium (Lu)	2
21	Scandium (Sc)	2	72	Hafnium (Hf)	2
22	Titanium (Ti)	2	73	Tantalum (Ta)	2
23	Vanadium (V)	2	74	Tungsten (W)	2
24	Chromium (Cr)	1	75	Rhenium (Re)	2
25	Manganese (Mn)	2	76	Osmium (Os)	2
26	Iron (Fe)	2	77	Iridium (Ir)	2
27	Cobalt (Co)	2	78	Platinum (Pt)	1
28	Nickel (Ni)	2	79	Gold (Au)	1
29	Copper (Cu)	1	80	Mercury (Hg)	2
30	Zinc (Zn)	2	81	Thallium (Tl)	3
31	Gallium (Ga)	3	82	Lead (Pb)	4
32	Germanium (Ge)	4	83	Bismuth (Bi)	5
33	Arsenic (As)	5	84	Polonium (Po)	6
34	Selenium (Se)	6	85	Astatine (At)	7
35	Bromine (Br)	7	86	Radon (Rn)	8
36	Krypton (Kr)	8	87	Francium (Fr)	1
37	Rubidium (Rb)	1	88	Radium (Ra)	2
38	Strontium (Sr)	2	89	Actinium (Ac)	2
39	Yttrium (Y)	2	90	Thorium (Th)	2
40	Zirconium (Zr)	2	91	Protactinium (Pa)	2
41	Niobium (Nb)	1	92	Uranium (U)	2
42	Molybdenum (Mo)	1	93	Neptunium (Np)	2
43	Technetium (Tc)	1	94	Plutonium (Pu)	2
44	Ruthenium (Ru)	1	95	Americium (Am)	2
45	Rhodium (Rh)	1	96	Curium (Cm)	2
46	Palladium (Pd)	—	97	Berkelium (Bk)	2
47	Silver (Ag)	1	98	Californium (Cf)	2
48	Cadmium (Cd)	2	99	Einsteinium (Es)	2
49	Indium (In)	3	100	Fermium (Fm)	2
50	Tin (Sn)	4	101	Mendelevium (Md)	2
51	Antimony (Sb)	5	102	Nobelium (No)	2

Key:
- Elements found in energy-yielding nutrients, vitamins, and water.
- Major minerals.
- Trace minerals.

Each type of atom has a characteristic number of protons in its nucleus. The hydrogen atom (symbol H) is the simplest of all. It possesses a single proton, with a single electron associated with it:

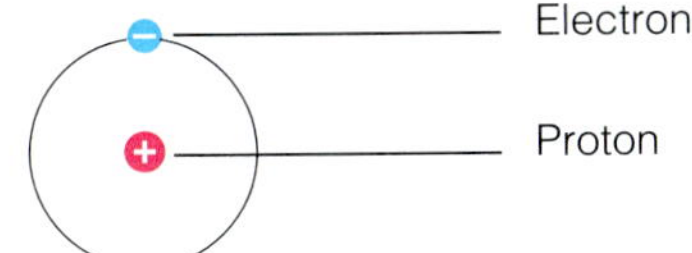

Hydrogen atom (H), atomic number 1.

Just as hydrogen always has one proton, helium always has two, lithium three, and so on. The atomic number of each element is the number of protons in the nucleus of that atom, and this never changes in a chemical reaction; it gives the atom its identity. The atomic numbers for the known elements are listed in Table B–1.

Besides hydrogen, the atoms most common in living things are carbon (C), nitrogen (N), and oxygen (O), whose atomic numbers are 6, 7, and 8, respectively. Their structures are more complicated than that of hydrogen, but each of them possesses the same number of electrons as there are protons in the nucleus. These electrons are found in orbits, or shells:

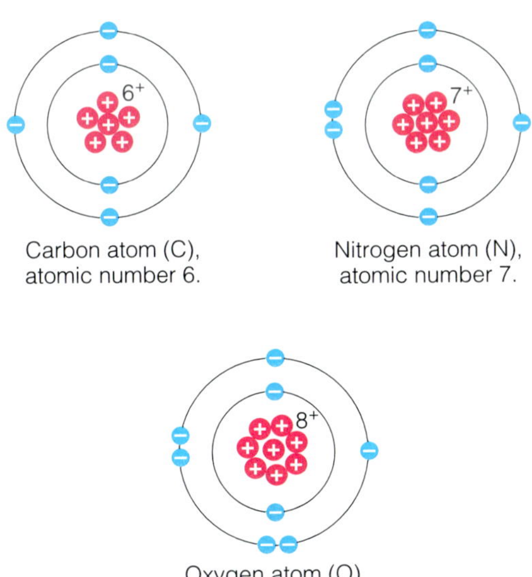

Carbon atom (C), atomic number 6.

Nitrogen atom (N), atomic number 7.

Oxygen atom (O), atomic number 8.

In these and all diagrams of atoms that follow, only the protons and electrons are shown. The neutrons, which contribute only to atomic weight, not to charge, are omitted.

The most important structural feature of an atom for determining its chemical behavior is the number of electrons in its outermost shell. The first, or innermost, shell is full when it is occupied by two electrons; so an atom with two or more electrons has a filled first shell. When the first shell is full, electrons begin to fill the second shell.

The second shell is completely full when it has eight electrons. A substance that has a full outer shell tends not to enter into chemical reactions. Atomic number 10, neon, is a chemically inert substance because its outer shell is complete. Fluorine, atomic number 9, has a great tendency to draw an electron from other substances to complete its outer shell, and thus it is highly reactive. Carbon has a half-full outer shell, which helps explain its great versatility; it can combine with other elements in a variety of ways to form a large number of compounds.

Atoms seek to reach a state of maximum stability or of lowest energy in the same way that a ball will roll down a hill until it reaches the lowest place. An atom achieves a state of maximum stability:

- By gaining or losing electrons to either fill or empty its outer shell.
- By sharing its electrons through bonding together with other atoms and thereby completing its outer shell.

The number of electrons determines how the atom will chemically react with other atoms. Hence the atomic number, not the weight, is what gives an atom its chemical nature.

CHEMICAL BONDING

Atoms often complete their outer shells by sharing electrons with other atoms. In order to complete its outer shell, a carbon atom requires four electrons. A hydrogen atom requires one. Thus, when a carbon atom shares electrons with four hydrogen atoms, each completes its outer shell (as shown on the next page).

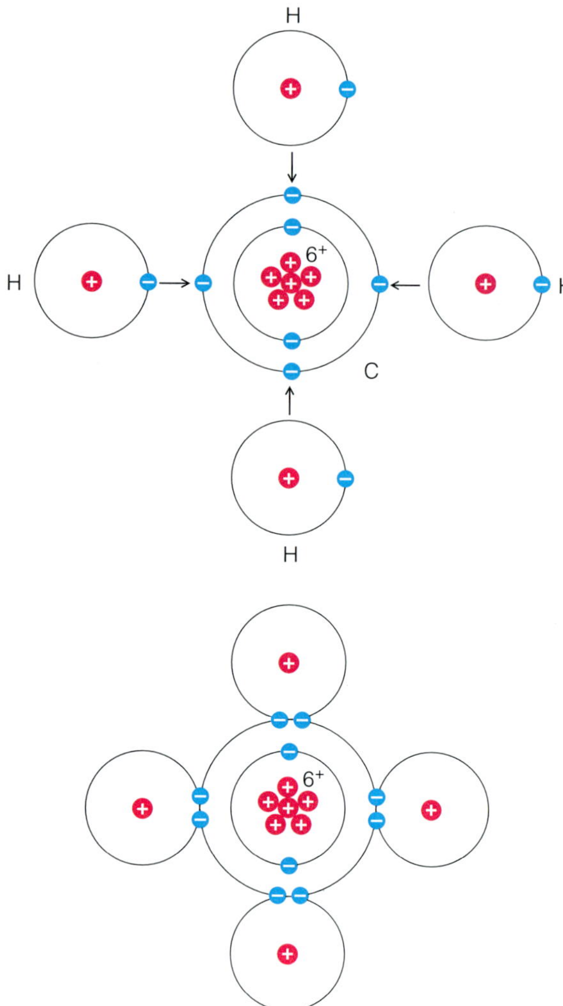

Methane molecule. The chemical formula for methane is CH_4. Note that by sharing electrons, every atom achieves a filled outer shell.

Electron sharing binds the atoms together and satisfies the conditions of maximum stability for the molecule. The outer shell of each atom is complete, since hydrogen effectively has the required two electrons in its first (outer) shell, and carbon has eight electrons in its second (outer) shell; and the molecule is electrically neutral, with a total of ten protons and ten electrons.

Bonds that involve the sharing of electrons, like the bond between carbon and hydrogen, are the most stable kind of association that atoms can form with one another. They are sometimes called covalent bonds, and the resulting combinations of atoms are called molecules. A single pair of shared electrons forms a single bond. A simplified way to represent a single bond is with a single line. Thus the structure of methane (CH_4) could be represented like this (ignoring the inner-shell electrons, which do not participate in bonding):

H
|
H—C—H
|
H

Methane (CH_4).

Similarly, one nitrogen atom and three hydrogen atoms can share electrons to form one molecule of ammonia (NH_3):

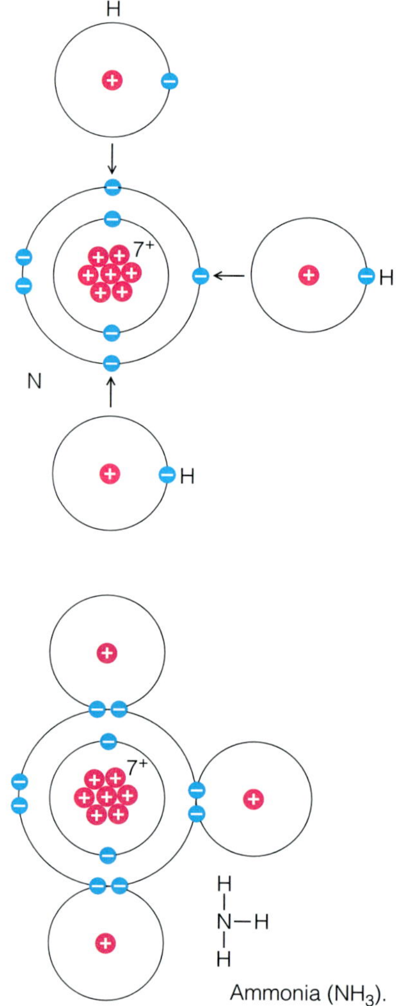

Ammonia molecule (NH_3). Count the electrons in each atom's outer shell to confirm that it is filled.

One oxygen atom may be bonded to two hydrogen atoms to form one molecule of water (H_2O):

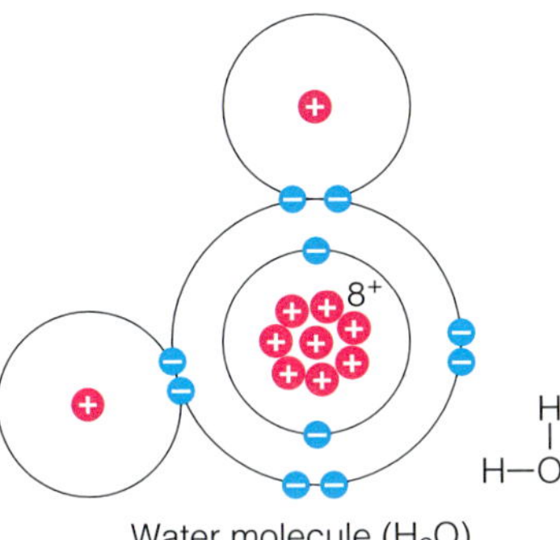

Water molecule (H_2O).

When two oxygen atoms form a molecule of oxygen, they must share two pairs of electrons. This double bond may be represented as two single lines:

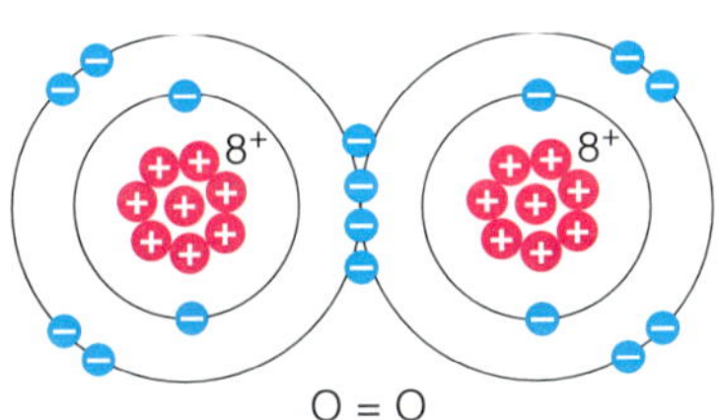

Oxygen molecule (O_2).

Small atoms form the tightest, most stable bonds. H, O, N, and C are the smallest atoms capable of forming one, two, three, and four electron-pair bonds (respectively). This is the basis for the statement in Chapter 4 that in drawings of compounds containing these atoms, hydrogen must always have one, oxygen two, nitrogen three, and carbon four bonds radiating to other atoms:

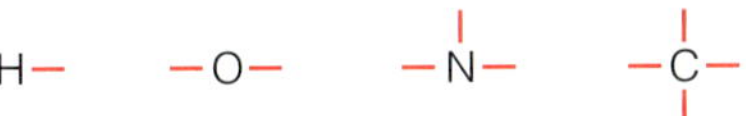

The stability of the associations between these small atoms and the versatility with which they can combine make them very common in living things. Interestingly, all cells, whether they come from animals, plants, or bacteria, contain the same elements in very nearly the same proportions. The atomic elements commonly found in living things are shown in Table B–2.

Table B–2
Elemental Composition of Living Cells

Element	Chemical Symbol	Composition by Weight (%)
Oxygen	O	65
Carbon	C	18
Hydrogen	H	10
Nitrogen	N	3
Calcium	Ca	1.5
Phosphorus	P	1.0
Sulfur	S	0.25
Sodium	Na	0.15
Magnesium	Mg	0.05
Total		99.30[a]

[a]The remaining 0.70 percent by weight is contributed by the trace elements: copper (Cu), zinc (Zn), selenium (Se), molybdenum (Mo), fluorine (F), chlorine (Cl), iodine (I), manganese (Mn), cobalt (Co), and iron (Fe). Cells may also contain variable traces of some of the following: lithium (Li), strontium (Sr), aluminum (Al), silicon (Si), lead (Pb), vanadium (V), arsenic (As), bronium (Br), and others.

FORMATION OF IONS

An atom such as sodium (Na, atomic number 11) cannot easily fill its outer shell by sharing. Sodium possesses a filled first shell of two electrons and a filled second shell of eight; there is only one electron in its outermost shell:

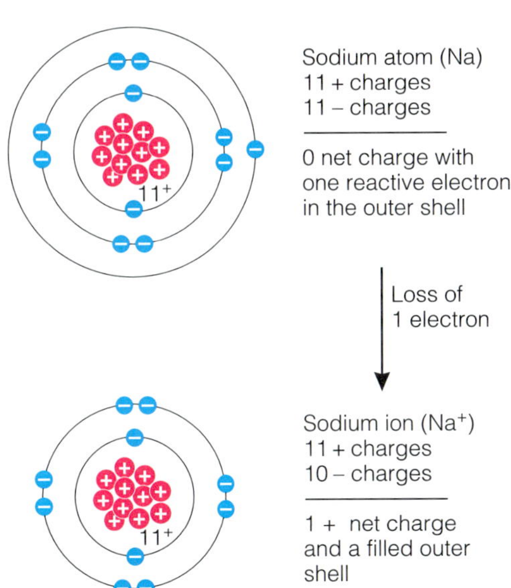

If sodium loses this electron, it satisfies one condition for stability: a filled outer shell (now its second shell counts as the outer shell). However, it is not electrically neutral. It has 11 protons (positive) and only 10 electrons (negative). It therefore has a net positive charge. An atom or molecule that has lost or gained one or more electrons and so is electrically charged is called an ion.

An atom such as chlorine (Cl, atomic number 17), with seven electrons in its outermost shell, can share electrons to fill its outer shell, or it can gain one electron to complete its outer shell and thus give it a negative charge:

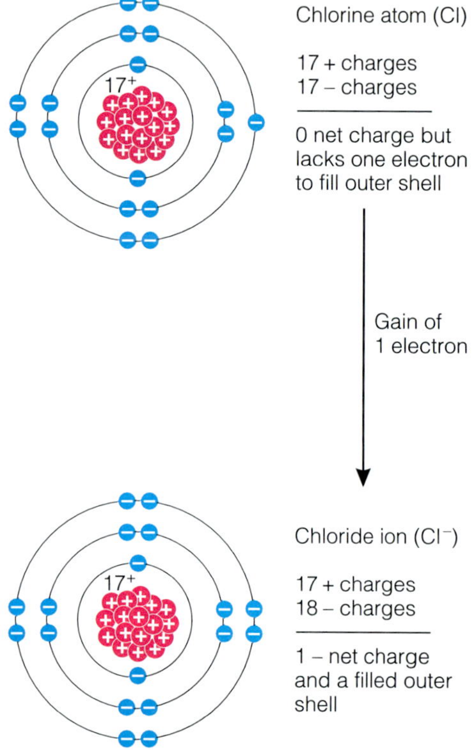

A positively charged ion such as sodium ion (Na^+) is called a cation; a negatively charged ion such as a chloride ion (Cl^-) is called an anion. Cations and anions attract one another to form salts:

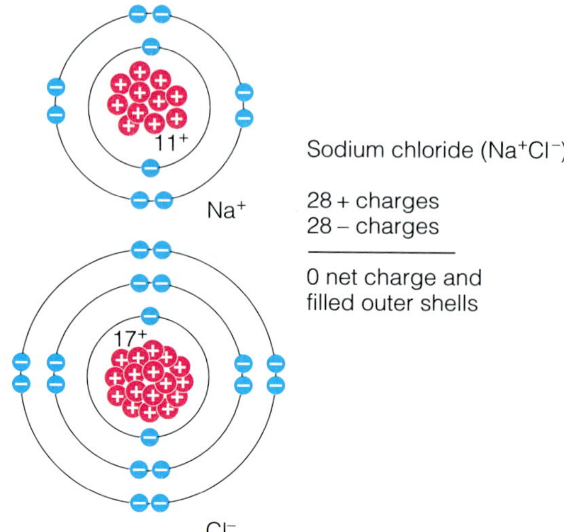

With all its electrons, sodium is a shiny, highly reactive metal; chlorine is the poisonous greenish-yellow gas that was used in World War I. But after sodium and chlorine have transferred electrons, they form the stable white salt familiar to you as table salt, or sodium chloride (Na^+Cl^-). The dramatic difference illustrates how profoundly the electron arrangement can influence the nature of a substance. The wide distribution of salt in nature attests to the stability of the union between the ions. Each meets the other's needs (a good marriage).

When dry, salt exists as crystals; its ions are stacked very regularly into a lattice, with positive and negative ions alternating in a three-dimensional checkerboard structure. In water, however, the salt quickly dissolves, and its ions separate from one another, forming an electrolyte solution in which they move about freely. Covalently bonded molecules rarely dissociate like this in a water solution. The most common exception is when they behave like acids and release H^+ ions, as discussed in the next section.

An ion can also be a group of atoms bound together in such a way that the group has a net charge and enters into reactions as a single unit. Many such groups are active in the fluids of the body. The bicarbonate ion is composed of five atoms—one H, one C, and three O—and has a net charge of -1 (HCO_3^-). Another important ion of this type is a phosphate ion with one H, one P, and four O, and a net charge of −2 (HPO_4^{-2}).

Whereas many elements have only one configuration in the outer shell and thus only one way to bond with other elements, some elements have the possibility of varied configurations. Iron is such an element. Under some conditions iron loses two electrons, and under other circumstances it loses three. If iron loses two electrons, it then has a net charge of +2, and we call it ferrous iron (Fe^{++}). If it donates three electrons to another atom, it becomes the +3 ion, or ferric iron (Fe^{+++}).

Ferrous iron (Fe^{++}) (had 2 outer-shell electrons but has lost them)	Ferric iron (Fe^{+++}) (had 3 outer-shell electrons but has lost them)
26 + charges	26 + charges
24 − charges	23 − charges
2 + net charge	3 + net charge

It is important to remember that a positive charge on an ion means that negative charges—electrons—have been lost and not that positive charges have been added to the nucleus.

WATER, ACIDS, AND BASES

Water The water molecule is electrically neutral, having equal numbers of protons and electrons. However, when a hydrogen atom shares its electron with oxygen, that electron will spend most of its time closer to the positively charged oxygen nucleus. This leaves the positive proton (nucleus of the hydrogen atom) exposed on the outer part of the water molecule. We know, too, that the two hydrogens both bond toward the same side of the oxygen. These two facts explain why water molecules are polar: they have regions of more positive and more negative charge.

Polar molecules like water are drawn to one another by the attractive forces between the positive polar areas of one and the negative poles of another. These attractive forces, sometimes known as polar bonds or hydrogen bonds, occur among many molecules and also within the different parts of single large molecules. Although very weak in comparison with covalent bonds, polar bonds may occur in such abundance that they become exceedingly important in determining the structure of such large molecules as proteins and DNA.

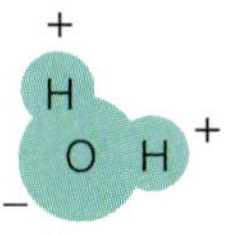

This diagram of the polar water molecule shows displacement of electrons toward the O nucleus; thus the negative region is near the O and the positive regions are near the Hs.

Water molecules have a slight tendency to ionize, separating into positive (H^+) and negative (OH^-) ions. In pure water, a small but constant number of these ions is present, and the number of positive ions exactly equals the number of negative ions.

Acids An acid is a substance that releases H^+ ions (protons) in a water solution. Hydrochloric acid (HCl) is such a substance because it dissociates in a water solution into H^+ and Cl^- ions. Acetic acid is also an acid because it dissociates in water to acetate ions and free H^+:

$$CH_3COOH \longrightarrow CH_3COO^- + H^+$$

Acetic acid dissociates into an acetate ion and a hydrogen ion.

The more H^+ ions released, the stronger the acid.

pH Chemists define degrees of acidity by means of the pH scale, which runs from 0 to 14. The pH expresses the concentration of H^+ ions: a pH of 1 is extremely acidic, 7 is neutral, and 13 is very basic. There is a tenfold difference in the concentration of H^+ ions between points on this scale. A solution with pH 3, for example, has *ten times* as many H^+ ions as a solution with pH 4. At pH 7, the concentrations of free H^+ and OH^- are exactly the same—1/10,000,000 moles per liter (10^{-7} moles per liter).* At pH 4, the concentration of free H^+ ions is 1/10,000 (10^{-4}) moles per liter. This is a higher concentration of H^+ ions, and the solution is therefore acidic.

*A mole is a certain number (about 6×10^{23}) of molecules. The pH of a solution is defined as the negative logarithm of the hydrogen ion concentration of the solution. Thus, if the concentration is 10^{-2} (moles per liter), the pH is 2; if 10^{-8}, the pH is 8; and so on.

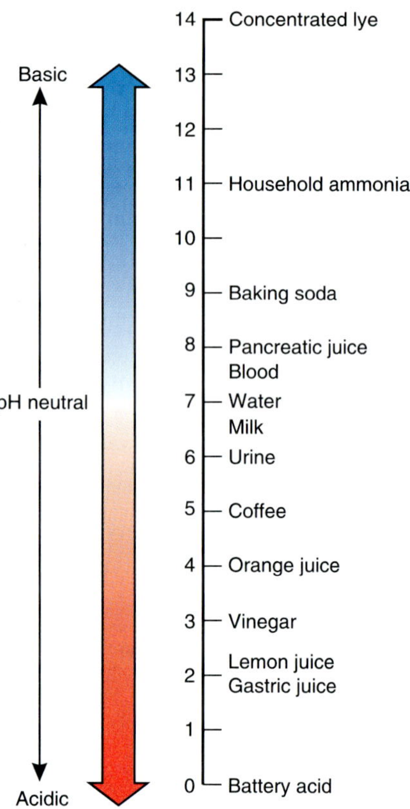

The pH scale.

Note: Each step is ten times as concentrated in base (1/10 as much acid, H^+) as the one below it.

Bases A base is a substance that can soak up, or combine with, H^+ ions, thus reducing the acidity of a solution. The compound ammonia is such a substance. The ammonia molecule has two electrons that are not shared with any other atom; a hydrogen ion (H^+) is just a naked proton with no shell of electrons at all. The proton readily combines with the ammonia molecule to form an ammonium ion; thus a free proton is withdrawn from the solution and no longer contributes to its acidity. Many compounds containing nitrogen are important bases in living systems. Acids and bases neutralize each other to produce substances that are neither acid nor base.

$$\begin{array}{c} \mathrm{H} \\ | \\ \mathrm{:N{-}H} \\ | \\ \mathrm{H} \end{array} + \mathrm{H^+} \longrightarrow \begin{array}{c} \mathrm{H} \\ | \\ \mathrm{H{-}N^+{-}H} \\ | \\ \mathrm{H} \end{array}$$

Ammonia captures a hydrogen ion from water. The two dots here represent the two electrons not shared with another atom. These are ordinarily not shown in chemical structure drawings. Compare this with the earlier diagram of an ammonia molecule (p. B–4).

CHEMICAL REACTIONS

A chemical reaction, or chemical change, results in the breakdown of substances and the formation of new ones. Almost all such reactions involve a change in the bonding of atoms. Old bonds are broken, and new ones are formed. The nuclei of atoms are never involved in chemical reactions—only their outer-shell electrons take part. At the end of a chemical reaction, the number of atoms of each type is always the same as at the beginning. For example, two hydrogen molecules ($2H_2$) can react with one oxygen molecule (O_2) to form two water molecules ($2H_2O$). In this reaction two substances (hydrogen and oxygen) disappear, and a new one (water) is formed, but at the end of the reaction there are still four H atoms and two O atoms, just as there were at the beginning. Because the atoms are now linked in a different way, their characteristics or properties have changed.

In many instances chemical reactions involve not the relinking of molecules but the exchanging of electrons or protons among them. In such reactions the molecule that gains one or more electrons (or loses one or more hydrogen ions) is said to be reduced; the molecule that loses electrons (or gains protons) is oxidized. A hydrogen ion is equivalent to a proton. Oxidation and reduction take place simultaneously because an electron or proton that is lost by one molecule is accepted by another. The addition of an atom of oxygen is also oxidation because oxygen (with six electrons in the outer shell) accepts two electrons in becoming bonded. Oxidation, then, is loss of electrons, gain of protons, or addition of oxygen (with six electrons); reduction is the opposite—gain of electrons, loss of protons, or loss of oxygen. The addition of hydrogen atoms to oxygen to form water can thus be described as the reduction of oxygen *or* the oxidation of hydrogen.

If a reaction results in a net increase in the energy of a compound, it is called an endergonic, or "uphill," reaction (energy, *erg,* is added into, *endo,* the compound). An example is the chief result of photosynthesis, the making of sugar in a plant from carbon dioxide and water using the energy of sunlight. Conversely, the oxidation of sugar to carbon dioxide and water is an exergonic, or "downhill," reaction because the end products have less energy than the starting products. Oftentimes, but not always, reduction reactions are endergonic, resulting in an increase in the energy of the products. Oxidation reactions often, but not always, are exergonic.

Chemical reactions tend to occur spontaneously if the end products are in a lower energy state and therefore are more stable than the reacting compounds. These reactions often give off energy in the form of heat as they occur. The generation of heat by wood burning in a fireplace and the maintenance of human body warmth both depend on energy-

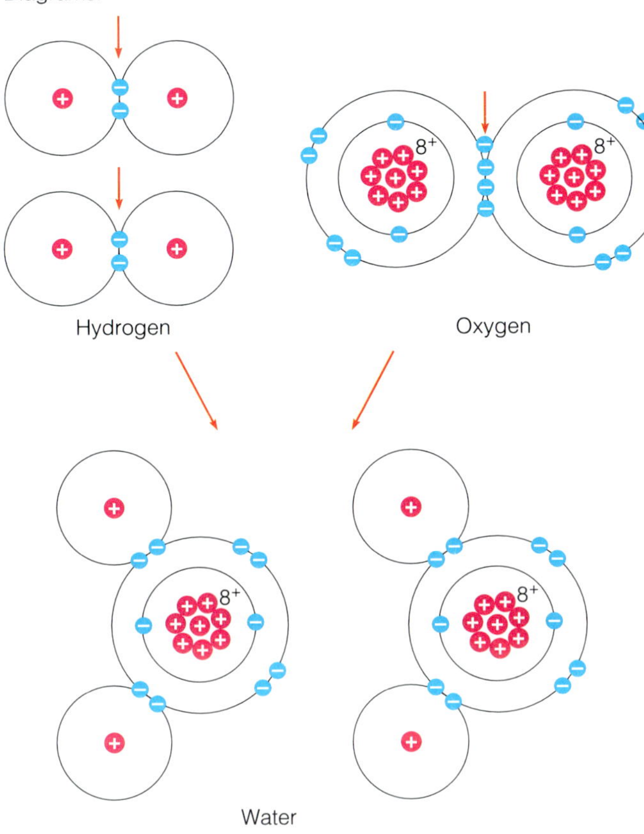

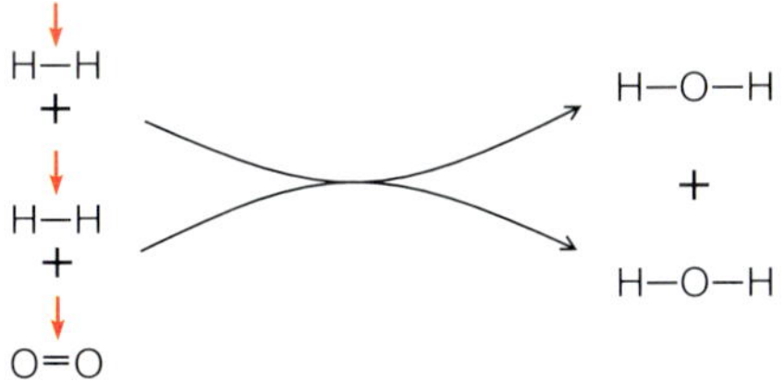

Formulas:

$$2H_2 + O_2 \longrightarrow 2H_2O$$

Hydrogen and oxygen react to form water.

yielding chemical reactions. These downhill reactions occur easily, although they may require some activation energy to get them started, just as a ball requires a push to start rolling downhill.

Uphill reactions, in which the products contain more energy than the reacting compounds started with, do not occur until an energy source is provided. An example of such an energy source is the sunlight used in photosynthesis, where carbon dioxide and water (low-energy compounds) are combined to form the sugar glucose (a higher-energy compound). Another example is the use of the energy in glucose to combine two low-energy compounds in the body into the high-energy compound ATP (see Chapter 7). The energy in ATP may be used to power many other energy-requiring, uphill reactions. Clearly, any of many different molecules can be used as a temporary storage place for energy.

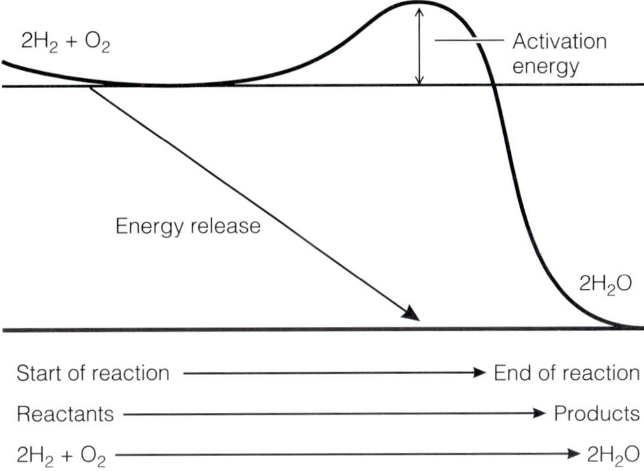

Neither downhill nor uphill reactions occur until something sets them off (activation) or until a path is provided for them to follow. The body uses enzymes as a means of providing paths and controlling chemical reactions (see Chapter 6). By controlling the availability and the action of its enzymes, the body can "decide" which chemical reactions to prevent and which to promote.

FORMATION OF FREE RADICALS

Normally, when a chemical reaction takes place, bonds break and re-form with some redistribution of atoms and rearrangement of bonds to form new, stable compounds. Normally, bonds don't split in such a way as to leave a molecule with an odd, unpaired electron. However, weak bonds can split this way, and when they do, free radicals are formed. Free radicals are highly unstable and quickly react with other compounds, forming more free radicals in a chain reaction.

H—O—O—H or R—O—O—H —(Heat or light)→ H—O· + ·O—H or R—O· + ·O—H

Hydrogen peroxide or any hydroperoxide (R is any carbon chain with appropriate numbers of H) — Free radical

Free radicals are formed. The dots represent single electrons that are available for sharing (the atom needs another electron to fill its outer shell).

A physical event such as the arrival of an energy-carrying particle of light or other radiation starts the process by breaking a weak bond so that free radicals are formed. A cascade may ensue in which many highly reactive radicals are generated, resulting finally in the disruption of a living structure such as a cell membrane.

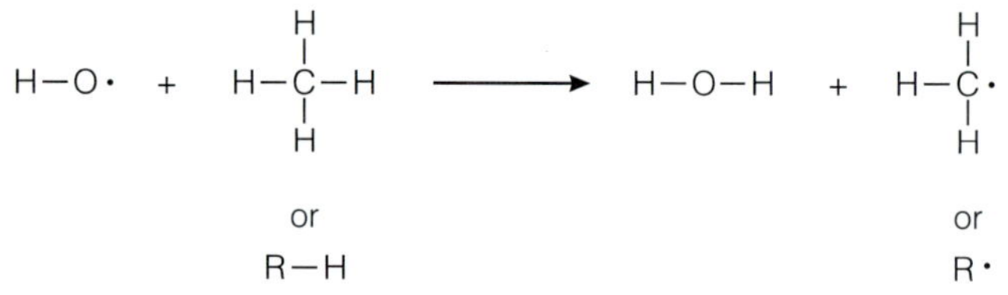

H—O· + H—C(H)(H)—H (or R—H) ⟶ H—O—H + H—C(H)(H)· (or R·)

Free radical — Compound with weak bond (perhaps an unsaturated fatty acid) — New stable compound (water or an alcohol) — Free radical

Destruction of biological compounds by free radicals. The free radical attacks a weak bond in a biological compound, disrupting it and forming a new stable molecule and another free radical. This can attack another biological compound, and so on.

Oxidation of some compounds can be induced by air at room temperature in the presence of light. Such reactions are thought to take place through the formation of compounds called peroxides:

Peroxides:

H—O—O—H	Hydrogen peroxide
R—O—O—H	Hydroperoxides (R is any carbon chain with appropriate numbers of H)
R—O—O—R	Peroxide

Some peroxides readily disintegrate into free radicals, initiating chain reactions like those just described.

Free radicals are of special interest in nutrition because the antioxidant properties of vitamins A, C, and E as well as the mineral selenium are thought to protect against the destructive effects of these free radicals (see Highlight 11). For example, vitamin E on the surface of the lungs reacts with, and is destroyed by, free radicals, thus preventing the radicals from reaching underlying cells and oxidizing the lipids in their membranes.

APPENDIX C

BIOCHEMICAL STRUCTURES AND PATHWAYS

Contents

The diagrams of nutrients presented here are meant to enhance your understanding of the most important organic molecules in the human diet. The names used are those agreed on by the American Institute of Nutrition and other scientific organizations in 1987.[1] Following the diagrams of nutrients are sections on the major metabolic pathways mentioned in Chapter 7—glycolysis, the TCA cycle, and the electron transport chain—and a description of how alcohol interferes with these pathways. Discussions of the urea cycle and the formation of ketone bodies complete the appendix.

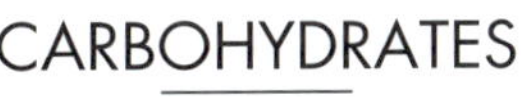

CARBOHYDRATES

MONOSACCHARIDES

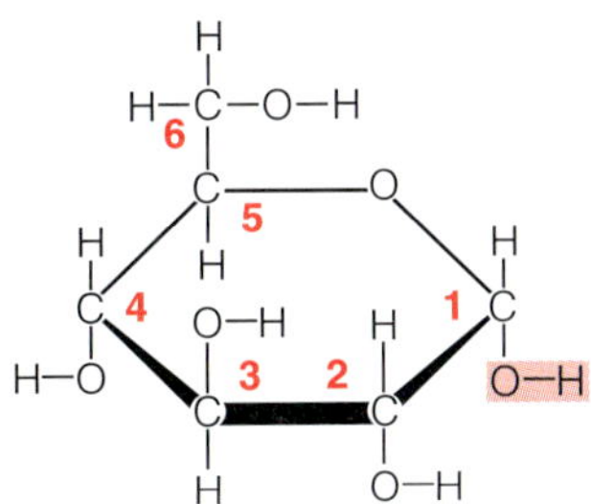

Glucose (alpha form). The ring would be at right angles to the plane of the paper. The bonds directed upward are above the plane; those directed downward are below the plane. This molecule is considered an alpha form because the OH on carbon 1 points downward.

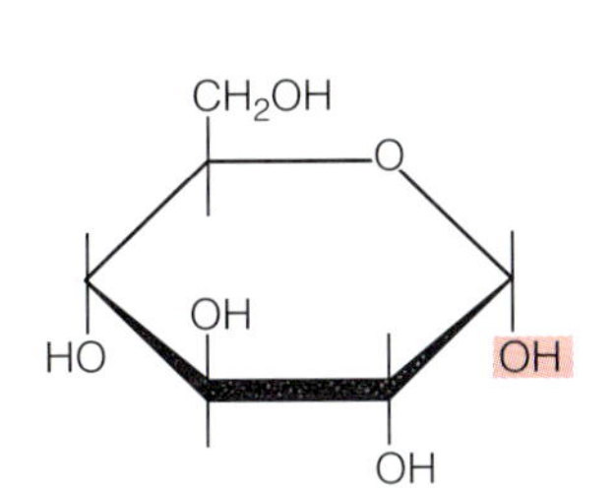

Glucose (alpha form) shorthand notation. This notation, in which the carbons in the ring and single hydrogens have been eliminated, will be used throughout this appendix.

Glucose (beta form). The OH on carbon 1 points upward.
Fructose, galactose: see Chapter 4.

DISACCHARIDES

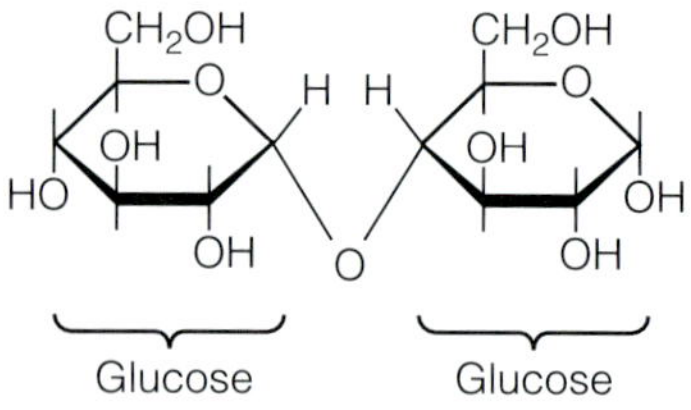

Maltose.

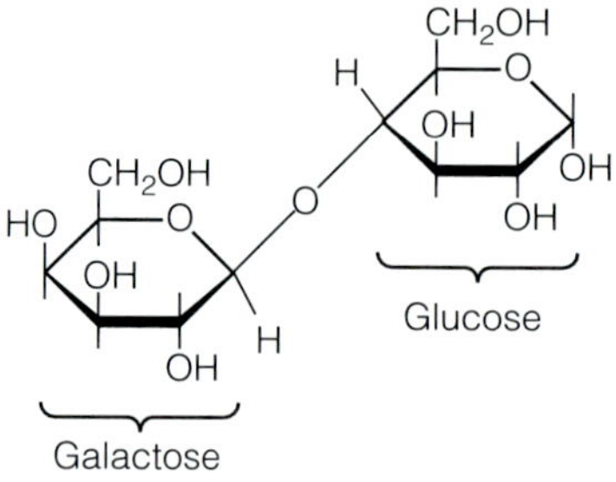

Lactose (alpha form).

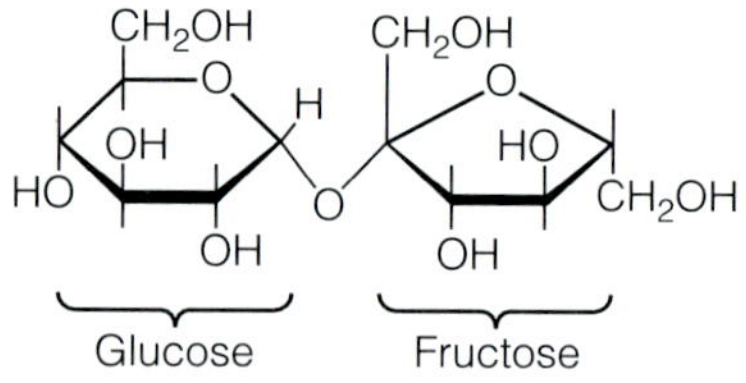

Sucrose.

POLYSACCHARIDES

As described in Chapter 4, starch, glycogen, and cellulose are all long chains of glucose molecules covalently linked together.

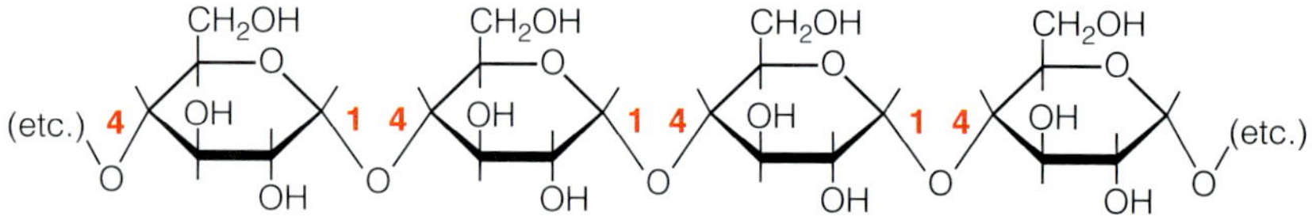

Amylose (unbranched starch)

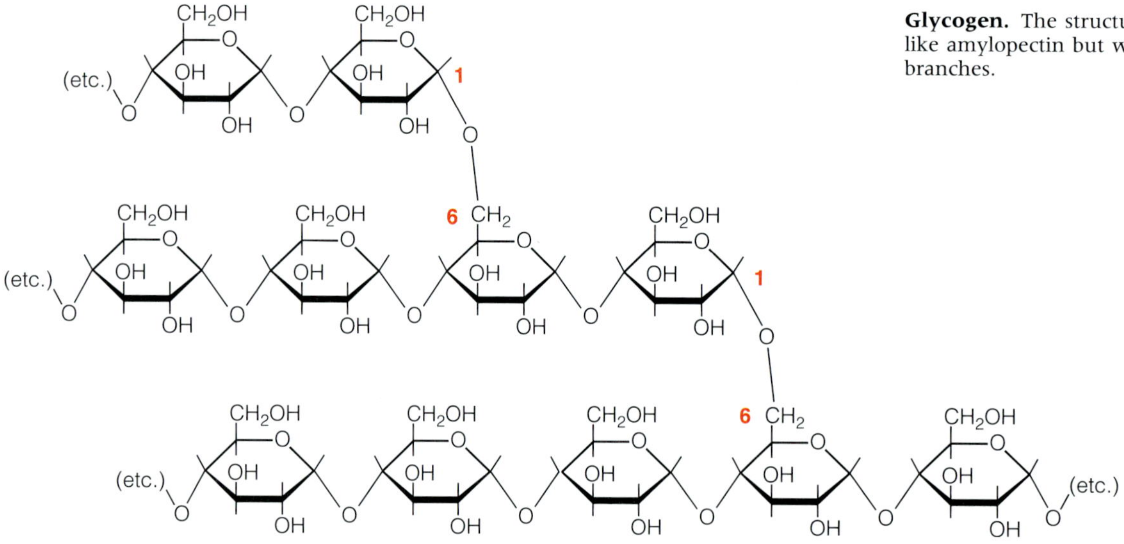

Amylopectin (branched starch)

Starch. Two kinds of covalent linkages occur between glucose molecules in starch, giving rise to two kinds of chains. Amylose is composed of straight chains, with carbon 1 of one glucose linked to carbon 4 of the next (α-1,4 linkage). Amylopectin is made up of straight chains like amylose but has occasional branches arising where the carbon 6 of a glucose is also linked to the carbon 1 of another glucose (α-1,6 linkage).

Glycogen. The structure of glycogen is like amylopectin but with many more branches.

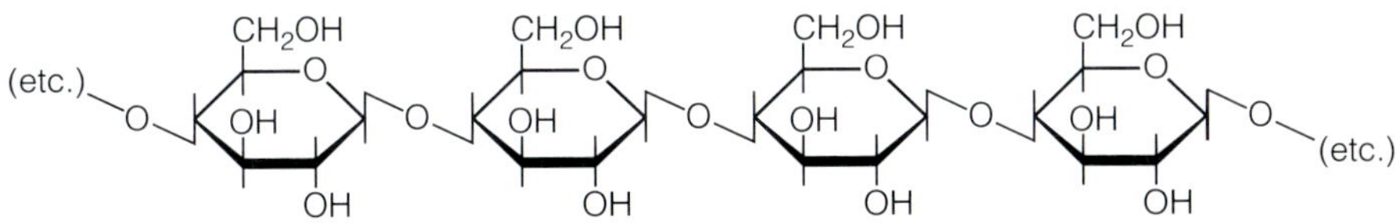

(etc.) (etc.)

Cellulose. Like starch and glycogen, cellulose is also made of chains of glucose units, but there is an important difference: in cellulose, the OH on carbon 1 is in the beta position (see p. C-1). When carbon 1 of one glucose is linked to carbon 4 of the next, it forms a β-1, 4 linkage, which cannot be broken by digestive enzymes in the human GI tract.

Monosaccharides in backbone chain

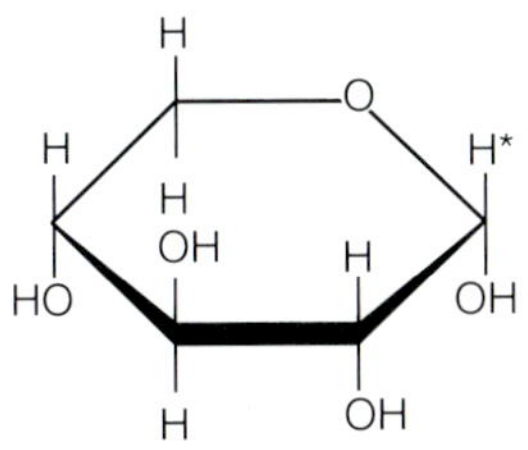

xylose

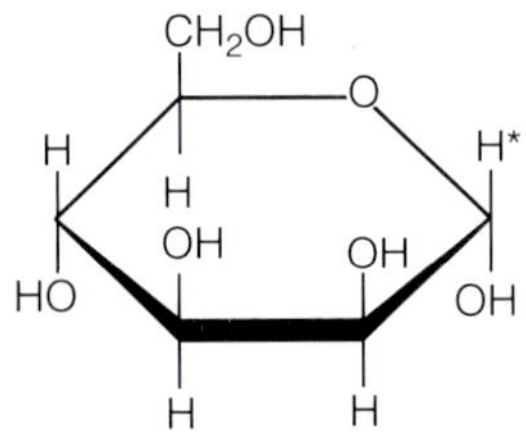

mannose

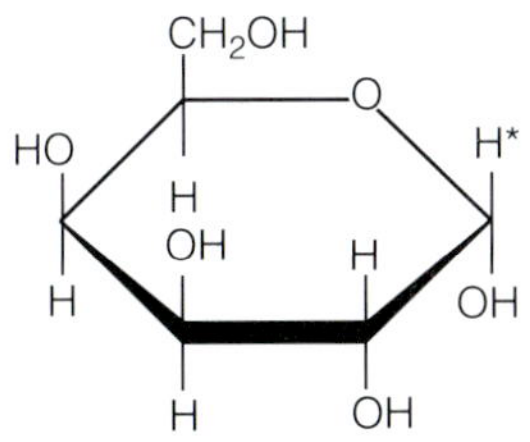

galactose

Monosaccharides in side chains

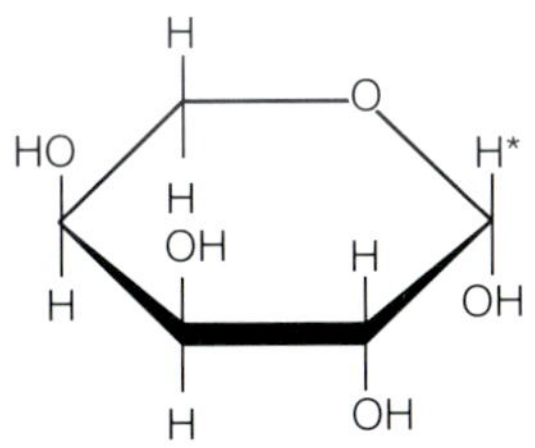

arabinose

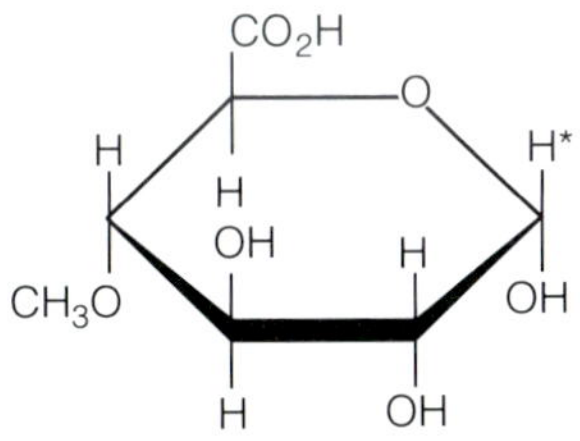

glucuronic acid

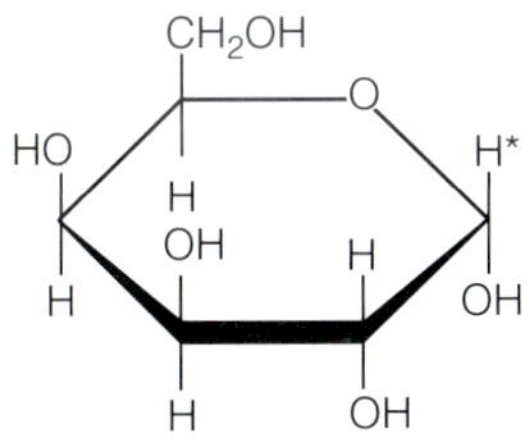

galactose

Hemicelluloses. The most common hemicelluloses are composed of a backbone chain of xylose, mannose, and galactose, with branching side chains of arabinose, glucuronic acid, and galactose.

*These structures are shown in the alpha form with the H on the carbon pointing upward and the OH pointing downward, but they may also appear in the beta form with the H pointing downward and the OH upward.

C

LIPIDS

Table C-1
Saturated Fatty Acids Found in Natural Fats

Saturated Fatty Acids	Chemical Formulas	Number of Carbons	Food Source
Butyric	C_3H_7COOH	4	Butterfat
Caproic	$C_5H_{11}COOH$	6	Butterfat
Caprylic	$C_7H_{15}COOH$	8	Coconut oil
Capric	$C_9H_{19}COOH$	10	Palm oil
Lauric	$C_{11}H_{23}COOH$	12	Coconut oil
Myristic[a]	$C_{13}H_{27}COOH$	14	Coconut oil, butterfat
Palmitic[a]	$C_{15}H_{31}COOH$	16	Animal and vegetable fat
Stearic[a]	$C_{17}H_{35}COOH$	18	Animal and some vegetable fat
Arachidic	$C_{19}H_{39}COOH$	20	Peanut oil

[a]Most common saturated fatty acids.

Table C-2
Unsaturated Fatty Acids Found in Natural Fats

Unsaturated Fatty Acids	Chemical Formulas	Number of Carbons	Number of Double Bonds	Standard Notation[b]	Omega Notation[b]	Food Source
Palmitoleic	$C_{15}H_{29}COOH$	16	1	16:1;9	16:1ω7	Butterfat
Oleic	$C_{17}H_{33}COOH$	18	1	18:1;9	18:1ω9	Olive oil
Linoleic	$C_{17}H_{31}COOH$	18	2	18:2;9,12	18:2ω6	Linseed oil
Linolenic	$C_{17}H_{29}COOH$	18	3	18:3;9,12,15	18:3ω3	Linseed oil
Arachidonic	$C_{19}H_{31}COOH$	20	4	20:4;5,8,11,14	20:4ω6	Lecithin
Eicosapentanoic	$C_{18}H_{29}COOH$	20	5	20:5;5,8,11,14,17	20:5ω3	Fish oils

Note: A fatty acid has two ends; designated the methyl (CH_3) end and the carboxyl, or acid (COOH), end.

[a]Standard chemistry notation begins counting carbons at the acid end. The number of carbons the fatty acid contains comes first, followed by a colon and another number that indicates the number of double bonds; next comes a semicolon followed by a number or numbers indicating the positions of the double bonds. Thus the notation for linoleic acid, an 18-carbon fatty acid with two double bonds between carbons 9 and 10 and between carbons 12 and 13, is 18:2;9,12.

[b]Because fatty acid chains are lengthened by adding carbons at the acid end of the chain, chemists use the omega system of notation to ease the task of identifying them. The omega system begins counting carbons at the methyl end. The number of carbons the fatty acid contains comes first, followed by a colon and the number of double bonds; next comes the omega symbol (ω) and number indicating the position of the double bond nearest the methyl end. Thus linoleic acid with its first double bond at the sixth carbon from the methyl end would be noted 18:2ω6 in the omega system.

PROTEIN: AMINO ACIDS

The common amino acids may be classified into the seven groups listed on the next page.[2] Amino acids marked with an asterisk (*) are essential because human beings cannot synthesize them.

1. Amino acids with aliphatic side chains, which consist of hydrogen and carbon atoms (hydrocarbons):

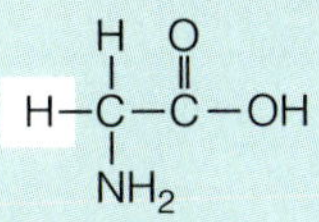
Glycine (Gly)

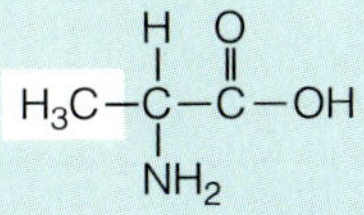
Alanine (Ala)

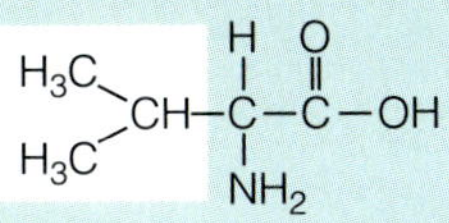
Valine* (Val)

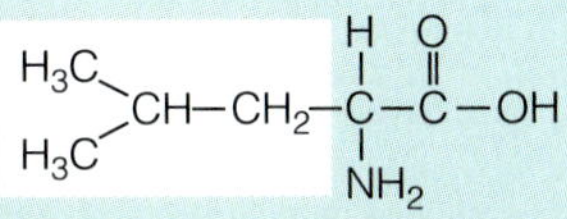
Leucine* (Leu)

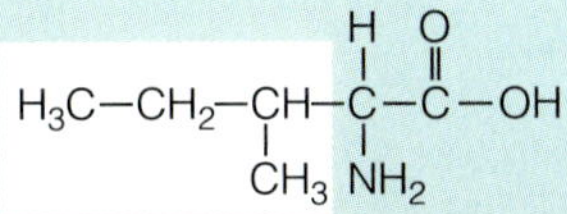
Isoleucine* (Ile)

2. Amino acids with hydroxyl (OH) side chains:

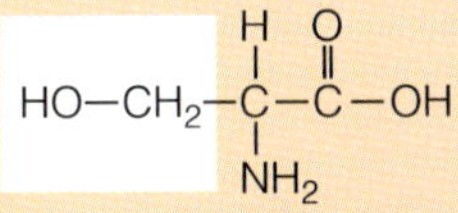
Serine (Ser)

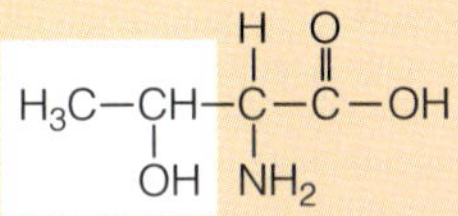
Threonine* (Thr)

3. Amino acids with side chains containing acidic groups or their amides, which contain the group NH_2:

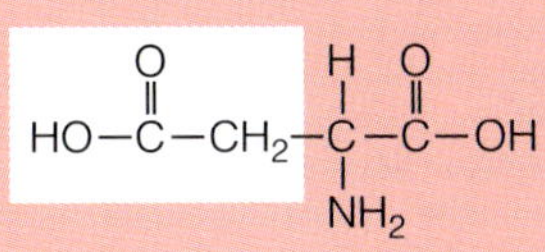
Aspartic acid (Asp)

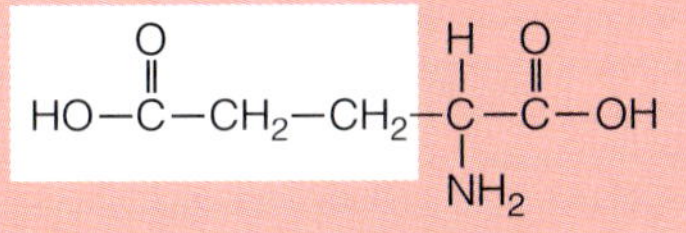
Glutamic acid (Glu)

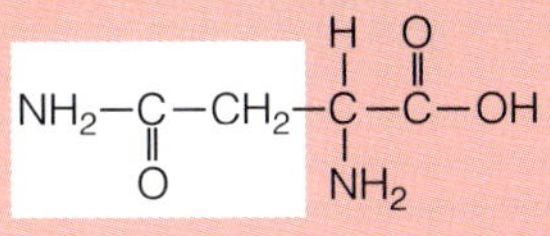
Asparagine (Asn)

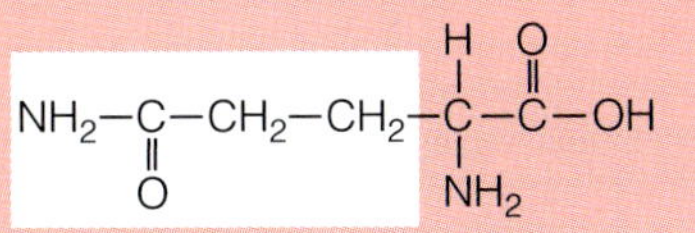
Glutamine (Gln)

4. Amino acids with basic side chains:

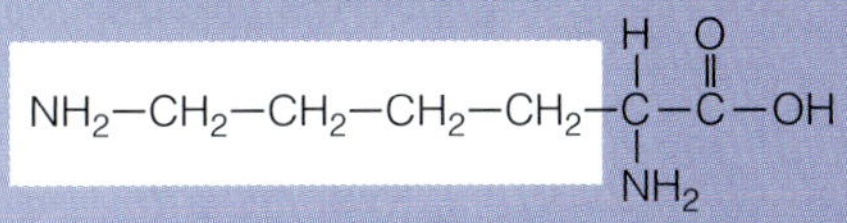
Lysine* (Lys)

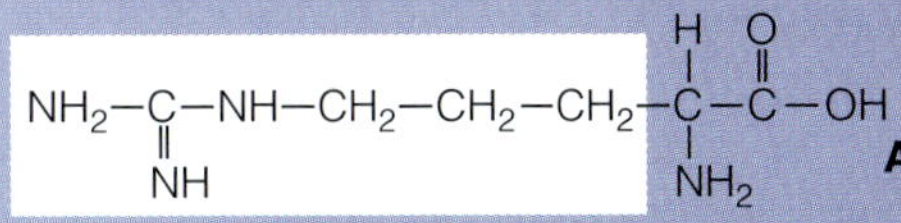
Arginine (Arg)

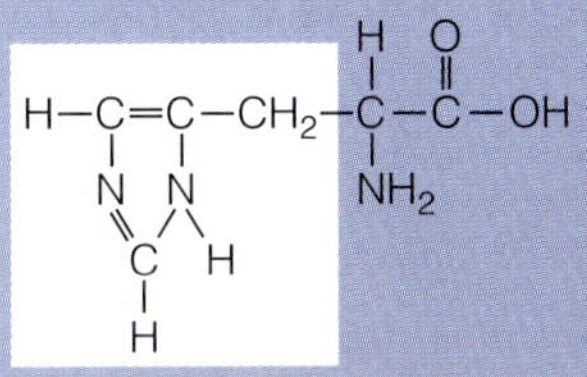
Histidine* (His)

5. Amino acids with aromatic side chains, which are characterized by the presence of at least one ring structure:

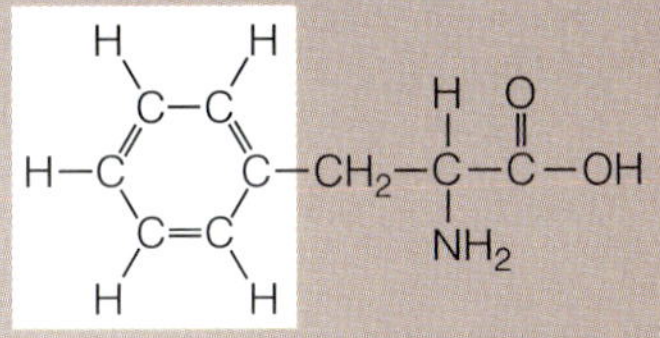
Phenylalanine* (Phe)

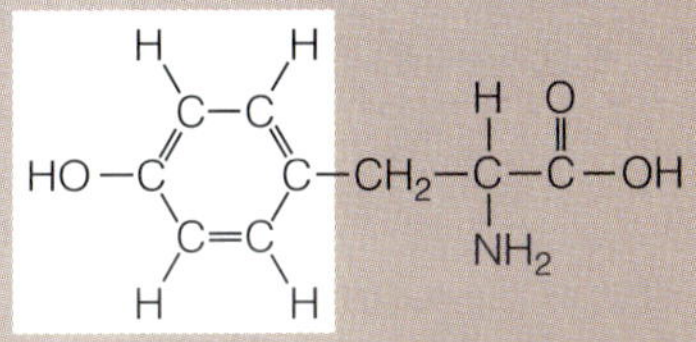
Tyrosine (Tyr)

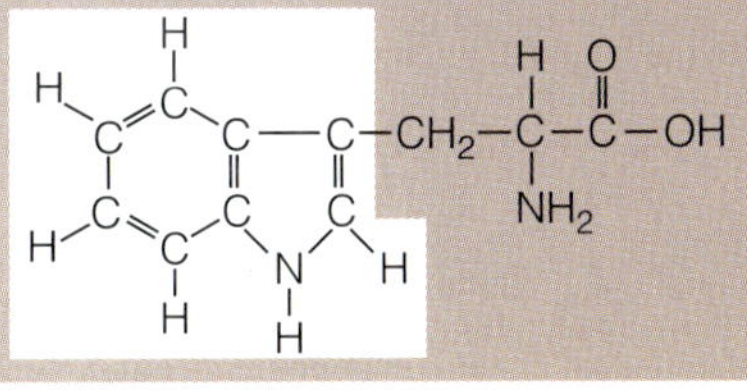
Tryptophan* (Trp)

6. Amino acids with side chains containing sulfur atoms:

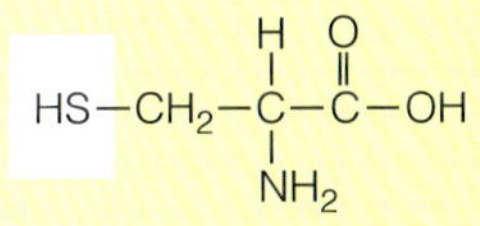
Cysteine (Cys)

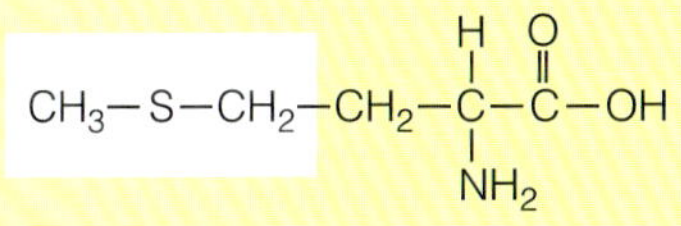
Methionine* (Met)

7. Imino acid:

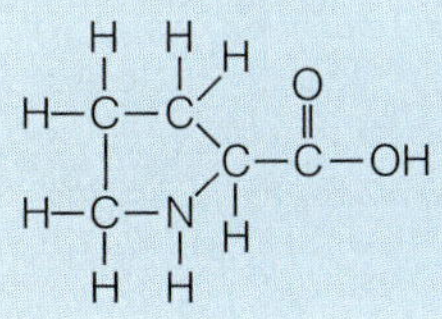
Proline (Pro)[a]

[a]Proline has the same $H_2N{-}C{-}COOH$ structure as the other amino acids, but its amino group has given up a hydrogen to form a ring.

C

VITAMINS AND COENZYMES

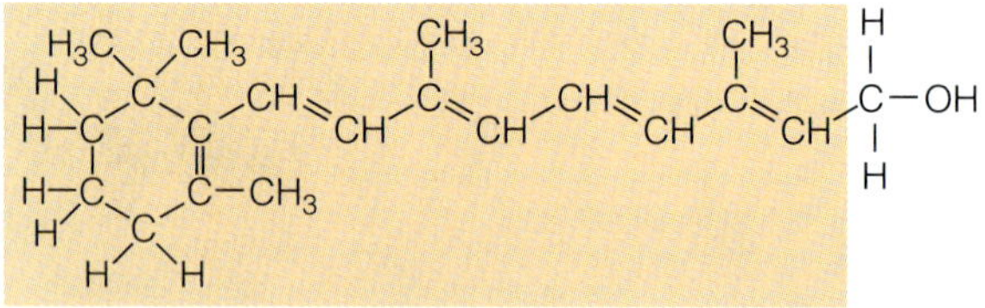

Vitamin A: retinol.

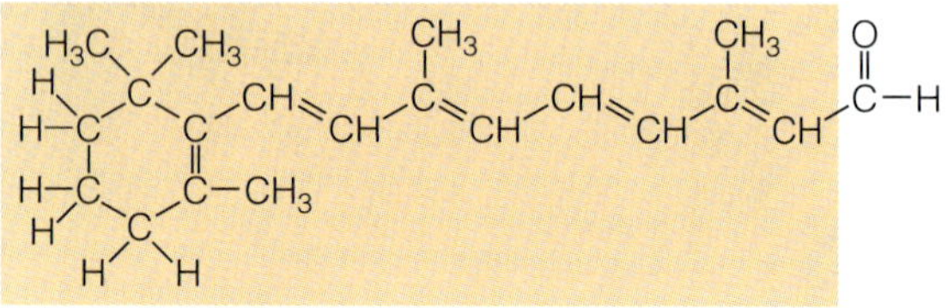

Vitamin A: retinal.

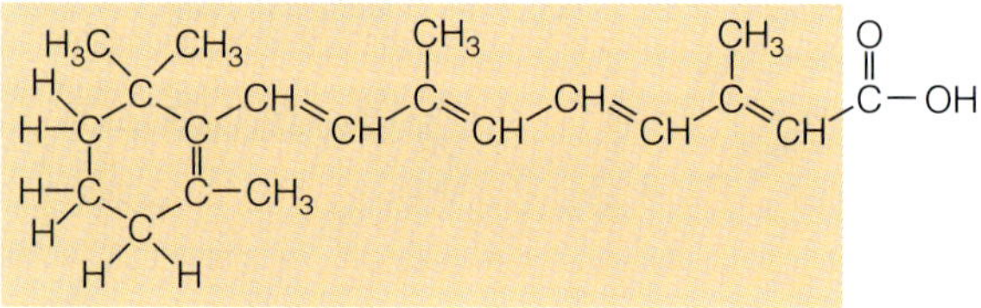

Vitamin A: retinoic acid.

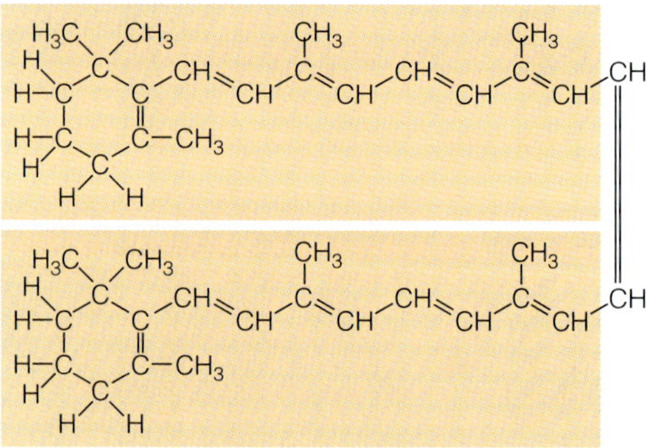

Vitamin A precursor: beta-carotene.

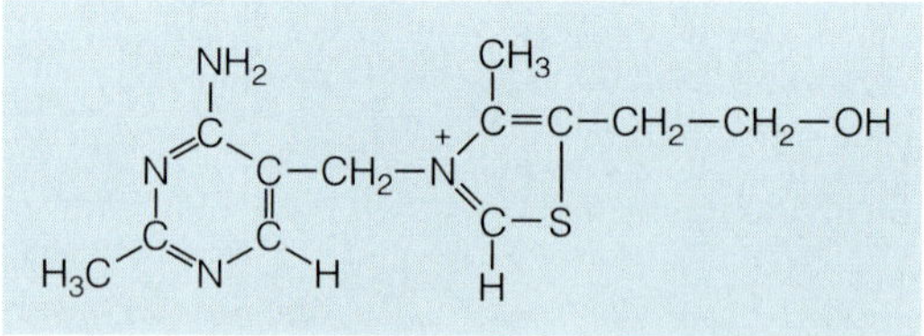

Thiamin. This molecule is part of the coenzyme thiamin pyrophosphate (TPP).

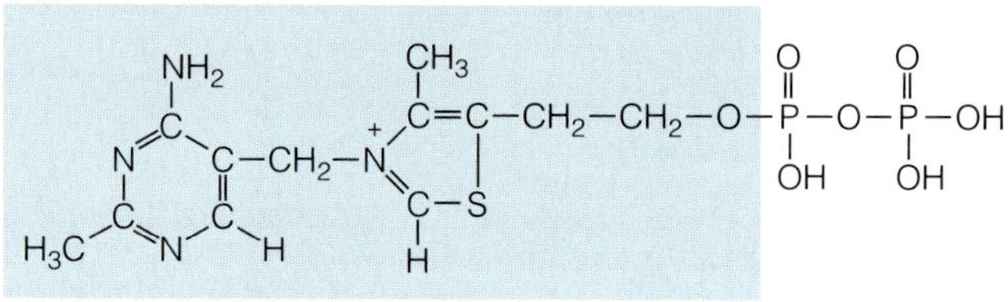

Thiamin pyrophosphate (TPP). TPP is a coenzyme that includes the thiamin molecule as part of its structure.

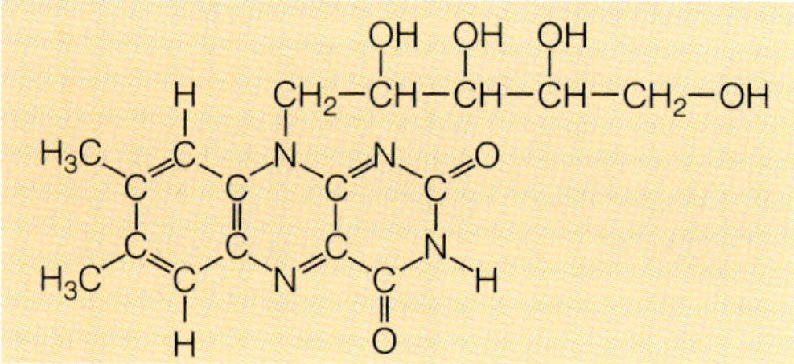

Riboflavin. This molecule is a part of two coenzymes—flavin mononucleotide (FMN) and flavin adenine dinucleotide (FAD).

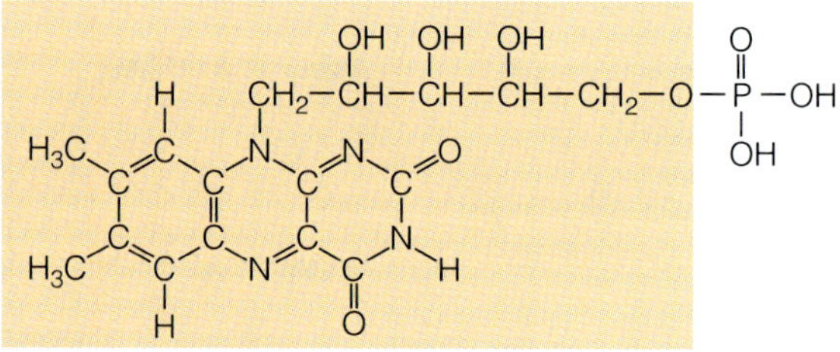

Flavin mononucleotide (FMN). FMN is a coenzyme that includes the riboflavin molecule as part of its structure.

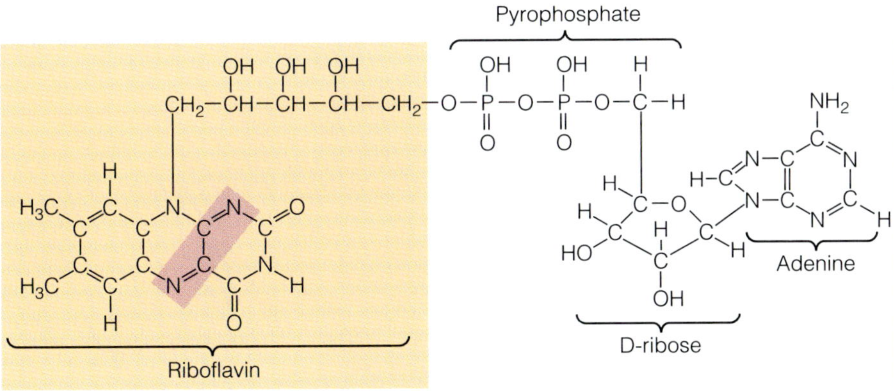

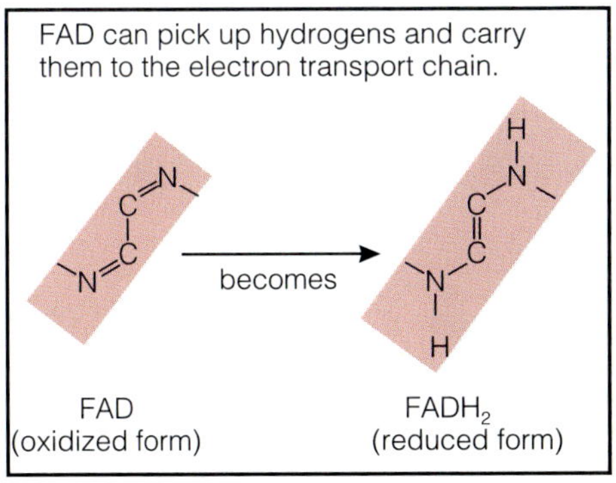

Pyrophosphate
Riboflavin
D-ribose
Adenine

FAD can pick up hydrogens and carry them to the electron transport chain.

FAD (oxidized form) becomes $FADH_2$ (reduced form)

Flavin adenine dinucleotide (FAD). FAD is a coenzyme that includes the riboflavin molecule as part of its structure.

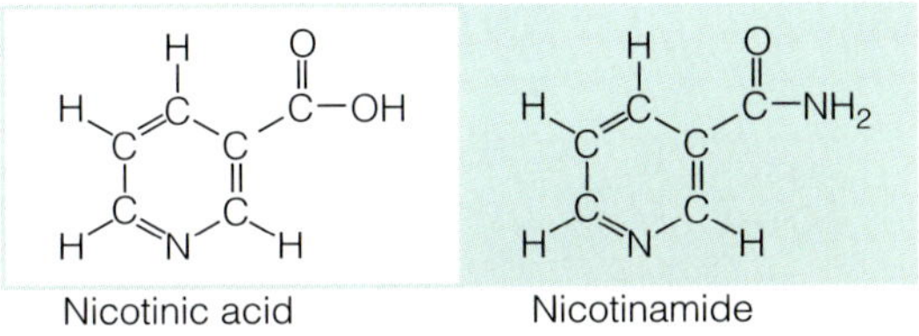

Nicotinic acid
Nicotinamide

Niacin (nicotinic acid and nicotinamide). These molecules are a part of two coenzymes—nicotinamide adenine dinucleotide (NAD^+) and nicotinamide adenine dinucleotide phosphate ($NADP^+$).

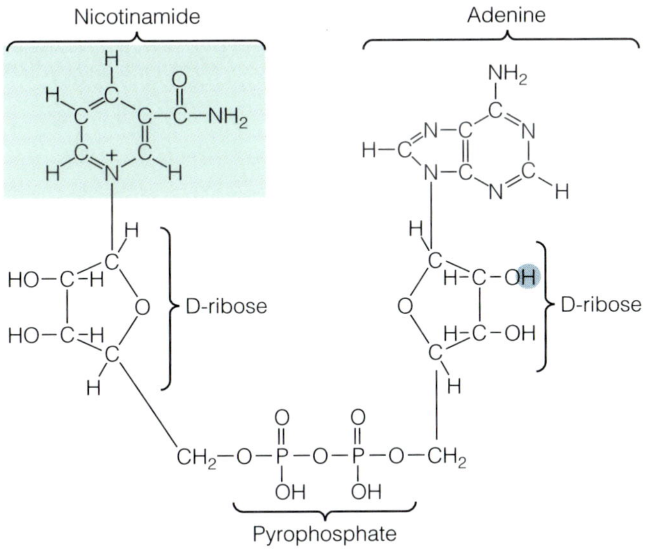

Nicotinamide
Adenine
D-ribose
D-ribose
Pyrophosphate

Nicotinamide adenine dinucleotide (NAD^+) and nicotinamide adenine dinucleotide phosphate ($NADP^+$). NADP has the same structure as NAD but with a phosphate group attached to the O instead of the H.

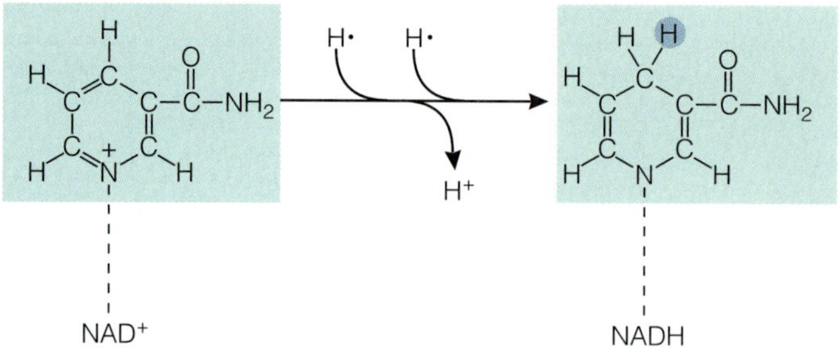

NAD$^+$ NADH

Reduced NAD$^+$ (NADH). When NAD$^+$ is reduced by the addition of H$^+$ and two electrons, it becomes the coenzyme NADH. (The dots on the H entering this reaction represent electrons—see Appendix B.)

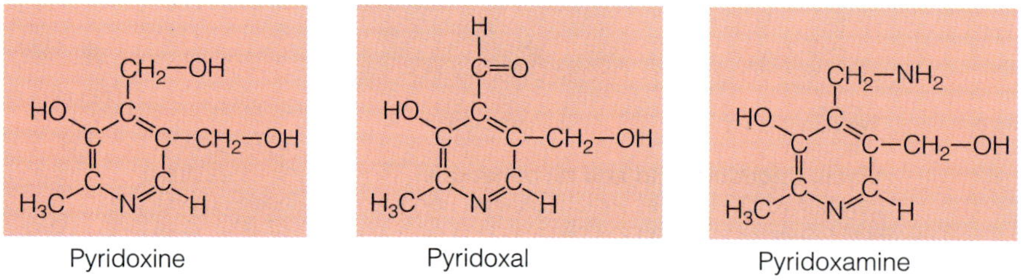

Pyridoxine Pyridoxal Pyridoxamine

Vitamin B_6 (a general name for three compounds—pyridoxine, pyridoxal, and pyridoxamine). These molecules are a part of two coenzymes—pyridoxal phosphate and pyridoxamine phosphate.

Pyridoxal phosphate Pyridoxamine phosphate

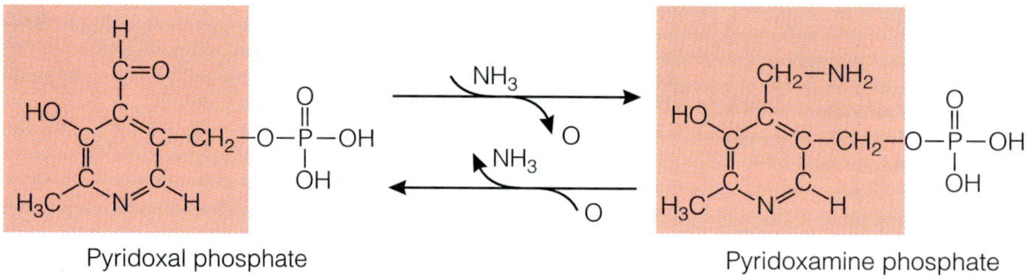

Pyridoxal phosphate (PLP) and pyridoxamine phosphate. These coenzymes are necessary for transamination and other important processes.

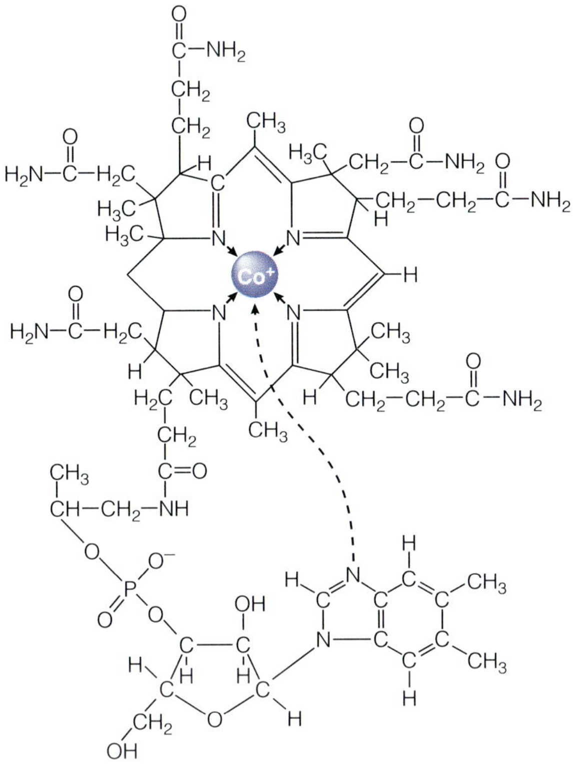

Vitamin B_{12} (cyanocobalamin). The arrows in this diagram indicate that the spare electron pairs on the nitrogens attract them to the cobalt.

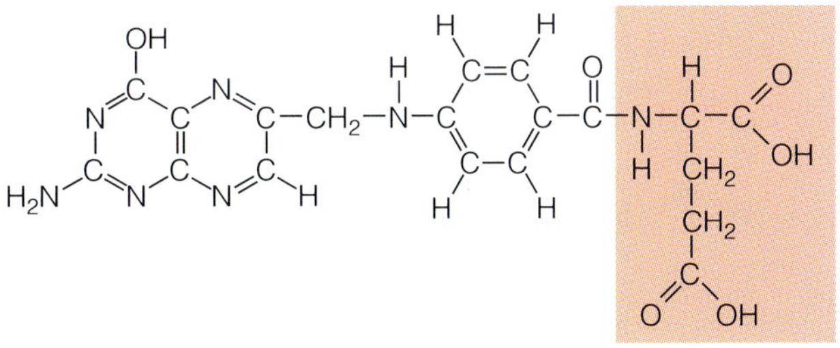

Folate (folacin or folic acid). This molecule consists of a double ring combined with a single ring and at least one glutamate (a nonessential amino acid marked in the box).

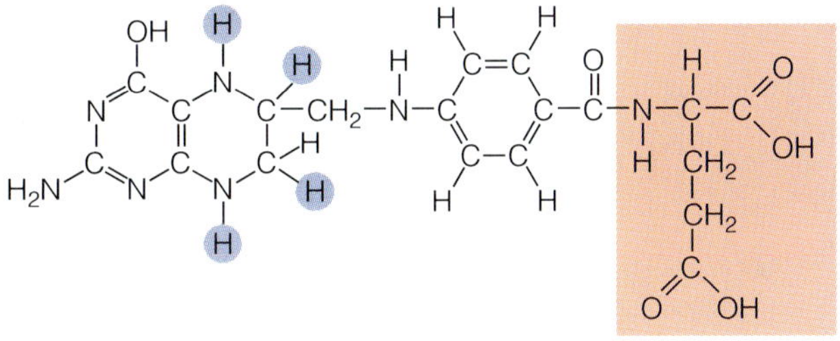

Tetrahydrofolic acid, the active coenzyme form of folate. This active form has four added hydrogens. An intermediate form, dihydrofolate, has two added hydrogens.

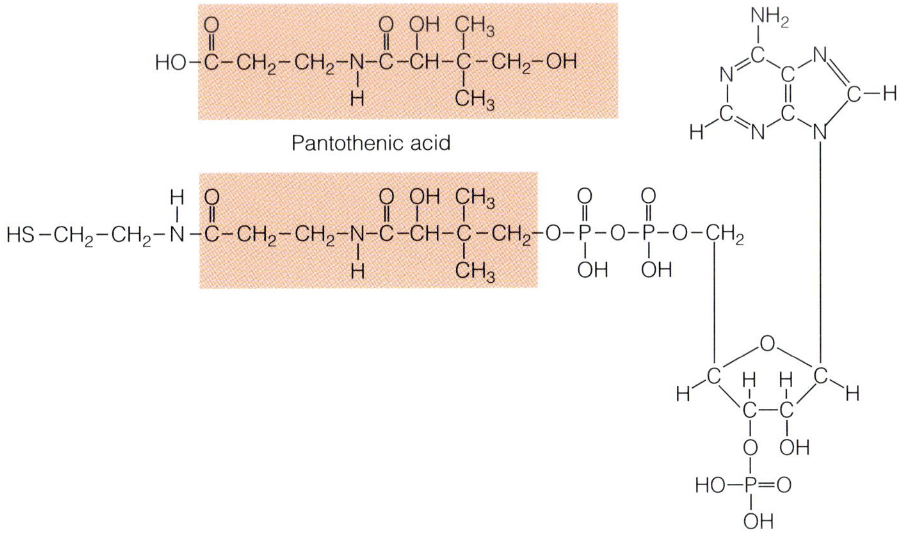

Pantothenic acid

Coenzyme A (CoA). This molecule is made up in part of pantothenic acid.

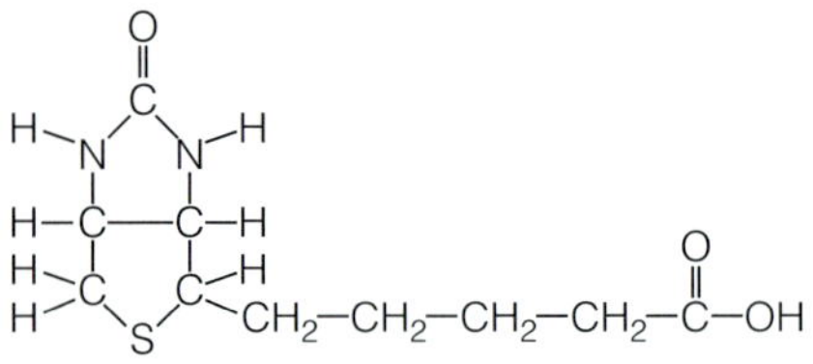

Biotin.

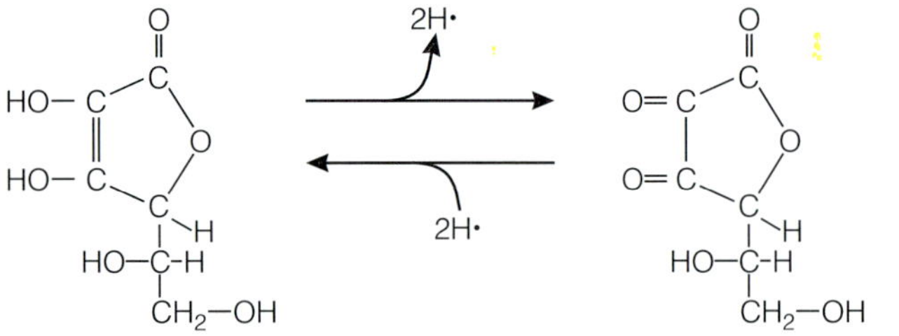

Ascorbic acid (reduced form) ⇌ Dehydroascorbic acid (oxidized form) ($2H\cdot$)

Vitamin C. The dots on the H indicate that two hydrogen atoms, complete with their electrons, are lost when ascorbic acid is oxidized and gained when it is reduced again.

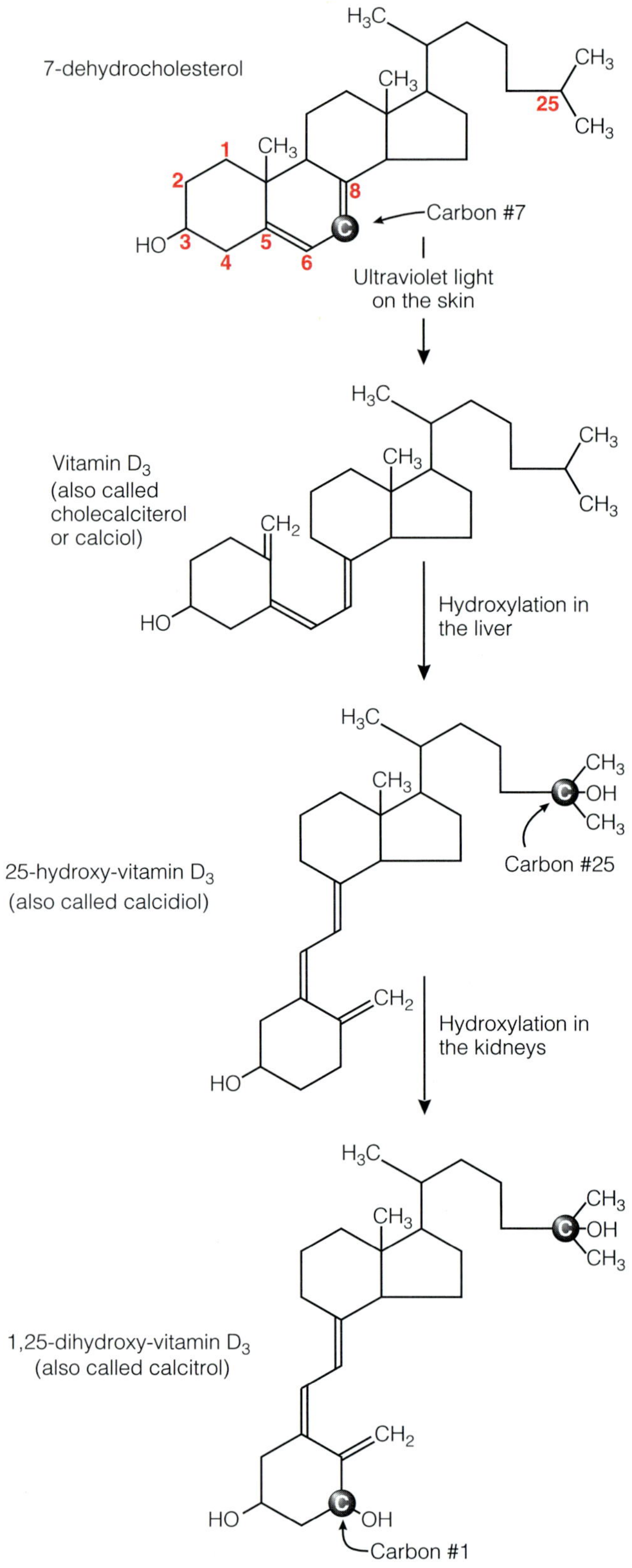

7-dehydrocholesterol

Carbon #7

Ultraviolet light on the skin

Vitamin D_3 (also called cholecalciterol or calciol)

Hydroxylation in the liver

25-hydroxy-vitamin D_3 (also called calcidiol)

Carbon #25

Hydroxylation in the kidneys

1,25-dihydroxy-vitamin D_3 (also called calcitrol)

Carbon #1

Active vitamin D and its precursors, beginning with 7-dehydrocholesterol. (The carbon atoms at which changes occur are numbered.)

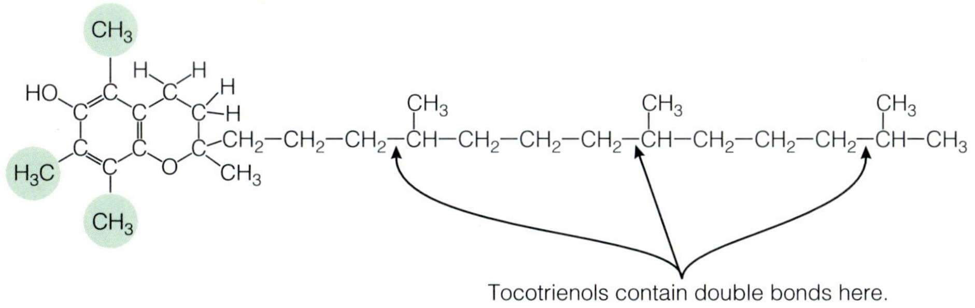

Tocotrienols contain double bonds here.

Vitamin E (alpha-tocopherol). The number and position of the methyl groups (CH_3) bonded to the ring structure differentiate among the tocopherols.

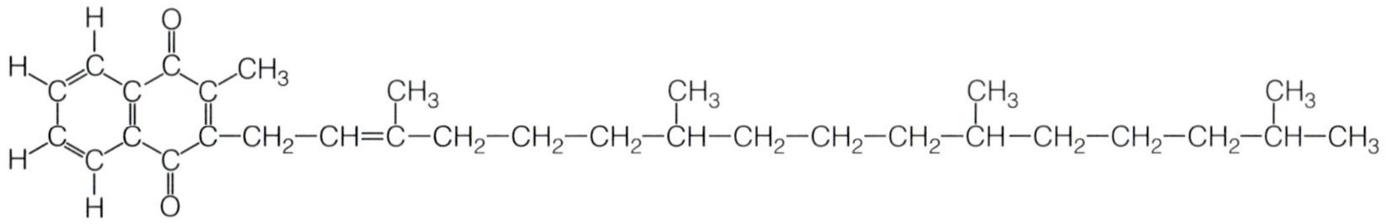

Vitamin K, a naturally occurring compound.

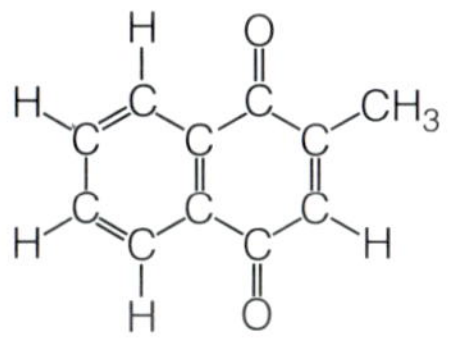

Menadione, a synthetic compound that has the same activity as natural vitamin K.

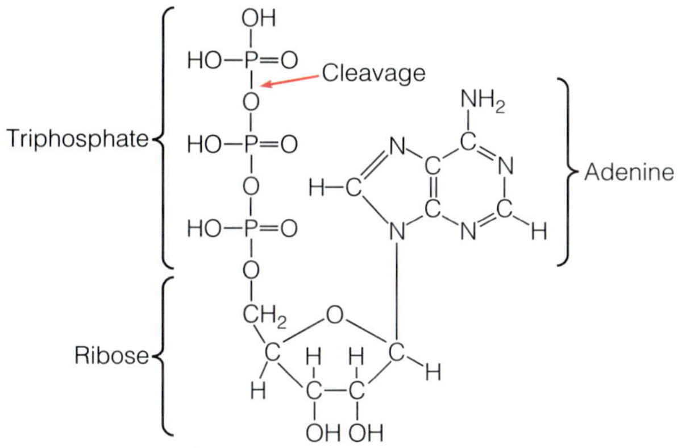

Triphosphate

Ribose

Adenine

Cleavage

Adenosine triphosphate (ATP), the energy carrier. The cleavage point marks the bond that is broken when ATP splits to become ADP + P.

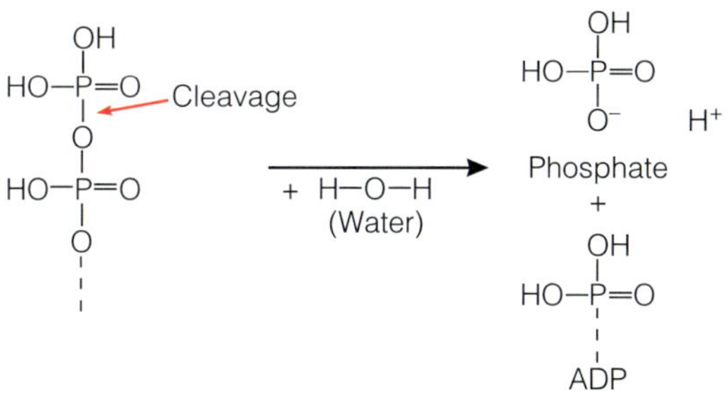

Cleavage

+ H—O—H (Water)

Phosphate + ADP

Adenosine diphosphate (ADP).

GLYCOLYSIS

Figure C–1 (on the next page) depicts the events of glycolysis. First, a phosphate is attached to glucose at the carbon that chemists call number 6. The product is called, logically enough, glucose-6-phosphate.

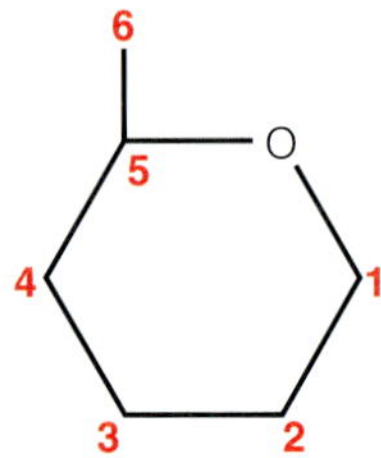

This is the way chemists number the carbons in a glucose molecule.

In the next couple of steps, glucose-6-phosphate is rearranged by an enzyme, and a phosphate is added in another coupled reaction with ATP. (A coupled reaction is a chemical event in which an enzyme complex catalyzes two reactions simultaneously. It often involves the breakdown of one compound and the synthesis of another.)

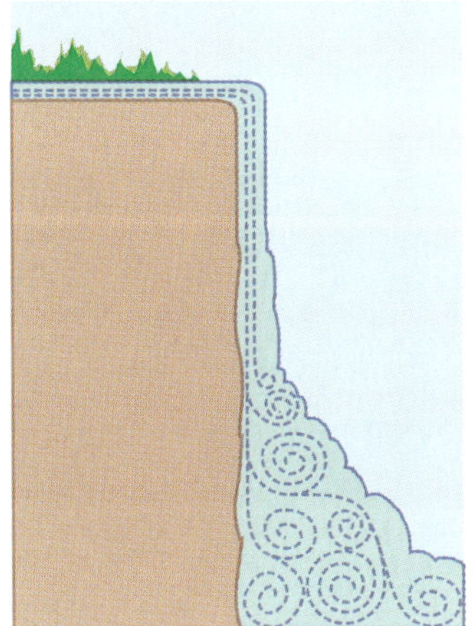

Falling water produces energy that is dissipated without doing work.

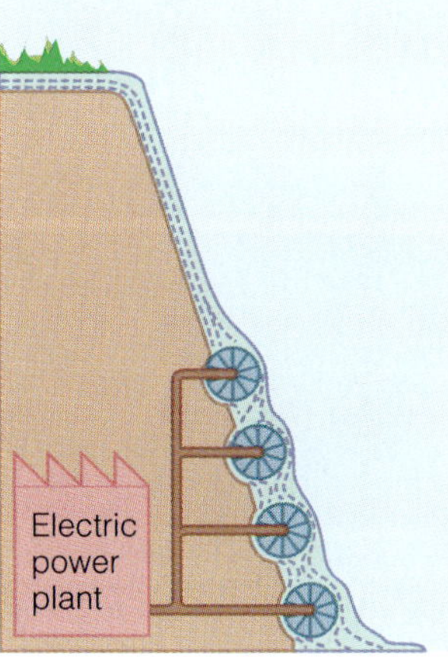

With the addition of a power plant (analogous to an enzyme), the energy of the falling water is coupled with a series of water wheels and turns them, producing energy.

A physical analogy of a coupled reaction. A coupled reaction often involves the breakdown of one compound and the synthesis of another. For example, the breakdown of glucose is coupled with the making of ATP, and the breakdown of ATP is coupled with the activation of glucose, or the making of glucose-P.

The product this time is fructose-1,6-diphosphate. At this point the six-carbon sugar has a phosphate group on its first and sixth carbons and is ready to break apart. Two ATP molecules have been used to accomplish this.

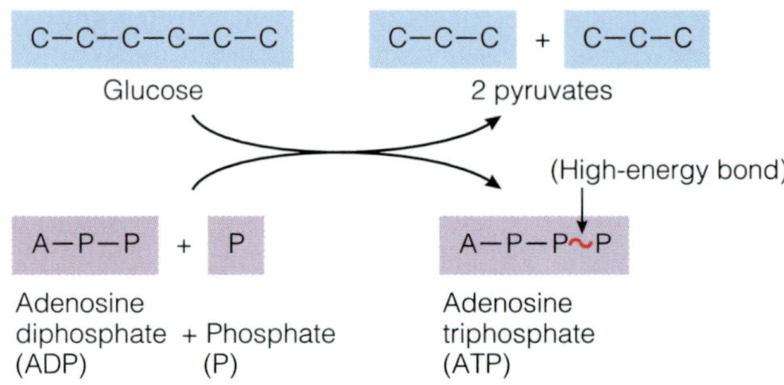

The breakdown of glucose is coupled with the making of ATP (simplified). Actually two ATP are used to prepare glucose for the reactions, and four ATP are gained in the breakdown of one glucose molecule to two molecules of pyruvate.

(From this point to the production of pyruvate, we will use letters in place of compound names. The names are in Figure C–1, for those who wish to know them.)

When fructose-1,6-diphosphate breaks in half, the two three-carbon compounds (A and A′) are not identical. Each has a phosphate group attached, but only one converts directly to pyruvate. The other compound, however, converts easily to the first. (Compound A′ is usually ignored, except for its role as the point of entry for the synthesis of glycerol; we say that two molecules of compound A are derived from one glucose molecule.)

In the step from compound A to compound B, enough energy is released to convert NAD^+ to NADH + H^+. Also, in the steps from B to C and from E to pyruvate, ATP is regenerated. Remember that in effect two molecules of compound A are produced from glucose; therefore, four ATP molecules are generated from each glucose molecule. Two ATP were needed to get the sequence started, so the net gain at this point is two ATP and two molecules of NADH + H^+.

So far, no oxygen has been used; the process has been anaerobic. But at this point, oxygen is needed. If oxygen is not immediately available, pyruvate converts to lactic acid to soak up the hydrogens from the NADH + H^+ that was generated. Lactic acid accumulates until oxygen becomes available. However, in the energy path from glucose to carbon dioxide, this side step usually is not necessary. As you will see later, each NADH + H^+ moves to the electron transport chain to unload its hydrogens onto oxygen. The associated energy produces two ATP, making a total yield of eight ATP for the process from glucose to pyruvate.

Figure C–1
Glycolysis

Notice that galactose and fructose enter at different places but all continue on the same pathway. Two molecules of compound A are produced (because compound A′ converts to A), and therefore two molecules of each succeeding compound.

- ◆ A = glyceraldehyde-3-phosphate.
- ◆ A′ = dihydroxyacetone phosphate.
- ◆ B = 1,3-diphosphoglyceric acid.
- ◆ C = 3-phosphoglyceric acid.
- ◆ D = 2-phosphoglyceric acid.
- ◆ E = phosphoenol pyruvic acid.

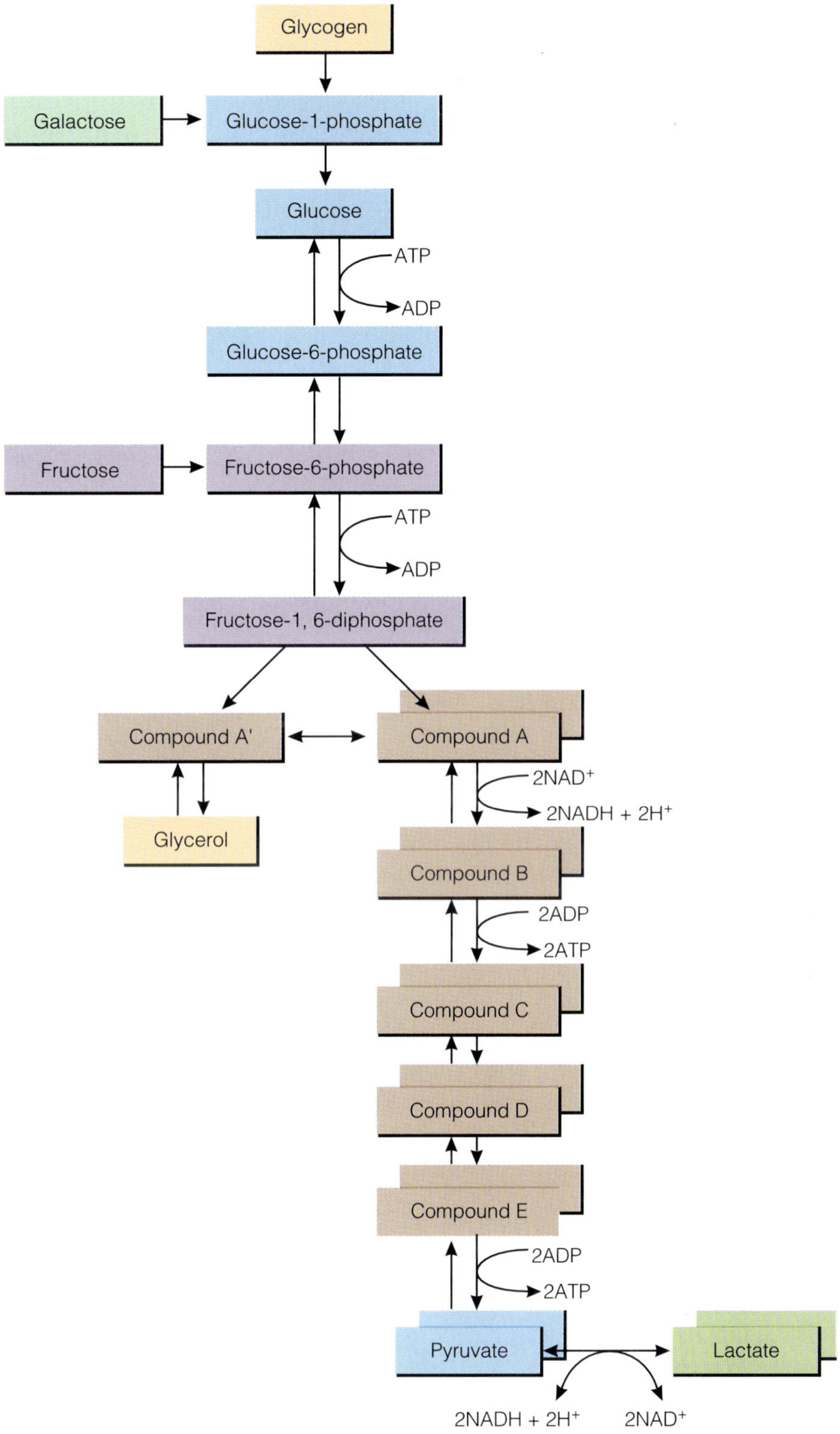

Glycogen
Galactose
Glucose-1-phosphate
Glucose
ATP
ADP
Glucose-6-phosphate
Fructose
Fructose-6-phosphate
ATP
ADP
Fructose-1, 6-diphosphate
Compound A'
Compound A
Glycerol
$2NAD^+$
$2NADH + 2H^+$
Compound B
2ADP
2ATP
Compound C
Compound D
Compound E
2ADP
2ATP
Pyruvate
Lactate
$2NADH + 2H^+$
$2NAD^+$

C

THE TCA CYCLE

The tricarboxylic acid, or TCA, cycle (Figure C–2 on p. C-15) is the name given to the set of reactions involving oxygen and leading from acetyl CoA to carbon dioxide (and water). To link glycolysis to the TCA cycle, pyruvate loses a carbon group and bonds with a molecule of CoA to become acetyl CoA. The TCA cycle is not restricted to the metabolism of carbohydrate. It also includes fat and protein. Any substance that can be converted to acetyl CoA directly, or indirectly through pyruvate, may enter the cycle.

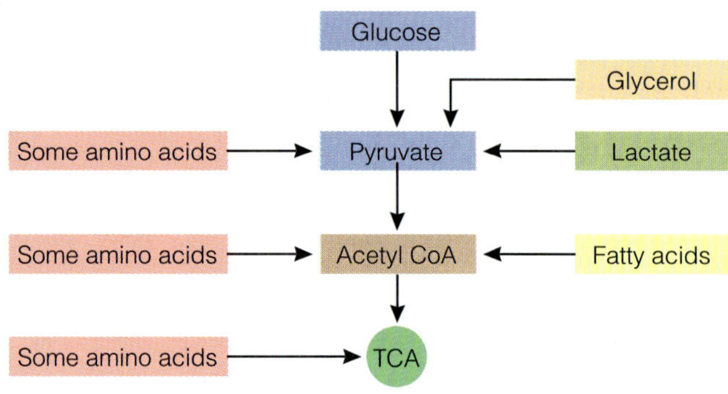

The step from pyruvate to acetyl CoA is exceedingly complex. We have included only those substances that will help you understand the transfer of energy from the nutrients. In the presence of oxygen, pyruvate loses a carbon to carbon dioxide and is attached to a molecule of CoA. In the process, NAD^+ picks up two hydrogens with their associated energy, becoming $NADH + H^+$.

As the acetyl CoA breaks down to carbon dioxide and water, its energy is captured in ATP. Let's follow the steps by which this occurs (see Figure C–2).

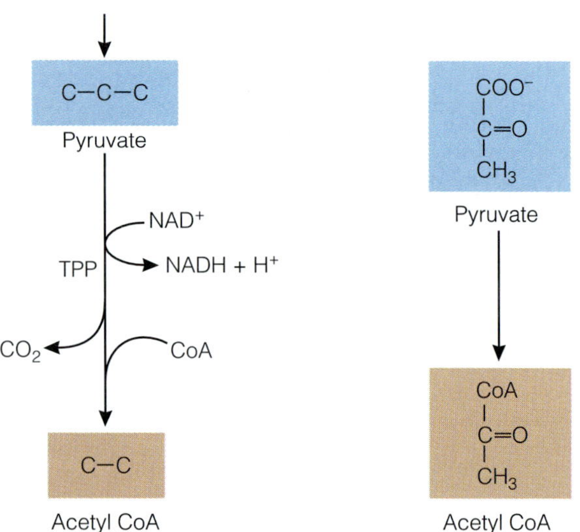

The step from pyruvate to acetyl CoA. (TPP and NAD are coenzymes containing the B vitamins thiamin and niacin, respectively.)

1. The two-carbon acetyl CoA combines with a four-carbon compound, oxaloacetate. The CoA comes off, and the product is a six-carbon compound, citrate.
2. The atoms of citrate are rearranged to form isocitrate.
3. Now NAD^+ reacts with isocitrate. Two H and two electrons are removed from the isocitrate. One H becomes attached to the NAD^+ with the two electrons; the other H is released as H^+. Thus NAD^+ becomes $NADH + H^+$. (Remember this $NADH + H^+$. It is carrying the H and the energy released from the last reaction. But let's follow the carbons first.) A carbon is combined with two oxygens, forming carbon dioxide (which diffuses away into the blood and is exhaled). What is left is the five-carbon compound alpha-ketoglutarate.
4. Now two compounds interact with alpha-ketoglutarate —a molecule of CoA and a molecule of NAD^+. In this complex reaction, a carbon and two oxygens are removed (forming carbon dioxide); two hydrogens are removed and go to NAD^+ (forming $NADH + H^+$); and the remaining four-carbon compound is attached to the CoA, forming succinyl CoA. (Remember this $NADH + H^+$ also. You will see later what happens to it.)
5. Now two molecules react with succinyl CoA—a molecule called GDP and one of phosphate (P). The CoA comes off, the GDP and P combine to form the high-energy compound GTP (similar to ATP), and succinate remains. (Remember this GTP.)
6. In the next reaction, two H with their energy are removed from succinate and are transferred to a molecule called FAD (an electron-hydrogen receiver like NAD^+) to form $FADH_2$. The product that remains is fumarate. (Remember this $FADH_2$.)
7. Next a molecule of water is added to fumarate, forming malate.
8. A molecule of NAD^+ reacts with the malate; two H with their associated energy are removed from the malate and form $NADH + H^+$. The product that remains is the four-carbon compound oxaloacetate. (Remember this $NADH + H^+$.)

We are back where we started. The oxaloacetate formed in this process can combine with another molecule of acetyl CoA (step 1), and the cycle can begin again. The whole scheme is shown in Figure C–2.

Figure C-2
The TCA Cycle

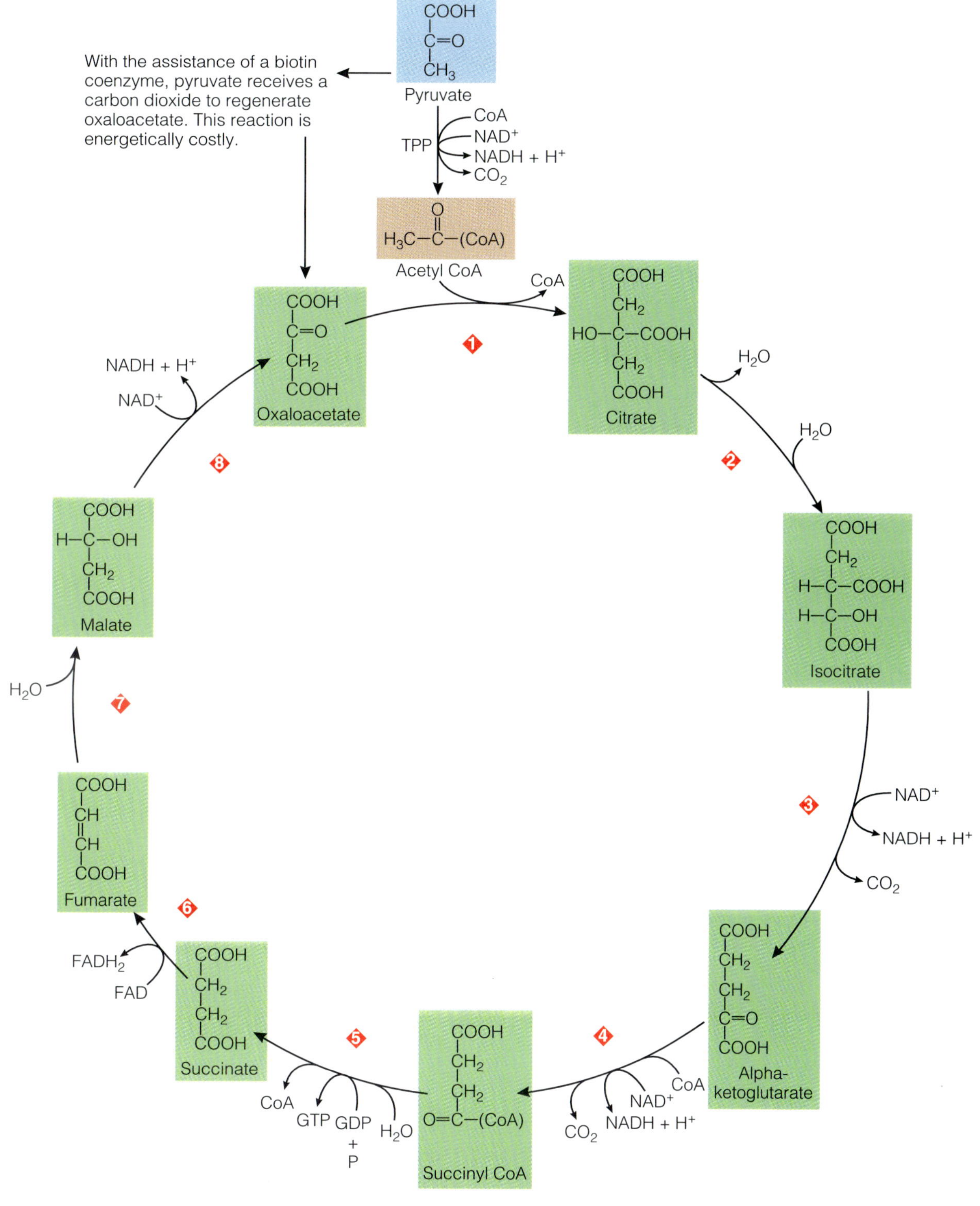

So far, we have seen two carbons brought in with acetyl CoA and two carbons ending up in carbon dioxide. But where are the energy and the ATP we promised?

Each time a pair of hydrogen atoms is removed from one of the compounds in the cycle, it includes a pair of electrons. Then the energy from this chemical bond is captured in the compound to which the H become attached. A review of the eight steps of the cycle shows that energy is transferred in this way into other compounds in steps 3, 4, 6, and 8. In step 5, energy is stored when GDP and P are bound together to form GTP. Thus the compounds NADH + H^+ (three molecules), $FADH_2$, and GTP store energy originally found in acetyl CoA. To see how this energy ends up in ATP, we must follow the electrons further. Let us take those attached to NAD^+ as an example.

THE ELECTRON TRANSPORT CHAIN

The six reactions described here are those of the electron transport chain, which is shown in Figure C–3. Since oxygen is required for these reactions, and ADP and P are combined to form ATP in several of them (ADP is phosphorylated), these reactions are also called oxidative phosphorylation.

An important concept to remember at this point is that an electron is not a fixed amount of energy. The electrons that bond the H to NAD^+ in NADH have a relatively large amount of energy. In the series of reactions that follow, they lose this energy in small amounts, until at the end they are attached (with H) to oxygen (O) to make water (H_2O). In some of the steps, the energy they lose is captured into ATP in coupled reactions.

1. In the first step of the electron transport chain, NADH reacts with a molecule called a flavoprotein, losing its electrons (and their H). The products are NAD^+ and reduced flavoprotein. A little energy is lost as heat in this reaction.
2. The flavoprotein passes on the electrons to a molecule called coenzyme Q. Again they lose some energy as heat, but ADP and P bond together and form ATP, storing much of the energy. This is a coupled reaction: ADP + P → ATP.
3. Coenzyme Q passes the electrons to cytochrome *b*. Again the electrons lose energy.
4. Cytochrome *b* passes the electrons to cytochrome *c* in a coupled reaction in which ATP is formed: ADP + P → ATP.
5. Cytochrome *c* passes the electrons to cytochrome *a*.
6. Cytochrome *a* passes them (with their H) to an atom of oxygen (O), forming water (H_2O). This is a coupled reaction in which ATP is formed: ADP + P → ATP.

Figure C–3
The Electron Transport Chain

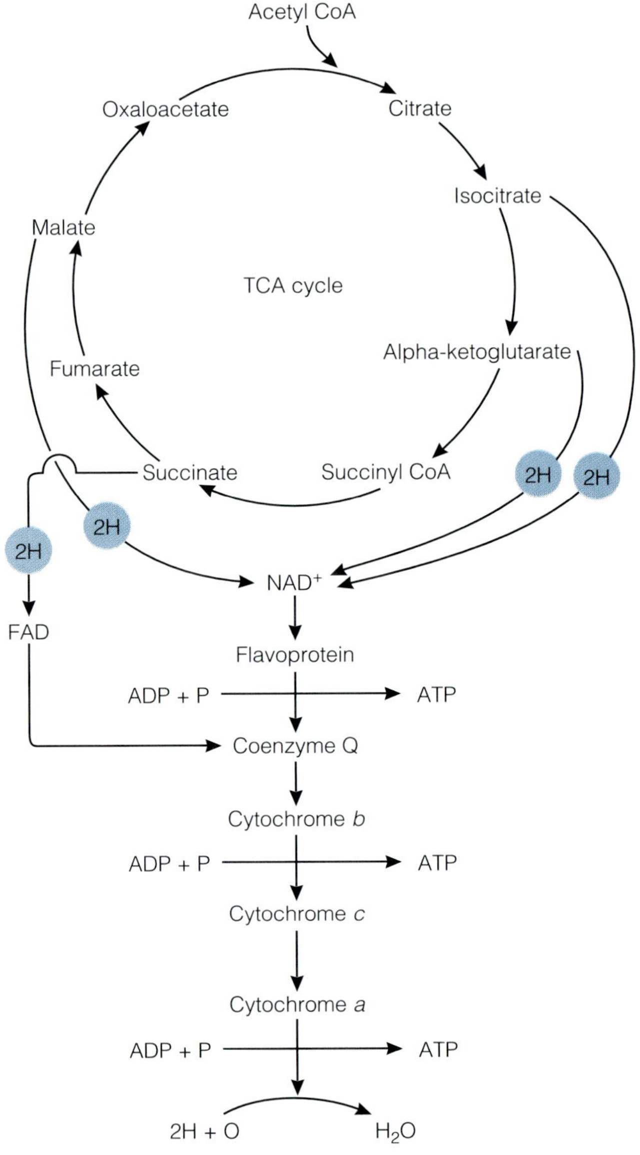

As Figure C–3 shows, each time NADH is oxidized (loses its electrons) by this means, the energy it loses is parceled out into three ATP molecules. When the electrons are passed on to water at the end, they are much lower in energy than they were originally. This completes the story of the electrons from NADH.

As for $FADH_2$, its electrons enter the electron transport chain at coenzyme Q. From coenzyme Q to water, ATP is generated in only two steps. Therefore, $FADH_2$ coming out of the TCA cycle yields just two ATP molecules.

Table C-3
Balance Sheet for Glucose Metabolism

	Expenditures	Income
Glycolysis:		
1 glucose	2 ATP	4 ATP
1 fructose-1,6-diphosphate		2 NADH + H^+
2 pyruvate		2 NADH + H^+
TCA cycle:		
2 isocitrate		2 NADH + H^+
2 alpha-ketoglutarate		2 NADH + H^+
2 succinyl CoA		2 GTP
2 succinate		2 $FADH_2$
2 malate		2 NADH + H^+
Total ATP collected:		
From glycolysis	2 ATP	4 ATP
From 2 NADH+ H^+		4–6 ATP[a]
From 8 NADH+ H^+		24 ATP
From 2 GTP		2 ATP
From 2 $FADH_2$		4 ATP
Totals:	2 ATP	38–40 ATP
Balance on hand from 1 molecule of glucose:		36–38 ATP

[a]Each NADH + H^+ from glycolysis can yield 2 or 3 ATP. See the accompanying text.

One energy-receiving compound of the TCA cycle (GTP) does not enter the electron transport chain but gives its energy directly to ADP in a simple phosphorylation reaction. This reaction yields one ATP.

It is now possible to draw up a balance sheet of glucose metabolism (see Table C–3). Glycolysis has yielded 4 NADH + H^+ and 4 ATP molecules and has spent 2 ATP. The 2 acetyl CoA going through the TCA cycle have yielded 6 NADH + H^+, 2 $FADH_2$, and 2 GTP molecules. After the NADH + H^+ and $FADH_2$ have gone through the electron transport chain, there are 34 ATP. Added to these are the 4 ATP from glycolysis and the 2 ATP from GTP, making the total 40 ATP generated from one molecule of glucose. After the expense of 2 ATP is subtracted, there is a net gain of 38 ATP.*

The TCA cycle and the electron transport chain are the body's major means of capturing the energy from nutrients in ATP molecules. Other means, such as anaerobic glycolysis, contribute, but the aerobic processes are the most efficient. Biologists and chemists understand much more about these processes than has been presented here.

*The total may sometimes be 36 or 37, rather than 38, ATP. The NADH + H^+ generated in the cytoplasm during glycolysis pass their electrons on to shuttle molecules, which move them into the mitochondria. One shuttle, malate, contributes its electrons to the electron transport chain before the first site of ATP synthesis, yielding 3 ATP. Another, glycerol phosphate, adds its electrons into the chain beyond that first site, yielding 2 ATP. Thus sometimes 3, and sometimes only 2, ATP result from the NADH + H^+ that arise from glycolysis. The amount depends on the cell.

ALCOHOL'S INTERFERENCE WITH ENERGY METABOLISM

Highlight 7 provides an overview of how alcohol interferes with energy metabolism. With an understanding of the TCA cycle, a few more details may be appreciated. During alcohol metabolism, the enzyme alcohol dehydrogenase oxidizes alcohol to acetaldehyde while it simultaneously reduces a molecule of NAD^+ to NADH + H^+. The related enzyme acetaldehyde dehydrogenase reduces another NAD^+ to NADH + H^+ while it oxidizes acetaldehyde to acetyl CoA, the compound that enters the TCA cycle to generate energy. Thus whenever alcohol is being metabolized in the body, NAD^+ diminishes, and NADH + H^+ accumulates. Chemists say that the body's "redox state" is altered, because NAD^+ can oxidize, and NADH + H^+ can reduce, many other body compounds. During alcohol metabolism, NAD^+ becomes unavailable for the multitude of reactions for which it is required.

As the previous sections just explained, for glucose to be completely metabolized, the TCA cycle must be operating, and NAD^+ must be present. If these conditions are not met (and when alcohol is present, they may not be), the pathway will be blocked, and traffic will back up—or an alternate route will be taken. Think about this as you follow the pathway shown in Figure C–4 on p. C-18.

In each step of alcohol metabolism in which NAD^+ is converted to NADH + H^+, hydrogen ions accumulate, resulting in a dangerous shift of the acid-base balance toward acid (Chapter 12 explains acid-base balance). The accumulation of NADH + H^+ depresses TCA cycle activity, so pyruvate and acetyl CoA build up. This condition favors the conversion of pyruvate to lactic acid, which serves as a temporary storage place for hydrogens from NADH + H^+. The conversion of pyruvate to lactic acid restores some NAD^+, but a lactic acid buildup has serious consequences of its own. It adds to the body's acid burden and interferes with the excretion of uric acid, causing goutlike symptoms. Molecules of acetyl CoA become building blocks for fatty acids or ketone bodies. The making of ketone bodies consumes acetyl CoA and generates NAD^+; but some ketone bodies are acids, so they push the acid-base balance further toward acid.

Figure C-4
Ethanol Enters the Metabolic Path

This is a simplified version of the glucose-to-energy pathway showing the entry of ethanol. The coenzyme NAD (which is the active form of the B vitamin niacin) is the only one shown here; however, many others are involved.

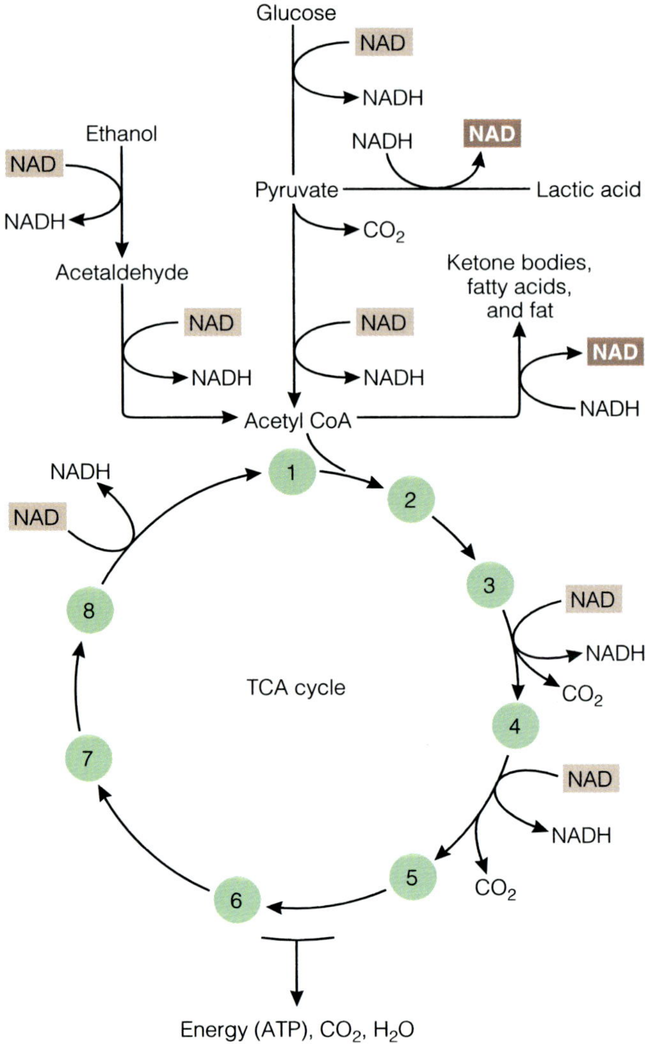

Thus alcohol cascades through the metabolic pathways, wreaking havoc along the way. These consequences have physical effects, which Highlight 7 describes.

THE UREA CYCLE

◆

Chapter 7 sums up the process by which waste nitrogen is eliminated from the body by stating that ammonia molecules combine with carbon dioxide to produce urea. This is true, but it is not the whole story. Urea is produced in a multistep process within the cells of the liver.

Ammonia, freed from an amino acid or other compound during metabolism anywhere in the body, arrives at the liver by way of the bloodstream and is taken into a liver cell. There, it is first combined with carbon dioxide and a phosphate group from ATP to form carbamyl phosphate:

$$\underset{\text{Carbon dioxide}}{CO_2} + \underset{\text{Ammonia}}{NH_3} \xrightarrow{2\text{ ATP} \rightarrow 2\text{ ADP} + \text{P}} \underset{\text{Carbamyl phosphate}}{H_2N-\overset{\overset{\large O}{\|}}{C}-\underbrace{O-\overset{\overset{\large O}{\|}}{\underset{\underset{\large O^-}{|}}{P}}-O^-}_{\text{Phosphate group}}}$$

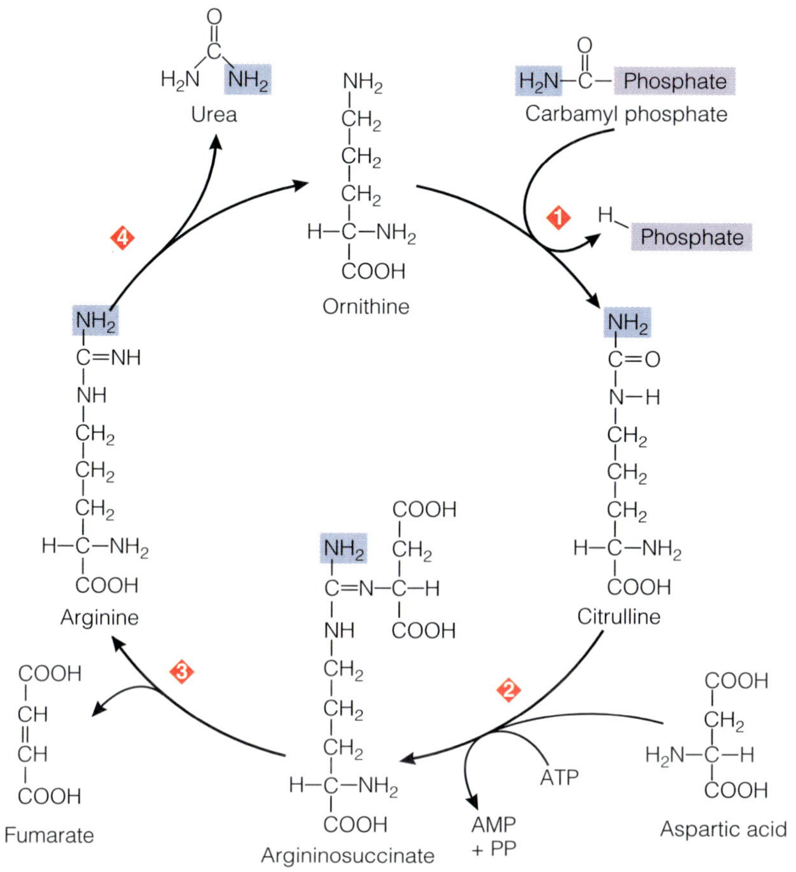

Figure C-5
The Urea Cycle

Figure C–5 shows the cycle of four reactions that follow. In the first step, carbamyl phosphate combines with the amino acid ornithine, losing its phosphate group. The compound formed is citrulline.

In the second step, citrulline combines with the amino acid aspartic acid, to form argininosuccinate. The reaction requires energy from ATP. (ATP was shown earlier losing one phosphorus atom in a phosphate group, P, to become ADP. In this reaction, it loses two phosphorus atoms joined together, PP, and becomes adenosine monophosphate, AMP.)

In the third step, argininosuccinate is split, forming another acid, fumarate, and the amino acid arginine.

In the fourth step, arginine loses its terminal carbon with two attached amino groups and picks up an oxygen from water. The end product is urea, which the kidneys excrete in the urine. The compound that remains is ornithine, identical to the ornithine with which this series of reactions began, and ready to react with another molecule of carbamyl phosphate and turn the cycle again.

FORMATION OF KETONE BODIES

Normally, fatty acid oxidation proceeds all the way to carbon dioxide and water. However, in ketosis (discussed in Chapter 7), an intermediate is formed from the condensation of two molecules of acetyl CoA: acetoacetyl CoA. Figure C–6 shows the formation of ketone bodies from that

Figure C-6
Formation of Ketone Bodies

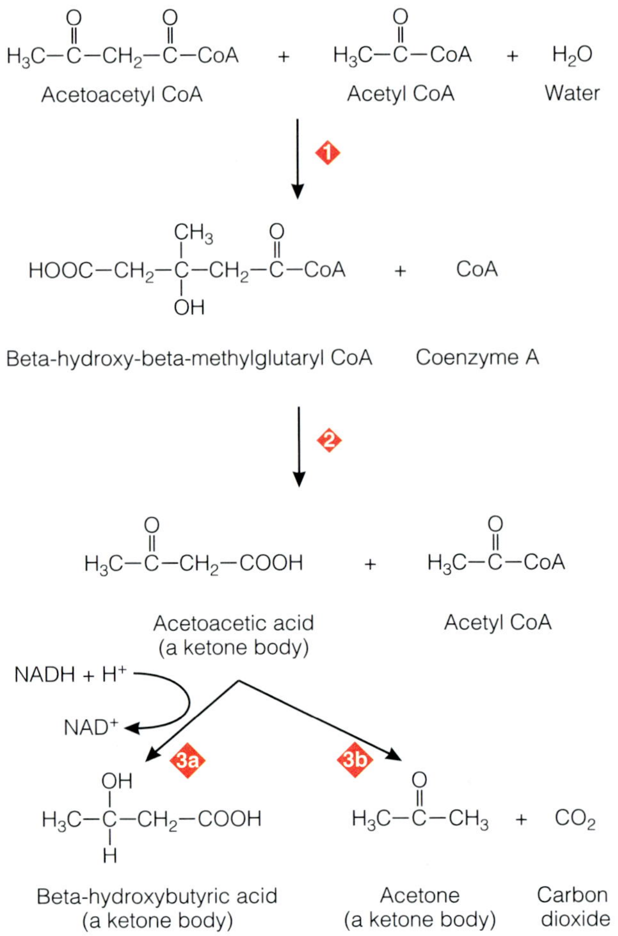

intermediate. In step 1, acetoacetyl CoA condenses with another acetyl CoA to form a six-carbon intermediate, beta-hydroxy-beta-methylglutaryl CoA. In step 2, this intermediate is cleaved to acetyl CoA and acetoacetic acid. This product can be metabolized either to beta-hydroxybutyric acid (step 3a) or to acetone (3b).

Acetoacetic acid, beta-hydroxybutyric acid, and acetone are the so-called ketone bodies of ketosis. Two are real ketones (they have a C=O group between two carbons); the other is an alcohol that has been produced during ketone formation—hence the term *ketone bodies,* rather than ketones, to describe the three of them. There are many other ketones in nature; these three are characteristic of ketosis in the body.

NOTES

1. Nomenclature policy: Generic descriptors and trivial names for vitamins and related compounds, *Journal of Nutrition* 117 (1987): 7–14; Nomenclature policy: Abbreviated designations of amino acids, *Journal of Nutrition* 117 (1987): 15.
2. A discussion of the designated abbreviations for the common amino acids presented here is found in Nomenclature policy: Abbreviated designations of amino acids, *Journal of Nutrition* 117 (1987): 15.

AIDS TO CALCULATION

Contents

Many mathematical problems have been worked out as examples at appropriate places in the text. This appendix aims to help with the use of the metric system and with problems not fully explained elsewhere.

CONVERSION FACTORS

Conversion factors are useful mathematical tools in everyday calculations, including those encountered in the study of nutrition. Skill in the use of conversion factors is especially desirable as the United States "goes metric."

A conversion factor is a fraction in which the numerator (top) and the denominator (bottom) express the same quantity in different units. For example, 2.2 pounds (lb) and 1 kilogram (kg) are equivalent; they express the same weight. The conversion factor used to change pounds to kilograms or vice versa is:

$$\frac{2.2\text{ lb}}{1\text{ kg}} \text{ or } \frac{1\text{ kg}}{2.2\text{ lb}}.$$

Because both factors equal 1, measurements can be multiplied by the factor without changing the value of the measurement. Thus the units can be changed.

To perform a conversion, use the factor with the unit you are seeking in the numerator (top) of the fraction. Following are two examples of problems commonly encountered in nutrition study; they illustrate the usefulness of conversion factors.

Example 1 Convert the weight of 130 pounds to kilograms.

1. Choose the conversion factor in which the unit you are seeking is on top:

$$\frac{1\text{ kg}}{2.2\text{ lb}}.$$

2. Multiply 130 pounds by the factor:

$$130\text{ lb} \times \frac{1\text{ kg}}{2.2\text{ lb}} = \frac{130\text{ kg}}{2.2} =$$

59 kg (rounded off to the nearest whole number).

Example 2 How many grams (g) of saturated fat are contained in a 3-ounce (oz) hamburger?

1. Consider a 4-ounce hamburger that contains 7 grams of saturated fat. You are seeking grams of saturated fat; therefore, the conversion factor is:

$$\frac{7\text{ g saturated fat}}{4\text{ oz hamburger}}.$$

2. Multiply 3 ounces of hamburger by the conversion factor:

$$3\text{ oz hamburger} \times \frac{7\text{ g saturated fat}}{4\text{ oz hamburger}} =$$

$$\frac{3 \times 7}{4} = \frac{21}{4}$$

= 5 g saturated fat (rounded off to the nearest whole number).

PERCENTAGES

A percentage is a comparison between a number of items (perhaps your intake of energy) and a standard number (perhaps the number of kcalories recommended for your age and sex—your energy RDA). The standard number is the number you divide by. The answer you get after the division must be multiplied by 100 to be stated as a percentage (*percent* means "per 100").

Example 3 What percentage of the RDA for energy is your energy intake?

1. Find your energy RDA (inside front cover, left). We'll use 2200 kcalories to demonstrate.
2. Total your energy intake for a day—for example, 1500 kcalories.
3. Divide your kcalorie intake by the RDA kcalories:

$$1500 \text{ kcal (your intake)} \div 2200 \text{ kcal (RDA)} = 0.68.$$

4. Multiply your answer by 100 to state it as a percentage:

$$0.68 \times 100 = 68 = 68\%.$$

In some problems in nutrition, the percentage may be more than 100. For example, suppose your daily intake of vitamin A is 3200 RE and your RDA (male) is 1000 RE. Your intake as a percentage of the RDA is more than 100 percent (that is, you consume more than 100 percent of your vitamin A RDA). The following calculations show your vitamin A intake as a percentage of the RDA:

$$3200 \div 1000 = 3.2.$$

$$3.2 \times 100 = 320\% \text{ of RDA.}$$

Sometimes the comparison is between a part of a whole (for example, your kcalories from protein) and the total amount (your total kcalories). In this case, the total number is the one you divide by.

Example 4 What percentages of your total kcalories for the day come from protein, fat, and carbohydrate?

1. Using Appendix H and your diet record, find the total grams of protein, fat, and carbohydrate you consumed—for example, 60 grams protein, 80 grams fat, and 310 grams carbohydrate.
2. Multiply the number of grams by the number of kcalories from 1 gram of each energy nutrient (conversion factors):

$$60 \text{ g protein} \times \frac{4 \text{ kcal}}{1 \text{ g protein}} = 240 \text{ kcal.}$$

$$80 \text{ g fat} \times \frac{9 \text{ kcal}}{1 \text{ g fat}} = 720 \text{ kcal.}$$

$$310 \text{ g carbohydrate} \times \frac{4 \text{ kcal}}{1 \text{ g carbohydrate}} = 1240 \text{ kcal.}$$

$$240 + 720 + 1240 = 2200 \text{ kcal.}$$

3. Find the percentage of total kcalories from each energy nutrient (see Example 3):

- Protein: $240 \div 2200 = 0.109 \times 100 = 10.9 = 11\%$ of kcal.
- Fat: $720 \div 2200 = 0.327 \times 100 = 32.7 = 33\%$ of kcal.
- Carbohydrate: $1240 \div 2200 = 0.563 \times 100 = 56.3 = 56\%$ of kcal.
- $11\% + 33\% + 56\% = 100\%$ of kcal (total).

The percentages total 100 percent, but sometimes they total 99 or 101 because of rounding off. This is a reasonable error.

RATIOS

A ratio is a comparison of two or three values in which one of the values is reduced to 1. A ratio compares identical units and so is expressed without units. For example, Figure 12–6 in Chapter 12 compares the milligrams of potassium to the milligrams of sodium in selected foods.

Example 5 Find the potassium-to-sodium ratio of your diet.

1. Using Appendix H and your diet record, find how many milligrams of potassium and sodium you consumed, say, 3000 milligrams potassium and 2500 milligrams sodium.
2. Divide the potassium milligrams by the sodium milligrams:

$$3000 \text{ mg potassium} \div 2500 \text{ mg sodium} = 1.2.$$

3. The potassium-to-sodium ratio is usually expressed as correct to one decimal point: 1.2.

The potassium-to-sodium ratio of your diet is 1.2:1 (read as "one point two to one" or simply "one point two"). A ratio greater than 1 means that the first value (in this case, milligrams of potassium) is greater than the second (sodium). When the second value is larger, the ratio is less than 1.

WEIGHTS AND MEASURES

Length

1 inch (in) = 2.54 centimeters (cm).
1 foot (ft) = 30.48 centimeters.
1 meter (m) = 39.37 inches.

Temperature

	Celsius*	Fahrenheit	
Steam	100°C	212°F	Steam
Body temperature	37°C	98.6°F	Body temperature
Ice	0°C	32°F	Ice

To find degrees Fahrenheit (t_F) when you know degrees Celsius (t_C), multiply by 9/5 and then add 32:

$$(9/5 \times t_C) + 32 = t_F.$$

To find degrees Celsius (t_C) when you know degrees Fahrenheit (t_F), multiply by 5/9 after subtracting 32:

$$5/9\ (t_F - 32) = t_C.$$

Volume

1 liter (L) = 1.06 quarts (qt) or 0.85 imperial quart.
1 liter = 1000 milliliters (mL).
1 milliliter = 0.03 fluid ounces.
30 milliliters = 1 fluid ounce.
1 gallon = 3.79 liters.
1 quart = 0.95 liter or 32 fluid ounces.
1 cup (c) = 8 fluid ounces or about 250 milliliters.
1 tablespoon (tbs) = 15 milliliters.
3 teaspoons (tsp) = 1 tablespoon.
1 teaspoon = about 5 g or 5 mL.
16 tablespoons = 1 cup.
4 cups = 1 quart.

Weight

1 ounce (oz) = approximately 28 grams (g).
16 ounces = 1 pound (lb).
1 pound = 454 grams.
1 kilogram (kg) = 1000 grams or 2.2 pounds.
1 gram = 1000 milligrams (mg).
1 milligram = 1000 micrograms (μg).

Energy units

1 kcalorie (kcal) = 4.2 kilojoules (kJ).
1 millijoule (mJ) = 240 kcal.
1 kJ = 0.24 kcal.
1 g carbohydrate = 4 kcal = 17 kJ.
1 g fat = 9 kcal = 37 kJ.
1 g protein = 4 kcal = 17 kJ.
1 g alcohol = 7 kcal = 29 kJ.

International Units (IU)

To convert IU to:

- μg RE, divide by 3.33 for retinol and by 10 for beta-carotene.
- μg vitamin D, divide by 40 or multiply by 0.025.
- mg α-TE, divide by 1.5.

*Also known as *centigrade*.

APPENDIX E

Contents

NUTRITION ASSESSMENT: SUPPLEMENTAL INFORMATION

Chapters 15 and 16 described the nutrition assessment techniques health care professionals commonly use to determine clients' nutrition status. From this assessment, they identify clients' nutrition needs and develop care plans for meeting those needs. This appendix provides additional details and alternative methods of assessing nutrition status to support a complete nutrition assessment.

DRUG HISTORY: NUTRITION AND DRUG INTERACTIONS

Chapter 15 described nutrient-drug interactions and Chapters 21 through 30 provided a series of "prescription pads," listing drugs used in the treatment of the specific diseases being discussed. Table E–1 provides examples of selected drugs, describes nutrition-related factors that affect drug administration, and lists the most common nutrition-related side effects.

Table E-1
Administration and Common Nutrition-Related Side Effects of Selected Drugs

Drug Classification and Examples	Administration	Common Nutrition-Related Side Effects[a]
Analgesics		
Narcotic: codeine, merperidine, morphine sulfate	Give with food to reduce GI distress.	N/V, GI distress, reduced GI motility, constipation, lethargy.
Nonnarcotic (also act as nonsteroidal anti-inflammatory agents): aspirin, ibuprofen, naproxen		N/V, GI distress, GI bleeding, constipation. Aspirin may lower blood folate and vitamin C.
Antacids	Give with fluids between meals or at bedtime.	
Al-containing (also act as phosphate binders): Al carbonate, Al hydroxide, Al phosphate	Give with meals when used as phosphate binder.	Constipation, phosphorus deficiency. Long-term use in renal failure may cause Al toxicity.
Ca-containing (also act as phosphate binders and Ca supplements): Ca carbonate and Ca gluconate	When used as a phosphate binder or supplement, give with meals and separately from foods high in fiber, oxalate, or phytate and iron or fluoride supplements.	Constipation, chalky taste. Concurrent use with vitamin D supplements may lead to elevated blood Ca.
Mg-containing (also act as laxatives): Mg hydroxide, Mg oxide, and Mg citrate	Give separately from iron and folate supplements.	Diarrhea, chalky taste. Long-term use in renal failure may lead to Mg toxicity.
Antianginals		
Amyl nitrate, isosorbide dinitrate, nitroglycerin (see also *Antihypertensives*)	Give oral forms on an empty stomach. Limit alcohol.	Nutrition-related side effects are uncommon.
Antianxiety Agents	Give with food to reduce GI distress.	
Alprazolam, chlordiazepoxide	Avoid alcohol.	Increased appetite, weight gain, nausea, drowsiness.
Diazepam, lorazepam, oxazepam	Limit caffeine and avoid alcohol.	Constipation, diarrhea, dry mouth, drowsiness.
Meprobamate	Avoid alcohol.	N/V, diarrhea, drowsiness.
Anticoagulants, oral		
Ticlopidine	Give with food to improve drug absorption and reduce GI distress.	N/V, GI pain, diarrhea.
Warfarin	Maintain consistent vitamin K intake, avoid high doses of vitamins A and E, which can reduce the anticoagulant effect. Avoid high doses of vitamin C, which can reduce drug absorption.	Nausea.
Anticonvulsants	Give with meals to reduce GI distress.	
Phenytoin	Tube feedings may interfere with drug absorption (see Chapter 23).	N/V, swollen gums. May cause folate-deficiency anemia. Increases metabolism of vitamins D and K.

[a]Note that many other medications not listed in this table also have nutrition-related side effects. In addition, nutrition-related side effects other than those listed may occur. For example, almost all medications cause nausea in some people. In this table, nausea is only listed as a side effect if it occurs with relative frequency or does not resolve with time. More detailed texts should be consulted for the medications you routinely encounter in clinical practice.

Abbreviations: N/V = nausea/vomiting; Al = aluminum; Ca = calcium; Mg = magnesium; K = potassium; GERD = gastroesophageal reflux disease; ACE = angiotensin-converting enzyme; H2 = histamine$_2$.

E

Table E–1
Administration and Common Nutrition-Related Side Effects of Selected Drugs (continued)

Drug Classification and Examples	Administration	Common Nutrition-Related Side Effects[a]
Anticonvulsants		
Primidone	Avoid alcohol.	N/V. May cause folate-deficiency anemia.
Valproic acid	Do not take tablets with milk or liquid form with carbonated beverages.	N/V, GI pain.
Antidepressants		
MAO inhibitors: phenelzine, tranylcypromine	Give with food to reduce GI distress. Avoid foods high in tyramine (see Chapter 15), alcohol, and tryptophan supplements. Limit caffeine.	Weight changes, dry mouth, constipation.
Tricyclic: amitriptyline, clomipramine, doxepin, imipramine, protriptyline	Give with food to reduce GI distress. Avoid alcohol and limit caffeine and high-fiber foods.	Dry mouth, constipation. Stimulates appetite, especially for sweets.
Other:		
bupropion	Give with food to reduce GI distress. Avoid alcohol.	Dry mouth, constipation.
fluoxetine	Give in morning without regard to food. Avoid tryptophan supplements.	Anorexia, weight loss, dry mouth, N/V, diarrhea.
nefazone	Food reduces drug absorption and bioavailability.	Dry mouth, N/V, constipation.
sertraline	Give at same time each day without regard to food. Avoid alcohol.	Dry mouth, N/V, constipation.
Antidiabetics		
Acarbose	Give at the start of each meal.	GI pain, flatulence, diarrhea, hypoglycemia.
Glipizide	Give 30 min before breakfast. Limit alcohol.	Hypoglycemia. GI side effects uncommon.
Glyburide	Give with breakfast. Limit alcohol.	Hypoglycemia. GI side effects uncommon.
Metformin	Give with meals to reduce GI distress. Limit alcohol.	N/V, bloating, flatulence, diarrhea. Lowers blood glucose, cholesterol, LDL, and triglycerides and raises HDL.
Troglitazone[c]	Give with meals.	Risk of hypoglycemia increases when used in combination with other antidiabetic agents. GI side effects uncommon.
Antidiarrheals		
Loperamide	Give without regard to food.	Nutrition-related side effects are uncommon.
Opium and paregoric	Give without regard to food.	N/V, constipation, sedation.

[a]Note that many other medications not listed in this table also have nutrition-related side effects. In addition, nutrition-related side effects other than those listed may occur. For example, almost all medications cause nausea in some people. In this table, nausea is only listed as a side effect if it occurs with relative frequency or does not resolve with time. More detailed texts should be consulted for the medications you routinely encounter in clinical practice.

Abbreviations: N/V = nausea/vomiting; Al = aluminum; Ca = calcium; Mg = magnesium; K = potassium; GERD = gastroesophageal reflux disease; ACE = angiotensin-converting enzyme; H2 = histamine$_2$.

[c]*Source:* Product advertisement in *Diabetes Care,* August 1977.

Table E-1
Administration and Common Nutrition-Related Side Effects of Selected Drugs (continued)

Drug Classification and Examples	Administration	Common Nutrition-Related Side Effects[a]
Antihypertensives	Avoid natural licorice.	
ACE inhibitors:		
benazepril, enalapril, lisopril, ramipril	Limit alcohol and avoid salt substitutes. Monitor use of K supplements.	May elevate blood K.
captopril	Give 1 hr before or 2 hr after meals. Limit alcohol and avoid salt substitutes. Monitor use of K supplements.	Mouth ulcers. May elevate blood K.
fosinopril	Give separately from Ca or Mg supplements. Limit alcohol and avoid salt substitutes. Monitor use of K supplements.	May elevate blood K.
Alpha-adrenergic blockers: doxazosin, prazosin, terazosin	Limit alcohol.	Weight gain, fatigue.
Beta-blockers (also act as antiarrythmics and antianginals):		May mask signs of hypoglycemia.
atenolol	Give with food to reduce GI distress. Give separately from Ca supplements or antacids.	Nausea, dizziness.
metoprolol	Give with food to enhance bioavailability.	Diarrhea, confusion, dizziness.
nadolol	Limit alcohol.	Nutrition-related side effects are uncommon.
propranolol	Give with food to enhance bioavailability. Avoid alcohol and give separately from Ca supplements or antacids.	Dizziness, drowsiness, weakness.
Ca-channel blockers (also act as antianginals):		
amlopidine, isradipine	Give without regard to food.	Edema, headache.
dilitiazem	Give tablets or extended release capsules before meals.	Edema, dizziness.
felopidine	Do not give with grapefruit juice.	Edema, headache.
nicarpidine, nisoldipine	Do not give with high-fat foods or grapefruit juice.	Edema, headache, dizziness.
Other:		
clonidine	Avoid alcohol.	Dry mouth, constipation, edema, drowsiness, dizziness.

[a]Note that many other medications not listed in this table also have nutrition-related side effects. In addition, nutrition-related side effects other than those listed may occur. For example, almost all medications cause nausea in some people. In this table, nausea is only listed as a side effect if it occurs with relative frequency or does not resolve with time. More detailed texts should be consulted for the medications you routinely encounter in clinical practice.

Abbreviations: N/V = nausea/vomiting; Al = aluminum; Ca = calcium; Mg = magnesium; K = potassium; GERD = gastroesophageal reflux disease; ACE = angiotensin-converting enzyme; H2 = histamine$_2$.

E

Table E–1
Administration and Common Nutrition-Related Side Effects of Selected Drugs (continued)

Drug Classification and Examples	Administration	Common Nutrition-Related Side Effects[a]
Antihypertensives (continued)		
guanfacine	Limit alcohol.	Dry mouth, constipation, drowsiness.
hydralazine	Give with food to enhance bioavailability. Limit alcohol.	Anorexia, N/V, edema, headache. Pyridoxine supplements correct drug-induced peripheral neuropathy.
methyldopa	Avoid alcohol. Do not give drug within 2 hr of giving iron supplements.	Dry mouth, headache, drowsiness, edema. High doses increase vitamin B_{12} and folate needs.
minoxidil		Bloating, edema.
Anti-Infectives		
Antibiotics:		
amoxicillin	Give without regard to food.	Diarrhea.
ampicillin	Give with 8 oz of water 1 hr before or 2 hr after meals.	Diarrhea.
cefaclor, cefoperazone, cefotaxime	Give parenterally. Avoid alcohol while using and for 3 days afterward. Give foods high in vitamin K or a vitamin K supplement with long-term use.	May interfere with bacterial vitamin K synthesis in intestine.
chloramphenicol	Give with 8 oz water 1 hr before or 2 hr after meals. Avoid alcohol. Limit use of iron supplements.	Increases risk of iron overload. Delays response to iron, folate, or vitamin B_{12}.
erythromycin	Give with 8 oz water 1 hr before or 2 hr after meals. Food decreases absorption of some forms (base and stearate), but may be given to reduce GI distress.	Epigastric pain, abdominal cramps.
ethambutol	Give with food to reduce GI distress.	Nutrition-related side effects are uncommon.
penicillin	Give penicillin K without regard to meals; penicillin G 1 hr before or 2 hr after meals. Use K supplements cautiously with penicillin K.	N/V, epigastric distress, mouth sores, diarrhea.
tetracycline	Give with water 1 hr before or 2 hr after meals. Separate the administration of Ca, iron, Mg, zinc, Al, or vitamin-mineral supplements or Al-, Ca-, or Mg-containing antacids by 3 hr.	N/V, diarrhea, cramps, dizziness.

[a]Note that many other medications not listed in this table also have nutrition-related side effects. In addition, nutrition-related side effects other than those listed may occur. For example, almost all medications cause nausea in some people. In this table, nausea is only listed as a side effect if it occurs with relative frequency or does not resolve with time. More detailed texts should be consulted for the medications you routinely encounter in clinical practice.

Abbreviations: N/V = nausea/vomiting; Al = aluminum; Ca = calcium; Mg = magnesium; K = potassium; GERD = gastroesophageal reflux disease; ACE = angiotensin-converting enzyme; H2 = histamine$_2$.

Table E-1
Administration and Common Nutrition-Related Side Effects of Selected Drugs (continued)

Drug Classification and Examples	Administration	Common Nutrition-Related Side Effects[a]
Anti-Infectives (continued)		
Antifungals:		
amphotericin	Give parenterally and encourage fluids.	Anorexia, N/V, weight loss, stomach pain, fever, headache, soreness.
clotrimazole	Dissolve lozenge slowly in mouth over 15–30 min.	N/V.
flucytosine	Give capsules slowly over 15 min to reduce GI distress.	N/V, diarrhea, lethargy, dizziness.
ketoconazole	Give with foods to enhance absorption. Give Ca or Mg separately by 2 hr.	N/V.
Antivirals:		
acyclovir	Encourage fluids.	Headache.
famciclovir	Give without regard to food.	Headache.
foscarnet	Give parenterally and encourage fluids.	Anorexia, N/V, abdominal pain, diarrhea, fever, headache, weakness, dizziness.
ganciclovir	Give with food and encourage fluids.	N/V, abdominal pain, headache, fever, weakness.
lamivudine (3TC)	Give without regard to food.	Nausea, GI pain, diarrhea, headache, fever.
saquinavir	Give within 2 hr of a full meal.	Nausea, GI pain, diarrhea, headache.
stavudine (d4T)	Give without regard to food.	N/V, diarrhea, fever.
zalcitabine (DDC)	Give on empty stomach, if possible, to enhance absorption.	Anorexia, weight loss, N/V, mouth ulcers.
zidovudine (AZT)	Give without regard to food.	Anorexia, N/V, headache, anemia.
Anti-Inflammatory Agents		
Corticosteroids (also act as immunosuppressants): cortisone, dexamethasone, hydrocortisone, prednisone	Give with food to reduce GI distress. Encourage high-protein, low-sodium diet. Avoid alcohol. May need supplements of or diets high in K, Ca, and phosphorus; vitamins A, C, and D; and pyridoxine and folate.	Edema, osteoporosis. Increase appetite and weight. Induce negative nitrogen and Ca balances.
Diclofenac	Give with food, milk, or water to reduce GI distress. Avoid alcohol.	Nausea, GI pain, constipation, diarrhea, headache, edema.
Diflunisal	Give with food or milk to reduce GI distress. Avoid alcohol.	Nausea, GI pain, diarrhea, headache.
Mesalamine, olsalazin	Give with food and 8 oz water.	Nutrition-related side effects are uncommon.
Salsalate	Give with food, milk or water. Limit alcohol and caffeine.	Nausea, dizziness.

[a]Note that many other medications not listed in this table also have nutrition-related side effects. In addition, nutrition-related side effects other than those listed may occur. For example, almost all medications cause nausea in some people. In this table, nausea is only listed as a side effect if it occurs with relative frequency or does not resolve with time. More detailed texts should be consulted for the medications you routinely encounter in clinical practice.

Abbreviations: N/V = nausea/vomiting; Al = aluminum; Ca = calcium; Mg = magnesium; K = potassium; GERD = gastroesophageal reflux disease; ACE = angiotensin-converting enzyme; H2 = histamine$_2$.

Table E–1
Administration and Common Nutrition-Related Side Effects of Selected Drugs (continued)

Drug Classification and Examples	Administration	Common Nutrition-Related Side Effects[a]
Anti-Inflammatory Agents (continued)		
Sulfasalazine (See also *Analgesics, nonnarcartic*)	Give with 8 oz water or food to reduce GI distress. Give folate supplement and encourage fluids.	Anorexia, N/V, GI pain, diarrhea, headache, dizziness. Lowers blood folate.
Antilipemics		
Cholestyramine	Give before meals. Mix powder form with water or fluids; never give dry or with carbonated beverages.	Nausea, belching, dyspepsia, constipation. May decrease absorption of fat, fat-soluble vitamins, folate, Ca, iron, zinc, and Mg.
Clofibrate	Give with food or milk to reduce GI distress.	Nausea, anemia.
Fluvastatin	Give without regard to food.	Nutrition-related side effects are uncommon.
Gemfibrozil	Give ½ hr before meals.	Taste alterations, dyspepsia, abdominal pain.
Lovastatin	Give with meals to enhance absorption. Give fiber, pectin, or oat bran separately by several hr. Avoid high doses of niacin and limit alcohol.	Constipation, headache.
Pravastatin, simvastatin	Avoid high doses of niacin and limit alcohol.	Nutrition-related side effects are uncommon.
Antinauseants, Antiemetics		
Dronabinol (marijuana derivative)	Give before lunch and dinner.	Stimulates appetite and causes weight gain. Euphoria.
Granisetron	Give without regard to food.	Constipation, headache, weakness.
Meclizine	Give without regard to food	Nutrition-related side effects are uncommon.
Metoclopramide	Give ½ hr before meals and at bedtime.	Nausea, diarrhea, lethargy.
Ondansetron	Give without regard to food.	Abdominal pain, constipation, headache, weakness.
Prochlorperazine	Give with food or milk. Avoid alcohol and limit caffeine.	Dry mouth, constipation. Stimulates appetite and causes weight gain. Increases urinary excretion of riboflavin.
Antineoplastics		
Aldesleukin	Give parenterally.	Anorexia, N/V, mouth inflammation, diarrhea, mental changes, dizziness, anemia, impaired renal function, fever, edema, infection.

[a]Note that many other medications not listed in this table also have nutrition-related side effects. In addition, nutrition-related side effects other than those listed may occur. For example, almost all medications cause nausea in some people. In this table, nausea is only listed as a side effect if it occurs with relative frequency or does not resolve with time. More detailed texts should be consulted for the medications you routinely encounter in clinical practice.

Abbreviations: N/V = nausea/vomiting; Al = aluminum; Ca = calcium; Mg = magnesium; K = potassium; GERD = gastroesophageal reflux disease; ACE = angiotensin-converting enzyme; H2 = histamine$_2$.

Table E-1
Administration and Common Nutrition-Related Side Effects of Selected Drugs (continued)

Drug Classification and Examples	Administration	Common Nutrition-Related Side Effects[a]
Antineoplastics (continued)		
Bleomyin	Give parenterally.	Anorexia, N/V, mouth inflammation, weight loss, fever, respiratory impairment.
Carboplatin	Give parenterally with adequate fluids to maintain hydration.	Anorexia, N/V, mouth inflammation, GI pain, diarrhea, constipation, weakness, infections, anemia. Lowers blood levels of sodium, K, Ca, and Mg.
Carmustine	Give parenterally with adequate fluids to maintain hydration.	N/V, mild liver impairment.
Cisplatin	Give parenterally with adequate fluids to maintain hydration.	Severe N/V, taste alterations, diarrhea, infections, impaired renal function, anemia. Lowers blood levels of sodium, K, Ca, phosphorus, Mg, and zinc.
Cyclophosphamide	Give oral forms with food only if GI distress occurs. Encourage fluids.	Anoerxia, N/V, mouth inflammation, delayed wound healing.
Cytarbine	Give parenterally and provide adequate liquids.	Anorexia, N/V, mouth inflammation, diarrhea, anal ulcers, weight loss, infection. Lowers blood levels of K and Ca.
Dactinomycin	Give parenterally and provide adequate fluids. Encourage high-kcalorie foods. Raises vitamin B_{12} needs.	Anorexia, severe N/V, dry mouth, mouth and tongue inflammation, taste alterations, severe esophagitis, dysphagia, GI pain, diarrhea, weight loss, fatigue, anemia. Reduces absorption of fat, Ca, and iron.
Daunorubicin, doxorubicin, idarubicin	Give parenterally and provide adequate fluids.	Anorexia, N/V, weight loss, dry mouth, mouth and esophageal inflammation, anemia.
Estramustine	Store capsules in refrigerator.	Anorexia, N/V, diarrhea, edema, lethargy, Impairs glucose tolerance.
Etoposide, teniposide	Give parenterally or orally (etoposide).	Anorexia, N/V, mouth inflammation, diarrhea.
Floxuridine	Give parenterally.	Anorexia, N/V, diarrhea, weakness, lethargy.
Fluorouracil	Give parenterally.	Anorexia, severe N/V, mouth and esophageal inflammation, taste alterations, intestinal inflammation, diarrhea, weakness, anemia. May increase pyridoxine needs.
Interferon alfa 2a and 2b	Give parenterally and provide adequate liquids.	Anorexia, N/V, dry mouth, taste alterations, mouth inflammation, abdominal pain, diarrhea, weight loss, dizziness, headache, fatigue.

[a]Note that many other medications not listed in this table also have nutrition-related side effects. In addition, nutrition-related side effects other than those listed may occur. For example, almost all medications cause nausea in some people. In this table, nausea is only listed as a side effect if it occurs with relative frequency or does not resolve with time. More detailed texts should be consulted for the medications you routinely encounter in clinical practice.

Abbreviations: N/V = nausea/vomiting; Al = aluminum; Ca = calcium; Mg = magnesium; K = potassium; GERD = gastroesophageal reflux disease; ACE = angiotensin-converting enzyme; H2 = histamine$_2$.

E

Table E–1
Administration and Common Nutrition-Related Side Effects of Selected Drugs (continued)

Drug Classification and Examples	Administration	Common Nutrition-Related Side Effects[a]
Antineoplastics (continued)		
Leuprolide	Give parenterally.	Anorexia, N/V, constipation, edema, headache, weakness, anemia.
Levamisole	Give without regard to food.	Nausea, taste alterations, diarrhea, fatigue.
Lomustine	Give on empty stomach to reduce GI distress. Provide adequate fluids.	N/V, anemia.
Mechlorethamine	Give adequate fluids.	Anorexia, severe N/V, anemia.
Megestrol acetate (see *Appetite Stimulants*)		
Melphalan	Give adequate fluids. Divide single daily dose if GI distress occurs (food reduces drug bioavailability).	Nutrition-related side effects are uncommon, but may include mild N/V and diarrhea.
Mercaptopurine	Give adequate fluids.	Anorexia, mild N/V, anemia.
Methotrexate	Give adequate fluids.	Anorexia, N/V, mouth and gum inflammation, weight loss, infection.
Mithramycin, plicamycin	Give parenterally.	Anorexia, N/V, mouth inflammation, diarrhea.
Mitomycin	Give parenterally.	Anorexia, N/V, weight loss, fever, weakness.
Mitoxantrone	Give parenterally.	N/V, mouth inflammation, GI bleeding, abdominal pain, diarrhea, fever.
Paclitaxel	Give parenterally.	N/V, mouth and esophageal inflammation, diarrhea, edema, fatigue, anemia.
Pegasparagase	Give parenterally.	N/V, fever, weakness.
Porfimer	Give parenterally.	N/V, dysphagia, abdominal pain, constipation, fever.
Streptozocin	Give parenterally.	N/V, renal and liver impairment.
Tamoxifen citrate	Give Ca and Mg supplements separately from enteric-coated tablet by 2 hr.	N/V.
Tretinoin	Give with meals. Do not give vitamin A supplements. Limit alcohol and fat.	N/V, abdominal pain, GI bleeding, respiratory impairment, elevated blood lipids, fever.
Antipsychotics		
Chlorpromazine (also acts as an antinauseant)	Give with food, milk, or water to reduce GI distress. Dilute oral concentrate in a 4 oz drink or soft food. Give Mg separately by 2 hr. Avoid alcohol.	Dry mouth, constipation, drowsiness, dizziness. May reduce vitamin B_{12} absorption.

[a]Note that many other medications not listed in this table also have nutrition-related side effects. In addition, nutrition-related side effects other than those listed may occur. For example, almost all medications cause nausea in some people. In this table, nausea is only listed as a side effect if it occurs with relative frequency or does not resolve with time. More detailed texts should be consulted for the medications you routinely encounter in clinical practice.

Abbreviations: N/V = nausea/vomiting; Al = aluminum; Ca = calcium; Mg = magnesium; K = potassium; GERD = gastroesophageal reflux disease; ACE = angiotensin-converting enzyme; H2 = histamine$_2$.

Table E–1
Administration and Common Nutrition-Related Side Effects of Selected Drugs (continued)

Drug Classification and Examples	Administration	Common Nutrition-Related Side Effects[a]
Antipsychotics (continued)		
Fluphenazine, perphenazine, trifluoperazine	Give with food to reduce GI distress. Do not mix concentrates with caffeinated drinks, tea, or apple juice. Avoid alcohol.	Stimulate appetite. Weight gain, dry mouth, constipation, drowsiness. May increase riboflavin needs.
Haloperidol	Give with food or milk to reduce GI distress. Do not mix concentrates with coffee, tea, or fruit juice. Avoid alcohol.	Stimulates appetite. Weight gain, dry mouth, constipation, drowsiness.
Loxapine	Give with food, milk, or water to reduce GI distress. Dilute concentrate with orange or grapefruit juice.	Dry mouth, drowsiness.
Prochlorperazine (see *Antinauseants*)		
Resperidone	Avoid alcohol.	Stimulates appetite. Weight gain, drowsiness.
Thioridazine	Give with food, milk, or water. Dilute concentrate in orange or grapefruit juice.	Stimulates appetite. Weight gain, dry mouth, constipation, drowsiness, dizziness. May increase riboflavin needs.
Antiulcer Agents		
Antisecretory agents (also act as anti-GERD): lanisoprazole, omeprazole	Give before a meal. Swallow capsules whole.	May reduce absorption of iron and vitamin B_{12}.
H2 blockers (also act as anti-GERD): cimetidine	Give iron supplements 1 hr before giving drug. Give Ca or Mg supplements separately by 2 hr. Limit caffeine, xanthine, and alcohol. Liquid form not compatible with tube feedings.	May reduce vitamin B_{12} absorption.
famotidine, nizatidine, rantidine	Limit caffeine, xanthine, and alcohol.	May reduce vitamin B_{12} absorption.
Other: sucralfate	Give with water on an empty stomach 1 hr before meals or at bedtime. Give Ca or Mg supplement separately by 30 min. Limit alcohol.	Nutrition-related side effects are uncommon. May cause Al-toxicity in people with end-stage renal failure.
Appetite Stimulants		
Dronabinol (see *Antinauseants*)		
Megestrol acetate, medroxy progesterone acetate	May take with food to reduce GI distress.	Increases appetite. Weight gain, edema. May increase blood sodium.
Appetite Suppressants		
Dexfenfluramine, fenfluramine, mazindol, phendimetrazine, phentermine	Give on empty stomach 1 hr before meals. Instruct client to follow a low-kcalorie diet.	Nausea, taste alterations, dry mouth, dizziness, drowsiness.

[a]Note that many other medications not listed in this table also have nutrition-related side effects. In addition, nutrition-related side effects other than those listed may occur. For example, almost all medications cause nausea in some people. In this table, nausea is only listed as a side effect if it occurs with relative frequency or does not resolve with time. More detailed texts should be consulted for the medications you routinely encounter in clinical practice.

Abbreviations: N/V = nausea/vomiting; Al = aluminum; Ca = calcium; Mg = magnesium; K = potassium; GERD = gastroesophageal reflux disease; ACE = angiotensin-converting enzyme; H2 = $histamine_2$.

E

Table E-1
Administration and Common Nutrition-Related Side Effects of Selected Drugs (continued)

Drug Classification and Examples	Administration	Common Nutrition-Related Side Effects[a]
Cardiac Glycosides		
Digitoxin, digoxin, digitalis	Give separately from high-fiber, high-pectin foods. Encourage low-salt, high-K diet. Mg supplements may decrease drug absorption. Avoid natural licorice and give Ca or vitamin D supplements cautiously. Hypokalemia, hypomagnesemia, hypoalbuminemia, and hypercalcemia increase drug effects.	Anorexia, N/V, weight loss, diarrhea.
Diuretics		
K–losing (thiazide, thiazide-related, and loop diuretics):		
bendroflumethiazide, chlorothalidone, chlorothiazide, hydrochlorothiazide, methyclothiazide, metolazone, quinethazone	Give with food or milk to reduce GI distress. Avoid natural licorice and limit alcohol. May need K or Mg supplements. Carefully monitor use of Ca and vitamin D supplements.	Lowers blood sodium, K, chloride, Mg. Raises blood Ca and glucose.
indapamide	Same as above.	Headache, dizziness, fatigue. Lowers blood K, sodium, chloride, Mg, and phosphorus. Raises blood Ca and glucose.
ethacrynic acid, furosemide	Give with food or milk to reduce GI distress. Avoid natural licorice and limit alcohol. May need K or Mg supplements.	Lowers blood K, sodium, chloride, Ca, Mg, and zinc. Raises blood glucose.
K-sparing:		
amiloride	Give with food or milk to reduce GI distress. Avoid natural licorice and alcohol. Avoid foods high in K, K supplements, and salt substitutes.	Anorexia, N/V. Lowers blood sodium and chloride. Raises blood K.
spironolactone	Same as above.	N/V, cramps, diarrhea. Lowers blood sodium and chloride. Raises blood K and Mg.
triamterene	Same as above.	Decreases the metabolism of folate. Lowers blood sodium, Mg, and folate. Raises blood K.
Immunosuppressants		
Azathioprine	Give with food to reduce GI distress.	N/V.

[a]Note that many other medications not listed in this table also have nutrition-related side effects. In addition, nutrition-related side effects other than those listed may occur. For example, almost all medications cause nausea in some people. In this table, nausea is only listed as a side effect if it occurs with relative frequency or does not resolve with time. More detailed texts should be consulted for the medications you routinely encounter in clinical practice.

Abbreviations: N/V = nausea/vomiting; Al = aluminum; Ca = calcium; Mg = magnesium; K = potassium; GERD = gastroesophageal reflux disease; ACE = angiotensin-converting enzyme; H2 = histamine$_2$.

Table E-1
Administration and Common Nutrition-Related Side Effects of Selected Drugs (continued)

Drug Classification and Examples	Administration	Common Nutrition-Related Side Effects[a]
Immunosuppressants (continued)		
Corticosteroids (see *Anti-Inflammatory Agents*)		
Cyclosporine	Mix liquid with milk or orange juice at room temperature; no grapefruit juice. Avoid K supplements or salt substitutes.	N/V, diarrhea, swollen gums, headache, impaired renal function, elevated blood pressure, elevated blood glucose. May raise blood K and lower Mg.
Muromonab-cd3	Give parenterally.	N/V, diarrhea, fever, infection.
Mycophenolate	Give with food to reduce GI distress.	N/V, diarrhea, constipation, impaired liver function, impaired kidney function, anemia, infection.
Tacrolimus	Give with food to reduce GI distress.	N/V, diarrhea, constipation, impaired liver function, impaired kidney function, headache.
Laxatives		
Bisacodyl	Give on empty stomach with water or juice. Encourage use of high-fiber foods and fluids.	Laxative dependency and low blood K and Ca with long-term use.
Docusate	Give syrup with milk or juice to mask taste. Encourage use of high-fiber foods and fluids.	Nausea, throat irritation. Long-term use may raise blood glucose and lower K.
Lactulose	Give with juice, milk, or water, or sweet food to improve palatability. Encourage use of high-fiber foods and fluids. Do not give to clients on lactose- or galactose-restricted diets. Dilute before using with tube feeding.	Belching, cramps, flatulence.
Magnesium salts (see *Antacids, Mg-containing*)		
Methycellulose	Give with fluids. Encourage use of high-fiber foods and fluids.	Increased peristalsis.
Mineral oil	Give 2 hr before or after eating. Encourage use of high-fiber foods and fluids.	May reduce absorption of fat-soluble vitamins.
Psyllium	Mix powder in water, juice, or milk. Encourage use of high-fiber foods and fluids.	Reduces blood cholesterol and LDL.
Senna	Give with water or juice. Encourage use of high-fiber foods and fluids.	Nausea, cramps.

[a]Note that many other medications not listed in this table also have nutrition-related side effects. In addition, nutrition-related side effects other than those listed may occur. For example, almost all medications cause nausea in some people. In this table, nausea is only listed as a side effect if it occurs with relative frequency or does not resolve with time. More detailed texts should be consulted for the medications you routinely encounter in clinical practice.

Abbreviations: N/V = nausea/vomiting; Al = aluminum; Ca = calcium; Mg = magnesium; K = potassium; GERD = gastroesophageal reflux disease; ACE = angiotensin-converting enzyme; H2 = histamine$_2$.

E

Table E-1
Administration and Common Nutrition-Related Side Effects of Selected Drugs (continued)

Drug Classification and Examples	Administration	Common Nutrition-Related Side Effects[a]
Phosphate Binders		
Al carbonate, Al hydroxide, Ca acetate, Ca carbonate, Ca citrate (see *Antacids, Al- and Ca-containing*)		
Miscellaneous		
Calcitonin (Ca regulator)	Give at bedtime to reduce GI distress.	N/V. Lowers blood Ca and phosphorus.
Calcitriol (Ca regulator)	Do not give with vitamin D, Mg supplements, or Mg–containing antacids. Avoid high-phosphorus foods.	Raises blood Ca levels.
Colchicine (antigout)	Give with low-purine diet during acute attacks of gout.	N/V, GI pain, diarrhea.
Dextroamphetamine (stimulant)	Limit caffeine.	Anorexia, weight loss, dizziness, headache, confusion.
Epoetin alfa (erythropoietin)	May need iron, folate, or vitamin B_{12} supplement.	Raises hemoglobin and hematocrit.
Lithium carbonate (antimanic)	Give with meals to reduce GI distress. Consistent sodium intake helps maintain drug levels. Give adequate fluids. Do not use syrup form with tube feedings.	N/V, thirst, weight gain, dry mouth, fatigue, weakness, edema, dizziness. Raises blood Ca, phosphorus, and Mg.
Oral contraceptives (hormone)	Give with food. Give foods high in folate, pyridoxine, and vitamin B_{12} and vitamin C supplements. Limit caffeine.	N/V, weight changes, appetite changes, bone loss, edema. Lowers blood folate, pyridoxine, and vitamin B_{12}.
Sodium polystyrene sulfonate (K exchange resin)	Mix powder with cool water or sorbitol. Mix with sorbitol-containing syrup to combat constipation. Avoid K supplements. Do not give Ca-containing supplements or antacids for at least several hours.	Anorexia, constipation. Lowers blood K, Ca, and Mg.

[a]Note that many other medications not listed in this table also have nutrition-related side effects. In addition, nutrition-related side effects other than those listed may occur. For example, almost all medications cause nausea in some people. In this table, nausea is only listed as a side effect if it occurs with relative frequency or does not resolve with time. More detailed texts should be consulted for the medications you routinely encounter in clinical practice.

Abbreviations: N/V = nausea/vomiting; Al = aluminum; Ca = calcium; Mg = magnesium; K = potassium; GERD = gastroesophageal reflux disease; ACE = angiotensin-converting enzyme; H2 = histamine$_2$.

Sources: Z. M. Pronsky, *Food Medication Interactions,* 9th ed. (Pottstown, Pa.: Food Medication Interactions, 1993); *Nursing Drug Guide* (Philadelphia: Lippincott-Raven Publishers, 1997).

GROWTH CHARTS AND ANTHROPOMETRIC DATA

Growth charts, shown in Figures E–1 through E–6, allow health care professionals to evaluate the growth and development of children from birth to 18 years of age. The assessor follows these steps to plot a weight measurement on a percentile graph:

- Select the appropriate chart based on age and gender. (When length is measured, use the chart for birth to 36 months; when height is measured, use the chart for 2 to 18 years.)
- Locate the child's age along the horizontal axis on the bottom or top of the chart.

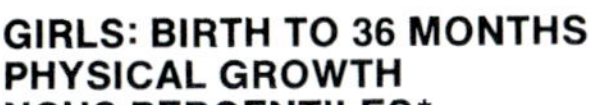

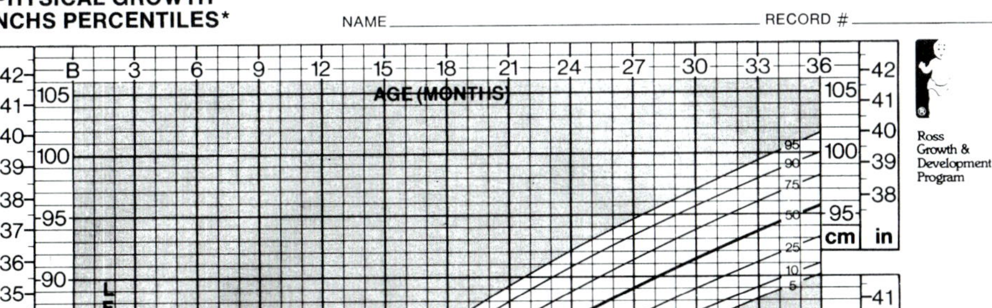

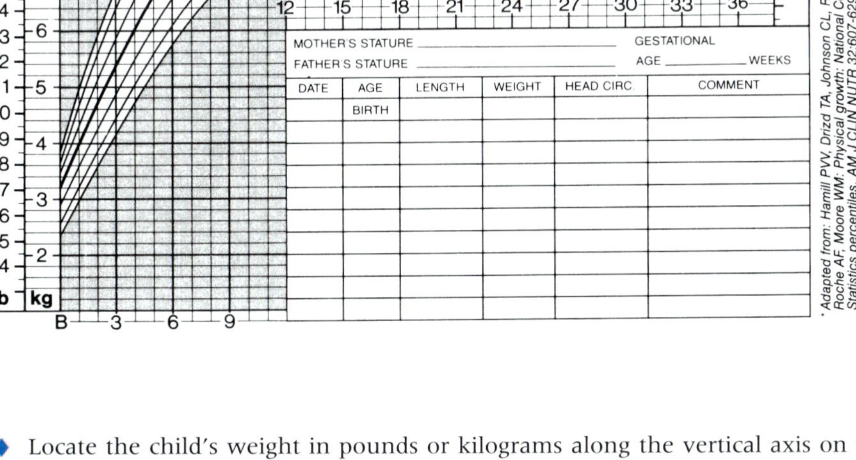

Figure E–1A
Girls: Birth to 36 Months Physical Growth NCHS Percentiles—Length and Weight for Age

- Locate the child's weight in pounds or kilograms along the vertical axis on the lower left or right side of the chart.
- Mark the chart where the age and weight lines intersect. Read the percentile.

To assess length, height, or head circumference, the assessor follows the same procedure, using the appropriate chart. Head circumference percentile should be similar to the child's height and weight percentiles.

Figure E-1B
Girls: Birth to 36 Months Physical Growth NCHS Percentiles—Head Circumference for Age and Weight for Length

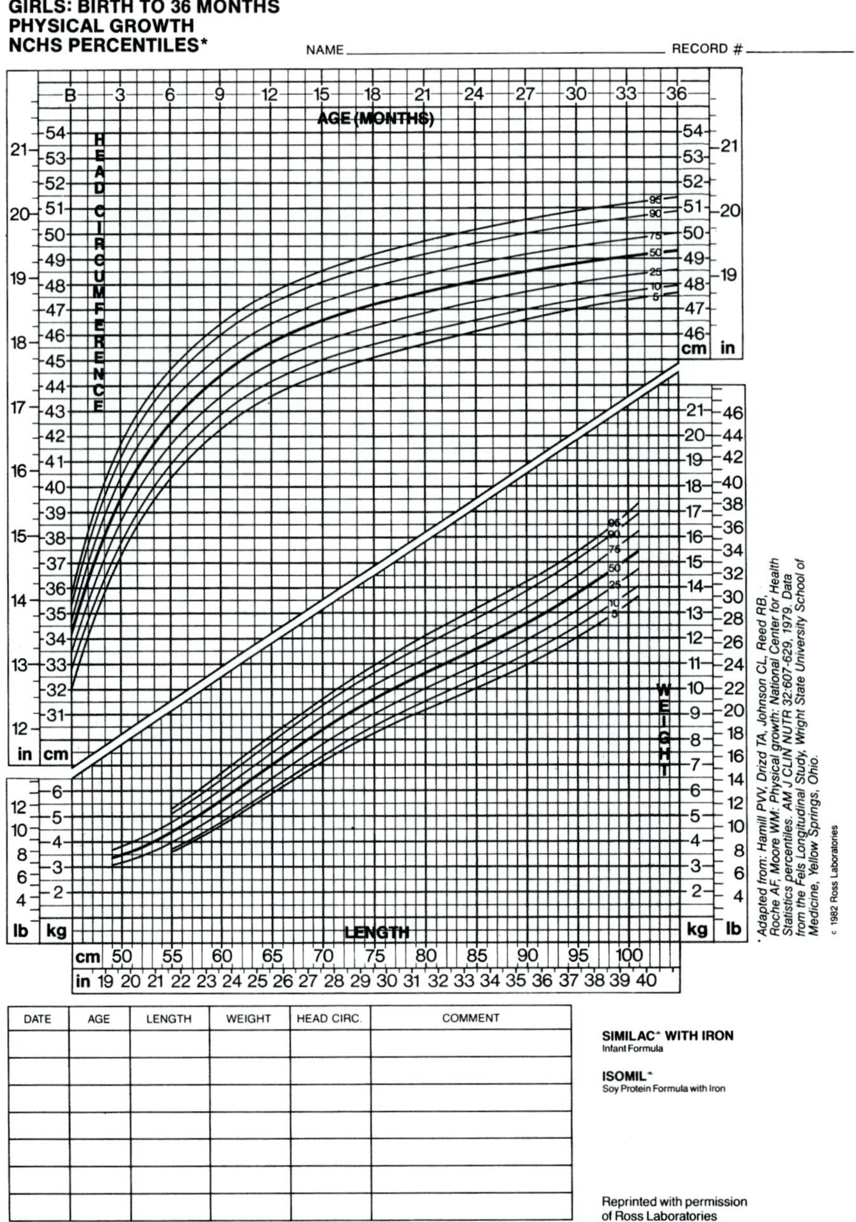

With height, weight, and head circumference measures plotted on growth percentile charts, a skilled clinician can begin to interpret the data. Percentile charts divide the measures of a population into 100 equal divisions. Thus half of the population falls above the 50th percentile, and half falls below. The use of percentile measures allows for comparisons among people of the same age and gender. For example, a six-month-old female infant whose weight is at the 75 percentile weighs more than 75 percent of the female infants her age.

(continued on p. E–19)

BOYS: BIRTH TO 36 MONTHS
PHYSICAL GROWTH
NCHS PERCENTILES*

NAME ______ RECORD # ______

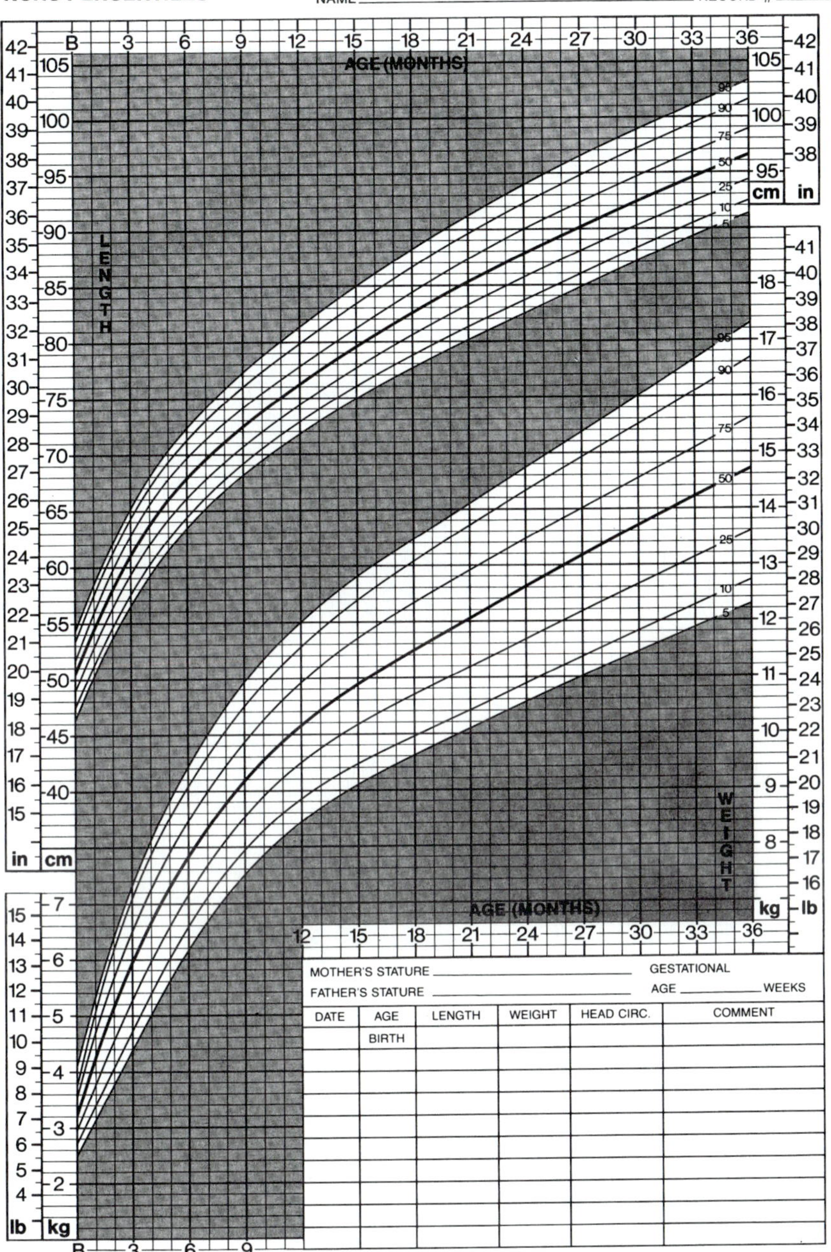

Ross Growth & Development Program

*Adapted from: Hamill PVV, Drizd TA, Johnson CL, Reed RB, Roche AF, Moore WM: Physical growth: National Center for Health Statistics percentiles. AM J CLIN NUTR 32:607-629, 1979. Data from the Fels Longitudinal Study, Wright State University School of Medicine, Yellow Springs, Ohio.

Figure E-2A
Boys: Birth to 36 Months Physical Growth NCHS Percentiles—Length and Weight for Age

E

Figure E–2B
Boys: Birth to 36 Months Physical Growth NCHS Percentiles—Head Circumference for Age and Weight for Length

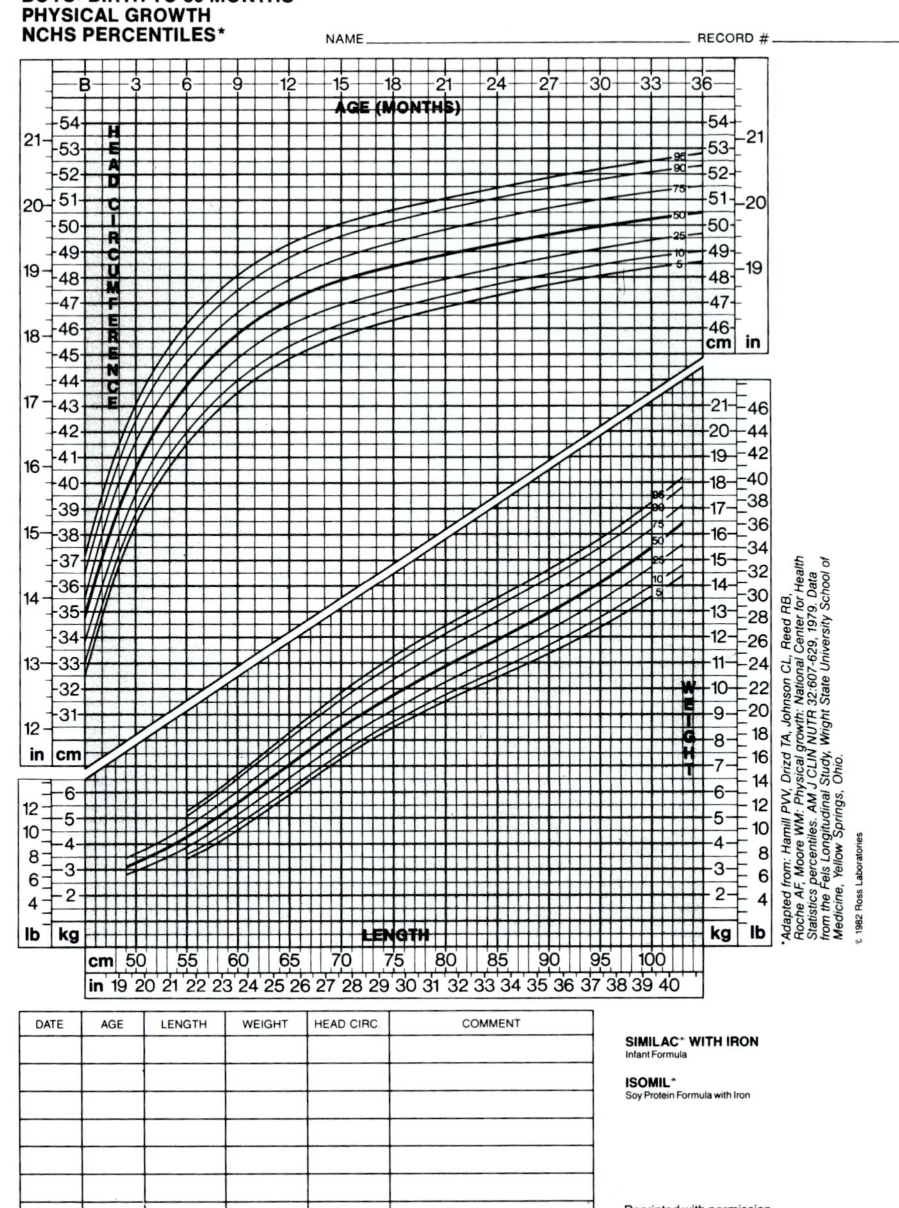

DATE	AGE	LENGTH	WEIGHT	HEAD CIRC	COMMENT

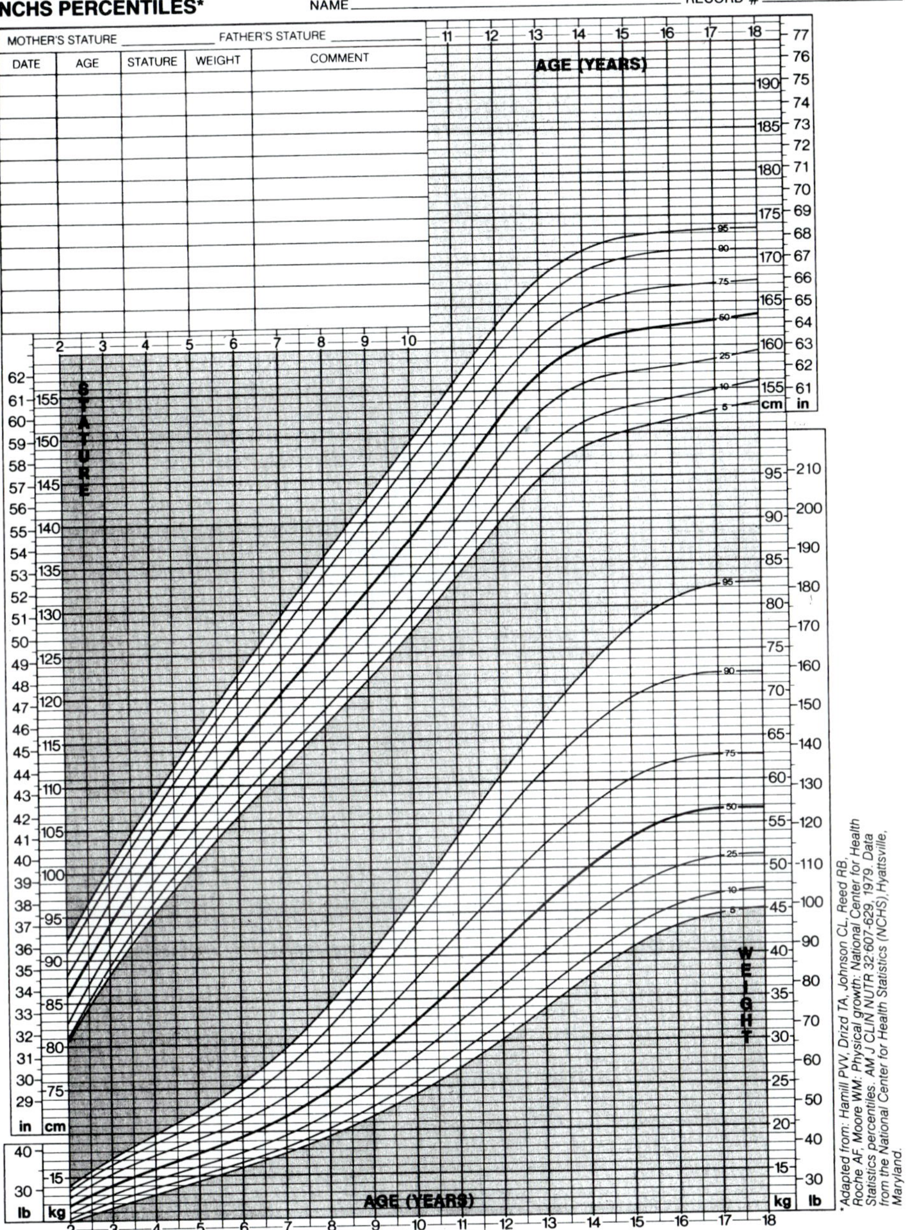

Figure E-3
Girls: 2 to 18 Years Physical Growth NCHS Percentiles—Height and Weight for Age

Figure E-4
Boys: 2 to 18 Years Physical Growth NCHS Percentiles—Height and Weight for Age

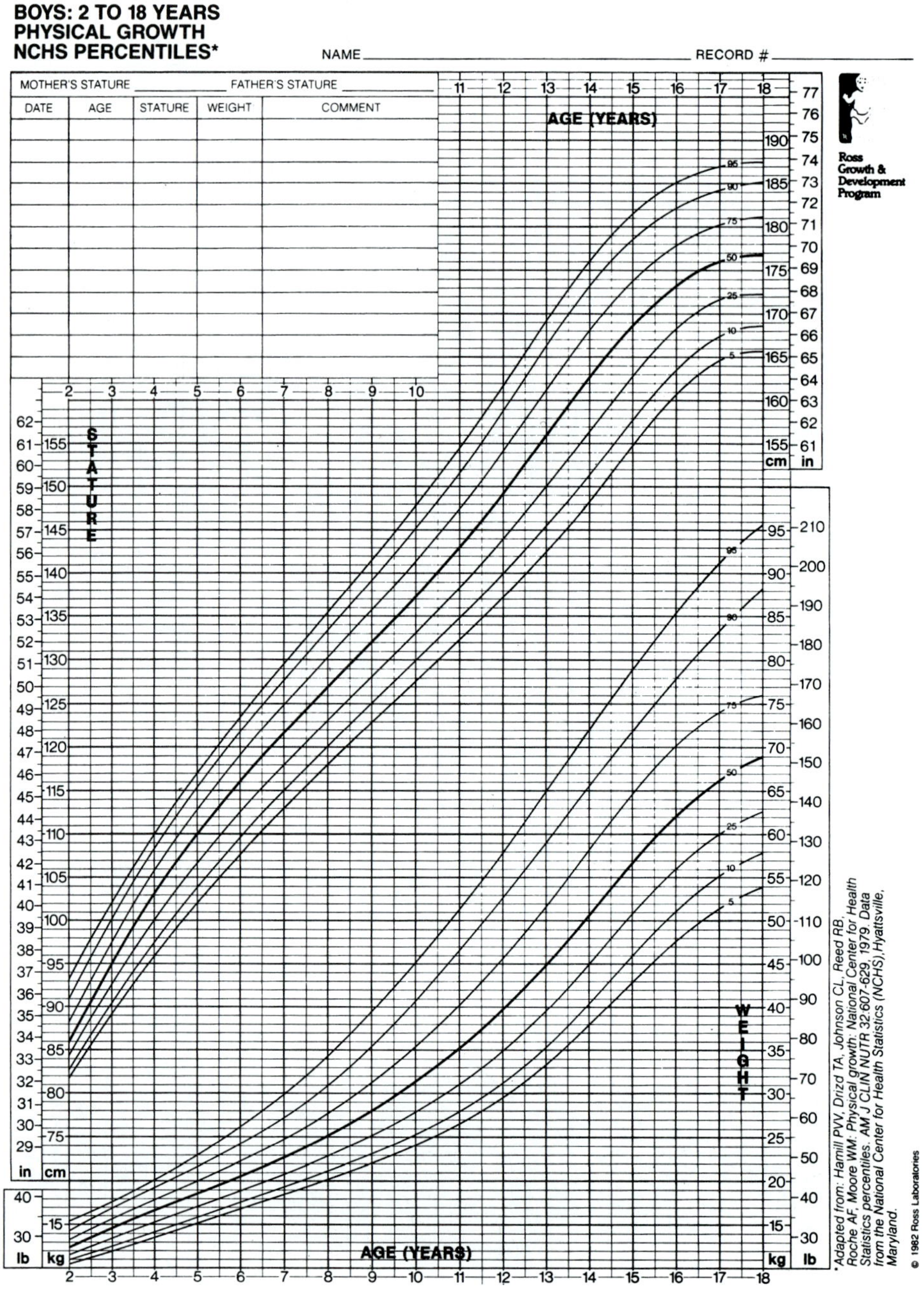
BOYS: 2 TO 18 YEARS
PHYSICAL GROWTH
NCHS PERCENTILES*
NAME
RECORD #
MOTHER'S STATURE
FATHER'S STATURE
DATE
AGE
STATURE
WEIGHT
COMMENT
AGE (YEARS)
STATURE
WEIGHT
in
cm
lb
kg
Ross Growth & Development Program
*Adapted from: Hamill PVV, Drizd TA, Johnson CL, Reed RB, Roche AF, Moore WM: Physical growth: National Center for Health Statistics percentiles. AM J CLIN NUTR 32:607-629, 1979. Data from the National Center for Health Statistics (NCHS), Hyattsville, Maryland.
© 1982 Ross Laboratories

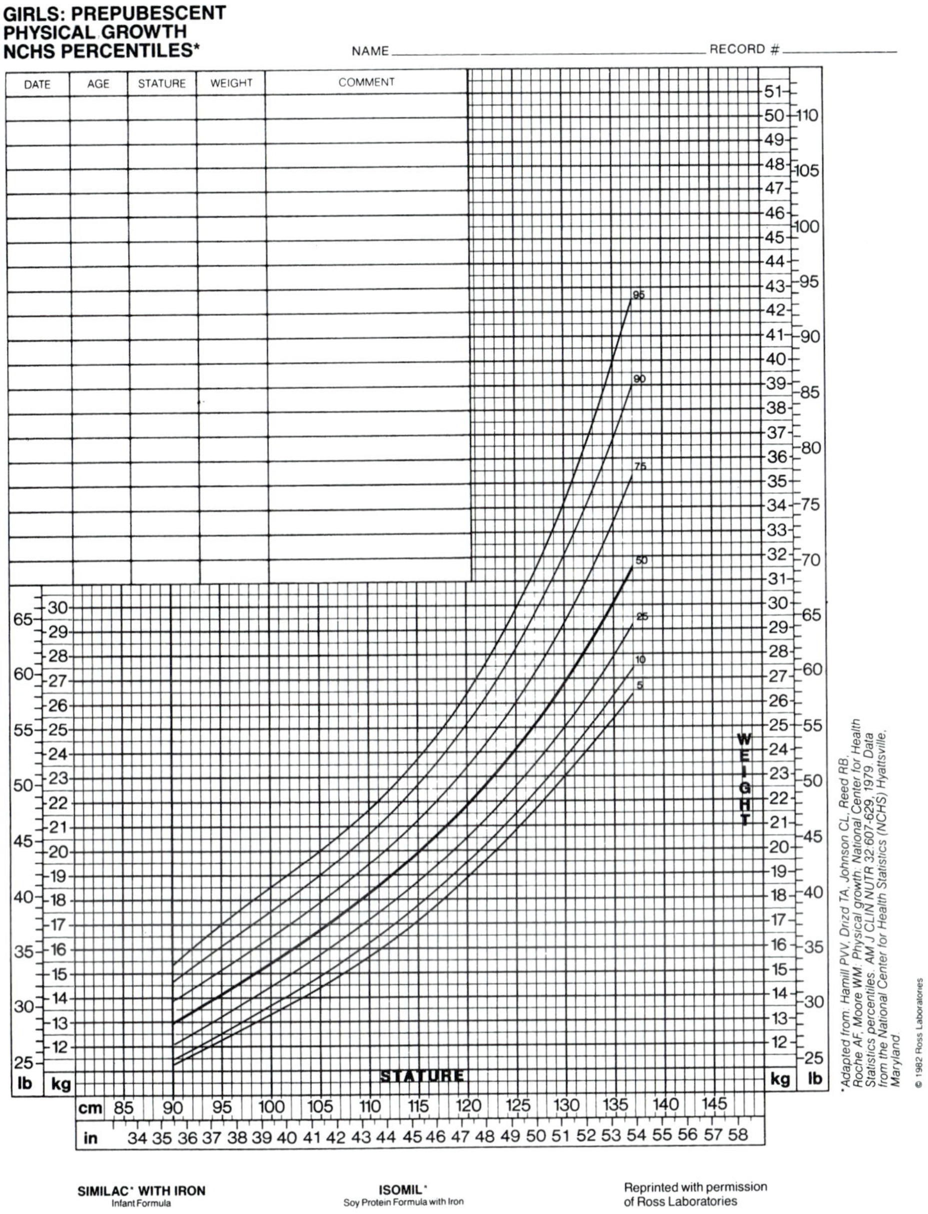
GIRLS: PREPUBESCENT PHYSICAL GROWTH NCHS PERCENTILES*
NAME
RECORD #
DATE
AGE
STATURE
WEIGHT
COMMENT
95
90
75
50
25
10
5
WEIGHT
STATURE
kg
lb
cm 85 90 95 100 105 110 115 120 125 130 135 140 145
in 34 35 36 37 38 39 40 41 42 43 44 45 46 47 48 49 50 51 52 53 54 55 56 57 58
*Adapted from: Hamill PVV, Drizd TA, Johnson CL, Reed RB, Roche AF, Moore WM: Physical growth: National Center for Health Statistics percentiles. AM J CLIN NUTR 32:607-629, 1979. Data from the National Center for Health Statistics (NCHS) Hyattsville, Maryland.
© 1982 Ross Laboratories
SIMILAC® WITH IRON
Infant Formula
ISOMIL®
Soy Protein Formula with Iron
Reprinted with permission of Ross Laboratories

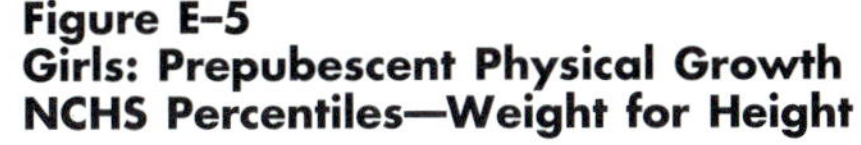

Figure E-5
Girls: Prepubescent Physical Growth NCHS Percentiles—Weight for Height

Chapter 8 described how assessors use the body mass index (BMI) to evaluate weight in adults. Assessors can also evaluate weight for height by comparing measures with population standards. To use the height-weight tables to assess body weight in adults, the assessor must determine the client's frame size. Figure E–7 shows how to measure the wrist to determine frame size (see Table E–2). Table E–3 (see p. E–21) presents another method of determining frame size, and Table E–4 shows the metropolitan height and weight standards. As noted, the BMI can also be used to assess body weight in adults. Figure E–8 on p. E–22 presents a nomogram for BMI. Figure E–9 on p. E–23 shows normal weight gains related to duration of pregnancy in weeks for women who start their pregnancies at normal weight, underweight, or overweight.

Figure E-6
Boys: Prepubescent Physical Growth NCHS Percentiles—Weight for Height

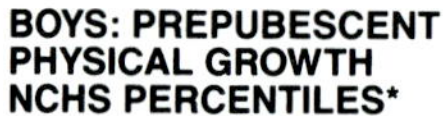

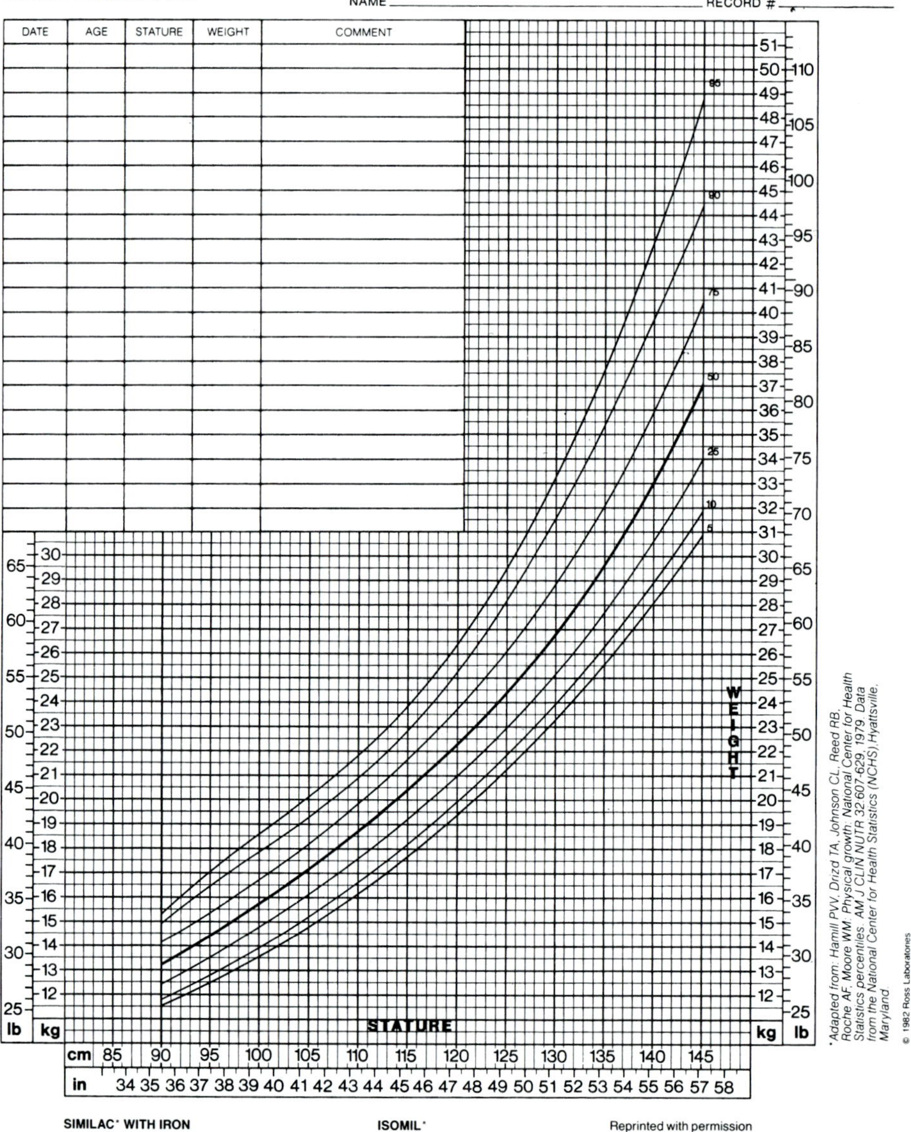

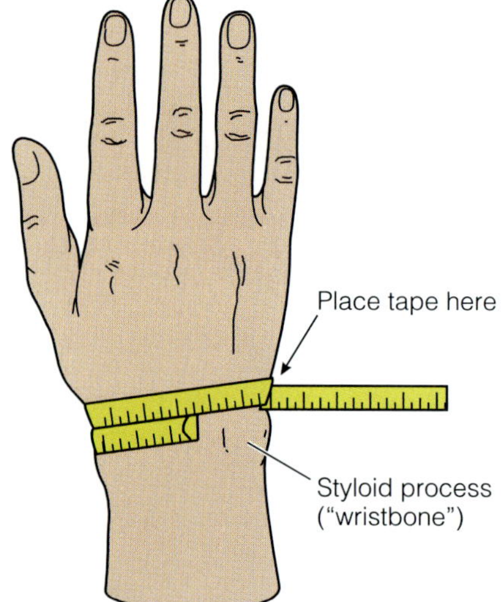

Figure E-7
Wrist Circumference

Table E-2
Frame Size from Height-Wrist Circumference Ratios (r)[a]

Frame Size	Male r Values	Female r Values
Small	>10.4	>11.0
Medium	9.6–10.4	10.1–11.0
Large	<9.6	<10.1

[a] $r = \frac{\text{height (cm)}}{\text{wrist circumference (cm)}}$. The wrist is measured where it bends (distal to the styloid process), on the right arm (see Figure E-7).

Table E-3
How to Determine Body Frame by Elbow Breadth

To make a simple approximation of frame size, do the following: Extend the arm, and bend the forearm upward at a 90° angle. Keep the fingers straight, and turn the inside of the wrist away from the body. Place the thumb and index finger on the two prominent bones on *either side* of the elbow. Measure the space between the fingers against a ruler or a tape measure.[a] Compare the measurements with the following standards.

These standards represent the elbow measurements for medium-framed men and women of various heights. Measurements smaller than those listed indicate a small frame, and larger measurements indicate a large frame.

Men		**Women**	
HEIGHT IN 1-INCH HEELS	ELBOW BREADTH	HEIGHT IN 1-INCH HEELS	ELBOW BREADTH
5 ft 2 in to 5 ft 3 in	2 1/2 to 2 7/8 in	4 ft 10 in to 4 ft 11 in	2 1/4 to 2 1/2 in
5 ft 4 in to 5 ft 7 in	2 5/8 to 2 7/8 in	5 ft 0 in to 5 ft 3 in	2 1/4 to 2 1/2 in
5 ft 8 in to 5 ft 11 in	2 3/4 to 3 in	5 ft 4 in to 5 ft 7 in	2 3/8 to 2 5/8 in
6 ft 0 in to 6 ft 3 in	2 3/4 to 3 1/8 in	5 ft 8 in to 5 ft 11 in	2 3/8 to 2 5/8 in
6 ft 4 in and over	2 7/8 to 3 1/4 in	6 ft 0 in and over	2 1/2 to 2 3/4 in

[a]For the most accurate measurement, measure elbow breadth with a caliper.

Source: Metropolitan Life Insurance Company.

Table E-4
1983 Metropolitan Height and Weight Tables

Men					**Women**				
Height		**Frame**			**Height**		**Frame**		
FEET	INCHES	SMALL	MEDIUM	LARGE	FEET	INCHES	SMALL	MEDIUM	LARGE
5	2	128–134	131–141	138–150	4	10	102–111	109–121	118–131
5	3	130–136	133–143	140–153	4	11	103–113	111–123	120–134
5	4	132–138	135–145	142–156	5	0	104–115	113–126	122–137
5	5	134–140	137–148	144–160	5	1	106–118	115–129	125–140
5	6	136–142	139–151	146–164	5	2	108–121	118–132	128–143
5	7	138–145	142–154	149–168	5	3	111–124	121–135	131–147
5	8	140–148	145–157	152–172	5	4	114–127	124–138	134–151
5	9	142–151	148–160	155–176	5	5	117–130	127–141	137–155
5	10	144–154	151–163	158–180	5	6	120–133	130–144	140–159
5	11	146–157	154–166	161–184	5	7	123–136	133–147	143–163
6	0	149–160	157–170	164–188	5	8	126–139	136–150	146–167
6	1	152–164	160–174	168–192	5	9	129–142	139–153	149–170
6	2	155–168	164–178	172–197	5	10	132–145	142–156	152–173
6	3	158–172	167–182	176–202	5	11	135–148	145–159	155–176
6	4	162–176	171–187	181–207	6	0	138–151	148–162	158–179

Note: To use the table, add an inch to your barefoot height (you are assumed to be wearing shoes with 1-inch heels), and adjust for clothing (the tables assume 5 pounds for clothes for men and 3 pounds for women). Weights are at age 25 to 29 based on lowest mortality, in pounds according to frame size.

Source: Reproduced courtesy of Metropolitan Life Insurance Company. Source of basic data: Society of Actuaries and Association of Life Insurance Medical Directors of America, *1979 Build Study*, 1980.

E

Figure E-8
Nomogram for Body Mass Index (BMI)

Weights and heights are without clothing. With clothes, add 5 pounds for men or 3 pounds for women, and 1 inch in height for shoes. Draw a straight line, or place a ruler, from your height (left) to your weight (right). At the point where it crosses the BMI line, read your BMI. The accompanying table in the margin indicates the BMI used to define the cutoff points in the graphs on the inside back covers.

	Men	Women
Underweight	<20.7	<19.1
Acceptable weight	20.7 to 27.8	19.1 to 27.3
Overweight	⩾27.8	⩾27.3
Severe overweight	⩾31.1	⩾32.3
Morbid obesity	⩾45.4	⩾44.8

Source: From the 1983 Metropolitan Life Insurance Company tables, designed by B. T. Burton and W. R. Roster, Health implications of obesity, and NIH Consensus Development Conference, *Journal of the American Dietetic Association* 85 (1985): 1117–1121.

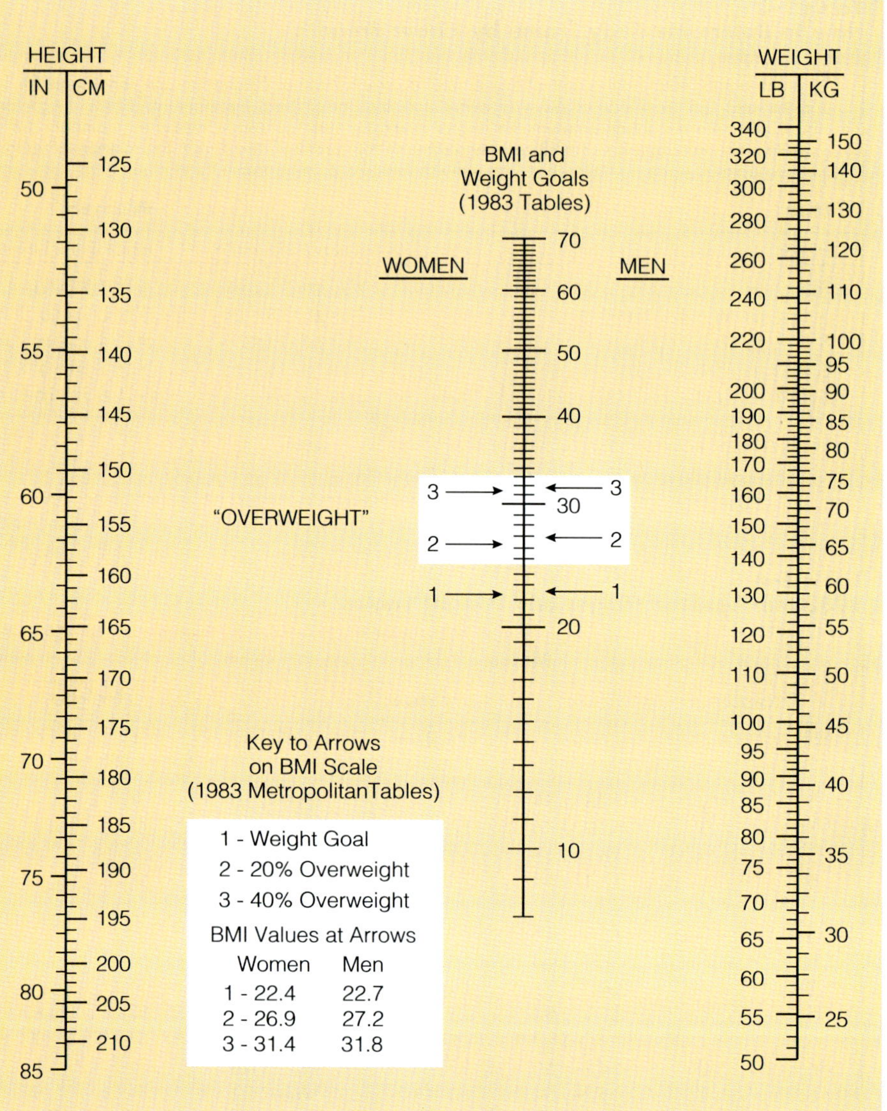

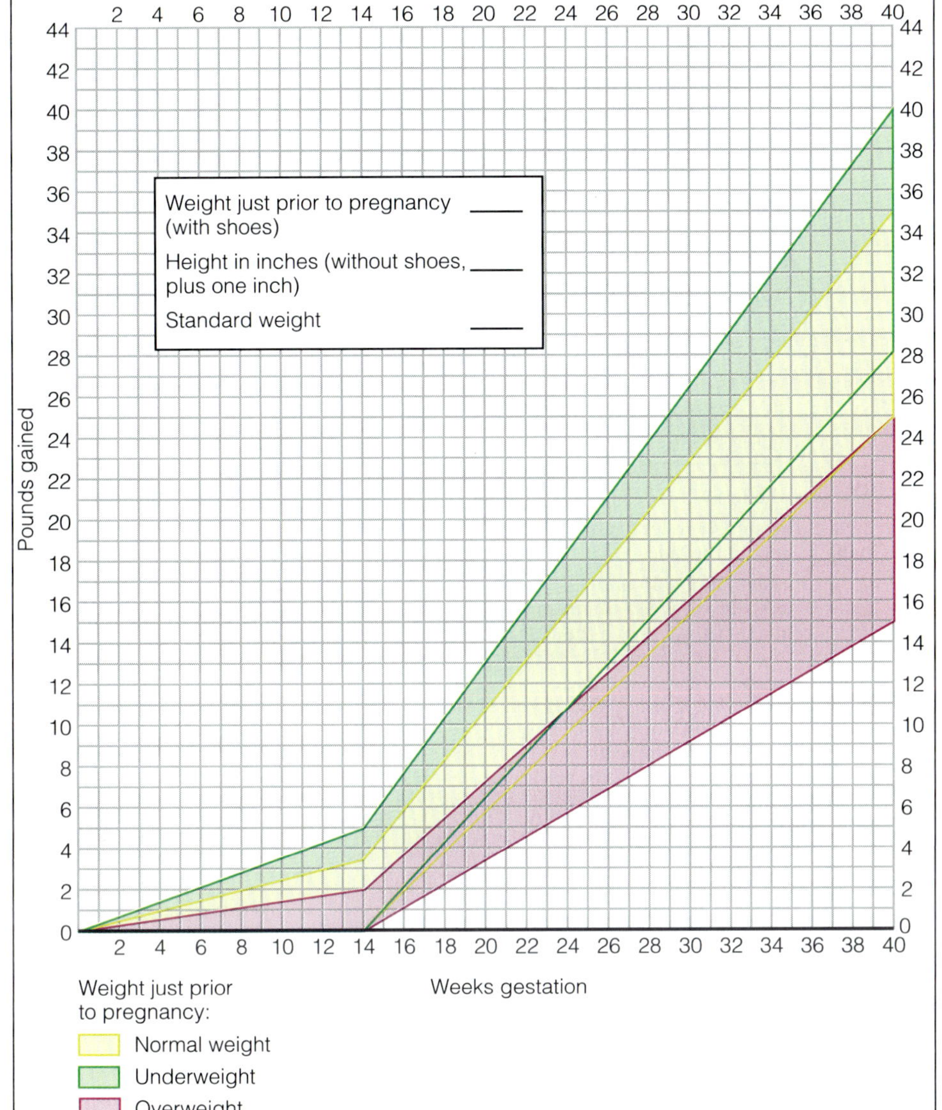

Figure E-9
Prenatal Weight-Gain Grid

A prenatal weight-gain grid plots the rate of weight gain during pregnancy. Normal-weight women should gain about $3^1/_2$ pounds in the first trimester and just under 1 pound/week thereafter, achieving a total gain of 25 to 35 pounds by term; underweight women should gain about 5 pounds in the first trimester and just over 1 pound/week thereafter, achieving a total gain of 28 to 40 pounds by term; and overweight women should gain about 2 pounds in the first trimester and $^2/_3$ pound/week thereafter, achieving a total gain of 15 to 25 pounds.

Fatfold measurements (see Figure E–10 on p. E–24) assist health care professionals in evaluating the composition of body weight. As already explained in Chapter 16, a lean tissue measure can be computed from the triceps fatfold measurement together with the midarm circumference measurement: the midarm muscle circumference (see Figures E–11 and E–12 on pp. E–24 and E–25). Table E–5 (p. E–25) gives triceps fatfold percentile standards. Table E–6 on p. E–26 shows the midarm muscle circumference percentile standards, and Figure E–13 (p. E–27) illustrates a nomogram method for determining midarm muscle circumference from these two measures.

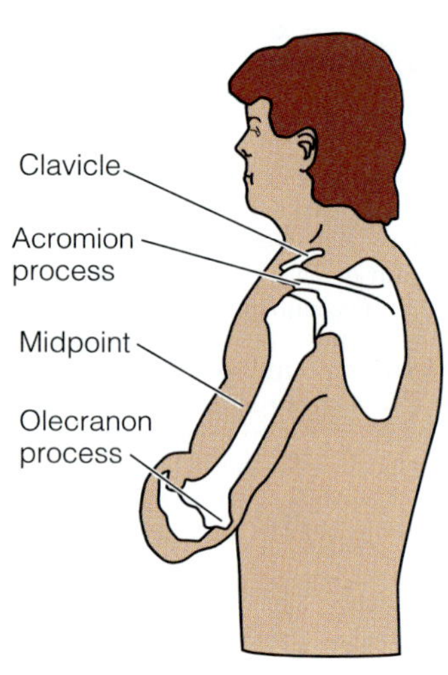

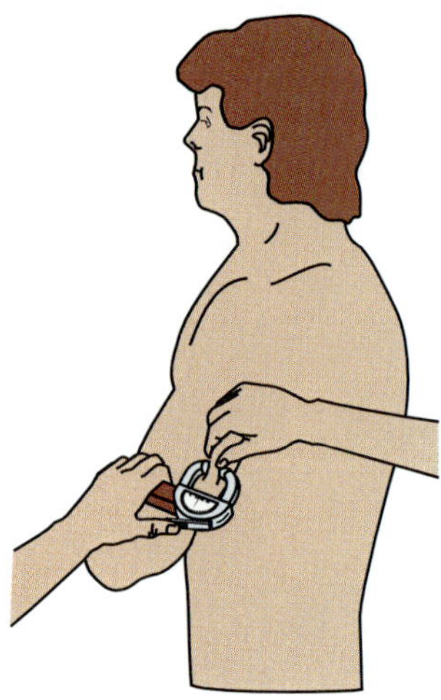

Figure E–10
How to Measure the Triceps Fatfold

A. Find the midpoint of the arm:

1. Ask the subject to bend his or her arm at the elbow and lay the hand across the stomach. (If he or she is right-handed, measure the left arm, and vice versa.)

2. Feel the shoulder to locate the acromion process. It helps to slide your fingers along the clavicle to find the acromion process. The olecranon process is the tip of the elbow.

3. Place a measuring tape from the acromion process to the tip of the elbow. Divide this measurement by 2, and mark the midpoint of the arm with a pen.

B. Measure the fatfold:

1. Ask the subject to let his or her arm hang loosely to the side.

2. Grasp the fold of skin and subcutaneous fat between the thumb and forefinger slightly above the midpoint mark. Gently pull the skin away from the underlying muscle. (This step takes a lot of practice. If you want to be sure you don't have muscle as well as fat, ask the subject to contract and relax the muscle. You should be able to feel if you are pinching muscle.)

3. Place the calipers over the fatfold at the midpoint mark, and read the measurement to the nearest 1.0 millimeter in two to three seconds. (If using plastic calipers, align pressure lines, and read the measurement to the nearest 1.0 millimeter in two to three seconds.)

4. Repeat steps 2 and 3 twice more. Add the three readings, and then divide by 3 to find the average.

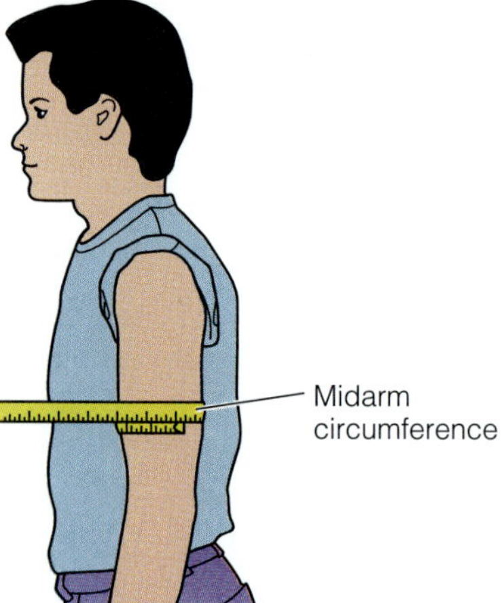

Figure E–11
How to Measure the Midarm Circumference

Ask the subject to let his or her arm hang loosely to the side. Place the measuring tape horizontally around the arm at the midpoint mark. This measurement is the midarm circumference.

Figure E–12
How to Derive the Midarm Muscle Circumference

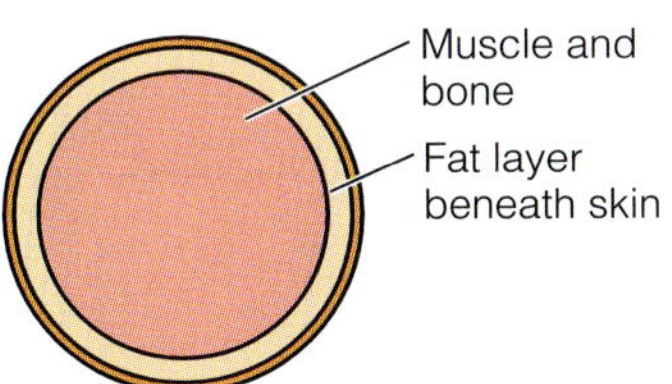

The arm is visualized as an inner circle of muscle and bone surrounded by an outer layer of fat and skin.

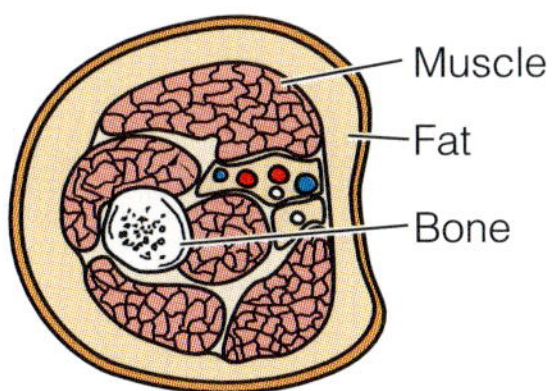

In reality, the arm is not circular, and there is some bone and blood vessels, but the simplified picture is approximately correct.

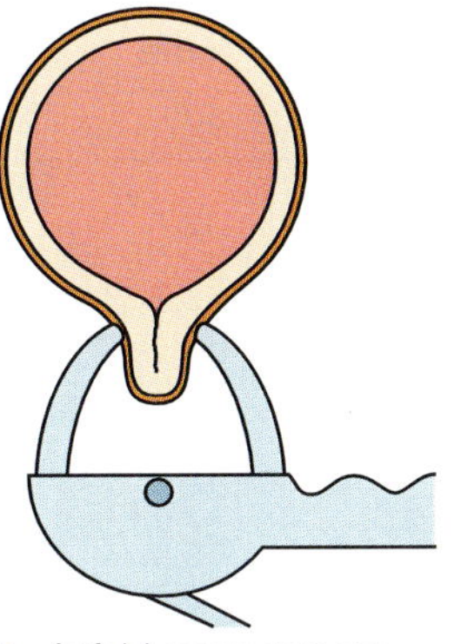

The fatfold measurement equals two times the thickness of the fat and skin.

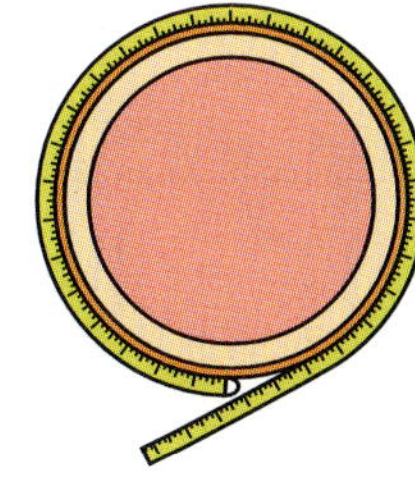

The midarm circumference measures the size of the arm and all of its components.

The following equation then derives the *circumference of the muscle*, an index of the body's total skeletal mass:
Midarm muscle circumference (cm) = midarm circumference (cm) – [0.314[a] × triceps fatfold (mm)].
[a]This factor converts the fatfold measurement to a circumference measurement and millimeters to centimeters.

Table E–5
Triceps Fatfold Percentiles (Millimeters)

Age	Male					Female				
	5TH	25TH	50TH	75TH	95TH	5TH	25TH	50TH	75TH	95TH
1–1.9	6	8	10	12	16	6	8	10	12	16
2–2.9	6	8	10	12	15	6	9	10	12	16
3–3.9	6	8	10	11	15	7	9	11	12	15
4–4.9	6	8	9	11	14	7	8	10	12	16
5–5.9	6	8	9	11	15	6	8	10	12	18
6–6.9	5	7	8	10	16	6	8	10	12	16
7–7.9	5	7	9	12	17	6	9	11	13	18
8–8.9	5	7	8	10	16	6	9	12	15	24
9–9.9	6	7	10	13	18	8	10	13	16	22
10–10.9	6	8	10	14	21	7	10	12	17	27
11–11.9	6	8	11	16	24	7	10	13	18	28
12–12.9	6	8	11	14	28	8	11	14	18	27
13–13.9	5	7	10	14	26	8	12	15	21	30
14–14.9	4	7	9	14	24	9	13	16	21	28
15–15.9	4	6	8	11	24	8	12	17	21	32
16–16.9	4	6	8	12	22	10	15	18	22	31
17–17.9	5	6	8	12	19	10	13	19	24	37
18–18.9	4	6	9	13	24	10	15	18	22	30
19–24.9	4	7	10	15	22	10	14	18	24	34
25–34.9	5	8	12	16	24	10	16	21	27	37
35–44.9	5	8	12	16	23	12	18	23	29	38
45–54.9	6	8	12	15	25	12	20	25	30	40
55–64.9	5	8	11	14	22	12	20	25	31	38
65–74.9	4	8	11	15	22	12	18	24	29	36

Note: If measurements fall between the percentiles shown here, the percentile can be estimated from the information in this table. For example, a measurement of 7 millimeters for a 27-year-old male would be about the 20th percentile.

Source: Adapted from A. R. Frisancho, New norms of upper limb fat and muscle areas for assessment of nutritional status. *American Journal of Clinical Nutrition* 34 (1981): 2540–2545.

E

Table E-6
Midarm Muscle Circumference Percentiles (Centimeters)

Age	Male 5TH	25TH	50TH	75TH	95TH	Female 5TH	25TH	50TH	75TH	95TH
1–1.9	11.0	11.9	12.7	13.5	14.7	10.5	11.7	12.4	13.9	14.3
2–2.9	11.1	12.2	13.0	14.0	15.0	11.1	11.9	12.6	13.3	14.7
3–3.9	11.7	13.1	13.7	14.3	15.3	11.3	12.4	13.2	14.0	15.2
4–4.9	12.3	13.3	14.1	14.8	15.9	11.5	12.8	13.6	14.4	15.7
5–5.9	12.8	14.0	14.7	15.4	16.9	12.5	13.4	14.2	15.1	16.5
6–6.9	13.1	14.2	15.1	16.1	17.7	13.0	13.8	14.5	15.4	17.1
7–7.9	13.7	15.1	16.0	16.8	19.0	12.9	14.2	15.1	16.0	17.6
8–8.9	14.0	15.4	16.2	17.0	18.7	13.8	15.1	16.0	17.1	19.4
9–9.9	15.1	16.1	17.0	18.3	20.2	14.7	15.8	16.7	18.0	19.8
10–10.9	15.6	16.6	18.0	19.1	22.1	14.8	15.9	17.0	18.0	19.7
11–11.9	15.9	17.3	18.3	19.5	23.0	15.0	17.1	18.1	19.6	22.3
12–12.9	16.7	18.2	19.5	21.0	24.1	16.2	18.0	19.1	20.1	22.0
13–13.9	17.2	19.6	21.1	22.6	24.5	16.9	18.3	19.8	21.1	24.0
14–14.9	18.9	21.2	22.3	24.0	26.4	17.4	19.0	20.1	21.6	24.7
15–15.9	19.9	21.8	23.7	25.4	27.2	17.5	18.9	20.2	21.5	24.4
16–16.9	21.3	23.4	24.9	26.9	29.6	17.0	19.0	20.2	21.6	24.9
17–17.9	22.4	24.5	25.8	27.3	31.2	17.5	19.4	20.5	22.1	25.7
18–18.9	22.6	25.2	26.4	28.3	32.4	17.4	19.1	20.2	21.5	24.5
19–24.9	23.8	25.7	27.3	28.9	32.1	17.9	19.5	20.7	22.1	24.9
25–34.9	24.3	26.4	27.9	29.8	32.6	18.3	19.9	21.2	22.8	26.4
35–44.9	24.7	26.9	28.6	30.2	32.7	18.6	20.5	21.8	23.6	27.2
45–54.9	23.9	26.5	28.1	30.0	32.6	18.7	20.6	22.0	23.8	27.4
55–64.9	23.6	26.0	27.8	29.5	32.0	18.7	20.9	22.5	24.4	28.0
65–74.9	22.3	25.1	26.8	28.4	30.6	18.5	20.8	22.5	24.4	27.9

Source: Adapted from A. R. Frisancho, New norms of upper limb fat and muscle areas for assessment of nutritional status, *American Journal of Clinical Nutrition* 34 (1981): 2540–2545.

LABORATORY TESTS OF NUTRITION STATUS

◆

As Chapter 16 pointed out, urine and blood tests provide valuable information in a nutrition assessment. Two urine tests—creatinine excretion and urine urea nitrogen—require a 24-hour urine collection and, therefore, are not routinely used.

Collecting a 24-hour urine sample presents many problems. Much effort is wasted if everyone involved does not conscientiously follow proper techniques. The collection of urine and recording of food intake data require client cooperation. The client must receive thorough instructions on how to collect and save all urine samples and must be advised to call for help if needed. Each urine sample is added to the collection container and refrigerated until the collection is complete. If even one urine sample is spilled or discarded, the test is invalid.

Most hospitals have a standard time for beginning urinary collections (often, between 6:00 A.M. and 6:00 P.M.). For nitrogen balance studies, food intake must also be recorded during the exact same time period. All nurses caring for the client on all shifts must record, or ensure that the client records, food intake data carefully.

To calculate the creatinine-height index (CHI) from the measured urinary creatinine and the client's height, use the following equation:

$$\text{CHI} = \frac{\text{measured urinary creatinine (24-hour sample)}}{\text{standard creatinine excretion for height and sex}} \times 100.$$

For example, to calculate the CHI in a man of medium frame, 5 feet 8 inches tall, who excretes 1090 milligrams of creatinine in 24 hours, follow these steps:

- Look up the standard creatinine excretion (Table E–7 on p. E–28).

In this example, the standard creatinine excretion is 1.56 grams or 1560 milligrams.

Figure E-13
Nomograms for Determination of Midarm Muscle Circumference

To obtain arm muscle circumference using either nomogram, lay a ruler between values of arm circumference and fatfold, and read off arm muscle circumference.

Source: Reproduced with permission from J. Gurney and D. Jelliffe, Arm anthropometry in nutritional assessment; nomogram for rapid calculation of muscle circumference and cross-sectional muscle and fat areas. *American Journal of Clinical Nutrition* 26 (1973): 912, as adapted by A. Grant, *Nutritional Assessment Guidelines,* 2nd ed., 1979.

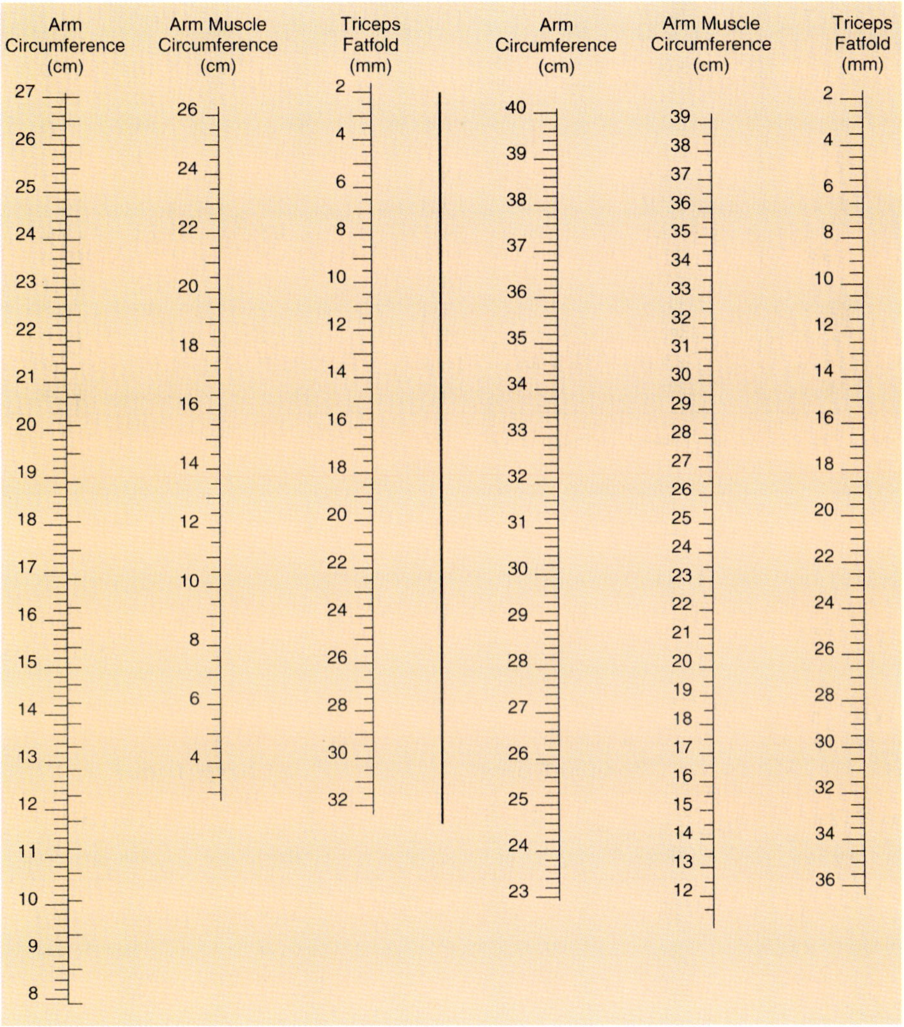

Arm Circumference (cm)
Arm Muscle Circumference (cm)
Triceps Fatfold (mm)
Arm Circumference (cm)
Arm Muscle Circumference (cm)
Triceps Fatfold (mm)

◆ Complete the CHI equation: $\text{CHI} = \dfrac{1090 \text{ mg}}{1560 \text{ mg}} \times 100 = 70\%.$

Based on the CHI, the man in this example has a skeletal muscle mass 70 percent of that considered typical for a man of his height. Table E–8 (p. E–28) shows the standard creatinine excretions for women.

Table E-7
Creatinine-Height Index Standards for Men

Height		Small Frame			Medium Frame			Large Frame		
			Creatinine			Creatinine			Creatinine	
in	cm	Ideal Weight (kg)	(g/24 h)	(mmol/d)	Ideal Weight (kg)	(g/24 h)	(mmol/d)	Ideal Weight (kg)	(g/24 h)	(mmol/d)
61	154.9	52.7	1.21	10.7	56.1	1.29	11.4	60.7	1.40	12.4
62	157.5	54.1	1.24	11.0	57.7	1.33	11.8	62.0	1.43	12.6
63	160.0	55.4	1.27	11.2	59.1	1.36	12.0	63.6	1.46	12.9
64	162.5	56.8	1.31	11.6	60.4	1.39	12.3	65.2	1.50	13.3
65	165.1	58.4	1.34	11.8	62.0	1.43	12.6	66.8	1.54	13.6
66	167.6	60.2	1.39	12.3	63.9	1.47	13.0	68.9	1.59	14.1
67	170.2	62.0	1.43	12.6	65.9	1.52	13.4	71.1	1.64	14.5
68	172.7	63.9	1.47	13.0	67.7	1.56	13.8	72.9	1.68	14.9
69	175.3	65.9	1.52	13.4	69.5	1.60	14.1	74.8	1.72	15.2
70	177.8	67.7	1.56	13.8	71.6	1.65	14.6	76.8	1.77	15.6
71	180.3	69.5	1.60	14.1	73.6	1.69	14.9	79.1	1.82	16.1
72	182.9	71.4	1.64	14.5	75.7	1.74	15.4	81.1	1.87	16.5
73	185.4	73.4	1.69	14.9	77.7	1.79	15.8	83.4	1.92	17.0
74	187.9	75.2	1.73	15.3	80.0	1.85	16.4	85.7	1.97	17.4
75	190.5	77.0	1.77	15.6	82.3	1.89	16.7	87.7	2.02	17.9

Note: To convert urinary creatinine measures (g/24 h) to standard international units (mmol/d) multiply by 8.840.

Source: A. Grant and S. DeHoog, *Nutritional Assessment and Support,* 3rd ed., 1985.

Table E-8
Creatinine-Height Index Standards for Women

Height		Small Frame			Medium Frame			Large Frame		
			Creatinine			Creatinine			Creatinine	
in	cm	Ideal Weight (kg)	(g/24 h)	(mmol/d)	Ideal Weight (kg)	(g/24 h)	(mmol/d)	Ideal Weight (kg)	(g/24 h)	(mmol/d)
56	142.2	43.2	0.79	7.0	46.1	0.83	7.3	50.7	0.91	8.0
57	144.8	44.3	0.80	7.1	47.3	0.85	7.5	51.8	0.93	8.2
58	147.3	45.4	0.82	7.2	48.6	0.88	7.8	53.2	0.96	8.5
59	149.8	46.8	0.84	7.4	50.0	0.90	8.0	54.5	0.98	8.7
60	152.4	48.2	0.87	7.7	51.4	0.93	8.2	55.9	1.01	8.9
61	154.9	49.5	0.89	7.9	52.7	0.95	8.4	57.3	1.03	9.1
62	157.5	50.9	0.92	8.1	54.3	0.98	8.7	58.9	1.06	9.4
63	160.0	52.3	0.94	8.3	55.9	1.01	8.9	60.6	1.09	9.6
64	162.5	53.9	0.97	8.6	57.9	1.04	9.2	62.5	1.13	10.0
65	165.1	55.7	1.00	8.8	59.8	1.08	9.5	64.3	1.16	10.3
66	167.6	57.5	1.04	9.2	61.6	1.11	9.8	66.1	1.19	10.5
67	170.2	59.3	1.07	9.5	63.4	1.14	10.1	67.9	1.22	10.8
68	172.7	61.4	1.11	9.8	65.2	1.17	10.3	70.0	1.26	11.1
69	175.2	63.2	1.14	10.1	67.0	1.21	10.7	72.0	1.30	11.5
70	177.8	65.0	1.17	10.3	68.9	1.24	11.0	74.1	1.33	11.8

Note: To convert urinary creatinine measures (g/24 h) to standard international units (mmol/d) multiply by 8.840.

Source: A. Grant and S. DeHoog, *Nutritional Assessment and Support,* 3rd ed., 1985.

Table E–9
Biochemical Tests Useful for Assessing Vitamin and Mineral Status

Nutrient	Assessment Tests
Vitamins	
Vitamin A	Retinol-binding protein, serum carotene
Thiamin	Erythrocyte (red blood cell) transketolase activity, urinary thiamin
Riboflavin	Erythrocyte glutathione reductase activity, urinary riboflavin
Vitamin B_6	Urinary xanthurenic acid excretion after tryptophan load test, urinary vitamin B_6, erythrocyte transaminase activity
Niacin	Urinary metabolites NMN (N-methyl nicotinamide) or 2-pyridone, or preferably both expressed as a ratio
Folate	Free folate in the blood, erythrocyte folate (reflects liver stores), urinary formiminoglutamic acid (FIGLU), vitamin B_{12} status (folate assessment tests alone do not distinguish between the two deficiencies)
Vitamin B_{12}	Serum vitamin B_{12}, erythrocyte vitamin B_{12}, urinary methylmalonic acid synthesis or DUMP test (from the abbreviation for the chemical name of DNA's raw material, deoxyuridine monophosphate) Schilling test
Biotin	Serum biotin, urinary biotin
Vitamin C	Serum or plasma vitamin C[a], leukocyte vitamin C, urinary vitamin C
Vitamin D	Serum alkaline phosphatase
Vitamin E	Serum tocopherol, erythrocyte hemolysis
Vitamin K	Blood clotting time (prothrombin time)
Minerals	
Potassium	Serum potassium
Magnesium	Serum magnesium
Iron	Hemoglobin, hematocrit, serum ferritin, total iron-binding capacity (TIBC), protoporphyrin, mean corpuscular volume (MCV), serum iron
Iodine	Serum protein-bound iodine, radioiodine uptake
Zinc	Plasma zinc, hair zinc

[a]Vitamin C shifts unpredictably between the plasma and the while blood cells known as leukocytes; thus a plasma or serum determination may not accurately reflect the body's pool. The appropriate clinical test may be a measurement of leukocyte vitamin C. A combination of both tests may be more reliable than either one alone.

Source: Adapted from A. Grant and S. DeHoog. *Nutritional Assessment and Support,* 3rd ed., 1985.

Table E–9 shows laboratory tests that help assess vitamin and mineral status. Some vitamin and mineral deficiencies, notably folate, vitamin B_{12}, and iron, can lead to anemia. Anemia, defined as a reduced number of red blood cells, can also result from many medical conditions unrelated to nutrition. Table E–10 shows the tests that help to define anemia and to distinguish among its major nutrition-related causes. Tables E–11 through E–15 provide standards for hemoglobin, hematocrit, serum ferritin, serum iron, percent transferrin saturation, and folate concentrations.

E

E

Table E–10
Laboratory Tests Useful in Evaluating Nutrition-Related Anemias

Test or Test Result	What It Reflects
General Tests for Anemia	
Hemoglobin (Hg)	Total amount of hemoglobin in the red blood cells (RBC)
Hematocrit (Hct)	Percentage of RBC in the total blood volume
Red blood cell (RBC) count	Number of RBC
Mean corpuscular volume (MCV)	RBC size; helps to determine if anemia is microcytic (iron deficiency) or macrocytic (folate or vitamin B_{12} deficiency)
Mean corpuscular hemoglobin concentration (MCHC)	Hemoglobin concentration within the average RBC; helps to determine if anemia is hypochromic (iron deficiency) or normochromic (folate or vitamin B_{12} deficiency)
Bone marrow aspiration	The manufacture of blood cells in different developmental states
Early Stages of Iron Deficiency	
↓ Serum ferritin	Early deficiency state with depleted iron stores
↓ Transferrin saturation	Progressing deficiency state with diminished transport iron
↑ Erythrocyte protoporphyrin	Later deficiency state with limited hemoglobin production
Folate-Deficiency Anemia	
↓ Serum Folate	Progressing deficiency state
↓ RBC Folate	Later deficiency state
Vitamin B_{12}–Deficiency Anemia	
↓ Serum vitamin B_{12}	Progressing deficiency state
Schilling test	Whether or not vitamin B_{12} is being absorbed

Table E–11
Standards for Hemoglobin Test Results

Age (yr)	Sex	Deficient (g/100 ml)	Acceptable (g/100 ml)
<2	M–F	<9.0	10.0 or >
2–5	M–F	<10.0	11.0 or >
6–12	M–F	<10.0	11.5 or >
13–16	M	<12.0	13.0 or >
	F	<10.0	11.5 or >
>16	M	<12.0	14.0 or >
	F	<10.0	12.0 or >
Pregnancy, 2nd trimester	F	<9.5	11.0 or >
Pregnancy, 3rd trimester	F	<9.0	10.5 or >

Note: To convert hemoglobin values (g/100 ml) to international standard units (g/L), multiply by 10.

Table E–12
Standards for Hematocrit Test Results

Age (yr)	Sex	Deficient (%)	Acceptable (%)
<2	M–F	<28	31 or >
2–5	M–F	<30	34 or >
6–12	M–F	<30	36 or >
13–16	M	<37	40 or >
	F	<31	36 or >
>16	M	<37	44 or >
	F	<31	38 or >
Pregnancy, 2nd trimester	F	<30	35 or >
Pregnancy, 3rd trimester	F	<30	33 or >

Note: To convert hematocrit values (%) to standard units, multiply by 0.01.

Table E-13
Standards for Serum Ferritin

Group	Deficient (ng/ml)
Children (3–14 years of age)	<10
Adolescents and adults	<12
Pregnant women	<10

Table E-14
Standards for Serum Iron

Age (yr)	Sex	Deficient		Acceptable	
		(μg/100 ml)	(μmol/L)	(μg/100 ml)	(μmol/L)
<2	M–F	<30	<5.3	30 or >	5.3 or >
2–5	M–F	<40	<7.1	40 or >	7.1 or >
6–12	M–F	<50	<8.9	50 or >	8.9 or >
<12	M	<60	<10.7	60 or >	10.7 or >
	F	<40	<7.1	40 or >	7.1 or >

Note: To convert mg/100 ml to international units, multiply by 0.1791.

Table E-15
Standards for Percent Transferrin Saturation

Age (yr)	Sex	Deficient %	Acceptable %
<2	M–F	<15	15 or >
2–12	M–F	<20	20 or >
≥13	M	<20	20 or >
	F	<15	15 or >

Table E-16
Standards for Folate Concentrations

Measurement	Deficient (ng/ml)	Borderline (ng/ml)	Acceptable (ng/ml)
Serum folate	<3.0	3.0–6.0	>6.0
Erythrocyte folate	<140	140–160	>160

Note: To convert folate values (ng/ml) to international standard units (nmol/L), multiply by 2.266.

APPENDIX F

NUTRITION RESOURCES

Contents

People interested in nutrition often want to know where they can find reliable nutrition information. Wherever you live, there are several sources you can turn to:

- The Department of Health may have a nutrition expert.
- The local extension agent is often an expert.
- The food editor of your local paper may be well informed.
- The dietitian at the local hospital had to fulfill a set of qualifications before he or she became an RD (see Highlight 1).
- There may be knowledgeable professors of nutrition or biochemistry at a nearby college or university.

In addition, you may be interested in building a nutrition library of your own. Books you can buy, journals you can subscribe to, and addresses you can write to for general information are given below.

BOOKS

For students seeking to establish a personal library of nutrition references, the authors of this text recommend the following books:

- *Present Knowledge in Nutrition,* 7th ed. (Washington, D.C.: International Life Sciences Institute—Nutrition Foundation, 1996).

This 646-page paperback has a chapter on each of 64 topics, including energy, obesity, each of the nutrients, several diseases, malnutrition, growth and its assessment, immunity, alcohol, fiber, exercise, drugs, and toxins. Watch for an update; new editions come out every few years.

- M. E. Shils, J. A. Olson, and M. Shike, eds., *Modern Nutrition in Health and Disease,* 8th ed. (Philadelphia: Lea & Febiger, 1994).

This two-volume set is a major technical reference book on nutrition topics. It contains encyclopedic articles on the nutrients, foods, the diet, metabolism, malnutrition, age-related needs, and nutrition in disease.

- Food and Nutrition Board, *Recommended Dietary Allowances,* 10th ed. (Washington, D.C.: National Academy Press, 1989).

This book reviews the function of each nutrient, dietary sources, and deficiency and toxicity symptoms as well as recommendations for intakes. The Canadian equivalent is *Nutrition Recommendations,* available by mail from the Canadian Government Publishing Centre, Supply and Services Canada, Ottawa, Ontario K1A OS9, Canada.

- Food and Nutrition Board, *Diet and Health: Implications for Reducing Chronic Disease Risk* (Washington, D.C.: National Academy Press, 1989).

This 749-page book presents the integral relationship between diet and chronic disease prevention. Its nutrient chapters provide evidence on how diet influences disease development, and its disease chapters review the dietary patterns implicated in each chronic disease.

- E. M. N. Hamilton and S. A. S. Gropper, *The Biochemistry of Human Nutrition: A Desk Reference* (St. Paul, Minn.: West, 1987).

This 324-page paperback presents the biochemical concepts necessary for an understanding of nutrition. It is a handy reference book for those who have forgotten the basics of biochemistry or for those who are learning biochemistry for the first time.

We also recommend three of our own books that explore current topics in nutrition, health, and the life span:

- E. N. Whitney, C. B. Cataldo, L. K. DeBruyne, and S. R. Rolfes, *Nutrition for Health and Health Care* (St. Paul, Minn.: West, 1995).
- F. S. Sizer and E. N. Whitney, *Nutrition: Concepts and Controversies,* 7th ed. (Belmont, Calif.: West/Wadsworth, 1997).
- S. R. Rolfes, L. K. DeBruyne, and E. N. Whitney, *Life Span Nutrition: Conception through Life* (St. Paul, Minn.: West, 1990).

JOURNALS

Nutrition Today is an excellent magazine for the interested layperson. It makes a point of raising controversial issues and providing a forum for conflicting opinions. Six issues per year are published. Order from Williams and Wilkins, 428 East Preston Street, Baltimore, MD 21202.

The *Journal of the American Dietetic Association,* the official publication of the ADA, contains articles of interest to dietitians and nutritionists, news of legislative action on food and nutrition, and a very useful section of abstracts of articles from many other journals of nutrition and related areas. There are twelve issues per year, available from the American Dietetic Association (see "Addresses," later).

Nutrition Reviews, a publication of the International Life Sciences Institute, does much of the work for the library researcher, compiling recent evidence on current topics and presenting extensive bibliographies. Twelve issues per year are available from Springer-Verlag New York, 175 Fifth Avenue, New York, NY 10010.

Nutrition and the M.D. is a monthly newsletter that provides up-to-date, easy-to-read, practical information on nutrition for health care providers. It is available from PM, Inc., 7100 Hayven Hurst Avenue, Suite 107, Van Nuys, CA 91406.

Other journals that deserve mention here are *Food Technology, Journal of Nutrition, American Journal of Clinical Nutrition, Nutrition Research,* and *Journal of Nutrition Education. FDA Consumer,* a government publication with many articles of interest to the consumer, is available from the Food and Drug Administration (see "Addresses," below). Many other journals of value are referred to throughout this book.

ADDRESSES

Many of the organizations listed below will provide publication lists free on request.

U.S. GOVERNMENT

- Federal Trade Commission (FTC)
  Public Reference Branch
  (202) 326-2222
  Internet address: http://www.ftc.gov
- Food and Drug Administration (FDA)
  Office of Consumer Affairs
  5600 Fishers Lane, HFE 88 Room 16–63
  Rockville, MD 20857
  (301) 443-3170 1 PM–3:30 PM EST
  Internet address: http://www.fda.gov
- FDA Office of Food Labeling (HFS-150)
  200 C Street SW
  Washington, DC 20204
  (202) 205-4561; fax: (202) 205-4564
- FDA Office of Plant and Dairy Foods
  and Beverages (HFS-300)
  200 C Street SW
  Washington, DC 20204
  (202) 205-4064; fax: (202) 205-4422
- FDA Office of Special Nutritionals (HFS-450)
  200 C Street SW
  Washington, DC 20204
  (202) 205-4168; fax: (202) 205-5295
- Food and Nutrition Information Center
  National Agricultural Library, Room 304
  10301 Baltimore Blvd.
  Beltsville, MD 20705-2351
  (301) 504-5719; fax: (301) 504-6409
  Internet address: http://www.nal.usda.gov/fnic
- Food Research and Action Center
  1875 Connecticut Avenue, NW, Suite 540
  Washington, DC 20009
  (202) 986-2200
- Superintendent of Documents
  Government Printing Office
  Washington, DC 20402
- U.S. Department of Agriculture (USDA)
  14th Street SW and Independence Avenue
  Washington, DC 20250
  (202) 720-2791
  Internet address: http://www.usda.gov
- USDA Center for Nutrition Policy and Promotion
  1120 20th Street, NW, Suite 200, North Lobby
  Washington, DC 20036
  (202) 418-2321
- U.S. Department of Education (DOE)
  Accreditation Agency Evaluation Branch
  7th and D Street SW, Building 3, Room 336
  Washington, DC 20202
  (202) 708-7417
- U.S. Environmental Protection Agency (EPA)
  Public Information Center, 3404
  401 M Street SW
  Washington, DC 20460
  (202) 260-2080

F

◆ U.S. Public Health Service Public Affairs Office
Hubert H. Humphrey Building, Room 725–H
200 Independence Avenue SW
Washington, DC 20201
(202) 245-6867

CANADIAN GOVERNMENT

◆ Bureau of Nutritional Sciences, Food Directorate
Health Protection Branch, Health Canada
Sir Frederick Banting Research Centre
Tunney's Pasture
Ottawa, Ontario K1A 0L2, Canada

◆ Food Production and Inspection Branch
Agriculture and Agri-Food Canada
59 Camelot Drive
Nepean, Ontario K1A 0Y9, Canada
Internet address: http//aceis.agr.ca

◆ Nutrition Programs Unit
Healthy Living and Disease Prevention Directorate
Health Promotion and Services Branch
Health Canada
Jeanne Mance Building
Tunney's Pasture
Ottawa, Ontario K1A 1B4, Canada
Internet address: http://hwc.ca

◆ Nutrition Specialist, Health Support Services
Indian and Northern Health Services
Health Canada
11th Flood, Jeanne Mance Building
Tunney's Pasture
Ottawa, Ontario K1A 0L3, Canada

INTERNATIONAL AGENCIES

◆ Food and Agriculture Organization of the United Nations (FAO), Liaison Office for North America
1001 22nd Street NW
Washington, DC 20437
(202) 653-2400

◆ World Health Organization (WHO)
Regional Office
525 23rd Street NW
Washington, DC 20037
(202) 861-3200
Internet address: http://www.who.ch

◆ International Food Information Council Foundation
Internet address: http://ificinfo.health.org

CONSUMER ORGANIZATIONS

◆ Center for Science in the Public Interest (CSPI)
1875 Connecticut Avenue NW, Suite 300
Washington, DC 20009

◆ Choice in Dying, Inc.
200 Varick Street, Suite 1001
New York, NY 10014
(212) 366-5540; fax: (212) 366-5337

◆ Consumer Information Center
Pueblo, CO 81009
Internet address: http://www.pueblo.gsa.gov

◆ Consumers Union of US Inc.
101 Truman Avenue
Yonkers, NY 10703–1057
(914) 378-2000

◆ National Council Against Health Fraud, Inc.
P.O. Box 1276
Loma Linda, CA 92354
Internet address: http://www.primenet.com/~nachf

FOOD SAFETY

◆ Alliance for Food & Fiber
Food Safety Hotline
(800) 266-0200

◆ FDA Seafood Hotline
(800) FDA-4010

◆ National Lead Information Center
(800) LEAD-FYI (532-3394)
(800) 424-LEAD (424-5323)

◆ National Pesticide Telecommunications Network
Oregon State University
Agricultural Chemistry Extension
Weniger Hall 333
Corvallis, OR 97331-6502

◆ USDA Meat and Poultry Hotline
(800) 535-4555

◆ U.S. EPA Safe Drinking Water Hotline
(800) 426-4791

INFANCY AND CHILDHOOD

◆ American Academy of Pediatrics
141 Northwest Point Boulevard
P.O. Box 927
Elk Grove Village, IL 60009–0927

◆ Association of Birth Defect Children, Inc.
827 Irma Street
Orlando, FL 32803
(407) 245-7035

◆ Canadian Pediatric Society
410 Smyth Road
Ottawa, Ontario K1H 8L1, Canada

- National Center for Education in Maternal & Child Health
2000 15th Street North, Suite 701
Arlington, VA 22201-2617
(703) 524-7802
- National Maternal and Child Health Clearinghouse
8201 Greensboro Drive
Suite 600
McLean, VA 22102
(703) 821-8955, Ext. 254 or 255
- Nurture/Center to Prevent Childhood Malnutrition
1840 18th Street, NW
Washington, DC 20009
(202) 797-9244; fax: (202) 797-9257

PROFESSIONAL NUTRITION ORGANIZATIONS

- American Dietetic Association (ADA)
216 West Jackson Boulevard, Suite 800
Chicago, IL 60606–6995
(312) 899-0040
Internet address: http://www.eatright.org
- ADA, National Center for Nutrition and Dietetics
(800) 366-1655
- American Institute of Nutrition
Internet address: http://www.nutrition.org/nutrition
- American Society for Clinical Nutrition
9650 Rockville Pike
Bethesda, MD 20814-3998
Internet address: http://www.faseb.org/ascn
- Dietitians of Canada
480 University Avenue, Suite 601
Toronto, Ontario M5G 1V2, Canada
(416) 596-0857
- National Academy of Sciences/National Research Council (NAS/NRC)
2101 Constitution Avenue NW
Washington, DC 20418
- National Institute of Nutrition
302-265 Carling Avenue
Ottawa, Ontario K1S 2E1, Canada
- Nutrition Foundation, Inc. (INACG)
1126 Sixteenth Street NW, Suite 111
Washington, DC 20036
- Nutrition Information Service
University of Alabama at Birmingham
Room 447 Webb Building
UAB Station
Birmingham, AL 35294-3360
- Society for Nutrition Education
2001 Killebrew Drive, Suite 340
Minneapolis, MN 55425-1882
(612) 854-6721
Internet address: http://www.uidaho.edu/~mswanson/sne.html

ALCOHOL AND DRUG ABUSE

- Al-Anon Family Group Headquarters
P.O. Box 862, Midtown Station
New York, NY 10018–0862
(800) 356-9996
- Alateen
1600 Corporate Landing Parkway
Virginia Beach, VA 23454
(800) 356-9996
- Alcohol & Drug Abuse Information Line
(800) 252-6465
- Alcoholics Anonymous (AA)
475 Riverside Drive
New York, NY 10115
(212) 870-3400
- Narcotics Anonymous (NA)
P.O. Box 9999
Van Nuys, CA 91409-9999
(818) 780-3951
- National Clearinghouse for Alcohol and Drug Information (NCADI)
P.O. Box 2345
Rockville, MD 20847-2345
(800) 729-6686
- National Council on Alcoholism and Drug Dependence, Inc.
12 West 21st Street
New York, NY 10010
(800) NCA-CALL

WEIGHT CONTROL AND EATING DISORDERS

- American Anorexia & Bulimia Association, Inc.
418 East 76th Street
New York, NY 10021
(212) 734-1114
- Anorexia Nervosa and Related Eating Disorders, Inc.
P.O. Box 5102
Eugene, OR 97405
(503) 344-1144
- National Association of Anorexia Nervosa and Associated Disorders, Inc. (ANAD)
P.O. Box 7
Highland Park, IL 60035
(708) 831-3438
- National Eating Disorder Information Centre
200 Elizabeth Street, College Wing 1-328
Toronto, Ontario M5G 2C4, Canada
- Overeaters Anonymous (OA)
383 Van Ness Avenue, Suite 1610
Torrance, CA 90501

- TOPS (Take Off Pounds Sensibly)
  P.O. Box 07360
  Milwaukee, WI 53207
  (800) 932-8677

FITNESS

- American College of Sports Medicine
  P.O. Box 1440
  Indianapolis, IN 46204
  (317) 637-9200
- President's Council on Physical Fitness and Sports
  701 Pennsylvania Avenue NW
  Suite 250
  Washington, DC 20004
  (202) 272-3421
- Sport Medicine and Science Council of Canada
  1600 James Naismith Drive
  Gloucester, Ontario K1B 5N4

PREGNANCY AND LACTATION

- American College of Obstetricians and Gynecologists
  409 12th Street SW
  Washington, DC 20024-2188
  (202) 638-5577
- La Leche League International, Inc.
  1400 N. Meacham Rd.
  P.O. Box 4079
  Schaumburg, IL 61068-4079
  (847) 519-7730
- March of Dimes Birth Defects Foundation
  (National Headquarters)
  1275 Mamaroneck Avenue
  White Plains, NY 10605

TRADE AND INDUSTRY ORGANIZATIONS

- Ralcorp Holdings, Inc.
  Beech-Nut Nutrition Corporation
  800 Market Street
  St. Louis, MO 63106
  (800) 523-6633
- Borden Farm Products, Product Publicity
  180 East Broad Street
  Columbus, OH 43215
- Campbell Soup Company, Food Service Division
  Campbell Place
  Camden, NJ 08103-1799
- Elan Pharma, Nutrition Division
  2 Thurber Blvd.
  Smithfield, RI 02917
- Kraft Foods
  Consumer Response and Information Center
  One Kraft Court
  Glenview, Illinois 60025
- General Mills, Inc., Nutrition Department
  Number One General Mills Boulevard
  Minneapolis, MN 55426
- Kellogg Company
  P.O. Box CAMB
  Battle Creek, MI 49016-1986
- Mead Johnson Nutritionals
  2400 West Lloyd Expressway
  Evansville, IN 47721
- Nabisco Consumer Affairs
  100 DeForest Avenue
  East Hanover, NJ 07936
  (800) 932-7800; (800) NABISCO
- National Dairy Council
  10255 West Higgins Road, Suite 900
  Rosemond, IL 60018
- The NutraSweet Company
  P.O. Box 830
  1751 Lake Cook Road
  Deerfield, IL 60015-5239
  (800) 323-5316
- Pillsbury Company, Consumer Relations
  P.O. Box 550
  Minneapolis, MN 55440-9843
- Procter and Gamble Company
  One Procter and Gamble Plaza
  Cincinnati, OH 45202
- Ross Laboratories, Abbot Laboratory
  625 Cleveland Avenue
  Columbus, OH 43216
- Sherwood Medical
  1915 Olive Street
  St. Louis, MO 63103
- Sunkist Growers, Consumer Affairs
  P.O. Box 7888
  Van Nuys, CA 91409-7888
- United Fresh Fruit and Vegetable Association
  727 North Washington Street
  Alexandria, VA 22314
  (703) 836-3410
- USA Rice Council
  P.O. Box 740121
  Houston, TX 77274
- Vitamin Nutrition Information Service (VNIS)
  Hoffmann-LaRoche, Inc.
  340 Kingsland Street
  Nutley, NJ 07110
- Weight Watchers® Food Company
  Consumer Affairs Department
  P.O. Box 10
  Boise, ID 83707–0010

F

WORLD HUNGER

- Bread for the World
1100 Wayne Ave., Ste 1000
Silver Spring, MD 20910

- Center on Hunger, Poverty and Nutrition Policy
Tufts University School of Nutrition
11 Curtis Avenue
Medford, MA 02155
(617) 627-3956

- Freedom from Hunger
P.O. Box 2000
1644 DaVinci Court
Davis, CA 95617
(916) 758-6200

- Oxfam America
115 Broadway
Boston, MA 02116

- SEEDS Magazine
P.O. Box 6170
Waco, TX 76706
(817) 755-7745

- Worldwatch Institute
1776 Massachusetts Avenue NW
Washington, DC 20036

HEALTH AND DISEASE

- Alzheimer's Association
919 North Michigan Avenue, Suite 1000
Chicago, IL 60611
(800) 272-3900

- Alzheimer's Disease Education and Referral Center
P. O. Box 8250
Silver Spring, Maryland 20907-8250
(800) 438-4380

- American Academy of Allergy, Asthma, and Immunology
611 East Wells Street
Milwaukee, WI 53202
(414) 272-6071; fax: (414) 276-3349

- American Cancer Society Information Center
2200 Lake Blvd.
Atlanta, GA 30319
(800) ACS-2345
Internet address: http://www.cancer.org

- American Council on Science and Health
1995 Broadway, 2nd Floor
New York, NY 10023-5860

- American Dental Association
Division of Communications
211 East Chicago Avenue
Chicago, IL 60611-2678

- American Diabetes Association
1660 Duke Street
Alexandria, VA 22314
(703) 549-1500; (800) 232-3472
Internet address: http://www.diabetes.org

- American Heart Association
Box BHG, National Center
7320 Greenville Avenue
Dallas, TX 75231
(800) 242-8721
Internet address: http://www.amhrt.org

- American Institute for Cancer Research
1759 R Street NW
Washington, DC 20009
Internet address: http://www.aicr.org

- American Medical Association
515 North State Street
Chicago, IL 60610
(312) 464-5000
Internet address: http://www.ama-assn.org

- American Public Health Association
1015 Fifteenth Street NW
Washington, DC 20005
Internet address: http://www.apha.org

- American Red Cross AIDS Education Office
1730 D Street NW
Washington, DC 20006
(202) 737-8300

- Canadian Diabetes Association
15 Toronto Street, Suite 1001
Toronto ON M5C 2E3
(416) 363-0177; fax: (416) 363-3393

- Canadian Public Health Association
Publications, Suite 400
1565 Carling Avenue
Ottawa, Ontario K1Z 8R1, Canada

- Centers for Disease Control (CDC)
Information Hotline
(404) 332-4555
Internet address: http://www.cdc.gov

- Disease Prevention and Health Promotion's National Health Information Center
(800) 336-4797

- The Food Allergy Network
10400 Eaton Place, Suite 107
Fairfax, VA 22030-5647
(703) 691-3179
(800) 929-4040

- National AIDS Hotline (CDC)
  (800) 342-AIDS (English)
  (800) 344-SIDA (Spanish)
  (800) 2437-TTY (Deaf)
  (900) 820-2437
- National Cancer Institute
  31 Center Drive MSC 2580
  Building 31, Room 10A16
  Bethesda, MD 20892-2580
  (800) 4–CANCER; (800) 422-6237
  Internet address: http://www.nci.nih.gov
- National Digestive Disease Information Clearinghouse
  2 Information Way
  Bethesda, MD 20892-3570
  (301) 654-3810
- National Heart, Lung, and Blood Institute
  National High Blood Pressure Education Program
  P.O. Box 30105
  Bethesda, MD 20824-0105
  (301) 951-3260
- National Institute of Allergy and Infectious Diseases
  Office of Communications, Building 31, Room 7A50
  31 Center Drive, MSC 2520
  Bethesda, MD 20892-2520
  (301) 496-5717
  Internet address: http://www.niaid.nih.gov
- National Institute of Dental Research (NIDR)
  Building 31, Room 2C35
  31 Center Drive, MSC 2290
  Bethesda, MD 20892
  (301) 496-4261
- National Institutes of Health (NIH)
  9000 Rockville Pike
  Bethesda, MD 20892
  (301) 496-2433
  Internet address: http://www.nih.gov
- National Osteoporosis Foundation
  1150 17th Street NW, Suite 500
  Washington, DC 20036
  (202) 223-2226
- Smoking and Health Office (CDC)
  Mail Stop K-12
  1600 Clifton Road NE
  Atlanta, GA 30333

F

APPENDIX G

UNITED STATES: RECOMMENDATIONS AND EXCHANGES

WORLD HEALTH ORGANIZATION: RECOMMENDATIONS

Contents

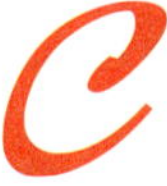hapters 1 and 2 introduced Recommended Dietary Allowances (RDA), Daily Values, Healthy People 2000, and exchange systems. This appendix provides additional details. (See Appendix I for Canada's nutrition recommendations and exchange system.)

RDA

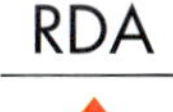

Some of the U.S. recommendations for nutrient intakes appear in the RDA table on the inside front cover, left. The remaining RDA are here, in Tables G–1, G–2, and G–3.

U.S. RDA AND DAILY VALUES

Food labels use another set of standards that derive from the RDA. From the late 1960s to the early 1990s, the set of standards used on food labels was called the U.S. RDA. The U.S. RDA were derived from the 1968 RDA and were established by the Food and Drug Administration (FDA) so that labels could express the nutrient contents of foods as percentages of those standards (see Table G–4). The intent was to help consumers evaluate the nutrient contents of foods for themselves and at the same time to spare them the burden of learning the different units in which nutrient amounts are expressed. Thus all nutrient amounts in a food, whether originally measured in micrograms, milligrams, grams, or RE, could be expressed as "percent of U.S. RDA."

With the new labeling regulations came a name change. The revised set of standards used on food labels—the Daily Values—are discussed fully in Chapter 2. With the exception of protein, the current Daily Values continue to use the same values as the old U.S. RDA. The FDA continues to consider their revision.

Table G-1
Estimated Safe and Adequate Daily Dietary Intakes of Additional Selected Vitamins and Minerals (United States)[a]

Age (yr)	Vitamins		Trace Elements[b]				
	Biotin (μg)	Pantothenic Acid (mg)	Chromium (μg)	Molybdenum (μg)	Copper (mg)	Manganese (mg)	Fluoride (mg)
Infants							
0–0.5	10	2	10–40	15–30	0.4–0.6	0.3–0.6	0.1–0.5
0.5–1	15	3	20–60	20–40	0.6–0.7	0.6–1.0	0.2–1.0
Children							
1–3	20	3	20–80	25–50	0.7–1.0	1.0–1.5	0.5–1.5
4–6	25	3–4	30–120	30–75	1.0–1.5	1.5–2.0	1.0–2.5
7–10	30	4–5	50–200	50–150	1.0–2.0	2.0–3.0	1.5–2.5
11+	30–100	4–7	50–200	75–250	1.5–2.5	2.0–5.0	1.5–2.5
Adults	30–100	4–7	50–200	75–250	1.5–3.0	2.0–5.0	1.5–4.0

[a]Less information is available on which to base allowances for these nutrients. Therefore, they are not included in the main table of the RDA, and the figures provided here are in the form of ranges of recommended intakes.
[b]The toxic levels for many trace elements may be only several times usual intakes, so the upper levels for the trace elements given in this table should not be habitually exceeded.
Source: Recommended Dietary Allowances, © 1989 by the National Academy of Sciences, National Academy Press, Washington, D.C.

Table G-2
Estimated Minimum Requirements of Sodium, Chloride, and Potassium

Age (yr)	Weight (kg)	Sodium[a] (mg)	Chloride (mg)	Potassium[b] (mg)
Infants				
0.0–0.5	4.5	120	180	500
0.5–1.0	8.9	200	300	700
Children				
1	11.0	225	350	1000
2–5	16.0	300	500	1400
6–9	25.0	400	600	1600
Adolescents	50.0	500	750	2000
Adults	70.0	500	750	2000

[a]Sodium requirements are based on estimates of needs for growth and for replacement of obligatory losses. They cover a wide variation of physical activity patterns and climatic exposure but do not provide for large, prolonged losses from the skin through sweat.
[b]Dietary potassium may benefit the prevention and treatment of hypertension, and recommendations to include many servings of fruits and vegetables would raise potassium intakes to about 3500 milligrams per day.
Source: Recommended Dietary Allowances, © 1989 by the National Academy of Sciences, National Academy Press, Washington, D.C.

Table G–3
Median Heights and Weights and Recommended Energy Intakes (United States)

Age (yr)	Weight		Height		Average Energy Allowance			
	kg	lb	cm	in	REE[a] (kcal/day)	MULTIPLES OF REE[b]	kcal/kg	kcal/day[c]
Infants								
0.0–0.5	6	13	60	24	320		108	650
0.5–1.0	9	20	71	28	500		98	850
Children								
1–3	13	29	90	35	740		102	1300
4–6	20	44	112	44	950		90	1800
7–10	28	62	132	52	1130		70	2000
Males								
11–14	45	99	157	62	1440	1.70	55	2500
15–18	66	145	176	69	1760	1.67	45	3000
19–24	72	160	177	70	1780	1.67	40	2900
25–50	79	174	176	70	1800	1.60	37	2900
51+	77	170	173	68	1530	1.50	30	2300
Females								
11–14	46	101	157	62	1310	1.67	47	2200
15–18	55	120	163	64	1370	1.60	40	2200
19–24	58	128	164	65	1350	1.60	38	2200
25–50	63	138	163	64	1380	1.55	36	2200
51+	65	143	160	63	1280	1.50	30	1900
Pregnant (2nd and 3rd trimesters)								+300
Lactating								+500

[a]REE (resting energy expenditure) represents the energy expended by a person at rest under normal conditions.

[b]Recommended energy allowances assume light-to-moderate activity and were calculated by multiplying the REE by an activity factor.

[c]Average energy allowances have been rounded.

Source: Recommended Dietary Allowances, © 1989 by the National Academy of Sciences, National Academy Press, Washington, D.C.

G

Table G-4
U.S. Recommended Daily Allowances (U.S. RDA)

Nutrient	Adults and Children over 4 Years	Infants	Children under 4 Years	Pregnant or Lactating Women
Protein (g)	45[a]	18[a]	20[a]	
Vitamin A (RE)	1000	300	500	1600
Vitamin D[b] (IU)	400	400	400	400
Vitamin E[b] (IU)	30	5.0	10	30
Vitamin C (mg)	60	35	40	60
Folate (mg)	0.4	0.1	0.2	0.8
Thiamin (mg)	1.5	0.5	0.7	1.7
Riboflavin (mg)	1.7	0.6	0.8	2.0
Niacin (mg)	20	8	9	20
Vitamin B_6[b] (mg)	2.0	0.4	0.7	2.5
Vitamin B_{12}[b] (μg)	6.0	2.0	3.0	8.0
Biotin[b] (mg)	0.3	0.5	0.15	0.3
Pantothenic acid[b] (mg)	10	3	5	10
Calcium (g)	1.0	0.6	0.8	1.3
Phosphorus[b] (g)	1.0	0.5	0.8	1.3
Iodine[b] (μg)	150	45	70	150
Iron (mg)	18	15	10	18
Magnesium[b] (mg)	400	70	200	450
Copper[b] (mg)	2.0	0.6	1.0	2.0
Zinc[b] (mg)	15	5	8	15

Note: Four sets of U.S. RDA were developed for different groups of people—infants, children, adults, and pregnant and lactating women. The most commonly used set was the U.S. RDA for adults. The one for infants was used for formulas. Supplements designed for children and for pregnant and lactating women used the U.S. RDA for these groups on their labels.

[a]If protein efficiency ratio of protein is equal to or better than that of casein.

[b]Optional for adults and children 4 years or over in vitamin and mineral supplements.

Source: U.S. Department of Health and Human Services, Public Health Service, Food and Drug Administration, Office of Public Affairs, 5600 Fishers Lane, Rockville, Maryland 20857, HHS publication no. (FDA) 81–2146, revised March 1981.

HEALTHY PEOPLE 2000

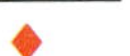

In 1990, the U.S. Department of Health and Human Services established a set of almost 300 health objectives for the nation called *Healthy People 2000.*[1] The 21 objectives that have a nutrition component were presented throughout this text wherever their topic was discussed. Table G–5 presents them in full.

Table G-5
Healthy People 2000 Nutrition Objectives

Health-Related Objectives
- Reduce coronary heart disease deaths to no more than 100 per 100,000 people.
- Reverse the rise in cancer deaths to achieve a rate of no more than 130 per 100,000 people.
- Reduce overweight to a prevalence of no more than 20% among people aged 20 years and older and maintain prevalence at no more than 15% among adolescents aged 12 through 19 years.
- Reduce growth retardation among low-income children aged five years and younger to less than 10%.

Nutrient Intake Objectives
- Reduce dietary fat intake to an average of 30% of energy or less and average saturated fat intake to less than 10% of energy among people aged two years and older.
- Increase complex carbohydrate and fiber-containing foods in the diets of adults to five or more daily servings for vegetables (including legumes) and fruits and to six or more daily servings for grain products.
- Increase to at least 50% the proportion of overweight people aged 12 years and older who have adopted sound dietary practices combined with regular physical activity to attain an appropriate body weight.
- Increase calcium intake, so that at least 50% of youth aged 12 through 24 years and 50% of pregnant and lactating women consume three or more servings of calcium-rich foods daily and at least 50% of people aged 25 years and older consume two or more servings of calcium-rich foods daily.
- Decrease salt and sodium intake so at least 65% of home meal preparers prepare foods without adding salt, at least 80% of people avoid using salt at the table, and at least 40% of adults regularly purchase foods modified or lower in sodium.
- Reduce iron deficiency to less than 3% among children aged 1 to 4 and women of childbearing age.
- Increase to at least 75% the proportion of mothers who breastfeed their babies in the early weeks and to at least 50% the proportion who continue breastfeeding until their babies are five to six months old.
- Increase to at least 75% the proportion of parents and caregivers who use feeding practices that prevent nursing bottle tooth decay.
- Increase to at least 85% the proportion of people aged 18 and older who use food labels to make nutritious food selections.

Services and Information Objectives
- Achieve useful and informative nutrition labeling for virtually all processed foods and at least 40% of fresh meats, poultry, fish, fruits, vegetables, baked goods, and ready-to-eat carry-away foods.
- Increase to at least 5000 brand items the number of processed food products that are reduced in fat and saturated fat.
- Increase to at least 90% the proportion of restaurants and institutional foodservice operations that offer identifiable low-fat, low-kcalorie food choices, consistent with the *Dietary Guidelines for Americans.*
- Increase to at least 90% the proportion of school lunch and breakfast services and increase to at least 50% the proportion of child care foodservices with menus that are consistent with the nutrition principles in the *Dietary Guidelines for Americans.*
- Increase to at least 80% the receipt of home foodservices by people aged 65 and older who have difficulty in preparing their own meals or are otherwise in need of home-delivered meals.
- Increase to at least 75% the proportion of the nation's schools that provide nutrition education from preschool through grade 12, preferably as part of quality school health education.
- Increase to at least 50% the proportion of worksites with 50 or more employees that offer nutrition education and/or weight management programs for employees.
- Increase to at least 75% the proportion of primary care providers who provide nutrition assessment and counseling and/or referral to qualified nutritionists or dietitians.

U.S. EXCHANGE LISTS FOR MEAL PLANNING

The U.S. exchange system groups together foods that have about the same amount of carbohydrate, protein, fat, and kcalories. Then any food on a list can be "exchanged" for any other food on that same list. Chapter 2 introduced the exchange lists and Tables G–6 through G–14 present the lists in detail.

Table G–6
U.S. Exchange System: Starch List

1 starch exchange = 15 g carbohydrate, 3 g protein, 0–1 g fat, and 80 kcal
Note: In general, a starch serving is ½ c cereal, grain, pasta, or starchy vegetable; 1 oz of bread; ¾ to 1 oz snack food.

Serving Size	Food
Bread	
½ (1 oz)	Bagels
2 slices (1½ oz)	Bread, reduced-kcalorie
1 slice (1 oz)	Bread, white (including French and Italian), whole-wheat, pumpernickel, rye
2 (⅔ oz)	Bread sticks, crisp, 4″ x ½″
½	English muffins
½ (1 oz)	Hot dog or hamburger buns
½	Pita, 6″ across
1 (1 oz)	Plain rolls, small
1 slice (1 oz)	Raisin bread, unfrosted
1	Tortillas, corn, 6″ across
1	Tortillas, flour, 7–8″ across
1	Waffles, 4½″ square, reduced-fat
Cereals and Grains	
½ c	Bran cereals
½ c	Bulgur, cooked
½ c	Cereals, cooked
¾ c	Cereals, unsweetened, ready-to-eat
3 tbs	Cornmeal (dry)
⅓ c	Couscous
3 tbs	Flour (dry)
¼ c	Granola, low-fat
¼ c	Grape nuts
½ c	Grits, cooked
½ c	Kasha
¼ c	Millet
¼ c	Muesli
½ c	Oats
½ c	Pasta, cooked
1½ c	Puffed cereals
½ c	Rice milk
⅓ c	Rice, white or brown, cooked
½ c	Shredded wheat
½ c	Sugar-frosted cereal
3 tbs	Wheat germ
Starchy Vegetables	
⅓ c	Baked beans
½ c	Corn
1 (5 oz)	Corn on cob, medium
1 c	Mixed vegetables with corn, peas, or pasta
½ c	Peas, green
½ c	Plantains
1 small (3 oz)	Potatoes, baked or boiled
½ c	Potatoes, mashed
1 c	Squash, winter (acorn, butternut)
½ c	Yams, sweet potatoes, plain
Crackers and Snacks	
8	Animal crackers
3	Graham crackers, 2½″ square
¾ oz	Matzoh
4 slices	Melba toast
24	Oyster crackers
3 c	Popcorn (popped, no fat added or low-fat microwave)
¾ oz	Pretzels
2	Rice cakes, 4″ across
6	Saltine-type crackers
15–20 (¾ oz)	Snack chips, fat-free (tortilla, potato)
2–5 (¾ oz)	Whole-wheat crackers, no fat added
Dried Beans, Peas, and Lentils	
½ c	Beans and peas, cooked (garbanzo, lentils, pinto, kidney, white, split, black-eyed)
⅔ c	Lima beans
3 tbs	Miso (sodium symbol)
Starchy Foods Prepared with Fat **Count as 1 starch + 1 fat exchange.**	
1	Biscuit, 2½″ across
½ c	Chow mein noodles
1 (2 oz)	Corn bread, 2″ cube
6	Crackers, round butter type
1 c	Croutons
16–25 (3 oz)	French-fried potatoes
¼ c	Granola
1 (1½ oz)	Muffin, small
2	Pancake, 4″ across
3 c	Popcorn, microwave
3	Sandwich crackers, cheese or peanut butter filling
⅓ c	Stuffing, bread (prepared)
2	Taco shell, 6″ across
1	Waffle, 4½″ square
4–6 (1 oz)	Whole-wheat crackers, fat added

(sodium symbol) = 400 mg or more of sodium per serving.

Table G–7
U.S. Exchange System: Fruit List

1 fruit exchange = 15 g carbohydrate and 60 kcal
Note: In general, a fruit serving is 1 small to medium fresh fruit; ½ c canned or fresh fruit or fruit juice; ¼ c dried fruit.

Serving Size	Food
1 (4 oz)	Apples, unpeeled, small
½ c	Applesauce, unsweetened
4 rings	Apples, dried
4 whole (5½ oz)	Apricots, fresh
8 halves	Apricots, dried
½ c	Apricots, canned
1 (4 oz)	Bananas, small
¾ c	Blackberries
¾ c	Blueberries
⅓ melon (11 oz) or 1 c cubes	Cantaloupe, small
12 (3 oz)	Cherries, sweet, fresh
½ c	Cherries, sweet, canned
3	Dates
1½ large or 2 medium (3½ oz)	Figs, fresh
1½	Figs, dried
½ c	Fruit cocktail
½ (11 oz)	Grapefruit, large
¾ c	Grapefruit sections, canned
17 (3 oz)	Grapes, small
1 slice (10 oz) or 1 c cubes	Honeydew melon
1 (3½ oz)	Kiwi
¾ c	Mandarin oranges, canned
½ (5½ oz) or ½ c	Mangoes, small
1 (5 oz)	Nectarines, small
1 (6½ oz)	Oranges, small
½ (8 oz) or 1 c cubes	Papayas
1 (6 oz)	Peaches, medium, fresh
½ c	Peaches, canned
½ (4 oz)	Pears, large, fresh
½ c	Pears, canned
¾ c	Pineapple, fresh
½ c	Pineapple, canned
2 (5 oz)	Plums, small
½ c	Plums, canned
3	Prunes, dried
2 tbs	Raisins
1 c	Raspberries
1¼ c whole berries	Strawberries
2 (8 oz)	Tangerines, small
1 slice (13½ oz) or 1¼ c cubes	Watermelon
Fruit Juice	
½ c	Apple juice/cider
⅓ c	Cranberry juice cocktail
1 c	Cranberry juice cocktail, reduced-kcalorie
⅓ c	Fruit juice blends, 100% juice
⅓ c	Grape juice
½ c	Grapefruit juice
½ c	Orange juice
½ c	Pineapple juice
⅓ c	Prune juice

Table G–8
U.S. Exchange System: Milk List

Serving Size	Food
Nonfat and Very Low-Fat Milk	
1 nonfat/low-fat milk exchange = 12 g carbohydrate, 8 g protein, 0–3 g fat, 90 kcal	
1 c	Nonfat milk
1 c	½% milk
1 c	1% milk
1 c	Nonfat or low-fat buttermilk
½ c	Evaporated nonfat milk
⅓ c dry	Dry nonfat milk
¾ c	Plain nonfat yogurt
1 c	Nonfat or low-fat fruit-flavored yogurt sweetened with aspartame or with a nonnutritive sweetener
Low-Fat Milk	
1 low-fat milk exchange = 12 g carbohydrate, 8 g protein, 5 g fat, 120 kcal	
1 c	2% milk
¾ c	Plain low-fat yogurt
1 c	Sweet acidophilus milk
Whole Milk	
1 whole milk exchange = 12 g carbohydrate, 8 g protein, 8 g fat, 150 kcal	
1 c	Whole milk
½ c	Evaporated whole milk
1 c	Goat's milk
1 c	Kefir

Table G-9
U.S. Exchange System: Other Carbohydrates List

1 other carbohydrate exchange = 15 g carbohydrate, or 1 starch, or 1 fruit, or 1 milk exchange

Food	Serving Size	Exchanges per Serving
Angel food cake, unfrosted	1/12 cake	2 carbohydrates
Brownies, small, unfrosted	2″ square	1 carbohydrate, 1 fat
Cake, unfrosted	2″ square	1 carbohydrate, 1 fat
Cake, frosted	2″ square	2 carbohydrates, 1 fat
Cookie, fat-free	2 small	1 carbohydrate
Cookies or sandwich cookies	2 small	1 carbohydrate, 1 fat
Cupcakes, frosted	1 small	2 carbohydrates, 1 fat
Cranberry sauce, jellied	¼ c	2 carbohydrates
Doughnuts, plain cake	1 medium, (1½ oz)	1½ carbohydrates, 2 fats
Doughnuts, glazed	3¾″ across (2 oz)	2 carbohydrates, 2 fats
Fruit juice bars, frozen, 100% juice	1 bar (3 oz)	1 carbohydrate
Fruit snacks, chewy (pureed fruit concentrate)	1 roll (¾ oz)	1 carbohydrate
Fruit spreads, 100% fruit	1 tbs	1 carbohydrate
Gelatin, regular	½ c	1 carbohydrate
Gingersnaps	3	1 carbohydrate
Granola bars	1 bar	1 carbohydrate, 1 fat
Granola bars, fat-free	1 bar	2 carbohydrates
Hummus	⅓ c	1 carbohydrate, 1 fat
Ice cream	½ c	1 carbohydrate, 2 fats
Ice cream, light	½ c	1 carbohydrate, 1 fat
Ice cream, fat-free, no sugar added	½ c	1 carbohydrate
Jam or jelly, regular	1 tbs	1 carbohydrate
Milk, chocolate, whole	1 c	2 carbohydrates, 1 fat
Pie, fruit, 2 crusts	⅙ pie	3 carbohydrates, 2 fats
Pie, pumpkin or custard	⅛ pie	1 carbohydrate, 2 fats
Potato chips	12–18 (1 oz)	1 carbohydrate, 2 fats
Pudding, regular (made with low-fat milk)	½ c	2 carbohydrates
Pudding, sugar-free (made with low-fat milk)	½ c	1 carbohydrate
Salad dressing, fat-free	¼ c	1 carbohydrate
Sherbet, sorbet	½ c	2 carbohydrates
Spaghetti or pasta sauce, canned	½ c	1 carbohydrate, 1 fat
Sweet roll or danish	1 (2½ oz)	2½ carbohydrates, 2 fats
Syrup, light	2 tbs	1 carbohydrate
Syrup, regular	1 tbs	1 carbohydrate
Syrup, regular	¼ c	4 carbohydrates
Tortilla chips	6–12 (1 oz)	1 carbohydrate, 2 fats
Yogurt, frozen, low-fat, fat-free	⅓ c	1 carbohydrate, 0–1 fat
Yogurt, frozen, fat-free, no sugar added	½ c	1 carbohydrate
Yogurt, low-fat with fruit	1 c	3 carbohydrates, 0–1 fat
Vanilla wafers	5	1 carbohydrate, 1 fat

= 400 mg or more sodium per exchange.

Table G–10

U.S. Exchange System: Vegetable List

1 vegetable exchange = 5 g carbohydrate, 2 g protein, 25 kcal

Note: In general, a vegetable serving is ½ c cooked vegetables or vegetable juice; 1 c raw vegetables. Starchy vegetables such as corn, peas, and potatoes are on the starch list.

Artichokes
Artichoke hearts
Asparagus
Beans (green, wax, Italian)
Bean sprouts
Beets
Broccoli
Brussels sprouts
Cabbage
Carrots
Cauliflower
Celery
Cucumbers
Eggplant
Green onions or scallions
Greens (collard, kale, mustard, turnip)
Kohlrabi
Leeks
Mixed vegetables (without corn, peas, or pasta)
Mushrooms
Okra
Onions
Pea pods
Peppers (all varieties)
Radishes
Salad greens (endive, escarole, lettuce, romaine, spinach)
Sauerkraut
Spinach
Summer squash (crookneck)
Tomatoes
Tomatoes, canned
Tomato sauce
Tomato/vegetable juice
Turnips
Water chestnuts
Watercress
Zucchini

= 400 mg or more sodium per exchange.

Table G–11

U.S. Exchange System: Meat and Meat Substitutes List

Note: In general, a meat serving is 1 oz meat, poultry, or cheese; ½ c dried beans (weigh meat and poultry and measure beans after cooking).

Serving Size	Food
Very Lean Meat and Substitutes	
1 very lean meat exchange = 7 g protein, 0–1 g fat, 35 kcal	
1 oz	Poultry: Chicken or turkey (white meat, no skin), Cornish hen (no skin)
1 oz	Fish: Fresh or frozen cod, flounder, haddock, halibut, trout; tuna, fresh or canned in water
1 oz	Shellfish: Clams, crab, lobster, scallops, shrimp, imitation shellfish
1 oz	Game: Duck or pheasant (no skin), venison, buffalo, ostrich
	Cheese with ≤ 1 g fat/oz:
¼ c	Nonfat or low-fat cottage cheese
1 oz	Fat-free cheese
	Other:
1 oz	Processed sandwich meats with ≤ 1 g fat/oz (such as deli thin, shaved meats, chipped beef 🧂, turkey ham)
2	Egg whites
¼ c	Egg substitutes, plain
1 oz	Hot dogs with ≤ 1 g fat/oz
1 oz	Kidney (high in cholesterol)
1 oz	Sausage with ≤ 1 g fat/oz 🧂
Count as one very lean meat and one starch exchange:	
½ c	Dried beans, peas, lentils (cooked)
Lean Meat and Substitutes	
1 lean meat exchange = 7 g protein, 3 g fat, 55 kcal	
1 oz	Beef: USDA Select or Choice grades of lean beef trimmed of fat (round, sirloin, and flank steak); tenderloin; roast (rib, chuck, rump); steak (T-bone, porterhouse, cubed), ground round
1 oz	Pork: Lean pork (fresh ham); canned, cured, or boiled ham; Canadian bacon 🧂; tenderloin, center loin chop
1 oz	Lamb: Roast, chop, leg
1 oz	Veal: Lean chop, roast
1 oz	Poultry: Chicken, turkey (dark meat, no skin), chicken white meat (with skin), domestic duck or goose (well-drained of fat, no skin)
	Fish:
1 oz	Herring (uncreamed or smoked)
6 medium	Oysters
1 oz	Salmon (fresh or canned), catfish
2 medium	Sardines (canned)
1 oz	Tuna (canned in oil, drained)
1 oz	Game: Goose (no skin), rabbit
	Cheese:
¼ c	4.5%-fat cottage cheese
2 tbs	Grated Parmesan
1 oz	Cheeses with ≤ 3 g fat/oz
	Other:
1½ oz	Hot dogs with ≤ 3 g fat/oz 🧂
1 oz	Processed sandwich meat with ≤ 3 g fat/oz (turkey pastrami or kielbasa)
1 oz	Liver, heart (high in cholesterol)
Medium-Fat Meat and Substitutes	
1 medium-fat meat exchange = 7 g protein, 5 g fat, and 75 kcal	
1 oz	Beef: Most beef products (ground beef, meatloaf, corned beef, short ribs, Prime grades of meat trimmed of fat, such as prime rib)
1 oz	Pork: Top loin, chop, Boston butt, cutlet
1 oz	Lamb: Rib roast, ground
1 oz	Veal: Cutlet (ground or cubed, unbreaded)
1 oz	Poultry: Chicken dark meat (with skin), ground turkey or ground chicken, fried chicken (with skin)
1 oz	Fish: Any fried fish product
	Cheese with ≤ 5 g fat/oz:
1 oz	Feta
1 oz	Mozzarella
¼ c (2 oz)	Ricotta
	Other:
1	Egg (high in cholesterol, limit to 3/week)
1 oz	Sausage with ≤ 5 g fat/oz
1 c	Soy milk
¼ c	Tempeh
4 oz or ½ c	Tofu
High-Fat Meat and Substitutes	
1 high-fat meat exchange = 7 g protein, 8 g fat, 100 kcal	
1 oz	Pork: Spareribs, ground pork, pork sausage
1 oz	Cheese: All regular cheeses (American 🧂, cheddar, Monterey Jack, swiss)
	Other:
1 oz	Processed sandwich meats with ≤ 8 g fat/oz (bologna, pimento loaf, salami)
1 oz	Sausage (bratwurst, Italian, knockwurst, Polish, smoked)
1 (10/lb)	Hot dog (turkey or chicken) 🧂
3 slices (20 slices/lb)	Bacon
Count as one high-fat meat plus one fat exchange:	
1 (10/lb)	Hot dog (beef, pork, or combination) 🧂
2 tbs	Peanut butter (contains unsaturated fat)

🧂 = 400 mg or more sodium per exchange.

Table G–12
U.S. Exchange System: Fat List

1 fat exchange = 5 g fat, 45 kcal
Note: In general, a fat serving is 1 tsp regular butter, margarine, or vegetable oil; 1 tbs regular salad dressing. Many fat-free and reduced fat foods are on the Free Foods List.

Serving Size	Food
Monounsaturated Fats	
⅛ medium (1 oz)	Avocadoes
1 tsp	Oil (canola, olive, peanut)
8 large	Olives, ripe (black)
10 large	Olives, green, stuffed
6 nuts	Almonds, cashews
6 nuts	Mixed nuts (50% peanuts)
10 nuts	Peanuts
4 halves	Pecans
2 tsp	Peanut butter, smooth or crunchy
1 tbs	Sesame seeds
2 tsp	Tahini paste
Polyunsaturated Fats	
1 tsp	Margarine, stick, tub, or squeeze
1 tbs	Margarine, lower-fat (30% to 50% vegetable oil)
1 tsp	Mayonnaise, regular
1 tbs	Mayonnaise, reduced-fat
4 halves	Nuts, walnuts, English
1 tsp	Oil (corn, safflower, soybean)
1 tbs	Salad dressing, regular
2 tbs	Salad dressing, reduced-fat
2 tsp	Mayonnaise type salad dressing, regular
1 tbs	Mayonnaise type salad dressing, reduced-fat
1 tbs	Seeds: pumpkin, sunflower
Saturated Fats*	
1 slice (20 slices/lb)	Bacon, cooked
1 tsp	Bacon, grease
1 tsp	Butter, stick
2 tsp	Butter, whipped
1 tbs	Butter, reduced-fat
2 tbs (½ oz)	Chitterlings, boiled
2 tbs	Coconut, sweetened, shredded
2 tbs	Cream, half and half
1 tbs (½ oz)	Cream cheese, regular
2 tbs (1 oz)	Cream cheese, reduced-fat
	Fatback or salt pork**
1 tsp	Shortening or lard
2 tbs	Sour cream, regular
3 tbs	Sour cream, reduced-fat

= 400 mg or more sodium per exchange
*Saturated fats can raise blood cholesterol levels.
** Use a piece 1″ × 1″ × ¼″ if you plan to eat the fatback cooked with vegetables. Use a piece 2″ × 1″ × ½″ when eating only the vegetables with the fatback removed.

G

Table G–13
U.S. Exchange System: Free Foods List

Note: A serving of free food contains less than 20 kcalories; those with serving sizes should be limited to three servings a day whereas those without serving sizes can be eaten freely.

Serving Size	Food
Fat-Free or Reduced-Fat Foods	
1 tbs	Cream cheese, fat-free
1 tbs	Creamers, nondairy, liquid
2 tsp	Creamers, nondairy, powdered
1 tbs	Mayonnaise, fat-free
1 tsp	Mayonnaise, reduced-fat
4 tbs	Margarine, fat-free
1 tsp	Margarine, reduced-fat
1 tbs	Mayonnaise type salad dressing, nonfat
1 tsp	Mayonnaise type salad dressing, reduced-fat
	Nonstick cooking spray
1 tbs	Salad dressing, fat-free
2 tbs	Salad dressing, fat-free, Italian
¼ c	Salsa
1 tbs	Sour cream, fat-free, reduced-fat
2 tbs	Whipped topping, regular or light
Sugar-Free or Low-Sugar Foods	
1 piece	Candy, hard, sugar-free
	Gelatin dessert, sugar-free
	Gelatin, unflavored
	Gum, sugar-free
2 tsp	Jam or jelly, low-sugar or light
	Sugar substitutes
2 tbs	Syrup, sugar-free
Drinks	
	Bouillon, broth, consommé
	Bouillon or broth, low-sodium
	Carbonated or mineral water
1 tbs	Cocoa powder, unsweetened
	Coffee
	Club soda
	Diet soft drinks, sugar-free
	Drink mixes, sugar-free
	Tea
	Tonic water, sugar-free
Condiments	
1 tbs	Catsup
	Horseradish
	Lemon juice
	Lime juice
	Mustard
1½ large	Pickles, dill
	Soy sauce, regular or light
1 tbs	Taco sauce
	Vinegar
Seasonings	
Flavoring extracts	
Garlic	
Herbs, fresh or dried	
Pimento	
Spices	
Hot pepper sauces	
Wine, used in cooking	
Worcestershire sauce	

= 400 mg or more sodium per exchange.

Table G–14
U.S. Exchange System: Combination Foods List

Food	Serving Size	Exchanges per Serving
Entrees		
Tuna noodle casserole, lasagna, spaghetti with meatballs, chili with beans, macaroni and cheese	1 c (8 oz)	2 carbohydrates, 2 medium-fat meats
Chow mein (without noodles or rice)	2 c (16 oz)	1 carbohydrate, 2 lean meats
Pizza, cheese, thin crust	¼ of 10″ (5 oz)	2 carbohydrates, 2 medium-fat meats, 1 fat
Pizza, meat topping, thin crust	¼ of 10″ (5 oz)	2 carbohydrates, 2 medium-fat meats, 2 fats
Pot pie	1 (7 oz)	2 carbohydrates, 1 medium-fat meat, 4 fats
Frozen entrees		
Salisbury steak with gravy, mashed potato	1 (11 oz)	2 carbohydrates, 3 medium-fat meats, 3–4 fats
Turkey with gravy, mashed potato, dressing	1 (11 oz)	2 carbohydrates, 2 medium-fat meats, 2 fats
Entree with less than 300 kcalories	1 (8 oz)	2 carbohydrates, 3 lean meats
Soups		
Bean	1 c	1 carbohydrate, 1 very lean meat
Cream (made with water)	1 c (8 oz)	1 carbohydrate, 1 fat
Split pea (made with water)	½ c (4 oz)	1 carbohydrate
Tomato (make with water)	1 c (8 oz)	1 carbohydrate
Vegetable beef, chicken noodle, or other broth-type	1 c (8 oz)	1 carbohydrate
Fast Foods		
Burritos with beef	2	4 carbohydrates, 2 medium-fat meats, 2 fats
Chicken nuggets	6	1 carbohydrate, 2 medium-fat meats, 1 fat
Chicken breast and wing, breaded and fried	1	1 carbohydrate, 4 medium-fat meats, 2 fats
Fish sandwich/tartar sauce	1	3 carbohydrates, 1 medium-fat meat, 3 fats
French fries, thin	20–25	2 carbohydrates, 2 fats
Hamburger, regular	1	2 carbohydrates, 2 medium-fat meats
Hamburger, large	1	2 carbohydrates, 3 medium-fat meats, 1 fat

G

Table G–14 (continued)
U.S. Exchange System: Combination Foods List

Food	Serving Size	Exchanges per Serving
Hot dog with bun	1	1 carbohydrate, 1 high-fat meat, 1 fat
Individual pan pizza	1	5 carbohydrates, 3 medium-fat meats, 3 fats
Soft serve cone	1 medium	2 carbohydrates, 1 fat
Submarine sandwich	1 (6″)	3 carbohydrates, 1 vegetable, 2 medium-fat meats, 1 fat
Taco, hard shell	1 (6 oz)	2 carbohydrates, 2 medium-fat meats, 2 fats
Taco, soft shell	1 (3 oz)	1 carbohydrate, 1 medium-fat meat, 1 fat

= 400 mg or more sodium per exchange.

NUTRITION RECOMMENDATIONS FROM WHO

Like the Committee on Diet and Health in the United States, the World Health Organization (WHO) has also assessed the relationships between diet and the development of chronic diseases.[2] Their recommendations are expressed in average daily ranges that represent the lower and upper limits:

- Total energy: sufficient to support normal growth, physical activity, and body weight (body mass index = 20–22).
- Total fat: 15 to 30 percent of total energy.
  - Saturated fatty acids: 0 to 10 percent total energy.
  - Polyunsaturated fatty acids: 3 to 7 percent total energy.
  - Dietary cholesterol: 0 to 300 milligrams per day.
- Total carbohydrate: 55 to 75 percent total energy.
  - Complex carbohydrates: 50 to 75 percent total energy.
  - Dietary fiber: 27 to 40 grams per day.
  - Refined sugars: 0 to 10 percent total energy.
- Protein: 10 to 15 percent total energy.
- Salt: upper limit of 6 grams/day (no lower limit set).

NOTES

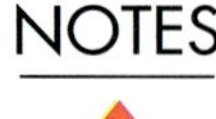

1. The Exchange Lists are the basis of a meal planning system designed by a committee of the American Diabetes Association and The American Dietetic Association. While designed primarily for people with diabetes and others who must follow special diets, the Exchange Lists are based on principles of good nutrition that apply to everyone. Copyright © 1995 by American Diabetes Association, Inc., and The American Dietetic Association.
2. *Healthy People 2000: National Health Promotion and Disease Prevention Objectives* (Washington, D.C.: U.S. Department of Health and Human Services, 1990).
3. Diet, nutrition and the prevention of chronic diseases: A report of the WHO Study Group on Diet, Nutrition and Prevention of Noncommunicable Diseases, *Nutrition Reviews* 49 (1991): 291–301.

TABLE OF FOOD COMPOSITION

APPENDIX H

This edition of the table of food composition contains more complete values for several nutrients than any comparable table.[1] These include dietary fiber; saturated, monounsaturated, and polyunsaturated fat; vitamin B_6; vitamin E; folate; magnesium; and zinc. The table includes a wide variety of foods from all food groups and is updated yearly to reflect current food patterns. For example, this edition includes many new nonfat items; several new ethnic items such as adzuki beans, tahitian taro, and gai choy chinese mustard; and a new selection of baby foods.

Sources of Data To achieve a complete and reliable listing of nutrients for all the foods, over 1200 sources of information are researched. Government sources are the primary base for all data for most foods. In addition to USDA data (from Release 11 and surveys), provisional USDA information—both published and unpublished—is included.

Even with all the government sources available, however, some nutrient values are still missing; and as the USDA updates various data, it sometimes reports conflicting values for the same items. To fill in the missing values and resolve discrepancies, other reliable sources of information are used. These sources include refereed journal articles, food composition tables from Canada and England, information from other nutrient data banks and publications, unpublished scientific data, and manufacturers' data.

The selection of brand foods are included as provided by the food manufacturers and the food chain restaurants. This information changes often because recipes and formulations are modified to meet consumer preferences, and the data is usually limited to those nutrients required for food labels. To provide more complete information, values for several nutrients have been estimated based on known values for major ingredients.

Accuracy The energy and nutrients in recipes and combination foods vary widely, depending on the ingredients. The amounts of various fatty acids and cholesterol are influenced by the type of fat used (the specific type of oil, vegetable shortening, butter, margarine, etc.).

Estimates of nutrient amounts for foods and nutrients include all possible adjustments in the interest of accuracy. When multiple values are reported for a nutrient, the numbers are averaged and weighted with consideration of the original number of analyses in the separate sources. Whenever water percentages are available, estimates of nutrient amounts are adjusted for water content. When no water is given, water percentage is assumed to be that shown in the table. Whenever a reported weight appeared inconsistent (cooked eggplant and collards, for example), many kitchen tests were made, and the average weight of the typical product was given as tested.

When estimates of nutrient amounts in cooked foods are derived from reported amounts in raw foods, published retention factors are applied. Data for combination foods are modified to include newer data for major ingredients.

Considerable effort has been made to report the most accurate data available and to eliminate missing values. The table is updated annually, and the authors welcome any suggestions or comments for future editions.

Average Values It is important to know that many different nutrient values can be reported for foods, even by reliable sources. Many factors influence the amounts of nutrients in foods, including the mineral content of the soil,

1. This food composition table has been prepared for West Publishing Company and is copyrighted by ESHA Research in Salem, Oregon—the developer and publisher of the Food Processor®, Genesis® R&D, and Computer Chef® nutrition software systems. The major sources for the data from the U.S. Department of Agriculture are supplemented by more than 1200 additional sources of information. Because the list of references is so extensive, it is not provided here, but it is available from the publisher.

the method of processing, genetics, the diet of the animal or the fertilizer of the plant, the season of the year, methods of analysis, the difference in moisture content of the samples analyzed, the length and method of storage, and methods of cooking the food.

Although each nutrient is presented as a single number, each number is actually an average of a range of data. More detailed reports from the USDA, for example, indicate the number of samples and the standard deviation of the data. One can also find different reported values for foods as older data is replaced with newer data from more recent publications and newer analytical techniques. Therefore, nutrient data should be viewed and used only as a guide, a close approximation of nutrient content.

Dietary Fiber There can be many different reported values for dietary fiber in foods, because information is dependent on the type of analytical technique used. The data in this table are primarily from the USDA/ARS Human Nutrition Information Service in Hyattsville, Maryland; Composition of Foods by Southgate and Paul (England); and many journal articles.

Vitamin A Vitamin A is reported in retinol equivalents. The amount of this vitamin can vary by the season of the year and the maturity of the plant. Reported values in both dairy products and plants are higher in summer and early fall than in winter. The values reported here represent year-round averages. The organ meats of all animal products (liver especially) contain large amounts of vitamin A, which vary widely, depending on the background of the animal. The vitamin is also present in very small amounts in regular meat and is often reported as a trace.

Vitamin E Vitamin E values are newly added to this Composition of Foods Table, reflecting the importance of this vitamin in human health. Vitamin E is actually a combination of various forms of this nutrient, and the measure of alpha tocopherol equivalents (α-TE) summarizes the activity of the various types of tocopherols and tocotrienols into on measure.

Fats Total fats, as well as the breakdown of total fats to saturated, monounsaturated, and polyunsaturated fats, are listed in the table. The fatty acids seldom add up to the total. This is due to rounding, to other fatty acid components that are not included in these basic categories, *trans*-fatty acids and glycerol. Trans-fatty acids can comprise a large share of the total fat in margarine and shortening (hydrogenated oils) and in any foods that include them as ingredients.

Brand Name Foods from Manufacturers The information for brand name foods from manufacturers will change from time to time as recipes and formulations change to meet consumer preferences. In addition, the data provided is usually limited to those nutrients required to meet label requirements. Additional values for magnesium, phosphorus, zinc, thiamin, riboflavin, niacin, vitamin B6, folate, some of the fatty acids, and percent water are estimates calculated from known values for major ingredients.

Niacin Niacin values are for preformed niacin and do not include additional niacin that may form in the body from the conversion of tryptophan.

Using the Table The items in this table have been organized into several categories, which are listed at the head of each right-hand page. As the key shows, each group has been color-coded to make it easier to find individual items.

In an effort to conserve space, the following abbreviations have been used in the food descriptions and nutrient breakdowns:

- diam = diameter
- ea = each
- enr = enriched
- f/ = from
- g = grams
- liq = liquid
- pce = piece
- pkg = package
- w/ = with
- w/o = without
- t = trace
- 0 = zero (no nutrient value)
- — = information not available

Caffeine Sources Caffeine occurs in several plants, including the familiar coffee bean, the tea leaf, and the cocoa bean from which chocolate is made. Most human societies use caffeine regularly, most often in beverages, for its stimulant effect and flavor. Caffeine contents of beverages vary depending on the plants they are made from, the climates and soils where the plants are grown, the grind or cut size, the method and duration of brewing, and the amounts served. The accompanying table shows that in general, a cup of coffee contains the most caffeine; a cup of tea, less than half as much; and cocoa or chocolate, less still. As for cola beverages, they are made from kola nuts which contain caffeine, but most of their caffeine is added, using the purified compound obtained from decaffeinated coffee beans.

The FDA lists caffeine as a multipurpose GRAS substance that may be added to foods and beverages. Drug industries in developed countries use caffeine in many kinds of drugs: stimulants, pain relievers, cold remedies, diuretics, and weight-loss aids.

1. This food composition table has been prepared for West Publishing Company and is copyrighted by ESHA Research in Salem, Oregon—the developer and publisher of the Food Processor®, Genesis® R&D and the Computer Chef® nutrition software systems. The major sources for the data are from the USDA, supplemented by more than 1100 additional sources of information. Because the list of references is so extensive, it is not provided here, but is available from the publisher.

Caffeine Content of Beverages, Foods, and Over-the-Counter Drugs

Beverages and Foods	Average (mg)	Range(mg)
Coffee (5-oz cup)		
Brewed, drip method	130	110–150
Brewed, percolator	94	64–124
Instant	74	40–108
Decaffeinated, brewed or instant	3	1–5
Tea (5-oz cup)		
Brewed, major U.S. brand	40	20–90
Brewed, imported brands	60	25–110
Instant	30	25–50
Iced (12-oz can)	70	67–76
Soft drinks (12-oz can)		
Dr. Pepper		40
Colas and cherry cola		
Regular		30–46
Diet		2–58
Caffeine-free		0–trace
Jolt		72
Mountain Dew, Mello Yello		52
Fresca, Hires Root Beer, 7-Up, Sprite, Squirt, Sunkist Orange		0
Cocoa beverage (5-oz cup)	4	2–20
Chocolate milk beverage (8 oz)	5	2–7
Milk chocolate candy (1 oz)	6	1–15
Dark chocolate, semisweet (1 oz)	20	5–35
Baker's chocolate (1 oz)	26	26
Chocolate flavored syrup (1 oz)	4	4
Drugs[a]		
Cold remedies (standard dose)		
Dristan	0	
Coryban-D, Triaminicin	30	
Diuretics (standard dose)		
Aqua-ban, Permathene H_2Off	200	
Pre-Mens Forte	100	
Pain relievers (standard dose)		
Excedrin	130	
Midol, Anacin	65	
Aspirin, plain (any brand)	0	
Stimulants		
Caffedrin, NoDoz, Vivarin	200	
Weight-control aids (daily dose)		
Prolamine	280	
Dexatrim, Dietac	200	

Note: A pharmacologically active dose of caffeine is defined as 200 milligrams.

[a]Because products change, contact the manufacturer for an update on products you use regularly.

H

Table H-1
Food Composition

Computer Code Number	Food Description	Measure	Wt (g)	H_2O (%)	Ener (kcal)	Prot (g)	Carb (g)	Dietary Fiber (g)	Fat (g)	Fat Breakdown (g) Sat	Mono	Poly
	BEVERAGES											
	Alcoholic:											
	Beer:											
1	Regular (12 fl oz)	1½ c	356	92	146	1	13	3	0	0	0	0
2	Light (12 fl oz)	1½ c	354	95	99[1]	1	5	1	0	0	0	0
1506	Nonalcoholic (12 fl oz)	1 ea	360	98	32	1	5	0	0	0	0	0
	Gin, rum, vodka, whiskey:											
3	80 proof	1½ fl oz	42	67	97	0	0	0	0	0	0	0
4	86 proof	1½ fl oz	42	64	105	0	<1	0	0	0	0	0
5	90 proof	1½ fl oz	42	62	110	0	0	0	0	0	0	0
	Liqueur:											
1359	Coffee liqueur, 53 proof	1½ fl oz	52	31	175	<1	24	0	<1	.1	<.1	.1
1360	Coffee & cream liqueur, 34 proof	1½ fl oz	47	46	154	1	10	0	7	4.5	2.1	.3
1361	Crème de menthe, 72 proof	1½ fl oz	50	28	186	0	21	0	<1	<.1	<.1	.1
	Wine:											
6	Dessert (4 fl oz)	½ c	118	72	181[2]	<1	14	0	0	0	0	0
7	Red	3½ fl oz	103	88	74	<1	2	0	0	0	0	0
8	Rosé	3½ fl oz	103	89	73	<1	1	0	0	0	0	0
9	White medium	3½ fl oz	103	90	70	<1	1	0	0	0	0	0
1592	Nonalcoholic	1 c	232	98	14	1	3	0	0	0	0	0
1593	Nonalcoholic light	1 c	251	98	15	1	3	0	0	0	0	0
1409	Wine cooler, bottle (12 fl oz)	1½ c	340	90	169	<1	20	<1	<1	<.1	<.1	<.1
1595	Wine cooler, cup	1 c	227	90	113	<1	13	<1	<1	<.1	<.1	<.1
	Carbonated:[3]											
10	Club soda (12 fl oz)	1½ c	355	100	0	0	0	0	0	0	0	0
11	Cola beverage (12 fl oz)	1½ c	370	89	152	0	38	0	0	0	0	0
12	Diet cola w/aspartame (12 fl oz)	1½ c	355	100	4	<1	<1	0	0	0	0	0
13	Diet cola w/saccharin (12 fl oz)	1½ c	355	100	0	0	<1	0	0	0	0	0
14	Ginger ale (12 fl oz)	1½ c	366	91	124	0	32	0	0	0	0	0
15	Grape soda (12 fl oz)	1½ c	372	89	160	0	42	0	0	0	0	0
16	Lemon-lime (12 fl oz)	1½ c	368	90	147	0	38	0	0	0	0	0
17	Orange (12 fl oz)	1½ c	372	88	179	0	46	0	0	0	0	0
18	Pepper-type soda (12 fl oz)	1½ c	368	89	151	0	38	0	<1	.1	0	0
19	Root beer (12 fl oz)	1½ c	370	89	152	0	39	0	0	0	0	0
20	Coffee,[3] brewed	1 c	240	99	5[4]	<1	1	0	<1	t	0	t
21	Coffee,[3] prepared from instant	1 c	240	99	5[4]	<1	1	0	<1	t	0	0
	Fruit drinks, noncarbonated:[5]											
22	Fruit punch drink, canned	½ c	126	88	59	0	15	0	<1	0	0	0
1358	Gatorade	1 c	240	94	60	0	15	0	0	0	0	0
23	Grape drink, canned	½ c	125	87	63	<1	16	<1	0	0	0	0
1304	Kool-Aid, with sugar	1 c	240	90	89	0	23	0	<1	<.1	<.1	<.1
1356	Kool-Aid, with NutraSweet	1 c	240	95	43	0	11	0	0	0	0	0

(1) kCalories can vary from 78 to 131 for 12 fl. oz.

(2) Values are for sweet dessert wine. Dry dessert wines contain 149 kcal and 5 g of carbohydrate.

(3) Mineral content varies depending on water source.

(4) kCalorie values vary from 1 to 5 kcal per cup.

(5) Usually less than 10% fruit juice.

PAGE KEY: H–4 = BEV H–6 = DAIRY H–12 = EGGS H–14 = FAT/OIL H–18 = FRUIT H–26 = BAKERY H–36 = GRAIN H–44 = FISH H–48 = MEATS H–50 = POULTRY H–54 = SAUSAGE H–56 = MIXED/FAST H–64 = NUTS/SEEDS H–68 = SWEETS H–70 = VEG/LEG H–84 = MISC H–88 = SOUPS/SAUCES H–90 = FAST H–106 = FRZN ENTREE H–112 = BABY FOODS

Chol (mg)	Calc (mg)	Iron (mg)	Magn (mg)	Pota (mg)	Sodi (mg)	Zinc (mg)	VT-A (RE)	Thia (mg)	VT-E (α-TE)	Ribo (mg)	Niac (mg)	V-B6 (mg)	Fola (µg)	VT-C (mg)
0	18	.11	21	89	18	.07	0	.04	0	.11	1.60	.18	21	0
0	18	.14	18	64	11	.11	0	.04	0	.11	1.38	.11	15	0
0	25	.04	32	90	18	.04	0	.02	0	.09	1.63	.18	22	0
0	0	.02	0	1	<1	.02	0	<.01	0	0	0	0	0	0
0	0	.02	0	1	<1	.02	0	<.01	0	0	0	0	0	0
0	0	.02	0	1	<1	.02	0	<.01	0	0	0	0	0	0
0	1	.03	2	16	4	.02	0	<.01	0	.01	.07	0	0	0
7	8	.06	1	15	43	.08	20	0	.09	.03	.04	.01	0	0
0	0	.04	0	0	3	.02	0	0	0	0	<.01	0	0	0
0	9	.28	11	108	11	.08	0	.02	0	.02	.25	0	<1	0
0	8	.44	13	116	5	.09	0	.01	0	.03	.08	.03	2	0
0	8	.39	10	102	5	.06	0	0	0	.02	.07	.02	1	0
0	9	.33	10	83	5	.07	0	0	0	.01	.07	.01	<1	0
0	21	.93	23	204	16	.19	0	0	0	.02	.23	.05	2	0
0	23	1	25	221	18	.2	0	0	0	.03	.25	.05	3	0
0	19	.92	18	152	29	.2	<1	.02	.02	.02	.15	.04	4	6
0	13	.61	12	102	19	.13	<1	.01	.02	.02	.10	.03	3	4
0	18	.04	4	7	75	.36	0	0	0	0	0	0	0	0
0	11	.11	4	4	15	.04	0	0	0	0	0	0	0	0
0	14	.11	4	0	21[6]	.28	0	.02	0	.08	0	0	0	0
0	14	.14	4	7	57	.18	0	0	0	0	0	0	0	0
0	11	.66	4	4	26	.18	0	0	0	0	0	0	0	0
0	11	.3	4	4	56	.26	0	0	0	0	0	0	0	0
0	7	.26	4	4	40	.18	0	0	0	0	.06	0	0	0
0	19	.22	4	7	45	.37	0	0	0	0	0	0	0	0
0	11	.15	0	4	37	.15	0	0	0	0	0	0	0	0
0	19	.19	4	4	48	.26	0	0	0	0	0	0	0	0
0	5	.12	12	130	5	.05	0	0	0	0	.53	0	<1	0
0	7	.12	10	86	7	.07	0	0	0	<.01	.68	0	0	0
0	10	.26	3	32	28	.15	2	0	0	.03	.03	0	2	37
0	0	.12	2	26	96	.05	0	.01	0	0	0	0	0	0
0	4	.13	5	44	1	.04	0	.01	0	.01	.13	.03	1	20
0	38	.12	2	2	34	.07	0	0	0	<.01	<.01	0	<1	28
0	17	.65	5	50	50	.26	2	.02	0	.05	.05	0	5	77

[6]Value for product sweetened with aspartame only; sodium is 32 mg if a blend of aspartame and sodium saccharin is used.

(For purposes of calculations, use "0" for t, <1, <.1, <.01, etc.)

H

Table H–1
Food Composition

Computer Code Number	Food Description	Measure	Wt (g)	H_2O (%)	Ener (kcal)	Prot (g)	Carb (g)	Dietary Fiber (g)	Fat (g)	Fat Breakdown (g) Sat	Mono	Poly
	BEVERAGES—Cont.											
	Fruit drinks, noncarbonated—Cont.											
26	Lemonade, frozen concentrate (6-oz can)	¾ c	219	52	396	1	103	1	<1	.1	t	.1
27	Lemonade, from concentrate	1 c	248	89	99	<1	26	<1	<1	t	t	t
28	Limeade, frozen concentrate (6-oz can)	¾ c	218	50	408	<1	107	1	<1	t	t	.1
29	Limeade, from concentrate	1 c	247	89	101	0	27	<1	<1	0	0	t
24	Pineapple grapefruit, canned	1 c	250	88	118	<1	29	<1	<1	t	t	.1
25	Pineapple orange, canned	1 c	250	87	125	3	30	<1	0	0	0	0
	Fruit and vegetable juices: see Fruit and Vegetable sections											
	Slim Fast:[1]											
1612	Chocolate malt with nonfat milk	1 c	273	82	190	14	32	2	1	.3	.1	<.1
1613	Strawberry with nonfat milk	1 c	273	82	190	14	32	2	1	.3	.1	<.1
1611	Vanilla with nonfat milk	1 c	273	82	190	14	32	2	1	.3	.1	<.1
	Ultra Slim Fast:[1]											
1616	Chocolate with nonfat milk	1 c	278	81	200	14	36	5	1	.3	.1	<.1
1614	French vanilla with nonfat milk	1 c	278	81	190	14	36	4	1	.3	.1	<.1
1615	Strawberry Supreme with nonfat milk	1 c	278	81	190	14	36	4	1	.3	.1	t
1357	Water, bottled: Perrier (6½ fl oz)	1 ea	192	100	0	0	0	0	0	0	0	0
1594	Water, bottled: Tonic water	1½ c	366	91	124	0	32	0	0	0	0	0
	Tea:[2]											
30	Brewed, regular	1 c	240	100	2	0	1	0	<1	t	0	t
1662	Brewed, herbal	¾ c	178	100	2	0	<1	0	<1	<.1	<.1	<.1
32	From instant, sweetened	1 c	262	91	89	<1	22	0	<1	t	0	t
31	From instant, unsweetened	1 c	237	100	2	<1	<1	0	0	0	0	0
	DAIRY											
	Butter: see Fats and Oils, #158,159,160											
	Cheese, natural:											
33	Blue	1 oz	28	42	100	6	1	0	8	5.3	2.2	.2
34	Brick	1 oz	28	41	105	7	1	0	8	5.3	2.4	.2
35	Brie	1 oz	28	48	95	6	<1	0	8	4.9	2.3	.2
36	Camembert	1 oz	28	52	85	6	<1	0	7	4.3	2	.2
37	Cheddar:	1 oz	28	37	114	7	<1	0	9	6	2.7	.3
38	1" cube	1 ea	17	37	69	4	<1	0	6	3.6	1.6	.2
39	Shredded	1 c	113	37	455	28	1	0	37	24	10.6	1.1
1406	Low fat, low sodium	1 oz	28	65	49	7	1	0	2	1.3	0.6	.1
	Cottage:											
984	Low sodium, low fat	1 c	225	84	162	28	6	0	2	1.4	.6	.1
40	Creamed, large curd	1 c	225	79	232	28	6	0	10	6.4	2.9	.3
41	Creamed, small curd	1 c	210	79	216	26	6	0	9	6	2.7	.3
42	With fruit	1 c	226	72	280	22	30	0	8	4.9	2.2	.2
43	Low fat 2%	1 c	226	79	203	31	8	0	4	2.8	1.2	.1
44	Low fat 1%	1 c	226	82	164	28	6	0	2	1.5	.7	.1
46	Cream	1 oz	28	54	99	2	1	0	10	6.2	2.8	.4
983	Cream, low fat	1 oz	28	64	65	3	2	0	5	3.1	1.6	.2
47	Edam	1 oz	28	42	101	7	<1	0	8	5	2.3	.2
48	Feta	1 oz	28	55	75	4	1	0	6	4.2	1.3	.2

(1)See Chapter 9 for healthy weight loss strategies. The formulas for these products change periodically; these data reflect nutrient values as of our publication date.

(2)Mineral content varies depending on water source.

(Computer code number is for West Diet Analysis program)

PAGE KEY: H–4 = BEV H–6 = DAIRY H–12 = EGGS H–14 = FAT/OIL H–18 = FRUIT H–26 = BAKERY H–36 = GRAIN H–44 = FISH H–48 = MEATS H–50 = POULTRY H–54 = SAUSAGE H–56 = MIXED/FAST H–64 = NUTS/SEEDS H–68 = SWEETS H–70 = VEG/LEG H–84 = MISC H–88 = SOUPS/SAUCES H–90 = FAST H–106 = FRZN ENTREE H–112 = BABY FOODS

Chol (mg)	Calc (mg)	Iron (mg)	Magn (mg)	Pota (mg)	Sodi (mg)	Zinc (mg)	VT-A (RE)	Thia (mg)	VT-E (α-TE)	Ribo (mg)	Niac (mg)	V-B6 (mg)	Fola (µg)	VT-C (mg)
0	15	1.58	11	146	9	.18	22	.06	0	.21	.16	.05	22	39[3]
0	7	.4	5	37	7	.1	5	.01	0	.05	.04	.01	5	10[3]
0	11	.22	9	128	0	.09	0	.02	0	.02	.22	0	9	26
0	7	.07	2	32	5	.05	0	0	0	0	.05	0	2	7
0	18	.78	15	152	35	.15	9	.08	0	.04	.67	.1	26	115
0	13	.68	15	115	7	.15	13	.08	0	.05	.52	.12	27	56
4	450	6.3	140	690	230	5.25	350	.53	5	.59	7	.7	120	21
4	450	6.3	140	720	220	5.25	350	.53	5	.59	7	.7	120	21
4	450	6.31	140	721	220	5.24	350	.53	5	.59	7	.7	120	21
<1	450	6.3	140	800	230	5.25	350	.53	10	.59	7	.7	120	21
<1	450	6.3	140	730	250	5.25	350	.53	10	.59	7	.7	120	21
<1	450	6.3	140	710	250	5.25	350	.52	10	.59	7	.7	120	21
0	27	0	0	0	2	0	0	0	0	0	0	0	0	0
0	4	.04	0	0	15	.37	0	0	0	0	0	0	0	0
0	0	.05	7	89	7	.05	0	0	0	.03	0	0	12	0
0	4	.14	2	16	2	.07	0	.02	0	.01	0	0	1	0
0	5	.05	5	50	8	.08	0	0	0	.05	.09	.01	10	0
0	5	.05	5	47	7	.07	0	0	0	<.01	.09	0	1	0
21	150	.09	6	73	395	.75	65	.01	.18	.11	.29	.05	10	0
27	191	.12	7	39	159	.74	86	0	.14	.1	.03	.02	6	0
28	52	.14	6	43	178	.67	52	.02	.18	.15	.11	.07	18	0
20	110	.09	6	53	239	.67	71	.01	.18	.14	.18	.06	18	0
30	204	.19	8	28	176	.88	86	.01	.1	.11	.02	.02	5	0
18	123	.12	5	17	106	.53	51	0	.06	.06	.01	.01	3	0
119	815	.77	31	111	702	3.51	342	.03	.41	.43	.09	.08	21	0
6	197	.2	8	32	6	.87	17	.01	.05	.01	.03	.02	5	0
9	137	.32	11	194	29	.86	25	.05	.25	.36	.3	.16	27	0
33	135	.32	12	190	911	.83	108	.05	.28	.37	.28	.15	27	0
31	126	.29	11	177	851	.78	101	.04	.26	.34	.26	.14	26	0
25	108	.25	9	151	915	.65	81	.04	.21	.29	.23	.12	22	0
19	155	.36	14	217	918	.95	45	.05	.13	.42	.33	.17	30	0
10	138	.32	12	193	918	.86	25	.05	.25	.37	.29	.15	28	0
31	23	.34	2	34	84	.15	124	0	.26	.06	.03	.01	4	0
16	32	.47	2	47	83	.22	62	.01	.13	.08	.04	.02	5	0
25	207	.12	8	53	274	1.07	72	.01	.21	.11	.02	.02	5	0
25	140	.18	5	18	316	.82	36	.04	.01	.24	.28	.12	9	0

(3)Vitamin C can range from 5 to 72 mg in a small can of frozen concentrate, and from 1 to 18 mg in 1 c of prepared lemonade.

(For purposes of calculations, use "0" for t, <1, <.1, <.01, etc.)

H

Table H-1
Food Composition

Computer Code Number	Food Description	Measure	Wt (g)	H_2O (%)	Ener (kcal)	Prot (g)	Carb (g)	Dietary Fiber (g)	Fat (g)	Fat Breakdown (g) Sat	Mono	Poly
	DAIRY—Cont.											
	Cheese—Cont.											
49	Gouda	1 oz	28	42	101	7	1	0	8	5	2.2	.2
50	Gruyère	1 oz	28	33	117	8	<1	0	9	5.4	2.8	.5
51	Gorgonzola	1 oz	28	39	111	7	0	0	9	5.5	2.4	.5
52	Liederkranz	1 oz	28	53	87	5	<1	0	8	5.3	2.2	.2
1676	Limburger	1 oz	28	48	92	6	<1	0	8	4.7	2.4	.1
53	Monterey Jack	1 oz	28	41	106	7	<1	0	9	5.4	2.5	.3
54	Mozzarella, whole milk	1 oz	28	54	80	6	1	0	6	3.7	1.9	.2
55	Mozzarella, part-skim milk, low moisture	1 oz	28	49	79	8	1	0	5	3.1	1.4	.1
56	Muenster	1 oz	28	42	104	7	<1	0	9	5.4	2.5	.2
1399	Nonfat (Kraft Singles)	1 oz	28	61	44	6	4	0	0	0	0	0
	Parmesan, grated:											
57	Cup, not pressed down	1 c	100	18	456	42	4	0	30	20	8.7	.7
58	Tablespoon	1 tbs	5	18	23	2	<1	0	2	1	.4	t
59	Ounce	1 oz	28	18	128	12	1	0	8	5.5	2.4	.2
60	Provolone	1 oz	28	41	100	7	1	0	8	4.9	2.1	.2
61	Ricotta, whole milk	1 c	246	72	428	28	7	0	32	20.4	8.9	1
62	Ricotta, part-skim milk	1 c	246	74	339	28	13	0	19	12.1	5.7	.6
63	Romano	1 oz	28	31	109	9	1	0	8	4.8	2.2	.2
64	Swiss	1 oz	28	37	107	8	1	0	8	5	2.1	.3
976	Swiss, low fat	1 oz	28	60	50	8	1	0	1	.9	.4	<.1
	Pasteurized processed cheese products:											
65	American	1 oz	28	39	106	6	<1	0	9	5.6	2.5	.3
66	Swiss	1 oz	28	42	94	7	1	0	7	4.6	2	.2
67	American cheese food, jar	1 oz	28	43	93	6	2	0	7	4.4	2	.2
68	American cheese spread	1 oz	28	48	82	5	2	0	6	3.8	1.8	.2
982	Velveeta cheese spread, low fat, low sodium	1 oz	28	63	51	7	1	0	2	1.3	0.6	0.1
69	Cream, sweet:	1 c	242	81	315	7	10	0	28	17.3	8	1
	Half & half (cream & milk):											
70	Tablespoon	1 tbs	15	81	19	<1	1	0	2	1.1	.5	.1
71	Light, coffee or table:	1 c	240	74	468	6	9	0	46	28.8	13.4	1.7
72	Tablespoon	1 tbs	15	74	29	<1	1	0	3	1.8	.8	.1
73	Light whipping cream, liquid:[1]	1 c	239	64	698	5	7	0	74	46.1	21.7	2.1
74	Tablespoon	1 tbs	15	64	44	<1	<1	0	5	2.9	1.4	.1
75	Heavy whipping cream, liquid:[1]	1 c	238	58	821	5	7	0	88	54.7	25.5	3.3
76	Tablespoon	1 tbs	15	58	52	<1	<1	0	6	3.4	1.6	.2
77	Whipped cream, pressurized:	1 c	60	61	154	2	8	0	13	8.3	3.8	.5
78	Tablespoon	1 tbs	4	61	10	<1	<1	0	1	.6	.3	t
79	Cream, sour, cultured:	1 c	230	71	492	7	10	0	48	29.9	13.9	1.8
80	Tablespoon	1 tbs	14	71	30	<1	1	0	3	1.8	.8	.1
	Cream products—imitation and part dairy:											
81	Coffee whitener, frozen or liquid	1 tbs	15	77	20	<1	2	0	2	1.4	t	0
82	Coffee whitener, powdered	1 tsp	2	2	11	<1	1	0	1	.6	t	t
83	Dessert topping, frozen, nondairy:	1 c	75	50	239	1	17	0	19	16.4	1.2	.4
84	Tablespoon	1 tbs	5	50	16	<1	1	0	1	1.1	.1	t
85	Dessert topping, mix with whole milk:	1 c	80	67	151	3	13	0	10	8.6	.7	.2
86	Tablespoon	1 tbs	5	67	9	<1	1	0	1	.5	t	t

[1]For whipped cream, (non-pressurized), double the liquid cream volume of codes 73, 74 or 75, 76. One tablespoon liquid cream becomes 2 tablespoons when "whipped."

(Computer code number is for West Diet Analysis program)

PAGE KEY: H–4 = BEV H–6 = DAIRY H–12 = EGGS H–14 = FAT/OIL H–18 = FRUIT H–26 = BAKERY H–36 = GRAIN H–44 = FISH H–48 = MEATS H–50 = POULTRY H–54 = SAUSAGE H–56 = MIXED/FAST H–64 = NUTS/SEEDS H–68 = SWEETS H–70 = VEG/LEG H–84 = MISC H–88 = SOUPS/SAUCES H–90 = FAST H–106 = FRZN ENTREE H–112 = BABY FOODS

Chol (mg)	Calc (mg)	Iron (mg)	Magn (mg)	Pota (mg)	Sodi (mg)	Zinc (mg)	VT-A (RE)	Thia (mg)	VT-E (α-TE)	Ribo (mg)	Niac (mg)	V-B6 (mg)	Fola (μg)	VT-C (mg)
32	198	.07	8	34	232	1.11	49	.01	.1	.09	.02	.02	6	0
31	286	.05	10	23	95	1.11	85	.02	.1	.08	.03	.02	3	0
25	149	.12	8	26	512	.57	103	.01	.22	.09	.2	.04	9	0
21	110	.12	7	68	389	.7	91	.01	.21	.18	.1	.04	34	0
25	140	.04	6	36	224	.6	89	.02	.18	.14	.04	.02	16	0
25	211	.2	8	23	152	.85	72	0	.1	.11	.03	.02	5	0
22	146	.05	5	19	105	.63	68	0	.1	.07	.02	.02	2	0
15	207	.07	7	27	149	.89	54	.01	.13	.1	.03	.02	3	0
27	203	.12	8	38	178	.8	90	0	.13	.09	.03	.02	3	0
4	221	0	–	81	427	–	126	–	0	.10	–	–	–	0
79	1375	.95	51	107	1861	3.19	173	.04	.8	.39	.31	.1	8	0
4	69	.05	3	5	93	.16	9	0	.04	.02	.02	.01	<1	0
22	385	.27	14	30	521	.9	48	.01	.22	.11	.09	.03	2	0
20	215	.15	8	39	249	.92	75	.01	.1	.09	.04	.02	3	0
124	509	.93	28	258	206	2.85	330	.03	.86	.48	.26	.11	30	0
76	669	1.08	36	308	308	3.3	278	.05	.53	.45	.19	.05	32	0
30	302	.22	12	25	341	.73	40	.01	.2	.1	.02	.02	2	0
26	273	.05	10	31	74	1.1	72	.01	.14	.1	.03	.02	2	0
10	269	.05	10	31	73	1.11	18	.01	.05	.1	.03	.02	2	0
27	175	.11	6	46	406	.85	82	.01	.13	.1	.02	.02	2	0
24	219	.17	8	61	389	1.03	65	0	.19	.08	.01	.01	2	0
18	163	.24	9	79	338	.85	62	.01	.2	.13	.04	.04	2	0
16	159	.09	8	69	380	.73	54	.01	.2	.12	.04	.03	2	0
10	191	.12	7	50	2	.93	18	.01	.14	.11	.02	.02	3	0
89	254	.17	25	315	98	1.23	259	.08	.27	.36	.19	.09	6	2
6	16	.01	2	19	6	.08	16	.01	.02	.02	.01	.01	<1	<1
158	231	.1	21	293	95	.65	437	.08	.36	.35	.14	.08	6	2
10	14	.01	1	18	6	.04	27	.01	.02	.02	.01	0	<1	<1
265	166	.07	17	231	82	.6	705	.06	1.43	.3	.1	.07	9	1
17	10	0	1	15	5	.04	44	.01	.09	.02	.01	0	1	<1
326	154	.07	17	179	89	.55	1001	.05	1.5	.26	.09	.06	9	1
21	10	0	1	11	6	.03	63	0	.1	.02	.01	0	1	<1
46	61	.03	6	88	78	.22	124	.02	.36	.04	.04	.02	2	0
3	4	0	<1	6	5	.01	8	0	.02	0	0	0	<1	0
102	267	.14	26	331	123	.62	449	.08	1.3	.34	.15	.04	25	2
6	16	.01	2	20	7	.04	27	0	.45	.02	.01	0	2	<1
0	1	<.01	<1	29	12	0	1	0	.24	0	0	0	0	0
0	<1	.02	<1	16	4	.01	<1	0	.01	0	0	0	0	0
0	5	.09	1	14	19	.02	64[2]	0	.14	0	0	0	0	0
0	<1	.01	<1	1	1	0	4[2]	0	.01	0	0	0	0	0
8	72	.03	8	120	53	.22	39[2]	.02	.11	.09	.05	.02	3	1
<1	5	0	<1	8	3	.01	2[2]	0	.01	.01	0	0	<1	<1

(2) Vitamin A value is from beta-carotene used for coloring.

(For purposes of calculations, use "0" for t, <1, <.1, <.01, etc.)

H

Table H–1
Food Composition

Computer Code Number	Food Description	Measure	Wt (g)	H_2O (%)	Ener (kcal)	Prot (g)	Carb (g)	Dietary Fiber (g)	Fat (g)	Fat Breakdown (g) Sat	Mono	Poly
DAIRY—Cont.												
88	Dessert topping, pressurized:	1 c	70	60	185	1	11	0	16	13.3	1.3	.2
87	Tablespoon	1 tbs	4	60	11	<1	1	0	1	.8	.1	t
91	Sour cream, imitation:	1 c	230	71	478	6	15	0	45	40.9	1.3	.1
92	Tablespoon	1 tbs	14	71	29	<1	1	0	3	2.5	.1	t
89	Sour dressing, part dairy:	1 c	235	75	418	8	11	0	39	31.3	4.6	1.1
90	Tablespoon	1 tbs	15	75	27	<1	1	0	2	2	.3	.1
	Milk, fluid:											
93	Whole milk	1 c	244	88	150	8	11	0	8	5.1	2.7	.3
94	2% low-fat milk	1 c	244	89	121	8	12	0	5	2.9	1.4	.2
95	2% milk solids added[1]	1 c	245	89	125	9	12	0	5	2.9	1.4	.2
96	1% low-fat milk	1 c	244	90	102	8	12	–	3	1.6	.8	.1
97	1% milk solids added[1]	1 c	245	90	104	9	12	0	2	1.5	.7	.1
98	Nonfat milk, vitamin A added	1 c	245	91	86	8	12	0	<1	.3	.12	t
99	Nonfat milk solids added[1]	1 c	245	90	90	9	12	0	1	.4	.2	t
100	Buttermilk, nonfat	1 c	245	90	99	8	12	0	2	1.3	.6	.1
	Milk, canned:											
101	Sweetened condensed	1 c	306	27	982	24	166	0	27	16.8	7.4	1
103	Evaporated, nonfat	1 c	255	79	199	19	29	0	1	.3	.2	t
	Milk, dried:											
104	Buttermilk, sweet	1 c	120	3	464	41	59	0	7	4.3	2	.3
105	Instant, nonfat, envelope[2]	1 ea	91	4	325	32	47	0	1	.4	.2	t
106	Instant nonfat, cup	1 c	68	4	243	24	35	0	<1	.3	.1	t
107	Goat milk	1 c	244	87	167	9	11	0	10	6.5	2.7	.4
108	Kefir, 2% milkfat[3]	1 c	233	82	122	9	9	0	5	2.9	1.2	.1
	Milk beverages and powdered mixes:											
	Chocolate:											
109	Whole	1 c	250	82	208	8	26	2	8	5.3	2.5	.3
110	2% fat	1 c	250	83	178	8	26	1	5	3.1	1.5	.2
111	1% fat	1 c	250	85	157	9	26	3	3	1.5	.8	.1
	Chocolate-flavored beverages:											
112	Powder containing nonfat dry milk:	1 oz	28	2	102	3	22	<1	1	.7	.4	t
113	Prepared with water	¾ c	206	86	100	4	23	<1	1	.7	.4	t
114	Powder without nonfat dry milk:	¾ oz	22	1	76	1	20	1	1	.4	.2	t
115	Prepared with whole milk	1 c	266	81	226	9	31	1	9	5.5	2.6	.3
116	Eggnog, commercial	1 c	254	74	343	10	34	0	19	11.3	5.7	.9
974	2% low-fat eggnog	1 c	254	85	189	12	17	0	8	3.8	2.7	.7
1027	Instant Breakfast, envelope, powder only:	1 ea	37	7	131	7	24	<1	1	.3	.1	<.1
1028	Prepared with whole milk	1 c	281	77	280	15	36	<1	9	5.4	2.5	.3
1029	Prepared with 2% milk	1 c	281	78	252	15	36	<1	5	3.3	1.5	.2
1283	Prepared with 1% milk	1 c	281	80	215	16	36	<1	1	.7	.3	<.1
1284	Prepared with nonfat milk	1 c	281	80	215	16	36	<1	1	.7	.3	<.1
117	Malted milk, chocolate, powder:	¾ oz	21	1	79	1	18	<1	1	.5	.2	.1
118	Prepared with whole milk	1 c	265	81	228	9	30	<1	9	5.5	2.6	.4
1661	Ovaltine with whole milk	1 c	265	81	225	9	29	<1	9	5.5	2.6	.4
119	Malted mix powder, natural	¾ oz	21	2	87	2	16	<1	2	.9	.4	.3
121	Milk shakes, chocolate (10 fl oz)	1¼ c	283	72	359	10	58	2	10	6.5	3.1	.4

(1)Milk solids added, label claims less than 10 g protein per cup.

(2)Yields 1 qt fluid milk when reconstituted according to package directions.

(3)Most values provided by product labeling.

(Computer code number is for West Diet Analysis program)

Chol (mg)	Calc (mg)	Iron (mg)	Magn (mg)	Pota (mg)	Sodi (mg)	Zinc (mg)	VT-A (RE)	Thia (mg)	VT-E (α-TE)	Ribo (mg)	Niac (mg)	V-B6 (mg)	Fola (μg)	VT-C (mg)
0	4	.01	1	13	43	.01	33[4]	.0	.12	0	0	0	0	0
0	<1	0	<1	1	2	0	2[4]	0	.01	0	0	0	0	0
0	6	.9	15	370	235	2.71	0	0	.34	0	0	0	0	0
0	<1	.05	1	23	14	.16	0	0	.02	0	0	0	0	0
13	266	.07	23	381	113	.87	5[4]	.09	.29	.38	.17	.04	28	2
1	17	0	1	24	7	.06	<1[4]	.01	.02	.02	.01	0	2	<1
33	290	.12	33	371	120	.93	76	.09	.24	.39	.2	.1	12	2
18	298	.12	33	376	122	.95	139	.09	.17	.4	.21	.1	12	2
18	311	.12	35	397	128	.98	140	.1	.17	.42	.22	.11	13	2
10	300	.12	34	381	123	.95	144	.09	.1	.41	.21	.1	12	2
10	314	.12	35	397	128	.98	145	.1	.1	.42	.22	.11	13	2
4	301	.1	28	407	126	.98	149	.09	.1	.34	.22	.1	13	2
5	316	.12	35	419	130	1	149	.1	.1	.43	.22	.11	13	2
9	284	.12	27	370	257	1.03	20	.08	.15	.38	.14	.08	12	2
104	869	.58	79	1135	389	2.88	248	.27	.65	1.27	.64	.16	34	8
9	740	.74	69	847	293	2.29	298	.11	.01	.79	.44	.14	22	3
83	1421	.36	132	1910	620	4.82	65	.47	.48	1.9	1.05	.41	57	7
17	1119	.28	106	1551	500	4.01	646[5]	.38	.02	1.58	.81	.31	45	5
12	836	.21	80	1159	373	3	483[5]	.28	.01	1.18	.61	.23	34	4
28	327	.12	34	498	122	.73	137	.12	.22	.34	.68	.11	1	3
10	350	.5	28	205	50	.9	155	.45	.12	.44	.3	.09	23	<1
30	280	.6	33	418	149	1.03	73	.09	.23	.41	.31	.1	12	2
17	285	.6	33	423	151	1.03	143	.09	.13	.41	.32	.1	12	2
7	288	.6	33	425	152	1.03	148	.09	.07	.42	.32	.1	12	2
1	93	.34	24	202	143	.41	1	.03	.04	.16	.17	.03	0	1
1	89	.28	23	223	139	1.25	1	.03	.08	.17	.18	.04	3	1
0	8	.68	21	128	45	.33	<1	.01	.09	.03	.11	<.01	1	<1
32	301	.8	53	497	165	1.28	77	.1	.22	.43	.32	.1	12	2
149	330	.51	47	419	138	1.17	203	.09	.58	.48	.27	.13	2	4
194	270	.71	32	367	155	1.26	197	.11	1.01	.55	.21	.15	30	2
4	106	4.74	84	350	143	3.16	554	.31	5.31	.07	5.27	.42	106	28
38	396	4.86	117	719	262	4.09	630	.41	5.51	.47	5.46	.52	118	31
23	401	4.86	118	726	264	4.12	693	.41	5.41	.48	5.46	.53	118	31
9	406	4.82	112	752	267	4.13	701	.4	5.28	.42	5.45	.52	118	31
9	406	4.82	112	752	267	4.13	701	.4	5.28	.42	5.47	.52	118	31
1	13	.48	15	129	53	.17	4	.04	.08	.04	.42	.03	4	<1
34	305	.61	48	498	172	1.09	80	.13	.27	.44	.62	.13	16	3
34	385	4	53	620	244	1.17	901	.74	.32	1.26	10.9	1.02	32	34
4	63	.15	20	159	104	.21	18	.11	.08	.19	1.1	.09	10	1
37	320	.88	48	566	275	1.16	65	.16	.19	.69	.46	.14	10	1

(4)Vitamin A value is from beta-carotene used for coloring.

(5)With added vitamin A.

Table H–1
Food Composition

Computer Code Number	Food Description	Measure	Wt (g)	H_2O (%)	Ener (kcal)	Prot (g)	Carb (g)	Dietary Fiber (g)	Fat (g)	Fat Breakdown (g) Sat	Mono	Poly
	DAIRY—Cont.											
122	Milk shakes, vanilla (10 fl oz)	1¼ c	283	75	314	10	51	1	8	5.3	2.4	.3
	Milk desserts:											
134	Custard, baked	1 c	265	79	278	14	28	0	12	6.2	4	1
1548	Low-fat frozen dessert bars	1 ea	81	72	89	2	18	0	1	.2	.1	.4
	Ice cream, vanilla (about 10% fat):											
123	Hardened: ½ gallon	1 ea	1064	61	2138	37	251	0	117	72.4	33.8	4.4
124	Cup	1 c	133	61	267	5	31	0	15	9	4.2	.6
125	Fluid ounces	3 oz	50	61	100	2	12	0	6	3.4	1.6	.2
126	Soft serve	1 c	173	60	372	7	38	0	22	12.9	6	.8
	Ice cream, rich vanilla (16% fat):											
127	Hardened: ½ gallon	1 ea	1188	60	2554	49	264	0	154	88.9	41.5	5.5
128	Cup	1 c	148	57	357	5	33	0	24	14.8	6.9	.9
1724	Ben & Jerry's	½ c	106	64	226	4	21	0	17	10	–	–
	Ice milk, vanilla (about 4% fat):											
129	Hardened: ½ gallon	1 ea	1048	68	1456	40	238	0	45	27.7	12.9	1.7
130	Cup	1 c	131	68	182	5	30	0	6	3.5	1.6	.2
131	Soft serve (about 3% fat)	1 c	175	70	221	9	38	0	5	2.8	1.3	.2
	Pudding, canned (5-oz can = .55 cup):											
135	Chocolate	1 ea	142	69	189	4	32	1	6	1	2.4	2
136	Tapioca	1 ea	142	74	169	3	27	<1	5	.9	2.2	1.9
137	Vanilla	1 ea	142	71	185	3	31	<1	5	.8	2.2	1.9
	Puddings, dry mix with whole milk:											
138	Chocolate, instant	1 c	260	75	289	8	49	3	8	4.8	2.4	.5
139	Chocolate, regular, cooked	½ c	130	74	144	4	23	1	4	2.7	1.3	.2
140	Rice, cooked	½ c	132	72	161	4	28	<1	4	2.3	1.1	.2
141	Tapioca, cooked	½ c	130	74	148	4	25	0	4	2.3	1.1	.1
142	Vanilla, instant	½ c	130	74	148	4	26	0	4	2.3	1.1	.2
143	Vanilla, regular, cooked	½ c	130	75	144	4	24	0	4	2.4	1.1	.2
132	Sherbet (2% fat): ½ gallon	1 ea	1542	66	2127	17	469	8	31	17.9	8.3	1.2
133	Cup	1 c	193	66	266	2	59	1	4	2.2	1	.2
144	Soy milk	1 c	240	93	79	7	4	3	5	.7	1	3.6
2301	Soy milk, fortified, fat free[2]	1 c	240	88	110	6	22	1	0	0	0	0
1584	Yogurt, frozen, low-fat	½ c	87	65	138	3	21	0	5	3	1.4	.2
1512	Scoop	1 ea	79	74	78	4	16	0	<1	.1	<.1	0
	Yogurt, low-fat:											
1172	Fruit added with low-calorie sweetener	1 c	241	86	122	12	19	1	<1	.2	.1	<.1
145	Fruit added[1]	1 c	227	75	232	10	43	<1	2	1.6	.7	.1
146	Plain	1 c	227	85	144	12	16	0	4	2.3	1	.1
147	Vanilla or coffee flavor	1 c	227	79	194	12	31	0	3	1.8	.8	.1
148	Yogurt, made with nonfat milk	1 c	227	85	127	14	17	0	<1	.3	.1	t
149	Yogurt, made with whole milk	1 c	227	88	139	9	11	0	7	4.8	2	.2
	EGGS											
	Raw, large:											
150	Whole, without shell	1 ea	50	75	74	6	1	0	5	1.5	1.9	.7
151	White	1 ea	33	88	17	3	<1	0	0	0	0	0
152	Yolk	1 ea	17	49	61	3	<1	0	5	1.6	1.9	.7

(1)Carbohydrate and kcalories vary widely—consult label if more precise values are needed.

(2)Nutrients will vary according to manufacturer—consult label.

PAGE KEY: H–4 = BEV H–6 = DAIRY H–12 = EGGS H–14 = FAT/OIL H–18 = FRUIT H–26 = BAKERY H–36 = GRAIN H–44 = FISH H–48 = MEATS H–50 = POULTRY H–54 = SAUSAGE H–56 = MIXED/FAST H–64 = NUTS/SEEDS H–68 = SWEETS H–70 = VEG/LEG H–84 = MISC H–88 = SOUPS/SAUCES H–90 = FAST H–106 = FRZN ENTREE H–112 = BABY FOODS

Chol (mg)	Calc (mg)	Iron (mg)	Magn (mg)	Pota (mg)	Sodi (mg)	Zinc (mg)	VT-A (RE)	Thia (mg)	VT-E (α-TE)	Ribo (mg)	Niac (mg)	V-B6 (mg)	Fola (μg)	VT-C (mg)
31	345	.25	34	492	232	1.02	91	.13	.17	.52	.52	.15	9	2
231	297	.79	37	405	204	1.4	159	.09	.64	.6	.22	.13	27	1
1	82	.07	10	111	47	.26	38	.03	.07	.11	.06	.03	3	1
468	1362	.96	149	2117	851	7.34	1245	.44	0	2.55	1.23	.51	53	6
59	170	.12	19	265	106	.92	156	.05	0	.32	.15	.06	7	1
22	64	.04	7	100	40	.34	59	.02	0	.12	.06	.02	3	<1
157	227	.36	21	306	106	.9	266	.08	.64	.31	.16	.08	16	1
1081	1556	2.49	143	2102	725	6.18	1829	.58	4.4	2.16	1.13	.57	107	10
90	173	.07	16	235	83	.59	272	.06	0	.24	.12	.06	7	1
93	147	.36	–	–	54	–	225	–	0	–	–	–	–	0
147	1457	1.05	157	2211	891	4.61	493	.61	0	2.78	.94	.68	63	8
18	182	.13	20	276	111	.58	62	.08	0	.35	.12	.08	8	1
21	275	.1	25	387	123	.93	51	.09	0	.35	.21	.08	11	2
4	128	.72	30	256	183	.6	16	.04	.18	.22	.49	.04	4	3
1	119	.33	11	148	168	.38	0	.03	.13	.14	.44	.14	6	1
10	125	.18	11	160	192	.35	9	.03	.18	.2	.36	.02	0	0
29	265	.75	47	432	738	1.09	55	.09	.16	.37	.25	.1	10	2
16	144	.47	20	212	134	.58	34	.04	.08	.23	.13	.05	5	1
15	136	.5	17	165	140	.6	26	.1	.07	.18	.6	.04	5	1
16	135	.08	16	172	157	.44	35	.04	.1	.18	.09	.05	5	1
14	131	.09	16	166	372	.43	33	.04	.08	.18	.1	.05	5	1
16	139	.06	17	177	208	.45	35	.04	.08	.18	.1	.04	5	1
77	833	2.16	123	1480	709	7.4	216	.39	.88	1.05	1.48	.52	62	66
10	104	.27	15	185	89	.93	27	.05	.11	.13	.18	.07	8	8
0	10	1.39	46	338	29	.55	7	.39	.02	.17	.35	.1	4	0
0	400	1.44	46	20	60	.5	0	.075	.02	.102	3	.1	4	0
2	124	.26	12	184	76	.36	50	.03	.04	.19	.25	.07	5	1
1	137	.07	13	175	53	.67	1	.03	<.01	.16	.09	.04	8	1
3	370	.61	41	550	140	1.83	6	.1	.17	.45	.5	.11	32	26
10	345	.16	33	443	133	1.68	25	.08	.07	.4	.22	.09	21	2
14	415	.18	40	531	159	2.02	36	.1	.1	.49	.26	.11	25	2
11	388	.16	37	497	149	1.88	30	.09	.08	.46	.24	.1	24	2
4	452	.2	43	579	174	2.2	5	.11	.01	.53	.28	.12	28	2
29	275	.11	26	352	105	1.34	68	.07	.2	.32	.17	.07	17	1
213	25	.72	5	61	63	.55	96	.03	.53	.25	.04	.07	24	0
0	2	.01	4	47	54	0	0	<.01	0	.15	.03	0	1	0
218	23	.6	2	16	7	.52	99	.03	.54	.11	<.1	.06	25	0

(For purposes of calculations, use "0" for t, <1, <.1, <.01, etc.)

Table H-1
Food Composition

Computer Code Number	Food Description	Measure	Wt (g)	H_2O (%)	Ener (kcal)	Prot (g)	Carb (g)	Dietary Fiber (g)	Fat (g)	Fat Breakdown (g) Sat	Mono	Poly
	EGGS—Cont.											
	Cooked:											
153	Fried in margarine	1 ea	46	69	92	6	1	0	7	1.9	2.8	1.3
154	Hard-cooked, shell removed	1 ea	50	75	78	6	1	0	5	1.6	2	.7
155	Hard-cooked, chopped	1 c	136	75	211	17	2	0	14	4.5	5.6	1.9
156	Poached, no added salt	1 ea	50	75	75	6	1	0	5	1.6	1.9	.7
157	Scrambled with milk & margarine	1 ea	61	73	101	7	1	0	7	2.2	2.9	1.3
1681	Egg substitute, liquid	½ c	126	83	106	17	1	0	4	.8	1.1	2
1254	Egg Beaters, Fleischmann's	¼ c	61	–	30	6	1	0	0	0	0	0
1262	Eggs, Second Nature, prepared	⅓ c	69	80	66	9	1	0	3	.5	.7	1.3
	FATS and OILS											
158	Butter: Stick	½ c	113	16	810	1	<1	0	92	57.2	27.1	3.4
159	Tablespoon	1 tbs	14	16	100	<1	<1	0	11	7.1	3.4	.4
160	Pat (about 1 tsp)[1]	1 ea	5	16	36	<1	<1	0	4	2.5	1.2	.2
1682	Whipped	1 tsp	3	16	22	<1	<1	0	2	1.5	.7	.1
	Fats, cooking:											
1363	Bacon fat	1 tbs	14	0	125	<1	0	0	14	6.4	5.9	1.1
1362	Beef fat/tallow	1 c	205	0	1849	0	0	0	205	103	87.3	8.2
1364	Chicken fat	1 c	205	<1	1845	0	0	0	205	61.1	91.6	42.8
161	Vegetable shortening:	1 c	205	0	1812	0	0	0	205	52.1	91.2	53.5
162	Tablespoon	1 tbs	13	0	115	0	0	0	13	3.3	5.8	3.4
163	Lard:	1 c	205	0	1849	0	0	0	205	80.4	92.5	28
164	Tablespoon	1 tbs	13	0	117	0	0	0	13	5.1	5.5	1.8
	Margarine:											
165	Imitation (about 40% fat), soft:	1 c	227	58	783	1	1	0	88	14.5	33	37
166	Tablespoon	1 tbs	14	58	49	<1	<1	0	6	1	2.2	2
167	Regular, hard (about 80% fat):	½ c	113	16	812	1	1	0	91	14.8	42	29.6
168	Tablespoon	1 tbs	14	16	101	<1	<1	0	11	1.8	5	3.6
169	Pat	1 ea	5	16	36	<1	<1	0	4	.8	1.8	1.3
170	Regular, soft (about 80% fat):	1 c	227	16	1625	2	1	0	183	30.7	83	61
171	Tablespoon	1 tbs	14	16	100	<1	<1	0	11	1.9	4	4.8
2056	Saffola, unsalted	1 tbs	14	20	100	0	0	0	11	2	3	4.5
2057	Saffola, reduced fat	1 tbs	14	37	60	0	0	0	8	1.3	2.7	4.4
172	Spread (about 60% fat), hard:	½ c	113	37	610	1	0	0	69	15.9	29.4	20.5
173	Tablespoon	1 tbs	14	37	76	<1	0	0	9	2	3.6	2.5
174	Pat[1]	1 ea	5	37	27	<1	0	0	3	.7	1.2	1
175	Spread (about 60% fat), soft:	1 c	227	37	1226	1	0	0	138	29.3	71.5	31.3
176	Tablespoon	1 tbs	14	37	76	<1	0	0	9	1.8	4.4	1.9
2160	Touch of Butter (47% fat)	1 tbs	14	36	60	0	0	0	7	1.5	3.1	1.5
	Oils:											
1585	Canola:	1 c	218	0	1927	0	0	0	218	15.5	128	64.5
1586	Tablespoon	1 tbs	14	0	124	0	0	0	14	1	8.2	4.1
177	Corn:	1 c	218	0	1927	0	0	0	218	29.4	54.1	130.8
178	Tablespoon	1 tbs	14	0	124	0	0	0	14	1.8	3.5	8.4

(1)Pat is 1" square, ⅓" thick; about 1 tsp; 90 per lb.

(Computer code number is for West Diet Analysis program)

PAGE KEY: H–4 = BEV H–6 = DAIRY H–12 = EGGS H–14 = FAT/OIL H–18 = FRUIT H–26 = BAKERY H–36 = GRAIN H–44 = FISH H–48 = MEATS H–50 = POULTRY H–54 = SAUSAGE H–56 = MIXED/FAST H–64 = NUTS/SEEDS H–68 = SWEETS H–70 = VEG/LEG H–84 = MISC H–88 = SOUPS/SAUCES H–90 = FAST H–106 = FRZN ENTREE H–112 = BABY FOODS

Chol (mg)	Calc (mg)	Iron (mg)	Magn (mg)	Pota (mg)	Sodi (mg)	Zinc (mg)	VT-A (RE)	Thia (mg)	VT-E (α-TE)	Ribo (mg)	Niac (mg)	V-B6 (mg)	Fola (μg)	VT-C (mg)
211	25	.72	5	61	162	.55	114	.03	.75	.24	.04	.07	17	0
212	25	.59	5	63	62	.53	84	.03	.53	.26	.03	.06	22	0
577	68	1.62	14	171	169	1.43	228	.09	1.43	.7	.09	.17	60	0
212	25	.72	5	60	140	.55	95	.02	.53	.22	.03	.06	18	0
215	43	.73	7	84	171	.61	119	.03	.8	.27	.05	.07	18	<1
1	67	2.65	11	416	223	1.64	272	.14	.61	.38	.14	<.01	19	0
0	40	1.08	–	85	100	–	–	–	.3	–	–	–	–	–
1	42	1.65	7	260	139	1.02	170	.07	.38	.22	.08	<.01	9	0
247	27	.18	2	29	933[2]	.06	852[3]	.01	1.79	.04	.05	<.01	3	0
31	3	.02	<1	4	117[2]	.01	107[3]	<.01	.22	<.01	.01	0	<1	0
11	1	.01	<1	1	41[2]	<.01	38[3]	0	.08	<.01	<.01	0	<1	0
7	1	<.01	<1	1	25[2]	<.01	23[3]	<.01	.05	<.01	<.01	0	<1	0
14	<1	<.01	<1	<1	76	<.01	0	0	.31	0	0	0	0	0
224	0	0	0	<1	<1	0	0	0	3.08	0	0	0	0	0
174	0	0	0	0	0	0	351	0	5.54	0	0	0	0	0
0	0	0	0	0	0	0	0	0	17	0	0	0	0	0
0	0	0	0	0	0	0	0	0	1.08	0	0	0	0	0
195	<1	0	<1	<1	<1	.23	0	0	2.46	0	0	0	0	0
12	<1	0	<1	<1	<1	.01	0	0	.16	0	0	0	0	0
0	40	0	4	57	800	0	1814[4]	.01	5.29	.05	.03	.01	2	<1
0	3	0	<1	4	136	0	114[4]	<.01	.33	<.01	<.01	<.01	<1	<1
0	34	0	3	48	1065	.23	903[4]	.01	14.5	.04	.03	.01	1	<1
0	4	0	<1	6	132	.03	112[4]	<.01	1.8	<.01	<.01	<.01	<1	<1
0	2	0	<1	2	47	.01	40[4]	<.01	.64	<.01	<.01	0	<1	<1
0	60	0	5	86	2447	0	1814[4]	.02	27.2	.07	.04	.02	2	<1
0	4	0	<1	5	151	0	112[4]	<.01	1.68	<.01	<.01	<.01	<1	<1
–	0	0	–	–	0	–	51	–	–	–	–	–	–	0
–	0	0	–	–	115	–	51	–	.14	–	–	–	–	0
0	24	0	2	34	1123	.17	903[4]	.01	5.65	.03	.02	.01	1	<1
0	3	0	<1	4	139	0	112[4]	<.01	.7	<.01	<.01	<.01	<1	<1
0	1	0	<1	1	50	0	40[4]	0	.25	<.01	<.01	0	<1	<1
0	47	0	4	68	2256	0	1814[4]	.02	20.5	.06	.04	.01	2	<1
0	3	0	<1	4	139	0	112[4]	<.01	1.26	<.01	<.01	<.01	<1	<1
0	0	0	<1	0	110	0	100	<.01	1.27	<.01	<.01	<.01	<1	<.1
0	0	0	0	0	0	0	0	0	45.8	0	0	0	0	0
0	0	0	0	0	0	0	0	0	2.94	0	0	0	0	0
0	0	0	0	0	0	0	0	0	46	0	0	0	0	0
0	0	0	0	0	0	0	0	0	2.95	0	0	0	0	0

(2)For salted butter, unsalted butter contains 12 mg sodium per stick or ½ c, 1.5 mg/tbs, or .5 mg/pat.

(3)Values for vitamin A are a year-round average.

(4)Based on average vitamin A content of fortified margarine. Federal specifications require a minimum of 15,000 IU/lb.

(For purposes of calculations, use "0" for t, <1, <.1, <.01, etc.)

H

Table H–1
Food Composition

Computer Code Number	Food Description	Measure	Wt (g)	H_2O (%)	Ener (kcal)	Prot (g)	Carb (g)	Dietary Fiber (g)	Fat (g)	Fat Breakdown (g) Sat	Mono	Poly
	FATS and OILS—Cont.											
	Oils—Cont.											
179	Olive:	1 c	216	0	1909	0	0	0	216	29.4	159	21.3
180	Tablespoon	1 tbs	14	0	124	0	0	0	14	1.9	10.3	1.4
1683	Olive, extra virgin	1 tbs	14	<1	126	0	0	0	14	1.96	10.8	1.3
181	Peanut:	1 c	216	0	1909	0	0	0	216	40	99.8	71.3
182	Tablespoon	1 tbs	14	0	124	0	0	0	14	2.6	6.5	4.6
183	Safflower:	1 c	218	0	1927	0	0	0	218	19.8	26.4	162
184	Tablespoon	1 tbs	14	0	124	0	0	0	14	1.3	1.7	10.4
185	Soybean:	1 c	218	0	1927	0	0	0	218	32	50.8	126
186	Tablespoon	1 tbs	14	0	124	0	0	0	14	2.1	3.3	8.1
187	Soybean/cottonseed:	1 c	218	0	1927	0	0	0	218	40	64.3	105
188	Tablespoon	1 tbs	14	0	124	0	0	0	14	2.5	4.1	6.7
189	Sunflower:	1 c	218	0	1927	0	0	0	218	25	42.5	143
190	Tablespoon	1 tbs	14	0	124	0	0	0	14	1.6	2.7	9.2
	Salad dressings/sandwich spreads:											
191	Blue cheese, regular	1 tbs	15	32	75	1	1	<1	8	1.5	1.9	4.4
1040	Low calorie	1 tbs	15	80	15	1	<1	<1	1	.2	.5	.4
1684	Caesar's	1 tbs	12	36	55	1	<1	<1	5	.9	3.7	.5
192	French, regular	1 tbs	16	38	67	<1	3	<1	9	1.5	1.2	3.4
193	Low calorie	1 tbs	16	71	21	<1	3	0	1	.1	.2	.5
194	Italian, regular	1 tbs	15	38	70	<1	1	<1	9	1	1.6	4.1
195	Low calorie	1 tbs	15	82	8	<1	1	<1	1	.1	.1	.2
	Kraft, Deliciously Right											
2150	1000 Island	2 tbs	32	–	70	0	8	0	4	1	–	–
2153	Bacon & tomato	2 tbs	31	–	60	1	3	0	5	1	–	–
2154	Cucumber ranch	2 tbs	31	–	60	0	2	0	5	1	–	–
2151	French	2 tbs	32	–	50	0	6	0	3	.5	–	–
2152	Ranch	2 tbs	31	–	100	0	5	0	9	1.5	–	–
199	Mayo type, regular	1 tbs	15	40	58	<1	4	0	5	.8	1.4	2.7
1030	Low calorie	1 tbs	15	54	39	<1	4	0	3	.4	.8	1.5
	Mayonnaise:											
197	Imitation, low calorie	1 tbs	15	63	35	<1	2	0	3	.5	.7	1.6
196	Regular (soybean)	1 tbs	14	17	100	<1	<1	0	11	1.7	3.1	5.7
1488	Regular, low calorie, low sodium	1 tbs	14	63	32	<1	2	0	3	.5	.6	1.4
1493	Regular, low calorie	1 tbs	16	63	37	<1	3	0	3	.5	.7	1.7
198	Ranch, regular	½ c	119	35	436	4	5	0	45	6.7	19.4	17
2251	Low calorie	2 tbs	28	70	60	0	2	0	5	1	–	–
1685	Russian	1 tbs	15	35	74	<1	2	0	8	1.1	1.8	4.4
1502	Salad dressing, low calorie, oil free	1 tbs	15	88	4	<1	1	<1	<1	<.1	0	<.1
	Salad dressing, no cholesterol											
1605	(Miracle Whip)	1 tbs	15	57	48	0	2	0	4	1.1	1.1	2.1
203	Salad dressing, from recipe, cooked[1]	1 tbs	16	69	25	1	2	<1	2	.5	.6	.3
200	Tartar sauce, regular	1 tbs	14	34	74	<1	1	<1	8	1.5	2.6	4.1
1503	Low calorie	1 tbs	14	63	31	<1	2	<1	2	.4	.6	1.3
201	Thousand island, regular	1 tbs	16	46	60	<1	2	<1	6	1	1.3	3.2
202	Low calorie	1 tbs	15	69	25	<1	3	<1	2	.2	.4	.9
204	Vinegar & oil	1 tbs	16	47	72	0	<1	0	8	1.5	2.4	3.9

(1)Fatty acid values apply to product made with regular margarine.

(Computer code number is for West Diet Analysis program)

PAGE KEY: H–4 = BEV H–6 = DAIRY H–12 = EGGS H–14 = FAT/OIL H–18 = FRUIT H–26 = BAKERY H–36 = GRAIN H–44 = FISH H–48 = MEATS H–50 = POULTRY H–54 = SAUSAGE H–56 = MIXED/FAST H–64 = NUTS/SEEDS H–68 = SWEETS H–70 = VEG/LEG H–84 = MISC H–88 = SOUPS/SAUCES H–90 = FAST H–106 = FRZN ENTREE H–112 = BABY FOODS

Chol (mg)	Calc (mg)	Iron (mg)	Magn (mg)	Pota (mg)	Sodi (mg)	Zinc (mg)	VT-A (RE)	Thia (mg)	VT-E (α-TE)	Ribo (mg)	Niac (mg)	V-B6 (mg)	Fola (μg)	VT-C (mg)
0	<1	.82	<1	0	<1	.13	0	0	26.8	0	0	0	0	0
0	<1	.05	<1	0	<1	.01	0	0	1.74	0	0	0	0	0
0	–	–	–	–	–	–	0	0	1.74	0	0	0	0	0
0	<1	.06	<1	<1	<1	.02	0	0	27.9	0	0	0	0	0
0	<1	0	<1	0	<1	0	0	0	1.81	0	0	0	0	0
0	0	0	0	0	0	0	0	0	94	0	0	0	0	0
0	0	0	0	0	0	0	0	0	6.03	0	0	0	0	0
0	<1	.04	<1	0	0	0	0	0	39.7	0	0	0	0	0
0	<1	<.01	<1	0	0	0	0	0	2.55	0	0	0	0	0
0	0	0	0	0	0	0	0	0	61.5	0	0	0	0	0
0	0	0	0	0	0	0	0	0	3.95	0	0	0	0	0
0	0	0	0	0	0	0	0	0	110	0	0	0	0	0
0	0	0	0	0	0	0	0	0	7.08	0	0	0	0	0
3	12	.03	0	6	164	0	10	<.01	1.4	.02	.02	.01	1	<1
<1	13	.08	1	1	180	.04	<1	<.01	.14	.02	.01	<.01	<1	<1
12	22	.19	3	20	203	.12	6	<.01	.7	.02	.49	.01	2	1
9	2	.06	1.6	2	188	.01	3	<.01	1.63	<.01	<.01	<.01	1	0
0	2	.06	0	13	126	.03	21	0	.19	0	0	0	0	0
0	2	.03	<1	5	118	.02	4	<.01	1.56	<.01	0	<.01	1	0
0	<1	.03	0	2	120	.02	0	0	.68	0	0	0	0	0
5	0	0	–	55	320	–	0	–	.38	–	–	–	–	0
3	0	0	–	40	300	–	0	–	1.45	–	–	–	–	0
0	0	0	–	20	450	–	0	–	1.41	–	–	–	–	0
0	0	0	–	15	260	–	100	–	.85	–	–	–	–	0
0	0	0	–	10	320	–	0	–	2.54	–	–	–	–	0
4	2	.03	<1	1	107	.03	13	<.01	.6	<.01	<.01	<.01	1	0
4	2	.03	<1	1	107	.03	10	<.01	.65	<.01	0	<.01	1	0
4	<1	0	<1	2	75	.02	0	0	.97	0	0	0	0	0
8	3	.07	<1	5	80	.02	12	0	1.7	0	<.01	.08	1	0
3	0	0	0	1	15	.02	1	0	.53	<.01	0	0	<1	0
4	<1	0	<1	2	80	02	0	0	1.03	0	0	0	0	0
47	119	.31	12	158	522	.44	86	.04	4.76	.17	.08	.05	6	1
10	20	0	–	–	240	–	0	–	1.41	–	–	–	–	0
3	3	.1	.23	24	130	.06	31	.01	1.53	.01	.1	<.01	1.59	1
0	1	.04	2	7	256	<.01	<1	<.01	<.01	<.01	<.01	<.01	<1	<1
0	0	<.01	0	0	102	0	2	0	.65	0	0	0	0	0
9	13	.08	0	19	117	0	20	.01	.3	.02	.04	0	0	<1
7	3	.13	<1	11	99	.02	9	<.01	2.24	<.01	0	.01	1	<1
3	2	.09	<1	5	83	.02	2	<.01	.83	<.01	.01	<.01	<1	<1
4	2	.09	<1	18	110	.02	15	<.01	1.14	<.01	<.01	<.01	1	0
2	2	.09	<1	17	153	.02	14	<.01	1.19	<.01	<.01	<.01	1	<1
0	0	0	0	1	<1	0	0	0	1.41	0	0	0	0	0

(For purposes of calculations, use "0" for t, <1, <.1, <.01, etc.)

Table H-1
Food Composition

Computer Code Number	Food Description	Measure	Wt (g)	H_2O (%)	Ener (kcal)	Prot (g)	Carb (g)	Dietary Fiber (g)	Fat (g)	Fat Breakdown (g) Sat	Mono	Poly
	FATS and OILS—Cont.											
	Salad dressings/sandwich spreads—Cont.											
	Wishbone											
2180	Creamy Italian, lite	1 tbs	15	–	26	<1	2	–	2	.4	–	.7
2166	Italian, lite	1 tbs	16	79	6	0	1	–	<1	0	–	.1
	FRUITS and FRUIT JUICES											
	Apples:											
	Fresh, raw, with peel:											
205	2 ¾" diam (about 3 per lb w/cores)	1 ea	138	84	81	<1	21	3	<1	.1	t	.1
206	3 ¼" diam (about 2 per lb w/cores)	1 ea	212	84	125	<1	32	6	1	.1	t	.2
207	Raw, peeled slices	1 c	110	85	63	<1	16	2	<1	.1	t	.1
208	Dried, sulfured	10 ea	64	32	155	1	42	6	<1	t	t	.1
209	Apple juice, bottled or canned	1 c	248	88	116	<1	29	<1	<1	<1	t	<.1
210	Applesauce, sweetened	1 c	255	80	193	<1	51	3	<1	.1	t	.1
211	Applesauce, unsweetened	1 c	244	88	104	<1	28	3	<1	<1	t	t
	Apricots:											
212	Raw, w/o pits (about 12 per lb w/pits)	3 ea	106	86	51	1	12	3	<1	t	.2	.1
	Canned (fruit and liquid):											
213	Heavy syrup	1 c	258	78	214	1	55	4	<1	t	.1	t
214	Halves	3 ea	85	78	70	<1	18	1	<1	t	t	t
215	Juice pack	1 c	248	87	119	2	30	4	<1	t	t	t
216	Halves	3 ea	84	87	40	1	10	1	<1	t	t	t
217	Dried, halves	10 ea	35	31	83	1	22	3	<1	t	.1	t
218	Dried, cooked, unsweetened, w/liquid	1 c	250	76	212	3	55	8	<1	t	.2	.1
219	Apricot nectar, canned	1 c	251	85	140	1	36	2	<1	t	.1	t
	Avocados, raw, edible part only:											
220	California (2 lb with refuse)	1 ea	173	73	306	4	12	8	30	4.5	19.6	3.5
221	Florida (1 lb with refuse)	1 ea	304	80	340	5	27	16	27	5.3	14.8	4.5
222	Mashed, fresh, average	1 c	230	74	370	5	17	12	35	5.6	22.1	4.5
	Bananas, raw, without peel:											
223	Whole, 8¾" long (175 g w/peel)	1 ea	114	74	104	1	27	3	1	.2	t	.1
224	Slices	1 c	150	74	137	2	35	4	1	.3	.1	.1
1285	Bananas, dehydrated slices	1 oz	28	3	97	1	25	2	1	.2	<.1	.1
225	Blackberries, raw	1 c	144	86	75	1	18	8	1	<.1	.1	.3
	Blueberries:											
226	Fresh	1 c	145	85	81	1	20	4	1	t	.1	.2
227	Frozen, sweetened	10 oz	284	77	230	1	62	6	<1	t	.1	.2
228	Frozen, thawed	1 c	230	77	186	1	50	5	<1	t	t	.1
	Cherries:											
229	Sour, red pitted, canned water pack	1 c	244	90	88	2	22	3	<1	.1	.1	.1
230	Sweet, red pitted, raw	10 ea	68	81	49	1	11	2	1	.1	.2	.2
231	Cranberry juice cocktail	1 c	253	85	144	0	36	<1	<1	t	t	.1
1411	Cranberry juice, low calorie	¾ c	178	95	34	0	8	<1	0	0	0	0
232	Cranberry-apple juice	1 c	253	83	169	<1	43	<1	0	0	0	0

(Computer code number is for West Diet Analysis program)

PAGE KEY: H–4 = BEV H–6 = DAIRY H–12 = EGGS H–14 = FAT/OIL H–18 = FRUIT H–26 = BAKERY H–36 = GRAIN H–44 = FISH H–48 = MEATS H–50 = POULTRY H–54 = SAUSAGE H–56 = MIXED/FAST H–64 = NUTS/SEEDS H–68 = SWEETS H–70 = VEG/LEG H–84 = MISC H–88 = SOUPS/SAUCES H–90 = FAST H–106 = FRZN ENTREE H–112 = BABY FOODS

Chol (mg)	Calc (mg)	Iron (mg)	Magn (mg)	Pota (mg)	Sodi (mg)	Zinc (mg)	VT-A (RE)	Thia (mg)	VT-E (α-TE)	Ribo (mg)	Niac (mg)	V-B6 (mg)	Fola (µg)	VT-C (mg)
<1	0	0	–	–	148	–	–	0	.56	0	0	–	–	0
0	1	0	–	–	255	–	–	0	.24	0	0	–	–	.2
0	10	.25	7	159	0	.05	7	.02	.44	.02	.11	.07	4	8
0	15	.38	11	244	0	.08	11	.04	.68	.03	.16	.1	6	12
0	4	.08	3	124	0	.04	4	.02	.09	.01	.1	.05	<1	4
0	9	.9	10	288	56	.13	4	0	.35	.1	.59	.08	0	2
0	17	.92	7	295	7	.07	<1	.05	.03	.04	.25	.07	<1	2
0	10	.89	8	155	8	.1	3	.03	.03	.07	.48	.07	2	4[1]
0	7	.29	7	183	5	.07	7	.03	.02	.06	.46	.06	1	3[1]
0	15	.57	8	313	1	.28	277	.03	.94	.04	.64	.06	9	11
0	23	.77	18	361	10	.28	317	.05	2.3	.06	.97	.14	4	8
0	8	.25	6	119	3	.09	105	.02	.76	.02	.32	.05	1	3
0	30	.74	25	409	10	.27	419	.04	2.21	.05	.85	.13	4	12
0	10	.25	8	139	3	.09	142	.01	.75	.02	.29	.04	1	4
0	16	1.65	16	482	4	.26	253	<.01	.53	.05	1.05	.05	4	1
0	40	4.18	42	1222	8	.66	590	.01	1.25	.07	2.36	.28	0	4
0	18	.95	13	286	8	.23	331	.02	.20	.03	.65	.05	3	2[2]
0	19	2.04	71	1096	21	.73	106	.19	2.32	.21	3.32	.48	113	14
0	33	1.61	103	1483	15	1.28	185	.33	2.37	.37	5.84	.85	162	24
0	25	2.34	90	1377	23	.97	140	.25	3.08	.28	4.42	.64	142	18
0	7	.35	33	451	1	.18	9	.05	.31	.11	.62	.66	22	10
0	9	.46	43	594	2	.24	12	.07	.41	.15	.81	.87	29	14
0	6	.33	30	418	1	.17	9	.05	0	.07	.79	.12	4	2
0	46	.82	29	282	0	.39	23	.04	1.02	.06	.58	.08	49	30
0	9	.25	7	129	9	.16	15	.07	1.45	.07	.52	.05	9	19
0	17	1.11	6	170	3	.17	11	.06	2.02	.15	.72	.17	19	3
0	14	.9	5	138	2	.14	9	.05	1.63	.12	.58	.14	15	2
0	27	3.34	15	239	17	.17	183	.04	.32	.1	.43	.11	19	5
0	10	.26	7	152	0	.04	14	.03	.09	.04	.27	.02	3	5
0	8	.38	5	45	5	.18	1	.02	0	.02	.09	.05	1	90[3]
0	16	.07	4	39	5	.04	1	.02	0	.02	.06	.03	<1	57
0	18	.15	5	68	5	.1	1	.01	0	.05	.15	.05	1	81[3]

(1)Value based on products without added vitamin C. Bottled apple juice with added vitamin C usually contains 41.6 mg/100 g, or 103 mg per cup. Check label for specific vitamin C values.

(2)Without added vitamin C. Products with added vitamin C contain 136 mg per cup. Check label.

(3)Nutrient added.

(For purposes of calculations, use "0" for t, <1, <.1, <.01, etc.)

H

Table H–1
Food Composition

Computer Code Number	Food Description	Measure	Wt (g)	H_2O (%)	Ener (kcal)	Prot (g)	Carb (g)	Dietary Fiber (g)	Fat (g)	Fat Breakdown (g) Sat	Mono	Poly
	FRUITS and FRUIT JUICES—Cont.											
233	Cranberry sauce, canned, strained	1 c	277	61	418	1	108	3	<1	t	<.1	.2
234	Dates, whole, without pits	10 ea	83	22	228	2	61	6	<1	.2	.1	t
235	Dates, chopped	1 c	178	22	490	4	130	13	1	.3	.3	<.1
236	Figs, dried	10 ea	187	28	477	6	122	17	2	.4	.5	1
	Fruit cocktail, canned, fruit and liq:											
237	Heavy syrup pack	1 c	255	80	186	1	48	3	<1	t	t	.1
238	Juice pack	1 c	248	87	114	1	30	2	<1	t	t	t
	Grapefruit:											
	Raw 3¾" diam (half w/rind = 241 g)											
239	Pink/red, half fruit, edible part	1 ea	123	91	37	1	9	2	<1	t	t	t
240	White, half fruit, edible part	1 ea	118	90	39	1	10	1	<1	t	t	t
241	Canned sections with light syrup	1 c	254	84	152	1	39	1	<1	t	t	.1
	Grapefruit juice:											
242	Fresh, raw	1 c	247	90	96	1	23	<1	<1	t	t	.1
243	Canned, unsweetened	1 c	247	90	94	1	22	<1	<1	t	t	.1
244	Sweetened	1 c	250	87	115	1	28	<1	<1	t	t	.1
	Frozen concentrate, unsweetened:											
245	Undiluted, 6-fl-oz can	¾ c	207	62	302	4	71	1	1	.1	.1	.2
246	Diluted with 3 cans water	1 c	247	89	101	1	24	<1	<1	.1	t	.1
	Grapes, raw European (adherent skin):											
247	Thompson seedless	10 ea	50	81	35	<1	9	<1	<1	.1	t	.1
248	Tokay/Emperor, seeded types	10 ea	57	81	40	<1	10	<1	<1	.1	t	.1
	Grape juice:											
249	Bottled or canned	1 c	253	84	154	1	38	2	<1	.1	t	.1
	Frozen concentrate, sweetened:											
250	Undiluted, 6-fl-oz can	¾ c	216	54	387	1	96	<1	1	.2	t	.2
251	Diluted with 3 cans water	1 c	250	87	127	<1	32	<1	<1	.1	t	.1
1410	Low calorie	1 c	250	84	153	1	38	<1	<1	.1	t	.1
252	Kiwi fruit, raw, peeled (88 g with peel)	1 ea	76	83	46	1	11	3	<1	t	t	.2
253	Lemons, raw, without peel and seeds (about 4 per lb whole)	1 ea	58	89	17	1	5	2	<1	t	t	.1
	Lemon juice:											
254	Fresh:	1 c	244	91	61	1	21	1	0	0	0	0
255	Tablespoon	1 tbs	15	91	4	<1	1	<1	0	0	0	0
256	Canned or bottled, unsweetened:	1 c	244	93	51	1	16	1	1	.1	t	.2
257	Tablespoon	1 tbs	15	93	3	<1	1	<1	<1	t	t	t
258	Frozen, single strength, unsweetened:	1 c	244	92	54	1	16	1	1	.1	t	.2
2298	Tablespoon	1 tbs	15	92	3	<1	1	<1	<1	t	t	t
	Lime juice:											
260	Fresh:	1 c	246	90	66	1	22	1	<1	t	t	.1
261	Tablespoon	1 tbs	15	90	4	<1	1	<1	<1	t	t	t
262	Canned or bottled, unsweetened	1 c	246	93	52	1	16	1	1	.1	.1	.2
263	Mangoes, raw, edible part (300 g w/skin & seeds)	1 ea	207	82	134	1	35	4	1	.1	.2	.1

(Computer code number is for West Diet Analysis program)

PAGE KEY: H–4 = BEV H–6 = DAIRY H–12 = EGGS H–14 = FAT/OIL H–18 = FRUIT H–26 = BAKERY H–36 = GRAIN H–44 = FISH H–48 = MEATS H–50 = POULTRY H–54 = SAUSAGE H–56 = MIXED/FAST H–64 = NUTS/SEEDS H–68 = SWEETS H–70 = VEG/LEG H–84 = MISC H–88 = SOUPS/SAUCES H–90 = FAST H–106 = FRZN ENTREE H–112 = BABY FOODS

Chol (mg)	Calc (mg)	Iron (mg)	Magn (mg)	Pota (mg)	Sodi (mg)	Zinc (mg)	VT-A (RE)	Thia (mg)	VT-E (α-TE)	Ribo (mg)	Niac (mg)	V-B6 (mg)	Fola (µg)	VT-C (mg)
0	11	.61	8	72	80	.14	6	.04	.28	.06	.28	.04	2	6
0	27	.95	29	541	2	.24	4	.07	.08	.08	1.83	.16	10	0
0	57	2.05	62	1160	5	.52	9	.16	.18	.18	3.92	.34	22	0
0	269	4.17	110	1331	21	.95	24	.13	9.35	.16	1.3	.42	14	2
0	15	.74	13	224	15	.2	51	.05	.74	.05	.95	.13	7	5
0	20	.52	17	235	10	.22	77	.03	.5	.04	1	.13	6	7
0	14	.15	10	159	0	.09	32[1]	.04	.31	.02	.23	.05	15	47
0	14	.07	11	175	0	.08	0	.04	.3	.02	.32	.05	12	39
0	36	1.02	25	328	5	.2	2	.1	.64	.05	.62	.05	22	54
0	23	.49	30	400	2	.12	2[2]	.1	.12	.05	.49	.11	25	94
0	17	.49	25	378	2	.22	2	.1	.12	.05	.57	.05	26	72
0	20	.9	25	405	5	.15	0	.1	.13	.06	.8	.05	26	67
0	56	1.01	79	1001	6	.37	6	.3	.37	.16	1.6	.32	26	248
0	20	.35	27	336	2	.12	2	.1	.12	.05	.54	.11	9	83
0	6	.13	3	92	1	.03	3	.05	.35	.03	.15	.05	2	5
0	6	.15	3	105	1	.03	4	.05	.4	.03	.17	.06	2	6
0	23	.61	25	334	8	.13	3	.07	0	.09	.66	.16	7	<1
0	28	.78	32	159	15	.28	6	.11	.38	.2	.93	.32	9	179[3]
0	10	.25	10	52	5	.1	3	.04	.13	.06	.31	.1	3	60[3]
0	23	.6	25	330	8	.13	3	.07	0	.09	.66	.16	7	<1
0	20	.31	23	252	4	.13	14	.01	.85	.04	.38	.07	29	74
0	15	.35	5	80	1	.03	2	.02	.14	.01	.06	.05	6	31
0	17	.07	15	303	2	.12	5	.07	.22	.02	.24	.12	31	112
0	1	0	1	19	<1	.01	<1	0	.01	0	.01	.01	2	7
0	27	.32	19	249	51	.15	5	.1	.22	.02	.48	.1	25	60
0	2	.02	1	15	3	.01	<1	.01	.01	0	.03	.01	2	4
0	19	.29	19	217	2	.12	2	.14	.22	.03	.33	.15	23	77
0	1	.02	1	13	<1	.01	<1	.01	.01	<.01	.02	.01	1	5
0	22	.07	15	268	2	.15	2	.05	.22	.02	.25	.11	20	72
0	1	0	1	16	<1	.01	<1	0	.01	0	.01	.01	1	4
0	29	.57	17	184	39[4]	.15	5	.08	.07	.01	.4	.07	19	16
0	21	.27	19	323	4	.08	805	.12	2.32	.12	1.21	.28	29	57

(1)Vitamin A in Texas red grapefruit would be 74 RE.

(2)This is vitamin A for white grapefruit juice; pink or red grapefruit juice = 109 RE per cup.

(3)With added vitamin C (ascorbic acid).

(4)Sodium benzoate and sodium bisulfite added as preservatives.

(For purposes of calculations, use "0" for t, <1, <.1, <.01, etc.)

H

Table H-1
Food Composition

Computer Code Number	Food Description	Measure	Wt (g)	H_2O (%)	Ener (kcal)	Prot (g)	Carb (g)	Dietary Fiber (g)	Fat (g)	Fat Breakdown (g) Sat	Mono	Poly
	FRUITS and FRUIT JUICES—Cont.											
	Melons, raw, without rind and contents:											
264	Cantaloupe, 5" diam (2⅓ lb whole with refuse), orange flesh	½ ea	267	90	93	2	22	2	1	.2	t	.3
265	Honeydew, 6½" diam (5¼ lb whole with refuse), slice = 1/10 melon	1 pce	129	90	45	1	12	1	<1	t	t	t
266	Nectarines, raw, w/o pits, 2½" diam	1 ea	136	86	67	1	16	2	1	.1	.2	.3
	Oranges, raw:											
267	Whole w/o peel and seeds, 2⅝" diam (180 g with peel and seeds)	1 ea	131	87	62	1	15	3	<1	t	t	t
268	Sections, without membranes	1 c	180	87	85	2	21	4	<1	t	t	t
	Orange juice:											
269	Fresh, all varieties	1 c	248	88	112	2	26	<1	<1	.1	.1	.1
270	Canned, unsweetened	1 c	249	89	105	1	25	<1	<1	t	.1	.1
271	Chilled	1 c	249	88	110	2	25	<1	1	.1	.1	.2
	Frozen concentrate:											
272	Undiluted (6-oz can)	¾ c	213	58	339	5	81	2	<1	.1	.1	.1
273	Diluted w/3 parts water by volume	1 c	249	88	112	2	27	<1	<1	t	t	t
1345	Orange juice, from dry crystals	1 c	248	88	114	0	29	0	0	0	0	0
274	Orange and grapefruit juice, canned	1 c	247	89	106	1	25	<1	<1	t	t	t
	Papayas, raw:											
275	½" slices	1 c	140	89	54	1	14	3	<1	.1	.1	t
276	Whole, 3½" diam by 5⅛" w/o seeds and skin (1 lb w/refuse)	1 ea	304	89	118	2	30	5	<1	.1	.1	.1
1031	Papaya nectar, canned	1 c	250	85	143	<1	36	2	<1	.1	.1	.1
	Peaches:											
277	Raw, whole, 2½" diam, peeled, pitted (about 4 per lb whole)	1 ea	87	88	37	1	10	2	<1	t	t	t
278	Raw, sliced	1 c	170	88	73	1	19	3	<1	t	.1	.1
	Canned, fruit and liquid:											
279	Heavy syrup pack:	1 c	256	79	189	1	51	3	<1	t	.1	.1
280	Half	1 ea	81	79	60	<1	16	1	<1	t	t	t
281	Juice pack:	1 c	248	88	109	2	29	3	<1	t	t	t
282	Half	1 ea	77	88	34	<1	9	1	<1	t	t	t
283	Dried, uncooked	10 ea	130	32	311	5	80	11	1	.1	.4	.5
284	Dried, cooked, fruit and liquid	1 c	258	78	198	3	51	7	1	.1	.2	.3
	Frozen, slice, sweetened:											
285	10-oz package	1 ea	284	75	267	2	68	5	<1	t	.1	.2
286	Cup, thawed measure	1 c	250	75	235	2	60	5	<1	t	.1	.2
1032	Peach nectar, canned	1 c	249	86	135	1	35	1	<1	t	t	t
	Pears:											
	Fresh, with skin, cored:											
287	Bartlett, 2½" diam (about 2½ per lb)	1 ea	166	84	98	1	25	4[1]	1	t	.1	.2
288	Bosc, 2 1/5" diam (about 3 per lb)	1 ea	141	84	83	1	21	3[1]	1	t	.1	.1
289	D'Anjou, 3" diam (about 2 per lb)	1 ea	200	84	118	1	30	5[1]	1	t	.2	.2
	Canned, fruit and liquid:											
290	Heavy syrup pack:	1 c	255	80	188	1	49	4[1]	<1	t	.1	.1
291	Half	1 ea	79	80	58	<1	15	1[1]	<1	t	t	t
292	Juice pack:	1 c	248	86	124	1	32	4[1]	<1	t	t	t
293	Half	1 ea	77	86	38	<1	10	1[1]	<1	t	t	t

(1) Dietary fiber data vary 2.4 to 3.4 g/100 g for fresh pears; 1.6 to 2.6 g/100 g for canned pears.

(Computer code number is for West Diet Analysis program)

PAGE KEY: H–4 = BEV H–6 = DAIRY H–12 = EGGS H–14 = FAT/OIL H–18 = FRUIT H–26 = BAKERY H–36 = GRAIN H–44 = FISH H–48 = MEATS H–50 = POULTRY H–54 = SAUSAGE H–56 = MIXED/FAST H–64 = NUTS/SEEDS H–68 = SWEETS H–70 = VEG/LEG H–84 = MISC H–88 = SOUPS/SAUCES H–90 = FAST H–106 = FRZN ENTREE H–112 = BABY FOODS

Chol (mg)	Calc (mg)	Iron (mg)	Magn (mg)	Pota (mg)	Sodi (mg)	Zinc (mg)	VT-A (RE)	Thia (mg)	VT-E (α-TE)	Ribo (mg)	Niac (mg)	V-B6 (mg)	Fola (μg)	VT-C (mg)
0	29	.56	29	825	24	.43	860	.1	.4	.06	1.53	.31	45	113
0	8	.09	9	350	13	.1	5	.1	.19	.02	.77	.08	8	32
0	7	.2	11	288	0	.12	101	.02	1.21	.06	1.35	.03	5	7
0	52	.13	13	237	0	.09	28	.11	.31	.05	.37	.08	40	70
0	72	.18	18	326	0	.13	38	.16	.43	.07	.51	.11	54	96
0	27	.5	27	496	2	.12	50	.22	.22	.07	.99	.1	75	124
0	20	1.1	27	436	5	.17	45	.15	.22	.07	.78	.22	45	86
0	25	.42	27	473	3	.1	20[2]	.19	.47	.28	.05	.7	45[2]	82[2]
0	68	.75	72	1435	6	.38	60	.6	.68	.14	1.53	.33	330	294
0	22	.25	25	473	3	.12	20	.2	.47	.04	.5	.11	109	97
0	62	.2	2	50	12	.1	551	<.01	0	.04	0	0	143	121
0	20	1.14	25	390	7	.17	30	.14	.17	.07	.83	.06	35	72
0	34	.14	14	360	4	.1	39	.04	1.6	.04	.47	.03	53	86
0	73	.3	30	781	9	.21	85	.08	3.4	.1	1.03	.06	115	187
0	25	.85	8	78	13	.38	28	.01	.05	.01	.38	.02	5	8
0	4	.1	6	171	0	.12	47	.01	.61	.04	.86	.02	3	6
0	8	.19	12	335	0	.24	92	.03	1.2	.07	1.68	.03	6	11
0	8	.69	13	235	15	.23	84	.03	2.28	.06	1.57	.05	8	7
0	2	.22	4	74	5	.07	27	.01	.72	.02	.5	.01	3	2
0	15	.67	17	317	10	.27	94	.02	3.72	.04	1.44	.05	8	9
0	5	.21	5	99	3	.08	29	.01	1.2	.01	.45	.01	3	3
0	36	5.28	55	1293	9	.74	281	<.01	0	.28	5.69	.09	<1	6
0	23	3.38	33	825	5	.46	52	.01	0	.05	3.92	.1	<1	10
0	9	1.05	14	369	17	.14	80	.04	2.53	.1	1.85	.05	9	267[3]
0	8	.92	12	325	15	.12	70	.03	2.23	.09	1.63	.04	8	236[3]
0	12	.47	10	100	17	.2	65	.01	.2	.03	.72	.02	3	13
0	18	.41	10	208	0	.2	3	.03	.83	.07	.17	.03	12	7
0	16	.35	8	176	0	.17	3	.03	.71	.06	.14	.02	10	6
0	22	.5	12	250	0	.24	4	.04	1	.08	.2	.04	15	8
0	13	.56	10	165	13	.2	0	.03	1.28	.06	.62	.04	3	3
0	4	.17	3	51	4	.06	0	.01	.4	.02	.19	.01	1	1
0	22	.72	17	238	10	.22	2	.03	1.24	.03	.5	.03	3	4
0	7	.22	5	74	3	.07	1	.01	.39	.01	.15	.01	1	1

(2)Values for juice from California oranges indicate the following values for 1 c: 36 RE of vitamin A, 72 μg of folate, and 106 mg of vitamin C.

(3)With added vitamin C (ascorbic acid).

(For purposes of calculations, use "0" for t, <1, <.1, <.01, etc.)

H

Table H-1
Food Composition

Computer Code Number	Food Description	Measure	Wt (g)	H_2O (%)	Ener (kcal)	Prot (g)	Carb (g)	Dietary Fiber (g)	Fat (g)	Fat Breakdown (g) Sat	Mono	Poly
	FRUITS and FRUIT JUICES—Cont.											
294	Dried halves	10 ea	175	27	459	3	121	13	1	.1	.2	.3
1033	Pear nectar, canned	1 c	250	84	150	<1	40	2	<1	t	t	t
	Pineapple:											
295	Fresh chunks, diced	1 c	155	87	76	1	19	2	1	t	.1	.2
	Canned, fruit and liquid:											
	Heavy syrup pack:											
296	Crushed, chunks, tidbits	⅓ c	84	79	65	<1	17	1	<1	t	t	t
297	Slices	1 ea	58	79	45	<1	12	<1	<1	t	t	t
298	Juice pack, crushed, chunks, tidbits	1 c	250	84	150	1	39	2	<1	t	t	.1
299	Juice pack, slices	1 ea	58	84	35	<1	9	<1	<1	t	t	t
300	Pineapple juice, canned, unsweetened	1 c	250	86	140	1	35	<1	<1	t	t	.1
	Plantains, without peel:											
301	Raw slices (whole = 179 g w/o peel)	1 c	148	65	181	2	47	3[1]	1	.2	t	.1
302	Cooked, boiled, sliced	1 c	154	67	179	1	48	4	<1	.1	t	.1
	Plums:											
303	Fresh, medium, 2⅛" diam	1 ea	66	85	36	1	9	1	<1	t	.3	.1
304	Fresh, small, 1½" diam	1 ea	28	85	15	<1	4	<1	<1	t	.1	t
	Canned, purple, with liquid:											
305	Heavy syrup pack:	1 c	258	76	229	1	60	3	<1	t	.2	.1
306	Plums	3 ea	110	76	98	<1	26	1	<1	t	.1	t
307	Juice pack:	1 c	252	84	146	1	38	3	<1	t	t	t
308	Plums	3 ea	95	84	55	<1	14	1	<1	t	t	t
1698	Pomegranate, fresh	1 ea	154	81	105	1	27	1	<1	.1	.1	.1
	Prunes, dried, pitted:											
309	Uncooked (10 = 97 g w/pits, 84 g w/o pits)	10 ea	84	32	200	2	53	6[2]	<1	t	.3	.1
310	Cooked, unsweetened, fruit & liq (250 g w/pits)	1c	212	70	227	2	60	14	<1	t	.3	.1
311	Prune juice, bottled or canned	1c	256	81	182	2	45	3	1	t	.5	t
	Raisins, seedless:											
312	Cup, not pressed down	1 c	145	15	435	5	115	5	1	.2	t	.2
313	One packet, ½ oz	½ oz	14	15	42	<1	11	1	<1	t	t	t
	Raspberries:											
314	Fresh	1 c	123	87	60	1	14	8	1	t	.1	.4
315	Frozen, sweetened:	10 oz	284	73	293	2	74	13	<1	t	t	.3
316	Cup, thawed measure	1 c	250	73	258	2	66	11	<1	t	t	.2
317	Rhubarb, cooked, added sugar	1 c	240	68	278	1	75	5	<1	t	t	.1
	Strawberries:											
318	Fresh, whole, capped	1 c	149	92	45	1	10	3	1	t	.1	.3
	Frozen, sliced, sweetened:											
319	10-oz container	10 oz	284	73	272	2	74	5	<1	t	.1	.2
320	Cup, thawed measure	1 c	255	73	244	1	66	5	<1	t	t	.2
	Tangerines, without peel and seeds:											
321	Fresh (2⅜" whole) 116 g w/refuse	1 ea	84	88	37	1	9	2	<1	t	t	t
322	Canned, light syrup, fruit and liquid	1 c	252	83	153	1	41	2	<1	t	t	t
323	Tangerine juice, canned, sweetened	1 c	249	87	124	1	30	<1	<1	t	t	.1

(1) Dietary fiber value partially derived from data for bananas.

(2) Dietary fiber data can vary between 6 and 13 g for 10 prunes.

(Computer code number is for West Diet Analysis program)

PAGE KEY: H–4 = BEV H–6 = DAIRY H–12 = EGGS H–14 = FAT/OIL H–18 = FRUIT H–26 = BAKERY H–36 = GRAIN H–44 = FISH H–48 = MEATS H–50 = POULTRY H–54 = SAUSAGE H–56 = MIXED/FAST H–64 = NUTS/SEEDS H–68 = SWEETS H–70 = VEG/LEG H–84 = MISC H–88 = SOUPS/SAUCES H–90 = FAST H–106 = FRZN ENTREE H–112 = BABY FOODS

Chol (mg)	Calc (mg)	Iron (mg)	Magn (mg)	Pota (mg)	Sodi (mg)	Zinc (mg)	VT-A (RE)	Thia (mg)	VT-E (α-TE)	Ribo (mg)	Niac (mg)	V-B6 (mg)	Fola (µg)	VT-C (mg)
0	59	3.68	58	933	10	.68	1	.01	0	.25	2.4	.13	0	12
0	13	.65	8	33	10	.18	<1	<.01	.25	.03	.32	.04	3	3
0	11	.57	22	175	2	.12	3	.14	.16	.06	.65	.13	16	24
0	12	.32	13	87	1	.1	1	.08	.08	.02	.24	.06	4	6
0	8	.22	9	60	1	.07	1	.05	.06	.01	.17	.04	3	4
0	35	.7	35	305	3	.25	10	.24	.25	.05	.71	.18	12	24
0	8	.16	8	71	1	.06	3	.05	.06	.01	.16	.04	3	6
0	42	.65	32	335	3	.27	1	.14	.05	.05	.64	.24	58	27[3]
0	4	.89	55	739	6	.21	167[4]	.08	.4	.08	1.02	.44	33	27
0	3	.89	49	716	8	.2	140	.07	.22	.08	1.16	.37	40	17
0	3	.07	5	113	0	.07	21	.03	.4	.06	.33	.05	1	6
0	1	.03	2	48	0	.03	9	.01	.17	.03	.14	.02	1	3
0	23	2.17	13	234	49	.18	67	.04	1.81	.1	.75	.07	6	1
0	10	.92	5	100	21	.08	29	.02	.77	.04	.32	.03	3	<1
0	25	.86	20	388	3	.28	255	.06	1.76	.15	1.19	.07	7	7
0	10	.32	8	146	1	.1	96	.02	.67	.06	.45	.03	2	3
0	5	.46	5	399	5	.18	0	.05	.85	.05	.46	.16	9	9
0	43	2.08	38	625	3	.44	167	.07	1.22	.14	1.65	.22	3	3
0	49	2.35	42	708	4	.51	66	.05	<.01	.21	1.53	.46	<1	6
0	31	3	36	707	10	.54	1	.04	.03	.18	2	.56	1	11
0	71	3.02	48	1088	17	.39	1	.23	1.02	.13	1.19	.36	5	5
0	7	.29	5	105	2	.04	<1	.02	.1	.01	.11	.03	<1	<1
0	27	.7	22	186	0	.57	16	.04	.55	.11	1.11	.07	32	31
0	43	1.85	37	324	3	.51	17	.05	1.28	.13	.65	.1	74	47
0	37	1.63	32	285	3	.45	15	.05	1.13	.11	.57	.08	65	41
0	348	.5	29	230	2	.19	17	.04	.48	.05	.48	.05	13	8
0	21	.57	15	247	1	.19	4	.03	.21	.1	.34	.09	26	84
0	31	1.68	20	278	9	.17	6	.04	.4	.14	1.14	.08	42	117
0	28	1.51	18	250	8	.15	5	.04	.4	.13	1.02	.08	38	105
0	12	.08	10	132	1	.2	77	.09	.2	.02	.13	.06	17	26
0	18	.93	20	196	15	.6	212	.13	.9	.11	1.12	.11	12	50
0	45	.5	20	443	3	.07	105	.15	.22	.05	.25	.08	11	55

(3) If vitamin C is added, it contains 96 mg per cup.

(4) Vitamin A values range from 1.5 RE for white-fleshed varieties to 178 RE for yellow-fleshed varieties.

Table H–1
Food Composition

Computer Code Number	Food Description	Measure	Wt (g)	H_2O (%)	Ener (kcal)	Prot (g)	Carb (g)	Dietary Fiber (g)	Fat (g)	Fat Breakdown (g) Sat	Mono	Poly
	FRUITS and FRUIT JUICES—Cont.											
	Watermelon, raw, without rind & seeds:											
324	Piece, 1" by 10" diam (2 lb w/refuse or 926 g)	1 pce	482	91	154	3	35	1	2	.2	.5	.1
325	Diced	1 c	160	91	51	1	11	1	1	.1	.2	.2
	BAKED GOODS: BREADS, CAKES, COOKIES, CRACKERS, PIES											
326	Bagels, plain, enriched, 3½" diam	1 ea	68	33	187	7	36	2	1	.1	.1	.5
1663	Bagel, oat bran	1 ea	71	33	181	8	38	3	1	.1	.2	.3
	Biscuits:											
327	From home recipe	1 ea	28	29	100	2	13	<1	5	1.2	2	1.2
328	From mix	1 ea	28	29	95	2	14	1	3	.8	1.2	1.2
329	From refrigerated dough	1 ea	20	27	75	1	9	<1	4	2	1	.1
330	Bread crumbs, dry, grated (see #364, 365 for soft crumbs)	1 c	100	6	395	13	73	2	5	1.3	2.1	1.6
2087	Bread sticks, brown & serve	1 ea	57	34	150	7	28	1	2	.5	.5	.5
	Breads:											
331	Boston brown, canned, 3¼" slice	1 pce	45	47	88	2	19	2	1	.1	.1	.3
332	Cracked wheat (¼ cracked-wheat & ¾ enr wheat flour): 1-lb loaf	1 ea	454	36	1180	39	225	25	18	4.2	8.6	3.1
333	Slice (18 per loaf)	1 pce	25	36	65	2	12	1	1	.2	.5	.2
334	Slice, toasted	1 pce	21	30	59	2	11	1	1	.2	.4	.2
335	French/Vienna, enriched: 1-lb loaf	1 ea	454	34	1243	40	236	14	14	2.9	5.5	3.1
337	Slice, 4¾ x 4 x ½"	1 pce	25	34	68	2	13	1	1	.2	.3	.2
336	French, slice, 5 x 2½"	1 pce	35	34	96	3	18	1	1	.2	.4	.2
	French toast: see Mixed Dishes, and Fast Foods, #691											
2083	Honey Wheatberry	1 pce	39	3	100	3	18	2	2	0	.5	0
338	Italian, enriched: 1-lb loaf	1 ea	454	36	1230	40	227	12	16	3.9	3.7	6.3
339	Slice, 4½ x 3¼ x ¾"	1 pce	30	36	81	3	15	1	1	.3	.2	.4
340	Mixed grain, enriched: 1-lb loaf	1 ea	454	38	1135	45	211	29	17	3.7	6.9	4.2
341	Slice (18 per loaf)	1 pce	25	38	62	3	12	2	1	.2	.4	.2
342	Slice, toasted	1 pce	23	32	63	3	12	2	1	.2	.4	.2
343	Oatmeal, enriched: 1-lb loaf	1 ea	454	37	1221	38	220	18	20	3.2	7.2	7.7
344	Slice (18 per loaf)	1 pce	25	37	67	2	12	1	1	.2	.4	.4
345	Slice, toasted	1 pce	23	31	67	2	12	1	1	.2	.4	.4
346	Pita pocket bread, enr, 6½" round	1 ea	60	32	165	5	33	1	1	.1	.1	.3
347	Pumpernickel (⅔ rye & ⅓ enr wheat flour): 1-lb loaf	1 ea	454	38	1135	40	216	30	14	2	4.2	5.6
348	Slice, 5 x 4 x ⅜"	1 pce	32	38	80	3	15	2	1	.1	.3	.4
349	Slice, toasted	1 pce	29	32	80	3	15	2	1	.1	.3	.4
350	Raisin, enriched: 1-lb loaf	1 ea	454	34	1244	36	237	20	20	4.9	10.5	3.1
351	Slice (18 per loaf)	1 pce	25	34	68	2	13	1	1	.3	.6	.2
352	Slice, toasted	1 pce	21	28	62	2	12	1	1	.2	.5	.2
353	Rye, light (⅓ rye & ⅔ enr wheat flour): 1-lb loaf	1 ea	454	37	1177	39	219	26	15	2.9	6	3.6
354	Slice, 4¾ x 3¾ x 7/16"	1 pce	25	37	65	2	12	1	1	.2	.3	.2
355	Slice, toasted	1 pce	22	31	62	2	12	1	1	.2	.3	.2

(Computer code number is for West Diet Analysis program)

PAGE KEY: H–4 = BEV H–6 = DAIRY H–12 = EGGS H–14 = FAT/OIL H–18 = FRUIT H–26 = BAKERY H–36 = GRAIN H–44 = FISH H–48 = MEATS H–50 = POULTRY H–54 = SAUSAGE H–56 = MIXED/FAST H–64 = NUTS/SEEDS H–68 = SWEETS H–70 = VEG/LEG H–84 = MISC H–88 = SOUPS/SAUCES H–90 = FAST H–106 = FRZN ENTREE H–112 = BABY FOODS

Chol (mg)	Calc (mg)	Iron (mg)	Magn (mg)	Pota (mg)	Sodi (mg)	Zinc (mg)	VT-A (RE)	Thia (mg)	VT-E (α-TE)	Ribo (mg)	Niac (mg)	V-B6 (mg)	Fola (μg)	VT-C (mg)
0	39	.82	53	559	10	.34	178	.39	.72	.1	.96	.69	11	46
0	13	.27	18	186	3	.11	59	.13	.24	.03	.32	.23	4	15
0	50	2.42	20	69	363	.6	0	.37	.02	.21	3.1	.03	15	0
0	9	2.2	40	145	360	1.48	<1	.24	.17	.24	2.1	.14	33	<1
1	67	.82	5	34	165	.15	6	.1	.67	.09	.84	.01	3	<1
1	53	.58	7	53	271	.17	7	.1	.11	.1	.86	.02	2	<1
1	24	.44	2	23	158	.08	7	.07	.12	.05	.44	.01	2	0
0	227	6.12	46	221	862	1.22	<1	.76	.88	.43	6.85	.1	25	0
0	60	2.7	–	–	290	–	0	.225	–	.102	1.6	–	–	0
<1	31	.95	28	143	284	.22	5	.01	.13	.05	.5	.04	3	0
0	195	12.8	236	804	2442	5.62	0	1.63	2.6	1.09	16.7	1.38	177	0
0	11	.7	13	44	135	.31	0	.09	.14	.06	.92	.08	10	0
0	10	.64	12	40	123	.28	0	.07	.13	.05	.75	.06	6	0
0	341	11.5	123	513	2766	3.95	0	2.36	1.07	1.49	21.6	.19	141	0
0	19	.63	7	28	152	.22	0	.13	.06	.08	1.19	.01	8	0
0	26	.89	9	40	213	.3	0	.18	.08	.11	1.66	.01	11	0
0	20	.72	–	–	200	–	0	.12	.24	.07	.8	–	–	0
0	354	13.3	123	499	2651	3.9	0	2.15	1.26	1.33	19.9	.22	136	0
0	23	.88	8	33	175	.26	0	.14	.08	.09	1.31	.01	9	0
0	413	15.8	241	926	2210	5.76	0	1.85	2.79	1.55	19.8	1.51	218	1
0	23	.87	13	51	122	.32	0	.1	.15	.09	1.09	.08	12	<1
0	23	.87	13	51	122	.32	0	.08	.15	.08	.98	.07	9	<1
0	300	12.3	168	645	2724	4.63	9	1.81	1.56	1.09	14.3	.31	123	2
0	17	.68	9	36	150	.26	<1	.1	.09	.06	.78	.02	7	<1
0	17	.68	9	35	150	.26	<1	.08	.09	.05	.71	.01	5	<1
0	52	1.57	16	72	322	.5	0	.36	.02	.2	2.78	.02	14	0
0	309	13	245	944	3046	6.72	0	1.48	2.3	1.38	14	.57	155	0
0	22	.92	17	67	215	.47	0	.1	.16	.1	.99	.04	11	0
0	22	.91	17	66	214	.47	0	.08	.17	.09	.89	.04	8	0
0	300	13.2	118	1030	1770	3.27	<1	1.54	3.44	1.81	15.8	.31	154	2
0	17	.73	7	57	98	.18	0	.08	.19	.1	.87	.02	9	<1
0	15	.66	6	52	89	.16	<1	.06	.173	.08	.71	.01	5	<1
0	331	12.8	182	754	2996	5.17	2	1.97	2.51	1.52	17.3	.34	232	1
0	18	.71	10	42	165	.29	<1	.11	.14	.08	.95	.02	13	<1
0	18	.68	9	40	160	.28	0	.08	.13	.07	.83	.02	9	<1

(For purposes of calculations, use "0" for t, <1, <.1, <.01, etc.)

Table H–1
Food Composition

Computer Code Number	Food Description	Measure	Wt (g)	H_2O (%)	Ener (kcal)	Prot (g)	Carb (g)	Dietary Fiber (g)	Fat (g)	Fat Breakdown (g) Sat	Mono	Poly
	BAKED GOODS: BREADS, CAKES, COOKIES, CRACKERS, PIES—Cont.											
356	Wheat (enr wheat & whole-wheat flour):[1] 1-lb loaf	1 ea	454	37	1160	43	213	25	19	3.9	7.3	4.5
357	Slice (18 per loaf)	1 pce	25	37	64	2	12	1	1	.2	.4	.2
358	Slice, toasted	1 pce	23	32	65	2	12	1	1	.2	.4	.2
359	White, enriched: 1-lb loaf	1 ea	454	37	1210	38	222	12	18	5.6	6.5	4.2
360	Slice (18 per loaf)	1 pce	25	37	67	2	12	1	1	.3	.4	.2
361	Slice, toasted	1 pce	22	30	69	2	13	1	1	.2	.3	.1
362	Slice (22 per loaf)	1 pce	20	37	53	2	10	1	1	.2	.3	.2
363	Slice, toasted	1 pce	17	24	53	2	10	<1	1	.2	.2	.1
364	White bread cubes, soft	1 c	30	36	81	3	15	1	1	.4	.5	.2
365	White bread crumbs, soft	1 c	45	36	121	4	23	1	2	.6	.8	.4
366	Whole-wheat: 1-lb loaf	1 ea	454	38	1116	44	209	31	19	4.2	7.6	4.6
367	Slice (16 per loaf)	1 pce	28	38	69	3	13	2	1	.3	.5	.3
368	Slice, toasted	1 pce	25	30	69	3	13	2	1	.3	.5	.3
	Bread stuffing, prepared from mix:											
369	Dry type	1 c	140	65	249	5	30	4	12	2.4	5.3	3.6
370	Moist type, with egg and margarine	1 c	203	65	341	8	45	4	15	3	6.5	4.3
	Cakes, prepared from mixes:[1]											
	Angel food:											
371	Whole cake, 9¾" diam tube	1 ea	635	33	1638	38	367	10	5	.8	.5	2.3
372	Piece, 1/12 of cake	1 pce	53	33	137	3	31	1	<1	.1	t	.2
373	Boston cream pie, ⅛ of cake	1 pce	120	45	302	3	52	2	10	3	5.3	1.2
	Coffee cake:											
374	Whole cake, 7¾ x 5⅝ x 1¼"	1 ea	430	31	1367	24	227	5	41	8	16.7	13.6
375	Piece, ⅙ of cake	1 pce	72	31	229	4	38	1	7	1.3	2.8	2.3
	Devil's food, chocolate frosting:											
376	Whole cake, 2 layer, 8 or 9" diam	1 ea	1107	23	4062	45	604	31	182	52	99.6	21.1
377	Piece, 1/16 of cake	1 pce	69	23	253	3	38	2	11	3.2	6.2	1.3
378	Cupcake, 2½" diam	1 ea	42	23	154	2	23	1	7	2	3.8	.8
	Gingerbread:											
379	Whole cake, 8" square	1 ea	570	33	1764	23	289	7	58	14.9	32	7.6
380	Piece, 1/9 of cake	1 pce	63	33	195	3	32	1	6	1.6	3.5	.8
	Yellow, chocolate frosting, 2 layer:											
381	Whole cake, 8 or 9" diam	1 ea	1108	22	4199	42	613	20	193	53	107	23.2
382	Piece, 1/16 of cake	1 pce	69	22	262	3	38	1	12	3.3	6.7	1.4
	Cakes from recipes w/enr flour:											
	Carrot cake, cream cheese frosting:[2]											
383	Whole, 9 x 13" cake	1 ea	1536	21	6696	71	725	18	406	75.1	100	209
384	Piece, 1/16 of cake, 2¼ x 3¼" slice	1 pce	112	21	488	5	53	1	30	5.5	7.3	15.2
	Fruitcake, dark:											
386	Piece, 1/32 of cake, ⅔" arc	1 pce	43	25	139	1	26	2	4	.5	1.8	1.4
	Sheet, plain, no frosting:[3]											
387	Whole cake, 9" square	1 ea	777	23	2828	35	434	3	108	30	51.8	25.6
388	Piece, 1/9 of cake	1 pce	86	23	313	4	48	<1	12	3.3	5.7	2.8

(1)Excepting angel food cake, cakes were made from mixes containing vegetable shortening, and frostings were made with margarine. All mixes use enriched flour.

(2)Made with vegetable oil.

(3)Cake made with vegetable shortening.

(Computer code number is for West Diet Analysis program)

PAGE KEY: H–4 = BEV H–6 = DAIRY H–12 = EGGS H–14 = FAT/OIL H–18 = FRUIT H–26 = BAKERY H–36 = GRAIN H–44 = FISH H–48 = MEATS H–50 = POULTRY H–54 = SAUSAGE H–56 = MIXED/FAST H–64 = NUTS/SEEDS H–68 = SWEETS H–70 = VEG/LEG H–84 = MISC H–88 = SOUPS/SAUCES H–90 = FAST H–106 = FRZN ENTREE H–112 = BABY FOODS

Chol (mg)	Calc (mg)	Iron (mg)	Magn (mg)	Pota (mg)	Sodi (mg)	Zinc (mg)	VT-A (RE)	Thia (mg)	VT-E (α-TE)	Ribo (mg)	Niac (mg)	V-B6 (mg)	Fola (μg)	VT-C (mg)
0	572	15.8	209	627	2447	4.77	0	2	3	1.45	20.5	.5	204	0
0	32	.87	12	50	135	.26	0	.11	.17	.08	1.13	.03	11	0
0	26	.83	12	50	132	.26	0	.08	.14	.06	.93	.02	7	0
5	572	12.9	95	508	2334	2.81	0	2.13	1.3	1.4	17	.15	159	
<1	32	.71	5	28	129	.15	0	.12	.07	.09	.99	.01	9	0
<1	22	.73	5	28	130	.16	0	.08	.04	.06	.84	.01	9	0
<1	25	.57	4	22	103	.12	0	.09	.06	.06	.75	.01	7	0
<1	17	.56	4	21	101	.12	0	.06	.03	.05	.67	.01	7	0
<1	25	.84	6	32	151	.19	0	.12	.05	.1	1	.01	10	0
1	38	1.3	9	48	227	.28	0	.18	.08	.11	1.5	.15	16	0
0	327	15	390	1144	2382	8.8	0	1.59	4.72	.93	17.4	.81	227	0
0	20	.94	24	72	150	.55	0	.1	.29	.06	1.09	.05	14	0
0	20	.93	24	71	148	.55	0	.08	.23	.05	.97	.05	10	0
0	45	1.53	17	104	760	.39	113	.19	1.96	.15	2.07	.06	24	0
0	130	3.33	30	266	936	.65	140	.34	2.44	.29	3.23	.11	35	3
0	889	3.3	76	591	4756	.44	0	.65	.64	3.12	5.61	.2	19	0
0	74	.28	6	49	397	.04	0	.05	.05	.26	.47	.02	2	0
44	28	.46	7	47	173	.19	28	.49	1.27	.32	.23	.03	10	<1
211	585	6.15	77	482	1810	1.94	172	.72	7.14	.75	6.54	.21	52	1
35	98	1.03	13	81	303	.32	29	.12	1.2	.13	1.09	.04	9	<1
509	476	24.3	376	2214	3697	7.64	310	.3	18.7	1.47	6.39	.34	89	1
32	30	1.52	23	138	231	.48	19	.02	1.7	.09	.4	.02	6	<1
19	18	.93	14	84	140	.29	12	.01	.71	.06	.24	.01	3	<1
200	393	18.9	91	1373	2615	2.34	91	1.08	7.81	1.06	8.89	.22	57	1
22	43	2.09	10	152	289	.26	10	.12	.73	.12	.98	.02	6	<1
609	410	23.1	332	1972	3733	6.87	299	1.33	29.9	1.74	13.9	.32	89	1
38	25	1.44	21	123	233	.43	19	.08	1.86	.11	.86	.02	6	<1
829	384	19.2	276	1720	3778	7.53	5898	2.09	64.8	2.4	15.5	1.17	184	17
60	28	1.4	20	125	276	.55	480	.15	4.73	.17	1.13	.08	13	1
2	14	.89	7	66	116	.12	8	.02	1.34	.04	.34	.02	1	<1
505	497	11.7	108	613	2331	2.75	373	1.24	11.03	1.4	10.1	.26	54	2
56	55	1.3	12	68	258	.3	41	.14	1.22	.15	1.12	.03	6	<1

(For purposes of calculations, use "0" for t, <1, <.1, <.01, etc.)

Table H–1
Food Composition

Computer Code Number	Food Description	Measure	Wt (g)	H_2O (%)	Ener (kcal)	Prot (g)	Carb (g)	Dietary Fiber (g)	Fat (g)	Fat Breakdown (g) Sat	Mono	Poly
	BAKED GOODS: BREADS, CAKES, COOKIES, CRACKERS, PIES—Cont.											
	Sheet, plain, uncooked white frosting:[1]											
389	Whole cake, 9" square	1 ea	1096	22	4088	39	644	4	159	26.2	67.5	56.1
390	Piece, 1/9 of cake	1 pce	121	22	451	4	71	<1	18	2.9	7.4	6.2
	Cakes, commercial:											
	Cheesecake:											
401	Whole cake, 9" diam	1 ea	1110	46	3540	61	283	5	250	128	86	15.3
402	Piece, 1/12 of cake	1 pce	92	46	295	5	23	<1	21	10.6	7.1	1.3
	Pound cake:											
393	Loaf, 8½ x 3½ x 3"	1 ea	500	25	1948	27	244	2	99	56	27.9	5.4
394	Slice, 1/17 of loaf, 2" slice	1 pce	29	25	113	2	14	<1	6	3.2	1.6	.3
	Snack: 2 small cakes per package											
395	Chocolate w/creme filling (Ding Dong)	1 ea	28	20	107	1	17	<1	4	1.8	1.6	.4
396	Sponge w/creme filling (Twinkie)	1 ea	42	20	153	1	27	<1	5	1.1	1.9	1.5
1677	Sponge cake, 1/12 of 12" cake	1 pce	38	30	110	2	23	<1	1	.3	.4	.2
1678	Strawberry shortcake, fresh	1 ea	254	74	327	5	40	4	17	10.1	4.9	1
	White, white frosting, 2 layer:											
397	Whole cake, 8 or 9" diam	1 ea	1140	20	4272	38	718	11	154	68.4	60	15.5
398	Piece, 1/16 of cake	1 pce	71	20	266	2	45	1	10	4.3	3.8	1
	Yellow, chocolate frosting, 2 layer:											
399	Whole cake, 8 or 9" diam	1 ea	1108	22	4196	42	614	20	193	53	107	23.2
400	Piece, 1/16 of cake	1 pce	69	22	262	3	38	1	12	3.3	6.7	1.4
1332	Bagel chips	5 pce	70	3	298	6	52	6	7	1.3	2.1	3.4
2225	Bagel chips, onion garlic, toasted	½ oz	14	–	55	2	9	1	2	.5	1.5	0
1035	Cheese puffs/Cheetos	1 oz	28	2	155	2	15	<1	10	1.9	5.7	1.3
	Cookies made with enriched flour:											
	Brownies with nuts:											
403	Commercial w/frosting, 1½ x 1¾ x ⅞"	1 ea	25	14	101	1	16	1	4	1.1	2.1	.6
404	Home recipe, 1¾ x 1¾ x ⅞"[2]	1 ea	20	13	93	1	10	<1	6	1.5	2.2	1.9
1902	Fat free fudge, Entenmann's	1 pce	40	24	110	2	27	1	0	0	0	0
	Chocolate chip:											
405	Commercial, 2¼" diam	4 ea	42	12	192	2	25	1	10	3.1	5.5	1.1
406	Home recipe, 2¼" diam	4 ea	40	6	195	2	23	1	11	3.2	4.2	3.4
407	From refrigerated dough, 2¼" diam	4 ea	48	13	213	2	29	1	10	3.3	4.9	1
408	Fig bars	4 ea	56	16	195	2	40	3	4	.7	2.2	.7
2052	Fruit bar, no fat	1 ea	28	–	90	2	21	0	0	0	0	0
2162	Fudge, fat free, Snackwell	1 ea	16	14	53	1	12	<1	<1	.1	.1	<.1
409	Oatmeal raisin, 2⅝" diam	4 ea	52	6	226	3	36	2	8	1.7	3.6	2.6
410	Peanut butter, home recipe, 2⅝" diam[3]	4 ea	48	6	228	4	28	1	11	2.1	5.2	3.5
411	Sandwich-type, all	4 ea	40	2	189	2	28	1	8	1.7	4.7	1.1
412	Shortbread, commercial, small	4 ea	32	4	161	2	21	1	8	2	4.3	1
413	Shortbread, home recipe, large[4]	2 ea	28	3	155	2	16	<1	9	5.8	2.7	.4

(1) Made with margarine.
(2) Made with vegetable oil.
(3) Made with vegetable shortening.
(4) Made with butter.

(Computer code number is for West Diet Analysis program)

PAGE KEY: H–4 = BEV H–6 = DAIRY H–12 = EGGS H–14 = FAT/OIL H–18 = FRUIT H–26 = BAKERY H–36 = GRAIN H–44 = FISH H–48 = MEATS H–50 = POULTRY H–54 = SAUSAGE H–56 = MIXED/FAST H–64 = NUTS/SEEDS H–68 = SWEETS H–70 = VEG/LEG H–84 = MISC H–88 = SOUPS/SAUCES H–90 = FAST H–106 = FRZN ENTREE H–112 = BABY FOODS

Chol (mg)	Calc (mg)	Iron (mg)	Magn (mg)	Pota (mg)	Sodi (mg)	Zinc (mg)	VT-A (RE)	Thia (mg)	VT-E (α-TE)	Ribo (mg)	Niac (mg)	V-B6 (mg)	Fola (μg)	VT-C (mg)
614	680	11.7	66	581	3770	2.74	208	1.1	20.8	.77	5.48	.38	99	2
68	75	1.31	7	64	416	.3	23	.12	2.3	.08	.6	.04	11	<1
611	566	6.99	122	999	2297	5.66	1787	.31	11.7	2.14	2.16	.58	167	7
51	47	.58	10	83	190	.47	148	.03	.97	.18	.18	.05	14	1
1105	175	6.9	55	595	1983	2.3	779	.68	3.29	1.15	6.55	.17	55	1
64	10	.4	3	34	115	.13	45	.04	.19	.07	.38	.01	3	<1
5	21	.95	12	35	121	.16	1	.06	.56	.08	.69	.01	2	<1
7	19	.54	3	38	153	.13	2	.06	.82	.06	.51	.01	2	<1
39	27	1	4	38	93	.19	18	.09	.17	.1	.73	.02	5	0
53	209	2.33	29	359	510	.57	172	.29	.73	.33	2.26	.13	40	95
91	547	9.12	60	661	2668	1.77	369	1.14	20.5	1.48	10.3	.16	64	1
6	34	.57	4	41	166	.11	23	.07	1.28	.09	.64	.01	4	<1
609	410	23	332	1972	3734	6.87	299	1.33	29.9	1.74	13.9	.32	89	1
38	25	1.44	21	123	233	.43	19	.08	1.86	.11	.86	.02	6	<1
0	9	1.38	41	167	419	.9	0	.1	.47	.12	1.57	.19	58	0
0	0	.72	–	–	140	–	0	.11	<.01	.07	1	–	–	0
1	16	.66	5	47	294	.11	10	.07	1.43	.1	.9	.04	34	<1
4	7	.56	8	37	78	.18	5	.06	.53	.05	.43	.01	3	<1
15	11	.37	11	35	69	.19	40	.03	.58	.04	.2	.02	3	<1
0	0	1.08	–	90	140	–	0	–	.01	–	–	–	–	0
0	6	1.01	15	39	137	.19	<1	.05	1.22	.08	.68	.07	2	0
13	16	.98	22	90	144	.37	66	.07	1.16	.07	.54	.03	5	<1
11	12	1.08	11	86	100	.24	8	.09	.98	.09	.95	.02	4	0
0	36	1.62	15	116	196	.22	2	.09	.39	.12	1.05	.04	6	<1
0	0	.36	–	–	95	–	0	–	.01	–	–	–	–	0
0	3	.29	5	26	71	.08	–	.02	<.01	.02	.26	<.01	–	0
17	52	1.38	22	124	280	.45	85	.13	1.3	.09	.65	.04	6	<1
15	19	1.07	19	111	249	.39	75	.11	1.82	.1	1.68	.04	9	<1
0	10	1.56	18	70	242	.32	0	.03	1.21	.07	.83	.01	2	0
6	11	.88	5	32	146	.17	4	.11	.98	.1	1.07	.01	3	0
25	5	.74	4	20	132	.12	86	.1	.22	.07	.83	.01	3	0

(For purposes of calculations, use "0" for t, <1, <.1, <.01, etc.)

H

Table H–1
Food Composition

Computer Code Number	Food Description	Measure	Wt (g)	H_2O (%)	Ener (kcal)	Prot (g)	Carb (g)	Dietary Fiber (g)	Fat (g)	Fat Breakdown (g)		
										Sat	Mono	Poly
	BAKED GOODS: BREADS, CAKES, COOKIES, CRACKERS, PIES—Cont.											
414	Sugar, from refrigerated dough, 2" diam	4 ea	48	5	232	2	31	<1	11	2.8	6.2	1.4
1874	Vanilla sandwich, Snackwell's	2 ea	26	4	109	1	21	1	2	.5	.8	.2
415	Vanilla wafers	10 ea	40	5	176	2	29	1	6	1.4	2.4	1.5
416	Corn chips	1 oz	28	1	153	2	16	1	9	1.3	2.7	4.7
	Crackers:[1]											
1034	Armenian cracker bread	4 pce	28	4	115	5	19	4	2	.4	.7	1
417	Cheese	10 ea	10	3	50	1	6	<1	3	.9	.9	.5
418	Cheese with peanut butter	4 ea	30	4	145	4	17	<1	7	1.5	3.6	1.3
	Fat Free:											
2161	Cracked pepper, Snackwell	1 ea	15	2	60	2	13	<1	<1	.1	<.1	.1
2159	Wheat, Snackwell	7 ea	15	1	60	2	12	1	<1	.1	.1	.1
2075	Whole wheat, herb seasoned	½ oz	14	5	50	2	11	2	0	0	0	0
2077	Whole wheat, onion	½ oz	14	5	50	2	11	2	0	0	0	0
419	Graham	2 ea	14	4	59	1	11	<1	1	.4	.7	.2
420	Melba toast, plain	1 pce	5	5	19	1	4	<1	<1	<.1	<.1	<.1
1514	Rice cakes, unsalted	2 ea	18	6	70	1	15	<1	1	.1	.2	.2
421	Rye wafer, whole grain	2 ea	14	5	47	1	11	3	<1	<.1	<.1	<.1
422	Saltine®[2]	4 ea	12	4	52	1	9	<1	1	.3	.8	.2
1971	Saltine®, Unsalted Tops	2 ea	6	–	25	1	4	0	1	0	0	0
423	Snack-type, round like Ritz	3 ea	9	3	45	1	5	<1	2	.4	1	.7
424	Wheat, thin	4 ea	8	3	35	1	5	1	1	.5	.5	.4
425	Whole-wheat wafers	2 ea	8	3	35	1	5	1	1	.2	.8	.2
426	Croissants, 4½ x 4 x 1¾"	1 ea	57	23	231	5	26	1	12	6.7	3.2	.7
1699	Croutons, seasoned	½ c	15	4	53	2	11	<1	0	0	0	0
	Danish pastry:											
427	Packaged ring, plain, 12 oz	1 ea	340	21	1349	19	181	1	65	13.5	40.9	6.4
428	Round piece, plain, 4¼" diam, 1" high	1 ea	57	21	226	3	30	<1	11	2.3	6.9	1.1
429	Ounce, plain	1 oz	28	21	111	2	15	<1	5	1.1	3.4	.5
430	Round piece with fruit	1 ea	65	29	231	3	31	–	11	2.3	7	1.1
	Desserts, 3 x 3" piece:											
1348	Apple crisp	1 pce	78	62	127	1	25	–	3	.6	1.2	.9
1353	Apple cobbler	1 pce	104	57	200	2	35	2	6	1.2	2.8	2
1349	Cherry crisp	1 pce	138	77	146	2	24	1	5	1	2.5	1.8
1352	Cherry cobbler	1 pce	129	66	198	2	34	1	6	1.2	2.8	1.9
1350	Peach crisp	1 pce	139	75	155	2	27	2	5	1	2.4	1.7
1351	Peach cobbler	1 pce	130	64	204	3	36	2	6	1.2	2.8	1.9
	Doughnuts:											
431	Cake type, plain, 3¼" diam	1 ea	50	21	211	3	25	1	11	1.9	4.8	4.1
432	Yeast-leavened, glazed, 3¾" diam	1 ea	60	25	242	4	27	1	14	3.5	7.7	1.7
	English muffins:											
433	Plain, enriched	1 ea	57	42	134	4	26	2	1	.2	.2	.5
434	Toasted	1 ea	50	37	128	4	25	1	1	.1	.2	.5
1504	Whole wheat	1 ea	50	46	102	4	20	3	1	.2	.3	.4
1414	Granola bar, soft	1 ea	42	6	187	3	29	2	7	3	1.6	2.2
1415	Granola bar, hard	1 ea	28	4	132	3	18	1	6	.7	1.2	3.4

[1] Crackers made with enriched white (wheat) flour except for rye wafers and whole-wheat wafers.

[2] Made with lard.

(Computer code number is for West Diet Analysis program)

PAGE KEY: H–4 = BEV H–6 = DAIRY H–12 = EGGS H–14 = FAT/OIL H–18 = FRUIT H–26 = BAKERY H–36 = GRAIN H–44 = FISH H–48 = MEATS H–50 = POULTRY H–54 = SAUSAGE H–56 = MIXED/FAST H–64 = NUTS/SEEDS H–68 = SWEETS H–70 = VEG/LEG H–84 = MISC H–88 = SOUPS/SAUCES H–90 = FAST H–106 = FRZN ENTREE H–112 = BABY FOODS

Chol (mg)	Calc (mg)	Iron (mg)	Magn (mg)	Pota (mg)	Sodi (mg)	Zinc (mg)	VT-A (RE)	Thia (mg)	VT-E (α-TE)	Ribo (mg)	Niac (mg)	V-B6 (mg)	Fola (μg)	VT-C (mg)
15	43	.88	4	78	225	.13	5	.09	1.54	.06	1.16	.01	3	0
<1	17	.61	5	28	95	.16	–	.05	–	.07	.69	.01	–	0
23	19	.95	6	39	125	.14	7	.11	.54	.13	1.24	.03	4	0
0	36	.37	21	40	179	.36	3	.01	.38	.04	.33	.07[3]	6	<1
0	21	.44	40	76	140	.89	1	.06	1.11	.04	1.04	.03	12	2
1	15	.48	4	15	100	.11	3	.06	.1	.04	.47	.05	3	0
2	24	.88	17	73	298	.33	11	.12	1.33	.1	1.96	.45	8	0
<1	26	.73	4	19	148	.14	–	.05	–	.06	.78	.01	–	<1
<1	28	.58	7	43	169	.21	–	.04	–	.07	.73	.02	–	0
0	–	.36	–	70	80	–	100	.06	–	–	.4	–	–	2
0	–	.36	–	70	80	–	500	.06	–	–	.4	–	–	2
0	3	.52	4	19	85	.11	0	.03	.27	.04	.58	.01	2	0
0	5	.19	3	10	41	.1	0	.02	.01	.01	.21	<.01	1	0
0	2	.27	24	52	5	.54	1	.01	.02	.03	1.4	.03	4	0
0	6	.83	17	69	111	.39	<1	.06	.28	.04	.22	.04	6	<1
0	14	.65	3	15	156	.09	0	.07	.2	.05	.63	<.01	4	0
0	–	.36	–	5	50	–	–	–	.1	–	–	–	–	–
0	11	.32	2	12	76	.06	0	.03	.4	.03	.36	<.01	1	0
1	3	.25	6	17	69	.24	0	.04	.3	.03	.4	.01	3	0
0	4	.25	8	24	53	.17	0	.02	.31	.01	.36	.01	2	0
43	21	1.16	9	67	424	.43	78	.22	.25	.14	1.25	.03	16	<1
<1	15	.81	6	20	195	.16	1	.07	.24	.11	.9	<.01	<1	0
105	143	6.94	54	371	1261	1.87	20	.99	3.06	.75	8.5	.2	54	10
18	24	1.16	9	62	211	.31	3	.16	.51	.12	1.43	.03	9	2
9	12	.57	4	31	104	.16	2	.08	.25	.06	.7	.02	4	1
13	15	.97	10	76	230	.33	17	.2	.59	.14	1.24	.04	10	1
0	22	.59	5	76	142	.12	24	.07	–	.06	.6	.03	4	2
1	22	.79	6	106	288	.16	76	.1	1.1	.09	.74	.04	3	<1
0	26	2.14	11	154	74	.16	150	.06	.93	.08	.59	.06	11	3
1	28	1.81	9	133	294	.2	135	.1	1.01	.11	.85	.05	9	2
0	20	.95	1	189	70	.2	108	.06	1.13	.05	1.06	.03	6	5
1	24	.91	10	159	291	.23	105	.09	1.16	.09	1.19	.03	6	3
18	22	.98	10	63	273	.27	9	.11	1.73	.12	.92	.03	4	<1
4	26	1.22	13	65	205	.46	6	.22	1.75	.13	1.71	.03	13	0
0	99	1.43	12	75	265	.4	0	.25	.07	.16	2.21	.02	21	<1
0	94	1.36	11	71	252	.38	0	.19	.06	.14	1.9	.02	15	<1
0	133	1.23	36	105	319	.8	0	.15	.35	.07	1.71	.08	25	0
<1	44	1.08	31	137	117	.63	0	.12	.51	.07	.22	.04	10	0
0	17	.83	27	94	82	.57	4	.07	.37	.03	.44	.02	6	<1

(3)Vitamin B_6 values vary between brands. Check the label.

Table H–1
Food Composition

Computer Code Number	Food Description	Measure	Wt (g)	H_2O (%)	Ener (kcal)	Prot (g)	Carb (g)	Dietary Fiber (g)	Fat (g)	Fat Breakdown (g) Sat	Mono	Poly
	BAKED GOODS: BREADS, CAKES, COOKIES, CRACKERS, PIES—Cont.											
	Granola bar, fat free:											
1985	Blueberry	1 ea	43	11	143	2	36	3	0	0	0	0
2012	Chocolate chip	1 ea	43	11	143	2	36	3	0	0	0	0
1983	Date almond	1 ea	43	11	143	2	36	3	0	0	0	0
1984	Raisin	1 ea	43	11	143	2	36	3	0	0	0	0
2011	Strawberry	1 ea	43	11	143	2	36	3	0	0	0	0
	Muffins, 2½" diam, 1½" high:											
	From home recipe											
435	Blueberry[1]	1 ea	45	39	131	3	18	1	5	1.1	1.2	2.4
436	Bran, wheat[2]	1 ea	45	35	130	3	19	3	6	1.2	1.4	2.8
437	Cornmeal	1 ea	45	32	144	3	20	2	6	1.2	1.4	2.8
	From commercial mix:											
438	Blueberry	1 ea	45	36	135	2	22	<1	4	.7	1.6	1.4
439	Bran, wheat	1 ea	45	35	124	3	21	2	4	1.1	2.1	.6
440	Cornmeal	1 ea	45	30	144	3	22	1	5	1.3	2.4	.6
	Nabisco Newtons, fat free:											
1864	Cranberry	1 ea	23	–	69	1	16	–	0	0	0	0
1867	Fig	1 ea	23	–	69	1	16	–	0	0	0	0
1865	Raspberry	1 ea	23	–	69	1	16	–	0	0	0	0
1868	Strawberry	1 ea	23	–	69	1	16	–	0	0	0	0
	Pancakes, 4" diam:											
441	Buckwheat, from mix w/ egg and milk	1 ea	27	54	56	2	8	1	2	.5	.5	.8
442	Plain, from home recipe	1 ea	27	53	61	2	8	<1	3	.6	.7	1.2
443	Plain, from mix; egg, milk, oil added	1 ea	27	53	52	1	10	<1	1	.1	.2	.2
1468	Pan dulce, sweet roll w/topping	1 ea	79	21	291	5	48	1	9	2	3.9	2.7
	Piecrust, with enriched flour, vegetable shortening, baked:											
444	Home recipe, 9" shell	1 ea	180	10	949	12	85	3	62	15.5	27.4	16.4
	From mix:											
445	For 2-crust pie	1 ea	320	10	1686	21	152	5	111	27.6	48.6	29.2
446	1 pie shell	1 ea	180	11	902	12	91	3	55	13.9	31.1	6.9
	Pies, 9" diam; crust made with vegetable shortening, enriched flour:											
447	Apple: Whole pie	1 ea	945	52	2239	18	321	15	104	19.9	56.1	19.8
448	Piece, ⅙ of pie	1 pce	158	52	374	3	54	3	17	3.3	9.4	3.3
449	Banana cream: Whole pie	1 ea	1188	48	3195	52	391	8	162	44.7	68	39.2
450	Piece, ⅙ of pie	1 pce	198	48	533	9	65	1	27	7.4	11.3	6.5
451	Blueberry: Whole pie	1 ea	945	51	2315	25	317	13	112	27.6	48.4	29.1
452	Piece, ⅙ of pie	1 pce	158	51	387	4	53	2	19	4.6	8.1	4.9
453	Cherry: Whole pie	1 ea	945	46	2551	26	364	14	115	28.3	50.2	30.7
454	Piece, ⅙ of pie	1 pce	158	46	427	4	61	2	19	4.7	8.4	5.1
455	Chocolate cream:[3] Whole pie	1 ea	1194	63	2150	47	281	12	97	35	38	18.6
456	Piece, ⅙ of pie	1 pce	199	63	358	8	47	2	16	5.9	6.4	3.1
457	Custard:[3] Whole pie	1 ea	910	61	1911	50	189	15	106	25.3	52.4	17.5
458	Piece, ⅙ of pie	1 pce	152	61	319	8	32	2	18	4.2	8.8	2.9
459	Lemon meringue: Whole pie	1 ea	840	42	2251	13	396	10	73	13.1	30.5	24.3
460	Piece, ⅙ of pie	1 pce	140	42	375	2	66	2	12	2.2	5.1	4
461	Peach: Whole pie	1 ea	945	45	2546	22	377	13	111	26.4	47	31.8

(1) Made with vegetable shortening.

(2) Made with vegetable oil.

(3) Values based on recipe: pie crust, cooked chocolate pudding, whipped cream topping.

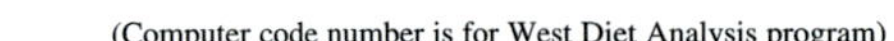
(Computer code number is for West Diet Analysis program)

Chol (mg)	Calc (mg)	Iron (mg)	Magn (mg)	Pota (mg)	Sodi (mg)	Zinc (mg)	VT-A (RE)	Thia (mg)	VT-E (α-TE)	Ribo (mg)	Niac (mg)	V-B6 (mg)	Fola (µg)	VT-C (mg)
0	0	3.7	–	120	5	–	512	.03	–	.07	.4	–	–	0
0	0	1.1	–	120	5	–	102	.03	–	.07	.4	–	–	0
0	0	3.7	–	120	5	–	102	.03	–	.07	.4	–	–	0
0	0	3.7	–	120	5	–	102	.03	–	.07	.4	–	–	0
0	20	1.1	–	120	5	–	102	.03	–	.07	.4	–	–	0
18	85	1.02	7	55	198	.24	13	.12	.81	.13	.99	.02	5	1
16	84	1.89	35	143	265	1.24	108	.15	1.04	.2	1.81	.14	23	4
20	116	1.18	10	65	263	.27	18	.14	.86	.14	1.07	.04	8	<1
21	11	.51	5	35	197	.17	10	.07	.63	.14	1.01	.03	5	<1
31	14	1.14	26	66	210	.51	14	.09	.68	.11	1.29	.08	7	0
28	34	.88	9	59	358	.29	20	.11	.68	.12	.94	.05	5	<1
–	–	–	–	–	77	–	–	–	–	–	–	–	–	–
–	–	–	–	–	77	–	–	–	–	–	–	–	–	–
–	–	–	–	–	77	–	–	–	–	–	–	–	–	–
–	–	–	–	–	77	–	–	–	–	–	–	–	–	–
18	69	.51	15	63	144	.32	18	.05	.56	.07	.36	.04	5	<1
16	59	.49	4	36	119	.15	15	.05	.26	.08	.42	.01	3	<1
3	34	.42	5	47	170	.1	2	.06	.23	.06	.46	.03	2	<1
26	13	1.82	10	57	140	.35	88	.23	1.35	.21	1.98	.04	22	<1
0	18	5.2	25	121	976	.79	0	.7	9.94	.5	5.96	.04	20	0
0	32	9.24	45	214	1734	1.41	0	1.25	17.7	.89	10.6	.08	35	0
0	108	3.87	27	112	1312	.7	0	.54	9.94	.33	4.27	.1	22	0
0	104	4.25	66	614	2513	1.51	284	.26	15.6	.25	2.49	.36	38	30
0	17	.71	11	103	420	.25	47	.04	2.61	.04	.42	.06	6	5
606	891	12.4	190	1960	2851	5.7	832	1.65	17.5	2.46	12.5	1.58	131	19
101	149	2.06	32	327	475	.95	139	.27	2.91	.41	2.08	.26	22	3
0	66	11.6	76	473	1748	1.89	38	1.45	19.8	1.25	11.2	.32	47	7
0	11	1.94	13	79	292	.32	6	.24	3.32	.21	1.88	.05	8	1
0	94	17.5	85	728	1804	1.89	454	1.4	18	1.18	12.1	.32	66	9
0	16	2.92	14	122	302	.32	76	.23	3	.2	2.02	.05	11	2
108.6	1028	8.8	170	1705	2085	4.9	235	1	11.4	2.4	7.34	.37	59	6
18	171	1.47	28	284	347.5	.82	39	.17	1.89	.4	1.22	.06	10	1
300	728	5.28	100	965	2184	4.73	455	.35	10.8	1.89	2.66	.44	182	3
50	122	.88	17	161	365	.79	76	.06	1.81	.32	.44	.07	30	<1
378	470	5.12	126	748	1226	4.12	437	.52	12	1.76	5.45	.25	67	27
63	78	.85	21	125	204	.69	73	.09	2	.29	.91	.04	11	4
0	50	10	68	891	1722	1.59	328	1.2	22.3	1	12.97	.17	49	501

(For purposes of calculations, use "0" for t, <1, <.1, <.01, etc.)

H

Table H-1
Food Composition

Computer Code Number	Food Description	Measure	Wt (g)	H_2O (%)	Ener (kcal)	Prot (g)	Carb (g)	Dietary Fiber (g)	Fat (g)	Fat Breakdown (g) Sat	Mono	Poly
	BAKED GOODS: BREADS, CAKES, COOKIES, CRACKERS, PIES—Cont.											
462	Piece, ⅙ of pie	1 pce	158	45	426	4	63	3	19	4.4	7.9	5.3
463	Pecan: Whole pie	1 ea	825	19	3400	34	486	30	157	32	91.8	25.5
464	Piece, ⅙ of pie	1 pce	138	19	552	6	79	5	26	5.2	14.9	4.1
465	Pumpkin: Whole pie	1 ea	1240	58	2604	48	339	33	118	25	62.1	19.8
466	Piece, ⅙ of pie	1 pce	206	58	433	8	56	6	20	4.2	10.3	3.3
467	Pies, fried, commercial: Apple	1 ea	85	40	266	2	33	2	14	6.5	5.8	1.2
468	Pies, fried, commercial: Cherry	1 ea	85	40	269	3	36	2	14	2	6	4.6
	Pretzels, made with enriched flour:											
469	Thin sticks, 2¼" long	10 ea	3	3	11	<1	2	<1	<1	t	t	t
470	Dutch twists, 2¾ x 2⅝"	1 ea	16	3	61	1	13	<1	1	.1	.2	.2
471	Thin twists, 3¼ x 2¼ x ¼"	10 ea	60	3	229	5	48	2	2	.4	.8	.7
	Rolls & buns, enriched, commercial:											
472	Cloverleaf rolls, 2½" diam, 2" high	1 ea	28	32	85	2	14	1	2	.5	1.1	.3
473	Hot dog buns	1 ea	40	34	114	3	20	1	2	.5	1	.4
474	Hamburger buns	1 ea	45	34	129	4	23	1	2	.5	1.1	.4
475	Hard roll, white, 3¾" diam, 2" high	1 ea	50	31	147	5	26	1	2	.3	.6	.9
476	Submarine rolls/hoagies, 11½ x 3 x 2½"	1 ea	135	31	392	12	75	4	4	.9	1.3	1.4
	Rolls & buns, enriched, home recipe:											
477	Dinner rolls 2½" diam, 2" high	1 ea	35	29	112	3	19	1	3	.7	1.1	.7
	Sports/fitness bar:											
2043	Forza energy bar	1 ea	70	18	231	11	45	4	1	–	–	–
2042	Power bar	1 ea	65	21	230	10	45	3	3	–	–	–
2041	Tiger sports bar	1 ea	65	17	229	11	40	4	2	–	–	–
478	Toaster pastries, fortified (Poptarts)	1 ea	54	12	212	3	38	1	6	.8	2.2	2.1
2132	Toaster strudel pastry—cream cheese	1 ea	53	32	184	3	24	<1	9	2.7	–	–
2134	Toaster strudel pastry—french toast	1 ea	53	31	184	3	24	<1	9	2.8	–	–
	Tortilla chips:											
1271	Plain	1 oz	28	7	140	2	18	2	7	1.4	4.3	1
1036	Nacho flavor	1 oz	28	2	139	2	17	1	7	1.4	4.3	1
1037	Taco flavor	1 oz	28	2	134	2	18	1	7	1.3	4	1
	Tortillas:											
479	Corn, enriched, 6" diam	1 ea	30	44	67	2	14	2	1	.1	.2	.3
480	Flour, 8" diam	1 ea	35	27	115	3	20	1	3	.4	1	1
1301	Flour, 10" diam	1 ea	57	27	185	5	32	2	4	.6	1.6	1.6
481	Taco shells	1 ea	14	4	63	1	9	1	3	.4	1.5	.6
	Waffles, 7" diam:											
482	From home recipe	1 ea	75	42	218	6	25	1	11	2.1	2.6	5.1
483	From mix, egg/milk added	1 ea	75	42	218	5	26	1	10	1.7	2.7	5.2
1510	Whole grain, prepared from frozen	1 ea	39	43	107	4	13	1	5	1.6	1.9	1
	GRAIN PRODUCTS: CEREAL, FLOUR, GRAIN, PASTA and NOODLES, POPCORN											
484	Barley, pearled, dry, uncooked	1 c	200	10	704	20	155	31	2	.5	.3	1.1
485	Barley, pearled, cooked	1 c	157	69	193	4	44	6	1	.1	.1	.3
	Breakfast bars, fat free:											
2009	Apple	1 ea	38	25	110	2	26	3	0	0	0	0
2005	Chocolate	1 ea	38	23	81	2	19	3	0	0	0	0
2003	Strawberry	1 ea	38	25	110	2	26	3	0	0	0	0

(Computer code number is for West Diet Analysis program)

PAGE KEY: H–4 = BEV H–6 = DAIRY H–12 = EGGS H–14 = FAT/OIL H–18 = FRUIT H–26 = BAKERY H–36 = GRAIN H–44 = FISH H–48 = MEATS H–50 = POULTRY H–54 = SAUSAGE H–56 = MIXED/FAST H–64 = NUTS/SEEDS H–68 = SWEETS H–70 = VEG/LEG H–84 = MISC H–88 = SOUPS/SAUCES H–90 = FAST H–106 = FRZN ENTREE H–112 = BABY FOODS

Chol (mg)	Calc (mg)	Iron (mg)	Magn (mg)	Pota (mg)	Sodi (mg)	Zinc (mg)	VT-A (RE)	Thia (mg)	VT-E (α-TE)	Ribo (mg)	Niac (mg)	V-B6 (mg)	Fola (μg)	VT-C (mg)
0	8	1.7	11	149	288	.27	55	.2	3.73	.17	2	.03	8	84
272	145	8.84	153	629	3604	4.8	400	.77	20.9	1.03	2.12	.18	51	9
44	23	1.45	25	102	585	.79	65	.13	3.49	.17	.34	.03	8	2
248	744	9.8	186	1909	3496	5.58	5951	.68	20	1.9	2.32	.71	186	19
41	124	1.63	31	317	581	.93	989	.11	3.32	.31	.38	.12	31	3
13	13	.88	8	51	325	.17	8	.1	.37	.08	.98	.03	4	2
0	19	1.03	9	55	318	.19	14	.1	.37	.09	1.2	.03	3	1
0	1	.13	1	4	51	.03	0	.01	.01	.02	.16	<.01	2	0
0	6	.69	6	23	274	.14	0	.07	.03	.1	.84	.02	13	0
0	22	2.59	21	88	1029	.51	0	.28	.13	.37	3.15	.07	50	0
<1	34	.89	6	38	148	.22	0	.14	.22	.09	1.14	.01	9	<1
0	56	1.27	8	56	224	.25	0	.19	.19	.12	1.57	.02	11	0
0	63	1.43	9	63	252	.28	0	.22	.21	.14	1.77	.02	12	0
0	48	1.64	14	54	272	.47	0	.24	.09	.17	2.12	.03	8	0
0	122	3.78	27	122	783	.85	0	.54	.1	.33	4.47	.05	41	0
13	21	1.04	7	53	145	.24	28	.14	.35	.14	1.21	.02	15	<1
0	300	6.3	160	220	65	5.25	–	1.5	20	1.7	20	2	400	60
–	300	5.4	140	150	110	5.25	–	1.5	–	1.7	20	2	400	60
–	349	4.5	140	279	100	–	50	1.5	20	1.7	20	2	400	60
0	14	1.89	10	60	226	.36	57[1]	.16	1	.2	2.13	.21	43	<1
12	12	.95	–	–	213	–	17	–	.99	–	–	–	–	0
12	12	.95	–	–	213	–	17	–	.99	–	–	–	–	0
0	43	.43	25	55	148	.43	6	.02	.38	.05	.36	.08	3	0
1	41	.4	23	60	198	.34	11	.04	.38	.05	.4	.08	4	1
1	44	.57	25	61	220	.36	25	.07	.38	.06	.56	.08	6	<1
0	52	.42	20	46	48	.28	7	.03	.05	.02	.45	.07	5	0
0	44	1.17	9	46	169	.25	0	.19	.44	.1	1.26	.02	4	0
0	71	1.88	15	74	273	.4	0	.3	.72	.17	2.03	.03	7	0
0	35	.35	15	34	25	.18	6	.04	.58	.02	.24	.04	4	0
52	191	1.74	14	119	383	.51	49	.2	1.73	.26	1.55	.04	11	<1
52	93	1.23	15	134	458	.35	20	.15	1.5	.2	1.23	.08	9	<1
39	84	.7	15	91	150	.46	25	.08	.53	.13	.75	.05	7	<1
0	58	5	158	560	18	4.26	4	.38	.26	.23	9.22	.52	46	0
0	17	2.09	34	146	5	1.29	2	.13	.08	.1	3.23	.18	25	0
0	20	.72	–	160	25	–	20	.09	–	.03	.4	–	–	1
0	20	1.3	–	160	22	–	74	.09	–	.03	.4	–	–	0
0	20	.72	–	160	25	–	20	.09	–	.03	.4	–	–	1

(1)Vitamin A values from label declarations vary.

(For purposes of calculations, use "0" for t, <1, <.1, <.01, etc.)

Table H–1
Food Composition

Computer Code Number	Food Description	Measure	Wt (g)	H_2O (%)	Ener (kcal)	Prot (g)	Carb (g)	Dietary Fiber (g)	Fat (g)	Fat Breakdown (g) Sat	Mono	Poly
	GRAIN PRODUCTS: CEREAL, FLOUR, GRAIN, PASTA and NOODLES, POPCORN—Cont.											
	Breakfast bar, Snackwell											
2165	Apple-cinnamon	1 ea	37	16	119	1	29	1	<1	0.1	<.1	.1
2164	Blueberry	1 ea	37	16	121	1	29	1	<1	<.1	<.1	.1
2163	Strawberry	1 ea	37	16	120	1	29	1	<1	<.1	<.1	.1
	Breakfast cereals, hot, cooked:											
	Corn grits (hominy) enriched:											
486	Regular and quick, prepared, yellow	1 c	242	85	145	3	31	5	<1	.1	.1	.2
487	Instant, prepared from packet, white	1 ea	137	82	89	2	21	1	<1	t	t	<.1
	Cream of wheat:											
488	Regular, quick, instant	1 c	244	87	132	5	27	1	<1	.1	.1	.2
489	Mix and eat, plain, packet	1 ea	142	82	102	3	21	<1	<1	t	t	.1
1664	Farina cereal, cooked	½ c	117	87	59	2	12	2	<1	<.1	<.1	<.1
490	Malt-O-Meal	1 c	240	88	122	4	26	1	<1	t	t	.1
494	Maypo	1 c	242	83	172	6	32	6	2	.4	.8	.1
	Oatmeal or rolled oats:											
491	Regular, quick, instant, nonfort	1 c	234	85	145	6	25	4	2	.4	.7	.9
	Instant, fortified:											
492	Plain, from packet	¾ c	177	85	104	5	18	3	2	.3	.6	.7
493	Flavored, from packet	¾ c	164	76	160	5	31	3	2	.3	.7	.8
	Breakfast cereals, ready to eat:											
495	All-Bran	⅓ c	28	4	77	4	21	10	1	.2	.2	.6
1306	Alpha Bits	1 c	28	1	110	2	24	1	1	.1	.2	.2
1307	Apple Jacks	1 c	28	3	108	1	25	1	<1	.1	.1	.2
1308	Bran Buds	1 c	84	3	232	8	67	34	2	.3	.4	1.3
1305	Bran Chex	1 c	49	2	156	5	39	8	1	.2	.3	.7
1309	Honey BucWheat Crisp	¾ c	28	5	109	3	23	2	1	.2	.2	.4
1310	C. W. Post, plain	1 c	97	2	421	9	73	7	13	1.7	6	4.7
1311	C. W. Post, with raisins	1 c	103	4	446	9	74	14	15	11	1.7	1.4
496	Cap'n Crunch	1 c	37	2	147	2	32	1	2	.5	.4	.3
1312	Cap'n Crunchberries	1 c	38	2	152	2	33	1	2	.5	.4	.3
1313	Cap'n Crunch, peanut butter	1 c	38	2	158	3	30	1	3	.7	1.2	.7
497	Cheerios	1 c	23	3	84	2	18	2	1	.3	.5	.2
1314	Cocoa Krispies	1 c	36	2	140	2	32	<1	1	.1	.2	.2
1316	Cocoa Pebbles	1 c	31	2	127	1	27	<1	2	1	.4	.1
1315	Corn Bran	1 c	36	3	120	2	30	6	1	.3	.3	.4
1317	Corn Chex	1 c	28	2	110	2	25	<1	1	.1	.2	<.1
498	Corn Flakes, Kellogg's	1¼ c	28	3	102	2	24	1	<1	t	t	t
499	Corn Flakes, Post Toasties	1¼ c	28	3	108	2	24	1	<1	t	t	t
1340	Corn Pops	1 c	28	3	107	1	26	<1	<1	.1	.1	<.1
1318	Cracklin' Oat Bran	1 c	60	4	245	5	44	7	8	3.2	3.5	.8
1038	Crispy Wheat 'N Raisins	1 c	43	7	150	3	35	3	1	.1	.1	.2
1319	Fortified Oat Flakes	1 c	48	3	181	8	36	1	1	.2	.3	.4
500	40% Bran Flakes, Kellogg's	1 c	39	3	127	4	31	6	1	.1	.1	.5
501	40% Bran Flakes, Post	1 c	47	3	152	5	37	9	1	.12	.1	.3
502	Froot Loops	1 c	28	2	111	1	25	1	1	.3	.2	.2
518	Frosted Flakes	1 c	35	3	132	1	32	1	<1	t	t	t
1320	Frosted Mini-Wheats	4 ea	31	5	105	3	26	3	<1	.1	.1	.3
1321	Frosted Rice Krispies	1 c	28	3	106	1	25	<1	<1	.1	.1	.1
1324	Fruit & Fibre w/dates	½ c	28	9	95	2	21	4	1	.2	.6	.5
1325	Fruitful Bran	¾ c	34	1	111	3	27	5	<1	<.1	<.1	.1

(Computer code number is for West Diet Analysis program)

Chol (mg)	Calc (mg)	Iron (mg)	Magn (mg)	Pota (mg)	Sodi (mg)	Zinc (mg)	VT-A (RE)	Thia (mg)	VT-E (α-TE)	Ribo (mg)	Niac (mg)	V-B6 (mg)	Fola (μg)	VT-C (mg)
<1	17	5	6	68	103	3.88	–	.39	–	.44	5.2	.52	–	<1
<1	14	4.83	5	44	107	3.85	–	.39	–	.44	5.2	.52	–	<1
<1	14	4.82	6	47	102	3.83	–	.39	–	.44	5.2	.52	–	2
0	0	1.55[1]	10	53	0[2]	.17	15[3]	.24[1]	.12	.14[1]	1.96[1]	.06	2	0
0	8	8.19[1]	11	29	289	.21	0	.15[1]	.03	.08[1]	1.3[1]	.05	1	0
0	51[1]	10.5[1]	12	46	141[4]	.34	0	.24[1]	.03	0[1]	1.46[1]	.03	10	0
0	20[1]	8.09[1]	7	38	241[5]	.24	376[1]	.43[1]	.02	.28[1]	4.97[1]	.57	101	0
0	2	.59	2	15	0[5]	.08	0	.09	.02	.06	.64	.01	2	0
0	5	9.6[1]	5	31	2[5]	.17	0	.48[1]	.03	.24[1]	5.76[1]	.02	5	0
0	126	8.47	51	213	261	1.5	709	.73	1.7	.73	9.44	.97	10	29
0	19	1.59	56	131	2[5]	1.15	5	.26	.23	.05	.3	.05	9	0
0	162[1]	6.3[1]	42	99	285[1]	.87	453[1]	.53[1]	.21	.28[1]	5.47[1]	.74	150	0
0	168[1]	7[1]	51	137	254[1]	1	460[1]	.53[1]	.21	.38[1]	5.9[1]	.76	150	0
0	100	4.26[1]	122	284	261	3.6	213[1]	.37[1]	.52	.39[1]	5[1]	.48	100	14[1]
0	8	2.7	17	54	178	1.48	371	.37	.02	.42	5	.5	99	0
0	3	4.2	8	23	125	3.5	210	.37	.05	.39	5	.48	99	14
0	56	12.6	234	755	559	18.06	631	1.09	1.33	1.2	14.03	1.43	252	42
0	29	14	69	216	346	6.5	11	.64	.56	.26	8.62	.88	173	26
0	40	8.12	32	105	266	.5	673	.67	6.62	.76	9	1.4	8	27
<1	47	15.4	67	198	167	1.64	1284	1.26	.68	1.46	17.1	1.75	342	0
<1	50	16.4	74	261	161	1.64	1363	1.34	.72	1.55	18.1	1.85	363	0
0	7	6.18[1]	13	47	285	5	5[1]	.5[1]	.18	.58[1]	6.85[1]	1	137	0
0	10	6.6	14	54	278	5.85	7	.55	.27	.62	7.3	.73	146	<1
0	4	6	26	87	287	5.28	5	.53	.21	.6	7.03	.7	141	0
0	42	6.2[1]	25	68	218	2.87	288	.28[1]	.16	.33[1]	3.84[1]	.38	77	12[1]
0	5	2.09	13	70	244	1.7	261	.43	.17	.5	5.8	.58	108	17
0	5	1.95	13	51	175	1.64	410	.4	.04	.47	5.5	.56	109	0
0	27	10	19	75	338	5	5	.1	.19	.6	6.7	.67	134	0
0	3	8	4	23	306	.1	14	.37	.07	.07	5	.5	99	15
0	1	8.68[1]	3	25	298	.16	210[1]	.36[1]	.03	.39[1]	4.68[1]	.48	99	15[1]
0	1	.74[1]	4	32	293	.08	371[1]	.36[1]	.07	.42[1]	4.93[1]	.5	99	0
0	2	1.7	2	20	111	1.4	210	.36	.03	.39	5	.48	99	14
0	27	2.2	83	278	213	1.8	276	.5	.4	.5	6.12	.6	167	18
0	54	3.52	33	180	223	.85	293	.29	.45	.33	3.9	.39	78	0
0	68	13.7	58	228	220	2.5	636	.62	.34	.72	8.45	.86	169	0
0	19	11[1]	81	236	304	5.03	488[1]	.51[1]	7.22	.58[1]	6.7[1]	.66	138	20
0	21	13.44[1]	102	251	431	2.49	622[1]	.61[1]	.54	.7[1]	8.27[1]	.85	166	0
0	3	4[1]	8	30	133	3.55	200[1]	.37[1]	.1	.4[1]	5[1]	.48	85	13[1]
0	1	5.25[1]	3	23	228	.18	263[1]	.45[1]	.05	.49[1]	5.85[1]	.6	124	18[1]
0	11	9.15	31	103	1	.84	0	.2	.28	.25	2.8	.28	58	0
0	2	1.93	7	22	205	.34	243	.39	.03	.45	5	.53	112	16
0	15	5	40	165	132	1.48	356	.37	.65	.42	5	.5	99	0
0	18	4	52	212	203	1	208	.35	.61	.4	5	.46	92	<1

(1)Nutrient added (values sometimes based on label declaration).

(2)Cooked without salt. If salt is added according to label recommendation, sodium content is 540 mg.

(3)Value for yellow corn grits; cooked white corn grits contain 0 RE of vitamin A.

(4)Values for quick cereal.

(5)Cooked without salt. If added according to label recommendations, sodium content is 390 mg for Cream of Wheat; 324 mg for Malt-O-Meal; 374 mg for oatmeal; 385 mg for Farina.

(For purposes of calculations, use "0" for t, <1, <.1, <.01, etc.)

H

Table H-1
Food Composition

Computer Code Number	Food Description	Measure	Wt (g)	H_2O (%)	Ener (kcal)	Prot (g)	Carb (g)	Dietary Fiber (g)	Fat (g)	Fat Breakdown (g) Sat	Mono	Poly
	GRAIN PRODUCTS: CEREAL, FLOUR, GRAIN, PASTA and NOODLES, POPCORN—Cont.											
	Breakfast cereals, ready to eat—Cont.											
1322	Fruity Pebbles	1 c	32	3	130	1	28	<1	2	1.4	.1	.1
503	Golden Grahams	1 c	39	3	150	2	33	1	1	.2	.4	.2
504	Granola, homemade	½ c	61	5	285	9	32	6	15	2.9	4.8	6.5
1670	Granola, low fat, commercial	½ c	47	5	173	4	37	3	2	1	1	1
505	Grape Nuts	½ c	57	3	203	7	47	6	<1	t	t	.1
1326	Grape Nuts Flakes	1 c	32	3	118	4	26	3	1	.1	.1	.2
1665	Heartland Natural with raisins	1 c	101	5	429	10	70	6	14	3.7	3.9	5.7
1327	Honey & Nut Corn Flakes	1 c	38	4	154	3	32	1	2	.3	.7	.6
506	Honey Nut Cheerios	1 c	33	2	128	3	27	2	1	.3	.5	.2
1328	HoneyBran	1 c	35	3	119	3	29	4	1	.3	.1	.3
1329	HoneyComb	1 c	22	1	86	1	20	<1	<1	.2	.1	.1
1330	King Vitaman	1 c	19	2	73	1	16	1	1	.2	.3	.2
1039	Kix	1 c	19	2	73	1	16	<1	<1	.1	.1	<.1
1331	Life	1 c	43	4	163	4	34	3	2	.3	.6	.8
507	Lucky Charms	1 c	32	2	124	2	27	1	1	.2	.4	.2
1323	Mueslix Five Grain	1 c	82	5	279	7	63	7	3	.5	1	1.2
1416	Granola, low-fat	⅓ c	31	3	119	3	25	2	2	0	–	–
508	Nature Valley Granola	1 c	113	4	510	12	74	7	20	2.6	13	3.8
1666	Nutri Grain Almond Raisin	⅔ c	40	6	147	3	31	3	3	.1	1	1.2
1333	Nutri-Grain—corn	1 c	42	3	160	3	35	3	1	.1	.5	.2
1336	100% Bran	1 c	66	3	178	8	48	20	3	.6	.6	1.9
509	100% Natural cereal, plain	½ c	57	3	252	6	39	4	9	4	4.1	1.2
1337	100% Natural with apples & cinnamon	1 c	104	2	477	11	70	7	20	15.5	1.8	1.3
1338	100% Natural with raisins & dates	1 c	110	3	496	11	72	7	20	13.6	3.7	1.7
510	Product 19	1 c	33	4	121	3	28	1	<1	t	.1	.2
1339	Quisp	1 c	30	3	121	2	25	<1	2	.5	.4	.2
511	Raisin Bran, Kellogg's	1 c	49	9	158	5	38	6	1	.12	.1	.3
512	Raisin Bran, Post	1 c	56	9	172	5	42	8	1	.2	.1	.5
1667	Raisin Squares	½ c	28	10	95	2	22	3	1	.1	.1	.3
1041	Rice Chex	¾ c	19	3	75	1	17	<1	1	<.1	.2	<.1
513	Rice Krispies, Kellogg's	1 c	29	2	114	2	26	<1	<1	t	t	t
514	Rice, puffed	1 c	14	4	53	1	12	<1	<1	t	t	t
515	Shredded Wheat	1 c	43	5	154	5	34	4	1	.1	.1	.4
516	Special K	1 c	21	3	78	4	15	1	<1	t	t	.1
517	Super Golden Crisp	1 c	33	1	123	3	30	<1	<1	t	t	.1
519	Honey Smacks	1 c	38	3	144	2	33	1	1	.4	.1	.3
1341	Tasteeos	1 c	24	2	94	3	19	3	1	.2	.2	.2
1342	Team	1 c	42	4	164	3	36	<1	1	.1	.2	.3
520	Total, wheat, with added calcium	1 c	33	3	116	3	26	3	1	.1	.1	.1
521	Trix	1 c	28	2	114	1	24	<1	2	.4	.9	.3
1344	Wheat Chex	1 c	46	2	169	5	38	4	1	.2	.1	.5

(Computer code number is for West Diet Analysis program)

PAGE KEY: H–4 = BEV H–6 = DAIRY H–12 = EGGS H–14 = FAT/OIL H–18 = FRUIT H–26 = BAKERY H–36 = GRAIN H–44 = FISH H–48 = MEATS H–50 = POULTRY H–54 = SAUSAGE H–56 = MIXED/FAST H–64 = NUTS/SEEDS H–68 = SWEETS H–70 = VEG/LEG H–84 = MISC H–88 = SOUPS/SAUCES H–90 = FAST H–106 = FRZN ENTREE H–112 = BABY FOODS

Chol (mg)	Calc (mg)	Iron (mg)	Magn (mg)	Pota (mg)	Sodi (mg)	Zinc (mg)	VT-A (RE)	Thia (mg)	VT-E (α-TE)	Ribo (mg)	Niac (mg)	V-B6 (mg)	Fola (μg)	VT-C (mg)
0	4	2.02	9	24	178	1.7	424	.42	.03	.48	5.6	.58	113	0
0	19	5.86[1]	12	69	357	4.88	293[1]	.49[1]	.29	.55[1]	6.5[1]	.7	130	19[1]
0	49	2.56[1]	109	328	15	2.47	2	.45	7.87	.17	1.25	.2	52	1
0	21	1.65	39	133	106	2.96	176	.28	4.74	.33	3.9	.38	94	0
0	5	16[1]	38	190	396	1.25	755[1]	.74[1]	.14	.85[1]	10.03[1]	1.03	201	0
0	13	9.15	35	114	181	.64	424	.42	.08	.48	5.6	.58	113	0
0	61	3.7	129	381	207	2.6	6	.29	.71	.13	1.41	.18	40	1
0	4	3.12	3	41	256	.27	159	.27	.1	.3	3.46	.34	76	10
0	23	5	33	95	288	4.17	250[1]	.42[1]	.34	.5[1]	5.57[1]	.6	111	17[1]
0	16	5.57	46	151	202	.9	463	.46	.81	.53	6.16	.63	23	19
0	4	2.09	7	25	124	1.17	291	.29	.09	.33	3.87	.4	78	0
0	2	5.36	16	52	159	2.39	192	.24	1.29	.27	3.2	.32	64	8
0	28	5.13	6	26	167	2.34	238	.24	.05	.27	3.17	.32	63	10
0	131	12	42	106	234	5.4	2	.54	.22	.61	7.2	.71	144	0
0	35	4.79[1]	21	58	217	4	240	.4[1]	.14	.45[1]	5.34[1]	.53	107	16[1]
0	38	8.94	82	369	107	7.46	747	.75	8.94	.84	9.84	.99	197	1
0	–	1.8	24	94	60	3.72	149	.37	4.99	.42	4.96	.5	100	–
0	85	3.53	107	375	183	2.27	0	.4	7.97	.12	1.25	.16	17	0
0	122	1	9	143	142	2.72	0	.28	4	.32	4	.36	80	0
0	1	.89	27	98	276	5.54	556	.55	11.1	.63	7.39	.76	148	22
0	46	8.12	312	652	457	5.74	0	1.58	1.53	1.78	20.9	2.11	47	63
<1	55	1.7	60	281	15	1.36	<1	.2	.65	.09	1	.1	14	<1
1	157	2.9	72	514	52	2	6	.33	.73	.57	1.87	.11	17	1
1	159	3.12	124	537	47	2.11	6	.31	.77	.65	2.09	.16	45	0
0	3	20[1]	14	57	310	16.5	248[1]	1.65[1]	24.4	1.88[1]	22[1]	2.21	466	66[1]
0	6	5.1	15	40	216	4.26	4	.42	.16	.48	5.67	.56	113	0
0	32	4[1]	72	281	314	3	200[1]	.34[1]	.45	.39[1]	4.46[1]	.44	91	0
0	26	8.9[1]	95	355	365	2.97	741[1]	.73[1]	1.3	.84[1]	9.86[1]	1.01	197	0
0	10	8.6[1]	24	132	2	.78	0	.2	.15	.22	3	.3	56	0
0	3	5.4[1]	5	22	159	.26	1	.25	.02	.01	3.34	.34	67	10
0	5	.73[1]	12	28	213	.49	384[1]	.54[1]	.03	.6[1]	7.16[1]	.72	143	15[1]
0	1	.4[1]	4	16	<1	.15	0	.01[1]	.01	.01[1]	.38[1]	0	1	0
0	16	1.8	57	155	4	1.41	0	.11	.23	.12	2.26	.11	22	0
0	3	5.69[1]	12	37	196	2.5	153[1]	.35[1]	.05	.39[1]	4.75	.48	63	10[1]
0	7	2.08[1]	20	48	51	1.75	437[1]	.43[1]	.12	.49[1]	5.81[1]	.59	117	0
0	4	2.53[1]	22	59	71	.49	316[1]	.53[1]	.2	.6	7[1]	.72	140	21[1]
0	11	6.86[1]	26	71	182	.69	318	.31	.17	.36	4.22	.43	85	13
0	6	12[1]	12	71	260	.58	556	.55	.1	.63	7.39	.76	7	22
0	284	20[1]	35	107	219	16.5	413[1]	1.65[1]	25.8	1.87[1]	22.1	2.2	440	66
0	30	4.2[1]	3	17	184	3.49	210[1]	.35[1]	.56	.39[1]	5[1]	.47	93	14[1]
0	18	13.16[1]	58	173	308	1.23	0	.6	.17	.17	8.1	.83	162	24

(1)Nutrient added (values sometimes based on label declaration).

(For purposes of calculations, use "0" for t, <1, <.1, <.01, etc.)

Table H-1
Food Composition

Computer Code Number	Food Description	Measure	Wt (g)	H_2O (%)	Ener (kcal)	Prot (g)	Carb (g)	Dietary Fiber (g)	Fat (g)	Fat Breakdown (g) Sat	Mono	Poly
	GRAIN PRODUCTS: CEREAL, FLOUR, GRAIN, PASTA and NOODLES, POPCORN—Cont.											
1043	Wheat cereal, puffed, fortified	1 c	12	4	44	2	10	1	<1	<.1	<.1	.1
522	Wheaties	1 c	29	3	106	3	23	2	1	.1	.2	.1
	Buckwheat flour:											
523	Dark	1 c	98	11	328	12	69	10	3	.7	.9	.9
524	Light	1 c	98	12	340	6	78	6	1	.2	.4	.4
525	Buckwheat, whole grain, dry	1 c	175	10	600	23	125	18	6	1.3	1.8	1.8
526	Bulgar, dry, uncooked	1 c	140	9	479	17	106	26	2	.3	.2	.8
527	Bulgar, cooked	1 c	182	78	151	6	34	8	<1	<.1	<.1	.2
	Cornmeal:											
528	Whole-ground, unbolted, dry	1 c	122	10	442	10	94	10	4	.6	1.2	2
529	Bolted, nearly whole, dry	1 c	122	10	441	10	94	12	4	.6	1.2	2
530	Degermed, enriched, dry	1 c	138	12	505	12	107	10	2	.3	.6	1
531	Degermed, enriched, cooked	1 c	240	78	209	5	44	4	1	.1	.2	.4
	Macaroni, cooked:											
532	Enriched	1 c	140	66	197	7	40	2	1	.1	.1	.4
533	Whole wheat	1 c	140	67	174	7	37	4	1	.1	.1	.3
534	Vegetable, enriched	1 c	134	68	172	6	36	2	<1	t	t	.1
535	Millet, cooked	½ c	120	71	143	4	28	2	1	.2	.2	.6
	Noodles (see also Pasta and Spaghetti)											
1507	Cellophane noodles, cooked	1 c	190	79	160	<1	39	<1	<1	<.1	<.1	<.1
1995	Cellophane noodles, dry	½ c	70	13	246	<1	60	<1	<1	<.1	<.1	<.1
537	Chow mein, dry	1 c	45	1	237	4	26	2	14	2	3.5	7.8
536	Egg noodles, cooked, enriched	1 c	160	69	213	8	40	2	2	.5	.7	.7
538	Spinach noodles, dry	3½ oz	100	8	372	13	75	11	2	.2	.2	.6
1343	Oat bran, dry	¼ c	23	7	57	4	15	4	2	.3	.6	.6
	Pasta, cooked:											
1418	Fresh	2 oz	57	69	75	3	14	1	1	.1	.1	.2
1417	Linguini	1 c	140	66	197	7	40	4	1	.1	.1	.4
1598	Rotini	1 c	140	66	197	7	40	2	1	.1	.1	.4
	Popcorn:											
539	Air popped, plain	1 c	8	4	31	1	6	1	<1	<.1	.1	.2
1042	Microwaved, low fat, low sodium	1 c	6	3	24	1	4	1	1	.1	.2	.3
540	Popped in vegetable oil/salted	1 c	11	2	55	1	6	1	3	.5	.9	1.5
541	Sugar-syrup coated	1 c	35	2	151	1	28	2	4	1.3	1	1.6
	Rice:											
542	Brown rice, cooked	1 c	195	73	216	5	45	4	2	.4	.6	.6
2215	Mexican rice, cooked	½ c	113	–	410	8	90	3	15	2	.1	.1
2216	Spanish rice, cooked	½ c	123	85	65	2	14	1	1	–	–	–
	White, enriched, all types:											
543	Regular/long grain, dry	1 c	185	11	675	13	148	2	1	.3	.4	.3
544	Regular/long grain, cooked	1 c	205	68	267	6	58	1	<1	.2	.2	.2
545	Instant, prepared without salt	1 c	165	76	161	3	35	1	<1	.1	.1	.1

(Computer code number is for West Diet Analysis program)

PAGE KEY: H–4 = BEV H–6 = DAIRY H–12 = EGGS H–14 = FAT/OIL H–18 = FRUIT H–26 = BAKERY H–36 = GRAIN H–44 = FISH H–48 = MEATS H–50 = POULTRY H–54 = SAUSAGE H–56 = MIXED/FAST H–64 = NUTS/SEEDS H–68 = SWEETS H–70 = VEG/LEG H–84 = MISC H–88 = SOUPS/SAUCES H–90 = FAST H–106 = FRZN ENTREE H–112 = BABY FOODS

Chol (mg)	Calc (mg)	Iron (mg)	Magn (mg)	Pota (mg)	Sodi (mg)	Zinc (mg)	VT-A (RE)	Thia (mg)	VT-E (α-TE)	Ribo (mg)	Niac (mg)	V-B6 (mg)	Fola (μg)	VT-C (mg)
0	3	.57	17	44	1	.37	<.1	.05	.08	.03	1.4	.02	4	0
0	53	7.83[1]	31	101	215	.69	218[1]	.36[1]	.36	.41[1]	4.8[1]	.48	97	15[1]
0	40	3.98	246	566	11	3.06	0	.41	1.01	.19	6.03	.57	53	0
0	11	1	47	314	1	2.56	0	.09	.5	.05	.47	.09	100	0
0	31	3.85	404	805	2	4.2	0	.18	1.8	.74	12.3	.37	52	0
0	49	3.44	230	574	24	2.7	0	.32	.22	.16	7.15	.48	38	0
0	18	1.75	58	124	9	1.04	0	.1	.05	.05	1.82	.15	33	0
0	7	4.21	155	350	43	2.22	57	.47	.82	.24	4.43	.37	31	0
0	7	4.21	154	350	43	2.22	57	.37	.96	.1	2.3	.37	31	0
0	7	5.7	55	224	4	.99	57	.99	.46	.56	6.94	.35	66	0
0	3	2.35	22	91	1	.41	23	.3	.21	.21	2.42	.12	22	0
0	10	1.96	25	43	1	.74	0	.29	.04	.14	2.34	.05	10	0
0	21	1.48	42	62	4	1.13	0	.15	.14	.06	.99	.11	7	0
0	15	.66	25	42	8	.59	7	.15	.05	.08	1.43	.03	8	0
0	4	.76	53	74	2	1.09	0	.13	.22	.1	1.6	.13	23	0
0	14	1	3	5	9	.23	0	.07	.06	0	.09	.02	1	0
0	18	1.52	2	7	7	.29	0	.11	.09	0	.14	.04	1	0
0	18	2.13	23	54	198	.63	4	.26	.07	.19	2.7	.05	10	0
53	19	2.54	30	45	11	.99	10	.3	.08	.13	2.38	.06	11	0
0	58	2.13	174	376	36	2.76	46	.37	.04	.2	4.55	.32	48	0
0	13	1.27	54	130	1	.72	0	.27	.39	.05	.22	.04	12	0
19	3	.65	10	14	3	.32	3	.12	.09	.09	.56	.02	4	0
0	10	1.96	25	43	1	.74	0	.29	.08	.14	2.34	.05	10	0
0	10	1.96	25	43	1	.74	0	.29	.04	.14	2.34	.05	10	0
0	1	.21	11	24	<1	.27	2	.02	.01	.02	.15	.02	2	0
0	1	.14	9	14	29	.22	1	.02	.06	.01	.12	.01	1	0
0	1	.31	12	25	97	.29	2	.01	.03	.01	.17	.02	2	<1
2	15	.61	12	38	72	.2	4	.02	.42	.02	.77	.01	1	0
0	20	.82	84	84	10	1.23	0	.19	5.3	.05	2.98	.28	8	0
0	150	4.5	–	–	1350	–	–	–	–	–	–	–	–	48
0	–	.36	–	–	670	–	–	–	–	–	–	–	–	–
0	52	8	46	213	9	2.02	0	1.07	.24	.09	7.75	.3	15	0
0	20	2.46	25	72	2	1	0	.33	.1	.03	3.03	.19	6	0
0	13	1.04	8	7	5[2]	.4	0	.12	.08	.08	1.45	.02	7	0

(1)Nutrient added (values sometimes based on label declaration).

(2)If prepared with salt according to label recommendation, sodium would be 608 mg.

(Computer code number is for West Diet Analysis program)

Table H-1
Food Composition

Computer Code Number	Food Description	Measure	Wt (g)	H_2O (%)	Ener (kcal)	Prot (g)	Carb (g)	Dietary Fiber (g)	Fat (g)	Fat Breakdown (g) Sat	Mono	Poly
	GRAIN PRODUCTS: CEREAL, FLOUR, GRAIN, PASTA and NOODLES, POPCORN—Cont.											
	Parboiled/converted rice:											
546	Raw, dry	1 c	185	10	686	13	151	3	1	.3	.3	.3
547	Cooked	1 c	175	73	200	4	43	1	<1	.1	.1	.1
1486	Sticky rice (glutinous), cooked	1 c	241	77	234	5	51	2	<1	.1	.2	.2
548	Wild rice, cooked	1 c	164	73	166	7	35	3	1	.1	.1	.4
1700	Rice and pasta (Rice-a-Roni), cooked	½ c	109	72	133	3	23	1	3	.6	1.2	1
549	Rye flour, medium	1 c	102	10	361	10	79	15	2	.2	.2	.8
1044	Soy flour, low-fat	1 c	88	2	325	45	30	9	6	.9	1.3	3.3
	Spaghetti pasta:											
550	Without salt, enriched	1 c	140	66	197	7	40	4	1	.1	.1	.4
551	With salt, enriched	1 c	140	66	197	7	40	2	1	.1	.1	.4
552	Whole-wheat spaghetti, cooked	1 c	140	67	174	7	37	6	1	.1	.1	.3
1302	Tapioca, pearl, dry	1 c	152	11	544	<1	134	1	<1	.01	.01	.01
553	Wheat bran, crude	½ c	30	10	65	5	19	13	1	.2	.2	.7
554	Wheat germ, raw	1 c	100	11	360	23	52	13	10	1.7	1.4	6
555	Wheat germ, toasted	1 c	113	5	432	33	56	15	12	2.1	1.7	7.5
1669	Wheat germ, with brown sugar & honey	½ c	57	3	212	15	33	6	4	.8	.6	2.8
556	Rolled wheat, cooked	1 c	240	83	149	5	33	4	1	.1	.1	.5
557	Whole-grain wheat, cooked	⅓ c	50	86	28	1	7	1	<1	t	t	.1
	Wheat flour (unbleached):											
	All-purpose white, enriched:											
558	Sifted	1 c	115	11	419	12	88	3	1	.2	.1	.5
559	Unsifted	1 c	125	11	455	13	95	3	1	.2	.1	.5
560	Cake or pastry, enriched, sifted	1 c	96	12	348	8	75	2	1	.1	.1	.4
561	Self-rising, enriched, unsifted	1 c	125	11	443	12	93	3	1	.2	.1	.5
562	Whole wheat, from hard wheats	1 c	120	10	406	16	87	15	2	.4	.3	.9
	MEATS: FISH and SHELLFISH											
1045	Bass, baked or broiled	4 oz	113	69	165	27	0	0	5	1.4	1.5	2.3
1046	Bluefish, baked or broiled	4 oz	113	63	180	29	0	0	6	1.4	2	2.7
1047	Bluefish, fried in bread crumbs	4 oz	113	61	232	26	5	<1	11	2.4	4.9	2.8
1686	Catfish, breaded/flour fried	4 oz	113	49	325	21	14	1	20	5	9	5
	Clams:											
563	Raw meat only	4 oz	113	81	84	14	3	0	1	.2	.3	.5
564	Canned, drained	4 oz	113	72	168	29	6	0	2	.5	.6	1.1
1290	Steamed, meat only	20 ea	90	64	133	23	5	0	2	.4	.5	.8
	Cod:											
565	Baked with butter	4 oz	113	75	150	26	0	0	4	.4	.3	.6
566	Batter fried	4 oz	113	76	196	20	8	<1	9	2.2	3.6	2.6
567	Poached, no added fat	4 oz	113	77	116	25	0	0	1	.2	.1	.3
	Crab, meat only:											
1048	Blue crab, cooked	4 oz	113	77	115	23	0	0	2	.3	.3	.8
1049	Dungeness crab, cooked	4 oz	113	73	124	25	1	0	1	.2	.2	.5
568	Blue crab, canned	4 oz	113	76	112	23	0	0	1	.3	.2	.5
1587	Crab, imitation, from surimi	4 oz	113	74	115	14	12	0	1	.3	.2	.8
569	Fish sticks, breaded pollock	2 ea	57	46	155	9	14	<1	7	1.8	2.9	1.8
	Flounder/sole, baked w/lemon juice:											
570	With butter	4 oz	113	73	160	21	<1	0	8	4.3	2	.7
571	With margarine	4 oz	113	73	160	21	<1	0	8	1.6	3.1	2.5

(Computer code number is for West Diet Analysis program)

PAGE KEY: H–4 = BEV H–6 = DAIRY H–12 = EGGS H–14 = FAT/OIL H–18 = FRUIT H–26 = BAKERY H–36 = GRAIN H–44 = FISH H–48 = MEATS H–50 = POULTRY H–54 = SAUSAGE H–56 = MIXED/FAST H–64 = NUTS/SEEDS H–68 = SWEETS H–70 = VEG/LEG H–84 = MISC H–88 = SOUPS/SAUCES H–90 = FAST H–106 = FRZN ENTREE H–112 = BABY FOODS

Chol (mg)	Calc (mg)	Iron (mg)	Magn (mg)	Pota (mg)	Sodi (mg)	Zinc (mg)	VT-A (RE)	Thia (mg)	VT-E (α-TE)	Ribo (mg)	Niac (mg)	V-B6 (mg)	Fola (μg)	VT-C (mg)
0	111	6.6	57	222	9	1.78	0	1.1	.24	.13	6.71	.65	31	0
0	33	1.98	21	65	5	.54	0	.44	.09	.03	2.45	.03	7	0
0	5	.34	12	24	12	.99	0	.05	.1	.03	.7	.06	2	0
0	5	.98	52	166	5	2.2	0	.08	.38	.14	2.12	.22	43	0
1	9	1.02	13	46	619	.31	0	.13	.15	.08	1.94	.11	8	<1
0	24	2.16	76	347	3	2.03	0	.29	1.4	.12	1.76	.27	19	0
0	165	5.27	201	2261	16	1.04	4	.33	.2	.25	1.9	.46	361	0
0	10	1.96	25	43	1	.74	0	.29	.08	.14	2.34	.05	10	0
0	10	1.96	25	43	140	.74	0	.29	.38	.14	2.34	.05	10	0
0	21	1.48	42	62	4	1.13	0	.15	.07	.06	.99	.11	7	0
0	30	2.4	2	17	2	.18	0	.01	0	0	0	.01	6	0
0	22	3.18	183	355	1	2.18	0	.16	.7	.17	4.08	.39	24	0
0	39	6.26	239	892	12	12.3	0	1.88	18	.5	6.81	1.3	281	0
0	51	10.3	362	1070	5	18.8	0	1.89	20.5	.93	6.32	1.11	398	7
0	29	4.59	155	550	6	7.92	6	.76	12.54	.39	2.7	.29	190	0
0	17	1.49	53	170	0	1.15	0	.17	.48	.12	2.14	.17	26	0
0	3	.29	12	33	<1	.24	0	.04	.1	.01	.5	.03	4	0
0	17	5.34	25	123	2	.8	0	.9	.07	.57	6.79	.05	30	0
0	19	5.8	27	133	2	.87	0	.98	.08	.62	7.38	.05	32	0
0	13	7	15	101	2	.6	0	.36	.06	.4	6.5	.03	18	0
0	422	5.84	24	155	1588	.77	0	.84	.08	.52	7.29	.06	53	0
0	41	4.66	166	486	6	3.52	0	.54	1.48	.26	7.64	.41	53	0
98	116	2.16	43	515	102	.94	40	.1	.84	.1	1.72	.16	19	2
86	10	.7	47	539	87	1.18	156	.08	.71	.11	8.19	.52	2	0
68	9	.6	42	468	76	1.02	136	.07	2.6	.09	6.22	.41	2	<1
92	41	1.44	34	376	598	1.03	33	.4	2.48	.19	3.4	.21	19	1
38	52	15.9	10	355	63	1.54	102	.09	1.13	.24	2	.07	18	15
76	104	31.6	20	712	127	3.1	194	.17	2.15	.48	3.79	.12	33	25
60	83	25.2	16	565	101	2.46	154	.13	1.8	.38	3.02	.1	26	20
68	23	.56	48	277	254	.66	34	.1	.41	.09	2.85	.32	11	<1
64	43	.9	36	443	124	.61	17	.12	.92	.13	2.58	.23	10	1
61	23	.54	41	496	69	.64	14	.09	.32	.08	2.48	.28	8	1
113	118	1.03	37	367	315	4.79	2	.11	1.13	.06	3.74	.2	57	4
86	67	.49	66	461	427	6.21	35	.06	1.3	.23	4.11	.2	47	4
100	114	.95	44	423	376	4.56	2	.09	1.13	.09	1.55	.17	48	3
23	15	.44	49	102	951	.37	23	.04	.12	.03	.2	.03	2	0
64	11	.42	14	149	331	.38	18	.07	.78	.1	1.21	.03	10	0
91	21	.37	67	363	193	.71	72	.09	2.5	.13	2.47	.27	13	1
73	21	.37	67	364	201	.71	92	.09	3.12	.13	2.47	.27	13	1

(For purposes of calculations, use "0" for t, <1, <.1, <.01, etc.)

Table H–1
Food Composition

Computer Code Number	Food Description	Measure	Wt (g)	H_2O (%)	Ener (kcal)	Prot (g)	Carb (g)	Dietary Fiber (g)	Fat (g)	Fat Breakdown (g) Sat	Mono	Poly
	MEATS: FISH and SHELLFISH—Cont.											
572	Without added fat	4 oz	113	73	133	27	0	0	2	.5	.4	.9
1599	Grouper, baked or broiled	4 oz	113	73	133	28	0	0	1	.4	.4	.6
573	Haddock, breaded, fried[1]	4 oz	113	55	264	22	14	1	13	3.2	5.4	3.3
1050	Haddock, smoked	4 oz	113	72	131	28	0	0	1	.3	.3	.5
	Halibut:											
574	Baked with butter & lemon juice	4 oz	113	69	186	29	0	0	7	2.7	2.1	1.1
1051	Smoked	1 oz	28	49	63	6	0	0	4	.7	1.3	1.9
1054	Raw	4 oz	113	78	124	24	0	0	3	.7	.8	1.1
575	Herring, pickled	3 oz	85	55	223	12	8	0	15	3.3	8.3	3.6
1052	Lobster meat, cooked w/moist heat	1 c	145	76	142	30	2	0	1	.2	.2	.5
1687	Ocean perch, baked/broiled	4 oz	113	73	137	27	0	0	2	.4	1	.7
576	Ocean perch, breaded/fried	4 oz	113	59	249	22	9	<1	13	3.2	5.7	3.4
1056	Octopus, raw	4 oz	113	80	93	17	3	0	1	.3	.2	.3
	Oysters:											
577	Raw, Eastern	1 c	248	85	169	17	10	0	6	2	.9	2.9
578	Raw, Pacific	1 c	248	82	201	23	12	0	6	1.3	.9	2.2
	Cooked:											
579	Eastern, breaded, fried, medium	6 ea	88	65	173	8	10	<1	11	3.2	2	5.6
580	Western, simmered	4 oz	113	64	184	21	11	0	5	1.7	.8	2.4
581	Pollock, baked or broiled	4 oz	113	74	128	27	0	0	1	.3	.2	.6
1055	Pollock, moist heat, poached	4 oz	113	74	128	27	0	0	1	.3	.2	.6
	Salmon:											
582	Canned pink, solids and liquid	4 oz	113	69	157	22	0	0	7	1.7	2.1	2.3
583	Broiled or baked	4 oz	113	62	244	31	0	0	12	2.2	6	2.7
584	Smoked	4 oz	113	72	132	21	0	0	5	1	2.3	1.1
585	Atlantic sardines, canned, drained, 2 = 24 g	4 oz	113	60	235	28	0	0	13	1.9	4.4	6.4
586	Scallops, breaded, cooked from frozen	6 ea	93	58	199	17	9	<1	10	2.1	2.5	5.3
1588	Scallops, imitation, from surimi	4 oz	113	74	112	14	12	0	<1	.1	.1	.3
1688	Scallops, steamed/boiled	½ c	60	76	64	10	1	0	2	.3	.7	.6
	Shrimp:											
587	Cooked, boiled, 2 large = 11 g	16 ea	86	77	76	16	0	0	1	.2	.2	.4
588	Canned, drained	½ c	64	73	77	15	1	0	1	.3	.3	.7
589	Fried, 2 large = 15 g[1]	12 ea	90	53	218	19	10	<1	11	2	3	5.9
1057	Raw, large, about 7 g each	14 ea	100	76	106	20	1	0	2	.3	.4	1
1589	Shrimp, imitation, from surimi	4 oz	113	75	114	14	10	0	2	.3	.2	1
1053	Snapper, baked or broiled	4 oz	113	70	145	30	0	0	2	.4	.4	.7
1060	Squid, fried in flour[2]	4 oz	113	65	198	20	9	0	8	2.1	3.1	2.4
1590	Surimi[3]	4 oz	113	76	112	17	8	0	1	.2	.2	.6
1058	Swordfish, raw	4 oz	113	76	137	22	0	0	5	1.3	1.8	1
1059	Swordfish, baked or broiled	4 oz	113	69	175	29	0	0	6	1.7	2.2	1.3
590	Trout, baked or broiled	4 oz	113	71	170	26	0	0	7	1.8	2	2.2
	Tuna, light, canned, drained solids:											
591	Oil pack	3 oz	85	60	168	25	0	0	7	1.3	2.5	2.5
592	Water pack	3 oz	85	75	99	22	0	0	1	.2	.1	.3
1061	Bluefin tuna, fresh	4 oz	113	68	163	26	0	0	6	1.4	1.8	1.6

(1)Dipped in egg, bread crumbs, and flour; fried in vegetable shortening.

(2)Recipe is 94.6% squid, 4.9% flour, and 0.6% salt.

(3)Surimi is processed from Walleye (Alaska) pollock. Also see Imitation crab, shrimp, scallops.

(Computer code number is for West Diet Analysis program)

Chol (mg)	Calc (mg)	Iron (mg)	Magn (mg)	Pota (mg)	Sodi (mg)	Zinc (mg)	VT-A (RE)	Thia (mg)	VT-E (α-TE)	Ribo (mg)	Niac (mg)	V-B6 (mg)	Fola (μg)	VT-C (mg)
77	20	.39	66	390	119	.72	13	.09	2.6	.13	2.47	.27	10	2
53	24	1.29	42	537	60	.58	57	.09	.71	.01	.43	.4	12	0
96	63	1.93	46	346	524	.59	33	.08	1.56	.14	4.51	.28	19	<1
87	55	1.58	61	469	862	.57	25	.05	.57	.06	5.75	.45	17	0
54	66	1.17	116	636	112	.57	93	.08	1.27	.1	7.69	.43	16	5
28	13	.24	23	126	134	.12	13	.01	.27	.02	1.64	.09	1	<1
36	53	.95	94	509	61	.48	53	.07	.96	.08	6.62	.39	14	0
11	65	1.04	7	59	740	.45	219	.03	1.4	.12	2.81	.14	2	0
104	88	.57	51	510	551	4.23	38	.01	2.1	.1	1.55	.11	16	0
61	155	1	44	396	109	.7	16	.15	1.8	.15	2.76	.31	12	1
71	136	1.58	38	324	432	.67	23	.14	2.41	.18	2.69	.24	15	1
54	60	6.01	34	396	260	1.9	51	.03	1.36	.04	2.37	.41	18	6
131	112	16.5	117	387	523	225	74	.25	1.98	.24	3.42	.15	25	9
124	20	12.6	55	417	263	41.2	201	.17	2.11	.58	4.98	.12	25	20
71	55	6.12	51	214	367	76.6	79	.13	2.01	.18	1.45	.06	12	3
113	18	10.4	50	341	240	37.5	165	.14	2	.5	4.1	.1	17	14
109	7	.32	83	439	132	.68	26	.08	.32	.09	1.87	.08	4	0
109	7	.32	83	437	132	.68	26	.08	.32	.09	1.87	.08	4	0
62	241[4]	.95	38	368	626	1.04	19	.03	1.53	.21	7.42	.34	17	0
98	8	.62	35	425	75	.58	71	.24	1.42	.19	7.56	.25	6	0
26	12	.96	20	198	886	.35	29	.03	1.53	.11	5.33	.31	2	0
160	433[4]	3.3	44	449	571	1.5	76	.09	.34	.26	5.93	.19	13	0
57	39	.76	55	310	432	.99	20	.04	1.77	.1	1.4	.13	17	2
25	9	.35	49	116	898	.37	23	.01	.12	.02	.35	.03	2	0
19	15	.15	33	168	246	.55	27	.01	.81	.04	.6	.08	7	1
150	30	2.37	26	140	172	1.2	51	.02	.66	.03	1.99	.09	3	2
111	38	1.75	26	134	108	.8	12	.02	.6	.02	1.76	.07	1	1
159	60	1.13	36	203	310	1.24	50	.12	1.35	.12	2.76	.09	7	1
152	52	2.41	37	185	148	1.11	54	.03	.82	.03	2.55	.1	3	2
41	21	.68	49	101	797	.37	23	.03	.12	.04	.19	.03	2	0
53	45	.27	42	590	64	.5	40	.06	.7	<.01	.39	.52	7	2
294	44	1.14	43	315	346	1.97	12	.06	2.1	.52	2.94	.07	6	5
34	10	.29	49	127	162	.37	23	.02	.28	.02	.25	.03	2	0
44	5	.92	31	325	102	1.3	41	.04	.57	.11	11	.37	2	1
57	7	1.18	38	417	130	1.67	46	.05	.71	.13	13.3	.43	3	1
78	97	.43	35	506	63	.58	17	.17	.57	.11	6.52	.39	21	2
15	11	1.18	26	176	301	.77	20	.03	1.02	.1	10.5	.09	5	0
26	9	1.3	23	202	287	.65	14	.03	.45	.06	11.3	.3	3	0
43	9	1.15	57	285	44	.68	740	.27	1.13	.28	9.78	.51	2	0

(4)If bones are discarded, calcium value is greatly reduced.

(For purposes of calculations, use "0" for t, <1, <.1, <.01, etc.)

Table H-1
Food Composition

Computer Code Number	Food Description	Measure	Wt (g)	H_2O (%)	Ener (kcal)	Prot (g)	Carb (g)	Dietary Fiber (g)	Fat (g)	Fat Breakdown (g) Sat	Mono	Poly
	MEATS: BEEF, LAMB, PORK, and others											
	BEEF, cooked:[1]											
	Braised, simmered, pot roasted:											
	Relatively fat, choice chuck blade:											
593	Lean and fat, piece 2½ x 2½ x ¾"	4 oz	113	47	393	31	0	0	29	13	14.8	1.2
594	Lean only	4 oz	113	55	297	35	0	0	16	7.3	8.2	.7
	Relatively lean, like choice round:											
595	Lean and fat, pce 4⅛ x 2½ x ¾"	4 oz	113	52	311	32	0	0	19	8.6	9.7	.8
596	Lean only	4 oz	113	57	249	36	0	0	11	4.8	5.4	.5
	Ground beef, broiled, patty 3 x ⅝":											
597	Extra lean, about 16% fat	4 oz	113	54	300	32	0	0	18	8	9.1	.8
598	Lean, 21% fat	4 oz	113	53	316	32	0	0	20	8.9	10.1	.8
	Roasts, oven cooked, no added liquid:											
	Relatively fat, prime rib:											
601	Lean and fat, pce 4⅛ x 2¼ x ½"	4 oz	113	46	425	25	0	0	35	15.8	17.9	1.5
602	Lean only	4 oz	113	58	271	31	0	0	16	7	7.9	.7
	Relatively lean, choice round:											
603	Lean and fat, pce 2½ x 2½ x ¾"	4 oz	113	59	272	30	0	0	16	7.1	8.1	.7
604	Lean only	4 oz	113	65	198	33	0	0	6	2.9	3.3	.3
1701	Steak, rib, broiled, lean	4 oz	113	58	250	32	0	0	13	5.7	6.4	.5
	Steak, broiled, relatively lean, choice sirloin:											
606	Lean only	4 oz	113	62	228	34	0	0	9	4	4.6	.4
	Steak, broiled, relatively fat, choice T-bone:											
1063	Lean and fat	4 oz	113	53	349	26	0	0	26	11.8	13.3	1.1
1064	Lean only	4 oz	113	62	232	30	0	0	11	5.1	5.8	.5
	Variety meats:											
1086	Brains, panfried	4 oz	113	71	222	14	0	0	18	6.7	7	3.9
599	Heart, simmered	4 oz	113	64	198	33	<1	0	6	2.9	1.5	1.5
600	Liver, fried	4 oz	113	56	245	30	9	0	9	3	1.8	1.9
1062	Tongue, cooked	4 oz	113	56	320	25	<1	0	23	10.1	11	.9
607	Beef, canned, corned	4 oz	113	58	283	31	0	0	17	7.5	8.5	.7
608	Beef, dried, cured	1 oz	28	57	46	8	<1	0	1	.5	.5	.1
	LAMB, domestic, cooked:											
	Chop, arm, braised (5.6 oz raw w/bone):											
609	Lean and fat	1 ea	70	44	242	21	0	0	17	7.8	7.3	1.4
610	Lean only	1 ea	55	49	154	20	0	0	8	3.6	3.4	.6
	Chop, loin, broiled (4.2 oz. raw w/bone):											
611	Lean and fat	1 ea	64	52	202	16	0	0	15	6.8	6.4	1.2
612	Lean only	1 ea	46	61	99	14	0	0	4	2.1	2	.4
1067	Cutlet, avg of lean cuts, cooked	4 oz	113	54	330	28	0	0	23	10.9	10.2	2
	Leg, roasted, 3 oz = 4⅛ x 2¼ x ½":											
613	Lean and fat	4 oz	113	58	292	29	0	0	19	8.7	8.1	1.6
614	Lean only	4 oz	113	64	216	32	0	0	9	4.1	3.8	.7
615	Rib, roasted, lean and fat	4 oz	113	48	406	24	0	0	34	15.7	14.7	2.8
616	Rib, roasted, lean only	4 oz	113	60	262	30	0	0	15	7	6.6	1.3
1065	Shoulder, roasted, lean and fat	4 oz	113	56	312	25	0	0	23	10.5	9.9	1.9

(1)Outer layer of fat removed to about ⅛" of the lean. Deposits of fat within the cut remain.

(Computer code number is for West Diet Analysis program)

PAGE KEY: H–4 = BEV H–6 = DAIRY H–12 = EGGS H–14 = FAT/OIL H–18 = FRUIT H–26 = BAKERY H–36 = GRAIN H–44 = FISH H–48 = MEATS H–50 = POULTRY H–54 = SAUSAGE H–56 = MIXED/FAST H–64 = NUTS/SEEDS H–68 = SWEETS H–70 = VEG/LEG H–84 = MISC H–88 = SOUPS/SAUCES H–90 = FAST H–106 = FRZN ENTREE H–112 = BABY FOODS

Chol (mg)	Calc (mg)	Iron (mg)	Magn (mg)	Pota (mg)	Sodi (mg)	Zinc (mg)	VT-A (RE)	Thia (mg)	VT-E (α-TE)	Ribo (mg)	Niac (mg)	V-B6 (mg)	Fola (μg)	VT-C (mg)
112	11	3.46	22	275	67	7.57	0	.08	.26	.27	3.54	.32	10	0
120	15	4.16	26	297	80	11.6	0	.09	.16	.32	3.02	.33	7	0
109	7	3.53	25	319	57	5.55	0	.08	.21	.27	4.22	.37	11	0
109	6	3.91	28	348	58	6.19	0	.08	.2	.29	4.61	.41	12	0
112	10	3.14	28	417	93	7.27	0	.08	.2	.36	6.61	.36	12	0
114	14	2.77	27	394	101	7.01	0	.07	.23	.27	6.77	.34	12	0
96	12	2.61	21	335	71	5.92	0	.08	.27	.19	3.8	.26	8	0
92	11	2.95	28	425	84	7.84	0	.09	.14	.24	4.64	.34	9	0
81	7	2.07	27	406	67	4.87	0	.09	.23	.18	3.92	.4	7	0
78	6	2.2	31	446	70	5.36	0	.1	.12	.19	4.24	.43	8	0
90	15	3	31	445	78	8	0	.11	.16	.25	5.42	.45	9	0
101	12	3.8	36	455	75	7.37	0	.15	.16	.33	4.84	.51	11	0
76	9	3.01	26	363	72	5.3	0	.1	.24	.24	4.64	.37	8	0
67	7	3.6	32	427	80	6.12	0	.12	.16	.28	5.23	.44	9	0
2254	10	2.51	17	400	179	1.53	0	.15	2.37	.29	4.27	.44	7	4
218	7	8.49	28	263	71	3.54	0	.16	.81	1.74	4.6	.24	2	2
545	12	7.1	26	411	120	6.16	12123[2]	.24	.72	4.68	16.3	1.62	249	26
121	8	3.83	19	203	68	5.42	0	.03	.4	.4	2.44	.18	6	1
97	14	2.35	16	154	1136	4.03	0	.02	.17	.17	2.75	.15	10	0
12	2	1.26	9	124	972	1.47	0	.02	.04	.06	1.53	.1	3	3
84	18	1.67	18	214	50	4.26	0	.05	.11	.18	4.67	.08	13	0
67	14	1.49	16	186	42	4.01	0	.04	.1	.15	3.48	.07	12	0
64	13	1.16	15	209	49	2.23	0	.06	.08	.16	4.54	.08	12	0
44	9	.92	13	173	39	1.9	0	.05	.07	.13	3.15	.07	11	0
110	12	2.26	25	340	77	4.68	0	.13	.15	.32	7.48	.16	19	0
105	12	2.24	27	354	75	4.97	0	.11	.17	.31	7.45	.17	23	0
101	9	2.4	29	382	77	5.6	0	.12	.2	.33	7.16	.19	26	0
110	25	1.81	23	306	82	3.94	0	.1	.11	.24	7.63	.12	17	0
99	24	2	24	356	92	5.05	0	.1	.17	.26	6.96	.17	25	0
104	23	2.23	26	284	75	5.91	0	.1	.16	.27	6.95	.15	24	0

(2)Value varies widely.

(For purposes of calculations, use "0" for t, <1, <.1, <.01, etc.)

H

Table H-1
Food Composition

Computer Code Number	Food Description	Measure	Wt (g)	H_2O (%)	Ener (kcal)	Prot (g)	Carb (g)	Dietary Fiber (g)	Fat (g)	Fat Breakdown (g) Sat	Mono	Poly
	MEATS: BEEF, LAMB, PORK, and others—Cont.											
1066	Shoulder, roasted, lean only	4 oz	113	63	231	28	0	0	12	5.7	5.3	1.1
	Variety meats:											
1069	Brains, panfried	4 oz	113	76	164	14	0	0	12	4.4	3.7	1.9
1068	Heart, braised	4 oz	113	64	209	28	2	0	9	3.9	2.7	1.1
1070	Sweetbreads, cooked	4 oz	113	60	264	26	0	0	17	8.2	6.6	1.4
1071	Tongue, cooked	4 oz	113	58	311	24	0	0	23	8.9	11.7	1.4
	PORK, cured, cooked (see also #669–672):											
617	Bacon, medium slices	3 pce	19	13	109	6	<1	0	9	3.3	4.5	1.1
1087	Breakfast strips, cooked	2 pce	23	27	106	7	<1	0	8	2.9	3.7	1.3
618	Canadian-style bacon	2 pce	47	62	87	11	1	0	4	1.3	1.9	.4
	Ham, roasted:											
619	Lean and fat, 2 pces 4⅛ x 2¼ x ¼"	4 oz	113	65	202	26	0	0	10	3.5	5.1	1.7
620	Lean only	4 oz	113	68	164	24	2	0	6	2	3	.6
621	Ham, canned, roasted, 8% fat	4 oz	113	69	154	24	1	0	6	1.8	2.8	.5
	PORK, fresh, cooked:											
	Chops, loin (cut 3 per lb with bone):											
1291	Braised, lean and fat	1 ea	71	58	170	19	0	0	10	3.6	4.3	1
1292	Braised, lean only	1 ea	55	61	112	16	0	0	5	1.9	2.3	.4
622	Broiled, lean and fat	1 ea	87	58	209	25	0	0	11	4.2	5	.9
623	Broiled, lean only	1 ea	72	61	146	22	0	0	6	2	2.6	.4
624	Panfried, lean and fat	1 ea	89	53	247	27	0	0	15	5.4	6.3	1.7
625	Panfried, lean only	1 ea	67	59	161	17	0	0	10	3.5	4	1.3
626	Leg, roasted, lean and fat	4 oz	113	55	310	30	0	0	20	7	9	2
627	Leg, roasted, lean only	4 oz	113	61	234	35	0	0	9	3	4	1
628	Rib, roasted, lean and fat	4 oz	113	56	289	31	0	0	17	6.7	7.9	1.5
629	Rib, roasted, lean only	4 oz	113	59	253	33	0	0	13	4.9	6	1
630	Shoulder, braised, lean and fat	4 oz	113	48	373	32	0	0	26	9.6	11.8	2.6
631	Shoulder, braised, lean only	4 oz	113	54	281	37	0	0	14	4.7	6.6	1.3
1088	Spareribs, cooked, yield from 1 lb raw with bone	4 oz	113	40	450	33	0	0	34	12.6	15	3
1095	Rabbit, roasted (1 cup meat = 140 g)	4 oz	113	61	223	33	0	0	9	4	2	3
	VEAL, cooked:											
632	Cutlet, braised or broiled, 4⅛ x 2¼ x ½"	4 oz	113	52	322	34	0	0	20	7.6	7.6	1.3
633	Rib roasted, lean, 2 pieces 4⅛ x 2¼ x ¼"	4 oz	113	60	259	27	0	0	16	6.1	6.2	1.1
634	Liver, panfried	4 oz	113	67	187	25	3	0	8	3.3	1.9	2.2
1096	Venison (deer meat), roasted	4 oz	113	65	179	34	0	0	4	1.4	1	.7
	MEATS: POULTRY and POULTRY PRODUCTS											
	CHICKEN, cooked:											
	Fried, batter dipped:[1]											
635	Breast (5.6 oz with bones)	1 ea	140	52	364	35	13	<1	19	5	7.6	4.3
636	Drumstick (3.4 oz with bones)	1 ea	72	53	193	16	6	<1	11	3	4.7	2.7
637	Thigh	1 ea	86	52	238	19	8	<1	14	3.8	5.9	3.4
638	Wing	1 ea	49	46	159	10	5	<1	11	2.9	4.5	2.5
	Fried, flour coated:[1]											
639	Breast (4.2 oz with bones)	1 ea	98	57	218	31	2	<1	9	2.5	3.5	1.9

(1)Fried in vegetable shortening.

(Computer code number is for West Diet Analysis program)

PAGE KEY: H–4 = BEV H–6 = DAIRY H–12 = EGGS H–14 = FAT/OIL H–18 = FRUIT H–26 = BAKERY H–36 = GRAIN H–44 = FISH H–48 = MEATS H–50 = POULTRY H–54 = SAUSAGE H–56 = MIXED/FAST H–64 = NUTS/SEEDS H–68 = SWEETS H–70 = VEG/LEG H–84 = MISC H–88 = SOUPS/SAUCES H–90 = FAST H–106 = FRZN ENTREE H–112 = BABY FOODS

Chol (mg)	Calc (mg)	Iron (mg)	Magn (mg)	Pota (mg)	Sodi (mg)	Zinc (mg)	VT-A (RE)	Thia (mg)	VT-E (α-TE)	Ribo (mg)	Niac (mg)	V-B6 (mg)	Fola (μg)	VT-C (mg)
99	21	2.42	28	301	77	6.85	0	.1	.2	.29	6.53	.17	28	0
2309	14	1.91	16	232	152	1.54	0	.12	1.73	.27	2.8	.12	6	14
281	16	6.26	27	213	71	4.17	0	.19	.79	1.35	4.94	.34	2	8
452	14	2.4	21	328	59	3.04	0	.02	.77	.24	2.9	.06	15	23
213	11	2.99	18	179	76	3.39	0	.09	.36	.48	4.18	.19	3	8
16	2	.31	5	92	303	.62	0	.13	.1	.05	1.39	.05	1	0
24	3	.45	6	107	483	.83	0	.17	.08	.08	1.72	.08	1	0
27	5	.38	10	183	726	.8	0	.39	.16	.09	3.25	.21	2	0
67	9	1.52	25	464	1701	2.8	0	.83	.45	.37	6.97	.35	3	0
60	9	1.68	16	326	1364	3.3	0	.86	.29	.23	4.56	.45	3	0
34	7	1	24	395	1287	2.6	0	1.2	.29	.28	5.55	.51	6	0
57	15	.76	13	266	34	1.7	2	.43	.24	.18	3	.26	2	<1
43	10	.62	11	213	28	1.4	1	.36	.21	.15	2.52	.21	2	<1
71	29	.7	22	312	50	2	3	.93	.28	.25	4.56	.37	5	<1
59	22	.61	19	270	43	1.7	2	.83	.3	.22	3.99	.34	4	<1
82	24	.81	26	378	71	2	2	1	.37	.27	5	.4	5	<1
55	15	.7	17	245	52	2.6	1	.49	.32	.24	3.03	.27	3	<1
107	16	1.15	25	399	68	3.36	3	.72	.34	.35	5.18	.46	11	<1
109	8	1.29	33	443	74	3.41	3	.91	.46	.4	5.58	.38	3	<1
83	32	1.01	24	477	52	2.34	2	.82	.41	.34	7	.37	3	<1
81	30	1.11	25	496	53	2.4	2	.86	.55	.36	7	.39	3	<1
124	20	1.83	22	418	100	4.7	3	.61	.5	.35	6	.4	5	<1
129	9	2.21	25	459	116	5.64	3	.68	.59	.41	6.74	.47	6	<1
137	53	2.1	27	363	106	5.22	3	.46	.52	.43	6.2	.4	5	0
93	22	2.57	24	434	53	2.57	0	.1	.96	.24	9.56	.53	13	0
134	32	1.24	27	318	91	4.12	0	.05	.45	.34	10.24	.3	16	0
125	13	1.1	25	335	104	4.64	0	.06	.4	.31	7.92	.28	15	0
636	8	2.97	22	233	60	10.8	9127[2]	.15	.42	2.2	9.62	.56	861	35
127	8	5.07	27	380	61	3.12	0	.2	.28	.68	7.61	.43[3]	5[3]	0
119	28	1.75	34	281	385	1.33	28	.16	1.48	.2	14.7	.6	8	0
62	12	.97	14	134	194	1.68	19	.08	.88	.16	3.67	.19	7	0
80	16	1.25	18	165	247	1.75	25	.1	1.05	.2	4.92	.22	8	0
39	10	.63	8	68	157	.68	17	.05	.52	.08	2.58	.15	3	0
87	16	1.17	29	254	75	1.08	15	.08	.56	.13	13.43	.57	4	0

(2)Value varies widely.

(3)Values estimated from other game meat.

H

Table H–1
Food Composition

Computer Code Number	Food Description	Measure	Wt (g)	H_2O (%)	Ener (kcal)	Prot (g)	Carb (g)	Dietary Fiber (g)	Fat (g)	Fat Breakdown (g) Sat	Mono	Poly
	MEATS: POULTRY and POULTRY PRODUCTS—Cont.											
	CHICKEN—Cont.											
1212	Breast, without skin	1 ea	86	60	161	29	<1	<1	4	1.1	1.6	.9
640	Drumstick (2.6 oz with bones)	1 ea	49	57	120	13	1	<1	7	1.8	2.7	1.6
641	Thigh	1 ea	62	54	162	17	2	<1	9	2.5	3.7	2.1
1099	Thigh, without skin	1 ea	52	59	113	15	1	<1	5	1.4	2	1.3
642	Wing	1 ea	32	49	103	8	1	<1	7	2	2.9	1.6
	Roasted:											
643	All types of meat	1 c	140	64	266	41	0	0	10	2.9	3.9	2.4
644	Dark meat	1 c	140	63	287	38	0	0	14	3.7	5	3.2
645	Light meat	1 c	140	65	242	43	0	0	6	1.8	2.2	1.4
646	Breast, without skin	1 ea	86	65	142	27	0	0	3	.9	1.1	.7
647	Drumstick	1 ea	44	67	76	13	0	0	3	.7	.8	.6
1703	Leg, without skin	1 ea	95	65	163	26	0	0	5	1.4	2	1
648	Thigh	1 ea	62	59	153	15	0	0	10	2.7	3.8	2.1
1100	Thigh, without skin	1 ea	52	63	108	13	0	0	6	1.6	2.2	1.3
649	Stewed, all types:	1 c	140	67	248	38	0	0	9	2.6	3.3	2.2
656	Canned, boneless chicken	4 oz	113	69	187	25	0	0	9	2.5	3.6	2
1102	Gizzards, simmered	3 ea	66	67	101	18	1	0	2	.7	.6	.7
1101	Hearts, simmered	8 ea	25	65	45	6	<1	0	2	.6	.5	.6
2300	Liver, simmered: Ounce	3 oz	85	68	133	21	1	0	5	1.6	1.1	.8
1098	Liver, simmered: Piece = 20 g	6 ea	120	68	188	29	1	0	7	2.2	1.6	1.1
	DUCK, roasted:											
1293	Meat with skin, about 2.7 cups	½ ea	382	52	1288	73	0	0	109	37	49.3	13.9
651	Meat only, about 1.5 cups	½ ea	221	64	444	52	0	0	25	9.2	8.2	3.2
	GOOSE, domesticated, roasted:											
1294	Meat only, 4.2 cups	½ ea	591	57	1407	173	0	0	75	23.6	40	10.9
1295	Meat with skin, about 5.5 cups	½ ea	774	52	2360	195	0	0	170	53.2	80.5	24.8
	TURKEY:											
	Roasted, meat only:											
652	Dark meat	4 oz	113	63	212	33	0	0	8	2.7	1.9	2.5
653	Light meat	4 oz	113	66	178	34	0	0	4	1.2	.6	1
654	All types, chopped or diced	1 c	140	65	238	42	0	0	7	2.3	1.5	2
655	All types, sliced	4 oz	113	65	193	34	0	0	6	1.9	1.2	1.6
1103	Ground, cooked	4 oz	113	59	267	31	0	0	15	4.2	5.6	3.7
1106	Gizzard, cooked	2 ea	134	65	218	39	1	0	5	1.5	1	1.5
1107	Heart, cooked	4 ea	64	64	113	17	1	0	4	1.1	.8	1.1
1108	Liver, cooked	1 ea	75	66	127	18	3	0	5	1.4	1.1	.8
	POULTRY FOOD PRODUCTS (see also items in Sausages and Lunchmeats section):											
1567	Chicken patty, breaded, cooked	1 ea	75	49	213	12	11	<1	13	4	6	1.7
659	Turkey and gravy, frozen package	3 oz	85	85	57	5	4	<1	2	.8	.8	.4
	Turkey breast, Louis Rich:											
1104	Barbecued	2 oz	57	40	58	12	2	0	1	.2	.2	.1
1943	Hickory smoked	1 pce	80	–	80	16	2	0	1	0	–	–

(Computer code number is for West Diet Analysis program)

PAGE KEY: H–4 = BEV H–6 = DAIRY H–12 = EGGS H–14 = FAT/OIL H–18 = FRUIT H–26 = BAKERY H–36 = GRAIN H–44 = FISH H–48 = MEATS H–50 = POULTRY H–54 = SAUSAGE H–56 = MIXED/FAST H–64 = NUTS/SEEDS H–68 = SWEETS H–70 = VEG/LEG H–84 = MISC H–88 = SOUPS/SAUCES H–90 = FAST H–106 = FRZN ENTREE H–112 = BABY FOODS

Chol (mg)	Calc (mg)	Iron (mg)	Magn (mg)	Pota (mg)	Sodi (mg)	Zinc (mg)	VT-A (RE)	Thia (mg)	VT-E (α-TE)	Ribo (mg)	Niac (mg)	V-B6 (mg)	Fola (μg)	VT-C (mg)
78	14	.98	27	237	68	.93	6	.07	.36	.11	12.7	.55	3	0
44	6	.66	11	112	44	1.42	12	.04	.41	.11	2.96	.17	4	0
60	9	.92	16	147	55	1.56	18	.06	.52	.15	4.31	.2	5	0
53	7	.76	14	135	49	1.45	11	.05	.3	.13	3.7	.2	5	0
26	5	.4	6	57	25	.56	12	.02	.18	.04	2.14	.13	1	0
125	21	1.69	35	340	120	2.94	22	.1	.58	.25	12.8	.66	8	0
130	21	1.86	32	336	130	3.92	31	.1	.81	.32	9.17	.5	11	0
119	21	1.48	38	346	108	1.72	13	.09	.37	.16	17.4	.84	6	0
73	13	.89	25	220	64	.86	5	.06	.33	.1	11.8	.52	3	0
41	5	.57	11	108	42	1.4	8	.03	.26	.1	2.68	.17	4	0
88	11	1.26	23	234	90	3.03	18	.07		.22	5.8	.35	9	0
58	7	.83	14	137	52	1.46	30	.04		.13	3.95	.19	4	0
49	6	.68	12	123	46	1.34	10	.04		.12	3.39	.18	4	0
116	20	1.64	29	252	98	2.79	21	.07		.23	8.55	.36	8	0
70	16	1.79	14	155	570	1.6	39	.02		.15	7.18	.4	5	2
128	7	2.74	13	118	44	2.89	37	.02		.16	2.63	.08	35	1
61	5	2.22	5	33	12	1.8	2	.01		.18	.69	.08	20	<1
536	12	7.23	18	119	42	3.68	4177	.13		1.49	3.78	.5	655	13
757	17	10.2	25	168	61	5.21	5895	.18	2.04	2.1	5.34	.7	924	19
321	42	10.3	61	779	225	7.1	241	.67	2.5	1.03	18.45	.69	23	0
197	27	5.97	44	557	144	5.75	51	.57	1.55	1.04	11.3	.55	22	0
568	83	17	148	2293	449	18.7	71	.54	9.16	2.3	24.1	2.78	71	0
704	101	21.9	170	2547	542	20.3	163	.6	13.47	2.5	32.3	2.86	16	0
96	36	2.64	27	329	90	5.06	0	.07	.95	.28	4.14	.41	10	0
78	22	1.53	32	346	73	2.31	0	.07	.12	.15	7.76	.61	7	0
106	35	2.49	36	417	98	4.34	0	.09	.59	.25	7.62	.64	10	0
86	28	2.02	29	338	79	3.52	0	.07	.48	.21	6.17	.52	8	0
116	28	2.2	27	306	121	3.24	0	.06	.45	.19	5.47	.44	8	0
311	20	7.29	26	283	72	5.57	74	.04	.27	.44	4.11	.16	70	2
145	8	4.4	14	117	35	3.37	5	.05	.13	.57	2.08	.2	51	1
470	8	5.85	11	146	48	2.32	2805	.04	2.41	1.07	4.46	.39	500	1
45	12	.94	15	185	399	.78	23	.07	1.46	.1	5.04	.23	8	<1
15	12	.79	7	52	472	.6	11	.02	.3	.11	1.53	.09	3	0
25	14	.6	16	178	608	.6	0	.02	–	.06	5.45	.22	2	0
35	0	.72	–	–	1060	–	0	–	–	–	–	–	–	0

(For purposes of calculations, use "0" for t, <1, <.1, <.01, etc.)

Table H-1
Food Composition

Computer Code Number	Food Description	Measure	Wt (g)	H_2O (%)	Ener (kcal)	Prot (g)	Carb (g)	Dietary Fiber (g)	Fat (g)	Fat Breakdown (g) Sat	Mono	Poly
MEATS:	POULTRY and POULTRY PRODUCTS											
	TURKEY—Cont.											
1947	Honey roasted	1 pce	80	–	80	16	3	0	1	.5	–	–
1945	Oven roasted	1 pce	80	–	70	16	–	0	1	0	–	–
661	Turkey patty, breaded, fried	2 oz	57	50	161	8	9	<1	10	2.7	4.2	2.7
662	Turkey, frozen, roasted, seasoned	4 oz	113	68	176	25	4	0	7	2.2	1.4	1.9
1704	Turkey roll, light meat	1 pce	28	72	41	5	<1	0	2	.6	.7	.5
MEATS:	SAUSAGES and LUNCHMEATS (see also Poultry Food Products)											
1072	Beerwurst/beer salami, beef	1 oz	28	53	93	4	<1	0	9	3.7	4	.3
1074	Beerwurst/beer salami, pork	1 oz	28	62	68	4	1	0	5	1.8	2.6	.7
1075	Berliner sausage	1 oz	28	61	65	4	1	0	5	1.7	2.3	.5
	Bologna:											
1297	Beef	1 pce	23	55	72	3	<1	0	7	2.8	3.2	.3
2115	Beef, light, Oscar Mayer	1 pce	28	65	56	3	2	0	4	1.6	2	.1
663	Beef & pork	1 pce	28	54	90	3	1	0	8	3	3.8	.7
2155	Healthy Favorites	2 ea	46	–	45	7	2	0	1	0	–	–
1298	Pork	1 pce	23	61	57	4	<1	0	5	1.6	2.3	.5
2114	Regular, light, Oscar Mayer	1 pce	28	65	56	3	2	0	4	1.6	2.1	.4
664	Turkey	1 pce	28	65	56	4	<1	0	4	1.4	1.4	1.2
1970	Turkey, Louis Rich	1 pce	28	67	58	3	1	0	5	1.5	1.8	1.3
665	Braunschweiger sausage	2 pce	57	48	205	8	2	0	18	6.2	8.5	2.1
1073	Bratwurst, link	1 ea	70	51	226	10	2	0	20	7	9.3	2
666	Brown & serve sausage links, cooked	2 ea	26	45	102	4	1	0	10	3.4	4.4	1
1089	Cheesefurter/cheese smokie	2 ea	86	53	281	12	1	0	25	9	11.8	2.6
2157	Chicken breast, Healthy Favorites	4 pce	52	–	40	9	1	0	0	0	0	0
1556	Chorizo, pork & beef	3 oz	85	32	387	22	2	0	33	12.2	15.6	2.9
1950	Coldcuts, fat free, deli thin	1 pce	13	77	11	2	1	0	<1	t	t	t
1090	Corned beef loaf, jellied	1 pce	28	69	43	7	0	0	2	.7	.8	.1
	Frankfurters:											
1077	Beef, large link, 8/package	1 ea	57	55	180	7	1	0	16	6.9	7.9	.8
1078	Beef and pork, large link, 8/package	1 ea	57	54	182	6	1	0	17	6.2	8	1.6
667	Beef and pork, small link, 10/pkg	1 ea	45	54	144	5	1	0	13	4.9	6.3	1.2
668	Turkey frankfurter, 10/package	1 ea	45	63	102	6	1	0	8	2.7	2.5	2.3
1968	Turkey/chicken frank 8/pkg	1 ea	43	–	80	6	1	0	6	2	–	–
	Ham:											
669	Ham lunchmeat, canned, 3 x 2 x ½"	1 pce	21	52	70	3	<1	0	6	2.3	3	.8
670	Chopped ham, packaged	2 pce	42	64	96	3	0	0	7	2.4	3	.8
2156	Honey ham, Healthy Favorites	4 pce	52	73	55	9	2	0	2	.5	–	.1
2113	Oscar Mayer lower sodium ham	1 pce	21	46	23	4	1	0	1	.3	.4	.1
673	Turkey ham lunchmeat	2 pce	57	71	73	11	<1	0	3	1	.7	.9
1091	Kielbasa sausage	1 pce	26	54	81	4	1	0	7	2.6	3.4	.8
1092	Knockwurst sausage, link	1 ea	68	56	210	8	1	0	19	6.9	8.7	2
1093	Mortadella lunchmeat	2 pce	30	52	93	5	1	0	8	2.9	3.4	.9
1097	Olive loaf lunchmeat	2 pce	57	58	134	7	5	<.01	9	3.3	4.5	1.1

(Computer code number is for West Diet Analysis program)

PAGE KEY: H–4 = BEV H–6 = DAIRY H–12 = EGGS H–14 = FAT/OIL H–18 = FRUIT H–26 = BAKERY H–36 = GRAIN H–44 = FISH H–48 = MEATS H–50 = POULTRY H–54 = SAUSAGE H–56 = MIXED/FAST H–64 = NUTS/SEEDS H–68 = SWEETS H–70 = VEG/LEG H–84 = MISC H–88 = SOUPS/SAUCES H–90 = FAST H–106 = FRZN ENTREE H–112 = BABY FOODS

Chol (mg)	Calc (mg)	Iron (mg)	Magn (mg)	Pota (mg)	Sodi (mg)	Zinc (mg)	VT-A (RE)	Thia (mg)	VT-E (α-TE)	Ribo (mg)	Niac (mg)	V-B6 (mg)	Fola (μg)	VT-C (mg)
35	0	.72	–	–	940	–	0	–	–	–	–	–	–	0
35	0	–	–	–	910	–	0	–	–	–	–	–	–	0
35	8	1.25	9	156	454	.82	6	.06	1.4	.11	1.3	.11	5	0
60	6	1.85	25	338	771	2.88	0	.05	.43	.19	7.11	.31	6	0
12	11	.36	5	70	137	.44	0	.02	.04	.06	1.96	.09	1	0
17	3	.43	3	49	291	.69	0	.02	.05	.03	.96	.05	1	0
17	2	.22	4	72	352	.49	0	.16	.06	.05	.92	.1	1	0
13	3	.33	4	80	368	.7	0	.11	.06	.06	.88	.06	1	0
13	3	.38	3	36	226	.5	0	.01	.04	.03	.55	.04	1	0
13	4	.34	4	44	314	.53	0	–	–	–	–	–	–	0
16	3	.43	3	51	289	.55	0	.05	.06	.04	.73	.05	1	0
15	–	.36	–	–	510	–	–	–	–	–	–	–	–	–
14	3	.18	3	65	272	.47	0	.12	.06	.04	.9	.06	1	0
15	14	.39	6	46	312	.45	0	–	–	–	–	–	–	0
28	24	.43	4	56	249	.49	0	.02	.15	.05	1	.06	2	0
22	34	.45	5	52	242	.57	0	.02	–	.05	1.08	.05	–	0
89	5	5.34	6	113	652	1.6	2405	.14	.2	.87	4.77	.19	25	0
44	34	.72	11	197	779	1.47	0	.18	.19	.16	2.31	.09	4	0
16	2	.62	4	70	248	.3	0	.21	.06	.09	.96	.06	1	0
58	50	.93	11	177	931	1.94	33	.21	.27	.14	2.5	.11	3	0
25	–	.72	–	–	620	–	–	–	–	–	–	–	–	–
75	7	1.35	15	338	1049	2.9	0	.54	.19	.26	4.36	.45	2	0
4	1	.15	4	27	155	.11	0	–	–	–	–	–	–	0
13	3	.58	3	29	270	1.16	0	0	.05	.03	.5	.03	2	0
35	11	.81	2	95	585	1.24	0	.03	.11	.06	1.38	.07	2	0
29	6	.66	6	95	638	1.05	0	.11	.14	.07	1.5	.07	2	0
23	5	.52	5	75	504	.83	0	.09	.11	.05	1.18	.06	2	0
48	48	.83	6	81	642	1.4	0	.02	.28	.08	1.86	.1	4	0
40	60	1.08	–	–	480	–	0	–	–	–	–	–	–	0
13	1	.15	2	45	271	.31	0	.08	.06	.04	.66	.04	1	<1
21	3	.35	7	134	576	.8	0	.27	.11	.09	1.63	.15	<1	0
24	6	.7	18	144	635	1.02	–	–	–	–	–	–	–	0
9	1	.3	5	197	175	.42	0	–	–	–	–	–	–	0
32	6	1.57	9	185	568	1.68	0	.03	.37	.14	2.01	.14	3	0
17	11	.38	4	71	280	.53	0	.06	.06	.06	.75	.05	1	0
40	8	.62	7	135	687	1.13	0	.23	.39	.1	1.86	.12	1	0
17	5	.42	3	49	374	.63	0	.04	.07	.05	.8	.04	1	0
22	62	.31	11	169	846	.79	11	.17	.14	.15	1.05	.13	1	0

(For purposes of calculations, use "0" for t, <1, <.1, <.01, etc.)

H

Table H–1
Food Composition

Computer Code Number	Food Description	Measure	Wt (g)	H_2O (%)	Ener (kcal)	Prot (g)	Carb (g)	Dietary Fiber (g)	Fat (g)	Fat Breakdown (g) Sat	Mono	Poly
MEATS:	SAUSAGES and LUNCHMEATS (see also Poultry Food Products)—Cont.											
1952	Turkey breast, fat free	1 pce	28	77	22	4	1	0	<1	<.1	<.1	<.1
1080	Turkey pastrami	2 pce	57	71	80	11	1	0	4	1	1.2	.9
1969	Turkey salami	1 pce	28	72	41	4	<1	0	3	1	1	.8
1081	Pepperoni sausage	2 pce	11	27	55	2	<1	0	5	1.8	2.3	.5
1094	Pickle & pimento loaf	2 pce	57	57	149	7	3	<.01	12	4.5	5.5	1.5
1082	Polish sausage	1 oz	28	53	92	4	<1	0	8	2.9	3.9	.9
674	Pork sausage, cooked,[1] link, small	2 ea	26	45	96	5	<1	0	8	2.8	4	1
1079	Pork sausage, cooked, patty	4 oz	113	45	418	22	1	0	35	12.2	17.8	3.3
675	Salami, pork and beef	2 pce	57	60	142	8	1	0	11	4.6	5.2	1.1
676	Salami, turkey	2 pce	57	66	112	9	<1	0	8	2.3	2.6	2
677	Beef & pork, dry	3 pce	30	35	125	7	1	0	10	3.7	5.1	1
	Sandwich spreads:											
1300	Ham salad spread	1 c	240	63	518	21	26	0	37	12.2	17.3	6.5
678	Pork and beef	2 tbs	30	60	71	2	4	<1	5	1.8	2.3	.8
1296	Chicken/turkey	2 tbs	26	66	52	3	2	0	4	.9	.8	1.6
1084	Smoked link sausage, beef and pork	1 ea	68	52	229	9	1	0	21	7.2	9.7	2.2
1083	Smoked link sausage, pork	1 ea	68	39	265	15	1	0	22	7.7	9.9	2.6
1085	Summer sausage	2 pce	46	51	154	7	<1	0	14	5.5	6	.6
1076	Turkey breakfast sausage	1 pce	28	60	65	6	0	0	5	1.6	1.8	1.2
679	Vienna sausage, canned	2 ea	32	60	89	3	1	0	8	3	4	.5
MIXED DISHES and FAST FOODS												
	MIXED DISHES:											
1445	Almond chicken	1 c	242	77	275	20	18	4	14	2	5.3	5.9
1981	Baked beans, fat free, honey	½ c	120	74	110	7	24	7	0	0	0	0
1454	Bean cake	1 ea	32	23	130	2	16	1	7	1	2.9	2.6
680	Beef stew w/ vegetables, homemade	1 c	245	82	218	16	15	2	11	5	4.5	.5
1109	Beef stew w/ vegetables, canned	1 c	245	83	194	14	17	3	8	2.5	3.1	.4
1116	Beef, macaroni, tomato sauce casserole	1 c	226	76	255	16	26	3	10	3.8	4.1	.5
2295	Beef fajita	1 ea	189	63	347	14	39	3	15	4.3	6.4	3.3
1265	Beef flauta	1 ea	113	49	360	17	13	2	27	4.9	11.6	9.1
681	Beef pot pie, homemade[2]	1 pce	210	55	517	21	40	3	31	8.4	14.7	7.4
1898	Broccoli, batter fried	1 c	85	74	123	3	9	2	9	1.3	2.2	4.9
1462	Buffalo wings/spicy chicken wings	2 ea	32	53	98	8	<1	<1	7	1.8	2.8	1.6
1675	Carrot raisin salad	½ c	88	58	204	1	21	2	14	2	3.9	7.3
2248	Cheeseburger deluxe	1 ea	219	53	563	28	38	–	33	15	12.6	2
682	Chicken à la king, homemade	1 c	245	68	468	27	12	1	34	12.7	14.3	6.2
683	Chicken & noodles, homemade	1 c	240	71	367	22	26	2	19	5.9	7.1	3.5
684	Chicken chow mein, canned	1 c	250	89	95	7	18	2	1	0	.1	.8
685	Chicken chow mein, homemade	1 c	250	78	255	31	10	1	10	2.4	4.3	3.1
1266	Chicken fajitas	1 ea	223	61	405	22	50	4	13	2.5	6	3.5
1264	Chicken flauta	1 ea	113	53	343	14	13	2	27	4.3	11.1	9.6
686	Chicken pot pie, homemade (⅓)	1 pce	232	57	545	23	43	4	31	10.9	14.5	5.8
1672	Chili con carne	½ c	127	77	128	12	11	2	4	1.7	1.7	.3
1112	Chicken salad with celery	½ c	78	53	268	11	3	<1	25	3.1	4.5	15.8
1382	Chicken teriyaki, breast	1 pce	128	67	176	26	7	<1	4	.9	1	.9
687	Chili with beans, canned	1 c	255	76	286	15	30	11	14	6	6	.9
1479	Chinese pastry	1 oz	28	46	67	1	13	<1	2	.2	.4	.8
688	Chop suey with beef & pork	1 c	250	63	483	25	35	4	28	5.7	9.8	10.5

(1)Cooked weight is half the weight of raw sausage.

(2)Crust made with vegetable shortening and enriched flour.

(Computer code number is for West Diet Analysis program)

PAGE KEY: H–4 = BEV H–6 = DAIRY H–12 = EGGS H–14 = FAT/OIL H–18 = FRUIT H–26 = BAKERY H–36 = GRAIN H–44 = FISH H–48 = MEATS H–50 = POULTRY H–54 = SAUSAGE H–56 = MIXED/FAST H–64 = NUTS/SEEDS H–68 = SWEETS H–70 = VEG/LEG H–84 = MISC H–88 = SOUPS/SAUCES H–90 = FAST H–106 = FRZN ENTREE H–112 = BABY FOODS

Chol (mg)	Calc (mg)	Iron (mg)	Magn (mg)	Pota (mg)	Sodi (mg)	Zinc (mg)	VT-A (RE)	Thia (mg)	VT-E (α-TE)	Ribo (mg)	Niac (mg)	V-B6 (mg)	Fola (μg)	VT-C (mg)
9	3	.34	8	59	387	.24	0	–	–	–	–	–	–	0
31	5	.95	8	148	596	1.23	0	.03	.12	.14	2.01	.15	3	0
21	11	.35	6	61	281	.65	0	–	–	–	–	–	–	0
9	1	.15	2	38	224	.28	0	.03	.02	.04	.55	.03	<1	0
21	54	.58	10	194	792	.8	4	.17	.14	.15	1.17	.11	3	0
20	3	.41	4	67	248	.55	0	.14	.07	.04	.98	.05	1	<1
22	8	.32	4	94	336	.65	0	.19	.07	.07	1.18	.09	<1	<1
94	36	1.42	19	409	1467	2.85	0	.84	.3	.29	5.13	.37	2	2
37	7	1.51	9	112	604	1.21	0	.14	.13	.21	2.01	.12	1	0
47	11	.92	9	139	572	1.03	0	.04	.33	.1	2.01	.14	2	0
24	2	.45	5	113	558	.97	0	.18	.08	.09	1.46	.15	<1	0
89	19	1.42	24	360	2188	2.64	0	1.04	4.18	.29	5.04	.36	2	0
11	4	.24	2	33	304	.31	3	.05	.52	.04	.52	.04	<1	0
8	3	.16	3	48	98	.27	11	.01	.57	.02	.43	.03	1	<1
48	7	.99	8	129	643	1.44	0	.18	.15	.12	2.2	.12	1	0
46	20	.79	13	229	1020	1.92	0	.48	.17	.18	3.08	.24	3	1
35	6	1.17	6	125	571	1.18	0	.07	.1	.15	1.98	.12	1	0
23	5	.52	6	76	191	.97	0	.03	.14	.08	1.42	.08	1	0
17	3	.28	2	32	305	.51	0	.03	.07	.03	.51	.04	1	0
35	81	2	59	551	615	1.54	76	.09	2.64	.19	8.59	.4	32	11
0	40	2.7	–	–	135	–	900	–	–	–	–	–	–	14
0	3	.67	6	58	55	.16	0	.07	1.14	.05	.49	.02	9	0
64	29	2.94	40	613	292	5.29	568	.15	.49	.17	4.66	.28	37	17
34	29	2.21	39	426	1006	4.24	262	.07	.34	.12	2.45	.2	31	7
39	26	2.7	40	522	862	3.14	97	.22	.57	.22	4.31	.29	20	14
22	64	3	32	362	721	2	44	.39	1.77	.26	4	.27	21	24
45	50	2.15	29	292	187	4.18	15	.07	4.01	.15	2.13	.25	10	14
44	29	3.78	6	334	596	3.17	519	.29	3.78	.29	4.83	.24	29	6
16	67	.94	20	242	62	.38	102	.08	2.1	.13	.75	.11	43	53
26	5	.4	6	59	61	.56	17	.01	.24	.04	2.06	.13	1	<1
10	26	.75	14	317	118	.19	1462	.08	5.03	.05	.64	.22	9	5
88	206	4.67	44	445	1108	5	129	.39	1.18	.46	7.4	.29	29	8
186	127	2.45	20	404	760	1.8	272	.1	.98	.42	5.39	.23	11	12
96	26	2.16	26	149	600	1.53	10	.05	–	.17	4.32	.19	10	0
8	45	1.25	14	418	725	1.3	28	.05	.05	.1	1	.09	12	13
78	58	2.5	28	473	718	2.12	50	.08	.75	.23	4.25	.41	19	10
41	83	3.7	51	532	439	1.77	56	.48	2.05	.37	6.6	.35	41	22
37	53	.97	28	243	189	1.18	22	.05	4.06	.1	3.21	.22	8	14
72	70	3.02	25	343	594	2	735	.33	3.25	.33	4.87	.46	29	5
67	34	2.6	23	347	505	1.8	84	.06	.81	.57	1.25	.17	15	<1
48	16	.62	11	138	201	.8	31	.03	6.27	.07	3.28	.34	9	1
80	27	1.76	36	309	1866	1.94	16	.08	.35	.2	8.69	.46	13	3
43	120	8.75	115	931	1331	5.1	87	.12	1.87	.27	.91	.34	58	4
0	8	.51	6	28	3	.2	<1	.04	.26	<.01	.42	.02	1	0
52	45	4.7	61	586	930	4	153	.42	2.07	.42	6.4	.51	50	23

(For purposes of calculations, use "0" for t, <1, <.1, <.01, etc.)

H

Table H-1
Food Composition

Computer Code Number	Food Description	Measure	Wt (g)	H_2O (%)	Ener (kcal)	Prot (g)	Carb (g)	Dietary Fiber (g)	Fat (g)	Fat Breakdown (g) Sat	Mono	Poly
	MIXED DISHES and FAST FOOD—Cont.											
	MIXED DISHES—Cont.											
690	Coleslaw[1]	1 c	120	74	178	2	16	2	13	2	2.9	7.8
689	Corn pudding[2]	1 c	250	76	273	11	32	4	13	6.3	4.3	1.8
1110	Corned beef hash, canned	1 c	220	67	398	19	24	1	25	11.9	10.9	.9
1255	Deviled egg (½ egg + filling)	1 ea	31	69	63	4	<1	0	5	1.24	1.8	1.5
	Egg foo yung patty:											
1467	Meatless	1 ea	86	78	113	6	3	<1	8	1.9	3.4	2.1
1458	With beef	1 ea	86	74	129	9	3	<1	9	2.2	3.2	2.4
1465	With chicken	1 ea	86	74	130	9	4	<1	9	2.1	3.1	2.5
1602	Egg roll, meatless	1 ea	64	70	102	3	10	1	6	1.3	2.5	1.6
1550	Egg roll, with meat	1 ea	64	66	115	5	9	1	6	1.5	2.8	1.6
1113	Egg salad	1 c	183	57	586	17	3	0	57	10.6	17.4	24.2
691	French toast w/wheat bread, homemade[3]	1 pce	65	54	151	5	16	<1	7	2	3	1.7
1355	Green pepper, stuffed	1 ea	172	75	229	11	20	2	12	5.1	4.9	.5
1487	Hot & sour soup (Chinese)	1 c	244	88	133	12	5	<1	6	2	2.5	1.2
2242	Hamburger deluxe	1 ea	110	49	279	13	27	–	14	4.1	5.3	2.6
1997	Hummous/hummus	¼ c	62	65	106	3	13	3	5	.8	2.2	2
	Lasagna:											
1346	With meat, homemade	1 pce	245	67	382	22	39	3	15	7.8	5	.9
1111	Without meat, homemade	1 pce	218	70	298	15	39	3	9	5.4	2.5	.6
1117	Frozen entree	1 pce	205	75	235	15	25	3	9	4	3.3	.5
1606	Lo mein, meatless	1 c	200	82	134	6	27	3	1	.1	.1	.3
1607	Lo mein, with meat	1 c	200	70	285	17	32	2	10	1.9	2.9	4.5
692	Macaroni & cheese, canned[4]	1 c	240	80	228	9	26	1	10	4.2	3.1	1.4
693	Macaroni & cheese, homemade[5]	1 c	200	58	430	17	40	1	22	8.9	8.8	3.6
1115	Macaroni salad, no cheese	1 c	177	60	461	5	28	2	37	4.1	6.1	25.5
1120	Meat loaf, beef	1 pce	87	63	182	16	4	<1	11	4	4.7	.5
1119	Meat loaf, beef and pork (⅓)	1 pce	87	60	205	15	5	<1	14	5.2	6.3	.9
1303	Moussaka (lamb & eggplant)	1 c	250	82	236	16	13	4	13	4.6	5.4	1.9
1899	Mushrooms, batter fried	5 ea	70	66	148	2	8	1	12	2.1	3	6.4
715	Potato salad with mayonnaise and eggs[6]	½ c	125	76	179	3	14	2	10	1.8	3.1	4.7
1674	Pizza, combination, 1/12 of 12" round	1 pce	53	48	123	9	14	–	4	1	1.7	.6
1673	Pizza, pepperoni, 1/12 of 12" round	1 pce	47	47	121	7	13	–	5	1.5	2.1	.8
694	Quiche Lorraine, ⅛ of 8" quiche[7]	1 pce	176	54	508	20	20	1	39	18	13.8	4.9
1449	Ramen noodles, cooked	1 c	227	82	156	6	29	3	2	.4	.5	.5
1671	Ravioli, meat	½ c	125	76	122	14	19	1	4	1	2.3	1
1597	Fried rice (meatless)	1 c	166	68	264	5	34	1	12	1.7	3	6.3
2142	Roast beef hash	½ c	95	66	187	8	9	1	13	5.7	4.7	2.6
	Spaghetti (enriched) in tomato sauce:											
	With cheese:											
695	Canned	1 c	250	80	190	6	39	3	2	0	.4	.5
696	Homemade	1 c	250	77	260	9	37	3	9	2	5.4	1.2

(1)Recipe: 41% cabbage; 12% celery; 12% table cream; 12% sugar; 7% green pepper; 6% lemon juice; 4% onion; 3% pimento; 3% vinegar; 2% each for salt, dry mustard, and white pepper.

(2)Recipe: 55% yellow corn, 23% whole milk, 14% egg, 4% sugar, 3% salt, and 1% pepper.

(3)Recipe: 35% whole milk, 32% white bread, 29% egg, and cooked in 4% margarine.

(4)Made with corn oil.

(5)Made with margarine.

(6)Recipe: 62% potatoes; 12% egg; 8% mayonnaise; 7% celery; 6% sweet pickle relish; 2% onion; 1% each for green pepper, pimento, salt, and dry mustard.

(7)Crust made with vegetable shortening and enriched flour.

(Computer code number is for West Diet Analysis program)

H

PAGE KEY: H–4 = BEV H–6 = DAIRY H–12 = EGGS H–14 = FAT/OIL H–18 = FRUIT H–26 = BAKERY H–36 = GRAIN H–44 = FISH H–48 = MEATS H–50 = POULTRY H–54 = SAUSAGE H–56 = MIXED/FAST H–64 = NUTS/SEEDS H–68 = SWEETS H–70 = VEG/LEG H–84 = MISC H–88 = SOUPS/SAUCES H–90 = FAST H–106 = FRZN ENTREE H–112 = BABY FOODS

Chol (mg)	Calc (mg)	Iron (mg)	Magn (mg)	Pota (mg)	Sodi (mg)	Zinc (mg)	VT-A (RE)	Thia (mg)	VT-E (α-TE)	Ribo (mg)	Niac (mg)	V-B6 (mg)	Fola (μg)	VT-C (mg)
6[8]	41	.88	11	215	324	.24	60	.05	4.8	.04	.1	.13	47	10
250	100	1.4	38	403	138	1.25	90	1.03	.53	.32	2.47	.3	63	7
73	29	4.4	36	440	1188	3.3	0	.02	.48	.2	4.62	.43	20	0
121	15	.35	3	37	94	.3	49	.02	.86	.14	.02	.05	13	0
184	31	1.1	12	118	310	.7	86	.05	1.57	.26	.44	.1	30	5
180	26	1.1	12	145	184	1.16	92	.05	1.79	.24	.74	.16	22	3
182	28	.85	12	145	187	.81	95	.05	1.87	.25	.96	.13	23	3
30	12	.76	9	98	306	.25	15	.08	.81	.11	.81	.06	13	3
37	13	.78	10	124	304	.5	14	.17	.79	.13	1.31	.1	9	2
574	74	1.8	13	180	666	1.42	260	.08	8.87	.66	.09	.47	62	0
76	64	1.09	11	87	311	.44	81	.13	.31	.21	1.06	.05	15	<1
34	16	1.77	21	233	201	2.3	44	.15	.75	.1	2.74	.3	17	55
23	29	1.83	27	351	1562	1.17	2	.19	.12	.22	4.58	.15	12	1
26	63	2.63	22	227	504	2	9	.23	.83	.2	3.7	.12	18.7	2
0	31	.97	18	108	151	.68	1	.06	.62	.03	.25	.25	37	5
57	258	3.22	50	461	745	3.25	158	.23	1.15	.33	4	.21	19	16
31	252	2.5	44	375	714	1.77	156	.23	1.07	.27	2.49	.17	17	15
33	158	2.08	39	453	496	2.23	149	.16	2.08	.23	3.06	.2	17	25
0	48	2.06	33	389	623	.92	130	.23	.35	.24	2.83	.19	49	13
30	25	2.11	40	246	276	1.63	6	.37	1.51	.24	4.25	.28	41	8
24	199	.96	31	139	730	1.2	73	.12	.14	.24	.96	.02	8	<1
42	362	1.8	37	240	1086	1.2	234	.2	.12	.4	1.8	.05	10	1
27	31	1.56	20	170	352	.53	44	.18	10.31	.1	1.43	.33	21	4
84	29	1.61	14	187	145	3.23	24	.05	.31	.22	2.61	.15	11	1
84	34	1.42	14	213	381	2.68	24	.2	.32	.22	2.68	.17	10	1
97	68	1.79	40	556	431	2.55	105	.15	.81	.31	4.13	.23	45	6
14	54	.77	8	180	121	.42	10	.07	.92	.22	1.65	.05	8	1
85	24	.81	19	318	661	.39	41	.1	2.33	.08	1.11	.18	8	13
14	68	1.02	12	119	255	.74	68	.14	1.05	.12	1.31	.06	18	1
10	43	.62	6	102	178	.35	36	.09	1.09	.16	2.03	.04	35	1
205	201	1.9	27	271	549	1.66	243	.23	1.91	.44	4.71	.2	17	3
38	20	1.89	24	51	1349	.77	204	.22	.09	.1	1.75	.06	9	<1
88	23	1.17	23	306	498	.76	22	.1	–	.09	1.9	.16	12	7
42	30	1.84	24	134	286	.89	21	.21	2.46	.11	2.25	.15	22	4
32	8	.73	18	294	564	2.43	0	.08	–	.1	1.89	.25	10	0
8	40	2.75	21	303	955	1.12	120	.35	2.13	.28	4.5	.13	6	10
8	80	2.25	26	408	955	1.3	140	.25	2.75	.18	2.25	.2	8	13

(8)From dairy cream in recipe.

Table H–1
Food Composition

Computer Code Number	Food Description	Measure	Wt (g)	H_2O (%)	Ener (kcal)	Prot (g)	Carb (g)	Dietary Fiber (g)	Fat (g)	Fat Breakdown (g) Sat	Mono	Poly
	MIXED DISHES and FAST FOODS—Cont.											
	MIXED DISHES—Cont.											
	With meatballs:											
697	Canned	1 c	250	78	258	12	29	6	10	2.2	3.9	3.9
698	Homemade	1 c	248	70	332	19	39	8	12	3.3	6.3	2.2
716	Spinach soufflé[1]	1 c	136	74	219	12	3	4	20	9.6	5.7	2.2
1553	Sweet & sour pork	1 c	226	77	231	15	25	1	8	2.2	2.9	2.5
1263	Sweet & sour chicken breast	1 ea	131	79	117	8	15	1	3	.6	.8	1.5
1515	Three bean salad	1 ea	340	82	316	9	31	7	19	2.8	4.3	11.1
717	Tuna salad[2]	1 c	205	63	383	33	19	0	19	3.2	5.9	8.5
1121	Tuna noodle casserole, homemade	1 c	202	75	238	17	26	1	7	1.9	1.5	3.2
1270	Waldorf salad	1 c	137	58	408	4	13	2	40	4.2	7.3	27
	FAST FOODS and SANDWICHES (see end of this appendix for additional Fast Foods):											
699	Burrito,[3] beef & bean	1 ea	175	52	385	17	50	4	14	6.3	5.3	.9
700	Burrito, bean	1 ea	174	53	358	11	57	7	11	5.5	3.8	1
2106	Burrito, chicken con queso	1 ea	306	77	280	12	53	5	6	1.5	–	–
701	Cheeseburger with bun, regular	1 ea	112	55	261	13	21	–	15	6.7	5.2	1.1
702	Cheeseburger with bun, 4-oz patty	1 ea	194	51	487	25	41	–	25	10.2	9.1	3.1
703	Chicken patty sandwich	1 ea	157	47	444	21	33	1	25	7.4	9	7.2
704	Corndog	1 ea	111	47	292	11	35	–	12	3.3	5.8	2.2
1922	Corndog, chicken	1 ea	113	59	271	13	26	–	13	–	–	–
705	Enchilada	1 ea	230	63	451	14	40	–	27	15	8.9	1.2
706	English muffin with egg, cheese, bacon	1 ea	138	49	362	19	30	1	19	8.6	6.4	2
	Fish sandwich:											
707	Regular, with cheese	1 ea	140	45	400	16	36	<1	22	6.2	6.8	7.2
708	Large, no cheese	1 ea	170	47	464	18	44	<1	25	5.6	8.3	8.9
709	Hamburger with bun, regular	1 ea	98	46	252	13	30	1	9	3.2	3.4	1.6
710	Hamburger with bun, 4-oz patty	1 ea	174	51	466	26	31	–	26	9.7	11.4	2.3
711	Hot dog/frankfurter with bun	1 ea	85	54	210	9	16	–	13	4.4	5.9	1.5
	Lunchables:											
2129	Bologna & American cheese	1 ea	128	–	450	18	19	0	34	15	–	–
2130	Ham & cheese	1 ea	128	–	320	22	19	0	17	8	–	–
2117	Honey ham & Amer. w/choc pudding	1 ea	176	–	390	18	34	<1	20	9	–	–
2118	Honey turkey & cheddar w/Jello	1 ea	163	–	320	17	27	1	16	9	–	–
2131	Pepperoni & American cheese	1 ea	128	–	480	20	19	0	36	17	–	–
2125	Salami & American cheese	1 ea	128	–	430	18	18	0	32	15	–	–
2127	Turkey & cheddar cheese	1 ea	128	–	360	20	20	1	22	11	–	–
712	Pizza, cheese, ⅛ of 15" round[4]	1 pce	120	49	268	15	39	2	6	2.9	1.9	.9
	SANDWICHES:											
	Avocado, cheese, tomato, & lettuce:											
1276	On white bread, firm	1 ea	210	58	478	15	41	5	29	8.7	11.3	7.3
1278	On part whole wheat	1 ea	201	59	444	15	35	7	29	8.6	11.4	7.4
1277	On whole wheat	1 ea	214	58	468	16	40	8	30	8.7	11.6	7.5

(1)Recipe: 29% whole milk, 26% spinach, 13% egg white, 13% cheddar cheese, 7% egg yolk, 7% butter, 4% flour, 1% salt and pepper.

(2)Made with drained chunk light tuna, celery, onion, pickle relish, and mayonnaise-type salad dressing.

(3)Made with a 10½"-diameter flour tortilla.

(4)Crust made with vegetable shortening and enriched flour.

(Computer code number is for West Diet Analysis program)

PAGE KEY: H–4 = BEV H–6 = DAIRY H–12 = EGGS H–14 = FAT/OIL H–18 = FRUIT H–26 = BAKERY H–36 = GRAIN H–44 = FISH H–48 = MEATS H–50 = POULTRY H–54 = SAUSAGE H–56 = MIXED/FAST H–64 = NUTS/SEEDS H–68 = SWEETS H–70 = VEG/LEG H–84 = MISC H–88 = SOUPS/SAUCES H–90 = FAST H–106 = FRZN ENTREE H–112 = BABY FOODS

Chol (mg)	Calc (mg)	Iron (mg)	Magn (mg)	Pota (mg)	Sodi (mg)	Zinc (mg)	VT-A (RE)	Thia (mg)	VT-E (α-TE)	Ribo (mg)	Niac (mg)	V-B6 (mg)	Fola (μg)	VT-C (mg)
23	53	3.25	20	245	1220	2.39	100	.15	1.5	.18	2.25	.12	5	5
74	124	3.72	40	665	1009	2.45	159	.25	1.64	.3	3.97	.2	10	22
184	230	1.35	38	201	763	1.29	675	.09	1.22	.3	.48	.12	62	3
38	28	1.36	34	390	1219	1.5	28	.55	.62	.21	3.6	.41	11	20
23	16	.8	21	187	732	.66	20	.06	.39	.08	3.06	.18	6	13
0	80	3.21	57	508	1164	1.22	52	.16	4.43	.21	.91	.1	120	10
27	35	2.05	39	365	824	1.15	55	.06	1.95	.14	13.7	.17	15	5
41	34	2.3	31	183	776	1.21	13	.18	1.19	.15	7.82	.2	10	1
21	43	.89	39	270	234	.63	40	.1	8.67	.05	.36	.37	27	6
37	81	3.71	63	497	1011	2.91	49	.4	1.05	.63	4.1	.28	56	1
4	91	3.62	70	524	790	1.22	26	.5	1.39	.49	3.25	.24	94	2
10	40	.72	–	–	600	–	40	–	–	–	–	–	–	15
38	132	1.93	19	167	710	1.9	51	.24	.97	.17	4.64	.11	16	2
70	200	4	35	392	1228	4.07	76	.41	–	.33	9.41	.21	27	2
52	52	4.04	30	305	826	1.62	27	.28	.47	.2	5.87	.17	25	8
50	64	3.92	11	167	617	.83	23	.18	.44	.44	2.64	.06	38	0
64	–	–	–	–	668	–	–	–	–	–	–	–	–	–
62	458	1.86	71	338	1106	3.54	262	.12	2.07	.6	2.69	.55	48	1
221	196	3.11	32	202	741	1.71	149	.46	.57	.5	3.71	.15	41	1
52	141	2.67	28	270	718	.9	74	.35	1.4	.32	3.23	.08	24	2
60	90	2.81	36	366	661	1.07	32	.36	.94	.24	3.66	.12	48	3
39	47	2.25	21	197	517	1.88	12	.24	.39	.29	4.3	.12	16	2
84	75	4.49	37	426	600	4.7	4	.28	1.31	.33	5.45	.3	37	1
38	20	2.01	11	124	581	1.72	0	.2	.24	.24	3.16	.04	26	<1
85	300	2.7	–	–	1620	–	60	–	–	–	–	–	–	0
60	300	1.8	–	–	1770	–	80	–	–	–	–	–	–	–
55	250	2.7	–	–	1540	–	–	–	–	–	–	–	–	–
50	20	6	–	–	1360	–	–	–	–	–	–	–	–	–
95	250	2.7	–	–	1840	–	–	–	–	–	–	–	–	–
80	250	2.7	–	–	1740	–	60	–	–	–	–	–	–	–
70	300	1.8	–	–	1650	–	60	–	–	–	–	–	–	–
18	222	1.1	30	209	640	1.55	140	.35	–	.31	4.73	.08	112	2
34	294	3.06	54	581	550	1.7	140	.37	4.55	.39	3.77	.32	80	11
31	291	3.1	67	617	525	1.91	140	.35	4.55	.39	3.94	.35	80	11
31	281	3.53	102	679	593	2.68	140	.36	4.17	.37	4.3	.42	92	11

(For purposes of calculations, use "0" for t, <1, <.1, <.01, etc.)

Table H–1
Food Composition

Computer Code Number	Food Description	Measure	Wt (g)	H_2O (%)	Ener (kcal)	Prot (g)	Carb (g)	Dietary Fiber (g)	Fat (g)	Fat Breakdown (g) Sat	Mono	Poly
	FAST FOODS and SANDWICHES (see end of this appendix for additional Fast Foods)—Cont.											
	SANDWICHES—Cont.											
	Bacon, lettuce & tomato:											
1137	On white bread, soft	1 ea	124	53	308	10	28	2	18	4.5	6.1	6.1
1139	On part whole wheat	1 ea	124	54	303	11	27	4	18	4.3	6.2	6.1
1138	On whole wheat	1 ea	137	53	328	12	32	5	18	4.4	6.5	6.3
	Cheese, grilled:											
1140	On white bread, soft	1 ea	118	37	399	18	30	1	24	13.1	7.5	2
1142	On part whole wheat	1 ea	118	37	394	18	28	3	24	12.9	7.5	2.07
1141	On whole wheat	1 ea	132	38	421	20	33	4	25	13.1	7.9	2.2
1596	Chicken fillet	1 ea	182	47	515	24	39	1	30	8.5	10.4	8.4
	Chicken salad:											
1143	On white bread, soft	1 ea	110	40	369	11	31	1	23	3.7	6	12
1145	On part whole wheat	1 ea	110	41	364	11	29	4	23	4	6	12
1144	On whole wheat	1 ea	123	41	387	13	35	5	24	3.6	6.4	12
1146	Corned beef & swiss on rye	1 ea	154	49	420	28	22	<1	26	9.4	7.4	6.3
	Egg salad:											
1147	On white bread, soft	1 ea	116	43	379	10	31	1	25	4.4	6.8	12
1149	On part whole wheat	1 ea	116	43	374	10	29	3	25	4.1	6.8	12.1
1148	On whole wheat	1 ea	130	43	400	12	35	5	25	4.3	7.1	12.2
	Ham:											
1279	On rye bread	1 ea	150	60	283	22	21	<1	14	2.4	3.8	6
1151	On white bread, soft	1 ea	156	55	333	22	30	1	14	3	4.4	5.9
1153	On part whole wheat	1 ea	156	55	328	22	28	3	14	2.7	4.4	6
1152	On whole wheat	1 ea	169	54	352	24	34	5	15	2.9	4.7	6.1
	Ham & cheese:											
1280	On white bread, soft	1 ea	156	49	402	23	30	1	22	8.4	5.9	6.1
1282	On part whole wheat	1 ea	156	50	397	23	28	3	22	8.1	5.9	6.2
1281	On whole wheat	1 ea	170	49	423	24	34	5	22	8.3	6.2	6.3
1150	Ham & swiss on rye	1 ea	150	54	339	22	22	<1	19	6.5	5.1	6
	Ham salad:											
1154	On white bread, soft	1 ea	131	47	362	11	37	1	20	4.8	6.8	7.4
1156	On part whole wheat	1 ea	131	48	357	11	35	3	20	4.6	6.8	7.5
1155	On whole wheat	1 ea	144	47	380	13	40	5	20	4.7	7.1	7.6
1157	Patty melt: Ground beef & cheese on rye	1 ea	182	46	561	37	22	3	37	13.3	11.7	8.4
	Peanut butter & jelly:											
1158	On white bread, soft	1 ea	101	26	351	12	47	3	15	3.1	6.7	3.9
1160	On part whole wheat	1 ea	101	27	346	12	45	5	15	2.9	6.7	4
1159	On whole wheat	1 ea	114	29	370	13	50	6	16	3	7	4.1
1161	Reuben, grilled: Corned beef, swiss cheese, sauerkraut on rye	1 ea	237	64	461	28	25	2	29	9.9	9.5	7.1
	Roast beef:											
713	On a bun	1 ea	150	49	374	23	36	–	15	3.9	7.4	1.9
1162	On white bread, soft	1 ea	156	46	403	29	34	1	17	3.4	4.2	8.2
1164	On part whole wheat	1 ea	156	47	398	29	32	3	17	3.2	4.3	8.3
1163	On whole wheat	1 ea	169	46	422	31	38	4	17	3.3	4.5	8.4
	Tuna salad:											
1165	On white bread, soft	1 ea	122	46	327	14	35	2	15	2.5	3.8	7.9
1167	On part whole wheat	1 ea	122	47	322	14	33	4	15	2.2	3.9	8

(Computer code number is for West Diet Analysis program)

PAGE KEY: H–4 = BEV H–6 = DAIRY H–12 = EGGS H–14 = FAT/OIL H–18 = FRUIT H–26 = BAKERY H–36 = GRAIN H–44 = FISH H–48 = MEATS H–50 = POULTRY H–54 = SAUSAGE H–56 = MIXED/FAST H–64 = NUTS/SEEDS H–68 = SWEETS H–70 = VEG/LEG H–84 = MISC H–88 = SOUPS/SAUCES H–90 = FAST H–106 = FRZN ENTREE H–112 = BABY FOODS

Chol (mg)	Calc (mg)	Iron (mg)	Magn (mg)	Pota (mg)	Sodi (mg)	Zinc (mg)	VT-A (RE)	Thia (mg)	VT-E (α-TE)	Ribo (mg)	Niac (mg)	V-B6 (mg)	Fola (μg)	VT-C (mg)
22	52	1.99	18	234	590	.96	31	.35	2.34	.19	3.2	.14	34	12
20	63	2.27	33	283	604	1.2	31	.37	2.7	.21	3.62	.17	37	12
20	55	2.68	64	342	670	1.9	31	.4	2.36	.2	4	.24	48	12
55	398	1.81	25	154	1139	2.05	211	.24	1.13	.34	1.91	.06	24	<1
53	410	2.11	39	208	1154	2.3	211	.25	1.52	.36	2.38	.1	28	<1
54	403	2.55	73	271	1229	3.08	212	.26	1.15	.35	2.74	.17	40	<1
60	60	4.68	35	353	957	1.88	31	.33	.55	.24	6.81	.2	29	9
32	60	2.04	18	139	460	.8	24	.25	6.16	.18	3.7	.25	26	<1
31	73	2.35	33	195	475	1.06	24	.26	6.57	.2	4.2	.29	30	<1
30	63	2.79	68	259	543	1.85	24	.27	6.14	.19	4.5	.36	42	<1
82	268	3.11	28	225	1391	3.64	81	.19	2.58	.33	2.7	.17	19	1
157	70	2.17	16	113	524	.74	76	.26	4.51	.31	1.97	.2	37	0
155	83	2.47	31	170	539	1	76	.27	4.91	.33	2.45	.23	41	0
155	74	2.92	66	234	611	1.8	76	.28	4.53	.32	2.82	.3	53	0
47	48	2.3	26	364	1566	2.11	8	.99	2.36	.31	5.45	.48	15	23
47	60	2.39	29	367	1615	2.04	8	1.02	2.34	.33	5.98	.47	24	22
45	72	2.68	43	421	1630	2.29	8	1.03	2.7	.35	6.45	.5	27	22
45	62	3.1	77	483	1696	3.05	8	1.04	2.34	.33	6.78	.57	39	22
60	232	2.28	30	314	1616	2.34	90	.76	2.53	.36	4.63	.36	25	15
59	244	2.58	45	368	1630	2.59	90	.77	2.93	.39	5.09	.39	28	15
59	235	3.01	79	431	1702	3.36	90	.78	2.55	.37	5.45	.46	40	15
57	258	2.25	29	344	1602	2.59	79	.72	2.52	.36	4.06	.35	16	15
31	56	2.07	19	160	921	1.06	8	.51	3.29	.22	3.26	.17	22	4
29	69	2.4	34	216	936	1.32	8	.52	3.69	.24	3.74	.21	26	4
29	59	2.82	69	279	1001	2.11	8	.53	3.29	.23	4.1	.28	38	4
113	222	4.19	36	391	701	7.11	123	.25	3.5	.46	6.14	.35	25	<1
2	60	2.25	56	245	293	1.07	<1	.27	.12	.17	5.33	.13	40	<1
0	72	2.55	71	299	308	1.32	<1	.28	.51	.19	5.8	.17	44	<1
0	63	2.97	104	361	375	2.09	<1	.29	.14	.17	6.14	.24	56	<1
80	288	4.24	38	361	1945	3.72	130	.21	4.45	.34	3	.27	38	13
56	59	4.56	33	341	855	3.66	23	.41	.21	.33	6.33	.29	44	2
45	60	3.97	28	431	1592	3.77	12	.29	3.3	.3	6.38	.39	30	12
43	62	4.3	43	485	1607	4.02	12	.31	3.69	.32	6.84	.42	34	12
43	62	4.7	77	547	1672	4.79	12	.31	3.31	.31	7.18	.49	46	12
16	60	2.24	23	161	567	.67	22	.25	2.72	.18	5.53	.12	25	1
13	73	2.55	37	217	582	.93	22	.26	3.12	.2	6.01	.16	29	1

(For purposes of calculations, use "0" for t, <1, <.1, <.01, etc.)

Table H–1
Food Composition

Computer Code Number	Food Description	Measure	Wt (g)	H_2O (%)	Ener (kcal)	Prot (g)	Carb (g)	Dietary Fiber (g)	Fat (g)	Fat Breakdown (g) Sat	Mono	Poly
	FAST FOODS and SANDWICHES (see end of this appendix for additional Fast Foods)—Cont.											
1166	On whole wheat	1 ea	135	46	346	16	39	5	16	2.4	4.1	8.1
	Turkey:											
1168	On white bread, soft	1 ea	156	54	346	24	29	1	15	2.4	3.2	8.3
1170	On part whole wheat	1 ea	156	54	341	25	27	3	15	2.2	3.2	8.3
1169	On whole wheat	1 ea	169	53	365	26	33	4	15	2.3	3.5	8.5
	Turkey ham:											
1272	On rye bread	1 ea	150	60	280	21	20	<1	14	2.5	2.8	6.9
1273	On white bread, soft	1 ea	156	55	331	21	30	1	14	3	3.4	6.8
1275	On part whole wheat	1 ea	156	56	326	22	28	3	14	3	4.2	5.6
1274	On whole wheat	1 ea	169	55	350	23	33	5	15	2.9	3.7	7
714	Taco	1 ea	78	58	169	9	12	–	9	5.2	3	.4
	Tostada:											
1114	With refried beans	1 ea	157	66	243	11	29	8	11	5.9	3.3	.8
1118	With beans & beef	1 ea	192	70	284	14	25	3	15	9.8	3	.5
1354	With beans & chicken	1 ea	156	68	248	20	18	3	11	5.3	3.9	1.6
	Vegetarian foods:											
1511	Baked beans, canned	½ c	127	73	118	6	26	6	1	.2	t	.3
1175	Breakfast links	1 ea	34	60	31	6	1	1	2	.4	.5	.96
1171	Nuteena	1 pce	67	58	198	7	7	2	16	6.3	7.1	2.1
1173	Redi-burger	1 pce	68	59	88	13	4	4	8	1.2	1.9	4.6
1174	Vege-burger	½ c	108	71	130	21	5	4	3	.9	1.2	1
	Vegetarian foods, Worthington											
1846	Chik slices, canned	2 pce	60	78	62	6	<1	<1	4	.6	.9	.2.3
1833	Chili, canned	½ c	106	73	136	9	10	4	7	1.1	1.7	4.1
1835	Choplets, canned slices	2 pce	92	72	94	17	3	2	2	.9	.3	.3
1831	Country stew, canned	1 c	240	73	208	13	20	5	9	1.6	2.3	4.9
1838	Numete, canned slices	1 pce	68	58	164	8	6	4	12	2.9	5.4	3.3
1839	Prime stakes, canned	1 pce	92	71	136	9	4	4	9	1.4	2.9	4.9
1840	Protose, canned slices	1 pce	76	53	181	18	7	4	9	1.3	4.2	3.3
1842	Saucettes, canned links	2 pce	67	62	152	10	2	2	11	1.9	2.8	6.7
1844	Savory slices, canned	2 pce	56	66	97	7	4	2	6	2.4	2.6	1.1
1847	Turkee slices, canned	2 pce	63	64	129	9	2	1	9	1.6	3.6	4
	NUTS, SEEDS, and PRODUCTS											
	Almonds:											
1365	Dry roasted, salted	1 c	138	3	810	23	33	19	71	6.8	46.2	14.9
718	Slivered, packed, unsalted	1 c	135	4	795	27	28	15[1]	71	6.7	45.8	14.9
719	Whole, dried, unsalted:	1 c	142	4	836	28	29	16[1]	74	7	48.1	15.6
720	Ounce	1 oz	28	4	165	6	6	3[1]	15	1.4	9.5	3.1
721	Almond butter	1 tbs	16	1	101	2	3	<1	10	.9	6.1	2
722	Brazil nuts, dry (about 7)	1 oz	28	3	184	4	4	2	19	4.5	6.4	6.8
	Cashew nuts, salted:											
723	Dry roasted:	1 c	137	2	786	21	45	4	64	12.8	37.4	10.7
724	Ounce	1 oz	28	2	161	4	9	1	13	2.6	7.6	2.2

(1)Values reported for dietary fiber in almonds vary from 7.0 to 14.3 g/100 g.

Chol (mg)	Calc (mg)	Iron (mg)	Magn (mg)	Pota (mg)	Sodi (mg)	Zinc (mg)	VT-A (RE)	Thia (mg)	VT-E (α-TE)	Ribo (mg)	Niac (mg)	V-B6 (mg)	Fola (μg)	VT-C (mg)
13	63	2.98	73	280	649	1.72	22	.27	2.71	.19	6	.23	41	1
45	56	2.01	29	302	1585	1.33	12	.26	3.46	.23	9	.4	24	0
43	68	2.3	43	356	1600	1.58	12	.27	3.85	.25	9.44	.44	28	0
43	59	2.73	77	418	1665	2.35	12	.28	3.47	.23	9.77	.51	40	0
55	51	4.06	25	342	1185	3	8	.22	2.8	.33	4.3	.29	17	<1
55	62	4.09	28	346	1248	2.9	8	.27	2.75	.35	4.87	.28	25	0
53	74	4.37	42	400	1262	3.15	8	.28	3.57	.37	5.34	.32	29	0
53	65	4.81	76	462	1329	3.91	8	.29	2.76	.35	5.68	.39	41	0
26	101	1.1	32	216	366	1.79	67	.07	.86	.2	1.47	.11	11	1
33	229	2.06	64	440	592	2.07	93	.11	1.26	.36	1.44	.17	82	1
63	161	2.09	58	419	743	2.71	148	.08	1.54	.42	2.44	.21	83	4
53	168	1.79	47	365	433	2.28	86	.11	1.87	.2	4.52	.32	54	4
0	64	.37	41	376	504	1.78	22	.19	.67	.08	.54	.17	30	4
1	11	1.62	12	44	255	.27	0	5.25	–	.16	3.92	.25	9	0
0	11	.33	40	202	145	.56	0	.13	–	.43	1.27	.55	60	0
<1	10	.85	13	97	364	.88	0	.11	–	.24	1.52	.41	17	0
0	15	.98	24	59	224	1.1	0	.39	–	.49	1.52	.61	29	0
<1	9	.73	–	111	257	.26	0	.06	–	.05	.37	.08	–	0
0	20	1.5	–	196	523	.57	0	.02	–	.03	1.04	.31	–	0
0	6	.37	–	40	500	.65	0	.05	–	.06	0	.06	–	0
2	51	5.09	–	270	826	1.03	432	1.85	–	.29	4.22	.86	–	0
0	12	1.39	–	192	337	.69	0	.1	–	.08	.67	.25	–	0
2	12	.4	–	82	445	.38	0	.12	–	.13	2	.38	–	0
<1	1	2.55	–	69	391	.99	0	.24	–	.18	1.85	.33	–	0
1	16	2.03	–	44	361	.46	0	1.05	–	.13	.17	.23	–	0
1	1	.94	–	27	357	.17	0	.16	–	.11	.96	.21	–	0
1	5	.91	–	31	388	.21	0	2.2	–	.1	.74	.16	–	0
0	389	5.24	420	1062	1076	6.76	0	.18	7.66	.83	3.89	.1	88	1
0	359	4.94	400	988	15	3.94	0	.29	32.4	1.05	4.54	.15	79	1
0	378	5.2	420	1039	16[2]	4.15	0	.3	34.08	1.11	4.77	.16	83	1
0	75	1.03	83	205	3[2]	.82	0	.06	6.72	.22	.94	.03	16	<1
0	43	.59	49	121	2[3]	.49	0	.02	3.25	.1	.46	.01	10	<1
0	49	.95	63	168	1	1.3	0	.28	2.13	.03	.45	.07	1	<1
0	62	8.22	356	774	877[4]	7.67	0	.27	.78	.27	1.92	.35	95	0
0	13	1.7	73	158	179[4]	1.59	0	.06	.16	.06	.4	.07	19	0

(2)Salted almonds contain 1108 mg sodium per cup, 221 mg per ounce.

(3)Salted almond butter contains 72 mg sodium per tablespoon.

(4)Dry-roasted cashews without salt contain 21 mg sodium per cup, or 4 mg per ounce.

(For purposes of calculations, use "0" for t, <1, <.1, <.01, etc.)

Table H-1
Food Composition

Computer Code Number	Food Description	Measure	Wt (g)	H_2O (%)	Ener (kcal)	Prot (g)	Carb (g)	Dietary Fiber (g)	Fat (g)	Fat Breakdown (g) Sat	Mono	Poly
	NUTS, SEEDS, and PRODUCTS—Cont.											
725	Oil roasted:	1 c	130	4	749	23	37	5	63	12.6	36.9	10.6
726	Ounce	1 oz	28	4	161	5	8	1	14	2.7	8	2.3
1366	Cashew nuts, unsalted, dry roasted	1 c	137	2	786	21	45	6	64	12.8	37.4	10.7
1367	Cashew nuts, unsalted, oil roasted	1 c	130	4	749	21	37	5	63	12.6	36.9	10.6
727	Cashew butter, unsalted	1 tbs	16	3	94	3	4	1	8	1.6	4.7	1.3
728	Chestnuts, European, roasted (1 cup = approx 17 kernels)	1 c	143	41	350	5	76	7	3	.6	1.1	1.2
	Coconut, raw:											
729	Piece 2 x 2 x ½"	1 pce	45	47	159	2	7	4	15	13.6	.6	.2
730	Shredded/grated, unpacked[1]	½ c	40	47	142	2	6	4	13	12	.6	.2
	Coconut, dried, shredded/grated:											
731	Unsweetened	1 c	78	3	515	6	19	13	50	45.1	2.2	.6
732	Sweetened	1 c	93	13	466	3	44	4	33	29.6	1.4	.4
733	Filberts/hazelnuts, chopped:	1 c	115	5	727	15	18	7	72	5.3	56.5	6.9
734	Ounce	1 oz	28	5	177	4	4	2	18	1.3	13.8	1.7
735	Macadamias, oil roasted, salted:	1 c	134	2	962	10	17	13	103	15.4	80.9	1.8
736	Ounce	1 oz	28	2	201	2	4	3	21	3.2	16.9	.4
1368	Macadamias, oil roasted, unsalted	1 c	134	2	962	10	17	13	103	15.4	80.9	1.8
	Mixed nuts:											
737	Dry roasted, salted	1 c	137	2	814	24	35	12	71	9.5	43	14.8
738	Oil roasted, salted	1 c	142	2	876	24	30	13	80	12.4	45	18.9
1369	Oil roasted, unsalted	1 c	142	2	876	27	30	14	80	12.4	45	18.9
	Peanuts:											
1370	Oil roasted, unsalted	1 c	144	2	837	38	27	10	71	9.9	35.3	22.5
741	Dried, salted:	1 c	146	2	854	35	31	12	73	10.1	36.1	22.9
742	Ounce	1 oz	28	2	164	7	6	2	14	1.9	6.9	4.4
1371	Peanut butter	2 tbs	32	1	190	8	6	2	16	3.6	7.8	4.4
744	Pecan halves, dried, unsalted:	1 c	108	5	720	9	20	8	73	5.9	45.6	18
745	Ounce	1 oz	28	5	187	2	5	2	19	1.5	11.8	4.7
1372	Pecan halves, dry roasted, salted	¼ c	28	1	185	2	6	3	18	1.5	11.3	4.5
746	Pine nuts/piñons, dried	1 oz	28	6	176	3	5	3	17	2.6	6.4	7.2
747	Pistachios, dried, shelled	1 oz	28	4	162	6	7	3	14	1.8	9.2	2.1
1373	Pistachios, dry roasted, salted, shelled	1 c	128	2	776	19	35	14	68	8.8	45.7	10.2
748	Pumpkin kernels, dried, unsalted	1 oz	28	7	152	7	5	1	13	2.4	4	5.9
1374	Pumpkin kernels, roasted, salted	1 c	227	7	1184	75	30	9	96	18.1	29.7	43.6
749	Sesame seeds, hulled, dried	¼ c	38	5	223	10	4	4	21	2.9	7.9	9.1
	Sunflower seed kernels:											
750	Dry	¼ c	36	5	205	8	7	4	18	1.9	3.4	11.8
751	Oil roasted	¼ c	34	3	209	7	5	2	20	2.1	3.7	12.9
752	Tahini (sesame butter)	1 tbs	15	3	91	3	3	1	9	1.2	3.2	3.7
1334	Trail Mix w/chocolate chips	1 c	146	7	707	21	66	8	47	9.3	19.8	16.5
753	Black walnuts, chopped:	1 c	125	4	759	31	15	6	71	4.8	15.9	46.9

[1]½ cup packed = 65 g.

(Computer code number is for West Diet Analysis program)

Chol (mg)	Calc (mg)	Iron (mg)	Magn (mg)	Pota (mg)	Sodi (mg)	Zinc (mg)	VT-A (RE)	Thia (mg)	VT-E (α-TE)	Ribo (mg)	Niac (mg)	V-B6 (mg)	Fola (µg)	VT-C (mg)
0	53	5.33	332	689	814[2]	6.18	0	.55	2.03	.23	2.34	.33	88	0
0	12	1.15	71	148	175[2]	1.33	0	.12	.44	.05	.5	.07	19	0
0	62	8.22	356	774	22	7.67	0	.27	.78	.27	1.92	.35	95	0
0	53	5.33	332	689	22	6.18	0	.55	2.03	.23	2.34	.33	88	0
0	7	.8	41	87	2[3]	.83	0	.05	.25	.03	.26	.04	11	0
0	42	1.3	47	847	3	.82	3	.35	1.72	.25	1.92	.71	100	37
0	6	1.09	14	160	9	.5	0	.03	.33	.01	.24	.02	12	2
0	6	.97	13	142	8	.44	0	.03	.29	.01	.22	.02	11	1
0	20	2.59	70	424	29	1.57	0	.05	1.05	.08	.47	.23	7	1
0	14	1.79	47	313	244	1.69	0	.03	1.26	.02	.44	.25	8	1
0	216	3.76	328	512	4	2.76	8	.58	27.49	.13	1.31	.7	83	1
0	53	.92	80	125	1	.67	2	.14	6.69	.03	.32	.17	20	<1
0	60	2.41	157	441	348[4]	1.47	1	.29	.55	.15	2.71	.27	21	0
0	13	.5	33	92	73[4]	.31	<1	.06	.12	.03	.57	.06	4	0
0	60	2.41	157	441	9	1.47	1	.29	.55	.15	2.71	.27	21	0
0	96	5.07	308	818	917[5]	5.21	1	.27	8.22	.27	6.44	.41	69	1
0	153	4.56	334	825	926[5]	7.21	3	.71	8.52	.32	7.19	.34	118	1
0	153	4.56	334	825	16	7.21	3	.71	8.52	.32	7.19	.34	118	1
0	127	2.64	266	982	9	9.55	0	.36	10.67	.16	20.6	.37	181	0
0	79	3.3	257	961	1186	4.83	0	.64	10.82	.14	19.7	.37	212	0
0	15	.63	49	184	228	.93	0	.12	2.08	.03	3.78	.07	41	0
0	12	.59	51	214	149[6]	.93	0	.03	3.2	.03	4.29	.15	24	0
0	39	2.3	138	423	1[7]	5.91	14	.92	3.35	.14	.96	.2	42	2
0	10	.6	36	110	<1[7]	1.53	4	.24	.87	.04	.25	.05	11	1
0	10	.61	37	104	218	1.59	4	.09	.84	.03	.26	.06	11	1
0	2	.86	66	176	20	1.2	1	.35	.98	.06	1.22	.03	16	1
0	38	1.9	44	306	2[8]	.38	6	.23	1.46	.05	.3	.07	16	2
0	90	4.06	166	1241	998	1.74	31	.54	8.26	.32	1.81	.33	76	9
0	12	4.2	150	226	5[9]	2.09	11	.06	.28	.09	.49	.06	16	1
0	98	33.8	1212	1829	1305	16.9	86	.48	2.27	.72	3.95	.2	130	4
0	50	2.96	132	155	15	3.91	3	.27	.86	.03	1.78	.06	37	0
0	42	2.44	127	248	1[10]	1.82	2	.82	18.11	.09	1.62	.28	82	1
0	19	2.28	43	164	1[10]	1.77	2	.11	17.1	.1	1.4	.27	80	<1
0	21	.95	53	69	<1	1.58	1	.24	.34	.02	.85	.02	15	0
5.84	159	4.95	235	946	177	4.58	7	.6	15.62	.33	6.44	.38	95	2
0	73	3.84	253	655	1	4.28	38	.27	3.28	.14	.86	.69	82	4

(2)Oil-roasted cashews without salt contain 22 mg sodium per cup, or 5 mg per ounce.

(3)Salted cashew butter contains 98 mg sodium per tablespoon.

(4)Macadamia nuts without salt contain 9 mg sodium per cup, or 2 mg per ounce.

(5)Mixed nuts without salt contain about 15 mg sodium per cup.

(6)Peanut butter without added salt contains 3 mg sodium per tablespoon.

(7)Salted pecans contain 816 mg sodium per cup, or 214 mg per ounce.

(8)Salted pistachios contain approx 221 mg sodium per ounce.

(9)Salted pumpkin/squash kernels contain approximately 163 mg sodium per ounce.

(10)Unsalted sunflower seeds contain 1 mg sodium per ¼ cup.

(For purposes of calculations, use "0" for t, <1, <.1, <.01, etc.)

Table H-1
Food Composition

Computer Code Number	Food Description	Measure	Wt (g)	H_2O (%)	Ener (kcal)	Prot (g)	Carb (g)	Dietary Fiber (g)	Fat (g)	Fat Breakdown (g)		
										Sat	Mono	Poly
	NUTS, SEEDS, and PRODUCTS—Cont.											
754	Ounce	1 oz	28	4	170	7	3	1	16	1.1	3.6	10.5
755	English walnuts, chopped:	1 c	120	4	770	17	22	6	74	7.2	17	46.9
756	Ounce	1 oz	28	4	180	4	5	1	17	1.7	4	11
	SWEETENERS and SWEETS (see also Dairy [milk desserts] and Baked Goods)											
757	Apple butter	2 tbs	35	52	64	<1	17	<1	<1	t	t	t
1124	Butterscotch topping	2 tbs	41	32	103	1	27	<1	<1	t	t	0
1125	Caramel topping	2 tbs	41	32	103	1	27	<1	<1	t	t	0
	Cake frosting, creamy vanilla:											
1127	Canned	2 tbs	31	13	130	<1	22	<1	5	1.5	2.7	.7
1123	From mix	2 tbs	31	12	131	<1	22	<1	5	1	2.1	1.8
	Cake frosting, lite:											
2061	Milk chocolate	1 tbs	29	18	105	<1	21	1	2	.7	–	–
2062	Vanilla	1 tbs	29	15	110	0	22	<1	2	.6	–	–
	Candy:											
1128	Almond Joy candy bar	1 oz	28	8	130	1	16	1	8	4.7	1.5	.7
2069	Butterscotch morsels	¼ c	43	1	246	0	29	0	13	12.5	–	–
758	Caramel, plain or chocolate	1 oz	28	8	107	1	22	<1	2	1.9	.2	.1
1961	Chewing gum, sugarless	1 pce	3	–	5	0	2	–	0	–	0	0
	Chocolate (see also #784, 785, 971):											
	Milk chocolate:											
759	Plain	1 oz	28	1	144	2	17	1	9	5.2	2.8	.3
760	With almonds	1 oz	28	2	147	3	15	2	10	4.8	3.8	.6
761	With peanuts	1 oz	28	1	155	5	12	2	12	3.4	5.1	2.6
762	With rice cereal	1 oz	28	2	139	2	18	1	7	4.5	2.4	.2
763	Semisweet chocolate chips	1 c	170	1	814	7	107	10	51	30.3	17	1.7
764	Sweet dark chocolate (candy bar)	1 oz	28	1	133	1	17	2	9	4.8	2.8	.3
1133	SKOR English toffee candy bar	1 ea	32	4	169	1	18	<1	11	7.1	2.5	.3
765	Fondant candy, uncoated (mints, candy corn, other)	1 oz	28	7	100	0	26	0	0	0	0	0
1697	Fruit Roll-up (small)	1 ea	14	11	49	<1	12	<1	<1	t	t	.1
766	Fudge, chocolate	1 oz	28	10	107	<1	22	<1	2	1.5	.7	.1
767	Gumdrops	1 oz	28	1	108	0	28	0	0	0	0	0
768	Hard candy, all flavors	1 oz	28	1	104	0	28	0	0	0	0	0
769	Jellybeans	1 oz	28	6	103	0	26	0	<1	t	t	t
1134	M&M's plain chocolate candy	1 pkg	48	2	236	2	34	1	10	6	3	.3
1135	M&M's peanut chocolate candy	1 pkg	47	2	243	5	28	2	12	4.8	5.2	2
1130	Mars almond bar	1 ea	50	5	234	4	31	1	12	2.7	5.6	2.8
1129	Milky Way candy bar	1 ea	60	6	254	3	43	1	10	4.7	3.6	.4
1708	Milk chocolate-coated peanuts	½ c	85	2	441	11	42	4	29	12.4	11.1	3.7
1709	Peanut brittle, recipe	½ c	74	2	335	6	51	2	14	3.7	6.3	3.5
1132	Reese's peanut butter cup	2 ea	45	6	222	5	22	2	14	6.4	4.4	1.8
1131	Snickers candy bar (2.2oz)	1 ea	61	6	292	5	36	2	15	5.5	6.4	3
1482	Fruit juice bar (2.5 fl oz)	1 ea	77	78	63	1	16	0	<1	t	0	t
771	Gelatin dessert/Jello, prepared	½ c	120	85	71	2	17	0	0	0	0	0
1702	SugarFree	½ c	113	98	8	1	1	0	0	0	0	0
772	Honey:	1 c	339	17	1030	1	279	<1	0	0	0	0
773	Tablespoon	1 tbs	21	17	64	<1	17	<1	0	0	0	0

(Computer code number is for West Diet Analysis program)

PAGE KEY: H–4 = BEV H–6 = DAIRY H–12 = EGGS H–14 = FAT/OIL H–18 = FRUIT H–26 = BAKERY H–36 = GRAIN H–44 = FISH H–48 = MEATS H–50 = POULTRY H–54 = SAUSAGE H–56 = MIXED/FAST H–64 = NUTS/SEEDS H–68 = SWEETS H–70 = VEG/LEG H–84 = MISC H–88 = SOUPS/SAUCES H–90 = FAST H–106 = FRZN ENTREE H–112 = BABY FOODS

Chol (mg)	Calc (mg)	Iron (mg)	Magn (mg)	Pota (mg)	Sodi (mg)	Zinc (mg)	VT-A (RE)	Thia (mg)	VT-E (α-TE)	Ribo (mg)	Niac (mg)	V-B6 (mg)	Fola (μg)	VT-C (mg)
0	16	.86	57	147	<1	.96	8	.06	.73	.03	.2	.16	18	1
0	113	2.93	203	602	12	3.28	14	.46	3.14	.18	1.25	.67	79	4
0	26	.68	47	141	3	.76	3	.11	.73	.04	.29	.16	19	1
0	2	.05	1	32	0	.02	0	<.01	.01	<.01	.03	.01	0	1
<1	22	.08	3	34	143	.08	11	<.01	0	.04	.02	.01	1	<1
<1	22	.08	3	34	143	.08	11	<.01	0	.04	.02	.01	1	<1
0	1	.03	<1	15	28	0	70	0	.62	<.01	<.01	0	0	0
0	3	.07	1	7	69	.03	33	.01	.62	.01	.11	<.01	0	0
0	3	.44	–	–	72	–	0	–	–	–	–	–	–	0
0	1	.03	–	–	53	–	0	–	–	–	–	–	–	0
1	22	.34	19	104	38	.22	1	.01	.63	.04	.13	.02	2	<1
0	0	0	–	80	46	–	0	.03	–	.04	.03	–	–	0
2	39	.04	5	61	69	.12	2	<.01	–	.05	.07	.01	1	<1
–	–	–	–	0	0	–	–	–	–	–	–	–	–	–
6	54	.39	17	108	23	.39	15	.02	.35	.08	.09	.01	2	<1
5	63	.46	25	124	21	.38	4	.02	.53	.12	.21	.01	3	<1
3	32	.52	35	150	11	.69	6	.08	1.3	.05	2.12	.05	23	0
5	48	.21	14	96	41	.31	3	.02	.35	.08	.13	.02	3	<1
0	54	5.32	196	621	19	2.75	3	.09	2.02	.15	.73	.06	5	0
0	5	.59	32	95	3	.42	1	.01	.28	.07	.19	.01	1	0
20	36	.13	11	76	74	.24	22	.01	.44	.11	.03	.01	2	<1
0	1	.02	<1	5	11	.01	0	<.01	0	<.01	<.01	<.01	0	0
0	5	.14	3	41	9	.03	2	<.01	.04	<.01	.01	.04	1	<1
4	12	.13	7	29	17	.11	13	<.01	.03	.02	.03	<.01	1	<1
0	1	.11	<1	1	12	0	0	0	0	<.01	<.01	0	0	0
0	1	.08	1	1	11	<.01	0	<.01	0	<.01	<.01	<.01	0	0
0	1	.31	1	10	7	.01	0	0	0	0	0	0	0	0
7	50	.53	20	128	29	.46	25	.03	.41	.1	.11	.01	2	<1
4	48	.54	29	162	23	.63	11	.07	1.01	.1	.95	.04	20	<1
5	84	.55	36	163	85	.56	23	.02	.3	.16	.47	.03	7	1
8	78	.46	20	145	144	.43	34	.02	.39	.13	.21	.03	5	1
8	88	1.11	77	427	35	1.6	0	.1	2.17	.15	3.61	.18	7	0
10	22	1.02	37	154	335	.72	35	.14	1.21	.04	2.59	.08	52	0
5	35	.5	38	180	131	.63	8	.02	.6	.1	1.79	.04	13	<1
8	57	.46	42	206	162	.9	24	.13	.93	.1	2.23	.07	45	<1
0	4	.15	3	41	3	.04	2	.01	0	.01	.12	.02	5	7
0	2	.04	1	1	50	.04	0	0	0	<.01	<.01	<.01	0	0
0	2	.01	1	0	54	.03	0	0	0	<.01	<.01	<.01	0	0
0	20	1.42	7	176	14	.75	0	0	0	.13	.41	.08	7	2
0	1	.09	<1	11	1	.05	0	0	0	.01	.03	.01	<1	<1

(For purposes of calculations, use "0" for t, <1, <.1, <.01, etc.)

Table H–1
Food Composition

Computer Code Number	Food Description	Measure	Wt (g)	H_2O (%)	Ener (kcal)	Prot (g)	Carb (g)	Dietary Fiber (g)	Fat (g)	Fat Breakdown (g)		
										Sat	Mono	Poly
	SWEETENERS and SWEETS (see also Dairy [milk desserts] and Baked Goods)—Cont.											
774	Jams or preserves:	1 tbs	20	29	54	<1	14	<1	<1	0	t	t
775	Packet	1 ea	14	35	34	<1	9	<1	<1	t	t	0
776	Jellies:	1 tbs	18	28	49	<1	13	<1	<1	t	t	t
777	Packet	1 ea	14	28	38	<1	10	<1	<1	t	t	t
1136	Marmalade	2 tbs	40	33	98	<1	27	<1	0	0	0	0
770	Marshmallows	4 ea	28	16	89	1	23	<1	<1	t	t	t
1126	Marshmallow creme topping	3 tbs	50	18	155	1	40	<1	<1	t	t	t
778	Popsicle/ice pops	1 ea	95	80	68	0	18	0	0	0	0	0
	Sugars:											
779	Brown sugar	1 c	220	2	827	0	214	0	0	0	0	0
780	White sugar, granulated:	1 c	200	0	774	0	200	0	0	0	0	0
781	Tablespoon	1 tbs	12	0	46	0	12	0	0	0	0	0
782	Packet	1 ea	6	0	23	0	6	0	0	0	0	0
783	White sugar, powdered, sifted	1 c	100	<1	389	0	100	0	<1	t	t	t
	Sweeteners:											
1711	Equal, packet	1 ea	1	12	4	<1	1	0	t	t	t	t
1712	Sweet 'N Low, packet	1 ea	1	<1	4	0	1	0	0	0	0	0
	Syrups:											
	Chocolate:											
785	Hot fudge type	2 tbs	38	22	132	2	22	<1	5	2.2	1.4	1.2
784	Thin type	2 tbs	38	29	93	1	25	1	<1	.3	.2	<.1
786	Molasses, blackstrap[1]	2 tbs	40	29	94	0	24	0	0	0	0	0
1710	Light cane	1 tbs	21	24	53	0	14	0	0	0	0	0
787	Pancake table syrup (corn and maple)	¼ c	79	24	227	0	60	0	0	0	0	0
	VEGETABLES and LEGUMES											
788	Alfalfa sprouts	1 c	33	91	10	1	1	1	<1	t	t	.1
1815	Amaranth leaves, raw, chopped	1 c	28	92	7	1	1	<1	<1	<.1	<.1	<.1
1816	Amaranth leaves, raw, each	1 ea	14	92	4	<1	1	<1	<1	<.1	<.1	<.1
1817	Amaranth leaves, cooked	1 c	132	92	28	3	5	2	<1	.1	.1	.1
1987	Arugula, raw, chopped	5 ea	10	92	3	<1	<1	<1	<.1	<.1	<.1	<.1
789	Artichokes, cooked globe (300 g w/refuse)	1 ea	120	84	60	4	13	7	<1	t	t	.1
1177	Artichoke hearts, cooked from frozen	9 oz	240	87	108	8	22	11	1	.3	t	.5
1176	Artichoke hearts, marinated	6 oz	170	59	168	4	13	8	14	2	3	7.7
2021	Artichoke hearts, in water	⅔ c	101	87	44	2	10	6	<1	<.1	<.1	.1
	Asparagus, green, cooked:											
	From fresh:											
790	Cuts and tips	½ c	90	92	22	2	4	1	<1	.1	t	.1
791	Spears, ½" diam at base	6 ea	90	92	22	2	4	1	<1	.1	t	.1
	From frozen:											
792	Cuts and tips	½ c	90	91	25	3	4	1	<1	.1	t	.2
793	Spears, ½" diam at base	6 ea	90	91	25	3	4	1	<1	.1	t	.2
794	Canned, spears, ½" diam at base	6 ea	120	94	23	3	3	2	1	.2	t	.3
795	Bamboo shoots, canned, drained slices	1 c	131	94	25	2	4	2	1	.1	t	.2
1795	Bamboo shoots, raw slices	1 c	151	91	41	4	8	3	<1	.1	<.1	.2
1798	Bamboo shoots, cooked slices	1 c	120	96	14	2	2	1	<1	.1	<.1	.1

[1] Light molasses would contain about 66 mg calcium, 2.1 mg iron, 18 mg magnesium, and 366 mg potassium for 2 tbsp.

Chol (mg)	Calc (mg)	Iron (mg)	Magn (mg)	Pota (mg)	Sodi (mg)	Zinc (mg)	VT-A (RE)	Thia (mg)	VT-E (α-TE)	Ribo (mg)	Niac (mg)	V-B6 (mg)	Fola (μg)	VT-C (mg)
0	4	.2	1	18	2	.01	<1	<.01	.02	<.01	.04	<.01	2	<1
0	3	.07	1	11	6	.01	<1	0	0	<.01	.01	<.01	5	1
0	1	.04	1	12	7	.01	<1	<.01	0	<.01	.01	<.01	<1	<1
0	1	.03	1	9	5	.01	<1	<.01	0	<.01	.01	<.01	<1	<1
0	15	.06	1	15	22	.02	2	<.01	0	<.01	.02	.01	14	2
0	1	.06	1	1	13	.01	<1	<.01	0	<.01	.02	<.01	<1	0
0	2	.11	1	3	23	.02	<1	<.01	0	<.01	.04	<.01	1	0
0	0	0	1	4	11	.02	0	0	0	0	0	0	0	0
0	187	4.2	64	761	86	.4	0	.02	0	.02	.18	.06	2	0
0	2	.12	0	4	2	.06	0	0	0	.04	0	0	0	0
0	<1	.01	0	<1	<1	<.01	0	0	0	<.01	0	0	0	0
0	<1	<.01	0	<1	<1	<.01	0	0	0	<.01	0	0	0	0
0	1	.06	0	2	1	.03	0	0	0	0	0	0	0	0
0	<1	<.01	<1	<1	<1	0	0	0	0	0	0	0	0	0
0	0	0	<1	3	4	–	0	0	–	0	–	0	–	0
5	38	.46	18	82	49	.3	8	.01	0	.08	.08	.01	2	<1
0	5	.5	25	183	58	.28	494	<.01	.01	.31	.13	<.01	2	<1
0	344[1]	7[1]	86[1]	997[1]	22	.4	0	.01	0	.02	.43	.28	<1	0
0	35	.9	51	193	3	.06	0	.02	0	.01	.04	.14	0	0
0	1	.07	2	2	66	.03	0	.01	0	.01	.02	0	0	0
0	11	.32	9	26	2	.3	5	.03	.01	.04	.16	.01	12	3
0	60	.65	15	171	6	.25	82	.01	.22	.04	.18	.05	24	12
0	30	.33	8	86	3	.13	41	<.01	.11	.02	.09	.03	12	6
0	276	2.98	73	846	28	1.16	366	.03	.66	.18	.74	.23	75	54
0	16	.15	5	37	3	.05	24	<.01	.04	.01	.03	.01	10	2
0	54	1.55	72	425	114	.59	22	.08	.23	.08	1.2	.13	61	12
0	50	1.34	74	634	127	.86	39	.15	.46	.38	2.2	.21	286	12
0	39	1.62	48	439	899	.54	28	.06	1.87	.17	1.38	.15	149	52
0	40	1.36	40	266	66	.3	15	.06	.2	.05	.6	.09	45	8
0	18	.66	9	144	10	.38	49	.11	.34	.11	.97	.11	131	10
0	18	.66	9	144	10	.38	49	.11	.34	.11	.97	.11	131	10
0	21	.58	12	196	4	.5	74	.06	1.13	.09	.94	.02	122	22
0	21	.58	12	196	4	.5	74	.06	1.13	.09	.94	.02	122	22
0	19	2.2	12	206	344[2]	.48	64	.07	.52	.12	1.15	.13	115	22
0	11	.42	5	105	9	.85	1	.03	.5	.03	.18	.18	4	1
0	20	.76	5	805	6	1.66	3	.23	1.51	.11	.91	.36	11	6
0	14	.29	4	640	5	.56	0	.02	.8	.06	.36	.12	3	0

(2)Low sodium pack contains 3 mg sodium.

(For purposes of calculations, use "0" for t, <1, <.1, <.01, etc.)

Table H–1
Food Composition

Computer Code Number	Food Description	Measure	Wt (g)	H_2O (%)	Ener (kcal)	Prot (g)	Carb (g)	Dietary Fiber (g)	Fat (g)	Fat Breakdown (g) Sat	Mono	Poly
	VEGETABLES AND LEGUMES—Cont.											
	Beans (see also alphabetical listing in this section):											
1990	Adzuki beans, cooked	½ c	115	66	147	9	29	1	<1	.04	.01	.02
796	Black beans, cooked	½ c	86	66	114	8	20	8	<1	.1	t	.2
	Canned beans (white/navy):											
803	With pork and tomato sauce	½ c	126	73	124	7	24	6	1	.5	.6	.2
804	With sweet sauce	1 c	253	71	281	13	53	11	4	1.4	1.6	.5
805	With frankfurters	1 c	253	69	359	17	39	18	17	6	7.2	2.1
	Lima beans:											
797	Thick seeded (Fordhooks), cooked from frozen	½ c	85	74	85	5	16	5	<1	.1	t	.1
798	Thin seeded (Baby), cooked from frozen	½ c	90	72	95	6	18	5	<1	.1	t	.1
799	Cooked from dry, drained	½ c	94	70	108	7	20	7	<1	.1	t	.2
1998	Red Mexican, cooked f/dry	1 c	224	70	252	16	47	18	1	.2	.2	.3
	Snap bean/green string beans cuts and french style:											
800	Cooked from fresh	½ c	62	89	22	1	5	2	<1	t	t	.1
801	Cooked from frozen	½ c	67	91	19	1	4	2	<1	t	t	.1
802	Canned, drained	½ c	67	93	13	1	3	1	<1	t	t	t
1713	Snap bean, yellow, cooked f/fresh	½ c	63	89	22	1	5	2	<1	t	t	.1
	Bean sprouts (mung):											
806	Raw	1 c	104	90	31	3	6	2	<1	.1	t	.1
807	Cooked, stir-fried	1 c	124	84	62	5	13	2	<1	.1	.1	.1
808	Cooked, boiled, drained	1 c	124	93	26	3	5	1	<1	t	t	t
1788	Canned, drained	1 c	125	96	15	2	3	1	<1	<.1	<.1	<.1
	Beets, cooked from fresh:											
809	Sliced or diced	½ c	85	87	37	1	9	2	<1	t	t	.1
810	Whole beets, 2" diam	2 ea	100	87	44	2	10	2	<1	t	t	.1
	Beets, canned:											
811	Sliced or diced	½ c	85	91	26	1	6	2	<1	t	t	t
812	Pickled slices	½ c	114	82	74	1	19	2	<1	t	t	t
813	Beet greens, cooked, drained	½ c	72	89	19	2	4	2	<1	t	t	.1
	Broccoli, raw:											
817	Chopped	1 c	88	91	25	3	5	3	<1	.1	t	.2
818	Spears	1 ea	151	91	42	5	8	5	1	.1	t	.3
	Broccoli, cooked from fresh:											
819	Spears	1 ea	180	91	50	5	9	5	1	.1	t	.3
820	Chopped	1 c	156	91	44	5	8	5	1	.1	t	.3
	Broccoli, cooked from frozen:											
821	Spear, small piece	3 ea	90	91	25	3	5	3	<1	t	t	.1
822	Chopped	1 c	184	91	52	6	10	6	<1	t	t	.1
1603	Broccoflower, steamed	3½ oz	100	90	32	3	6	3	<1	t	t	.1
823	Brussels sprouts, cooked from fresh	½ c	78	87	30	2	7	3	<1	.1	t	.2
824	Brussels sprouts, cooked from frozen	½ c	77	87	32	3	6	3	<1	.1	t	.2
	Cabbage, common varieties:											
825	Raw, shredded or chopped	1 c	70	92	18	1	4	2	<1	t	t	.1

(Computer code number is for West Diet Analysis program)

PAGE KEY: H–4 = BEV H–6 = DAIRY H–12 = EGGS H–14 = FAT/OIL H–18 = FRUIT H–26 = BAKERY H–36 = GRAIN H–44 = FISH H–48 = MEATS H–50 = POULTRY H–54 = SAUSAGE H–56 = MIXED/FAST H–64 = NUTS/SEEDS H–68 = SWEETS H–70 = VEG/LEG H–84 = MISC H–88 = SOUPS/SAUCES H–90 = FAST H–106 = FRZN ENTREE H–112 = BABY FOODS

Chol (mg)	Calc (mg)	Iron (mg)	Magn (mg)	Pota (mg)	Sodi (mg)	Zinc (mg)	VT-A (RE)	Thia (mg)	VT-E (α-TE)	Ribo (mg)	Niac (mg)	V-B6 (mg)	Fola (µg)	VT-C (mg)
0	32	2.3	60	612	9	2	1	.13	.12	.07	.83	.11	139	0
0	23	1.81	60	305	1	.96	1	.21	.07	.05	.43	.06	128	0
9	71	4.13	44	378	554	7.4	15	.07	.68	.06	.63	.09	28	4
18	154	4.23	86	673	850	3.82	29	.12	–	.15	.89	.22	95	8
15	121	4.38	71	595	1087	4.73	38	.15	1.19	.14	2.28	.12	76	6
0	19	1.16	29	347	45	.37	16	.06	.25	.05	.91	.1	18	11
0	25	1.76	50	370	26	.5	15	.06	.58	.05	.69	.1	14	5
0	16	2.25	40	478	2	.89	0	.15	.17	.05	.4	.15	78	0
0	84	3.72	96	738	481	1.74	1	.27	.16	.13	.75	.23	188	4
0	29	.79	16	185	2	.22	42	.05	.09	.06	.38	.03	21	6
0	33	.59	16	84	6	.32	27	.02	.09	.06	.26	.04	15	3
0	17	.6	9	73	176	.19	24	.01	.09	.04	.14	.03	21	3
0	29	.8	16	188	2	.23	5	.05	.18	.06	.39	.04	21	6
0	14	.95	22	155	6	.43	2	.09	.03	.13	.78	.09	63	14
0	16	2.36	41	272	11	1.12	4	.17	.02	.22	1.49	.16	86	20
0	15	.81	17	125	12	.58	1	.06	.01	.13	1.01	.07	36	14
0	18	.54	11	34	175	.35	3	.04	.01	.09	.28	.04	12	<1
0	14	.67	20	259	66	.3	3	.02	.26	.03	.28	.06	68	3
0	16	.79	23	305	77	.35	4	.03	.3	.04	.33	.07	80	4
0	13	1.55	15	126	165	.18	1	.01	.26	.03	.13	.05	26	4
0	13	.47	17	169	301	.3	1	.01	.15	.06	.29	.06	30	3
0	82	1.37	49	655	174	.36	367	.08	.22	.21	.36	.1	10	18
0	42	.77	22	286	24	.35	136[1]	.06	1.46	.1	.56	.14	63	82
0	73	1.33	38	491	41	.6	233[1]	.1	2.51	.18	.96	.24	107	141
0	83	1.51	43	526	47	.68	250[1]	.1	3.04	.2	1.03	.26	90	134
0	73	1.31	37	456	41	.59	217[1]	.09	2.64	.18	.9	.22	78	116
0	46	.55	18	162	22	.27	170[1]	.05	.93	.07	.41	.12	27	36
0	94	1.12	37	331	44	.55	348[1]	.1	3.04	.15	.84	.24	104	74
0	32	.7	20	322	23	.5	7	.07	.3	.1	.76	.18	49	63
0	28	.94	16	247	16	.26	56	.08	.66	.06	.47	.14	47	48
0	19	.57	19	250	18	.28	45	.08	.45	.09	.41	.22	78	35
0	33	.41	11	172	13	.13	9	.04	.07	.03	.21	.07	30	23

[1] Vitamin A for whole plant: leaves are 1600 RE/100 g raw; flower clusters are 300/100 g raw; stalks are 40 RE/100 g raw.

Table H–1
Food Composition

Computer Code Number	Food Description	Measure	Wt (g)	H_2O (%)	Ener (kcal)	Prot (g)	Carb (g)	Dietary Fiber (g)	Fat (g)	Fat Breakdown (g) Sat	Mono	Poly
	VEGETABLES AND LEGUMES—Cont.											
826	Cooked, drained	1 c	150	94	33	2	7	4	1	.1	t	.3
	Cabbage, Chinese:											
1178	Bok choy, raw, shredded	1 c	70	95	9	1	2	1	<1	t	t	.1
827	Bok choy, cooked, drained	1 c	170	96	20	3	3	3	<1	t	t	.1
1937	Kim chee style	1 c	150	92	31	3	6	2	<1	<.1	<.1	.2
828	Pe tsai, raw, chopped	1 c	76	94	12	1	3	2	<1	t	t	.1
1796	Pe tsai, cooked	1 c	119	95	17	2	3	3	<1	<.1	<.1	.1
	Cabbage, red, coarsely chopped:											
829	Raw	1 c	70	92	19	1	4	1	<1	t	t	.1
830	Cooked, drained	½ c	75	94	16	1	4	2	<1	t	t	.1
831	Cabbage, savoy, coarsely chopped, raw	1 c	70	91	19	1	4	2	<1	t	t	t
1785	Cabbage, savoy, cooked	1 c	145	92	35	3	8	4	<1	<.1	<.1	.1
1896	Capers	1 tsp	5	86	0	0	0	0	0	–	–	–
	Carrots, raw:											
832	Whole, 7½ x 1⅛"	1 ea	72	88	31	1	7	2	<1	t	t	.1
833	Grated	½ c	55	88	24	1	6	2	<1	t	t	t
	Carrots, cooked, sliced, drained:											
834	From fresh	½ c	78	87	35	1	8	3	<1	t	t	.1
835	From frozen	½ c	73	90	26	1	6	3	<1	t	t	t
836	Carrots, canned, sliced, drained	½ c	73	93	17	<1	4	1	<1	t	t	.1
837	Carrot juice, canned	½ c	123	89	49	1	11	1	<1	t	t	.1
	Cauliflower, flowerets:											
838	Raw	½ c	50	92	13	1	3	1	<1	t	t	.1
839	Cooked from fresh, drained	½ c	62	93	14	1	3	2	<1	.1	t	.1
840	Cooked, from frozen, drained	½ c	90	94	17	1	3	2	<1	t	t	.1
	Celery, pascal type, raw:											
841	Large outer stalk, 8 x 1½" (root end)	1 ea	40	95	6	<1	2	1	<1	t	t	t
842	Diced	1 c	120	95	19	1	4	2	<1	t	t	.1
1789	Celeriac/celery root, cooked	3½ oz	99	92	25	1	6	1	<1	<.1	<.1	.1
1179	Chard, swiss, raw, chopped	1 c	36	93	7	1	1	1	<1	t	t	t
1180	Chard, swiss, cooked	1 c	175	93	35	3	7	4	<1	t	t	.1
1855	Chayote fruit, raw	1 ea	203	93	49	2	11	6	1	.1	.1	.3
1856	Chayote fruit, cooked	1 c	160	93	38	1	8	5	1	.2	.1	.3
	Chickpeas (see Garbanzo Beans #854)											
	Collards, cooked, drained:											
843	From fresh	½ c	64	92	17	1	4	2	<1	t	t	.1
844	From frozen	½ c	85	89	31	3	6	3	<1	.1	t	.2
	Corn, cooked, drained:											
845	From fresh, on cob, 5" long	1 ea	77	73	72	3	17	2	1	.1	.2	.3
846	From frozen, on cob, 3½" long	1 ea	63	73	59	2	14	2	<1	.1	.1	.2
847	Kernels, cooked from frozen	½ c	82	77	66	2	16	2	<1	.1	.1	.2
	Corn, canned:											
848	Cream style	½ c	128	79	92	2	23	3	1	.1	.2	.3
849	Whole kernel, vacuum pack	½ c	105	77	83	3	20	2	1	.1	.2	.3
	Cowpeas (see Black-eyed peas #814–816)											
850	Cucumber slices with peel	7 pce	28	96	4	<1	1	<1	<1	t	t	t
1948	Cucumber, kim chee style	1 c	150	91	32	2	7	2	<1	.1	0	.1

(Computer code number is for West Diet Analysis program)

PAGE KEY: H–4 = BEV H–6 = DAIRY H–12 = EGGS H–14 = FAT/OIL H–18 = FRUIT H–26 = BAKERY H–36 = GRAIN H–44 = FISH H–48 = MEATS H–50 = POULTRY H–54 = SAUSAGE H–56 = MIXED/FAST H–64 = NUTS/SEEDS H–68 = SWEETS H–70 = VEG/LEG H–84 = MISC H–88 = SOUPS/SAUCES H–90 = FAST H–106 = FRZN ENTREE H–112 = BABY FOODS

Chol (mg)	Calc (mg)	Iron (mg)	Magn (mg)	Pota (mg)	Sodi (mg)	Zinc (mg)	VT-A (RE)	Thia (mg)	VT-E (α-TE)	Ribo (mg)	Niac (mg)	V-B6 (mg)	Fola (μg)	VT-C (mg)
0	47	.26	12	146	12	.14	20	.09	.16	.08	.42	.17	30	30
0	74	.56	13	176	46	.13	210	.03	.08	.05	.35	.14	46	32
0	158	1.77	19	631	58	.29	437	.05	.2	.11	.73	.28	69	44
0	145	1.28	28	375	995	.35	426	.07	.24	.1	.76	.34	88	80
0	59	.24	10	181	7	.18	91	.03	.09	.04	.3	.18	60	21
0	38	.36	12	268	11	.21	115	.05	.14	.05	.6	.21	64	19
0	36	.34	11	144	8	.15	3	.04	.07	.02	.21	.15	15	40
0	28	.26	8	105	6	.11	2	.03	.09	.02	.15	.1	10	26
0	25	.28	20	161	20	.19	70	.05	.07	.02	.21	.13	56	22
0	44	.55	35	267	35	.33	129	.07	.15	.03	.04	.22	67	25
0	2	.05	–	–	105	–	1	–	–	–	–	–	–	0
0	19	.36	11	233	25	.14	2025	.07	.33	.04	.67	.11	10	7
0	15	.28	8	178	19	.11	1547	.05	.25	.03	.51	.08	8	5
0	24	.48	10	177	52	.23	1914	.03	.33	.04	.4	.19	11	2
0	20	.34	7	115	43	.18	1292	.02	.31	.03	.32	.09	8	2
0	18	.47	6	131	177[1]	.19	1005	.01	.31	.02	.4	.08	7	2
0	30	.57	17	359	36	.22	3167	.11	.01	.07	.5	.27	5	11
0	11	.22	8	152	15	.14	1	.03	.02	.03	.26	.11	29	23
0	10	.2	6	88	9	.11	1	.03	.03	.03	.25	.11	27	28
0	15	.37	8	125	16	.12	2	.03	–	.05	.28	.08	37	28
0	16	.16	4	115	35	.05	5	.02	.14	.02	.13	.03	11	3
0	48	.48	13	344	104	.16	16	.06	.43	.05	.39	.1	34	8
0	26	.43	12	171	60	.2	0	.03	.2	.04	.42	.1	3	4
0	18	.65	29	136	77	.13	119	.01	.68	.03	.14	.04	5	11
0	102	3.96	151	961	313	.58	550	.06	3.31	.15	.63	.15	15	32
0	39	.81	28	305	8	.71	12	.06	.24	.08	1.02	.27	56	22
0	21	.35	19	277	2	.5	8	.04	.19	.06	.67	.19	29	13
0	15	.1	5	84	10	.07	175	.01	.56	.03	.19	.03	4	8
0	179	.95	26	213	43	.23	508	.04	.43	.1	.54	.1	65	22
0	2	.47	22	193	3	.49	16[2]	.13	.07	.05	1.17	.17	24	4
0	2	.38	18	158	3	.4	13[2]	.11	.06	.04	.96	.14	19	3
0	3	.29	16	121	4	.33	18[2]	.07	.07	.06	1.07	.11	25	3
0	4	.49	22	172	365[3]	.68	13[2]	.03	.12	.07	1.23	.08	57	6
0	5	.44	24	195	286[4]	.48	25[2]	.04	.1	.08	1.23	.06	52	9
0	4	.07	3	40	1	.06	6	.01	.02	.02	.06	.02	4	2
0	14	7.23	12	176	1531	.77	50	.05	.24	.05	.69	.17	35	5

(1)Low sodium pack contains 31 mg sodium.

(2)For yellow varieties; white varieties contain only a trace of vitamin A.

(3)Low sodium pack contains 4 mg sodium per ½ cup.

(4)Low sodium pack contains 6 mg sodium per cup.

(For purposes of calculations, use "0" for t, <1, <.1, <.01, etc.)

H

Table H–1
Food Composition

Computer Code Number	Food Description	Measure	Wt (g)	H_2O (%)	Ener (kcal)	Prot (g)	Carb (g)	Dietary Fiber (g)	Fat (g)	Fat Breakdown (g) Sat	Mono	Poly
	VEGETABLES AND LEGUMES—Cont.											
	Dandelion greens:											
851	Raw	1 c	55	86	25	2	5	2	<1	.1	t	.2
852	Chopped, cooked, drained	1 c	105	90	35	2	7	3	1	.2	t	.3
853	Eggplant, cooked	1 c	160	92	45	1	11	4	<1	.1	t	.2
1714	Endive, fresh, chopped	¼ c	13	94	2	<1	<1	<1	<1	t	t	t
856	Escarole/curly endive, chopped	1 c	50	94	9	1	2	2	<1	t	t	t
854	Garbanzo beans (chickpeas), cooked	1 c	164	60	269	15	45	13	4	.4	1	1.9
1939	Grape leaves, raw	10 g	10	79	7	<1	1	–	<1	–	–	–
855	Great northern beans, cooked	1 c	177	69	209	15	37	12	1	.3	t	.3
857	Jerusalem artichoke, raw slices	1 c	150	78	114	3	26	2	<1	0	t	t
1794	Jicama	1 c	120	90	46	1	11	6	<1	<.1	<.1	.1
	Kale, cooked, drained:											
858	From fresh	½ c	65	91	21	1	4	1	<1	t	t	.1
859	From frozen	½ c	65	91	20	2	3	1	<1	t	t	.2
860	Kidney beans, canned	1 c	256	77	218	13	40	16	1	.1	.1	.5
1181	Kohlrabi, raw slices	1 c	140	91	38	2	9	5	<1	t	t	.1
861	Kohlrabi, cooked	1 c	165	90	48	3	11	2	<1	t	t	.1
1183	Leeks, raw, chopped	1 c	104	83	63	2	15	2	<1	t	t	.2
1182	Leeks, cooked, chopped	½ c	52	91	16	<1	4	<1	<1	t	t	.1
862	Lentils, cooked from dry	½ c	99	70	115	9	20	9	<1	.1	.1	.2
1288	Lentils, sprouted, stir-fried	4 oz	113	69	114	10	24	4	1	.1	.1	.2
1289	Lentils, sprouted, raw	1 c	77	67	82	7	17	3	<1	t	.1	.2
	Lettuce:											
	Butterhead/Boston types:											
863	Head, 5" diameter	¼ ea	41	96	5	1	1	<1	<1	t	t	.1
864	Leaves, inner or outer	4 ea	30	96	4	<1	1	<1	<1	t	t	t
	Iceberg/crisphead:											
865	Head, 6" diameter	¼ ea	135	96	16	1	3	2	<1	t	t	.1
866	Wedge, ¼ head	1 ea	135	96	16	1	3	2	<1	t	t	.1
867	Chopped or shredded	1 c	56	96	7	1	1	1	<1	t	t	.1
868	Looseleaf, chopped	½ c	28	94	5	<1	1	<1	<1	t	t	t
869	Romaine, chopped	½ c	28	95	5	<1	1	<1	<1	t	t	t
870	Romaine, inner leaf	3 ea	30	95	5	<1	1	<1	<1	t	t	t
1930	Luffa, cooked (Chinese okra)	1 c	178	89	57	3	13	6	<1	.1	.1	.1
	Mushrooms:											
871	Raw, sliced	½ c	35	92	9	1	2	<1	<1	t	t	.1
872	Cooked from fresh, pieces	½ c	78	91	21	2	4	2	<1	t	t	.1
1962	Stir fried, shitake slices	1 c	145	84	80	2	21	3	<1	.1	.1	<.1
873	Canned, drained	½ c	78	91	19	2	4	2	<1	t	t	.1
1951	Mushroom caps, pickled	8 ea	47	92	11	1	2	1	<1	<.1	<.1	.1
	Mustard greens:											
874	Cooked from fresh	½ c	70	95	11	2	2	1	<1	t	.1	t
875	Cooked from frozen	½c	75	94	14	2	2	2	<1	t	.1	t
876	Navy beans, cooked from dry	1 c	182	63	258	16	48	12	1	.3	.1	.5
	Okra, cooked:											
877	From fresh pods	8 ea	85	90	27	2	6	2	<1	t	t	t
878	From frozen slices	½ c	92	91	34	2	5	3	<1	.1	.1	.1
1236	Batter fried from fresh	1 c	92	69	175	3	12	2	13	2.1	3.5	7.2
1930	Chinese, (Luffa), cooked	1 c	178	89	57	3	13	6	<1	.1	.1	.1

(Computer code number is for West Diet Analysis program)

H

PAGE KEY: H–4 = BEV H–6 = DAIRY H–12 = EGGS H–14 = FAT/OIL H–18 = FRUIT H–26 = BAKERY H–36 = GRAIN H–44 = FISH H–48 = MEATS H–50 = POULTRY H–54 = SAUSAGE H–56 = MIXED/FAST H–64 = NUTS/SEEDS H–68 = SWEETS H–70 = VEG/LEG H–84 = MISC H–88 = SOUPS/SAUCES H–90 = FAST H–106 = FRZN ENTREE H–112 = BABY FOODS

Chol (mg)	Calc (mg)	Iron (mg)	Magn (mg)	Pota (mg)	Sodi (mg)	Zinc (mg)	VT-A (RE)	Thia (mg)	VT-E (α-TE)	Ribo (mg)	Niac (mg)	V-B6 (mg)	Fola (µg)	VT-C (mg)
0	103	1.71	20	218	42	.23	770	.11	1.38	.14	.44	.14	15	19
0	147	1.89	25	244	46	.29	1228	.14	2.63	.18	.54	.17	13	19
0	10	.56	21	397	5	.24	10	.12	.48	.03	.96	.14	23	2
0	7	.10	2	41	3	.1	27	.01	.06	.01	.05	<.01	19	1
0	26	.42	8	157	11	.4	103	.04	.22	.04	.2	.01	71	3
0	80	4.74	79	477	12	2.51	5	.19	.57	.1	.86	.23	282	2
0	72	.69	–	26	2	–	270	.02	–	.01	.12	–	–	1
0	120	3.77	89	692	4	1.56	<1	.28	.53	.1	1.21	.21	181	2
0	21	5.1	26	644	6	.18	3	.3	.29	.09	1.95	.12	20	6
0	14	.72	14	180	5	.19	2	.02	5.48	.04	.24	.05	14	24
0	47	.59	12	148	15	.16	481	.04	.55	.05	.33	.09	9	27
0	90	.61	12	209	10	.12	413	.03	.12	.07	.44	.06	9	16
0	61	3.23	72	658	873	1.41	0	.27	.13	.23	1.17	.06	130	3
0	34	.56	27	490	28	.04	6	.07	.67	.03	.56	.21	23	87
0	41	.66	31	561	35	.51	7	.07	2.76	.03	.64	.25	20	89
0	61	2.18	29	187	21	.13	10	.06	.96	.03	.42	.24	67	13
0	16	.57	7	45	5	.03	3	.01	.32	.01	.1	.06	13	2
0	19	3.3	36	365	2	1.26	1	.17	.11	.07	1.05	.18	179	2
0	16	3.5	40	321	11	1.81	5	.25	.1	.1	1.36	.19	76	14
0	19	2.47	29	248	9	1.16	4	.18	.07	.1	.87	.15	77	13
0	13	.12	5	105	2	.07	40	.03	.18	.03	.12	.02	30	3
0	10	.09	4	77	2	.05	29	.02	.13	.02	.09	.02	22	2
0	26	.68	12	213	12	.3	45	.06	.38	.04	.25	.05	76	5
0	26	.68	12	213	12	.3	45	.06	.38	.04	.25	.05	76	5
0	11	.28	5	89	5	.12	19	.03	.16	.02	.1	.02	31	2
0	19	.39	3	74	3	.08	53	.01	.12	.02	.11	.02	14	5
0	10	.31	2	81	2	.07	73	.03	.12	.03	.14	.01	38	7
0	11	.33	2	87	2	.08	78	.03	.13	.03	.15	.01	41	7
0	112	.8	101	570	420	.97	103	.23	1.22	.1	1.54	.33	81	29
0	2	.43	4	130	1	.26	0	.04	.04	.16	1.44	.03	7	1
0	5	1.36	9	278	2	.68	0	.06	.09	.23	3.48	.07	14	3
0	4	.64	20	170	6	1.93	0	.05	.17	.25	2.18	.23	30	.44
0	9	.62	12	101	332	.56	0	.07	.09	.02	1.24	.05	10	0
0	2	.5	5	139	95	.28	0	.03	.05	.16	1.42	.03	6	1
0	52	.49	11	141	11	.08	212	.03	1.41	.04	.3	.07	51	18
0	76	.84	10	104	19	.15	335	.03	1.31	.04	.19	.08	52	10
0	127	4.51	107	670	2	1.93	<1	.37	.73	.11	.97	.3	255	2
0	54	.38	49	274	4	.47	49	.11	.59	.05	.74	.16	39	14
0	88	.62	47	215	3	.57	47	.09	.64	.11	.72	.04	134	11
15	104	.77	37	214	137	.5	43	.13	3.09	.1	.75	.13	38	10
0	112	.8	101	570	420	.97	103	.23	1.22	.1	1.54	.33	81	29

(For purposes of calculations, use "0" for t, <1, <.1, <.01, etc.)

H

Table H–1
Food Composition

Computer Code Number	Food Description	Measure	Wt (g)	H_2O (%)	Ener (kcal)	Prot (g)	Carb (g)	Dietary Fiber (g)	Fat (g)	Fat Breakdown (g) Sat	Mono	Poly
	VEGETABLES AND LEGUMES—Cont.											
	Onions:											
879	Raw, chopped	1 c	160	90	61	2	14	3	<1	<.1	<.1	.1
880	Raw, sliced	1 c	115	90	44	1	10	2	<1	<.1	<.1	.1
881	Cooked, drained, chopped	½ c	105	88	46	1	11	1	<1	<.1	<.1	.1
882	Dehydrated flakes	¼ c	14	4	45	1	12	1	<1	<.1	<.1	<.1
1934	Onions, pearl, cooked	1 c	185	87	81	3	19	3	<1	.1	.1	.1
	Spring/green onions, chopped:											
883	Bulb and top	½ c	50	90	16	1	4	1	<1	<.1	<.1	<.1
1185	Green tops only	1 c	100	92	34	2	6	3	<1	.1	.1	.2
1184	White part only	½ c	50	92	25	1	5	1	<1	<.1	<.1	<.1
884	Onion rings, breaded, heated f/frozen	2 ea	20	29	81	1	8	<1	5	1.7	2.2	1
1917	Palm hearts, cooked slices	1 c	146	70	150	4	39	2	<1	.1	.1	<.1
	Parsley:											
885	Raw, chopped	½ c	30	88	11	1	2	1	<1	<.1	.1	<.1
886	Raw, sprigs	5 ea	5	88	2	<1	<1	<1	<1	<.1	<.1	<.1
888	Parsnips, sliced, cooked	½ c	78	78	63	1	15	3	<1	<.1	.1	<.1
	Peas:											
	Black-eyed, cooked:											
814	From dry, drained	½ c	85	70	99	7	18	3	<1	.1	<.1	.2
815	From fresh, drained	½ c	82	76	80	3	17	4	<1	.1	<.1	.1
816	From frozen, drained	½ c	85	66	112	7	20	5	1	.1	.1	.2
889	Edible pod peas, cooked	1 c	160	89	67	5	11	4	<1	.1	<.1	.2
890	Green, canned, drained	½ c	85	82	59	4	11	3	<1	.1	<.1	.1
891	Green, cooked from frozen	½ c	80	80	62	4	11	4	<1	t	t	.1
1786	Snow peas, raw	1 c	145	89	61	4	11	4	<1	.1	<.1	.1
1787	Snow peas, raw	10 ea	29	89	12	1	2	1	<1	<.1	<.1	<.1
892	Split, green, cooked from dry	½ c	98	70	116	8	21	3	<1	.1	.1	.2
1187	Peas & carrots, cooked from frozen	½ c	80	86	38	2	8	3	<1	.1	t	.2
1186	Peas & carrots, canned w/liquid	½ c	128	88	49	3	11	4	<1	.1	t	.2
	Peppers, hot:											
893	Hot green chili, canned	½ c	68	93	14	1	4	1	<1	t	t	t
894	Hot green chili, raw	1 ea	45	88	18	1	4	1	<1	t	t	.1
1715	Hot red chili, raw, diced	1 tbs	9	88	4	<1	1	<1	<1	t	t	t
1988	Jalapeno, raw	2 oz	57	90	25	–	–	–	–	–	–	–
895	Jalapeno, chopped, canned	½ c	68	90	16	1	3	1	<1	<.1	<.1	.2
1918	Jalapeno wheels, in brine (Ortega)	2 tbs	29	90	10	<1	2	1	<1	<.1	<.1	.1
	Peppers, sweet, green:											
896	Whole pod (90 g with refuse), raw	1 ea	74	92	20	1	5	1	<1	t	t	.1
897	Cooked, chopped (1 pod cooked = 73 g)	½ c	68	92	19	1	5	1	<1	t	t	.1
	Peppers, sweet, red:											
1286	Raw, chopped	1 c	100	92	27	1	6	2	<1	t	t	.1
1807	Raw, each	1 ea	74	92	20	1	5	2	<1	<.1	<.1	.1
1287	Cooked, chopped	½ c	68	92	19	1	5	1	<1	t	t	.1
	Peppers, sweet, yellow:											
1872	Raw, large	1 ea	186	92	50	2	12	2	<1	<.1	<.1	.2
1873	Strips	10 pce	52	92	14	1	3	1	<1	<.1	<.1	.1
898	Pinto beans, cooked from dry	½ c	85	64	117	7	22	7	<1	t	.1	.2

(Computer code number is for West Diet Analysis program)

Chol (mg)	Calc (mg)	Iron (mg)	Magn (mg)	Pota (mg)	Sodi (mg)	Zinc (mg)	VT-A (RE)	Thia (mg)	VT-E (α-TE)	Ribo (mg)	Niac (mg)	V-B6 (mg)	Fola (μg)	VT-C (mg)
0	32	.35	16	251	5	.3	0	.07	.21	.03	.24	.19	30	10
0	23	.25	12	181	3	.22	0	.05	.15	.02	.17	.13	22	7
0	23	.25	12	174	3	.22	0	.04	.14	.02	.17	.14	16	5
0	36	.22	13	227	3	.26	0	.07	.19	.01	.14	.22	23	11
0	41	.44	20	305	433	.39	0	.08	.24	.04	.30	.24	28	10
0	36	.74	10	138	8	.2	20	.03	.07	.04	.26	.03	32	9
0	56	2.2	21	260	7	.22	40	.07	.3	.1	.6	0	80	51
0	20	.45	8	115	4	.13	<1	.03	.06	.02	.17	.05	18	13
0	6	.34	4	26	75	.08	5	.06	.14	.03	.72	.01	3	<1
0	26	2.47	15	2637	20	5.45	10	.07	.73	.25	1.25	1.06	30	10
0	41	1.86	15	166	17	.32	156	.03	.54	.03	.39	.03	46	40
0	7	.31	2	27	2	.04	26	<.01	.09	<.01	.04	<.01	9	5
0	29	.45	23	286	8	.2	0	.06	.78	.04	.56	.07	45	10[1]
0	20	2.13	45	236	3	1.1	2	.17	.24	.05	.42	.09	177	<1
0	105	.92	43	343	3	.85	65	.08	.18	.12	1.15	.05	104	2
0	20	1.8	43	319	4	1.21	7	.22	.33	.05	.62	.08	120	2
0	67	3.15	42	384	6	.59	21	.2	.62	.12	.86	.23	47	77
0	17	.81	14	147	214[2]	.6	65	.1	.32	.07	.62	.05	38	8
0	19	1.26	23	134	70	.75	54	.23	.14	.08	1.18	.09	47	8
0	62	3.02	35	290	6	.39	20	.22	.57	.12	.87	.23	61	87
0	13	.6	7	58	1	.08	4	.04	.11	.02	.17	.05	12	17
0	14	1.26	35	355	2	.98	1	.19	.38	.05	.87	.05	64	<1
0	18	.75	13	126	54	.36	621	.18	.26	.05	.92	.07	21	6
0	29	.96	18	128	332	.74	739	.09	.54	.07	.74	.11	23	8
0	5	.34	10	127	798	.12	42[3]	.01	.47	.03	.54	.1	7	46
0	8	.54	11	153	3	.14	35[3]	.04	.31	.04	.43	.13	11	109
0	2	.11	2	31	1	.03	97	.01	.06	.01	.09	.03	2	22
–	–	–	–	3	3	–	39	–	.47	–	–	–	–	66
0	18	1.9	8	93	995	.13	116	.02	.47	.03	.34	.14	9	9
0	8	.8	4	55	390	–	49	.01	.2	.01	.14	.06	4	21
0	7	.34	7	131	2	.09	47	.05	.51	.02	.38	.18	16	66
0	6	.31	7	113	1	.08	40	.04	.47	.02	.32	.16	11	51
0	9	.46	10	177	2	.12	570	.07	.69	.03	.51	.25	22	190
0	7	.34	7	131	2	.09	422	.05	.51	.02	.38	.18	16	141
0	6	.31	7	113	1	.08	256	.04	.47	.02	.32	.16	11	116
0	21	.86	22	394	4	.32	45	.05	1.28	.05	1.66	.31	48	342
0	6	.24	6	110	1	.09	13	.02	.36	.01	.46	.09	14	96
0	41	2.22	47	398	2	.92	<1	.16	.8	.08	.34	.13	146	2

(1) Value for Vitamin C is highest right after harvest and drops after that.

(2) Low sodium pack contains 1.7 mg sodium.

(3) Data is for green chili peppers; red varieties contain 809 RE vitamin A per ½ cup; 484 RE per whole pepper.

(For purposes of calculations, use "0" for t, <1, <.1, <.01, etc.)

Table H–1
Food Composition

Computer Code Number	Food Description	Measure	Wt (g)	H_2O (%)	Ener (kcal)	Prot (g)	Carb (g)	Dietary Fiber (g)	Fat (g)	Fat Breakdown (g)		
										Sat	Mono	Poly
	VEGETABLES AND LEGUMES—Cont.											
1191	Poi, two finger	¼ c	60	72	67	<1	16	<1	<1	<.1	<.1	<.1
	Potatoes:[1]											
	Baked in oven, 4¾" x 2⅓" diam:											
899	With skin	1 ea	202	71	220	5	51	5	<1	.1	<.1	.1
900	Flesh only	1 ea	156	75	145	3	34	2	<1	<.1	<.1	.1
901	Skin only	1 ea	58	47	115	2	27	5	<1	<.1	<.1	<.1
	Baked in microwave, 4¾" x 2⅓" diam:											
902	With skin	1 ea	202	72	212	5	49	5	<1	.1	<.1	.1
903	Flesh only	1 ea	156	74	156	3	36	2	<1	<.1	<.1	.1
904	Skin only	1 ea	58	64	77	3	17	3	<1	<.1	<.1	<.1
	Boiled, about 2½" diam:											
905	Peeled after boiling	1 ea	136	77	118	3	27	2	<1	<.1	<.1	.1
906	Peeled before boiling	1 ea	135	78	116	2	27	2	<1	<.1	<.1	.1
	French fried, strips 2–3½" long:											
907	Oven heated	10 pce	50	35	167	2	20	2	9	3	5.7	.7
908	Fried in vegetable oil	10 ea	50	40	155	2	19	2	8	2.5	4	1.2
1188	Fried in veg and animal oil	10 ea	50	38	158	2	20	2	8	1.9	4.7	.7
909	Hashed browns from frozen	1 c	156	56	340	5	44	3	18	7	8	2.1
	Mashed:											
910	Home recipe with whole milk[2]	½ c	105	79	81	2	18	2	1	.4	.2	.1
911	Home recipe with milk and marg	½ c	105	76	111	2	18	2	4	1.1	1.9	1.3
912	Prepared from flakes; water, milk, margarine, salt added	½ c	110	76	124	2	17	3	6	1.6	2.5	1.7
	Potato products, prepared:											
	Au gratin:											
913	From dry mix	½ c	122	79	114	3	16	1	5	3.5	1.4	.2
914	From home recipe[3]	½ c	122	74	161	7	14	2	9	4.8	3.2	1.3
	Scalloped:											
915	From dry mix	½ c	122	79	114	3	16	1	5	3.2	1.5	.2
916	From home recipe[4]	½ c	122	81	105	4	13	2	5	1.7	1.7	.9
	Potato salad (see Mixed Dishes #715)											
1192	Potato puffs, cooked from frozen	½ c	62	53	138	2	19	2	7	3.2	2.7	.5
918	Pumpkin, cooked from fresh, mashed	1 c	245	94	49	2	12	4	<1	.1	<.1	<.1
919	Pumpkin, canned	½ c	123	90	42	1	10	4	<1	.2	<.1	<.1
1891	Radicchio, raw, shredded	½ c	20	93	5	<1	1	<1	<1	<.1	<.1	<.1
1894	Radicchio, raw, leaf	10 ea	80	93	18	1	4	<1	<1	<.1	<.1	<.1
920	Red radishes	10 ea	45	95	8	<1	2	<1	<1	<.1	<.1	<.1
1793	Daikon radishes (Chinese) raw	½ c	44	95	8	<1	2	1	<1	<.1	<.1	<.1
921	Refried beans, canned	½ c	126	76	118	7	20	7	2	.6	.7	.2
1375	Rutabaga, cooked cubes	½ c	85	89	33	1	7	2	<1	<.1	<.1	.1
922	Sauerkraut, canned with liquid	½ c	118	93	22	1	5	3	<1	<.1	<.1	.1
923	Seaweed, kelp, raw	1 oz	28	82	12	<1	3	<1	<1	.1	<.1	<.1
924	Seaweed, spirulina, dried	1 oz	28	5	81	16	7	1	2	.7	.2	.6
1866	Shallots, raw, chopped	1 tbs	10	80	7	<1	2	<1	<1	<.1	<.1	<.1

(1)Vitamin C varies with length of storage. After 3 months of storage approximately two-thirds of the ascorbic acid remains; after 6 to 7 months, about one-third remains.

(2)Recipe: 84% potatoes, 15% whole milk, 1% salt.

(3)Recipe: 55% potatoes, 30% whole milk, 9% cheddar cheese, 3% butter, 2% flour, 1% salt.

(4)Recipe: 59% potatoes, 36% whole milk, 2% butter, 2% flour, 1% salt.

(Computer code number is for West Diet Analysis program)

PAGE KEY: H–4 = BEV H–6 = DAIRY H–12 = EGGS H–14 = FAT/OIL H–18 = FRUIT H–26 = BAKERY H–36 = GRAIN H–44 = FISH H–48 = MEATS H–50 = POULTRY H–54 = SAUSAGE H–56 = MIXED/FAST H–64 = NUTS/SEEDS H–68 = SWEETS H–70 = VEG/LEG H–84 = MISC H–88 = SOUPS/SAUCES H–90 = FAST H–106 = FRZN ENTREE H–112 = BABY FOODS

Chol (mg)	Calc (mg)	Iron (mg)	Magn (mg)	Pota (mg)	Sodi (mg)	Zinc (mg)	VT-A (RE)	Thia (mg)	VT-E (α-TE)	Ribo (mg)	Niac (mg)	V-B6 (mg)	Fola (μg)	VT-C (mg)
0	10	.53	14	110	7	.13	1	.08	.11	.02	.66	.16	13	2
0	20	2.75	55	844	16	.65	0	.22	.1	.07	3.33	.7	22	26[1]
0	8	.55	39	610	8	.45	0	.16	.06	.03	2.18	.47	14	20[1]
0	20	4.08	25	332	12	.28	0	.07	.02	.06	1.78	.36	13	8[1]
0	22	2.5	55	903	16	.73	0	.24	.1	.06	3.45	.69	24	31[1]
0	8	.64	39	641	11	.51	0	.2	.06	.04	2.54	.5	19	24[1]
0	27	3.45	21	377	9	.3	0	.04	.02	.04	1.29	.29	10	9[1]
0	7	.42	30	515	5	.41	0	.14	.07	.03	1.96	.41	14	18[1]
0	11	.42	27	443	7	.36	0	.13	.07	.03	1.77	.36	12	10[1]
0	6	.83	12	270	307	.2	0	.04	.25	.02	1.34	.11	11	3
0	8	.68	17	356	82	.26	1	.07	.25	.02	1.14	.12	17	3
7	10	.38	17	366	108	.19	0	.09	.25	.01	1.63	.12	15	5
0	23	2.36	27	680	53	.5	0	.17	.3	.03	3.78	.2	10	10
2	27	.28	19	314	318	.3	6	.09	.05	.04	1.18	.24	9	7[1]
2[5]	27	.27	19	304	310	.28	21	.09	.32	.04	1.13	.24	8	6[1]
4[5]	54	.24	20	256	365	.2	23	.12	.77	.06	.74	.01	8	11
18	101	.39	18	267	536	.29	38	.02	1.5	.1	1.15	.05	8	4
18[6]	145	.78	24	483	528	.84	46	.08	.64	.14	1.21	.21	10	12
13	44	.47	17	248	416	.31	26	.02	.18	.07	1.26	.05	12	4
7[7]	70	.7	23	461	409	.49	23	.08	.4	.11	1.28	.22	11	13
0	19	.97	12	236	463	.19	1	.12	.03	.04	1.3	.14	10	4
0	37	1.4	22	564	2	.56	2651	.08	2.6	.19	1.01	.11	21	12
0	32	1.71	28	253	6	.21	2713	.03	1.3	.07	.45	.07	15	5
0	4	.11	3	60	4	.12	1	<.01	.45	.01	.05	.01	12	2
0	15	.45	10	242	18	.5	2	.01	1.81	.02	.2	.05	48	6
0	9	.13	4	104	11	.14	<1	<.01	<.01	.02	.14	.03	12	10
0	12	.18	7	100	9	.07	0	.01	<.01	.01	.09	.02	12	10
10	44	2.09	42	336	377	1.47	0	.03	.39	.02	.4	.18	14	8
0	41	.45	20	277	17	.3	48	.07	.13	.03	.61	.09	13	16
0	35	1.74	15	201	780	.22	2	.02	.12	.03	.17	.15	28	17
0	47	.8	34	25	65	.34	3	.01	.24	.04	.13	<.01	50	1
0	34	8	55	382	293	.56	16	.67	1.4	1.03	3.6	.1	26	3
0	4	.12	2	33	1	.04	125	.01	.01	<.01	.02	.03	3	1

(5)Data is for margarine; if butter is used, cholesterol = 25 mg for 29 total mg.

(6)Data is for butter; if margarine is used, cholesterol = 37 mg.

(7)Data is for butter; if margarine is used cholesterol = 15 mg.

(For purposes of calculations, use "0" for t, <1, <.1, <.01, etc.)

H

Table H–1
Food Composition

Computer Code Number	Food Description	Measure	Wt (g)	H_2O (%)	Ener (kcal)	Prot (g)	Carb (g)	Dietary Fiber (g)	Fat (g)	Fat Breakdown (g)		
										Sat	Mono	Poly
	VEGETABLES AND LEGUMES—Cont.											
1557	Snow peas, stir-fried	1 c	165	89	69	5	12	4	<1	.1	<.1	.1
925	Soybeans, cooked from dry	½ c	86	63	149	15	9	5	8	1.1	1.7	4.4
1996	Soybeans, dry roasted	½ c	86	1	387	34	28	7	19	2.7	4.1	10.6
	Soybean products:											
	Soy milk, see Dairy											
926	Miso	½ c	138	46	282	16	39	7	8	1.2	1.9	4.7
927	Tofu (soybean curd, regular)	½ c	124	85	94	10	2	1	6	.9	1.3	3.4
	Spinach:											
928	Raw, chopped	1 c	56	92	12	2	2	2	<1	<.1	<.1	.1
929	Cooked, from fresh, drained	½ c	90	91	21	3	3	2	<1	<.1	<.1	.1
930	Cooked from frozen (leaf)	½ c	95	90	27	3	5	3	<1	<.1	<.1	.1
931	Canned, drained solids	½ c	107	92	25	3	4	3	1	.1	<.1	.2
	Spinach soufflé (see Mixed Dishes)											
	Squash, summer varieties, cooked:											
932	Varieties averaged	½ c	90	94	18	1	4	1	<1	.1	<.1	.1
933	Crookneck	½ c	90	94	18	1	4	2	<1	.1	<.1	.1
934	Zucchini	½ c	90	95	14	1	4	1	<1	<.1	<.1	<.1
	Squash, winter varieties, cooked:											
	Average of all varieties, baked:											
935	Mashed	1 c	245	89	96	2	21	7	2	.3	.1	.6
936	Cubes	1 c	205	89	80	2	18	6	1	.3	.1	.5
937	Acorn, baked, mashed	½ c	122	83	68	1	18	5	<1	<.1	<.1	.1
1218	Acorn, boiled, mashed	½ c	122	90	41	1	11	3	<1	<.1	<.1	<.1
	Butternut:											
938	Baked cubes	1 c	205	88	82	2	22	6	<1	<.1	<.1	.1
1219	Baked, mashed	½ c	122	88	49	1	13	3	<1	<.1	<.1	<.1
1193	Cooked from frozen	½ c	120	88	47	1	12	3	<1	<.1	<.1	<.1
1194	Hubbard, baked, mashed	½ c	120	85	60	3	13	3	1	.2	.1	.3
1195	Hubbard, boiled, mashed	½ c	118	91	35	2	8	3	<1	.1	<.1	.2
1196	Spaghetti, baked or boiled	½ c	77	92	22	1	5	1	<1	<.1	<.1	.1
1189	Succotash, cooked from frozen	½ c	85	74	79	4	17	4	1	.1	.1	.4
	Sweet potatoes:											
939	Baked in skin, peeled, 5 x 2" diam	1 ea	114	73	117	2	28	3	<1	<.1	<.1	.1
940	Boiled without skin, 5 x 2" diam	1 ea	151	73	159	3	37	4	<1	.1	<.1	.2
941	Candied, 2½ x 2"	1 pce	105	67	144	1	29	3	3	1.4	.7	.2
	Canned:											
942	Solid pack	½ c	128	74	129	3	30	3	<1	.1	<.1	.1
943	Vacuum pack, mashed	½ c	127	76	116	2	27	3	<1	.1	<.1	.1
944	Vacuum pack, 3¾ x 1"	2 pce	80	76	73	1	17	2	<1	<.1	<.1	.1
1940	Taro shoots, cooked slices	1 c	140	95	20	1	4	1	<1	<.1	<.1	<.1
1941	Taro, tahitian, cooked slices	1 c	137	87	60	6	9	1	1	.19	.08	.39
	Tomatillos:											
1877	Raw, each	1 ea	34	92	11	<1	2	1	<1	<.1	.1	.1
1875	Raw, chopped	½ c	66	92	21	1	4	1	1	.1	.1	.3
	Tomatoes:											
945	Raw, whole, 2⅗" diam	1 ea	123	94	26	1	6	1	<1	.1	.1	.2
946	Raw, chopped	1 c	180	94	38	2	8	2	1	.1	.1	.2

(Computer code number is for West Diet Analysis program)

PAGE KEY: H–4 = BEV H–6 = DAIRY H–12 = EGGS H–14 = FAT/OIL H–18 = FRUIT H–26 = BAKERY H–36 = GRAIN H–44 = FISH H–48 = MEATS H–50 = POULTRY H–54 = SAUSAGE H–56 = MIXED/FAST H–64 = NUTS/SEEDS H–68 = SWEETS H–70 = VEG/LEG H–84 = MISC H–88 = SOUPS/SAUCES H–90 = FAST H–106 = FRZN ENTREE H–112 = BABY FOODS

Chol (mg)	Calc (mg)	Iron (mg)	Magn (mg)	Pota (mg)	Sodi (mg)	Zinc (mg)	VT-A (RE)	Thia (mg)	VT-E (α-TE)	Ribo (mg)	Niac (mg)	V-B6 (mg)	Fola (μg)	VT-C (mg)
0	71	3.43	40	330	7	.45	21	.22	.64	.13	.94	.25	55	84
0	88	4.42	74	443	1	.99	1	.13	1.68	.25	.34	.2	46	1
0	232	3.4	196	1173	2	4.1	2	.37	3.96	.65	.91	.19	176	4
0	92	3.76	58	226	5014	4.57	12	.13	.01	.34	1.19	.3	46	0
0	130	6.65	128	150	9	.99	11	.1	.01	.06	.24	.06	19	<1
0	55	1.52	44	313	44	.3	376	.04	1.06	.11	.4	.11	109	16
0	122	3.21	78	419	63	.68	737	.09	.86	.21	.44	.22	131	9
0	139	1.44	66	283	82	.67	739	.06	.91	.16	.4	.14	103	12
0	136	2.46	81	370	29[1]	.49	940	.02	1.39	.15	.42	.11	105	15
0	24	.32	22	173	1	.35	26[2]	.04	.11	.04	.46	.06	18	5
0	24	.32	22	173	1	.35	26[2]	.04	.11	.04	.46	.08	18	5
0	12	.31	20	228	3	.16	22[2]	.04	.11	.04	.39	.07	15	4
0	34	.81	20	1070	2	.64	872	.21	.29	.06	1.72	.18	69	24
0	29	.68	16	896	2	.53	730	.17	.25	.05	1.44	.15	57	20
0	54	1.14	52	533	5	.21	52	.2	.15	.02	1.08	.24	23	13
0	32	.68	32	321	4	.13	32	.12	.15	.01	.65	.14	14	8
0	84	1.23	59	582	8	.27	1435	.15	.35	.03	1.99	.25	39	31
0	50	.73	35	347	5	.16	854	.09	.2	.02	1.19	.15	23	18
0	23	.7	11	160	2	.14	401	.06	.16	.05	.56	.08	20	4
0	20	.56	26	430	10	.18	725	.09	.14	.06	.67	.21	19	11
0	12	.33	15	253	6	.12	473	.05	.14	.03	.39	.12	11	8
0	16	.26	8	90	14	.15	8	.03	.09	.02	.63	.08	6	3
0	13	.76	20	225	38	.38	20	.06	.31	.06	1.11	.08	28	5
0	32	.51	23	397	11	.33	2487	.08	.32	.14	.69	.27	26	28
0	32	.85	15	278	20	.41	2574	.08	.42	.21	.97	.37	17	26
8[3]	27	1.19	12	199	74	.16	440	.02	3.99	.04	.41	.04	12	7
0	38	1.7	31	269	96	.27	1936	.03	.35	.12	1.22	.3	14	7
0	28	1.13	28	396	67	.23	1013	.05	.32	.07	.94	.24	21	34
0	18	.71	18	250	42	.14	638	.03	.2	.05	.59	.15	13	21
0	20	.57	11	482	3	.76	7	.05	1.4	.07	1.13	.16	4	26
0	204	2.14	70	854	74	.14	241	.06	3.7	.27	.66	.16	9.9	52
0	2	.21	7	91	<1	.07	4	.02	.13	.01	.63	.02	2	4
0	5	.41	13	177	1	.15	7	.03	.25	.02	1.22	.04	5	8
0	6	.55	14	273	11	.11	76	.07	.47	.06	.77	.1	18	23[4]
0	9	.81	20	400	16	.16	112	.11	.68	.09	1.13	.14	27	34[4]

(1) Dietary pack contains 58 mg sodium.

(2) Applies to squash including skin; flesh has no appreciable vitamin A value.

(3) For recipe using butter.

(4) Year-round average. From June through October, ascorbic acid is approximately 32 mg and 47 mg, respectively, for one tomato and 1 c chopped tomato. From November through May, market samples average around 12 and 18 mg, respectively.

(For purposes of calculations, use "0" for t, <1, <.1, <.01, etc.)

H

Table H-1
Food Composition

Computer Code Number	Food Description	Measure	Wt (g)	H_2O (%)	Ener (kcal)	Prot (g)	Carb (g)	Dietary Fiber (g)	Fat (g)	Fat Breakdown (g) Sat	Mono	Poly
	VEGETABLES AND LEGUMES—Cont.											
	Tomatoes—Cont.:											
947	Cooked from raw	1 c	240	92	65	3	14	2	1	.1	.2	.4
948	Canned, solids and liquid	1 c	240	94	46	2	10	2	<1	<.1	.1	.1
1879	Tomatoes, sundried:	1 c	54	15	139	8	30	7	2	.2	.3	.6
1881	Pieces	10 pce	20	15	52	3	11	2	1	.1	.1	.2
1885	Oil pack, drained	33 ea	100	54	213	5	23	6	14	1.9	8.7	2.1
2020	Tomato, raw	1 ea	123	94	26	1	6	1	<1	.1	.1	.2
949	Tomato juice, canned	1 c	244	94	41	2	10	1	<1	<.1	<.1	.1
	Tomato products, canned:											
950	Paste, no added salt	1 c	262	74	215	10	51	11	1	.2	.2	.6
951	Puree, no added salt	1 c	250	88	100	4	24	5	<1	.1	.1	.2
952	Sauce	1 c	245	89	74	3	18	3	<1	.1	.1	.2
953	Turnips, cubes, cooked from fresh	½ c	78	94	14	1	4	2	1	<.1	<.1	<.1
	Turnip greens, cooked:											
954	From fresh, leaves and stems	1 c	144	93	29	2	6	5	<1	.1	<.1	.1
955	From frozen, chopped	1 c	164	90	49	6	8	6	1	.2	<.1	.3
956	Vegetable juice cocktail, canned	½ c	121	94	23	1	6	1	<1	<.1	<.1	<.1
	Vegetables, mixed:											
957	Canned, drained	½ c	81	87	38	2	8	2	<1	<.1	<.1	.1
958	Frozen, cooked, drained	½ c	91	83	54	3	12	4	<1	<.1	<.1	.1
1818	Water chestnuts, Chinese, raw	½ c	62	74	66	1	15	2	<1	<.1	<.1	<.1
959	Water chestnuts, canned, slices	½ c	70	86	35	1	9	2	<1	<.1	<.1	<.1
960	Water chestnuts, canned, whole	4 ea	28	86	14	<1	3	1	<1	<.1	<.1	<.1
1190	Watercress, fresh, chopped	½ c	17	95	2	<1	<1	<1	<1	<.1	<.1	<.1
	MISCELLANEOUS											
	Baking powders for home use:											
	Sodium aluminum sulfate:											
962	With monocalcium phosphate monohydrate	1 tsp	3	2	4	<1	1	0	0	0	0	0
963	With monocalcium phosphate monohydrate, calcium sulfate	1 tsp	3	5	2	0	1	<1	0	0	0	0
964	Straight phosphate	1 tsp	4	4	2	<1	1	<1	0	0	0	0
965	Low sodium	1 tsp	4	6	4	<1	2	<1	<1	<.1	<.1	<.1
1204	Baking soda	1 tsp	3	<1	0	0	0	0	0	0	0	0
966	Basil, dried	1 tbs	4	6	10	1	2	2	<1	<.1	<.1	.1
2068	Cajun seasoning	1 tsp	3	5	6	<1	1	<1	<1	–	–	–
961	Carob flour	1 c	103	4	185	5	92	41	1	.1	.2	.2
967	Catsup:	¼ c	61	67	64	1	17	1	<1	<.1	<.1	.1
968	Tablespoon	1 tbs	15	67	16	<1	4	<1	<1	<.1	<.1	<.1
1200	Cayenne/red pepper	1 tbs	5	8	16	1	3	1	1	.2	.1	.4
969	Celery seed	1 tsp	2	6	8	<1	1	<1	1	<.1	.3	.1
1203	Chili powder:	1 tbs	8	8	25	1	4	3	1	.3	.3	.6
970	Teaspoon	1 tsp	3	8	9	<1	2	1	<1	.1	.1	.2
	Chocolate:											
971	Baking, unsweetened, square	1 oz	28	1	146	3	8	4	15	9.1	5.2	.5

(Computer code number is for West Diet Analysis program)

PAGE KEY: H–4 = BEV H–6 = DAIRY H–12 = EGGS H–14 = FAT/OIL H–18 = FRUIT H–26 = BAKERY H–36 = GRAIN H–44 = FISH H–48 = MEATS H–50 = POULTRY H–54 = SAUSAGE H–56 = MIXED/FAST H–64 = NUTS/SEEDS H–68 = SWEETS H–70 = VEG/LEG H–84 = MISC H–88 = SOUPS/SAUCES H–90 = FAST H–106 = FRZN ENTREE H–112 = BABY FOODS

Chol (mg)	Calc (mg)	Iron (mg)	Magn (mg)	Pota (mg)	Sodi (mg)	Zinc (mg)	VT-A (RE)	Thia (mg)	VT-E (α-TE)	Ribo (mg)	Niac (mg)	V-B6 (mg)	Fola (μg)	VT-C (mg)
0	14	1.34	34	670	26	.26	178	.17	.91	.14	1.8	.23	31	55
0	72[1]	1.32	29	530	355[2]	.38	144	.11	.77	.07	1.76	.22	19	34
0	59	4.91	105	1850	1131	1.08	47	.29	.01	.26	4.89	.18	37	21
0	22	1.82	39	685	419	.4	17	.11	<.01	.1	1.81	.07	14	8
0	47	2.68	81	1565	266	.78	129	.19	.53	.38	3.63	.32	23	102
0	6	.55	14	273	11	.11	76	.07	.47	.06	.77	.1	18	23
0	22	1.42	27	537	881[3]	.34	137	.11	2.22	.08	1.64	.27	49	45
0	92	5.08	134	2454	231	2.1	639	.41	11.3	.5	8.44	1	59	111
0	43	3.1	60	1065	85	.55	320	.18	6.3	.14	4.3	.38	28	26
0	34	1.89	47	909	1482[4]	.61	240	.16	3.43	.14	2.82	.38	23	32
0	17	.17	6	105	39	.16	0	.02	.02	.02	.23	.05	7	9
0	197	1.15	32	292	42	.2	792	.06	2.48	.1	.59	.26	170	39
0	249	3.18	43	367	25	.67	1308	.09	4.79	.12	.77	.11	65	36
0	13	.51	13	234	327	.24	142	.05	.39	.03	.88	.17	26	34
0	22	.85	13	236	121	.33	944	.04	.49	.04	.47	.06	19	4
0	23	.75	20	154	32	.45	390	.06	.33	.11	.77	.07	17	3
0	7	.04	14	362	9	.31	0	.09	.74	.12	.62	.20	10	2
0	3	.61	4	83	6	.27	0	.01	.35	.02	.25	.11	4	1
0	1	.24	1	33	2	.11	0	<.01	.14	.01	.1	.04	2	<1
0	20	.03	4	56	7	.02	80	.02	.17	.02	.03	.02	2	7
0	58	0	<1	5	328	0	0	0	–	0	0	0	0	0
0	176	.33	1	1	318	<.01	0	0	0	0	0	0	0	0
0	295	.45	2	<1	316	<.01	0	0	0	0	0	0	0	0
0	173	.33	1	404	4	.03	0	0	<.01	0	0	0	0	0
0	0	0	0	0	821	0	0	0	0	0	0	0	0	0
0	85	1.68	17	137	1	.23	38	.01	.07	.01	.28	.05	11	2
–	–	–	–	29	474	–	–	–	–	–	–	–	–	–
0	358	3.03	56	852	36	.95	1	.05	.65	.47	1.96	.38	30	<1
0	12	.43	13	293	724	.14	62	.05	.9	.04	.84	.11	9	9
0	3	.1	3	72	178	.03	15	.01	.22	.01	.21	.03	2	2
0	7	.39	8	101	2	.12	208	.02	.24	.05	.44	.1	5	4
0	35	.9	9	28	3	.14	<1	.01	.02	.01	.1	.01	<1	<1
0	22	1.14	14	153	81	.21	279	.03	.08	.06	.63	.15	8	5
0	8	.43	5	57	30	.08	105	.01	.03	.02	.2	.06	3	2
0	21	1.77	87	233	4	1.12	3	.02	.34	.05	.31	.03	2	0

(1)Calcium is added as a firming agent.

(2)Dietary pack contains 31 mg sodium.

(3)If no salt is added, sodium content is 24 mg.

(4)With salt added.

H

Table H–1
Food Composition

Computer Code Number	Food Description	Measure	Wt (g)	H_2O (%)	Ener (kcal)	Prot (g)	Carb (g)	Dietary Fiber (g)	Fat (g)	Fat Breakdown (g) Sat	Mono	Poly
	MISCELLANEOUS—Cont.											
	For other chocolate items, see Sweeteners & Sweets											
972	Cilantro/coriander, fresh	1 tbs	1	93	<1	<1	<1	<1	<1	<.1	<.1	<.1
1197	Cornstarch	1 tbs	8	8	30	<1	7	<1	<1	<.1	<.1	<.1
2239	Curry powder	1 tsp	2	10	7	<1	1	.1	<1	<.1	.1	.1
1202	Dill weed, dried	1 tbs	3	7	8	1	2	<1	<1	<.1	.1	<.1
1705	Dip, french onion	1 tbs	14	70	30	<1	1	<1	3	1.8	.8	.1
975	Garlic cloves	1 ea	3	59	4	<1	1	<1	<1	<.1	<.1	<.1
2238	Garlic powder	1 tsp	3	6	10	1	2	<1	<1	<.1	<.1	<.1
977	Gelatin, dry, unsweetened: Envelope	1 ea	7	13	23	6	0	0	<1	<.1	<.1	<.1
978	Ginger root, slices, raw	2 pce	4	82	3	<1	1	<1	<1	<.1	<.1	<.1
1198	Horseradish, prepared	1 tbs	15	87	6	<1	1	<1	<1	<.1	<.1	<.1
1997	Hummous/hummus	1 c	246	65	421	12	50	13	21	3.1	8.8	7.8
1909	Mustard, country dijon	1 tsp	5	–	5	<1	0	0	0	0	0	0
2019	Mustard, gai choy chinese	1 tbs	15.6	94	33	2	6	–	.27	–	–	–
979	Mustard, prepared (1 packet = 1 tsp)	1 tsp	5	80	4	<1	<1	<1	<1	<.1	.2	<.1
	Miso (see #926 under Vegetables and Legumes, Soybean products)											
2067	No MSG seasoned salt	1 tsp	5	5	4	<1	1	<1	<1	–	–	–
980	Olives, green	5 ea	19	78	22	<1	<1	<1	2	.3	1.8	.2
981	Olives, ripe, pitted	5 ea	22	80	25	<1	1	1	2	.3	1.7	.2
2237	Oregano, ground	1 tsp	1	7	3	<1	1	<1	<1	<.1	<.1	.1
2066	Oriental seasoning blend	1 tsp	3	5	10	<1	2	<1	<1	–	–	–
2236	Paprika	1 tsp	2	10	6	<1	1	<1	<1	<.1	<.1	.2
887	Parsley, freeze dried	¼ c	1	2	3	<1	<1	<1	<1	<.1	<.1	<.1
	Parsley, fresh (see #885 and #886)											
985	Pepper, black	1 tsp	2	11	5	<1	1	1	<1	<.1	<.1	<.1
	Pickles:											
986	Dill, medium, 3¾ x 1¼" diam	1 ea	65	92	12	<1	3	1	<1	<.1	<.1	.1
987	Fresh pack, slices, 1½" diam x ¼"	2 pce	15	79	11	<1	3	<1	<1	0	<.1	<.1
988	Sweet, medium	1 ea	35	65	41	<1	11	<1	<1	<.1	<.1	<.1
989	Pickle relish, sweet	2 tbs	30	63	41	<1	10	1	<1	<.1	<.1	.1
	Popcorn (see Grain Products #539–541)											
917	Potato chips	14 ea	28	2	150	2	15	1	10	3.1	2.8	3.4
1201	Sage, ground	1 tsp	1	8	3	<1	1	<1	<1	.1	<.1	<.1
1347	Salsa, from recipe	1 tbs	14	93	3	<1	1	<1	<1	<.1	<.1	<.1
2218	Salsa, pico de gallo, medium	2 tbs	30	92	5	0	2	<1	0	0	0	0
990	Salt	1 tsp	5	<1	0	0	0	0	0	0	0	0
	Salt substitutes:											
1205	Morton, salt substitute	1 tsp	2	2	<1	0	<1	0	0	0	0	0
1207	Morton, light salt	1 tsp	6	0	0	0	0	0	0	0	0	0
991	Vinegar, cider	½ c	120	94	17	0	7	0	0	0	0	0
2172	Balsamic	1 tbs	15	64	21	0	5	0	0	0	0	0
2176	Malt	1 tbs	15	90	5	0	<1	0	0	0	0	0
2182	Tarragon	1 tbs	15	95	3	0	<1	0	0	0	0	0
2181	White wine	1 tbs	15	89	5	0	<1	0	0	0	0	0

(Computer code number is for West Diet Analysis program)

H

PAGE KEY: H–4 = BEV H–6 = DAIRY H–12 = EGGS H–14 = FAT/OIL H–18 = FRUIT H–26 = BAKERY H–36 = GRAIN H–44 = FISH H–48 = MEATS H–50 = POULTRY H–54 = SAUSAGE H–56 = MIXED/FAST H–64 = NUTS/SEEDS H–68 = SWEETS H–70 = VEG/LEG H–84 = MISC H–88 = SOUPS/SAUCES H–90 = FAST H–106 = FRZN ENTREE H–112 = BABY FOODS

Chol (mg)	Calc (mg)	Iron (mg)	Magn (mg)	Pota (mg)	Sodi (mg)	Zinc (mg)	VT-A (RE)	Thia (mg)	VT-E (α-TE)	Ribo (mg)	Niac (mg)	V-B6 (mg)	Fola (μg)	VT-C (mg)
0	1	.02	<1	5	<1	<.01	3	<.01	.25	<.01	.01	<.01	<1	<1
0	<1	.04	<1	<1	1	<.01	0	0	0	0	0	0	0	0
0	10	.59	5	31	1	.08	2	.01	.01	.01	.07	.01	3	<1
0	54	1.46	14	99	6	.1	18	.01	–	.01	.08	.04	–	2
6	16	.01	2	21	27	.04	27	.01	.08	.02	.02	<.01	2	<1
0	5	.05	1	12	1	.03	0	.01	<.01	<.01	.02	.04	<1	1
0	2	.08	2	33	1	.08	0	.01	<.01	<.01	.02	.08	<1	<1
0	4	.08	2	1	14	.01	0	<.01	0	.02	.01	<.01	2	0
0	1	.02	2	17	1	.01	0	<.01	.01	<.01	.03	.01	<1	<1
0	9	.13	4	44	14	.18	0	0	<.01	0	0	.01	2	0
0	123	4	71	428	600	2.7	5	.23	2.46	.13	1	.98	146	19
0	–	–	–	10	120	–	–	–	–	–	–	–	–	–
–	–	–	–	–	–	–	–	–	–	–	–	–	–	–
0	4	.1	2	7	63	.03	0	0	.09	0	0	<.01	0	0
–	–	–	–	15	1542	–	–	–	–	–	–	–	–	–
0	12	.3	4	10	456	.01	6	0	.57	0	0	<.01	<1	0
0	19	.73	1	2	192	.05	9	<.01	.66	0	.01	<.01	0	<1
0	16	.44	3	17	<1	.04	7	<.01	.02	<.01	.06	.01	3	1
–	–	–	–	12	107	–	–	–	–	–	–	–	–	–
0	4	.5	4	47	1	.08	121	.01	.01	.03	.3	.04	2	1
0	2	.54	4	63	4	.06	63	.01	.06	.02	.1	.01	15	1
0	9	.58	4	25	1	.03	<1	<.01	.02	<.01	.02	.01	<1	<1
0	6	.34	7	75	833	.09	21	.01	.1	.02	.04	.01	1	1
0	5	.27	1	30	101	0	2	0	.02	<.01	0	<.01	0	1
0	1	.21	1	11	329	.03	5	<.01	.06	.01	.06	.01	<1	<1
0	6	.24	1	60	214	.02	3	0	.05	.01	0	<.01	0	2
0	7	.46	19	357	166[1]	.31	0	.05	1.37	.06	1.07	.19	13	9
0	17	.28	4	11	<1	.05	6	.01	.02	<.01	.06	.01	3	<1
0	1	.06	1	23	55	.02	21	.01	.04	<.01	.06	.01	2	5
0	–	–	–	–	260	–	–	–	–	–	–	–	–	–
0	1	.02	<1	<1	1937	0	0	0	0	0	0	0	0	0
0	11	–	<1	1006	<1	–	0	–	–	–	–	–	–	–
0	3	0	4	1500	1099	0	0	0	0	0	0	0	0	0
0	7	.7	26	120	1	0	0	0	0	0	0	0	0	0
–	2	.08	–	11	3	–	–	.08	–	.08	.08	–	–	<1
–	2	.08	–	14	5	–	–	.08	–	.08	.08	–	–	2
–	<1	.08	–	2	1	–	–	.08	–	.08	.08	–	–	<1
–	1	.08	–	12	1	–	–	.08	–	.08	.08	–	–	<1

(1) If no salt added, sodium = 2 mg.

(For purposes of calculations, use "0" for t, <1, <.1, <.01, etc.)

H

Table H-1
Food Composition

Computer Code Number	Food Description	Measure	Wt (g)	H_2O (%)	Ener (kcal)	Prot (g)	Carb (g)	Dietary Fiber (g)	Fat (g)	Fat Breakdown (g) Sat	Mono	Poly
	MISCELLANEOUS—Cont.											
	Yeast:											
992	Baker's, dry, active, package	1 ea	7	8	21	3	3	2	<1	<.1	.2	<.1
993	Brewer's, dry	1 tbs	8	5	23	3	3	3	<1	<.1	<.1	0
	SOUPS, SAUCES, AND GRAVIES											
	SOUPS, canned, condensed:											
	Unprepared, condensed:											
1210	Cream of celery	1 c	251	85	181	3	18	2	11	2.8	2.6	5
1215	Cream of chicken	1 c	251	82	233	7	19	1	15	4.2	6.6	3
1216	Cream of mushroom	1 c	251	81	259	4	19	1	19	5.1	3.6	8.9
1220	Onion	1 c	246	86	113	8	16	2	4	.5	1.5	1.3
	Prepared w/equal volume whole milk:											
994	Clam chowder, New England	1 c	248	85	164	9	17	1	7	3	2.3	1.1
1209	Cream of celery	1 c	248	87	164	6	15	1	10	3.9	2.5	2.7
995	Cream of chicken	1 c	248	85	191	8	15	<1	11	4.6	4.5	1.6
996	Cream of mushroom	1 c	248	85	203	6	15	<1	14	5.1	3	4.6
1214	Cream of potato	1 c	248	87	149	6	17	<1	6	3.8	1.7	.6
1213	Oyster stew	1 c	245	89	135	6	10	0	8	5	2.1	.3
997	Tomato	1 c	248	85	161	6	22	3	6	2.9	1.6	1.1
	Prepared with equal volume of water:											
998	Bean with bacon	1 c	253	84	172	8	23	9	6	1.5	2.2	1.8
999	Beef broth/bouillon/consommé	1 c	240	98	17	3	<1	0	1	.3	.2	<.1
1000	Beef noodle	1 c	244	92	83	5	9	1	3	1.1	1.2	.5
1001	Chicken noodle	1 c	241	92	75	4	9	1	2	.7	1.1	.6
1002	Chicken rice	1 c	241	94	60	4	7	1	2	.5	.9	.4
1208	Chili beef	1 c	250	85	170	7	21	10	7	3.4	2.8	.3
1003	Clam chowder, Manhatten	1 c	244	92	78	2	12	1	2	.4	.4	1.3
1004	Cream of chicken	1 c	244	91	117	3	9	<1	7	2.1	3.3	1.5
1005	Cream of mushroom	1 c	244	90	129	2	9	<1	9	2.4	1.7	4.2
1006	Minestrone	1 c	241	91	82	4	11	1	3	.6	.7	1.1
1211	Onion	1 c	241	93	58	4	8	1	2	.3	.7	.7
1007	Split pea & ham	1 c	253	82	190	10	28	2	4	1.8	1.8	.6
1008	Tomato	1 c	244	90	85	2	17	<1	2	.4	.4	1
1009	Vegetable beef	1 c	244	92	78	6	10	<1	2	.9	.8	.1
1010	Vegetarian vegetable	1 c	241	92	72	2	12	<1	2	.3	.8	.7
1707	Ready to serve											
	Chunky chicken soup	½ c	126	84	89	7	9	<1	3	1	1.5	.7
	SOUPS, dehydrated:											
	Unprepared, dry products:											
1011	Beef bouillon, packet	1 ea	6	3	14	1	1	0	1	.3	.2	<.1
1012	Onion soup, packet	1 ea	34	4	100	4	18	4	2	.5	1.2	.2
	Prepared with water:											
1299	Beef broth/bouillon	1 c	244	97	20	1	2	0	1	.3	.3	<.1
1376	Chicken broth	1 c	244	97	22	1	1	0	1	.3	.4	.4
1013	Chicken noodle	1 c	251	94	53	3	8	<1	1	.3	.5	.3
1122	Cream of chicken	1 c	261	91	107	2	13	1	5	3.4	1.2	.4
1014	Onion	1 c	246	96	27	1	5	<1	1	.1	.3	.1
1217	Split pea	1 c	255	87	125	7	21	3	1	.4	.7	.3
1015	Tomato vegetable	1 c	252	94	55	2	10	1	1	.4	.3	.1

(Computer code number is for West Diet Analysis program)

H

PAGE KEY: H–4 = BEV H–6 = DAIRY H–12 = EGGS H–14 = FAT/OIL H–18 = FRUIT H–26 = BAKERY H–36 = GRAIN H–44 = FISH H–48 = MEATS H–50 = POULTRY H–54 = SAUSAGE H–56 = MIXED/FAST H–64 = NUTS/SEEDS H–68 = SWEETS H–70 = VEG/LEG H–84 = MISC H–88 = SOUPS/SAUCES H–90 = FAST H–106 = FRZN ENTREE H–112 = BABY FOODS

Chol (mg)	Calc (mg)	Iron (mg)	Magn (mg)	Pota (mg)	Sodi (mg)	Zinc (mg)	VT-A (RE)	Thia (mg)	VT-E (α-TE)	Ribo (mg)	Niac (mg)	V-B6 (mg)	Fola (μg)	VT-C (mg)
0	4	1.16	7	140	4	.45	<1	.17	.01	.38	2.79	.11	164	<1
0	17	1.38	18	151	10	.63	0	1.25	–	.34	3.03	.4	313	0
28	80	1.26	13	246	1900	.3	60	.06	.38	.1	.67	.03	5	1
20	68	1.2	5	176	1972	1.26	113	.06	.33	.12	1.64	.03	3	<1
3	65	1.05	10	168	1736	1.19	0	.06	2.6	.17	1.62	.03	8	2
0	54	1.35	5	138	2115	1.23	0	.07	.57	.05	1.21	.1	31	2
22	186	1.49	22	300	992	.8	40	.07	.15	.24	1.03	.13	10	3
32	186	.69	22	310	1009	.2	67	.07	.97	.25	.44	.06	8	1
27	181	.67	17	273	1046	.67	94	.07	.24	.26	.92	.07	8	1
20	179	.6	20	270	918	.64	37	.08	1.34	.28	.91	.06	10	2
22	166	.55	17	322	1061	.67	67	.08	.1	.24	.64	.09	9	1
32	167	1.05	20	235	1041	10.3	44	.07	.49	.23	.34	.06	10	4
17	159	1.81	22	449	744	.29	109	.13	2.6	.25	1.52	.16	21	68
3	81	2.05	46	402	951	1.03	89	.09	.08	.03	.57	.04	32	2
0	14	.41	5	130	782	0	0	<.01	0	.05	1.87	.02	5	0
5	15	1.1	5	100	952	1.54	63	.07	.02	.06	1.07	.04	4	<1
7	17	.77	5	55	1106	.4	72	.05	.07	.06	1.39	.03	2	<1
7	17	.75	0	101	815	.26	65	.02	.05	.02	1.13	.02	1	<1
13	43	2.13	30	525	1035	1.4	150	.06	.18	.08	1.07	.16	18	4
2	27	1.64	12	188	578	.98	98	.03	.73	.04	.82	.1	10	4
10	34	.61	2	88	986	.63	56	.03	.2	.06	.82	.02	2	<1
2	46	.51	5	100	881	.59	0	.05	1.24	.09	.72	.01	5	1
2	34	.92	7	313	911	.74	234	.05	.07	.04	.94	.1	16	1
0	27	.67	2	67	1053	.61	0	.03	.29	.02	.6	.05	15	1
8	23	2.28	48	400	1006	1.32	45	.15	.15	.08	1.48	.07	3	2
0	12	1.76	7	264	695	.24	68	.09	2.49	.05	1.42	.11	15	66
5	17	1.12	5	173	791	1.55	190	.04	.32	.05	1.03	.08	10	2
0	22	1.09	7	210	822	.46	301	.05	.8	.05	.92	.05	11	1
15	13	.87	4	88	446	.5	66	.04	.09	.09	2.21	.03	2	1
1	4	.06	3	27	1018	0	<1	<.01	.01	.01	.27	.01	2	0
2	48	.51	22	227	3045	.2	1	.1	.37	.21	1.73	.03	6	1
0	10	.02	7	37	1361	.07	<1	<.01	.02	.02	.36	0	0	0
0	15	.07	5	24	1483	.01	12	.01	.02	.03	.2	0	2	0
3	32	.5	7	31	1277	.2	5	.07	.03	.06	.88	.01	2	<1
3	76	.26	5	214	1184	1.57	123	.1	.15	.2	2.61	.05	5	1
0	12	.15	5	64	849	.06	<1	.03	.103	.06	.48	0	1	<1
3	20	.94	43	224	1147	.56	5	.21	.13	.14	1.26	.05	40	0
0	8	.63	20	104	1141	.17	20	.06	.81	.05	.79	.05	10	7

(For purposes of calculations, use "0" for t, <1, <.1, <.01, etc.)

Table H-1
Food Composition

Computer Code Number	Food Description	Measure	Wt (g)	H_2O (%)	Ener (kcal)	Prot (g)	Carb (g)	Dietary Fiber (g)	Fat (g)	Fat Breakdown (g) Sat	Mono	Poly
	SAUCES											
	From dry mixes, prepared with milk:											
1016	Cheese sauce	1 c	279	77	307	17	23	1	17	9.3	5.3	1.6
1017	Hollandaise	1 c	259	84	240	5	14	<1	20	11.6	5.9	.9
1018	White sauce	1 c	264	82	240	10	21	<1	13	6.4	4.7	1.7
	From home recipe:											
1019	White sauce, medium[1]	1 c	250	77	356	9	20	<1	27	7.8	10.8	7
1206	Lowfat cheese sauce	¼ c	61	73	85	6	4	<1	5	2.1	1.9	.9
	Ready to serve:											
2202	Alfredo sauce, reduced fat	¼ c	69	–	170	5	16	0	10	6	–	–
1020	Barbeque sauce	1 tbs	16	81	10	<1	1	<1	<1	t	.1	.1
1706	Chili sauce, tomato base	1 tbs	17	68	18	<1	4	<1	<1	<.1	<.1	<.1
2126	Creole sauce	¼ c	62	89	25	1	4	1	1	.1	.2	.3
2124	Hoisin sauce	2 tbs	34	47	70	1	14	0	2	0	–	–
2199	Pesto sauce	2 tbs	29	–	150	4	1	0	15	3.3	9.8	1.2
1021	Soy sauce	1 tbs	18	71	10	1	2	<1	<1	<.1	<.1	<.1
2123	Szechuan sauce	2 tbs	31	71	40	<1	6	<1	2	.2	.5	.8
1380	Teriyaki sauce	1 tbs	18	68	15	1	3	<1	0	0	0	0
	Spaghetti sauce, canned:											
1377	Plain	1 c	249	75	271	5	40	8	12	1.7	6.1	3.3
1378	With meat	1 c	257	74	308	9	38	8	15	2.8	7.2	3.3
1379	With mushrooms	½ c	123	75	108	2	13	1	3	.4	1.5	.8
	GRAVIES											
	Canned:											
1022	Beef	1 c	233	88	124	9	11	1	5	2.7	2.2	.2
1023	Chicken	1 c	238	85	188	5	13	1	14	3.4	6.1	3.6
1024	Mushroom	1 c	238	89	119	3	13	1	6	1	2.8	2.4
1025	From dry mix, brown	1 c	258	92	75	2	13	<1	2	.8	.7	.1
1026	From dry mix, chicken	1 c	260	91	83	3	14	<1	2	.5	.9	.4
	FAST FOOD RESTAURANTS											
	ARBY'S											
1402	Bac'n cheddar deluxe	1 ea	226	59	501	21	38	<1	31	8.5	12.4	9.9
	Roast beef sandwiches:											
1403	Regular	1 ea	147	47	363	21	34	1	17	6.6	7.6	3.3
1404	Junior	1 ea	86	48	225	11	22	<1	10	4	5	2.4
1405	Super	1 ea	234	58	509	22	50	1	26	7	11	7.7
1407	Beef 'n cheddar	1 ea	197	51	472	32	39	1	21	9.7	10	1.3
1408	Chicken breast sandwich	1 ea	184	52	401	20	47	1	20	3	8.8	10.3
1412	Ham'n cheese sandwich	1 ea	156	54	328	23	32	<1	13	4.7	5.4	2.7
1726	Italian sub sandwich	1 ea	297	–	671	34	47	–	39	12.8	15.7	8.5
1413	Turkey sandwich, deluxe	1 ea	197	61	263	20	33	<1	6	1.6	2.3	2.4
1680	Turkey sub sandwich	1 ea	277	62	486	33	47	–	19	5.3	6	7
	Milk shakes:											
1419	Chocolate	1 ea	340	74	451	10	77	<1	12	2.8	7	1.7
1420	Jamocha	1 ea	326	75	368	9	59	0	11	2.5	6.4	1.6
1421	Vanilla	1 ea	312	75	330	11	46	0	12	3.9	5.3	2.3
1728	Salad, roast chicken	1 ea	400	89	204	24	12	–	7	3.3	.9	.9
1729	Sports drink, Upper Ten	1 ea	358	88	169	0	42	–	0	0	0	0

Source: Arby's Inc. for the basic nutrients. Values for some nutrients from known values of major ingredients.

[1]Made with enriched flour, margarine, and whole milk.

(Computer code number is for West Diet Analysis program)

Chol (mg)	Calc (mg)	Iron (mg)	Magn (mg)	Pota (mg)	Sodi (mg)	Zinc (mg)	VT-A (RE)	Thia (mg)	VT-E (α-TE)	Ribo (mg)	Niac (mg)	V-B6 (mg)	Fola (μg)	VT-C (mg)
53	569	.28	47	552	1565	.97	117	.15	.33	.56	.32	.14	13	2
52	124	.9	8	124	1564	.7	220	.05	.26	.18	.06	.5	22	<1
34	425	.26	264	444	797	.55	92	.08	1.58	.45	.53	.07	16	3
29	261	.74	32	346	286	.9	310	.19	3.4	.42	.98	.1	14	2
11	166	.25	10	100	389	.73	58	.03	.55	.14	.16	.03	4	<1
30	150	0	8	80	600	–	80	0	–	.1	0	–	–	0
0	3	.12	1	27	128	.03	14	<.01	.18	<.01	.06	.01	1	1
0	3	.14	2	63	227	.05	24	.02	.05	.01	.27	.02	1	3
0	35	.31	9	187	340	.1	24	.03	.6	.02	.5	.07	9	0
0	0	0	–	–	500	–	0	–	–	–	–	–	–	0
7	117	.17	11	28	234	.52	70	.01	–	.05	0	.04	.8	0
0	3	.36	6	32	1028	.07	0	.01	0	.02	.6	.03	3	0
0	3	.23	3	25	423	.04	19	<.01	.13	.01	.19	.02	1	<1
0	5	.31	11	41	690	.02	0	.01	0	.01	.23	.02	4	0
0	70	1.62	60	956	1235	.52	306	.14	4.98	.15	3.76	.88	54	28
16	69	2	61	978	1212	1.4	297	.14	6.08	.17	4.63	.9	54	27
0	15	1	15	332	495	.34	241	.08	1.35	.08	.93	.16	13	9
7	14	1.63	5	188	1304	2.33	0	.07	.15	.08	1.54	.02	5	0
5	48	1.12	5	259	1373	1.9	264	.04	.37	.1	1.05	.02	5	0
0	17	1.57	5	252	1356	1.67	0	.08	.19	.15	1.6	.05	29	0
3	67	.23	10	57	1075	.31	0	.04	.05	.09	.81	0	0	0
3	39	.26	10	62	1133	.32	0	.05	.05	.15	.78	.03	3	3
37	108	4.2	–	480	1070	3	39	.34	–	.45	9.4	–	–	11
41	57	4.6	15	400	888	3.56	1	.28	–	.45	10.4	.2	13	1
21	39	2.6	8	194	502	1.5	–	.17	–	.25	6.4	.1	7	–
40	83	6	23	491	1081	3.45	28	.36	–	.5	11.4	.3	19	8
74	297	4.6	26	429	1582	4.13	88	.23	–	.6	9	.24	21	0
41	54	2.6	27	298	919	.14	–	.2	–	.51	8	.34	16	5
51	157	2.7	29	353	1292	.83	37	.77	–	.34	7	.31	24	22
69	410	4.32	–	565	2062	–	100	.92	–	.49	8.2	–	–	11
33	131	3.5	30	357	1274	1.5	40	.08	–	.41	15.6	.52	20	12
51	400	4.68	–	500	2033	–	–	13.2	–	.54	18.8	–	–	–
36	250	.72	48	410	341	1.5	60	.12	–	.68	.8	.14	14	5
35	250	2.7	36	525	262	1.5	60	.12	–	.68	.8	.14	14	2
32	300	2.7	36	686	281	1.5	60	.12	–	.68	4	.14	37	2
43	170	1.98	–	877	508	–	485	.33	–	.54	5.6	–	–	51
0	–	–	–	0	40	–	–	–	–	–	–	–	–	–

Note for fast foods: Values for magnesium, phosphorus, zinc, thiamin, riboflavin, niacin, vitamin B_6, folate, some of the fatty acids, and percent water are estimates calculated from known values for major ingredients.

(For purposes of calculations, use "0" for t, <1, <.1, <.01, etc.)

Table H–1
Food Composition

Computer Code Number	Food Description	Measure	Wt (g)	H_2O (%)	Ener (kcal)	Prot (g)	Carb (g)	Dietary Fiber (g)	Fat (g)	Fat Breakdown (g) Sat	Mono	Poly
	BURGER KING											
	Croissant sandwiches:											
1423	Egg, sausage, & cheese	1 ea	163	46	556	20	23	1	43	14.8	20.5	5.1
	Whopper sandwiches:											
1425	Whopper	1 ea	265	58	628	27	44	3	38	10.8	10.8	12.8
1426	Whopper with cheese	1 ea	289	57	718	32	45	3	45	15.7	12.8	12.8
1427	Double beef	1 ea	351	57	870	46	45	3	56	19	19	13
1428	Double beef & cheese	1 ea	374	57	954	52	46	3	63	23.9	21.9	14
1431	Hamburger	1 ea	109	48	286	17	24	1	13	5	5	1
1432	Cheeseburger	1 ea	120	48	330	20	24	1	17	7.8	6.3	1
1433	Double cheeseburger with bacon	1 ea	159	48	467	32	20	1	28	13	12.9	2
1434	Chicken sandwich	1 ea	230	45	713	26	54	2	43	9	11	20.1
1629	BK broiler chicken sandwich	1 ea	248	59	550	30	41	2	29	6	–	–
1435	Chicken tenders	1 ea	95	50	248	17	15	2	13	3.2	5.3	3.2
1437	Ocean catch fish fillet	1 ea	189	51	519	19	42	2	30	4.4	5.8	12.7
1439	French fries (salted)	1 svg	74	38	236	3	27	2	13	3	6	1
1630	French toast sticks	1 svg	141	33	500	4	60	1	27	7	–	–
1440	Onion rings	1 svg	79	51	198	3	26	4	9	1.3	5.1	2.5
1441	Milk shakes, chocolate	1 ea	273	75	308	9	52	3	7	3.8	3.9	0
1442	Milk shakes, vanilla	1 ea	273	75	288	9	51	1	6	3.8	2.9	0
1443	Fried apple pie	1 ea	125	47	332	3	43	2	17	3.3	8.9	1
	Source: Burger King Corporation.											
	DAIRY QUEEN											
	Ice cream cones:											
1446	Small vanilla	1 ea	85	63	138	4	23	0	4	3	1	–
1447	Regular vanilla	1 ea	142	64	230	5	38	0	7	4.7	1	1
1448	Large vanilla	1 ea	213	65	345	8	55	0	10	7	1	1
1450	Chocolate dipped	1 ea	156	59	340	6	42	<1	17	9	4	3
1453	Chocolate sundae	1 ea	177	62	301	6	54	0	7	4.4	1	1
1455	Banana split	1 ea	383	68	529	8	100	3	12	8.3	3.1	.4
1456	Peanut Buster Parfait	1 ea	305	51	730	16	99	2	31	17	10	9
1457	Hot Fudge Brownie Delight	1 ea	266	53	619	10	89	1	25	12.2	10.5	1.7
1459	Buster bar	1 ea	149	45	450	10	41	2	28	12	10	8
1645	Breeze, strawberry, regular	1 ea	354	70	425	12	92	1	1	.9	0	0
1460	Dilly bar	1 ea	85	55	210	3	21	0	13	7	3	3
1461	DQ ice cream sandwich	1 ea	60	46	148	3	24	1	5	2	1	1
1463	Milk shakes, regular	1 ea	418	71	548	13	93	<1	15	8.4	2.1	2.1
1464	Milk shakes, large	1 ea	489	72	636	14	107	<1	17	10.6	2.1	2.1
1466	Milk shakes, malted	1 ea	418	68	610	13	106	<1	14	8	2	2
1470	Misty slush, small	1 ea	454	88	220	0	56	0	0	0	0	0
2250	Starkiss	1 ea	85	75	80	0	21	0	0	0	0	0

H

PAGE KEY: H–4 = BEV H–6 = DAIRY H–12 = EGGS H–14 = FAT/OIL H–18 = FRUIT H–26 = BAKERY H–36 = GRAIN H–44 = FISH H–48 = MEATS H–50 = POULTRY H–54 = SAUSAGE H–56 = MIXED/FAST H–64 = NUTS/SEEDS H–68 = SWEETS H–70 = VEG/LEG H–84 = MISC H–88 = SOUPS/SAUCES H–90 = FAST H–106 = FRZN ENTREE H–112 = BABY FOODS

Chol (mg)	Calc (mg)	Iron (mg)	Magn (mg)	Pota (mg)	Sodi (mg)	Zinc (mg)	VT-A (RE)	Thia (mg)	VT-E (α-TE)	Ribo (mg)	Niac (mg)	V-B6 (mg)	Fola (μg)	VT-C (mg)
241	139	3.33	–	–	1055	–	74	.37	–	.33	4.1	.12	–	0
88	79	4.4	–	–	854	–	98	.32	–	.4	6.87	.34	–	9
113	246	4.4	–	–	1327	–	147	.33	–	.47	6.88	.32	–	9
170	80	7.2	–	–	940	–	100	.34	–	.56	10	–	–	9
195	249	7.18	–	–	1416	–	150	.35	–	.63	9.97	–	–	9
48	35	1.6	–	–	559	–	17	.24	–	.27	4.23	–	–	0
57	87	2.35	–	–	670	–	52	.23	–	.29	4.17	–	–	0
106	146	3.28	–	–	904	–	58	.23	–	.3	4.38	–	–	0
60	100	3.62	–	–	1406	–	0	.45	–	.31	10	–	–	0
80	60	5.4	–	–	480	–	60	–	–	–	–	–	–	6
38	0	.78	–	–	572	–	0	.08	–	.08	7.56	–	–	0
67	44	2	–	–	726	–	15	.21	–	.2	2.96	–	–	1
0	0	.69	–	–	153	–	0	.06	–	.2	5	–	–	2
0	60	2.7	–	–	490	–	0	–	–	–	–	–	–	0
0	64	.92	–	–	516	–	0	.04	–	.03	.46	–	–	0
19	192	1.73	–	–	221	–	58	.13	–	.53	.13	–	–	0
19	288	0	–	–	221	–	58	.11	–	.55	.13	–	–	3
0	0	1.6	–	–	254	–	0	.27	–	.18	.6	–	–	7
12	120	.6	–	150	69	–	73	.03	–	.17	.06	–	–	<1
20	200	1.2	–	260	113	–	100	.06	–	.26	.11	.09	–	1.6
34	295	1.5	–	380	168	–	168	.1	–	.34	.17	–	–	2
20	200	1.2	–	290	133	–	100	.06	–	.25	.11	.09	–	1.6
22	184	1.1	–	289	154	–	110	.06	–	.25	.3	.14	–	0
31	260	1.9	–	893	187	–	208	.16	–	.27	.42	.21	–	16
35	300	1.8	–	660	400	–	150	.15	–	.51	3	.23	–	1
31	262	4.71	–	445	297	–	70	.1	–	.6	.26	.16	–	1
15	150	1.1	–	400	280	–	80	.09	–	.17	3	.09	–	0
9	416	2.5	–	490	250	–	0	.12	–	.67	–	–	–	8
10	100	.36	–	170	75	–	60	.03	–	.14	–	.06	–	0
5	59	.71	–	103	113	–	39	.03	–	.25	.39	.05	–	0
47	421	1.52	–	600	242	–	84	.13	–	.63	.84	.2	–	<1
53	477	1.53	–	700	276	–	212	.16	–	.72	.85	–	–	<1
45	400	1.44	–	570	230	–	80	.12	–	.6	.8	.19	–	<1
0	0	0	–	–	20	–	0	–	–	–	–	–	–	0
0	0	0	–	–	10	–	0	–	–	–	–	–	–	0

Note for fast foods: Values for magnesium, phosphorus, zinc, thiamin, riboflavin, niacin, vitamin B_6, folate, some of the fatty acids, and percent water are estimates calculated from known values for major ingredients.

(For purposes of calculations, use "0" for t, <1, <.1, <.01, etc.)

H

Table H-1
Food Composition

Computer Code Number	Food Description	Measure	Wt (g)	H_2O (%)	Ener (kcal)	Prot (g)	Carb (g)	Dietary Fiber (g)	Fat (g)	Fat Breakdown (g) Sat	Mono	Poly
	DAIRY QUEEN—Cont.											
	Yogurt:											
1641	Yogurt cone, regular	1 ea	142	66	187	6	39	0	1	.3	–	–
1643	Yogurt sundae, strawberry	1 ea	170	70	200	6	44	1	<1	.3	0	0
	Sandwiches:											
1474	Chicken	1 ea	202	56	455	25	39	2	21	4.2	7.4	8.5
1647	Chicken fillet, grilled	1 ea	184	64	310	24	30	3	10	3	2	3
1475	Fish fillet	1 ea	177	58	385	17	41	2	17	3.6	5.2	8.3
1476	Fish fillet with cheese	1 ea	191	56	436	20	42	2	22	6.2	7.3	8.3
1477	Hamburger, single	1 ea	148	56	311	18	31	2	13	5.4	6.4	1
1478	Hamburger, double	1 ea	210	62	436	30	29	2	22	9.9	11.7	2.1
1480	Cheeseburger, single	1 ea	162	55	362	21	31	2	18	8.5	7.3	1
1481	Cheeseburger, double	1 ea	239	55	589	38	33	2	34	17.5	13.7	2.1
	Hot dog:											
1483	Regular	1 ea	100	57	242	9	19	1	14	5.1	7.1	2
1484	With cheese	1 ea	114	55	293	12	20	1	18	8.1	8.1	2
1485	With chili	1 ea	128	53	323	11	26	2	19	7.1	8.1	2
1489	French fries, small	1 ea	71	38	210	3	29	3	10	2	5	3
1490	French fries, large	1 ea	113	38	344	4	46	5	16	3.5	7.1	5.3
1491	Onion rings	1 ea	85	46	240	4	29	2	12	2.5	5	4
	Source: International Dairy Queen.											
	HARDEE'S											
1734	Frisco burger hamburger	1 ea	242	–	760	36	43	–	50	18	–	–
1735	Frisco grilled chicken sandwich	1 ea	244	–	620	35	44	–	34	10	–	–
1736	Frisco grilled chicken salad	1 ea	278	–	120	18	2	–	4	1	–	–
1737	Peach shake	1 ea	345	–	390	10	77	–	4	3	–	–
	JACK IN THE BOX											
	Breakfast items:											
1492	Breakfast Jack sandwich	1 ea	126	50	312	19	31	0	13	5.2	5.2	2.6
1494	Sausage crescent	1 ea	156	39	580	22	28	0	43	15.5	21.5	5.7
1495	Supreme crescent	1 ea	146	40	506	22	32	0	31	9.5	18	7.4
1496	Pancake platter	1 ea	231	46	610	15	87	0	22	9	7.6	3.5
1497	Scrambled egg platter	1 ea	249	52	655	21	58	0	37	10.5	19.4	5.1
	Sandwiches:											
1654	Bacon cheeseburger	1 ea	242	49	710	35	41	0	45	15	15.7	8.7
1498	Hamburger	1 ea	98	39	283	13	31	0	11	4	5	2
1499	Cheeseburger	1 ea	113	39	339	16	33	0	15	6.2	6.1	2.4
1739	Chicken caesar pita sandwich	1 ea	237	59	520	27	44	4	26	6	–	–
1500	Jumbo Jack burger	1 ea	205	55	501	23	37	0	29	9	11.6	7.2
1501	Jumbo Jack burger with cheese	1 ea	246	55	620	29	42	0	37	12.2	15.3	9.1
1655	Chicken sandwich	1 ea	160	52	400	20	38	0	18	4	–	–
1505	Chicken supreme	1 ea	228	55	577	23	45	0	34	10.2	13.8	10.6

(Computer code number is for West Diet Analysis program)

H

Chol (mg)	Calc (mg)	Iron (mg)	Magn (mg)	Pota (mg)	Sodi (mg)	Zinc (mg)	VT-A (RE)	Thia (mg)	VT-E (α-TE)	Ribo (mg)	Niac (mg)	V-B6 (mg)	Fola (μg)	VT-C (mg)
3	200	1.2	–	190	113	–	0	.06	–	.25	–	–	–	1.6
3	200	1.2	–	235	120	–	0	.06	–	.33	–	–	–	4
58	42	1.9	–	370	804	–	0	.4	–	.36	12	–	–	0
50	200	2.7	–	330	1040	–	0	.3	–	1.02	12	–	–	0
47	42	1.9	–	292	656	–	0	.3	–	.23	3	–	–	0
62	104	1.9	–	301	882	–	83	.3	–	.27	5	–	–	0
48	64	2.9	–	270	676	–	43	.31	–	.26	4	–	–	4
89	59	4.5	–	440	674	–	59	.3	–	.45	7	–	–	6
59	160	3.84	–	280	906	–	64	.31	–	.35	4	–	–	4
126	273	4.9	–	465	1233	–	164	.3	–	.53	7.4	–	–	4
25	60	1.82	–	172	737	–	20	.23	–	.14	2	–	–	4
40	151	1.82	–	182	958	–	61	.23	–	.17	2	–	–	4
30	40	1.45	–	262	726	–	60	.23	–	.14	3	–	–	<1
0	0	.72	–	430	115	–	0	.09	–	.03	2	–	–	5
0	0	1.27	–	689	177	–	0	.13	–	.06	2.65	–	–	8
0	0	1.08	–	90	135	–	0	.09	–	.05	.4	–	–	0
70	–	–	–	–	1280	–	–	–	–	–	–	–	–	–
95	–	–	–	–	1730	–	–	–	–	–	–	–	–	–
60	–	–	–	–	520	–	–	–	–	–	–	–	–	–
25	–	–	–	–	290	–	–	–	–	–	–	–	–	–
193	208	2.8	–	229	927	–	83	.49	–	.43	3	–	–	9
185	150	2.7	–	260	1010	–	100	.6	–	.51	4.6	–	–	0
200	143	3.4	–	258	888	–	143	.62	–	.52	4	–	–	11
100	100	1.8	–	310	890	–	80	.03	–	.85	7	–	–	6
444	175	5.26	–	526	1239	–	175	–	–	.77	5.85	–	–	11
110	250	5.4	–	540	1240	–	80	.24	–	.48	8.8	.39	–	9
25	101	2.7	–	192	434	–	20	.15	–	.26	2	–	–	1
36	206	2.77	–	206	524	–	62	.24	–	.24	3.08	–	–	1
55	250	2.7	–	490	1050	–	80	–	–	–	–	–	–	2
58	90	4.03	–	403	627	–	36	.32	–	.26	1.66	–	–	5
81	203	5.49	–	468	793	–	61	.37	–	.45	1.63	–	–	6
45	150	1.8	–	180	1290	–	40	–	–	–	–	–	–	0
70	186	2.5	–	177	1414	–	93	.36	–	.3	10.2	–	–	2

Note for fast foods: Values for magnesium, phosphorus, zinc, thiamin, riboflavin, niacin, vitamin B_6, folate, some of the fatty acids, and percent water are estimates calculated from known values for major ingredients.

(For purposes of calculations, use "0" for t, <1, <.1, <.01, etc.)

Table H-1
Food Composition

Computer Code Number	Food Description	Measure	Wt (g)	H_2O (%)	Ener (kcal)	Prot (g)	Carb (g)	Dietary Fiber (g)	Fat (g)	Fat Breakdown (g) Sat	Mono	Poly
	JACK IN THE BOX—Cont.											
1656	Chicken sandwich, sourdough ranch	1 ea	225	73	205	14	41	7	0	0	0	0
1583	Double cheeseburger	1 ea	149	41	441	24	34	0	24	11.8	11.4	3.1
1651	Grilled sourdough burger	1 ea	223	48	670	32	39	0	43	16	17.8	7.9
1740	Monterey roast beef sandwich	1 ea	238	57	540	30	40	3	30	9	–	–
1508	Tacos, regular	1 ea	81	58	197	7	16	2	11	4.2	–	–
1509	Tacos, super	1 ea	135	59	300	13	24	3	18	6.4	–	–
	Teriyaki bowl:											
1668	Chicken	1 ea	440	62	580	28	115	6	2	–	–	–
1679	Beef	1 ea	440	62	640	28	124	7	3	1	–	–
1516	French fries	1 ea	109	38	350	4	45	4	17	4	11	.6
1517	Hash browns	1 ea	62	51	174	1	15	1	12	2.7	7.4	.3
1518	Onion rings	1 ea	108	34	398	5	40	0	24	6.3	15.9	.9
	Milk shakes:											
1519	Chocolate	1 ea	322	72	390	9	74	0	6	3.5	2.1	–
1520	Strawberry	1 ea	328	67	363	10	66	0	8	4.4	2.2	–
1521	Vanilla	1 ea	317	73	365	9	65	0	7	4.2	1.9	–
1522	Apple turnover	1 ea	119	34	379	3	52	0	21	4.3	11.5	1.6
	Source: Jack in the Box Restaurant, Inc.											
	KENTUCKY FRIED CHICKEN											
	Rotisserie Gold:											
1472	Dark qtr, no skin	1 ea	117	60	217	27	0	0	12	3.5	–	–
1473	Dark qtr, w/skin	1 ea	146	54	333	30	1	–	24	6.6	–	–
1513	White qtr with wing, w/skin	1 ea	176	59	335	40	1	–	19	5.4	–	–
1525	White qtr with wing, no skin	1 ea	117	20	199	37	0	0	6	1.7	–	–
	Original recipe:											
1253	Center breast	1 ea	95	52	240	23	8	<1	13	3.5	7.2	1.8
1251	Side breast	1 ea	69	47	204	15	7	<1	12	3.5	7.3	1.8
1250	Drumstick	1 ea	47	51	125	12	2	<1	7	1.8	3.4	1.1
1252	Thigh	1 ea	88	49	266	17	7	<1	19	4.9	8.7	2.9
1249	Wing	1 ea	42	41	136	10	4	<1	9	2.4	4.8	1.4
	Dinners:											
	Hot & spicy:											
1451	Center breast	1 ea	125	48	360	28	13	–	22	5	–	–
1452	Side breast	1 ea	120	43	400	22	16	–	28	6	–	–
1430	Thigh	1 ea	119	47	370	24	10	–	27	6	–	–
1471	Wing	1 ea	61	38	220	14	5	–	16	4	–	–
	Extra crispy recipe:											
1261	Center breast	1 ea	104	48	291	23	12	1	17	4.2	9.5	1.9
1259	Side breast	1 ea	84	40	290	15	14	<1	20	4	9.3	1.7
1258	Drumstick	1 ea	58	48	170	12	5	<1	11	3	6.9	1.5
1260	Thigh	1 ea	107	43	373	23	7	<1	29	7.6	15.7	4.1
1257	Wing	1 ea	53	32	216	12	7	<1	15	4	9.6	2.2
	Dinners:											

PAGE KEY: H–4 = BEV H–6 = DAIRY H–12 = EGGS H–14 = FAT/OIL H–18 = FRUIT H–26 = BAKERY H–36 = GRAIN H–44 = FISH H–48 = MEATS H–50 = POULTRY H–54 = SAUSAGE H–56 = MIXED/FAST H–64 = NUTS/SEEDS H–68 = SWEETS H–70 = VEG/LEG H–84 = MISC H–88 = SOUPS/SAUCES H–90 = FAST H–106 = FRZN ENTREE H–112 = BABY FOODS

Chol (mg)	Calc (mg)	Iron (mg)	Magn (mg)	Pota (mg)	Sodi (mg)	Zinc (mg)	VT-A (RE)	Thia (mg)	VT-E (α-TE)	Ribo (mg)	Niac (mg)	V-B6 (mg)	Fola (μg)	VT-C (mg)
0	0	4.91	–	–	136	–	341	–	–	–	–	–	–	82
74	245	3.5	–	314	882	–	98	.15	–	.33	5.9	–	–	0
110	200	4.5	–	510	1140	–	150	.65	–	.48	8	.33	–	6
75	300	3.6	–	500	1270	–	80	–	–	–	–	–	–	5
21	104	1.1	36	249	426	1.2	0	.07	–	.18	1	.14	–	0
32	161	1.9	48	396	771	1.9	0	.13	–	.09	1.5	.19	–	3
30	100	1.8	–	380	1220	–	1100	–	–	–	–	–	–	9
25	150	4.5	–	430	930	–	1000	–	–	–	–	–	–	6
0	0	1.1	–	690	190	–	0	.18	–	.03	3.8	–	–	24
0	0	.39	–	207	337	–	0	.05	–	–	1.09	–	–	7
0	21	1.9	–	136	472	–	0	.3	–	.18	2.73	–	–	3
25	300	.72	–	680	210	–	0	.15	–	.6	.4	–	–	0
33	330	0	–	605	198	–	0	.17	–	.47	.44	–	–	0
31	313	0	–	594	188	–	0	.16	–	.35	.4	–	–	0
0	0	1.95	–	87	498	–	0	.22	–	.13	1.95	–	–	10
128	10	.18	–	–	772	–	15	–	–	–	–	–	–	1
163	10	.18	–	–	980	–	15	–	–	–	–	–	–	1
157	10	.18	–	–	1104	–	15	–	–	–	–	–	–	1
97	10	.18	–	–	667	–	15	–	–	–	–	–	–	1
85	28	.66	–	–	562	–	14	.08	–	.16	10.6	–	–	–
65	57	1	–	–	502	–	12	.05	–	.1	5.74	–	–	–
62	17	.91	–	–	222	–	12	.04	–	.1	2.64	–	–	–
104	37	1	–	–	548	–	29	.07	–	.28	5.1	–	–	–
47	24	.43	–	–	304	–	12	.02	–	.06	2.93	–	–	–
80	20	.72	–	–	750	–	15	–	–	–	–	–	–	6
80	40	1.08	–	–	850	–	15	–	–	–	–	–	–	6
100	20	1.08	–	–	670	–	15	–	–	–	–	–	–	6
65	20	.72	–	–	440	–	30	–	–	–	–	–	–	–
66	29	.71	–	–	652	–	13	1	–	.1	11.6	–	–	–
54	14	.52	–	–	514	–	11	.07	–	.07	6.16	–	–	–
58	18	.32	–	–	277	–	27	.05	–	.1	3.3	–	–	–
88	48	1.18	–	–	511	–	29	1	–	.21	6.38	–	–	–
58	18	.32	–	–	288	–	27	–	–	.04	.05	2.96	–	–

Note for fast foods: Values for magnesium, phosphorus, zinc, thiamin, riboflavin, niacin, vitamin B_6, folate, some of the fatty acids, and percent water are estimates calculated from known values for major ingredients.

(For purposes of calculations, use "0" for t, <1, <.1, <.01, etc.)

Table H–1
Food Composition

Computer Code Number	Food Description	Measure	Wt (g)	H_2O (%)	Ener (kcal)	Prot (g)	Carb (g)	Dietary Fiber (g)	Fat (g)	Fat Breakdown (g) Sat	Mono	Poly
	KENTUCKY FRIED CHICKEN—Cont.											
1526	Breadstick	1 ea	33	10	110	3	17	0	3	0	–	–
1268	Corn-on-the-cob	1 ea	143	70	210	4	26	8	11	1.9	1	1.4
1527	Cornbread	1 pce	56	26	228	3	25	1	13	2	–	–
1269	Coleslaw	⅓ c	79	75	100	1	12	<1	5	.9	1.5	3
1429	Chicken, hot wings	1 svg	119	38	415	24	16	–	29	–	–	–
1381	Kentucky nuggets	6 ea	96	41	287	16	15	<1	18	4	8.7	2.2
	Kentucky nugget sauce:											
1386	Kentucky fries	1 svg	119	42	352	5	40	5	18	5	12.5	1.1
1534	Macaroni & cheese	1 svg	114	71	162	7	15	0	8	3	–	–
1387	Mashed potatoes & gravy	⅓ c	86	80	74	1	11	<1	4	.3	.4	.1
1388	Buttermilk biscuit	1 ea	75	28	271	6	32	<1	15	3.9	7.1	2.7
1530	Pasta salad	1 svg	108	78	135	2	14	1	8	1	–	–
1389	Potato salad	⅓ c	90	74	130	2	13	1	8	1.4	2	3.5
1383	Potato wedges	1 svg	92	55	192	3	25	3	9	3	–	–
1390	Baked beans	⅓ c	89	70	107	4	19	3	2	.8	.4	.2
1391	Chicken Little sandwich	1 ea	57	32	205	7	17	1	12	2.4	–	4.1
1535	Red beans & rice	1 svg	111	76	113	4	18	3	3	1	–	–
1529	Vegetable medley salad	1 ea	114	77	126	1	21	3	4	1	–	–
	Source: Kentucky Fried Chicken Corporation.											
	LONG JOHN SILVER'S											
	Fish, batter fried:											
1523	Fish & Fryes (fries), 3 piece	1 ea	350	54	893	28	84	–	46	10	26	9
1524	Fish & Fryes, 2 piece	1 ea	260	54	608	27	52	–	37	8	23	5
2240	Fish and lemon crumb dinner, 3 piece	1 ea	493	71.3	610	39	86	–	13	2.2	3.9	5.3
2241	Fish and lemon crumb dinner, 2 piece	1 ea	334	76.8	330	24	46	–	5	.9	1.6	1.2
	Chicken:											
1528	Chicken Plank dinner, 3 piece	1 ea	370	56	825	30	94	–	41	8.8	23	8.7
1531	Clam chowder	1 ea	185	86	131	10	9	1	6	1.7	2.3	1.6
1532	Clam dinner	1 ea	460	47	1261	31	145	–	66	14	40	13
1533	Fish & chicken dinner	1 ea	460	52	1013	38	109	–	52	11	31	10
2243	Oysters, breaded and fried	1 svg	139	48	368	13	40	1	18	4.6	6.9	4.6
1537	Shrimp dinner, batter fried	1 ea	300	54	761	16	80	–	43	8.8	24.7	8.2
	Salads:											
1539	Ocean chef salad	1 ea	320	89	150	16	18	3	1	.5	.5	.3
1540	Seafood salad	1 ea	480	89	656	26	21	3	54	8.8	14	30
1541	Coleslaw	1 ea	98	70	140	1	20	1	6	1	1.5	3.5
1542	Fryes (fries) serving	1 ea	85	43	250	3	28	1	15	2.5	7.4	5.1
1543	Hush puppies	1 ea	47	38	137	4	20	<1	4	.8	2.5	.4
	Source: Long John Silver's, Lexington, KY.											
	McDONALD'S											
	Sandwiches:											
1221	Big Mac	1 ea	215	53	508	25	46	3	26	9	7.4	4.1
1444	McChicken	1 ea	187	52	486	17	41	2	28	5.4	8.4	10.1
1591	McLean deluxe	1 ea	206	64	332	23	36	2	11	4	3.5	1.1
1438	McLean deluxe with cheese	1 ea	219	63	382	25	37	2	15	6.5	4.4	1.3

PAGE KEY: H–4 = BEV H–6 = DAIRY H–12 = EGGS H–14 = FAT/OIL H–18 = FRUIT H–26 = BAKERY H–36 = GRAIN H–44 = FISH H–48 = MEATS H–50 = POULTRY H–54 = SAUSAGE H–56 = MIXED/FAST H–64 = NUTS/SEEDS H–68 = SWEETS H–70 = VEG/LEG H–84 = MISC H–88 = SOUPS/SAUCES H–90 = FAST H–106 = FRZN ENTREE H–112 = BABY FOODS

Chol (mg)	Calc (mg)	Iron (mg)	Magn (mg)	Pota (mg)	Sodi (mg)	Zinc (mg)	VT-A (RE)	Thia (mg)	VT-E (α-TE)	Ribo (mg)	Niac (mg)	V-B6 (mg)	Fola (μg)	VT-C (mg)
0	30	.18	–	–	15	–	0	–	–	–	–	–	–	0
0	0	.34	–	72	–	–	19	.13	–	.1	1.7	–	–	2
42	60	.72	–	–	194	–	10	–	–	–	–	–	–	–
4	26	.32	–	–	155	–	28	.03	–	.03	.18	–	–	24
132	35	2.87	–	–	1084	–	13	–	–	–	–	–	–	5
67	2	.1	–		874	–	15	.02	–	.02	1	.05	–	<1
7	17	1.5	–	–	826	–	0	.23	–	.08	3.09	–	–	0
16	120	.72	–	–	531	–	–	–	–	–	–	–	–	0
<1	14	.3	–	–	278	–	11	–	–	.03	.86	–	–	–
3	49	2.2	–	–	652	–	32	.3	–	.23	3	–	–	–
1	20	1.08	–	–	663	–	110	–	–	–	–	–	–	7
8	7	1.6	11	184	305	.21	58	.05	–	.02	.4	.14	5	–
3	–	–	–	–	428	–	–	–	–	–	–	–	–	–
2	32	1.2	23	185	433	1.04	40	.05	–	.03	.4	.06	26	2
21	27	2.06	–	–	401	–	6	.19	–	.15	2.67	–	–	–
4	10	.71	–	–	312	–	–	–	–	–	–	–	–	–
0	20	.36	–	–	240	–	375	–	–	–	–	–	–	5
64	182	4	–	1020	1394	2.7	36	.41	–	.39	7.3	–	–	14
60	40	2	–	897	1474	1.2	–	.38	–	.34	8	–	–	9
125	200	5.4	–	990	1420	2.25	700	.75	–	.6	24	–	–	6
75	80	1.8	–	440	640	.9	1000	.3	–	.26	14	–	–	18
51	186	4	–	1084	1854	2.78	37	.49	–	.47	14.8	–	–	8
19	187	1.68	–	355	551	.56	140	.1	–	.24	1.87	–	–	–
96	255	5.73	–	1159	2331	3.8	51	.96	–	.54	15	–	–	15
80	213	4.8	–	1366	2230	3	43	.64	–	.64	15	–	–	10
108	28	4.46	24	182	677	15.7	108	.3	–	.35	4.4	.03	13	4
91	181	3.26	–	761	1477	2.7	36	.41	–	.4	8	–	–	8
55	137	5	–	130	998	.4	684	.16	–	.2	4	–	–	29
95	259	7.8	–	225	1692	1.6	345	.26	–	.44	5	–	–	36
15	60	.72	–	190	260	.6	40	.06	–	.07	2	–	–	–
0	200	.72	–	370	500	.3	–	.09	–	–	1.6	–	–	6
–	78	1.4	–	127	49	.6	–	.12	–	.07	1.6	–	–	–
76	201	4.3	45	454	928	4.8	–	.48	1.01	.44	6	.25	49	3
52	127	2.5	32	316	789	1	–	.9	6.1	.24	7.7	.38	36	1
57	127	4	38	517	780	4.7	–	.41	.6	.33	7	.28	42	8
70	134	4.1	42	537	1005	5.1	150	.4	.82	.38	7	2.8	45	8

Note for fast foods: Values for magnesium, phosphorus, zinc, thiamin, riboflavin, niacin, vitamin B_6, folate, some of the fatty acids, and percent water are estimates calculated from known values for major ingredients.

(For purposes of calculations, use "0" for t, <1, <.1, <.01, etc.)

H

Table H–1
Food Composition

Computer Code Number	Food Description	Measure	Wt (g)	H_2O (%)	Ener (kcal)	Prot (g)	Carb (g)	Dietary Fiber (g)	Fat (g)	Fat Breakdown (g) Sat	Mono	Poly
	McDONALD's—Cont.											
	Sandwiches—Cont.:											
1222	Quarter-pounder	1 ea	166	52	403	22	35	2	20	7.6	6.5	1.3
1223	Quarter-pounder with cheese	1 ea	194	50	507	27	36	2	28	12.3	8.5	1.6
1224	Filet-O-Fish	1 ea	142	49	357	13	40	1	16	3.6	3.8	5.5
1225	Hamburger	1 ea	102	49	251	12	33	2	8	3	2.7	.9
1226	Cheeseburger	1 ea	116	55	302	14	34	2	12	5.3	3.6	1
1227	French fries, small serving	1 ea	68	40	207	3	26	2	10	1.7	3.1	2.5
1228	Chicken McNuggets	6 ea	112	51	304	19	16	0	18	3.8	5.7	3.7
	Sauces (packet):											
1229	Hot mustard	1 ea	30	60	63	1	7	1	4	.47	1.1	2
1230	Barbecue	1 ea	32	58	53	<1	12	<1	<1	.1	.1	.2
1231	Sweet & sour	1 ea	32	57	55	<1	12	<1	<1	.1	.1	.3
	Low-fat (frozen yogurt) milk shakes:											
1232	Chocolate	1 ea	293	71	346	13	62	1	5	3.5	.1	.7
1233	Strawberry	1 ea	293	72	342	12	63	<1	5	3.4	.1	.6
1234	Vanilla	1 ea	293	75	308	12	54	<1	5	3.3	.1	.6
	Low-fat (frozen yogurt) sundaes:											
1237	Hot caramel	1 ea	168	56	283	6	58	1	3	1.8	.3	.9
1235	Hot fudge	1 ea	168	60	275	8	50	2	5	4.5	.1	.4
1267	Strawberry	1 ea	168	65	226	6	49	1	1	.7	.1	.2
1238	Vanilla	1 ea	80	68	105	4	21	<1	1	.4	.2	<.1
1239	Pie, apple	1 ea	83	47	220	2	31	1	10	2.5	4.5	2.8
	Muffins (fat-free)											
1240	Apple bran	1 ea	85	39	207	4	46	2	1	.2	.1	.4
1241	Cookies, McDonaldland	1 ea	56	3	258	<1	41	1	9	1.8	6.4	.8
1242	Cookies, Chocolaty chip	1 ea	56	3	282	3	36	1	14	3.9	4.4	1
	Breakfast items:											
1243	English muffin with spread	1 ea	59	33	177	5	28	2	5	2.3	1.4	1.3
1244	Egg McMuffin	1 ea	138	57	292	17	27	1	13	.7	4.5	1.6
1245	Hotcakes with marg & syrup	1 ea	176	44	442	7	80	2	11	1.9	3.7	4.6
1246	Scrambled eggs	1 ea	100	73	166	12	1	0	12	3.6	5.2	1.7
1247	Pork sausage	1 ea	48	45	193	7	<1	0	18	6.1	7.1	2.3
1248	Hashbrown potatoes	1 ea	53	55	130	1	14	1	8	1.3	2.3	1.9
1392	Sausage McMuffin	1 ea	117	42	377	13	28	2	24	8.6	8.5	2.9
1393	Sausage McMuffin with egg	1 ea	167	53	454	19	28	1	29	10.2	10.9	3.7
1394	Biscuit with biscuit spread	1 ea	75	32	257	4	31	1	13	3.7	3.7	.8
1395	Biscuit with sausage	1 ea	123	37	448	10	33	1	30	8.9	10.4	2.9
1396	Biscuit with sausage & egg	1 ea	180	48	548	17	35	1	37	11.1	13.5	3.9
1397	Biscuit with bacon, egg, cheese	1 ea	156	46	462	18	34	1	28	9	9	2
	Salads:											
1398	Chef salad	1 ea	283	86	186	18	8	3	10	3.8	2.7	1
1400	Garden salad	1 ea	213	92	77	5	6	2	4	1	1.3	.6
1401	Chunky chicken salad	1 ea	250	88	138	19	7	3	4	1.1	1.3	.8

Source: McDonald's Corporation.

(Computer code number is for West Diet Analysis program)

PAGE KEY: H–4 = BEV H–6 = DAIRY H–12 = EGGS H–14 = FAT/OIL H–18 = FRUIT H–26 = BAKERY H–36 = GRAIN H–44 = FISH H–48 = MEATS H–50 = POULTRY H–54 = SAUSAGE H–56 = MIXED/FAST H–64 = NUTS/SEEDS H–68 = SWEETS H–70 = VEG/LEG H–84 = MISC H–88 = SOUPS/SAUCES H–90 = FAST H–106 = FRZN ENTREE H–112 = BABY FOODS

Chol (mg)	Calc (mg)	Iron (mg)	Magn (mg)	Pota (mg)	Sodi (mg)	Zinc (mg)	VT-A (RE)	Thia (mg)	VT-E (α-TE)	Ribo (mg)	Niac (mg)	V-B6 (mg)	Fola (μg)	VT-C (mg)
68	123	4	33	394	672	4.5	40	.38	.35	.32	7	.24	27	3
94	139	4.4	–	–	1131	–	150	.38	.79	.42	7	.26	32	3
36	121	1.81	31	260	693	.7	20	.3	1.49	.22	2.53	.1	29	0
27	119	2.6	23	245	502	2.13	40	.31	.22	.24	3.6	.13	20	2
40	127	2.6	26	268	729	2.5	80	.3	.44	.3	3.6	.14	23	2
0	9	.53	26	469	135	.32	0	.05	.83	0	2	.24	26	8
65	15	1	26	323	542	1.05	0	.12	1.48	.17	8	.32	–	0
3	7	.8	–	29	85	–	2	.01	–	.01	.15	–	–	0
0	4	0	–	51	277	–	0	.01	–	.01	.17	–	–	4
0	2	.16	–	8	158	–	60	0	–	.01	.08	–	–	0
24	369	1.03	–	539	240	–	60	.12	–	.51	.4	.1	–	3
24	365	.29	–	540	169	–	60	.12	–	.51	.4	.11	–	3
24	360	.29	–	533	193	–	60	.12	–	.51	.31	–	–	3
7	227	.14	–	318	182	–	16	.08	–	.31	.25	–	–	1
5	242	.55	–	414	178	–	7	.08	–	.32	.27	–	–	2
5	209	.23	–	307	109	–	6	.06	–	.32	.24	–	–	2
3	118	.2	–	155	75	–	4	<.01	–	.01	.2	–	–	1
0	6	.93	6	66	175	.16	10	.12	1.58	.09	1.02	.03	3	1
0	39	1.46	15	88	243	.38	0	.16	0	.16	1.5	.03	6	1
0	10	1.73	11	62	267	.39	0	.24	.99	.16	2	.03	–	0
3	28	1.8	24	142	229	.4	0	.14	.92	.16	1.48	–	–	0
12	96	2	12	65	362	.4	31	.24	.12	.3	2.45	.03	16	1
235	152	2.46	24	200	735	1.6	101	.5	.86	.45	3.36	.15	33	2
9	86	1.57	22	226	592	.42	95	.2	.95	.21	1.48	.07	.1	<1
416	49	1.2	10	124	140	1	165	.06	.9	.5	.06	.12	43	0
36	7	.6	7	114	325	.87	0	.21	.29	.07	1.9	.1	–	0
0	7	.3	11	213	332	.15	0	.08	.58	.02	.9	.08	8	3
48	138	2.17	23	–	784	1.58	50	.59	.69	.29	3.92	14	16	0
264	160	2.86	27	257	841	2.12	120	.6	1.14	.5	3.88	.2	34	0
0	67	1.83	9	104	825	.29	0	.29	.8	.23	2.12	.03	5	0
34	78	2.43	16	214	1165	1.12	0	.49	1.11	.3	4.06	.12	5	0
259	106	3.12	22	286	1269	1.7	62	.54	1.62	.58	4.19	.19	29	0
244	105	2.7	21	252	1349	1.7	102	.4	1.53	.59	3.4	.13	31	0
161	142	1.64	36	547	657	1.96	1067	.3	1.31	.33	3.9	.32	90	20
127	48	1.22	22	370	55	.66	1014	.11	.87	.22	.6	.15	87	20
64	45	1.36	37	569	269	1.3	1666	.43	1.08	.17	7.15	.44	70	26

Note for fast foods: Values for magnesium, phosphorus, zinc, thiamin, riboflavin, niacin, vitamin B_6, folate, some of the fatty acids, and percent water are estimates calculated from known values for major ingredients.

(For purposes of calculations, use "0" for t, <1, <.1, <.01, etc.)

Table H–1
Food Composition

Computer Code Number	Food Description	Measure	Wt (g)	H_2O (%)	Ener (kcal)	Prot (g)	Carb (g)	Dietary Fiber (g)	Fat (g)	Fat Breakdown (g) Sat	Mono	Poly
	PIZZA HUT											
	Pan pizza:											
1657	Cheese	2 pce	205	52	495	23	53	4	21	9.5	6.5	3.2
1658	Pepperoni	2 pce	211	49	539	22	57	4	24	8.1	10.1	3.8
1659	Supreme	2 pce	255	56	581	28	52	6	28	11.2	11.2	3.9
1660	Super supreme	2 pce	257	57	580	27	50	5	31	10.8	3.8	2
	Thin 'n crispy:											
1649	Cheese pizza	2 pce	148	51	350	19	36	3	14	6.8	–	–
1623	Pepperoni pizza	2 pce	146	48	374	19	37	2	17	7	–	–
1622	Supreme pizza	2 pce	200	57	444	24	36	3	22	8.6	–	–
1620	Super supreme pizza	2 pce	203	57	445	23	36	3	23	9.9	–	–
	Hand tossed:											
1619	Cheese pizza	2 pce	220	53	479	26	59	4	14	8.1	–	–
1618	Pepperoni pizza	2 pce	197	51	452	23	55	4	15	7.6	–	–
1648	Supreme pizza	2 pce	239	56	498	28	53	5	21	8.8	–	–
1617	Super supreme pizza	2 pce	243	57	502	27	51	5	22	8.5	–	–
	Personal pan pizza:											
1610	Pepperoni	1 ea	256	50	639	27	69	5	28	10	11.8	4.5
1609	Supreme	1 ea	264	58	582	27	56	5	27	9.7	11.9	4.5
	Source: Pizza Hut.											
	TACO BELL											
	Breakfast burrito:											
1601	Bacon breakfast burrito	1 ea	99	48	291	11	23	–	17	4	–	–
1627	Country breakfast burrito	1 ea	113	53	281	10	26	–	16	5	–	–
1626	Fiesta breakfast burrito	1 ea	92	47	275	9	23	–	16	6	–	–
1625	Grande breakfast burrito	1 ea	177	52	457	14	46	–	24	8	–	–
1604	Sausage breakfast burrito	1 ea	106	49	303	11	23	–	19	6	–	–
	Burritos:											
1544	Bean with red sauce	1 ea	191	53	377	13	56	11	12	3.9	4.6	1.2
1545	Beef with red sauce	1 ea	191	57	417	21	41	4	18	7.7	6.5	.7
1546	Beef & bean with red sauce	1 ea	191	57	397	16	48	5	15	5.8	5.9	2
1569	Big beef supreme	1 ea	298	64	525	25	51	–	25	11	–	–
1552	Chicken burrito	1 ea	171	58	345	17	41	–	13	5	–	–
1547	Supreme with red sauce	1 ea	241	64	428	17	52	5	18	8.3	6.5	1.6
1571	7 layer burrito	1 ea	234	60	458	14	55	8	20	5.9	–	–
1538	Chilito	1 ea	156	49	391	17	41	–	18	9	–	–
1549	Chilito, steak	1 ea	257	62	496	26	47	–	23	10	–	–
	Tacos:											
1551	Taco	1 ea	78	58	180	10	11	1	11	4.6	4.5	.8
1554	Soft taco	1 ea	92	57	204	11	18	2	10	4.6	4.4	1
1536	Soft taco supreme	1 ea	124	60	262	13	20	2	15	7.3	–	–
1568	Soft taco, chicken	1 ea	128	65	223	14	20	–	10	4	–	–
1572	Soft taco, steak	1 ea	100	56	217	12	21	–	9	4	–	–
1555	Tostada with red sauce	1 ea	156	69	242	10	27	5	11	4.1	5.5	.8
1558	Mexican pizza	1 ea	223	55	574	19	40	2	38	12	16	10
1559	Taco salad with salsa	1 ea	595	72	956	36	71	11	61	17	31.9	12.1
1560	Nachos, regular	1 ea	107	41	348	7	37	3	18	6.1	9.9	2
1561	Nachos, Bellgrande	1 ea	287	59	633	22	61	–	34	12.3	19.2	2.5
1562	Pintos & cheese with red sauce	1 ea	128	69	190	9	19	7	9	3.6	4	.8

(Computer code number is for West Diet Analysis program)

PAGE KEY: H–4 = BEV H–6 = DAIRY H–12 = EGGS H–14 = FAT/OIL H–18 = FRUIT H–26 = BAKERY H–36 = GRAIN H–44 = FISH H–48 = MEATS H–50 = POULTRY H–54 = SAUSAGE H–56 = MIXED/FAST H–64 = NUTS/SEEDS H–68 = SWEETS H–70 = VEG/LEG H–84 = MISC H–88 = SOUPS/SAUCES H–90 = FAST H–106 = FRZN ENTREE H–112 = BABY FOODS

Chol (mg)	Calc (mg)	Iron (mg)	Magn (mg)	Pota (mg)	Sodi (mg)	Zinc (mg)	VT-A (RE)	Thia (mg)	VT-E (α-TE)	Ribo (mg)	Niac (mg)	V-B6 (mg)	Fola (μg)	VT-C (mg)
47	273	2.8	60	320	951	4.1	200	.56	–	.6	5.2	.17	–	7
49	209	3.3	56	405	1156	4.2	193	.63	–	.49	5.4	.17	0	8
56	219	4.3	76	580	1428	5.6	183	.81	–	.8	6	.31	–	10
61	212	3.95	72	532	1482	5.4	181	.75	–	.66	6.4	–	–	11
43	247	1.8	48	261	911	3.6	185	.39	–	.39	4.8	.16	–	5
44	181	1.9	44	287	1091	3.5	173	.42	–	.43	5.2	–	–	6
53	205	3.1	68	544	1371	4.7	170	.6	–	.49	5.4	–	–	10
58	196	2.8	60	463	1448	4.5	171	.59	–	.44	5.4	–	–	8
51	289	3.1	72	396	1265	4.7	202	.48	–	.49	5.4	–	–	10
46	192	3	60	415	1307	3.8	177	.54	–	.53	5.6	–	–	7
53	203	4	80	578	1548	5.7	168	.69	–	.53	7.2	–	–	12
58	197	3.7	76	516	1605	4.8	168	.71	–	.58	7.4	–	–	12
55	251	4	60	408	1344	3.8	234	.56	–	.66	8.2	.2	–	10
53	223	4.2	60	487	1419	3.8	194	.59	–	.66	8	.32	–	11
181	80	1.8	–	–	652	–	310	–	–	–	–	–	–	–
173	80	3.42	–	–	627	–	310	–	–	–	–	–	–	–
27	60	1.44	–	–	680	–	260	–	–	–	–	–	–	–
183	200	3.6	–	–	1053	–	630	–	–	–	–	–	–	1
183	80	1.8	–	–	661	–	320	–	–	–	–	–	–	–
5	183	3.47	–	478	1097	–	367	.04	–	1.95	1.91	.3	–	2
55	154	3.82	–	367	1256	–	511	.38	–	2.06	3.32	.31	–	1
31	164	3.65	48	426	1177	2.58	434	.47	–	.4	2.98	.57	37	1
72	200	4.5	–	–	1418	–	840	–	–	–	–	–	–	8
57	140	2.52	–	–	854	–	440	–	–	–	–	–	–	1
44	194	3.5	47	473	1146	–	777	.39	–	2	2.73	.33	–	9
17	85	2.29	–	–	984	–	297	–	–	–	–	–	–	5
47	300	3.06	–	–	980	–	950	–	–	–	–	–	–	–
78	200	2.70	–	–	1313	–	970	–	–	–	–	–	–	2
30	80	1.08	–	159	280	–	350	.05	–	.14	1.20	.12	–	1
28	56	1.7	–	196	502	–	186	.39	–	.22	2.74	1	–	0
44	78	1.74	–	–	533	–	291	–	–	–	–	–	–	2
58	60	1.44	–	–	553	–	540	–	–	–	–	–	–	2
31	50	1.08	–	–	569	–	130	–	–	–	–	–	–	–
14	170	1.44	–	401	593	–	660	.06	–	.17	.63	.26	–	3
50	310	4.5	80	408	1003	5.4	1090	.32	–	.33	2.96	1.11	60	8
89	167	6.01	–	1066	1801	–	1334	.52	–	.77	4.88	.57	–	30
9	232	.73	52	161	402	1.7	565	.17	–	.16	.69	.19	10	2
49	360	3.6	–	674	952	–	990	.1	–	.34	2.17	–	–	7
14	150	1.26	110	384	640	2.17	430	.05	–	.15	.40	.21	68	1

Note for fast foods: Values for magnesium, phosphorus, zinc, thiamin, riboflavin, niacin, vitamin B_6, folate, some of the fatty acids, and percent water are estimates calculated from known values for major ingredients.

(For purposes of calculations, use "0" for t, <1, <.1, <.01, etc.)

Table H–1
Food Composition

Computer Code Number	Food Description	Measure	Wt (g)	H_2O (%)	Ener (kcal)	Prot (g)	Carb (g)	Dietary Fiber (g)	Fat (g)	Fat Breakdown (g) Sat	Mono	Poly
	TACO BELL—Cont											
	Tacos–Cont.:											
1563	Taco sauce, packet	1 ea	4	94	1	1	<1	<1	<1	0	0	0
1564	Salsa	1 ea	10	23	27	1	6	–	<1	0	0	0
1565	Cinnamon twists	1 ea	47	5	187	1	27	1	8	0	7.1	.9
1628	Caramel roll	1 ea	85	19	353	6	46	–	16	4	–	–
	Border Light menu:											
1749	Bean burrito	1 ea	198	–	330	14	55	8	6	2	–	–
1750	Burrito supreme	1 ea	248	–	350	20	50	4	8	3	–	–
1744	7 layer burrito	1 ea	276	–	440	19	67	10	9	3.5	–	–
1745	Taco	1 ea	78	–	140	11	11	2	5	1.5	–	–
1746	Taco supreme	1 ea	106	–	160	13	14	2	5	1.5	–	–
1747	Soft taco	1 ea	99	–	180	13	19	2	5	2.5	–	–
1748	Soft taco supreme	1 ea	128	–	200	14	23	2	5	2.5	–	–
1742	Taco salad without chips	1 ea	464	–	330	30	35	10	9	4.5	–	–
1743	Taco salad with chips	1 ea	535	–	680	35	81	10	25	8	–	–
	Source: Taco Bell Corporation.											
	WENDY'S											
	Hamburgers:											
1566	Single on white bun, no toppings	1 ea	119	44	322	22	28	2	14	5.4	–	–
	Cheeseburgers:											
1570	Bacon cheeseburger	1 ea	147	54	355	19	29	2	18	6.9	9.8	1.3
1730	Chicken sandwich, grilled	1 ea	177	62	290	24	35	2	7	1.5	–	–
	Baked potatoes:											
1573	Plain	1 ea	250	71	273	6	63	6	0	0	0	0
1574	With bacon & cheese	1 ea	350	69	497	16	72	6	17	3.7	10.1	3.2
1575	With broccoli & cheese	1 ea	365	74	417	8	71	8	12	2.7	7.1	2.2
1576	With cheese	1 ea	350	68	521	13	71	6	21	8.2	8.9	4.4
1577	With chili & cheese	1 ea	400	69	565	18	76	8	22	8.2	12.8	1
1578	With sour cream & chives	1 ea	310	71	375	8	73	8	6	3.9	1.33	.8
1579	Chili	1 ea	256	81	237	17	24	6	8	2.8	–	–
1580	French fries	1 ea	106	43	310	4	38	4	15	3.3	9.7	2
1581	Frosty dairy dessert	1 c	216	68	302	8	51	3	9	4.4	3.6	1
1582	Chocolate chip cookies	1 ea	64	4	320	3	40	1	17	5.5	5.8	4.9
	Source: Wendy's International.											
	CONVENIENCE FOODS & MEALS											
	BUDGET GOURMET											
1695	Chicken cacciatore	1 ea	312	80	300	20	27	–	13	–	–	–
1694	Sweet & sour chicken with rice	1 ea	284	72	350	18	53	–	7	–	–	–
1689	Teriyaki chicken	1 ea	340	77	360	20	44	–	12	–	–	–
1692	Linguini & shrimp	1 ea	284	77	330	15	33	–	15	–	–	–
1691	Scallops & shrimp	1 ea	326	79	320	16	43	–	9	–	–	–
2245	Seafood Newburg	1 ea	284	74	350	17	43	–	12	–	–	–
1693	Sirloin tips with country gravy	1 ea	284	80	310	16	21	–	18	–	–	–
1690	Veal parmigiana	1 ea	340	75	440	26	39	–	20	–	–	–
1696	Yankee pot roast	1 ea	312	77	380	27	22	–	21	–	–	–
	Source: The All American Gourmet Company.											

(Computer code number is for West Diet Analysis program)

PAGE KEY: H–4 = BEV H–6 = DAIRY H–12 = EGGS H–14 = FAT/OIL H–18 = FRUIT H–26 = BAKERY H–36 = GRAIN H–44 = FISH H–48 = MEATS H–50 = POULTRY H–54 = SAUSAGE H–56 = MIXED/FAST H–64 = NUTS/SEEDS H–68 = SWEETS H–70 = VEG/LEG H–84 = MISC H–88 = SOUPS/SAUCES H–90 = FAST H–106 = FRZN ENTREE H–112 = BABY FOODS

Chol (mg)	Calc (mg)	Iron (mg)	Magn (mg)	Pota (mg)	Sodi (mg)	Zinc (mg)	VT-A (RE)	Thia (mg)	VT-E (α-TE)	Ribo (mg)	Niac (mg)	V-B6 (mg)	Fola (μg)	VT-C (mg)
0	1	.03	–	4	40	–	40	0	–	<.01	.02	<.01	–	<1
0	50	.6	–	376	709	–	168	.02	–	.14	0	–	–	10
1	37	.48	–	36	254	–	67	.14	–	.05	.96	.05	–	1
15	60	1.44	–	–	312	–	330	–	–	–	–	–	–	4
5	100	3.6	–	–	1340	–	400	–	–	–	–	–	–	2
25	80	2.7	–	–	1300	–	600	–	–	–	–	–	–	9
5	250	4.5	–	–	1430	–	350	–	–	–	–	–	–	5
20	0	0	–	–	280	–	40	–	–	–	–	–	–	0
20	0	0	–	–	340	–	100	–	–	–	–	–	–	2
25	40	1.08	–	–	550	–	40	–	–	–	–	–	–	0
25	40	1.08	–	–	610	–	100	–	–	–	–	–	–	2
50	100	2.7	–	–	1610	–	1200	–	–	–	–	–	–	27
50	250	3.6	–	–	1620	–	1800	–	–	–	–	–	–	27
58	89	4	–	265	412	–	0	.38	–	.34	6	–	–	0
52	130	3.1	33	332	787	5.1	69	.27	–	.28	5.7	.23	25	8
55	100	2.7	–	–	720	–	40	–	–	–	–	–	–	6
0	18	3.17	66	1360	22	.65	0	.27	–	.1	3.79	.7	68	32
18	184	4.1	80	1379	1317	2.53	92	.22	–	.18	4.64	.87	33	33
4	178	4	83	1549	417	.86	311	.3	–	.26	4	.86	66	64
27	366	4.1	78	1379	585	.61	137	.23	–	.26	3.3	.8	33	36
36	319	4.92	111	1589	711	3.78	182	.3	–	.26	4.1	.9	50	33
15	79	4.4	70	1419	39	.9	296	.23	–	.14	3	.79	32	47
34	90	3.05	–	565	902	–	90	.12	–	.17	3	–	–	4
0	16	.88	45	689	98	.51	0	.15	–	.03	2.94	.27	33	5
36	267	.96	43	518	194	.92	143	.11	–	.45	.31	.12	17	<1
5	10	1.09	15	518	178	.92	71	.11	–	.45	.31	.12	16	0
60	150	1.8	–	–	810	–	40	.23	–	.51	5	–	–	21
40	60	.72	–	–	640	–	80	.12	–	.34	3	–	–	2
55	80	1.4	–	–	610	–	300	.15	–	.34	6	–	–	12
75	10	3.6	–	–	1250	–	1000	.3	–	.17	3	–	–	2
70	150	.72	–	–	690	–	150	–	–	.26	3	–	–	12
70	100	.72	–	–	660	–	40	.23	–	.26	2	–	–	–
40	60	.36	–	–	570	–	150	.15	–	.17	4	.28	–	2
165	30	4.5	–	–	1160	–	1000	.45	–	.6	6	–	–	6
70	150	1.8	–	–	690	–	600	.15	–	.43	7	–	–	6

Note for fast foods: Values for magnesium, phosphorus, zinc, thiamin, riboflavin, niacin, vitamin B_6, folate, some of the fatty acids, and percent water are estimates calculated from known values for major ingredients.

(For purposes of calculations, use "0" for t, <1, <.1, <.01, etc.)

Table H–1
Food Composition

Computer Code Number	Food Description	Measure	Wt (g)	H_2O (%)	Ener (kcal)	Prot (g)	Carb (g)	Dietary Fiber (g)	Fat (g)	Fat Breakdown (g) Sat	Mono	Poly
	HAAGEN DAZS											
1755	Ice cream bar, vanilla almond	1 ea	107	–	371	6	26	–	27	14	10	3
	Sorbet:											
1758	Lemon	½ c	113	–	140	0	35	–	0	0	0	0
1760	Orange	½ c	113	–	140	0	36	–	0	0	0	0
1759	Raspberry	½ c	113	–	110	0	27	–	0	0	0	0
	Yogurt, frozen:											
1753	Chocolate	½ c	98	–	171	8	26	–	4	2	2	0
1754	Strawberry	½ c	98	–	171	6	27	–	4	2	2	0
	Yogurt extra, frozen:											
1752	Brownie nut	½ c	101	–	220	8	29	–	9	4	4	1
1751	Raspberry rendezvous	½ c	101	–	132	4	26	–	2	1	1	0
	HEALTHY CHOICE											
	Entrees:											
2112	Fish, lemon pepper	1 ea	303	78	290	14	47	7	5	1	–	–
1624	Lasagna	1 ea	284	76	289	19	44	7	4	1	–	–
2111	Meatloaf, traditional, entree	1 ea	340	79	320	16	46	7	8	4	–	–
2104	Zucchini lasagna	1 ea	397	80	330	20	58	11	2	1	–	–
	Dinners:											
2110	Pasta shells marinara	1 ea	340	74	360	25	59	5	3	1.5	–	–
	Low-fat ice milk:											
1608	Cookie & cream	½ c	113	62	191	5	33	1	3	2.4	–	0
1621	Vanilla	½ c	113	66	159	5	29	2	3	1	–	0
	Low-fat ice cream:											
973	Brownie	½ c	71	61	120	3	22	2	2	1	–	.7
650	Chocolate chip	½ c	71	62	120	3	21	1	2	1	–	0
259	Butter pecan	½ c	71	61	89	2	16	1	1	.7	–	.5
45	Rocky road	½ c	71	53	140	3	28	2	2	1	–	0
391	Vanilla fudge	½ c	71	62	120	3	21	1	2	1.5	–	.7
	Source: ConAgra Frozen Foods, Omaha, NE.											
	HEALTH VALLEY											
	Soups, fat-free:											
2001	Beef broth, no salt added	6.9 oz	196	98	15	4	0	0	0	0	0	0
2073	Beef broth, w/salt	6.9 oz	196	98	25	4	2	0	0	0	0	0
2016	Black bean & vegetable	7.5 oz	213	85	98	10	21	11	0	0	0	0
2017	Chicken broth	7.5 oz	213	97	27	5	0	0	0	0	0	0
2018	14 garden vegetable	7.5 oz	213	90	71	5	15	4	0	0	0	0
2015	Lentil & carrot	7.5 oz	213	85	80	9	22	12	0	0	0	0
2014	Split pea & carrot	7.5 oz	213	89	98	7	15	4	0	0	0	0
2013	Tomato vegetable	7.5 oz	213	90	71	5	15	4	0	0	0	0
	LA CHOY											
2100	Egg rolls, mini, chicken	1 svg	106	53	220	8	35	3	6	1.5	–	–
2099	Egg rolls, mini, shrimp	1 svg	106	56	210	7	35	3	4	1	–	–
	LEAN CUISINE											
	Dinners:											
1639	Baked cheese ravioli	1 ea	241	77	250	12	32	4	8	3	2	1

Chol (mg)	Calc (mg)	Iron (mg)	Magn (mg)	Pota (mg)	Sodi (mg)	Zinc (mg)	VT-A (RE)	Thia (mg)	VT-E (α-TE)	Ribo (mg)	Niac (mg)	V-B6 (mg)	Fola (μg)	VT-C (mg)
90	161	.39	–	222	85	–	161	–	–	.18	–	–	–	–
0	–	–	–	30	20	–	–	–	–	–	–	–	–	7
0	–	–	–	80	20	–	–	–	–	–	–	–	–	20
0	–	–	–	60	15	–	–	–	–	–	–	–	–	7
40	147	.71	–	241	45	–	20	–	–	.17	–	–	–	5
50	147	–	–	141	45	–	20	.03	–	.17	–	–	–	5
55	152	.73	–	250	60	–	20	–	–	.14	–	–	–	–
20	81	–	–	97	25	–	0	–	–	.1	–	–	–	5
25	20	1.08	–	–	360	–	100	–	–	–	–	–	–	30
11	111	2.7	–	37	408	–	74	.2	–	.2	1	–	–	4
35	40	1.8	–	–	460	–	150	–	–	–	–	–	–	54
10	200	2.7	–	–	310	–	250	–	–	–	–	–	–	0
25	400	1.8	–	–	390	–	100	–	–	–	–	–	–	4
4	159	–	–	404	143	–	96	.04	–	.24	–	–	–	4
8	159	–	–	404	80	–	96	.08	–	.36	–	–	–	4
3	80	0	–	268	55	–	40	–	–	–	–	–	–	0
3	100	0	–	240	50	–	40	–	–	–	–	–	–	0
2	74	0	–	156	44	–	30	–	–	–	–	–	–	0
3	100	0	–	168	60	–	40	.03	–	.15	–	–	–	0
3	100	0	–	296	50	–	40	–	–	–	–	–	–	0
0	–	–	–	160	60	–	–	–	–	–	.8	–	–	–
0	–	–	–	160	131	–	0	–	–	–	.8	–	–	4
0	36	3.2	–	600	249	–	1775	.3	–	.1	1.2	.2	120	8
0	18	1.6	–	130	151	–	0	–	–	.03	2.17	–	–	1
0	36	1.6	–	360	222	–	1775	.23	–	.07	2	.16	24	13
0	53	4.8	–	390	195	–	1775	.09	–	.14	5	.4	24	2
0	36	4.8	–	390	204	–	1775	.09	–	.14	5	.4	–	8
0	36	4.8	–	540	213	–	1775	.09	–	.07	2	.12	32	8
5	20	1.44	–	–	460	–	20	–	–	–	–	–	–	0
5	20	1.44	–	–	510	–	20	–	–	–	–	–	–	0
55	200	1.08	42	400	500	1.5	150	.06	–	.26	1.2	.2	48	6

(For purposes of calculations, use "0" for t, <1, <.1, <.01, etc.)

H

Table H-1
Food Composition

Computer Code Number	Food Description	Measure	Wt (g)	H_2O (%)	Ener (kcal)	Prot (g)	Carb (g)	Dietary Fiber (g)	Fat (g)	Fat Breakdown (g) Sat	Mono	Poly
	LEAN CUISINE—Cont.											
	Dinners—Cont.:											
1632	Chicken chow mein	1 ea	255	81	210	13	28	2	5	1	2	1
1633	Lasagna	1 ea	291	79	270	19	34	5	6	3	2	.5
1634	Macaroni & cheese	1 ea	255	78	270	13	39	2	7	4	1.5	.5
1631	Spaghetti w/meatballs	1 ea	269	74	290	17	40	4	7	2	3	1.5
	Pizza:											
1636	French bread sausage pizza	1 ea	170	50	420	19	41	4	20	5	13.89	1.11
	Source: Stouffer's Foods Corp, Solon, OH.											
	TASTE ADVENTURE SOUPS											
1905	Black bean	1 c	227	–	130	6	26	6	1	–	–	–
1904	Curry lentil	1 c	227	–	130	6	28	5	1	–	–	–
1906	Lentil chili	1 c	227	–	170	10	31	6	1	–	–	–
1903	Split pea	1 c	227	–	130	5	25	5	1	–	–	–
	WEIGHT WATCHERS											
	Cheese, fat-free slices:											
1978	Cheddar, sharp	2 pce	21	59	30	5	2	0	0	0	0	0
1980	Swiss	2 pce	21	58	30	5	2	0	0	0	0	0
1977	White	2 pce	21	58	30	5	2	0	0	0	0	0
1979	Yellow	2 pce	21	58	30	5	2	0	0	0	0	0
	Dinners:											
1646	Oven fried fish	1 ea	198	78	209	14	23	2	7	2.3	4.5	1.8
2029	Chicken chow mein	1 ea	255	81	200	12	34	3	2	.5	–	–
1972	Margarine, reduced fat	1 tbs	14	49	59	0	0	0	7	1.5	–	–
	Pizza:											
1653	Cheese pizza	1 ea	164	48	392	23	49	6	12	4	3	1
1650	Deluxe combination pizza	1 ea	200	56	409	25	50	6	12	3.8	5.4	2.2
1652	Pepperoni pizza	1 ea	171	48	422	25	50	4	13	4.3	5.4	2.2
	Desserts:											
1644	Chocolate brownie	1 ea	35	29	37	1	7	1	1	.2	.4	.2
2024	Chocolate eclair	1 ea	60	45	151	3	24	2	5	1.5	–	–
1642	Strawberry cheesecake	1 ea	109	62	177	7	28	2	5	2	1	2
2027	Triple chocolate cheesecake	1 ea	89	52	200	7	32	1	5	2.5	–	–
2247	Chocolate mousse	1 ea	78	44	190	6	33	3	4	1.5	–	–
	SWEET SUCCESS:											
	Drinks, prepared:											
1776	Chocolate chip	1 c	265	81	180	15	30	6	3	1.6	–	–
1777	Chocolate fudge	1 c	265	81	180	15	30	6	2	–	–	–
1774	Chocolate mocha	1 c	265	81	180	15	30	6	1	.6	–	–
1778	Milk chocolate	1 c	265	81	180	15	30	6	2	1	–	–
1775	Vanilla	1 c	265	81	180	15	33	6	1	.6	–	–
	Drinks, ready to drink:											
2147	Chocolate mint	1¼ c	284	82	179	11	34	5	3	0	–	–
2148	Strawberry	1¼ c	284	82	179	11	34	5	3	0	–	–
	Shakes:											
1771	Chocolate almond	1¼ c	313	82	197	12	38	6	3	0	2.7	.3
1773	Chocolate fudge	1¼ c	313	82	197	12	38	6	3	0	2.7	.3
1768	Chocolate mocha	1¼ c	313	82	197	12	38	6	3	0	.8	2.2
1769	Chocolate raspberry truffle	1¼ c	313	82	197	12	38	6	3	0	2.7	.3
1770	Vanilla creme	1¼ c	313	82	197	12	38	6	3	0	2.6	.4

(Computer code number is for West Diet Analysis program)

PAGE KEY: H–4 = BEV H–6 = DAIRY H–12 = EGGS H–14 = FAT/OIL H–18 = FRUIT H–26 = BAKERY H–36 = GRAIN H–44 = FISH H–48 = MEATS H–50 = POULTRY H–54 = SAUSAGE H–56 = MIXED/FAST H–64 = NUTS/SEEDS H–68 = SWEETS H–70 = VEG/LEG H–84 = MISC H–88 = SOUPS/SAUCES H–90 = FAST H–106 = FRZN ENTREE H–112 = BABY FOODS

Chol (mg)	Calc (mg)	Iron (mg)	Magn (mg)	Pota (mg)	Sodi (mg)	Zinc (mg)	VT-A (RE)	Thia (mg)	VT-E (α-TE)	Ribo (mg)	Niac (mg)	V-B6 (mg)	Fola (μg)	VT-C (mg)
35	20	.36	30	300	510	1.1	20	.15	–	.17	5	–	–	6
25	150	1.8	44	620	560	2.9	100	.15	–	.26	3	.32		12
20	250	.72	–	170	550	–	20	.12	–	.26	1.2	–	–	0
30	100	2.7	47	480	520	2.5	80	.15	–	.26	3	.2	–	4
35	250	2.7	39	340	900	2.2	80	.45	–	.51	5	.07	–	6
–	–	–	–	610	530	–	–	–	–	–	–	–	–	–
–	–	–	–	440	550	–	–	–	–	–	–	–	–	–
–	–	–	–	610	420	–	–	–	–	–	–	–	–	–
–	–	–	–	450	550	–	–	–	–	–	–	–	–	–
0	99	0	–	64	306	–	56	–	–	–	–	–	–	0
0	99	0	–	74	276	–	56	–	–	–	–	–	–	0
0	99	0	–	64	306	–	56	–	–	–	–	–	–	0
0	99	0	–	64	306	–	56	–	–	–	–	–	–	0
23	18	1.31	–	336	409	–	36	.08	–	.13	1.5	–	–	0
25	40	.72	–	360	430	–	300	–	–	–	–	–	–	36
0	0	0	–	5	128	–	49	–	–	–	–	–	–	0
35	704	1.8	–	292	594	–	80	.3	–	.51	3	.06	–	6
43	538	3.9	–	398	591	–	161	.3	–	.55	3	.2	–	5
49	487	1.9	–	346	704	–	87	.25	–	.55	3	–	–	5
1	15	.2	–	44	31	–	0	.01	–	.01	.03	.01	–	0
0	40	0	–	66	151	–	0	–	–	–	–	–	–	0
15	79	.35	–	113	226	–	39	.06	–	.07	1.6	–	–	2
10	80	1.08	–	169	199	–	0	–	–	–	–	–	–	0
5	60	1.8	–	320	150	–	0	–	–	–	–	–	–	0
6	500	6.3	140	600	288	5.25	–	.53	7.05	.6	7	.7	140	21
6	500	6.3	140	750	336	5.25	–	.53	7.05	.6	7	.7	140	21
6	500	6.3	140	830	312	5.25	–	.53	7.05	.6	7	.7	140	21
6	500	6.3	140	750	336	5.25	–	.53	7.05	.6	7	.7	140	21
6	500	6.3	140	830	312	5.25	–	.53	7.05	.6	7	.7	140	21
6	449	5.68	125	502	216	4.83	315	.48	6.28	.54	6.24	.62	125	19
6	449	5.68	125	332	187	4.83	315	.48	6.28	.54	6.24	.62	125	19
6	495	6.3	138	554	238	5.3	347	.53	6.92	.6	7	.7	138	21
6	495	6.3	138	554	219	5.3	347	.53	6.92	.6	7	.7	138	21
6	495	6.3	138	504	219	5.3	347	.53	6.92	.6	7	.7	138	21
6	480	6.3	138	554	219	5.3	347	.53	6.92	.6	7	.7	138	21
6	495	6.3	138	366	219	5.3	347	.53	6.92	.6	7	.7	138	21

(For purposes of calculations, use "0" for t, <1, <.1, <.01, etc.)

H

Table H–1
Food Composition

Computer Code Number	Food Description	Measure	Wt (g)	H_2O (%)	Ener (kcal)	Prot (g)	Carb (g)	Dietary Fiber (g)	Fat (g)	Fat Breakdown (g) Sat	Mono	Poly
	SWEET SUCCESS—Cont.											
	Snack bars:											
1767	Chocolate brownie	1 ea	33	9	120	2	23	3	4	2	.5	.6
1766	Chocolate chip	1 ea	33	9	120	2	23	3	4	2	.4	.5
1765	Peanut butter	1 ea	33	9	120	2	23	3	4	2	.6	.6
1921	Oatmeal raisin	1 ea	33	9	120	2	23	3	4	2	–	–
	Source: Foodway National Inc., Boise, ID.											
	BABY FOODS											
1720	Apple juice	4 fl oz	125	88	59	0	15	<1	<1	<.1	<.1	<.1
1721	Applesauce, strained	1 tbs	14	89	6	<1	2	<1	<1	<.1	<.1	<.1
1716	Carrots, strained	1 tbs	14	92	4	<1	1	<1	<1	<.1	<.1	<.1
1718	Cereal, mixed, millk added	1 tbs	14	75	16	1	2	<1	<1	.3	–	–
1719	Cereal, rice, milk added	1 tbs	14	75	16	<1	2	<1	1	.3	–	–
1723	Chicken and noodles, strained	1 tbs	14	89	7	<1	1	<1	<1	.1	.1	<.1
1722	Peas, strained	1 tbs	14	88	6	<1	1	<1	<1	<.1	<.1	<.1
1717	Teething biscuits	1 ea	11	6	43	1	8	<1	<1	.2	.2	.1

(Computer code number is for West Diet Analysis program)

PAGE KEY: H–4 = BEV H–6 = DAIRY H–12 = EGGS H–14 = FAT/OIL H–18 = FRUIT H–26 = BAKERY H–36 = GRAIN H–44 = FISH H–48 = MEATS H–50 = POULTRY H–54 = SAUSAGE H–56 = MIXED/FAST H–64 = NUTS/SEEDS H–68 = SWEETS H–70 = VEG/LEG H–84 = MISC H–88 = SOUPS/SAUCES H–90 = FAST H–106 = FRZN ENTREE H–112 = BABY FOODS

Chol (mg)	Calc (mg)	Iron (mg)	Magn (mg)	Pota (mg)	Sodi (mg)	Zinc (mg)	VT-A (RE)	Thia (mg)	VT-E (α-TE)	Ribo (mg)	Niac (mg)	V-B6 (mg)	Fola (μg)	VT-C (mg)
3	150	2.71	60	140	45	.6	150	.22	3.01	.25	3	.3	60	9
3	150	2.71	60	110	40	.6	150	.22	3.01	.25	3	.3	60	9
3	150	2.71	60	125	35	.6	150	.22	3.01	.25	3	.3	60	9
3	150	2.71	60	–	30	.6	150	.22	3.01	.25	3	.3	60	9
0	5	.71	4	114	4	.04	3	.01	.75	.02	.1	.04	<1	72
0	1	.03	<1	10	<1	<.01	<1	<.01	.08	<.01	.01	<.01	<1	6
0	3	.05	1	27	5	.02	160	<.01	.07	.01	.07	.01	2	1
2	31	1.46	4	28	7	.1	4	.06	–	.08	.81	.01	2	<1
1.6	33	1.71	6	27	6	.09	4	.07	–	.07	.73	.02	1	<1
3	3	.06	1	5	2	.04	16	<.01	.03	.01	.07	<.01	1	<1
0	3	.13	2	16	1	.05	8	.01	.07	.01	.14	.01	4	1
0	29	.39	4	36	40	.1	1	.03	.05	.06	.48	.01	2	1

(For purposes of calculations, use "0" for t, <1, <.1, <.01, etc.)

H

APPENDIX I

Contents

RNI

Canadian Choice System for Meal Planning

Food Labels

CANADA: RECOMMENDATIONS, CHOICES, AND LABELS

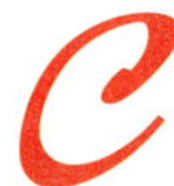

hapter 2 introduced Recommended Nutrient Intakes (RNI), exchange systems, and food labels. This appendix presents details for Canadians. Appendix F includes addresses of Canadian governmental agencies and professional organizations that may provide additional information.

Table I–1
Recommended Nutrient Intakes for Canadians, 1990

				Fat-Soluble Vitamins		
Age	**Sex**	**Weight (kg)**	**Protein (g/day)[a]**	VITAMIN A (RE/day)[b]	VITAMIN D (μg/day)[c]	VITAMIN E (mg/day)[d]
Infants (months)						
0–4	Both	6	12[f]	400	10	3
5–12	Both	9	12	400	10	3
Children and Adults (years)						
1	Both	11	13	400	10	3
2–3	Both	14	16	400	5	4
4–6	Both	18	19	500	5	5
7–9	M	25	26	700	2.5	7
	F	25	26	700	2.5	6
10–12	M	34	34	800	2.5	8
	F	36	36	800	5	7
13–15	M	50	49	900	5	9
	F	48	46	800	5	7
16–18	M	62	58	1000	5	10
	F	53	47	800	2.5	7
19–24	M	71	61	1000	2.5	10
	F	58	50	800	2.5	7
25–49	M	74	64	1000	2.5	9
	F	59	51	800	2.5	6
50–74	M	73	63	1000	5	7
	F	63	54	800	5	6
75+	M	69	59	1000	5	6
	F	64	55	800	5	5
Pregnancy (additional amount needed)						
1st trimester			5	0	2.5	2
2nd trimester			20	0	2.5	2
3rd trimester			24	0	2.5	2
Lactation (additional amount needed)			20	400	2.5	3

Note: Recommended intakes of energy and of certain nutrients are not listed in this table because of the nature of the variables upon which they are based. The figures for energy are estimates of average requirements for expected patterns of activity (see Table I–2). For nutrients not shown, the following amounts are recommended based on at least 2000 kcalories per day and body weights as given: thiamin, 0.4 milligrams per 1000 kcalories (0.48 milligrams/5000 kilojoules); riboflavin, 0.5 milligrams per 1000 kcalories (0.6 milligrams/5000 kilojoules); niacin, 7.2 niacin equivalents per 1000 kcalories (8.6 niacin equivalents/5000 kilojoules); vitamin B_6, 15 micrograms, as pyridoxine, per gram of protein. Recommended intakes during periods of growth are taken as appropriate for individuals representative of the midpoint in each age group. All recommended intakes are designed to cover individual variations in essentially all of a healthy population subsisting upon a variety of common foods available in Canada.

Source: Health and Welfare Canada, *Nutrition Recommendations: The Report of the Scientific Review Committee* (Ottawa: Canadian Government Publishing Centre, 1990), Table 20, p. 204.

RNI

The Canadian equivalent of the RDA is the Recommended Nutrient Intakes (RNI). The Canadian RNI are presented in Tables I–1 and I–2.

Table I-1 (continued)
Recommended Nutrient Intakes for Canadians, 1990

Water-Soluble Vitamins			Minerals					
VITAMIN C (mg/day)[e]	FOLATE (μg/day)	VITAMIN B_{12} (μg/day)	CALCIUM (mg/day)	PHOSPHORUS (mg/day)	MAGNESIUM (mg/day)	IRON (mg/day)	IODINE (μg/day)	ZINC (mg/day)
20	25	0.3	250	150	20	0.3[g]	30	2[h]
20	40	0.4	400	200	32	7	40	3
20	40	0.5	500	300	40	6	55	4
20	50	0.6	550	350	50	6	65	4
25	70	0.8	600	400	65	8	85	5
25	90	1.0	700	500	100	8	110	7
25	90	1.0	700	500	100	8	95	7
25	120	1.0	900	700	130	8	125	9
25	130	1.0	1100	800	135	8	110	9
30	175	1.0	1100	900	185	10	160	12
30	170	1.0	1000	850	180	13	160	9
40	220	1.0	900	1000	230	10	160	12
30	190	1.0	700	850	200	12	160	9
40	220	1.0	800	1000	240	9	160	12
30	180	1.0	700	850	200	13	160	9
40	230	1.0	800	1000	250	9	160	12
30	185	1.0	700	850	200	13[i]	160	9
40	230	1.0	800	1000	250	9	160	12
30	195	1.0	800	850	210	8	160	9
40	215	1.0	800	1000	230	9	160	12
30	200	1.0	800	850	210	8	160	9
0	200	0.2	500	200	15	0	25	6
10	200	0.2	500	200	45	5	25	6
10	200	0.2	500	200	45	10	25	6
25	100	0.2	500	200	65	0	50	6

[a]The primary units are expressed per kilogram of body weight. The figures shown here are examples.

[b]One retinol equivalent (RE) corresponds to the biological activity of 1 microgram of retinol, 6 micrograms of beta-carotene, or 12 micrograms of other carotenes.

[c]Expressed as cholecalciferol or ergocalciferol.

[d]Expressed as δ-α-tocopherol equivalents, relative to which β- and γ-tocopherol and α-tocotrienol have activities of 0.5, 0.1, and 0.3, respectively.

[e]Cigarette smokers should increase intake by 50 percent.

[f]The assumption is made that the protein is from breast milk or has the same biological value as breast milk and that, between 3 and 9 months, adjustment for the quality of the protein is made.

[g]Based on the assumption that breast milk is the source of iron.

[h]Based on the assumption that breast milk is the source of zinc.

[i]After menopause, the recommended intake is 8 milligrams per day.

Table I-2
Average Energy Requirements for Canadians

Age	Sex	Average Height (cm)	Average Weight (kg)	Requirements[a]					
				(kcal/kg)[b]	(MJ/kg)[b]	(kcal/day)	(MJ/day)	(kcal/cm)	(MJ/cm)
Infants (months)									
0–2	Both	55	4.5	120–100	0.50–0.42	500	2.0	9	0.04
3–5	Both	63	7.0	100–95	0.42–0.40	700	2.8	11	0.05
6–8	Both	69	8.5	95–97	0.40–0.41	800	3.4	11.5	0.05
9–11	Both	73	9.5	97–99	0.41	950	3.8	12.5	0.05
Children and Adults (years)									
1	Both	82	11	101	0.42	1100	4.8	13.5	0.06
2–3	Both	95	14	94	0.39	1300	5.6	13.5	0.06
4–6	Both	107	18	100	0.42	1800	7.6	17	0.07
7–9	M	126	25	88	0.37	2200	9.2	17.5	0.07
	F	125	25	76	0.32	1900	8.0	15	0.06
10–12	M	141	34	73	0.30	2500	10.4	17.5	0.07
	F	143	36	61	0.25	2200	9.2	15.5	0.06
13–15	M	159	50	57	0.24	2800	12.0	17.5	0.07
	F	157	48	46	0.19	2200	9.2	14	0.06
16–18	M	172	62	51	0.21	3200	13.2	18.5	0.08
	F	160	53	40	0.17	2100	8.8	13	0.05
19–24	M	175	71	42	0.18	3000	12.6		
	F	160	58	36	0.15	2100	8.8		
25–49	M	172	74	36	0.15	2700	11.3		
	F	160	59	32	0.13	1900	8.0		
50–74	M	170	73	31	0.13	2300	9.7		
	F	158	63	29	0.12	1800	7.6		
75+	M	168	69	29	0.12	2000	8.4		
	F	155	64	23	0.10	1500	6.3		

[a]Requirements can be expected to vary within a range of ±30 percent.

[b]First and last figures are averages at the beginning and end of the three-month period.

Source: Health and Welfare Canada, *Nutrition Recommendations: The Report of the Scientific Review Committee* (Ottawa: Canadian Government Publishing Centre, 1990), Tables 5 and 6, pp. 25, 27.

THE CANADIAN CHOICE SYSTEM

The *Good Health Eating Guide* is the Canadian choice system of meal planning.[1] It contains several features similar to those of the U.S. exchange system including the following:

- Foods are divided into lists according to carbohydrate, protein, and fat content.
- Foods are interchangeable within a group.
- Most foods are eaten in measured amounts.
- An energy value is given for each food group.

Tables I–3 through I–10 present the Canadian choice system.

[1] The tables for the Canadian choice system are adapted from the *Good Health Eating Guide Resource,* copyright 1994, with permission of the Canadian Diabetes Association.

Table I-3
Canadian Choice System: Starch Foods

1 starch choice = 15 g carbohydrate (starch), 2 g protein, 290 kJ (68 kcal)

Food	Measure	Mass (Weight)
Breads		
Bagels	½	30 g
Bread crumbs	50 mL (¼ c)	30 g
Bread cubes	250 mL (1 c)	30 g
Bread sticks	2	20 g
Brewis, cooked	50 mL (¼ c)	45 g
Chapati	1	20 g
Cookies, plain	2	20 g
English muffins, crumpets	½	30 g
Flour	40 mL (2 ½ tbs)	20 g
Hamburger buns	½	30 g
Hot dog buns	½	30 g
Kaiser rolls	½	30 g
Matzo, 15 cm	1	20 g
Melba toast, rectangular	4	15 g
Melba toast, rounds	7	15 g
Pita, 20-cm (8″) diameter	¼	30 g
Pita, 15-cm (6″) diameter	½	30 g
Plain rolls	1 small	30 g
Pretzels	7	20 g
Raisin bread	1 slice	30 g
Rice cakes	2	30 g
Roti	1	20 g
Rusks	2	20 g
Rye, coarse or pumpernickel	½ slice	30 g
Soda crackers	6	20 g
Tortillas, corn (taco shell)	1	30 g
Tortilla, flour	1	30 g
White (French and Italian)	1 slice	25 g
Whole-wheat, cracked-wheat, rye, white enriched	1 slice	30 g
Cereals		
Bran flakes, 100% bran	125 mL (½ c)	30 g
Cooked cereals, cooked	125 mL (½ c)	125 g
Dry	30 mL (2 tbs)	20 g
Cornmeal, cooked	125 mL (½ c)	125 g
Dry	30 mL (2 tbs)	20 g
Ready-to-eat unsweetened cereals	125 mL (½ c)	20 g
Shredded wheat biscuits, rectangular or round	1	20 g
Shredded wheat, bite size	125 mL (½ c)	20 g
Wheat germ	75 mL (⅓ c)	30 g
Cornflakes	175 mL (⅔ c)	20 g
Rice Krispies	175 mL (⅔ c)	20 g
Cheerios	200 mL (¾ c)	20 g
Muffets	1	20 g
Puffed rice	300 mL (1¼ c)	15 g
Puffed wheat	425 mL (1⅔ c)	20 g

(continued on the next page)

Table I-3 (continued)
Canadian Choice System: Starch Foods

Food	Measure	Mass (Weight)
Grains		
Barley, cooked	125 mL (½ c)	120 g
Dry	30 mL (2 tbs)	20 g
Bulgur, kasha, cooked, moist	125 mL (½ c)	70 g
Cooked, crumbly	75 mL (⅓ c)	40 g
Dry	30 mL (2 tbs)	20 g
Rice, cooked, brown & white (short & long grain)	125 mL (½ c)	70 g
Rice, cooked, wild	75 mL (⅓ c)	70 g
Tapioca, pearl and granulated, quick cooking, dry	30 mL (2 tbs)	15 g
Couscous, cooked moist	125 mL (½ c)	70 g
Dry	30 mL (tbs)	20 g
Quinoa, cooked moist	125 mL (½ c)	70 g
Dry	30 mL (2 tbs)	20 g
Pastas		
Macaroni, cooked	125 mL (½ c)	70 g
Noodles, cooked	125 mL (½ c)	80 g
Spaghetti, cooked	125 mL (½ c)	70 g
Starchy Vegetables		
Beans and peas, dried, cooked	125 mL (½ c)	80 g
Breadfruit	1 slice	75 g
Corn, canned, whole kernel	125 mL (½ c)	85 g
Corn on the cob	½ medium cob	140 g
Cornstarch	30 mL (2 tbs)	15 g
Plantains	⅓ small	50 g
Popcorn, air-popped, unbuttered	750 mL (3 c)	20 g
Potatoes, whole (with or without skin)	½ medium	95 g
Yams, sweet potatoes, (with or without skin)	½	75 g

Food	Choices per serving	Measure	Mass (Weight)
Note: Food items found in this category provide more than 1 starch choice:			
Bran flakes	1 starch + ½ sugar	150 mL (⅔ c)	24 g
Croissant, small	1 starch + 1½ fats	1 small	35 g
Large	1 starch + 1½ fats	½ large	30 g
Corn, canned creamed	1 starch + ½ fruits and vegetables	12 mL (½ c)	113 g
Potato chips	1 starch + 2 fats	15 chips	30 g
Tortilla chips (nachos)	1 starch + 1½ fats	13 chips	20 g
Corn chips	1 starch + 2 fats	30 chips	30 g
Cheese twists	1 starch + 1½ fats	30 chips	30 g
Cheese puffs	1 starch + 2 fats	27 chips	30 g
Tea biscuit	1 starch + 2 fats	1	30 g
Pancakes, homemade using 50 mL (¼ c) batter (6″ diameter)	1 ½ starches + 1 fat	1 medium	50 g
Potatoes, french fried (homemade or frozen)	1 starch + 1 fat	10 regular size	35 g
Soup, canned*, (prepared with equal volume of water)	1 starch	250 mL (1 c)	260 g
Waffles, packaged	1 starch + 1 fat	1	35 g

*Soup can vary according to brand and type. Check the label for Food Choice Values and Symbols or the core nutrient listing.

Table I-4
Canadian Choice System: Fruits and Vegetables

1 fruits and vegetables choice = 10 g carbohydrate, 1 g protein, 190 kJ (44 kcal)

Food	Measure	Mass (Weight)
Fruits (fresh, frozen, without sugar, canned in water)		
Apples, raw (with or without skin)	½ medium	75 g
Sauce unsweetened	125 mL (½ c)	120 g
Sweetened	see *Combined Food Choices*	
Apple butter	20 mL (4 tsp)	20 g
Apricots, raw	2 medium	115 g
Canned, in water	4 halves, plus 30 mL (2 tbs) liquid	110 g
Bake-apples (cloudberries), raw	125 mL (½ c)	120 g
Bananas, with peel	½ small	75 g
Peeled	½ small	50 g
Berries (blackberries, blueberries, boysenberries, huckleberries, loganberries, raspberries)		
Raw	125 mL (½ c)	70 g
Canned, in water	125 mL (½ c), plus 30 mL (2 tbs) liquid	100 g
Cantaloupe, wedge with rind	¼	240 g
Cubed or diced	250 mL (1 c)	160 g
Cherries, raw, with pits	10	75 g
Raw, without pits	10	70 g
Canned, in water, with pits	75 mL (⅓ c), plus 30 mL (2 tbs) liquid	90 g
Canned, in water, without pits	75 mL (⅓ c), plus 30 mL (2 tbs) liquid	85 g
Crabapples, raw	1 small	55 g
Cranberries, raw	250 mL (1 c)	100 g
Figs, raw	1 medium	50 g
Canned, in water	3 medium, plus 30 mL (2 tbs) liquid	100 g
Foxberries, raw	250 mL (1 c)	100 g
Fruit cocktail, canned, in water	125 mL (½ c), plus 30 mL (2 tbs) liquid	120 g
Fruit, mixed, cut-up	125 mL (½ c)	120 g
Gooseberries, raw	250 mL (1 c)	150 g
Canned, in water	250 mL (1 c), plus 30 mL (2 tbs) liquid	230 g
Grapefruit, raw, with rind	½ small	185 g
Raw, sectioned	125 mL (½ c)	100 g
Canned, in water	125 mL (½ c), plus 30 mL (2 tbs) liquid	120 g
Grapes, raw, slip skin	125 mL (½ c)	75 g
Raw, seedless	125 mL (½ c)	75 g
Canned, in water	75 mL (⅓ c), plus 30 mL (2 tbs) liquid	115 g
Guavas, raw	½	50 g
Honeydew melon, raw, with rind	½	225 g
Cubed or diced	250 mL (1 c)	170 g
Kiwis, raw, with skin	2	155 g
Kumquats, raw	3	60 g
Loquats, raw	8	130 g
Lychee fruit, raw	8	120 g
Mandarin oranges, raw, with rind	1	135 g
Raw, sectioned	125 mL (½ c)	100 g
Canned, in water	125 mL (½ c), plus 30 mL (2 tbs) liquid	100 g
Mangoes, raw, without skin and seed	⅓	65 g
Diced	75 mL (⅓ c)	65 g
Nectarines	½ medium	75 g
Oranges, raw, with rind	1 small	130 g
Raw, sectioned	125 mL (½ c)	95 g

(continued on the next page)

Table I-4 (continued)
Canadian Choice System: Fruits and Vegetables

1 fruits and vegetables choice = 10 g carbohydrate, 1 g protein, 190 kJ (44 kcal)

Food	Measure	Mass (Weight)
Papayas, raw, with skin and seeds	¼ medium	150 g
Raw, without skin and seeds	¼ medium	100 g
Cubed or diced	125 mL (½ c)	100 g
Peaches, raw, with seed and skin	1 large	100 g
Raw, sliced or diced	125 mL (½ c)	100 g
Canned in water, halves or slices	125 mL (½ c), plus 30 mL (2 tbs) liquid	120 g
Pears, raw, with skin and core	½	90 g
Raw, without skin and core	½	85 g
Canned, in water, halves	1 half plus 30 mL (2 tbs) liquid	90 g
Persimmons, raw, native	1	30 g
Raw, Japanese	¼	50 g
Pineapple, raw	1 slice	75 g
Raw, diced	125 mL (½ c)	75 g
Canned, in juice, diced	75 mL (⅓ c), plus 15 mL (1 tbs) liquid	55 g
Canned, in juice, sliced	1 slice, plus 15 mL (1 tbs) liquid	55 g
Canned, in water, diced	125 mL (½ c), plus 30 mL (2 tbs) liquid	100 g
Canned, in water, sliced	2 slices, plus 15 mL (1 tbs) liquid	100 g
Plums, raw	2 small	60 g
Damson	6	65 g
Japanese	1	70 g
Canned, in apple juice	2, plus 30 mL (2 tbs) liquid	70 g
Canned, in water	3, plus 30 mL (2 tbs) liquid	100 g
Pomegranates, raw	½	140 g
Strawberries, raw	250 mL (1 c)	150 g
Frozen/canned, in water	250 mL (1 c), plus 30 mL (2 tbs) liquid	240 g
Rhubarb	250 mL (1 c)	150 g
Tangelos, raw	1	205 g
Tangerines, raw	1 medium	115 g
Raw, sectioned	125 mL (½ c)	100 g
Watermelon, raw, with rind	1 wedge	310 g
Cubed or diced	250 mL (1 c)	160 g
Dried Fruit		
Apples	5 pieces	15 g
Apricots	4 halves	15 g
Banana flakes	30 mL (2 tbs)	15 g
Currants	30 mL (2 tbs)	15 g
Dates, without pits	2	15 g
Peaches	½	15 g
Pears	½	15 g
Prunes, raw, with pits	2	15 g
Raw, without pits	2	10 g
Stewed, no liquid	2	20 g
Stewed, with liquid	2, plus 15 mL (1 tbs) liquid	35 g
Raisins	30 mL (2 tbs)	15 g
Juices (no sugar added or unsweetened)		
Apricot, grape, guava, mango, prune	50 mL (¼ c)	55 g
Apple, carrot, papaya, pear, pineapple, pomegranate	75 mL (⅓ c)	80 g
Cranberry (see Sugars Section)		
Clamato (see Sugars Section)		
Grapefruit, loganberry, orange, raspberry, tangelo, tangerine	125 mL (½ c)	130 g

Table I-4 (continued)
Canadian Choice System: Fruits and Vegetables

1 fruits and vegetables choice = 10 g carbohydrate, 1 g protein, 190 kJ (44 kcal)

Food	Measure	Mass (Weight)
Tomato, tomato-based mixed vegetables	250 mL (1 c)	255 g
Vegetables (fresh, frozen, or canned)		
Artichokes, French, globe	2 small	50 g
Beets, diced or sliced	125 mL (½ c)	85 g
Carrots, diced, cooked or uncooked	125 mL (½ c)	75 g
Chestnuts, fresh	5	20 g
Parsnips, mashed	125 mL (½ c)	80 g
Peas, fresh or frozen	125 mL (½ c)	80 g
Canned	75 mL (⅓ c)	55 g
Pumpkin, mashed	125 mL (½ c)	45 g
Rutabagas, mashed	125 mL (½ c)	85 g
Sauerkraut	250 mL (1 c)	235 g
Snow peas	250 mL (1 c)	135 g
Squash, yellow or winter, mashed	125 mL (½ c)	115 g
Succotash	75 mL (⅓ c)	55 g
Tomatoes, canned	250 mL (1 c)	240 g
Tomato paste	50 mL (¼ c)	55 g
Tomato sauce*	75 mL (⅓ c)	100 g
Turnips, mashed	125 mL (½ c)	115 g
Vegetables, mixed	125 mL (½ c)	90 g
Water chestnuts	8 medium	50 g

*Tomato sauce varies according to brand name. Check the label or discuss with your dietitian.

Table I-5
Canadian Choice System: Milk

Type of Milk	Carbohydrate (g)	Protein (g)	Fat (g)	Energy
Nonfat (0%)	6	4	0	170 kJ (40 kcal)
1%	6	4	1	206 kJ (49 kcal)
2%	6	4	2	244 kJ (58 kcal)
Whole (4%)	6	4	4	319 kJ (76 kcal)

Food	Measure	Mass (Weight)
Buttermilk (higher in salt)	125 mL (½ c)	125 g
Evaporated milk	50 mL (¼ c)	50 g
Milk	125 mL (½ c)	125 g
Powdered milk, regular	30 mL (2 tbs)	15 g
Instant	50 mL (¼ c)	15 g
Plain yogurt	125 mL (½ c)	125 g

Note: Food items found in this category provide more than 1 milk choice:

Food	Exchanges per serving	Measure	Mass (Weight)
Milkshake	1 milk + 3 sugars + ½ protein	250 mL (1 c)	300 g
Chocolate milk, 2%	2 milks 2% + 1 sugar	250 mL (1 c)	300 g
Frozen yogurt	1 milk + 1 sugar	125 mL (½ c)	125 g

Table I-6
Canadian Choice System: Sugars

1 sugar choice = 10 g carbohydrate (sugar), 167 kJ (40 kcal)

Food	Measure	Mass (Weight)
Beverages		
Condensed milk	15 mL (1 tbs)	
Flavoured fruit crystals*	75 mL (⅓ c)	
Iced tea mixes*	75 mL (⅓ c)	
Regular soft drinks	125 mL (½ c)	
Sweet drink mixes*	75 mL (⅓ c)	
Tonic water	125 mL (½ c)	
*These beverages have been made with water.		
Miscellaneous		
Bubble gum (large square)	1 piece	5 g
Cranberry cocktail	75 mL (⅓ c)	80 g
Cranberry cocktail, light	350 mL (1⅓ c)	260 g
Cranberry sauce	30 mL (2 tbs)	
Hard candy mints	2	5 g
Honey, molasses, corn & cane syrup	10 mL (2 tsp)	15 g
Jelly bean	4	10 g
Licorice	1 short stick	10 g
Marshmallows	2 large	15 g
Popsicle	1 stick (½ popsicle)	
Powdered gelatin mix (Jello®) (reconstituted)	50 mL (¼ c)	
Regular jam, jelly, marmalade	15 mL (1 tbs)	
Sugar, white, brown, icing, maple	10 mL (2 tsp)	10 g
Sweet pickles	2 small	100 g
Sweet relish	30 mL (2 tbs)	

Food	Choices per Serving	Measures	Mass (Weight)
The following food items provide more than 1 sugar exchange:			
Brownie	1 sugar + 1 fat	1	20 g
Clamato juice	1½ sugars	175 mL (⅔ c)	
Fruit salad, light syrup	1 sugar + 1 fruits & vegetables	125 mL (½ c)	130 g
Aero® bar	2½ sugars + 2½ fats	1 bar	43 g
Smarties®	4½ sugars + 2 fats	1 box	60 g
Sherbet	3 sugars + ½ fat	125 mL (½ c)	95 g

Table I–7
Canadian Choice System: Protein Foods

1 protein choice = 7 g protein, 3 g fat, 230 kJ (55 kcal)

Food	Measure	Mass (Weight)
Cheese		
Low-fat cheese, about 7% milk fat	1 slice	30 g
Cottage cheese, 2% milkfat or less	50 mL (¼ c)	55 g
Ricotta, about 7% milkfat	50 mL (¼ c)	60 g
Fish		
Anchovies (see *Extras*, Table I–9)		
Canned, drained (e.g., mackerel, salmon, tuna packed in water)	(⅓ of 6.5 oz can)	30 g
Cod tongues, cheeks	75 mL (⅓ c)	50 g
Fillet or steak (e.g., Boston blue, cod, flounder, haddock, halibut, mackerel, orange roughy, perch, pickerel, pike, salmon, shad, snapper, sole, swordfish, trout, tuna, whitefish)	1 piece	30 g
Herring	⅓ fish	30 g
Sardines, smelts	2 medium or 3 small	30 g
Squid, octopus	50 mL (¼ c)	40 g
Shellfish		
Clams, mussels, oysters, scallops, snails	3 medium	30 g
Crab, lobster, flaked	50 mL (¼ c)	30 g
Shrimp, fresh	5 large	30 g
Frozen	10 medium	30 g
Canned	18 small	30 g
Dry pack	50 mL (¼ c)	30 g
Meat and Poultry (e.g., beef, chicken, goat, ham, lamb, pork, turkey, veal, wild game)		
Back, peameal bacon	3 slices, thin	30 g
Chop	½ chop, with bone	40 g
Minced or ground, lean or extra-lean	30 mL (2 tbs)	30 g
Sliced, lean	1 slice	30 g
Steak, lean	1 piece	30 g
Organ Meats		
Hearts, liver	1 slice	30 g
Kidneys, sweetbreads, chopped	50 mL (¼ c)	30 g
Tongue	1 slice	30 g
Tripe	5 pieces	60 g
Soyabean		
Bean curd or tofu	½ block	70 g
Eggs		
In shell, raw or cooked	1 medium	50 g
Without shell, cooked or poached in water	1 medium	45 g
Scrambled	50 mL (¼ c)	55 g

(continued on the next page)

Table I-7 (continued)
Canadian Choice System: Protein Foods

1 protein choice = 7 g protein, 3 g fat, 230 kJ (55 kcal)

Food	Choices per Serving	Measures	Mass (Weight)
Note: The following choices provide more than 1 protein exchange:			
Cheese			
Cheeses	1 protein + 1 fat	1 piece	25 g
Cheese, coarsely grated (e.g., Cheddar)	1 protein + 1 fat	50 mL (¼ c)	25 g
Cheese, dry, finely grated (e.g., parmesan)	1 protein + 1 fat	45 mL	15 g
Cheese, ricotta, high fat	1 protein + 1 fat	50 mL (¼ c)	55 g
Fish			
Eel	1 protein + 1 fat	1 slice	50 g
Meat			
Bologna	1 protein + 1 fat	1 slice	20 g
Canned lunch meats	1 protein + 1 fat	1 slice	20 g
Corned beef, canned	1 protein + 1 fat	1 slice	25 g
Corned beef, fresh	1 protein + 1 fat	1 slice	25 g
Ground beef, medium-fat	1 protein + 1 fat	30 mL (2 tbs)	25 g
Meat spreads, canned	1 protein + 1 fat	45 mL	35 g
Mutton chop	1 protein + 1 fat	½ chop, with bone	35 g
Paté (see *Fats and Oils* group, Table I–8)			
Sausages, garlic, Polish or knockwurst	1 protein + 1 fat	1 slice	50 g
Sausages, pork, links	1 protein + 1 fat	1 link	25 g
Spareribs or shortribs, with bone	1 protein + 1 fat	1 large	65 g
Stewing beef	1 protein + 1 fat	1 cube	25 g
Summer sausage or salami	1 protein + 1 fat	1 slice	40 g
Weiners, hot dog	1 protein + 1 fat	½ medium	25 g
Miscellaneous			
Blood pudding	1 protein + 1 fat	1 slice	25 g
Peanut butter	1 protein + 1 fat	15 mL (1 tbs)	15 g

Table I–8
Canadian Choice System: Fats and Oils

1 fat choice = 5 g fat, 190 kJ (45 kcal)

Food	Measure	Mass (Weight)
Avocado*	⅛	30 g
Bacon, side, crisp*	1 slice	5 g
Butter*	5 mL (1 tsp)	5 g
Cheese spread	15 mL (1 tbs)	15 g
Coconut, fresh*	45 mL (3 tbs)	15 g
Coconut, dried*	15 mL (1 tbs)	10 g
Cream, Half and half (cereal), 10%*	30 mL (2 tbs)	30 g
Light (coffee), 20%*	15 mL (1 tbs)	15 g
Whipping, 32 to 37%*	15 mL (1 tbs)	15 g
Cream cheese*	15 mL (1 tbs)	15 g
Gravy*	30 mL (2 tbs)	30 g
Lard*	5 mL (1 tsp)	5 g
Margarine	5 mL (1 tsp)	5 g
Nuts, shelled:		
Almonds	8	5 g
Brazil nuts	2	10 g
Cashews	5	10 g
Filberts, hazelnuts	5	10 g
Macadamia	3	5 g
Peanuts	10	10g
Pecans	5 halves	5 g
Pignolias, pine nuts	25 mL (5 tsp)	10 g
Pistachios, shelled	20	10 g
Pistachios, in shell	20	20 g
Pumpkin and squash seeds	20 mL (4 tsp)	10 g
Nuts (continued):		
Sesame seeds	15 mL (1 tbs)	10 g
Sunflower seeds		
Shelled	15 mL (1 tbs)	10 g
In shell	45 mL (3 tbs)	15 g
Walnuts	4 halves	10 g
Oil, cooking and salad	5 mL (1 tsp)	5 g
Olives, green	10	45 g
Ripe black	7	57 g
Pâté, liverwurst, meat spreads	15 mL (1 tbs)	15 g
Salad dressing: blue,	10 mL (2 tsp)	10 g
French, Italian, mayonnaise, Thousand Island	5 mL (1 tsp)	5 g
Salad dressing, low-calorie	30 mL (2 tbs)	30 g
Salt pork, raw or cooked*	5 mL (1 tsp)	5 g
Sesame oil	5 mL (1 tsp)	5 g
Sour cream		
12% milkfat	30 mL (2 tbs)	30 g
7% milkfat	60 mL (4 tbs)	60 g
Shortening*	5 mL (1 tsp)	

*These items contain higher amounts of saturated fat.

I

Table I-9
Canadian Choice System: Extras

Extras have no more than 2.5 g carbohydrate, 60 kJ (14 kcal)

Vegetables 125 mL (½ c)
Artichokes
Asparagus
Bamboo shoots
Bean sprouts, mung or soya
Beans, string, green, or yellow
Bitter melon (balsam pear)
Bok choy
Broccoli
Brussels sprouts
Cabbage
Cauliflower
Celery
Chard
Cucumbers
Eggplant
Endive
Fiddleheads
Greens: beet, collard, dandelion, mustard, turnip, etc.
Kale
Kohlrabi
Leeks
Lettuce
Mushrooms
Okra
Onions, green or mature
Parsley
Peppers, green, yellow or red
Radishes
Rapini
Rhubarb
Sauerkraut
Shallots
Spinach
Sprouts: alfalfa, radish, etc.
Tomato wedges
Watercress
Zucchini

Free Foods (may be used without measuring)
Artificial sweetener, such as cyclamate or aspartame
Baking powder, baking soda
Bouillon from cube, powder, or liquid
Bouillon or clear broth
Chowchow, unsweetened
Coffee, clear
Consommé
Dulse
Flavorings and extracts
Garlic
Gelatin, unsweetened
Ginger root
Herbal teas, unsweetened
Horseradish, uncreamed
Lemon juice or lemon wedges
Lime juice or lime wedges
Marjoram, cinnamon, etc.
Mineral water
Mustard
Parsley
Pimentos
Salt, pepper, thyme
Soda water, club soda
Soya sauce
Sugar-free Crystal Drink
Sugar-free Jelly Powder
Sugar-free soft drinks
Tea, clear
Vinegar
Water
Worcestershire sauce

Condiments

Food	**Measure**
Anchovies	2 fillets
Barbecue sauce	15 mL (1 tbs)
Bran, natural	30 mL (2 tbs)
Brewer's yeast	5 mL (1 tsp)
Carob powder	5 mL (1 tsp)
Catsup	5 mL (1 tsp)
Chili sauce	5 mL (1 tsp)
Cocoa powder	5 mL (1 tsp)
Cranberry sauce, unsweetened	15 mL (1 tbs)
Dietetic fruit spreads	5 mL (1 tsp)
Maraschino cherries	1
Nondairy coffee whitener	5 mL (1 tsp)
Nuts, chopped pieces	5 mL (1 tsp)
Pickles	
unsweetened dill	2
sour mixed	11
Sugar substitutes, granular	5 mL (1 tsp)
Whipped toppings	15 mL (1 tbs)

Table I-10
Canadian Choice System: Combined Food Choices

Food	Choices per serving	Measure	Mass (Weight)
Angel food cake	½ starch + 2½ sugars	1/12 cake	50 g
Apple crisp	½ starch + 1½ fruits & vegetables + 1 sugar + 1–2 fats	125 mL (½ c)	
Applesauce, sweetened	1 fruits & vegetables + 1 sugar	125 mL (½ c)	
Beans and pork in tomato sauce	1 starch + ½ fruits & vegetables + ½ sugar + 1 protein	125 mL (½ c)	135 g
Beef burrito	2 starches + 3 proteins + 3 fats		110 g
Brownie	1 sugar + 1 fat	1	20 g
Cabbage rolls*	1 starch + 2 proteins	3	310 g
Caesar salad	2–4 fats	20 mL dressing (4 tsp)	
Cheesecake	½ starch + 2 sugars + ½ protein + 5 fats	1 piece	80 g
Chicken fingers	1 starch + 2 proteins + 2 fats	6 small	100 g
Chicken and snow pea Oriental	2 starches + ½ fruits & vegetables + 3 proteins + 1 fat	500 mL (2 c)	
Chili	1½ starches + ½ fruits & vegetables + 3½ protein	300 mL (1¼ c)	325 g
Chips			
Potato chips	1 starch + 2 fats	15 chips	30 g
Corn chips	1 starch + 2 fats	30 chips	30 g
Tortilla chips	1 starch + 1½ fats	13 chips	
Cheese twist	1 starch + 1½ fats	30 chips	30 g
Chocolate bar			
Aero®	2½ sugars + 2½ fats	bar	43 g
Smarties®	4½ sugars + 2 fats	package	60 g
Chocolate cake (without icing)	1 starch + 2 sugars + 3 fats	1/10 of a 8″ pan	
Chocolate devil's food cake (without icing)	2 starches + 2 sugars + 3 fats	1/12 of a 9″ pan	
Chocolate milk	2 milks 2% + 1 sugar	250 mL (1 c)	300 g
Clubhouse (triple-decker) sandwich	3 starches + 3 proteins + 4 fats		
Cookies			
chocolate chip	½ starch + ½ sugar + 1½ fats	2	22 g
oatmeal	1 starch + 1 sugar + 1 fat	2	40 g
Donut (chocolate glazed)	1 starch + 1½ sugars + 2 fats	1	65 g
Egg roll	1 starch + ½ protein + 1 fat		75 g
Four bean salad	1 starch + ½ protein + 1 fat	125 mL (½ c)	
French toast	1 starch + ½ protein + 2 fats	1 slice	65 g
Fruit in heavy syrup	1 fruits & vegetables + 1½ sugars	125 mL (½ c)	
Granola bar	½ starch + 1 sugar + 1–2 fats		30 g
Granola cereal	1 starch + 1 sugar + 2 fats	125 mL (½ c)	45 g
Hamburger	2 starches + 3 proteins + 2 fats	junior size	
Ice cream and cone, plain flavour			
Ice cream	½ milk + 2–3 sugars + 1–2 fats		100 g
Cone	½ sugar		4 g
Lasagna			
regular cheese	1 starch + 1 fruits & vegetables + 3 proteins + 2 fats	3″ x 4″ piece	
low-fat cheese	1 starch + 1 fruits & vegetables + 3 proteins	3″ x 4″ piece	

* If eaten with sauce, add ½ fruits & vegetables exchange.

(continued on the next page)

Table I–10 (continued)
Canadian Choice System: Combined Food Choices

Food	Choices per serving	Measure	Mass (Weight)
Legumes			
Dried beans (kidney, navy, pinto, fava, chick peas)	2 starches + 1 protein	250 mL (1 c)	180 g
Dried peas	2 starches + 1 protein	250 mL (1 c)	210 g
Lentils	2 starches + 1 protein	250 mL (1 c)	210 g
Macaroni 'and cheese	2 starches + 2 proteins + 2 fats	250 mL (1 c)	210 g
Minestrone soup	1½ starches + ½ fruits & vegetables + ½ fat	250 mL (1 c)	
Muffin	1 starch + ½ sugar + 1 fat	1 small	45 g
Nuts (dry or roasted without any oil added).			
Almonds, dried sliced	½ protein + 2 fats	50 mL (¼ c)	22 g
Brazil nuts, dried unblanched	½ protein + 2½ fats	5 large	23 g
Cashew nuts, dry roasted	½ starch + ½ protein + 2 fats	50 mL (¼ c)	28 g
Filbert hazelnut, dry	½ protein + 3½ fats	50 mL (¼ c)	30 g
Macadamia nuts, dried	½ protein + 4 fats	50 mL (¼ c)	28 g
Peanuts, raw	1 protein + 2 fats	50 mL (¼ c)	30 g
Pecans, dry roasted	½ fruits & vegetables + 3 fats	50 mL (¼ c)	22 g
Pine nuts, pignolia dried	1 protein + 3 fats	50 mL (¼ c)	34 g
Pistachio nuts, dried	½ fruits & vegetables + ½ protein + 2 ½ fats	50 mL (¼ c)	27 g
Pumpkin seeds, roasted	2 proteins + 2½ fats	50 mL (¼ c)	47 g
Sesame seeds, whole dried	½ fruits & vegetables + ½ protein + 2½ fats	50 mL (¼ c)	30 g
Sunflower kernel, dried	½ protein + 1½ fats	50 mL (¼ c)	17 g
Walnuts, dried chopped	½ protein + 3 fats	50 mL (¼ c)	26 g
Perogies	2 starches + 1 protein + 1 fat	3	
Pie, fruit	1 starch + 1 fruits & vegetables + 2 sugars + 3 fats	1 piece	120 g
Pizza, cheese	1 starch + 1 protein + 1 fat	1 slice (⅛ of a 12″)	50 g
Pork stir fry	½ to 1 fruits & vegetables + 3 proteins	200 mL (¾ c)	
Potato salad	1 starch + 1 fat	125 mL (½ c)	130 g
Potatoes, scalloped	2 starches + 1 milk + 1–2 fats	200 mL (¾ c)	210 g
Pudding, bread or rice	1 starch + 1 sugar +1 fat	125 mL (½ c)	
Pudding, vanilla	1 milk + 2 sugars	125 mL (½ c)	
Raisin bran cereal	1 starch + ½ fruits & vegetables + ½ sugar	175 mL (⅔ c)	40 g
Rice krispie squares	½ starch + 1½ sugars + ½ fat	1 square	30 g
Shepherd's pie	2 starches + 1 fruits & vegetables + 3 proteins	325 mL (1⅓ c)	
Sherbet, orange	3 sugars + ½ fat	125 mL (½ c)	
Spaghetti and meat sauce	2 starches + 1 fruits & vegetables + 2 proteins + 3 fats	250 mL (1 c)	
Stew	2 starches + 2 fruits & vegetables + 3 proteins + ½ fat	200 mL (¾ c)	
Sundae	4 sugars + 3 fats	125 mL (½ c)	
Tuna casserole	1 starch + 2 proteins + ½ fat	125 mL (½ c)	
Yogurt, fruit bottom	1 fruits & vegetables + 1 milk + 1 sugar	125 mL (½ c)	125 g
Yogurt, frozen	1 milk + 1 sugar	125 mL (½ c)	125 g

FOOD LABELS

◆

Consumers can gather a lot of information from a nutrition label. Figure I–1 demonstrates the reading of a food label and Table I–11 defines terms.

Figure I-1

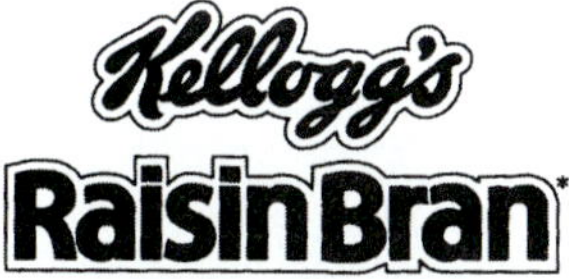

OUR COMMITMENT TO QUALITY

Kellogg's is committed to providing foods of outstanding quality and freshness. If this product in any way falls below the high standards you've come to expect from Kellogg's, please send your comments and both top flaps to:

Consumer Affairs
KELLOGG CANADA INC.
Etobicoke, Ontario M9W 5P2

IF IT DOESN'T SAY Kellogg's* ON THE BOX, IT'S NOT Kellogg's* IN THE BOX.
SI LE NOM Kellogg's* N'EST PAS SUR LA BOÎTE, CE N'EST PAS Kellogg's* DANS LA BOÎTE.

• HIGH IN FIBRE
• LOW IN FAT
• PRESERVATIVE FREE
• SOURCE ÉLEVÉE DE FIBRES
• FAIBLE EN MATIÈRES GRASSES
• SANS AGENT DE CONSERVATION

NUTRITION INFORMATION
APPORT NUTRITIONNEL

	Per 40 g serving cereal (175 mL, ¾ cup) Par ration de 40 g de céréale (175 mL, ¾ tasse)	Per 40 g serving cereal with 125 mL Partly Skimmed Milk (2%) Par ration de 40 g de céréale avec 125 mL de lait partiellement écrémé (2,0 %)	
ENERGY	130Cal 540kJ	195Cal 810kJ	ÉNERGIE
PROTEIN	3.0g	7.3g	PROTÉINES
FAT	0.4g	2.9g	MATIÈRES GRASSES
CARBOHYDRATE	32g	38g	GLUCIDES
SUGARS*	11g	18g	*SUCRES
STARCH	16g	16g	AMIDON
DIETARY FIBRE	4.6g	4.6g	FIBRES ALIMENTAIRES
SODIUM	235mg	300mg	SODIUM
POTASSIUM	240mg	440mg	POTASSIUM
% of Recommended Daily Intake % de l'apport quotidien conseillé			
VITAMIN A	0%	7%	VITAMINE A
VITAMIN D	0%	23%	VITAMINE D
VITAMIN B1	62%	66%	VITAMINE B1
VITAMIN B2	3%	16%	VITAMINE B2
NIACIN	13%	18%	NIACINE
VITAMIN B6	13%	16%	VITAMINE B6
FOLACIN	11%	14%	FOLACINE
VITAMIN B12	0%	25%	VITAMINE B12
PANTOTHENATE	9%	15%	PANTOTHÉNATE
CALCIUM	1%	15%	CALCIUM
PHOSPHORUS	12%	23%	PHOSPHORE
MAGNESIUM	20%	27%	MAGNÉSIUM
IRON	38%	39%	FER
ZINC	16%	22%	ZINC

*Approximately half of the sugars occur naturally in the raisins.
Environ la moitié des sucres se retrouvent à l'état naturel dans les fruits.

Canadian Diabetes Association Food Choice Values: 40 g (175 mL, ¾ cup) cereal. Système des choix d'aliments de l'Association canadienne du diabète : 40 g (175 mL, ¾ tasse) céréale = 1 [■] + ½ [◆] + ½ [✱] choices/choix

INGREDIENTS / INGRÉDIENTS

WHOLE WHEAT, RAISINS (COATED WITH SUGAR, HYDROGENATED VEGETABLE OIL), WHEAT BRAN, SUGAR/GLUCOSE-FRUCTOSE, SALT, MALT (CORN FLOUR, MALTED BARLEY), VITAMINS (THIAMIN HYDROCHLORIDE, PYRIDOXINE HYDROCHLORIDE, FOLIC ACID, d-CALCIUM PANTOTHENATE), MINERALS (IRON, ZINC OXIDE).

BLÉ ENTIER, RAISINS SECS (ENROBÉS DE SUCRE, D'HUILE VÉGÉTALE HYDROGÉNÉE), SON DE BLÉ, SUCRE/GLUCOSE-FRUCTOSE, SEL, MALT (FARINE DE MAÏS, ORGE MALTÉ), VITAMINES (CHLORHYDRATE DE THIAMINE, CHLORHYDRATE DE PYRIDOXINE, ACIDE FOLIQUE, PANTOTHÉNATE DE d-CALCIUM), MINÉRAUX (FER, OXYDE DE ZINC).

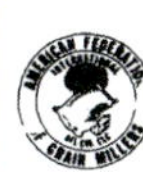

Made by / Produit par
KELLOGG CANADA INC.
ETOBICOKE, ONTARIO
CANADA M9W 5P2
*Registered trademark of /
*Marque déposée de
KELLOGG CANADA INC. © 1994
00094

WHAT YOU WILL FIND ON A LABEL:

Nutrition Claims

- in Canada, it is optional for a company to decide to use claims,
- when claims appear on a label, they must follow government laws

Nutrition Information

- gives detailed nutrition facts about the product, including serving size and core list
- does not have to appear by law on food products in Canada
- refers to the food as packaged, so if you add milk, eggs or other food, the nutritional content of the food you eat can be very different

Serving Size

- the amount of food for which the information is given
- check the serving size: the serving size on the label may not be the same as the serving size you would actually eat (for example, the serving size of cereal may be ¾ cup, much smaller than your regular serving

Core List

- the energy (in Calories and kilojoules), grams of protein, fat and carbohydrate for each serving
- some products break down fat into monounsaturates, polyunsaturates, saturates, and cholesterol (to find out what these mean, look at the Fats & Oils section)
- carbohydrates may include the amount of sugars, starch and fibre, or may list these items separately

Sodium and Potassium (in milligrams)

Vitamins and Minerals (as percent of your recommended daily intake)

Canadian Diabetes Association Food Choice Values and Symbols

- the Values and Symbols are tools to help you fit the food into your meal plan, they are not an endorsement by CDA
- it is up to the food company to decide if they want their foods analyzed and assigned symbols
- when they are on a label, they have been assigned by a dietitian working for CDA, so you can be sure the information is correct

Ingredients

- must be found on all food labels by law
- ingredients are listed in decreasing order by weight, so what you see first is what you get the most of

I

Table I-11
Terms on Food Labels

Energy
kcalorie reduced: 50% or fewer kcalories than the regular version. **light:** term may be used to describe anything (for example, light in colour, texture, flavour, taste, or kcalories); read the label to find out what is "light" about the product. **low kcalorie:** kcalorie-reduced and no more than 15 kcalories per serving.
Fat and Cholesterol
low cholesterol: no more than 3 mg of cholesterol per 100 g of the food and low in saturated fat; *does not* always mean low in total fat. **low fat:** no more than 3 g of fat per serving; *does not* always mean low in kcalories. **lower fat:** at least 25% less fat than the comparison food; be aware that 80% fat-free still means the food is 20% fat.
Carbohydrates: Fibre and Sugar
carbohydrate reduced: not more than 50% of the carbohydrate found in the regular version; *does not* always mean the product is lower in kcalories because other ingredients such as fat may have increased. **source of dietary fibre:** a product that provides 2–4 g of fibre. **high source of dietary fibre:** a product that provides 4–6 g of fibre. **very high source of fibre:** a product that provides 6 g (or more) of fibre. **sugar free:** low in carbohydrates and kcalories; can be used as an extra food in the exchange system. **unsweetened or no sugar added:** no sugar was added to the product; sugar may be found naturally in the food (for example, fruit canned in its own juice).

APPENDIX J

MEASURES OF PROTEIN QUALITY

♦

Contents

In a world where food is scarce and many people's diets contain marginal or inadequate amounts of protein, it is important to know which foods contain the highest-quality protein. Chapter 6 describes protein quality and the different measures researchers use to assess the quality of a food protein. This appendix provides a few more details.

AMINO ACID SCORING

♦

Amino acid, or chemical, scoring allows researchers to determine the amino acid composition of any protein relatively inexpensively, but unfortunately, it does not always accurately reflect the way the body will use a protein. The advantages of amino acid scoring are that it is simple and inexpensive, it identifies in one step the limiting amino acid, and it can be used to score mixtures of different proportions of two or more proteins mathematically without having to make up a mixture and test it. Its chief weaknesses are that it fails to predict the digestibility of a protein, which may strongly affect the protein's quality; it relies on a chemical procedure in which certain amino acids may be destroyed, making the pattern that is analyzed inaccurate; and it is blind to other features of the protein (such as the presence of substances that may inhibit the digestion or utilization of the protein) that would only be revealed by a test in living animals. Table J–1 shows how to use a reference pattern for the nine essential amino acids.

PDCAAS

♦

PDCAAS (protein-digestibility-corrected amino acid score) takes the amino acid scoring method a step further by correcting for the digestibility of the protein. To calculate the PDCAAS, researchers first determine the amino acid profile of the test protein (in this example, pinto beans). The second column of Table J–2 presents the essential amino acid profile for pinto beans. The third column presents the amino acid requirements of preschool-aged children for comparison. To determine how well the food protein meets human needs, researchers calculate the ratio by dividing the second column by the third column (for example, $30 \div 19 = 1.578$ or 1.58).

The amino acid with the lowest ratio is the first limiting amino acid—in this case, tryptophan. Its ratio is the amino acid score for the protein—in this case, 80. Remember, though, the amino acid score does not account for digestibility. Protein digestibility, as determined by rat balance studies, yields a value of 79 percent for pinto beans. Together, the amino acid score and the digestibility value determine the PDCAAS:

$$\text{PDCAAS} = \text{protein digestibility} \times \text{lowest amino acid ratio}.$$

$$\text{PDCAAS for pinto beans} = .79 \times .80 = 63\%.$$

Thus the PDCAAS for pinto beans is 63 percent (or 0.63).

The PDCAAS is used to determine the % Daily Value on food labels. To calculate the % Daily Value for protein for canned pinto beans, multiply the number of grams of protein in a standard serving (in this case, 7 grams per ½ cup) by the PDCAAS:

$$7 \text{ g} \times .63 = 4.41.$$

This value is then divided by the RDI for protein (for children over age four and adults, the RDI is 50 grams):

$$4.41 \div 50 = 0.088 \text{ (or } 8.8\%\text{)}.$$

The food label for this can of pinto beans would declare that one serving provides 7 grams protein, and if the label included a % Daily Value for protein, the value would be 9 percent.

BIOLOGICAL VALUE

♦

To determine the actual value of a protein as it is used by the body, it is necessary to measure both urinary and fecal losses of nitrogen

Table J–1
A Reference Pattern for Amino Acid Scoring of Proteins

Essential Amino Acids	Reference Protein (Whole Egg) Mg Amino Acid per G Nitrogen
Histidine	145
Isoleucine	340
Leucine	540
Lysine	440
Methionine + cystine[a]	355
Phenylalanine + tyrosine[b]	580
Threonine	294
Tryptophan	106
Valine	410
Total	3210

[a]Methionine is essential and is also used to make cystine. Thus the methionine requirement is lower if cystine is supplied.

[b]Phenylalanine is essential and is also used to make tyrosine if not enough of the latter is available. Thus the phenylalanine requirement is lower if tyrosine is also supplied.

Note: To interpret the table, read, "For every 3210 units of essential amino acids, 145 must be histidine, 340 must be isoleucine, 540 must be leucine," and so on. To compare a test protein with the reference protein, the experimenter first obtains a chemical analysis of the test protein's amino acids. Then, taking 3210 units of the amino acids, the experimenter compares the amount of each amino acid to the amount found in 3210 units of essential amino acids in egg protein. For example, suppose the test protein contained (per 3210 units) 360 units of isoleucine; 500 units of leucine; 350 of lysine; and for each of the other amino acids, more units than egg protein contains. The two amino acids that are low are leucine (500 as compared with 540 in egg) and lysine (350 versus 440 in egg). The ratio, amino acid in the test protein divided by amino acid in egg, is 500/540 (or about 0.93) for leucine and 350/440 (or about 0.80) for lysine. Lysine is the limiting amino acid (lowest ratio compared with egg), so the test protein receives a chemical score of 80.

J

when that protein is actually fed to human beings under test conditions. Even then, small additional losses from sweat, shed skin, hair, and fingernails will be missed. This kind of experiment determines the biological value (BV) of proteins, a measure used internationally.

In a test of biological value, two nitrogen balance studies are done. In the first, no protein is fed, and nitrogen (N) excretions in the urine and feces are measured. It is assumed that under these conditions, N lost in the urine is the amount the body always necessarily loses by filtration into the urine each day, regardless of what protein is fed (endogenous N). The N lost in the feces (called metabolic N in the equation) is the amount the body invariably loses into the intestine each day, whether or not food protein is fed. (To help you remember the terms: endogenous N is "urinary N on a zero-protein diet"; metabolic N is "fecal N on a zero-protein diet.")

In the second study, an amount of protein slightly below the requirement is fed. Intake and losses are measured; then the BV is derived using this formula:

Table J–2
An Example of PDCAAS

Essential Amino Acids	Amino Acid Profile of Pinto Beans (mg/g protein)	Amino Acid Requirements for 2–5 yr (mg/g protein)	Ratio
Histidine	30.0	19	1.58
Isoleucine	42.5	28	1.52
Leucine	80.4	66	1.22
Lysine	69.0	58	1.19
Methionine + cystine	21.1	25	0.84
Phenylalanine + tyrosine	90.5	63	1.44
Threonine	43.7	34	1.28
Tryptophan	8.8	11	0.80
Valine	50.1	35	1.43

$$\text{BV} = \frac{\text{food N} - (\text{fecal N} - \text{metabolic N}) - (\text{urinary N} - \text{endogenous N})}{\text{food N} - (\text{fecal N} - \text{metabolic N})} \times 100.$$

The denominator of this equation expresses the amount of nitrogen *absorbed:* food N minus fecal N (excluding the N the body would lose in the feces anyway, even without food). The numerator expresses the amount of N *retained* from the N absorbed: absorbed N (as in the denominator) minus the N excreted in the urine (excluding the N the body would lose in the urine anyway, even without food). Thus it can be more simply expressed:

$$\text{BV} = \frac{\text{N retained}}{\text{N absorbed}} \times 100.$$

This method has the advantages of being based on experiments with human beings (it can be done with animals, too, of course) and of measuring actual nitrogen retention. But it is also cumbersome, expensive, and often impractical, and it is based on several assumptions that may not be valid. For example, the physiology, normal environment, or typical food intake of the subjects used for testing may not be similar to those for whom the test protein may ultimately be used. For another example, the retention of protein in the body does not necessarily mean that it is being well utilized. Considerable exchange of protein among tissues (protein turnover) occurs, but is hidden from view when only N intake and output are measured. The test of biological value wouldn't detect if one tissue were shorted.

NET PROTEIN UTILIZATION

◆

Like measurements of BV, determinations of net protein utilization (NPU) involve two balance studies: one on zero nitrogen intake, and the other on submaximal intake. The formula for NPU is:

$$\text{NPU} = \frac{\text{food N} - (\text{fecal N} - \text{metabolic N}) - (\text{urinary N} - \text{endogenous N})}{\text{food N}} \times 100.$$

The numerator is the same as it is for BV, but the denominator represents food N intake only—not absorbed N. More simply exprssed:

$$\text{NPU} = \frac{\text{N retained}}{\text{N intake}} \times 100.$$

This method offers advantages similar to those of BV determinations and is used more frequently, with animals as the test subjects. A drawback is that if a low NPU is obtained, the test results offer no help in distinguishing between two possible causes: a poor amino acid composition of the test protein or poor digestibility. There is also a limit to the extent to which animal test results can be assumed to be applicable to human beings.

PROTEIN EFFICIENCY RATIO

◆

The protein efficiency ratio (PER) is a widely used procedure for evaluating protein quality. Young rats are fed a measured amount of protein and weighed periodically as they grow. The PER is expressed as:

$$\text{PER} = \frac{\text{weight gain (g)}}{\text{protein intake (g)}}.$$

This method has the virtues of economy and simplicity, but it also has many drawbacks. The experiments are time-consuming; the amino acid needs of rats are not the same as those of human beings; and the amino acid needs for growth are not the same as for the maintenance of adult animals (growing animals need more lysine, for example).

APPENDIX K

ENTERAL FORMULAS

The staggering number of enteral formulas available allows health care professionals to meet a variety of their client's medical needs, but also complicates the process of selecting an appropriate formula. The first step in narrowing the choice of formulas is to determine the client's ability to digest and absorb nutrients. Table K–1 lists examples of intact protein formulas for clients with the ability to digest and absorb nutrients and Table K–2 provides examples of hydrolyzed formulas for clients with limited ability to digest and absorb nutrients. Each formula is listed only once, although the formula may have more than one use. A high-protein formula, for example, may also be a fiber-containing formula. Tables K-3 through K-5 list modular formulas. Although this appendix provides many examples, the list of formulas is not complete. The information reflects the manufacturers literature and does not suggest endorsement by the authors. Be aware that formula composition changes periodically. Consult manufacturer's literature for updates. The following products are listed in this appendix:

- Braun Medical, Inc.[a]
  - Hepatic-Aid® II
  - Immune-Aid®
- Mead Johnson Nutritionals[b]
  - Casec®
  - Choice®
  - Comply®
  - Criticare HN®
  - Deliver® 2.0
  - Isocal®
  - Isocal® HN
  - Kindercal®
  - Lipisorb®
  - MCT Oil®
  - Microlipid®
  - Moducal®
  - Magnacal® Renal
  - Protain XL®
  - Respalor®
  - Sustacal®
  - Sustacal® Basic
  - Sustacal® with Fiber
  - Sustacal® Plus
  - Traumacal®
  - Ultracal®
- Nestlé Clinical Nutrition[c]
  - Crucial®
  - Entrition® HN
  - Glytrol®
  - Nutren ®1.0
  - Nutren® 1.0 with Fiber
  - Nutren® 1.5
  - Nutren® 2.0
  - Nutren® Junior
  - Nutren® Junior with Fiber
  - NutriHep®
  - NutriVent®
  - Peptamen®
  - Peptamen® Junior
  - Peptamen® VHP
  - ProBalance®
  - Reabilan®
  - Reabilan® HN
  - Replete®
  - Replete® with Fiber
- Novartis Nutrition Corporation[d]
  - Compleat® Modified
  - Compleat® Regular
  - Compleat® Pediatric
  - DiabetiSource®
  - FiberSource®
  - FiberSource® HN
  - Impact®
  - Impact® 1.5
  - Impact® with Fiber
  - IsoSource® Standard
  - IsoSource® HN
  - IsoSource® VHN
  - IsoSource® 1.5
  - Resource® Diabetic
  - Resource® Standard
  - Resource® Plus
  - SandoSource® Peptide
  - Tolerex®
  - Vivonex® Pediatric
  - Vivonex® Plus
  - Vivonex® T.E.N.
- Nutrition Medical[e]
  - Fiberlan®
  - Gluco-PRO®
  - Isolan®
  - L-Emental®
  - L-Emental® Hepatic
  - L-Emental® Pediatric
  - L-Emental® Plus
  - Nitrolan®
  - PRO-Peptide®
  - PRO-Peptide® for Kids
  - PRO-Peptide® VHN
  - Ultralan®
- Ross Laboratories[f]
  - Advera®
  - Alitraq®
  - Ensure®
  - Ensure® Plus
  - Ensure® Plus HN
  - Ensure® with Fiber
  - Glucerna®
  - Jevity®
  - Jevity® Plus
  - Nepro®
  - Osmolite®
  - Osmolite® HN
  - Osmolite® HN Plus
  - PediaSure®
  - PediaSure® with Fiber
  - Perative®
  - Polycose®
  - ProMod®
  - Promote®
  - Promote® with Fiber
  - Pulmocare®
  - Suplena®
  - TwoCal® HN
  - Vital® HN

---

[a] *Enteral Nutrition Products Ready Reference* (provided June, 1997), *Hepatic-Aid II Instant Drink* (1992), and *Immune-Aid* (1992), McGaw Inc., Irvine, CA 92714.

[b] *Enteral Product Handbook* (1994), *Choice* (1995), *Comply* (1996), *Magnacal Renal* (1996), and *Protain XL* (1996), Mead-Johnson Nutritionals, Evansville, IN 47721.

[c] *Enteral Product Reference Guide* (1997), Nestlé Clinical Nutrition, Deerfield, IL 60015.

[d] *Enteral Products Guide* (1995) and *Compleat Pediatric* (1997), Sandoz Nutrition, Minneapolis, MN 55416.

[e] *Enteral Formulary, Gluco-PRO* (1997), *L-Emental* (1994), *L-Emental Hepatic* (1996), *L-Emental Pediatric* (1996), *L-Emental Plus* (1997), *PRO-peptide* (1997), *PRO-Peptide for Kids* (1997), and *PRO-Peptide VHN* (1997), Nutrition Medical, Inc., Minneapolis, MN 55442.

[f] *Ross Medical Nutritional System* (1996), Ross Laboratories, Columbus, OH 43215.

Table K-1
Intact Protein Formulas

Product	Form	Volume to Meet 100% RDI (ml)	Energy (kcal/ml)	Protein or Amino Acids (g/L)	Carbohydrate (g/L)	Fat (g/L)	Osmolality (mOsm/kg)	Notes
Lactose-Free, Isotonic or Near-Isotonic Formulas								
Compleat® Modified	liquid	1500	1.07	43	140	37	300	4.4 g fiber/L
Isocal®	liquid	1890	1.06	34	135	44	270	Low-residue, 20% fat from MCT
Isolan®	liquid	1250	1.06	40	144	36	300	Low-residue
IsoSource Standard®	liquid	1500	1.20	43	170	41	360	Low-residue, 50% fat from MCT
Nutren® 1.0	liquid	1500	1.00	40	127	38	300	Low-residue, 24% fat from MCT
Osmolite®	liquid	1887	1.06	37	151	35	300	Low-residue, 20% fat from MCT
Low- to Moderate-Residue Formulas[a]								
Compleat® Regular	liquid	1500	1.07	43	130	43	450	Blenderized formula, contains lactose, 4.4 g fiber/1000 ml
Ensure®	liquid	948	1.06	37	145	37	555	Lactose-free
Resource® Standard	liquid	1890	1.10	37	140	37	430	Lactose-free
Sustacal Basic®	liquid	1080	1.01	61	140	23	650	Lactose-free
Lactose-Free, Fiber-Containing Formulas								
Ensure® with Fiber	liquid	1391	1.10	40	162	37	480	14 g fiber/L
Fiberlan®	liquid	1250	1.20	50	160	40	310	Near-isotonic 14 g fiber/L
FiberSource®	liquid	1500	1.20	43	170	41	390	10 g fiber/L
Impact® with Fiber	liquid	1500	1.00	56	140	28	375	10 g fiber/L, enriched with arginine, nucleic acids, and omega-3 fatty acids
Jevity®	liquid	1321	1.06	44	154	35	300	Isotonic, 14 g fiber/L
Nutren® 1.0 with Fiber	liquid	1500	1.00	40	127	38	303	Near-isotonic, 14 g fiber/L
ProBalance®	liquid	1000	1.20	45	130	34	350	10 g fiber/L
Promote® with Fiber	liquid	1000	1.00	63	139	28	370	14.4 g fiber/L
Replete® with Fiber	liquid	1000	1.00	63	113	34	300	Isotonic, 14 g fiber/L
Sustacal® with Fiber	liquid	1500	1.06	46	139	35	480	11 g fiber/L
Ultracal®	liquid	1250	1.06	44	123	45	310	Near isotonic, 14.4 g fiber/L
Lactose-Free, High-kCalorie, High-Protein Formulas								
Comply®	liquid	1250	1.50	60	180	61	60	
Ensure® Plus	liquid	1420	1.50	55	200	53	690	
Ensure® Plus HN	liquid	947	1.50	63	200	50	650	
Deliver® 2	liquid	1000	2.00	75	200	102	640	
IsoSource® 1.5 Cal	liquid	933	1.50	68	170	65	650	8.0 g fiber/L
Nutren® 1.5	liquid	1000	1.50	40	113	45	430	50% fat from MCT
Nutren® 2.0	liquid	750	2.00	40	98	53	720	75% fat from MCT

[a]These formulas are frequently used as oral supplements. All formulas listed under "Intact Formulas: Isotonic or Near-Isotonic Formulas" can be used as a low- to moderate-residue formula.

Table K-1
Intact Protein Formulas (continued)

Product	Form	Volume to Meet 100% RDI (ml)	Energy (kcal/ml)	Protein or Amino Acids (g/L)	Carbohydrate (g/L)	Fat (g/L)	Osmolality (mOsm/kg)	Notes
Lactose-Free, High-kCalorie, High-Protein Formulas								
Osmolite® HN Plus	liquid	1000	1.20	56	158	39	360	
Resource Plus®	liquid	1400	1.50	55	200	53	600	
Sustacal® Plus	liquid	1180	1.52	61	190	57	670	
TwoCal HN®	liquid	947	2.00	84	217	91	690	20% fat from MCT
Ultralan®	liquid	1000	1.50	60	202	50	540	50% fat from MCT
Lactose-Free, High-Protein Formulas								
Entrition® HN	liquid	1300	1.00	44	114	41	300	Isotonic, low-residue
FiberSource® HN	liquid	1500	1.20	53	160	41	390	7 g fiber/L
Isocal® HN	liquid	1250	1.06	44	123	46	270	Near-isotonic, low residue, 20% fat from MCT
IsoSource® HN	liquid	1500	1.20	53	160	41	330	Near-isotonic, low residue
IsoSource® VHN	liquid	1250	1.00	62	130	29	300	Isotonic, 10g fiber/L
Jevity® Plus	liquid	1000	1.20	56	175	39	450	12.0 g fiber/L
Libisorb®	liquid	1180	1.35	57	161	57	630	85% fat from MCT
Nitrolan	liquid	1250	1.24	60	160	40	310	Near-isotonic, 50% fat from MCT
Osmolite® HN	liquid	1321	1.06	44	144	35	300	Lactose-free, low-residue, 20% fat from MCT
Promote®	liquid	1000	1.00	63	130	26	340	Fat primarily from polyunsaturated and monounsaturated sources, 20% fat from MCT
Replete®	liquid	1500	1.00	63	113	33	350	Near-isotonic, lactose-free, low-residue
Sustacal®	liquid	1080	1.01	61	139	23	650	
Special Use Formulas: Pediatric (1 to 10 years)								
Compleat® Pediatric	liquid	900	1.00	38	126	39	N/A	Blenderized formula, 4.4 g fiber/L
Kindercal®	liquid	946	1.06	32	127	42	N/A	
Nutren Junior™	liquid	1000	1.00	30	128	42	350	
Nutren Junior™ with Fiber	liquid	1000	1.00	30	128	42	350	6.0 g fiber/L
PediaSure®	liquid	1000	1.00	30	110	50	345	
PediaSure® with Fiber	liquid	1000	1.00	30	114	50	345	5.0 g fiber/L
Special Use Formulas: Glucose Intolerance								
Choice dm™	liquid	948	1.06	45	106	51	440	13.6 g fiber/L, 25% kcalories from monounsaturated fat
DiabetiSource™	liquid	1500	1.00	50	90	49	360	4.4 g fiber/L

Table K–1
Intact Protein Formulas (continued)

Product	Form	Volume to Meet 100% RDI (ml)	Energy (kcal/ml)	Protein or Amino Acids (g/L)	Carbohydrate (g/L)	Fat (g/L)	Osmolality (mOsm/kg)	Notes
Special-Use Formulas: Glucose Intolerance								
Glucerna®	liquid	1422	1.00	42	96	54	355	14.4 g fiber/L, high in monounsaturated fat
Gluco-PRO™	liquid	1000	1.06	45	106	51	300	Isotonic, 14.4 g fiber/L
Glytrol®	liquid	1400	1.00	45	100	48	380	15 g fiber/L
Resource® Diabetic	liquid	1890	1.06	63	99	47	450	12 g fiber/L
Special Use Formulas: Immune System Support								
Immun-Aid®	powder	2000	1.00	80	120	22	460	Enriched with arginine, glutamine, branched-chain amino acids, nucleic acids, omega-3 fatty acids, vitamins A, C, E, and B_6 and trace elements
Impact®	liquid	1500	1.00	56	130	28	375	Enriched with arginine, nucleic acids, and omega-3 fatty acids
Impact® 1.5	liquid	1250	1.50	80	140	69	550	Same as above
Impact® with Fiber (see Fiber-Containing Formulas)								
Special Use Formulas: Renal Insufficiency								
Magnacal® Renal	liquid	N/A	2.00	75	200	101	570	High in monounsaturated fat, 20% fat from MCT; intended for use once hemodialysis has been instituted
Nepro®	liquid	947	2.00	70	215	96	635	Lactose-free, high-calcium, low phosphorus; intended for use once dialysis has been instituted
Suplena®	liquid	947	2.00	30	255	96	600	Lactose-free, low in electrolytes; intended for use before dialysis is instituted
Special Use Formulas: Respiratory Insufficiency								
NutriVent®	liquid	1000	1.50	68	100	94	450	Lactose-free, 55% kcal from fat, 40% fat from MCT
Pulmocare®	liquid	947	1.50	63	106	93	475	Lactose-free, 55% kcal from fat, 20% fat from MCT, enriched with antioxidant nutrients
Respalor™	liquid	1420	1.52	76	148	71	580	Lactose-free; 41% kcal from fat; 30% fat from MCT; enriched with vitamins C and E, B-complex vitamins, zinc and trace elements

K

Table K-1
Intact Protein Formulas (continued)

Product	Form	Volume to Meet 100% RDI (ml)	Energy (kcal/ml)	Protein or Amino Acids (g/L)	Carbohydrate (g/L)	Fat (g/L)	Osmolality (mOsm/kg)	Notes
Special Use Formulas: Wound Healing								
Protain XL®	liquid	1200	1.00	57	129	30	340	14 g fiber/L, 20% fat from MCT, enriched with vitamins A and C and zinc
Replete®	liquid	1000	1.00	63	113	34	320	Enriched with vitamins A and C and zinc
Replete® with Fiber (see Fiber-Containing Formulas)								
TraumaCal®	liquid	2000	1.50	83	145	69	560	Enriched with vitamins C, B-complex, and E and copper and zinc

Table K-2
Hydrolyzed Protein Formulas

Product	Form	Volume to Meet 100% RDI (ml)	Energy (kcal/ml)	Protein or Amino Acids (g/L)	Carbohydrate (g/L)	Fat (g/L)	Osmolality (mOsm/kg)	Notes
Formulas Containing 40 grams or Less Protein per Liter								
Criticare HN®	liquid	1890	1.06	38	220	5	650	50% free amino acids, 50% small peptides
L-Emental™	powder	N/A	1.00	38	205	3	630	100% free amino acids, enriched with glutamine
Peptamen	liquid	1500	1.00	40	127	39	325	Near-isotonic
PRO-Peptide™	liquid	1500	1.00	40	127	39	270	Isotonic, 70% fat from MCT, enriched with glutamine
Reabilan®	liquid	2000	1.00	32	132	53	350	50% fat from MCT
Tolerex®	powder	3160	1.00	21	230	1.5	550	100% free amino acids
Vivonex® T.E.N.	powder	2000	1.00	38	210	3.0	630	100% free amino acids, enriched with branched-chain amino acids
Formulas Containing More than 40 Grams Protein per Liter								
L-Emental™ Plus	powder	1800	1.00	45	190	7	650	100% free amino acids, enriched with glutamine
Peptamen VHP®	liquid	1500	1.00	63	105	39	365	70% fat from MCT
PRO-Peptide™ VHN	liquid	1500	1.00	62	104	39	300	Isotonic, 70% fat from MCT, enriched with glutamine
Reabilan® HN	liquid	1500	1.33	44	119	41	490	50% fat from MCT
SandoSource® Peptide	liquid	1750	1.00	50	160	17	490	60% free amino acids and small peptides
Vital® HN	powder	1500	1.00	42	185	11	500	87% hydrolyzed proteins, 13% essential amino acids
Special Use Hydrolyzed Formulas: Pediatric (1 to 10 years)								
L-Emental™ Pediatric	powder	1000* 1170**	0.8	24	130	24	360	100% free amino acids, contains glutamine
Peptamin Junior™	liquid	1000	1.0	30	138	39	310	60% fat from MCT
PRO-Peptide™ for Kids	liquid	1000**	1.0	30	138	39	360	40% fat from MCT, enriched with trace elements, taurine, and carnitine
Vivonex® Pediatric	powder	1000* 1170**	0.8	24	130	24	360	100% free amino acids

*Children 1 to 6 years old.
**Children 7 to 10 years old

K

K

Table K-2
Hydrolzed Protein Formulas (continued)

Product	Form	Volume to Meet 100% RDI (ml)	Energy (kcal/ml)	Protein or Amino Acids (g/L)	Carbohydrate (g/L)	Fat (g/L)	Osmolality (mOsm/kg)	Notes
Special Use Hydrolyzed Formulas: Hepatic Insufficiency								
Hepatic Aid® II	powder	—	1.20	44	169	36	560	Free amino acids, high in branched-chain amino acids, low in aromatic amino acids, no added vitamins or electrolytes.
L-Emental™ Hepatic	powder	N/A	1.20	44	169	36	560	Free amino acids, high in branched-chain amino acids, low in aromatic amino acids, contains vitamins and minimal electrolytes
NutriHep®	liquid	1000	1.50	40	290	21	690	Free amino acids, high in branched-chain amino acids, low in aromatic amino acids, contains vitamins and minimal electrolytes
Special Use Hydrolyzed Formulas: HIV Infection or AIDS								
Advera®	liquid	1184	1.28	60	216	23	680	78% hydrolyzed and 22% intact protein, low fat, fiber added,enriched with vitamins E, C, B_6, B_{12}, and folate
Special Use Hydrolyzed Formulas: Immune System Support								
Alitraq®	powder	1500	1.00	53	165	16	575	47% free amino acids, 42% small peptides, enriched with glutamine and arginine
Crucial®	liquid	1000	1.50	63	90	45	490	Enriched with arginine
Perative®	liquid	1155	1.30	67	177	37	385	Enriched with arginine and β-carotene
Vivonex® Plus	powder	1800	1.00	45	190	7	650	100% free amino acids, enriched with glutamine, arginine, and branched-chain amino acids

Table K–3
Protein Modules

Product	Form	Major Protein Source	Energy (kcal/g)	Protein (g/100 g)
Casec®	powder	Calcium caseinate	3.7	88
Pro Mod®	powder	Whey protein	4.2	75.8

Table K–4
Carbohydrate Modules

Product	Form	Major Carbohydrate Source	Energy (kcal/ml or g)
Moducal®	powder	Hydrolyzed corn starch	3.8 kcal/g
Polycose Liquid®	liquid	Hydrolyzed corn starch	2.0 kcal/ml
Polycose Powder®	powder	Hydrolyzed corn starch	3.8 kcal/g

Table K–5
Fat Modules

Product	Form	Major Fat Source	Energy (kcal/ml)	Fat (g/100 ml)
MCT Oil®	liquid	Derived from coconut oil	7.7	87
Microlipid®	liquid	Safflower oil	4.5	50

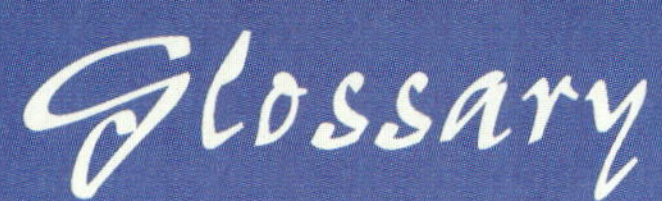

Many medical terms have their origins in Latin or Greek. By learning a few common derivations, you can glean the meaning of words you have never heard of before. For example, once you know that "hyper" means above normal, "glyc" means glucose, and "emia" means blood, you can easily determine that "hyperglycemia" means high blood glucose. The following derivations will help you to learn many terms presented in this glossary.

GENERAL

a or *an* = not or without
anti = against
di = two
dys or *mal* = bad
endo = inside or within
exo or *extra* = outside
genesis = gives rise to, making
homeo = the same
hyper = over, above normal, excessive
hypo = below normal, under, beneath
inter = between, in the midst
intra = within
-itis = infection or inflammation
-lysis = break
macro = large
micro = tiny
mono = one
neo = new
-osis = condition
peri = around
poly = many
pre or *pro* = before
-stasis = staying
tri = three

BODY

arterio = artery
cardiac or *cardio* = heart
cyte = cell
enteron = intestine
gastro = stomach
hemo or *-emia* = blood
hepatic = liver
myo = muscle
osteo = bone
pulmo = lung
renal = kidney
ure or *-uria* = urine
vaso = vessel
vena = vein

CHEMISTRY

-al = aldehyde
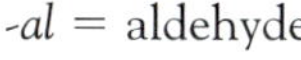
-ase = enzyme
-ate = salt
glyc or *gluc* = glucose
hydro or *hydrate* = water
lipo = lipid
-ol = alcohol
-ose = sugar
saccharide = sugar

abscess: an accumulation of pus, caused by a local infection, that builds up and may eventually burst.

absorption: the taking up of nutrients into the intestinal cells.

Acceptable Daily Intake: the amount of a sweetener that individuals can safely consume each day over the course of a lifetime without adverse effect. It includes a 100-fold safety factor.

accredited: approved; in the case of medical centers or universities, certified by an agency recognized by the U.S. Department of Education.

acesulfame potassium: a low-kcalorie sweetener recently approved by the FDA; also known as acesulfame-K, because K is the chemical symbol for potassium. Approved in Canada.

acetaldehyde: an intermediate in alcohol metabolism.

acetone breath: a distinctive fruity odor that can be detected on the breath of a person who is experiencing ketosis.

acetyl CoA: a 2-carbon compound (acetate, or acetic acid) to which a molecule of CoA is attached.

acid-base balance: the equilibrium in the body between acid and base concentrations.

acidosis: above-normal acidity in the blood and body fluids.

acids: compounds that release hydrogen ions in a solution.

acne: a chronic inflammation of the skin's follicles and oil-producing glands, which leads to an accumulation of oils inside the ducts that surround hairs; usually associated with the maturation of young adults.

acquired immune deficiency syndrome (AIDS): the end stage of HIV infection, in which severe complications are manifested.

active vitamin D: the 1,25-dihydroxy form of vitamin D that promotes calcium balance and bone mineralization.

acupuncture: a technique that involves piercing the skin with long thin needles at specific anatomical points to relieve pain or illness. Acupuncture sometimes uses heat, pressure, friction, suction, or electromagnetic energy to stimulate the points.

acute disease: a disease the develops quickly, produces sharp symptoms, and runs a short course.

acute PEM: protein-energy malnutrition caused by recent severe food restriction or hypermetabolism; characterized in children by thinness for height (wasting).

ADA: see *American Dietetic Association*.

adaptive thermogenesis: adjustments in energy expenditure related to changes in environment such as cold and to physiological events such as overfeeding, trauma, and changes in hormone status.

additives: substances not normally consumed as foods but added to food either intentionally or by accident.

adenomas: cancers that arise from glandular tissues.

adenosine triphosphate: see *ATP*.

adequacy (dietary): providing all the essential nutrients, fiber, and energy in amounts sufficient to maintain health.

ADH: see *antidiuretic hormone*.

ADI: see *Acceptable Daily Intake*.

adipose tissue: the body's fat tissue, which consists of masses of fat-storing cells.

adolescence: the period from the beginning of puberty until maturity.

adrenal glands: glands adjacent to, and just above, each kidney.

advance directive: the means by which competent adults record their preferences for future medical interventions. The living will and durable power of attorney are types of advance directives.

adverse reactions: unusual responses to food (including intolerances and allergies).

aerobic: requiring oxygen.

aflatoxin: potent cancer-causing toxin produced by the mold *Aspergillus flavus* that infects grains and peanuts. The USDA tests grains and peanuts grown in this country for aflatoxin contamination.

AIDS: see *acquired immune deficiency syndrome*.

AIDS enteropathies: the diarrhea and malabsorption associated with AIDS for which no known cause has been identified.

AIDS-related complex (ARC): the cluster of mild symptoms that sometimes occur early in the course of HIV infection.

albuminuria: loss of the protein albumin in the urine.

alcohol dehydrogenase: an enzyme that converts ethanol to acetaldehyde; see also *MEOS*.

alcohol: a class of organic compounds containing hydroxyl (OH) groups.

aldosterone: a hormone secreted by the adrenal glands that stimulates the reabsorption of sodium by the kidneys; aldosterone also regulates chloride and potassium concentrations.

alimentary (or postgastrectomy) hypoglycemia: the type of hypoglycemia that occurs following gastric surgery.

alitame: a compound of two amino acids (alanine and aspartic acid) that is 2000 times sweeter than sucrose; FDA approval pending.

alkalosis: above-normal alkalinity (base) in the blood and body fluids.

alpha-lactalbumin: the chief protein in human breast milk, as opposed to *casein*, the chief protein in cow's milk.

alpha-tocopherol: the most biologically active vitamin E compound.

alternative therapies: approaches to medical diagnosis and treatment that are not fully accepted by the established medical community; as such, they are not widely taught at U.S. medical schools or practiced in U.S. hospitals; also called *adjunctive*, *unconventional*, or *unorthodox* therapies.

alveoli: air sacs in the lungs; one sac is an *alveolus*.

Alzheimer's disease: see *senile dementia of the Alzheimer's type*.

amenorrhea: the absence of or cessation of menstruation. *Primary amenorrhea* is menarche delayed beyond 16 years of age. *Secondary amenorrhea* is the absence of three to six consecutive menstrual cycles.

American Dietetic Association: the professional organization of dietitians in the United States. The Canadian equivalent is the Dietitians of Canada (DC), which operates similarly.

amino acids: building blocks of proteins; each contains an amino group, an acid group, a hydrogen atom, and a distinctive side group attached to a central carbon atom.

amino acid scoring: a method of evaluating protein quality by comparing a test protein's amino acid pattern with that of a reference protein; sometimes called *chemical scoring*.

ammonia: a compound with the chemical formula NH_3; produced during the deamination of amino acids.

amniotic sac: the "bag of waters" in the uterus, in which the fetus floats.

amylase: an enzyme that hydrolyzes amylose (a form of starch). Amylase is a carbohydrase, an enzyme that breaks down carbohydrates.

anabolism: reactions in which small molecules are put together to build larger ones. Anabolic reactions require energy.

anaerobic: not requiring oxygen.

anemia: literally, "too little blood." Anemia is any condition in which too few red blood cells are present, or the red blood cells are immature (and therefore large) or too small or contain too little hemoglobin to carry the normal amount of oxygen to the tissues. It is not a disease itself but can be a symptom of many different disease conditions, including many nutrient deficiencies, bleeding, excessive red blood cell destruction, and defective red blood cell formation.

angina: a painful feeling of tightness or pressure, felt in the area in and around the heart, often radiating to the back, neck, and arms; caused by a lack of oxygen to an area of heart muscle.

angiotensin: a blood protein that helps to raise blood pressure.

angiotensinogen: precursor protein for angiotensin.

anions: negatively charged ions.

anorexia nervosa: an eating disorder characterized by a refusal to maintain a minimally normal body weight and a distortion in perception of body shape and weight, most commonly seen in teenage girls and young women.

antacids: acid-buffering agents used to counter excess acidity in the stomach.

antagonist: a competing factor that counteracts the action of another factor. When a drug displaces a vitamin from its site of action, the drug renders the vitamin ineffective and thus acts as a vitamin antagonist.

anthropometric: relating to measurement of the physical characteristics of the body, such as height and weight.

antibodies: large proteins of the blood and body fluids, produced by the immune system in response to the invasion of the body by foreign molecules (usually proteins called *antigens*); antibodies combine with and inactivate the foreign invaders, thus protecting the body.

antidiarrheal agents: drugs used to treat diarrhea.

antidiuretic hormone (ADH): a hormone produced by the pituitary gland in response to dehydration (or a high sodium concentration in the blood); it stimulates the kidneys to reabsorb more water and therefore to excrete less. This ADH should not be confused with the enzyme alcohol dehydrogenase, which is sometimes also abbreviated ADH.

antigen: a substance that elicits the formation of antibodies or an inflammation reaction from the immune system. A bacterium, a virus, a toxin, and a protein in food that causes allergy are all examples of foreign antigens.

antimicrobial agents: preservatives that prevent microorganisms from growing.

antioxidant: a compound that protects others from oxidation by being oxidized itself. An antioxidant donates electrons to another substance; that substance becomes reduced as the antioxidant simultaneously becomes oxidized. Chemists describe the antioxidant action of vitamin C as maintaining the "oxidation-reduction equilibrium," or "redox state."

antipromoters: factors that oppose the development of cancer.

antiscorbutic factor: the original name for vitamin C.

antisense gene: the chemical opposite of a native gene that adheres to the native working gene and blocks its production of proteins.

anuria: no urine excretion.

anus: the terminal sphincter of the GI tract.

appendix: a narrow blind sac extending from the beginning of the colon; a vestigial organ with no known function.

appetite: the psychological desire to eat or an interest in food; a positive sensation that accompanies the sight, smell, or thought of food.

arachidonic acid: an omega-6 polyunsaturated fatty acid with 20 carbons and four double bonds (20:4); synthesized from linoleic acid.

aroma therapy: a technique that uses oil extracts from plants and flowers (usually applied by massage or baths) to enhance physical, psychological, and spiritual health.

artery: a vessel that carries blood away from the heart.

artesian water: water that is drawn from a well that taps a confined aquifer in which the water level stands above the natural water table.

arthritis: a usually painful inflammation of a joint caused by many conditions, including infections, metabolic disturbances, or injury; joint structure is usually altered, with loss of function.

artificial colors: certified food colors added to enhance appearance. (*Certified* means approved by the FDA.)

artificial feeding: feeding by tube or by vein.

artificial flavors, flavor enhancers: chemicals that mimic natural flavors and those that enhance flavor.

artificial sweeteners: sugar substitutes that provide no energy; sometimes called *nonnutritive sweeteners*.

ascites: a type of edema characterized by the accumulation of fluid in the abdominal cavity.

ascorbic acid: one of the two active forms of vitamin C. Many people refer to vitamin C by this name.

-ase: a word ending denoting an enzyme. Enzymes are often identified by the place they come from and the compounds they work on; *gastric lipase*, for example, is a stomach enzyme that acts on lipids, whereas *pancreatic lipase* comes from the pancreas (and also works on lipids).

aspartame: a compound of two amino acids (phenylalanine and aspartic acid) that tastes like the sugar sucrose but is much sweeter. It provides 4 kcalories per gram, as does protein, but because so little is used, it is virtually kcalorie-free. In powdered form it is sometimes mixed with lactose, however, so a 1-gram packet may provide 4 kcalories. It is used in both the United States and Canada.

aspiration: to draw in by suction, as may occur when food or liquid is sucked into the lungs.

aspiration pneumonia: an infection of the lungs caused by inhaling fluids regurgitated from the stomach. Aspiration pneumonia can be a fatal complication of a tube feeding.

-ate: a word ending denoting a salt of the mineral.

atherosclerosis: a type of artery disease characterized by accumulations of lipid-containing material on the inner walls of the arteries.

atom: the smallest component of an element that has all of the properties of the element.

ATP (adenosine triphosphate): a common high-energy compound composed of a purine (adenine), a sugar (ribose), and three phosphate groups.

atrophic gastritis: chronic inflammation of the stomach accompanied by a diminished size and functioning of the mucosa and glands.

atrophy: of muscles, a decrease in size because of disuse, undernutrition, or wasting diseases.

attention deficit hyperactivity disorder (ADHD): hyperactivity accompanied by an inability to pay attention and poor impulse control.

autoimmune disorders: immune system disorders in which the body destroys its own tissues.

available carbohydrates: carbohydrates such as starch and sugar that human digestive enzymes make available to the body.

avidin: a protein in egg whites that binds biotin.

ayurveda: a traditional Hindu system of improving health by using herbs, diet, meditation, massage, and yoga to stimulate the body to make its own natural drugs.

balance (dietary): providing foods of a number of types in proportion to each other, such that foods rich in some nutrients do not crowd out foods that are rich in other nutrients.

basal metabolic rate (BMR): the rate of energy use for metabolism under basal conditions, usually expressed as kcalories per kilogram body weight per hour.

basal metabolism: the energy needed to maintain life when a body is at complete rest after a 12-hour fast (to exclude the thermic effect of the previous meal).

bases: compounds that accept hydrogen ions in a solution.

beer: an alcoholic beverage brewed by fermenting malt and hops.

behavior modification: the changing of behavior by the manipulation of *antecedents* (cues or environmental factors that trigger behavior), the *behavior* itself, and *consequences* (the penalties or rewards attached to behavior).

beikost: supplemental, or weaning, foods.

belch: the expulsion of gas from the stomach through the mouth.

benign: tumors that stop growing without intervention or can be removed surgically and pose no threat to health.

beriberi: the thiamin-deficiency disease; it pointed the way to discovery of the first vitamin, thiamin.

beta-carotene: an orange pigment and vitamin A precursor found in plants.

BGH: see *bovine growth hormone*.

BHA and **BHT:** preservatives commonly used to slow the development of off-flavors, odors, and color changes caused by oxidation.

bicarbonate: an alkaline secretion of the pancreas, part of the pancreatic juice. (Bicarbonate also occurs widely in all cell fluids.)

bifidus factors: factors in colostrum and breast milk that favor the growth of the "friendly" bacterium *Lactobacillus bifidus* in the infant's intestinal tract, so that other, less desirable intestinal inhabitants will not flourish.

bile: an emulsifier that prepares fats and oils for digestion; an exocrine secretion made by the liver, stored in the gallbladder, and released into the small intestine when needed.

bilirubin: a pigment in the bile whose concentration in the blood may rise as a result of some disorders.

binders: chemical compounds occurring in foods that can combine with nutrients (especially minerals) to form complexes the body cannot absorb. Examples of such binders include *phytic acid* and *oxalic acid*.

bioaccumulation: the accumulation of contaminants in the flesh of animals high on the food chain.

bioavailability: the rate and extent to which a nutrient is absorbed.

bioelectrical impedance: a method for estimating body fat using low-intensity electrical current.

bioelectromagnetic medical applications: the use of electrical energy, magnetic energy, or both to stimulate bone repair, wound healing, and tissue regeneration.

biofeedback: the use of special devices to convey information about heart rate, blood pressure, skin temperature, muscle relaxation, and the like to enable a person to learn how to consciously control these medically important functions.

biofield therapeutics: a manual healing method that directs a healing force from an outside source (commonly God or another supernatural being) through the practitioner and into the client's body; commonly known as "laying on of hands."

biological value (BV): the amount of protein nitrogen that is retained for growth and maintenance, expressed as a percentage of the protein nitrogen that has been digested and absorbed; a measure of protein quality.

biosensor: a genetically altered microbe that provides a rapid, low-cost, and accurate test for the products of spoilage in foods.

biotechnology: the use of biological systems or organisms to create or modify products; also called *biogenetic engineering*.

biotin: a B vitamin that functions as a coenzyme in the metabolism of carbohydrates and fats.

blind experiment: an experiment in which the subjects do not know whether they are members of the experimental group or the control group.

blood lipid profile: results of blood tests that reveal a person's total cholesterol, triglycerides, and various lipoproteins.

BMI: see *body mass index*.

BMR: see *basal metabolic rate*.

body composition: the proportions of muscle, bone, fat, and other tissue that make up a person's total body weight.

body mass index (BMI): an index of a person's weight in relation to height, determined by dividing the weight (in kilograms) by the square of the height (in meters).

bolus: a portion; with respect to food, the amount swallowed at one time.

bolus feeding: delivery of about 300 to 400 ml of a tube feeding over 10 minutes or less.

bomb calorimeter: an instrument that measures the *heat* energy released when foods are burned, thus providing an estimate of the potential energy of foods.

bone density: a measure of bone strength. When minerals fill the bone matrix, they give it strength.

bone marrow transplant: the replacement of diseased bone marrow in a recipient with healthy bone marrow from a donor; used as a treatment for breast cancer, leukemia, and other blood disorders.

borderline diabetes: impaired glucose tolerance.

botulin: the toxin responsible for botulism.

botulism: an often fatal food-borne illness caused by the ingestion of foods containing a toxin produced by bacteria that grow in improperly canned acidic foods.

bovine growth hormone (BGH): a hormone produced naturally in the pituitary gland of a cow that promotes growth and milk production; now produced for agricultural use by transgenic bacteria.

bran: the protective coating around the kernel similar in function to the shell of a nut; rich in nutrients and fiber.

bronchitis: inflammation of the lungs' air passages.

brown sugar: refined white sugar crystals to which manufacturers have added molasses syrup with natural flavor and color; 91 to 96 percent pure sucrose.

buffers: compounds that help keep a solution's acidity or alkalinity constant.

bulimia nervosa: an eating disorder characterized by repeated episodes of binge eating usually followed by self-induced vomiting, misuse of laxatives or diuretics, fasting, or excessive exercise.

calcitonin: a hormone from the thyroid gland that lowers blood calcium by inhibiting its release from bone.

calcitriol: the active form of supplemental vitamin D.

calcium: the most abundant mineral in the body, found primarily in the body's bones and teeth.

calcium-binding protein: a protein in the intestinal cells, made with the help of vitamin D, that facilitates calcium absorption.

calcium rigor: hardness or stiffness of the muscles caused by high blood calcium concentrations.

calcium tetany: intermittent spasm of the extremities due to nervous and muscular excitability caused by low blood calcium concentrations.

calmodulin: an inactive protein that becomes active when bound to calcium; then it becomes a messenger that tells other proteins what to do. The system serves as interpreter for hormone- and nerve-mediated messages arriving at cells.

calorie: a unit by which energy is measured. Food energy is measured in *kilocalories* (1000 calories equal 1 kilocalorie), abbreviated *kcalories* or *kcal*. A capitalized version is also sometimes used: *Calories*. One kcalorie is the amount of heat necessary to raise the temperature of 1 kilogram (kg) of water 1°C.

cancer cachexia syndrome: a syndrome that frequently accompanies many types of cancer; characterized by anorexia, inadequate intake of food, malnutrition, accelerated metabolism and wasting, and general ill health.

cancers: diseases that result from the unchecked growth of malignant tumors.

capillary: a small vessel that branches from an artery. Capillaries connect arteries to veins. Exchange of oxygen, nutrients, and waste materials takes place across capillary walls.

carbohydrase: an enzyme that hydrolyzes carbohydrates.

carbohydrate loading: a regimen of exhaustive exercise followed by the consumption of a high-carbohydrate diet that enables muscles to store glycogen beyond their normal capacity; also called *glycogen loading* or *glycogen supercompensation*.

carbohydrates: compounds composed of carbon, oxygen, and hydrogen arranged as monosaccharides or multiples of monosaccharides.

carbonic acid: a compound with the formula H_2CO_3 that results from the combination of carbon dioxide (CO_2) and water (H_2O), of particular importance in the body's buffer system.

carcinogens: agents that can give rise to cancer.

carcinomas: cancers that arise from epithelial tissues.

cardiac cachexia: chronic PEM that develops as a consequence of heart disease.

cardiac sphincter: the sphincter muscle at the junction between the esophagus and the stomach; also called the *lower esophageal sphincter* or the *gastroesophageal sphincter*.

cardiomegaly: enlargement of the heart.

cardiovascular disease (CVD): a general term for all diseases of the heart and blood vessels. Atherosclerosis is the main cause of CVD.

carotene: a vitamin A precursor found in plants; an orange pigment.

carotenoids: pigments commonly found in plants and animals, some of which have provitamin A activity. Carotenoids are among the best-known *phytochemicals*—plant chemicals that are not nutrients but have biological activity in the body.

carotid endartectomy: surgery to restore blood flow through the carotid artery to the brain.

carpal tunnel syndrome: a pinched nerve at the wrist, causing pain or numbness in the hand.

carrier: an individual who possesses one dominant and one recessive gene for a recessive trait, such as an inborn error of metabolism. Such a person may show no signs of the trait but can pass it on.

cartilage therapy: the use of cleaned and powdered connective tissue, such as collagen, to improve health.

cash crops: crops grown for cash, as opposed to crops grown for food; examples include cotton and tobacco.

catabolism: reactions in which large molecules are broken down to smaller ones. Catabolic reactions usually release energy.

catalyst: a compound that facilitates chemical reactions without itself being changed in the process.

cataracts: thickenings of the eye lenses that impair vision and can lead to blindness.

cathartic: a strong laxative.

cations: positively charged ions.

CCK: see *cholecystokinin*.

CDC: see *Centers for Disease Control*.

CD4+ T-lymphocyte: a type of circulating white blood cell that has the CD4+ protein on its surface and is a necessary component of the immune system.

celiac disease: a sensitivity to gliadin that causes flattening of the intestinal villi and generalized malabsorption; also called *gluten-sensitive enteropathy* or *celiac sprue*.

cellulite: supposedly, a lumpy form of fat; actually, a fraud. The lumpy appearance in fatty areas of the body is caused by strands of connective tissue that attach the skin to underlying muscles. These points of attachment may pull tight where the fat is thick, making lumps appear between them. The fat itself is not different from fat anywhere else in the body. So, if the fat in these areas is lost, the lumpy appearance disappears.

Centers for Disease Control: a branch of the Department of Health and Human Services that is responsible for, among other things, monitoring food-borne diseases.

central obesity: excess fat around the trunk of the body; also called *abdominal fat* or *upper-body fat*.

central total parenteral nutrition (TPN): a method for meeting all nutrient needs by infusing formula into a large-diameter central vein.

central veins: the large-diameter veins located close to the heart.

cerebral cortex: the outer surface of the cerebrum.

certification: the process in which a private laboratory inspects shipments of a product for selected chemicals and then, if the product is free of violative levels of those chemicals, issues a guarantee to that effect.

cesarean section: a surgically assisted birth involving removal of the fetus by an incision into the uterus, usually by way of the abdominal wall.

CHD: see *coronary heart disease*.

chelate: a substance that can grasp the positive ions of a metal.

chelation therapy: the use of ethylene diamine tetraacetic acid (EDTA) to bind with metallic ions, thus healing the body by removing toxic metals.

chemical scoring: see *amino acid scoring*.

chemotherapy: the use of drugs to arrest or destroy cancer cells. Drugs used for chemotherapy are called *chemotherapeutic* or *antineoplastic agents*.

CHF: see *congestive heart failure*.

Chinese restaurant syndrome: an intolerance reaction that may occur in 1 to 2 percent of the population 20 minutes after the ingestion of the additive MSG (monosodium glutamate). Symptoms include burning sensations, chest and facial flushing and pain, and throbbing headaches.

chiropractic: a manual healing method of manipulating vertebrae to relieve musculoskeletal pain suspected of causing problems with internal organs.

chloride: the major anion in the extracellular fluids of the body. Chloride is the ionic form of chlorine, Cl^-; see Appendix B for a description of the chlorine-to-chloride conversion.

chlorophyll: the green pigment of plants, which absorbs photons and transfers their energy to other molecules, thereby initiating photosynthesis.

cholecalciferol: vitamin D; also known as vitamin D_3.

cholecystokinin (CCK): a hormone produced by cells of the intestinal wall. Target organ: the gallbladder. Response: release of bile and slowing of GI motility.

cholesterol: one of the sterols.

choline: a nonessential nutrient that can be made in the body from an amino acid. Choline is used to make the phospholipid lecithin and the neurotransmitter acetylcholine.

chronic disease: a disease of long duration that progresses slowly, often characterized by deterioration of the body organs; also called *chronic, noncommunicable diseases (NCD)*. Examples include heart disease, cancer, and diabetes.

chronic obstructive pulmonary disease (COPD): one of several disorders, including emphysema and bronchitis, that interfere with respiration.

chronic PEM: protein-energy malnutrition caused by long-term food deprivation; characterized in children by short height for age (stunting).

chronological age: a person's age in years from his or her date of birth.

chylomicrons: the class of lipoproteins that transport lipids from the intestinal cells into the body.

chyme: the semiliquid mass of partly digested food expelled by the stomach into the duodenum.

cirrhosis: advanced liver disease in which liver cells turn orange, die, and harden, permanently losing their function; often associated with alcoholism.

clinically severe obesity: a BMI of 40 or greater or 100 pounds or more overweight for an average adult. A less preferred term used to describe the same condition is *morbid obesity*.

CoA: coenzyme A; the coenzyme derived from the B vitamin pantothenic acid and central to the energy metabolism of nutrients.

coenzymes: small organic molecules that work with enzymes to facilitate the enzymes' activity. Many coenzymes have B vitamins as part of their structures.

cofactor: a mineral element that, like a coenzyme, works with an enzyme to facilitate a chemical reaction. The cofactor maintains the structural integrity of the enzyme and may also facilitate the enzyme's catalytic activity.

collagen: the protein material from which connective tissues such as scars, tendons, ligaments, and the foundations of bones and teeth are made.

collaterals: small blood vessels that develop to divert blood flow away from an obstructed organ; also called *shunts*.

colon: see *large intestine*.

colonic irrigation: the popular, but potentially harmful practice of "washing" the large intestine with a powerful enema machine.

colostomate: a person who has a surgically formed opening from the colon to the outside of the body (a colostomy).

colostrum: a milklike secretion from the breast, present during the first day or so after delivery before milk appears; rich in protective factors.

comatose: in a state of deep unconsciousness from which the person cannot be aroused.

competent: having sufficient mental ability to understand a treatment, weigh its risks and benefits, and comprehend the consequences of refusing or accepting the treatment.

complementary proteins: two or more proteins whose amino acid assortments complement each other in such a way that the essential amino acids missing from one are supplied by the other.

complete formulas: enteral formulas designed to supply all needed nutrients when given in sufficient volume.

complete protein: a dietary protein containing all the amino acids essential in human nutrition in amounts adequate for human use.

complex carbohydrates (starches and fibers): polysaccharides composed of straight or branched chains of monosaccharides.

compound: a substance composed of two or more different atoms—for example, water (H_2O).

condensation: a chemical reaction in which two reactants combine to yield a larger product.

conditionally essential amino acid: an amino acid that is normally nonessential, but must be supplied by the diet in special circumstances when the need for it exceeds the body's ability to produce it.

cones: the cells of the retina that respond to bright light and are responsible for color vision.

confectioners' sugar: finely powdered sucrose; 99.9 percent pure.

congestive heart failure (CHF): a syndrome in which the heart can no longer adequately pump blood through the circulatory system.

congregate meal sites: nutrition programs that provide food for the elderly in a conveniently located setting such as a community center.

constipation: the condition of having painful or difficult bowel movements (elapsed time between movements is not relevant).

contaminant: a substance that does not normally occur in a food.

contamination iron: iron found in foods as the result of contamination by inorganic iron salts from iron cookware, iron-containing soils, and the like.

control group: a group of individuals similar in all possible respects to the experimental group except for the treatment. Ideally, the control group receives a placebo while the experimental group receives a real treatment.

COPD: see *chronic obstructive pulmonary disease*.

Cori cycle: the path from muscle glycogen to glucose to pyruvate to lactic acid (which travels to the liver) to glucose (which can travel back to the muscle) to glycogen; named after the scientist who elucidated this pathway.

corn sweeteners: corn syrup and sugars derived from corn.

corn syrup: a syrup produced by the action of enzymes on cornstarch; contains mostly glucose. See also *high-fructose corn syrup (HFCS)*.

cornea: the transparent membrane covering the outside of the eye.

coronary artery bypass graft (CABG): surgery to restore blood flow to the heart muscle to prevent a heart attack.

coronary heart disease (CHD): insufficient delivery of oxygen to the heart that occurs when the arteries that carry blood to the heart muscle become occluded.

correlation: the simultaneous increase, decrease, or change of two variables. If A increases as B increases, or if A decreases as B decreases, the correlation is positive. (This does not mean that A causes B or vice versa.) If A increases as B decreases, or if A decreases as B increases, the correlation is negative. (This does not mean that A prevents B or vice versa.) Some third factor may account for both A and B.

correspondence school: a school that offers courses and degrees by mail. Some correspondence schools are accredited; others are *diploma mills*.

cortical bone: the ivorylike outer bone layer that forms a shell surrounding trabecular bone and comprises the shaft of a long bone.

counterregulatory hormones: hormones such as glucagon, cortisol, and catecholamines that oppose insulin's actions and promote catabolism.

coupled reactions: pairs of chemical reactions in which energy released from the breakdown of one compound is used to create a bond in the formation of another compound.

covert: hidden, as if under covers.

cretinism: an iodine-deficiency disease characterized by mental and physical retardation.

critical periods: finite periods during development in which certain events may occur that will have irreversible effects on later developmental stages. In a body organ, a critical period is usually a period of rapid cell division.

Crohn's disease: inflammation and ulceration along the length of the GI tract, often with granulomas; also called *regional ileitis*.

crypts: tubular glands that lie between the intestinal villi and secrete intestinal juices into the small intestine.

cuisine: style of cooking or preparing food.

CVD: see *cardiovascular disease*.

cyanosis: a bluish discoloration of the skin caused by a lack of oxygen.

cyclamate: a 0-kcalorie sweetener; FDA approval pending in the United States; available in Canada on grocery-store shelves but only as a tabletop sweetener, not as an additive.

cystic fibrosis: a hereditary disorder characterized by the production of thick mucus that affects many organs, including the lungs, pancreas, liver, heart, gallbladder, and small intestine.

cystinuria: the presence of cystine in the urine; the symptom of an inherited metabolic disorder in which large amounts of the amino acids cystine, lysine, arginine, and ornithine are excreted in the urine. Cystinuria commonly results in kidney stone formation.

cytokines: immune system factors that help to control the inflammatory response.

D, L: *D* stands for *dextro*, or "right-handed," and *L*, for *levo*, or "left-handed," referring to the shapes of the molecules, which are mirror images of each other.

Daily Reference Values (DRV): a set of standards for nutrients and food components (such as fat and fiber) that have important relationships with health; used on food labels as part of the Daily Values.

Daily Values (DV): reference values developed by the FDA specifically for use on food labels. The Daily Values represent two sets of standards: Reference Daily Intakes (RDI) and Daily Reference Values (DRV).

dawn phenomenon: early morning hyperglycemia that develops in IDDM in response to counterregulatory hormones that act to raise glucose levels during an overnight fast.

deamination: removal of the amino (NH_2) group from a compound such as an amino acid.

death: permanent cessation of vital functions.

debridement: the removal of dead tissue resulting from burns and other wounds; speeds healing and helps prevent infection.

defecate: to move the bowels and eliminate waste.

deficient: the amount of a nutrient below which *almost all healthy people* can be expected, over time, to experience deficiency symptoms.

dehydration: the condition in which body water output exceeds water input.

Delaney Clause: a clause in the Food Additive Amendment to the Food, Drug, and Cosmetic Act that states that no substance that is known to cause cancer in animals or human beings at any dose level shall be added to foods.

denaturation: the change in a protein's shape brought about by heat, acid, base, alcohol, heavy metals, or other agents.

dental caries: decay of teeth.

dextrins: short chains of glucose that result from the breakdown of starch.

dextrose: an older name for glucose.

dextrose monohydrate: the form of glucose used in IV solutions. Dextrose solutions provide 3.4 kcal/g, whereas glucose provides 4 kcal/g.

DHEA (dehydroepiandrosterone): a hormone secreted by the adrenal glands. DHEA is available without prescription and is sold as an anti-aging remedy to improve energy, strength, and immunity. Proof of safety or effectiveness is lacking.

diabetes mellitus: a metabolic disorder characterized by altered blood glucose regulation and utilization, usually caused by insufficient or relatively ineffective insulin.

diabetic coma: unconsciousness precipitated by hyperglycemia, dehydration, ketosis, and acidosis in uncontrolled IDDM.

diagnosis: the disease a person has or is thought to have.

dialysis: removal of waste from the blood using the principles of simple diffusion and osmosis through a semipermeable membrane.

diarrhea: the frequent passage of watery bowel movements.

diet: the foods and beverages a person eats and drinks.

diet history: a record of eating behaviors and the foods a person eats.

diet manual: a book that describes the foods allowed and restricted on a diet, outlines the rationale and indications for use of each diet, and provides sample menus.

diet order: a physician's written statement in the medical record of what diet a client should receive.

Dietary Reference Intakes (DRI): the revised set of dietary recommendations that will replace the RDA; see inside front cover, left.

dietetic technician registered (DTR): a person with an associate's degree and training in nutrition, food science, and diet planning who works under the guidance of an RD (registered dietitian).

dietitian: a person trained in nutrition, food science, and diet planning. See also *registered dietitian*.

differentiation: development of specific functions different from those of the original.

digestion: the process by which food is broken down into absorbable units.

digestive enzymes: proteins found in digestive juices that act on food substances, causing them to break down into simpler compounds.

diglyceride: a molecule of glycerol with two fatty acids attached.

diketopiperazine (DKP): a product to which aspartame breaks down during metabolism.

dioxins: any of 75 structurally related compounds that contain both nitrogen and chlorine.

dipeptide: two amino acids bonded together.

direct calorimetry: the measurement of energy output as heat energy.

disaccharide: a pair of monosaccharides linked together.

dissociation: the physical separation of a compound into ions.

distilled liquor: an alcoholic beverage made by fermenting and distilling grains; sometimes called *distilled spirits* or *hard liquor*.

distilled water: water that has been vaporized and recondensed, leaving it free of dissolved minerals.

diuretics: a drug that promotes water excretion; popularly, a "water pill."

diuretic phase: the phase of renal failure characterized by large fluid and electrolyte losses in the urine.

diverticula: a sac or pouch that develops in the weakened areas of the intestinal wall (like bulges in an inner tube where the tire wall is weak).

diverticulitis: diverticula that have become infected or inflamed and may rupture.

diverticulosis: the condition of having diverticula.

docosahexaenoic acid (DHA): an omega-3 polyunsaturated fatty acid with 22 carbons and six double bonds (22:6); synthesized from linolenic acid.

dominant gene: a gene that has an observable effect on an organism even when it is paired with a normal gene; see also *recessive gene*.

double-blind experiment: an experiment in which neither the subjects nor the researchers know which subjects are members of the experimental group and which are serving as control subjects until after the experiment is over.

Down syndrome: a genetic abnormality that causes mental retardation, short stature, and flattened facial features.

DRI: see *Dietary Reference Intakes*.

drink: a dose of any alcoholic beverage that delivers ½ ounce of pure ethanol.

drug: a substance that can modify one or more of the body's functions.

drug history: a record of all the medications, over-the-counter and prescribed, that a person takes routinely.

DRV: see *Daily Reference Values*.

DTR: see *dietetic technician registered*.

dumping syndrome: the symptoms that result from the rapid emptying of undigested food into the jejunum: sweating, weakness, and diarrhea shortly after eating and hypoglycemia later. Dumping syndrome is common following pyloroplasties, vagotomies, total gastrectomies, and gastric bypass surgery.

duodenum: the top portion of the small intestine (about "12 fingers' breadth" long in ancient terminology).

durable power of attorney: a legal document in which one competent adult authorizes another competent adult to make decisions for her or him in the event of incapacitation. The phrase "durable power" means that the agent's authority survives the client's incompetence; "attorney" refers to an attorney-in-fact (not an attorney-at-law).

DV: see *Daily Values*.

dysentery: an infection of the digestive tract that causes diarrhea.

dyslipidemia: abnormal blood lipids; elevated LDL and low HDL are examples.

dyspepsia: vague abdominal pain; a symptom, not a disease.

dysphagia: difficulty in swallowing.

dysuria: painful or difficult urination.

eating disorder: a disturbance in eating behavior that jeopardizes a person's physical or psychological health.

eclampsia: a condition characterized by convulsions and coma that develops in some women with untreated preeclampsia.

edema: the swelling of body tissue caused by excessive amounts of fluid in the interstitial spaces; seen in protein deficiency (among other conditions).

edentulous: without teeth.

eicosanoids: derivatives of fatty acids; hormonelike compounds that regulate blood pressure, clotting, and other body functions. They include *prostaglandins*, *thromboxanes*, and *leukotrienes*.

eicosapentaenoic acid (EPA): an omega-3 polyunsaturated fatty acid with 20 carbons and five double bonds (20:5); synthesized from linolenic acid.

electrolyte solutions: solutions that can conduct electricity due to the presence of ions.

electrolytes: salts that dissolve in water and dissociate.

element: a substance composed of atoms that are alike—for example, iron (Fe).

embolism: the obstruction of a blood vessel by a blood clot or foreign substance causing sudden tissue death.

embolus: a blood clot or other undissolved mass traveling in the circulatory system.

embryo: the developing infant from two to eight weeks after conception.

emetic: an agent that causes vomiting.

emphysema: a type of COPD in which the lungs lose their elasticity and the victim has difficulty breathing; often occurs along with bronchitis.

empty-kcalorie food: a popular term used to denote foods that contribute energy but lack protein, vitamins, and minerals. Empty-kcalorie foods are *low–nutrient density foods*. The most notorious empty-kcalorie foods are sugar, fat, and alcohol.

emulsifier: a substance with both water-soluble and fat-soluble portions that promotes the mixing of oils and fats in a watery solution.

endocrine glands: glands that secrete juices "into" the blood.

endogenous: made in the body.

endogenous protein: the protein in the body. In contrast, protein in foods is *exogenous protein*.

endosperm: the bulk of the edible part of the kernel containing starch and proteins.

end-stage renal disease: the severe stage of renal failure in which dialysis or a kidney transplant is necessary to sustain life.

energy: the capacity to do work. The energy in food is chemical energy. The body can convert this chemical energy to mechanical, electrical, or heat energy.

energy metabolism: all the reactions by which the body obtains and spends the energy from food.

energy-yielding nutrients: the nutrients that break down to yield energy the body can use; carbohydrate, fat, protein.

enriched: the addition of nutrients to a food to meet a specified standard; often used interchangeably with *fortified*.

enteral formulas: liquid diets intended for oral use or for tube feedings.

enteric hyperoxaluria: a condition of excess oxalate absorption that comes about because calcium is unable to bind oxalate in the gut; may lead to kidney stone formation.

enterogastrone: a gastrointestinal hormone.

enterohepatic circulation (of bile): the recycling of cholesterol and bile through the intestine and liver.

enteropancreatic circulation: the circulatory route from the pancreas to the intestine and back to the pancreas.

enterostomal therapist (ET): a health care professional specially trained to assist ostomates in learning the proper methods of caring for ostomy sites and adjusting to the ostomy.

enterostomy: a gastric or jejunal opening made surgically or under local anesthesia through which a feeding tube can be passed.

Environmental Protection Agency: a federal agency that is responsible for, among other things, regulating pesticides and establishing water quality standards.

enzyme replacements: extracts of pork or beef pancreatic enzymes that are taken as supplements to help with digestion.

enzymes: proteins that facilitate chemical reactions without being changed in the process; protein catalysts.

EPA: see *Environmental Protection Agency*.

epigastric: the region of the body just above the stomach.

epiglottis: cartilage in the throat that guards the entrance to the trachea and prevents fluid or food from entering it when a person swallows.

epinephrine: a hormone of the adrenal gland that modulates the stress response; formerly called *adrenaline*.

epithelial cells: cells on the surface of the skin and mucous membranes.

epithelial tissues: the layers of the body that serve as selective barriers between the body's interior and the environment (examples are the cornea, the skin, the respiratory lining, and the lining of the digestive tract).

ergocalciferol: the plant version of vitamin D; also known as vitamin D_2.

erythrocyte: red blood cell.

erythrocyte hemolysis: the breaking open of red blood cells; a symptom of vitamin E–deficiency disease in human beings.

erythrocyte protoporphyrin: a precursor to hemoglobin.

erythropoietin: a hormone secreted by the kidneys in response to oxygen depletion or anemia that stimulates the bone marrow to produce red blood cells.

esophageal stricture: narrowing of the esophagus that occurs when scar tissue forms in response to the continuous reflux of gastric juice.

esophageal ulcers: lesions or sores in the lining of the esophagus.

esophageal varices: tangles of distended blood vessels that protrude into the esophagus.

esophagus: the food pipe; the conduit from the mouth to the stomach.

essential amino acids: amino acids that the body cannot synthesize in amounts sufficient to meet physiological needs. Some researchers refer to essential amino acids as *indispensable* and to nonessential amino acids as *dispensable*.

essential fatty acids: fatty acids needed by the body, but not made by the body in amounts sufficient to meet physiological needs.

essential (primary) hypertension: high blood pressure that develops without an identifiable cause.

essential nutrients: nutrients a person must obtain from food because the body cannot make them for itself in sufficient quantity to meet physiological needs; also called *indispensable nutrients*. About 40 nutrients are known to be essential for human beings.

ethanol: a particular type of alcohol found in beer, wine, and distilled spirits; also called *ethyl alcohol*. Ethanol is the most widely used—and abused—drug in our society. It is also the only legal, nonprescription drug that produces euphoria.

ethical: in accordance with moral principles or professional standards. Socrates described *ethics* as "how we ought to live."

ethnic diets: foodways and cuisines typical of national origins, cultural heritages, or geographic locations.

euphoria: a feeling of great well-being, which people often seek through the use of drugs such as alcohol.

exchange lists: diet-planning tools that organize foods by their proportions of carbohydrate, fat, and protein. Foods on any single list can be used interchangeably.

exocrine glands: glands that secrete juices "out" into the digestive tract or onto the surface of the skin.

exogenous: outside the body (from foods).

experimental group: a group of individuals similar in all possible respects to the control group except for the treatment. The experimental group receives the test treatment.

external cue theory: the theory that some people eat in response to such external factors as the presence of food or the time of day rather than to such internal factors as hunger.

exudate: the fluid containing plasma proteins, electrolytes, and immune factors that leaks out through the capillaries in response to injury.

FAE: see *fetal alcohol effects*.

faith healing: healing by invoking divine intervention without the use of medical, surgical, or other traditional therapy.

false negative: a test result indicating that a condition is *not* present (negative) when in fact it is present (therefore false).

false positive: a test result indicating that a condition is present (positive) when in fact it is not (therefore false).

FAO (Food and Agriculture Organization): an international agency (part of the United Nations) that has adopted standards to regulate pesticide use among other responsibilities.

FAS: see *fetal alcohol syndrome*.

fasting hypoglycemia: hypoglycemia that develops gradually and primarily affects the brain and central nervous system.

fat: the lipids in foods or body fat, both of which are composed mostly of triglycerides.

fatfold measure: a clinical estimate of total body fatness in which the thickness of a fold of skin on the back of the arm (over the triceps muscle), below the shoulder blade (subscapular), or in other places is measured with a caliper. (The older, less preferred, term is *skinfold test*.)

fatty acid: an organic compound composed of a carbon chain with hydrogens attached and an acid group (COOH) at one end.

fatty acid oxidation: the metabolic breakdown of fatty acids to acetyl CoA.

fatty liver: a symptom of liver dysfunction seen in several diseases, including kwashiorkor and alcoholic liver disease. Fatty liver is characterized by an accumulation of fat in the liver cells; also called *hepatic steatosis*.

FDA (Food and Drug Administration): a part of the Department of Health and Human Services' Public Health Service that is responsible for ensuring the safety and wholesomeness of all foods sold in interstate commerce except meat, poultry, and eggs (which are under the jurisdiction of the USDA); inspecting food plants and imported foods; and setting standards for food composition.

fermentation: the oxidation of carbohydrate in the absence of atmospheric oxygen, a process that yields alcohol as an end product.

ferric iron: the oxidized form of iron (Fe^{+++}).

ferritin: an iron storage protein.

ferrous iron: the reduced form of iron (Fe^{++}).

fertility: the capacity of a woman to produce a normal ovum periodically and of a man to produce normal sperm; the ability to reproduce.

fetal alcohol effects (FAE): a subclinical version of FAS, with hidden defects including learning disabilities, behavioral abnormalities, and motor impairments; also called *alcohol-related birth defects (ARBD)*.

fetal alcohol syndrome (FAS): the cluster of symptoms seen in an infant or child whose mother consumed excess alcohol during pregnancy, including retarded growth, impaired development of the central nervous system, and facial malformations.

fetor hepaticus: the odor that may develop in people with impending hepatic coma.

fetus: the developing infant from eight weeks after conception until term.

fever: an elevation of body temperatures above normal.

fiber: a general term denoting in plant foods the *nonstarch polysaccharides* that are not digested by *human* digestive enzymes, although some are digested by GI tract bacteria; fibers include cellulose, hemicelluloses, pectins, gums, and mucilages and the nonpolysaccharides lignins, cutins, and tannins.

fibrocystic breast disease: a harmless condition in which the breasts develop lumps, sometimes associated with caffeine consumption. In some, it responds to treatment by abstinence from caffeine; in others, it can be treated with vitamin E.

fibrosis: the condition in which damaged cells lose function and are replaced by fibrous connective tissue cells.

fibrous: composed of fibers.

filtrate: in the kidneys, the fluid that passes from the blood through the capillary walls of the glomeruli, eventually forming urine.

fistula: an abnormal opening between two organs or from an organ to the skin.

fitness: the characteristics that enable the body to perform physical activity; more broadly, the ability to meet routine physical demands with enough reserve energy to rise to a sudden challenge; or the body's ability to withstand stress of all kinds.

flapping tremor: uncontrolled movement of the muscle group that causes the outstretched arm and hand to flap like a wing; occurs in hepatic coma and other diseases that cause encephalopathy; also called *asterixis*.

fluid and electrolyte balance: maintenance of the proper types and amounts of fluid and minerals in each compartment of the body fluids.

fluorapatite: the stabilized form of bone and tooth crystal, in which fluoride has replaced the hydroxyl groups of hydroxyapatite.

fluoridated water: water that has been treated so as to contain at least 0.8 mg fluoride per liter.

fluorosis: discoloration of tooth enamel caused by excess fluoride.

folate: a B vitamin; also known as folic acid, folacin, or pteroylglutamic acid (PGA). The coenzyme forms are DHF (dihydrofolate) and THF (tetrahydrofolate).

food allergies: adverse reactions to foods that involve an immune response; also called *food-hypersensitivity reactions*.

food aversion: a strong desire to avoid a particular food.

food-borne illnesses: illnesses transmitted to human beings through food, caused by either an infectious agent (*food-borne infection*) or a poisonous substance (*food intoxication*); commonly known as *food poisoning*.

food chain: the sequence in which living things depend on other living things for food.

food consumption survey: a survey that measures the amounts and kinds of foods people consume (using diet histories), estimates the nutrient intakes, and compares them with a standard such as the RDA.

food craving: a deep longing for a particular food.

food frequency checklist: a checklist of foods on which a person can record the frequency with which he or she eats different types of foods.

food group plans: diet-planning tools that sort foods of similar origin and nutrient content into groups and then specify that people should eat certain numbers of servings from each group.

food insecurity: intermittent hunger caused by lack of money or lack of control over other resources needed to assure a reliable food supply; the predominant form of hunger in the United States today.

food intolerances: adverse reactions to foods that do not involve the immune system.

food record: an extensive, accurate log of all foods eaten over a period of several days or weeks.

foods: products derived from plants or animals that can be taken into the body to yield nutrients for the maintenance of life and the growth and repair of tissues.

Food Stamp Program: a federal food assistance program. The USDA issues food stamp coupons through state social services or welfare agencies to households—people who buy and prepare food together. The number of stamps a household receives depends on the household's size and income. Recipients may use the coupons like cash to purchase food and seeds, but not to buy tobacco, cleaning items, alcohol, or other nonfood items.

foodways: the sum of the food habits, customs, beliefs, and preferences of a culture.

fortified: the addition to a food of nutrients that were either not originally present or present in insignificant amounts. Fortification can be used to correct or prevent a widespread nutrient deficiency, to balance the total nutrient profile of a food, or to restore nutrients lost in processing.

fossil fuel: coal, oil, and natural gas; these are nonrenewable fuels that pollute. (Renewable or alternative fuels, such as solar and wind energy, pollute less or not at all.)

frame size: the size of a person's bones and musculature. Appendix E describes how to take measures to estimate body frame size and provides tables of standards used in assessment.

fraud or quackery: the promotion, for financial gain, of devices, treatments, services, plans, or products (including diets and supplements) that alter or claim to alter a human condition without proof of safety or effectiveness. (The word *quackery* comes from the term *quacksalver*, meaning a person who quacks loudly about a miracle product—a lotion or a salve.)

free radical: an atom or molecule that has one or more unpaired electron(s) in the outer orbital (see Appendix B for a review of basic chemistry concepts). This electron imbalance makes free radicals unstable and highly reactive. Radicals typically arise during oxidation reactions and readily attack other molecules with which they come in contact.

fructose: a monosaccharide; sometimes known as fruit sugar or levulose, fructose is found abundantly in fruits, honey, and saps.

galactose: a monosaccharide; part of the disaccharide lactose.

galactosemia: an inborn error of metabolism in which galactose cannot be metabolized normally to compounds the body can handle and an alternative metabolite accumulates in the tissues, causing damage.

gallbladder: the organ that stores and concentrates bile. When it receives the signal that fat is present in the duodenum, the gallbladder contracts and squirts bile through the bile duct into the duodenum.

galvanized: a term referring to metals that have been treated with a zinc-containing coating to prevent rust.

gangrene: death of tissue due to a deficient blood supply and/or infection.

garlic oil: extract of garlic; proof of effectiveness is lacking.

gastric glands: exocrine glands in the stomach wall that secrete gastric juice into the stomach.

gastric-inhibitory peptide: a hormone produced by the intestine. Target organ: the stomach. Response: slowing of the secretion of gastric juices and of GI motility.

gastric juice: the digestive secretion of the gastric glands of the stomach.

gastric partitioning: a surgical procedure used to treat clinically severe obesity. The operation limits food intake by reducing the size of the stomach and delays gastric emptying by restricting the outlet.

gastric residual: the volume of formula that remains in the stomach from a previous feeding. It is measured by gently withdrawing the gastric contents through the feeding tube using a syringe. If the measured gastric residual is acceptable, the residual is returned to the client through the feeding tube.

gastrin: a hormone secreted by cells in the stomach wall. Target organ: the stomach. Response: secretion of gastric juice.

gastritis: inflammation of the stomach lining.

gastronintestinal tract: see *GI tract*.

gastroparesis: delayed gastric emptying.

gastrostomy: an opening in the stomach made surgically or under local anesthesia through which a feeding tube can be passed.

gatekeepers: with respect to nutrition, key people who control other people's access to foods and thereby exert profound impacts on their nutrition. Examples are the spouse who buys and cooks the food, the parent who feeds the children, and the caretaker in a day-care center.

genes: the basic units of hereditary information, made of DNA, that are passed from parent to offspring in the chromosomes. Each gene codes for a protein.

geophagia: clay eating.

germ: the nutrient-rich inner part of a grain. The germ is the seed that grows into a wheat plant, so it is especially rich in vitamins and minerals to support new life.

gestation: the period from conception to birth; for human beings gestation lasts from 38 to 42 weeks.

gestational diabetes: the appearance of abnormal glucose tolerance during pregnancy, with subsequent return to normal postpartum.

GFR: see *glomerular filtration rate*.

GI tract: the gastrointestinal tract or digestive tract; the principal organs are the stomach and intestines.

gland: a cell or group of cells that secretes materials for special uses in the body.

gliadin: a fraction of the gluten protein.

gliomas: cancers that arise from glial cells of the central nervous system.

glomerular filtration rate (GFR): the rate at which the kidneys form filtrate. Normally, the GFR is between 90 and 120 ml/min.

glomerulonephritis: an inflammation of the glomerular capillaries.

glomerulus: a cup-shaped membrane enclosing a tuft of capillaries within a nephron. (The plural is *glomeruli*.)

glucagon: a hormone that is secreted by special cells in the pancreas in response to low blood glucose concentration and elicits release of glucose from storage.

gluconeogenesis: the making of glucose from a noncarbohydrate source.

glucose: a monosaccharide; sometimes known as *blood sugar* or *dextrose*.

glucose tolerance: the ability of the body to regulate its blood glucose concentration to either the intake of dietary carbohydrate or the release of glucose from cells during fasting or metabolic stress.

glucose tolerance factor (GTF): a small organic compound that enhances insulin's action.

glucosuria: see *glycosuria*.

gluten: a vegetable protein found in wheat, oats, rye, barley, and other grains that gives dough its structure and cohesiveness.

glycemic effect: a measure of the extent to which a food, as compared with pure glucose, raises the blood glucose concentration and elicits an insulin response.

glycerol: an alcohol composed of a three-carbon chain, which can serve as the backbone for a triglyceride.

glycogen: an animal polysaccharide composed of glucose; it is manufactured and stored in the liver and muscles as a storage form of glucose. Glycogen is not a significant food source of carbohydrate and is not counted as one of the complex carbohydrates in foods.

glycogen loading: see *carbohhdrate loading*.

glycolysis: the metabolic breakdown of glucose to pyruvate. Glycolysis does not require oxygen (anaerobic).

glycosuria or glucosuria: glucose in the urine, which generally occurs when blood glucose exceeds 180 mg/100 ml.

goblet cells: cells of the GI tract (and lungs) that secrete mucus.

goiter: an enlargement of the thyroid gland due to an iodine deficiency, malfunction of the gland, or overconsumption of a goitrogen. Goiter caused by iodine deficiency is *simple goiter*.

goitrogen: a thyroid antagonist found in food; causes *toxic goiter*. Goitrogens are found in such foods as cabbage, kale, brussels sprouts, cauliflower, broccoli, and kohlrabi.

gout: a metabolic disorder that results in excess uric acid in the blood and sometimes in the urine; characterized by acute arthritis and inflammation of the joints.

graft-versus-host disease (GVHD): destruction of healthy donor cells by the recipient's immune system, which recognizes the donor cells as foreign.

granulated sugar: crystalline sucrose; 99.9 percent pure.

granulomas: granular tumors or growths.

GRAS (generally recognized as safe) list: a list, established by the FDA in 1958, of food additives that had long been in use and were believed safe. The list is subject to revision as new facts become known.

grazing: a popular term to describe eating many small meals and snacks throughout the day.

GTF: see *glucose tolerance factor*.

GVHD: see *graft-versus-host disease*.

hair follicle: a group of cells in the skin from which a hair grows.

hard water: water with a high calcium and magnesium concentration.

hazard: source of danger; used to refer to circumstances in which toxicity is possible under normal conditions of use.

HDL (high-density lipoprotein): the type of lipoprotein that transports cholesterol back to the liver from peripheral cells; composed primarily of protein.

health care team: a group of professionals representing several disciplines who work together to resolve their clients' medical problems.

health claim: any statement that characterizes the relationship between any nutrient or other substance in a food and a disease or health-related condition.

health history: an account of the client's current and past health status and risk factors for disease. Traditionally, the health history has been called the *medical history*. The term *health history* now seems more appropriate, however, since the contents describe the client's health status, and current trends in the medical profession now emphasize health promotion and disease prevention.

health maintenance organization (HMO): a form of managed care that limits the subscriber's choice of health care professionals and controls access to services by directing care through a primary care physician.

Healthy People 2000: a report that sets national objectives in health promotion and disease prevention for the year 2000. The 21 nutrition-related priorities are listed in Appendix G.

heart attacks: sudden tissue death caused by blockages of vessels that feed the heart muscle; also called *myocardial infarction* or *cardiac arrest*.

heartburn: a burning sensation in the chest area caused by backflow of stomach acid into the esophagus.

heat stroke: the dangerous accumulation of body heat with accompanying loss of body fluid.

heavy metal: any of a number of mineral ions such as mercury and lead, so called because they are of relatively high atomic weight. Many heavy metals are poisonous.

Heimlich maneuver: a technique for removing an object from the trachea of a choking person.

hematocrit: measurement of the percentage of the red blood cells in a given volume of blood.

hematuria: blood in the urine.

heme: the iron-holding part of the hemoglobin and myoglobin proteins. About 40 percent of the iron in meat, fish, and poultry is bound into heme; the other 60 percent is nonheme iron.

hemlock: a poisonous herb having finely divided leaves and small white flowers.

hemochromatosis: a hereditary defect in iron metabolism characterized by deposits of iron-containing pigment in many tissues, with tissue damage.

hemodialysis: a method of eliminating waste products in kidney failure whereby a blood vessel is tapped, and the blood is routed through a dialysis machine where excess fluids and wastes are removed. Blood is then returned from the machine to the body.

hemoglobin: the globular protein of the red blood cells that carries oxygen from the lungs to the cells throughout the body.

hemolysis: bursting of red blood cells.

hemophilia: a hereditary disease in which the blood is unable to clot because it lacks the ability to synthesize certain clotting factors.

hemorrhagic disease: a disease characterized by excessive bleeding.

hemorrhoids: painful swelling of the veins surrounding the rectum.

hemosiderin: an iron storage protein.

hemosiderosis: a condition characterized by the deposition of hemosiderin in the liver and other tissues.

hepatic: of, like, or pertaining to the liver.

hepatic coma: a state of unconsciousness that results from severe liver disease; also called *hepatic encephalopathy* or *portal systemic encephalopathy*.

hepatitis: inflammation of the liver caused by a virus, alcohol, drug, or other toxin.

herbal medicine: the use of plants to treat disease or improve health; also known as *botanical medicine* or *phytotherapy*.

herpes virus: a virus that can lead to mouth lesions and may also affect the lower GI tract, causing diarrhea.

hexoses: simple sugars with six atoms of carbon and the formula $C_6H_{12}O_6$.

HFCS: see *high-fructose corn syrup*.

hiatal hernia: a protrusion of a portion of the stomach through the esophageal hiatus of the diaphragm. There are several types of hiatal hernias, but the *sliding hiatal hernia* is the most common.

hiatus: the opening in the diaphragm through which the esophagus passes.

hiccups: repeated cough-like sounds and jerks that are produced when an involuntary spasm of the diaphragm muscle sucks air down the windpipe; also spelled *hiccoughs*.

high-fructose corn syrup (HFCS): a corn-syrup sweetener made especially for use in processed foods and beverages, where it is the predominant sweetener. HFCS is mostly fructose; glucose makes up the balance.

high potency: a nutrient present in a supplement in an amount that provides 100 percent or more of the Daily Value per serving.

high-quality protein: an easily digestible, complete protein.

high-risk pregnancy: a pregnancy characterized by indicators that make it likely the birth will be surrounded by problems such as premature delivery, difficult birth, retarded growth, birth defects, and early infant death.

histamine: a substance produced by cells of the immune system as part of a local immune reaction to an antigen; participates in causing inflammation.

HIV: see *human immunodeficiency virus*.

homeopathic medicine: a practice based on the theory that "like cures like," that is, that substances that cause symptoms in healthy people can cure those symptoms when given in very dilute amounts.

homeostasis: the maintenance of constant internal conditions (such as blood chemistry, temperature, and blood pressure) by the body's control systems. A homeostatic system is constantly reacting to external forces so as to maintain limits set by the body's needs.

honey: sugar (mostly sucrose) formed from nectar gathered by bees. An enzyme splits the sucrose into glucose and fructose. Composition and flavor vary, but honey always contains a mixture of sucrose, fructose, and glucose.

hormones: chemical messengers. Hormones are secreted by a variety of glands in response to altered conditions in the body. Each hormone travels to one or more specific target tissues or organs, where it elicits a specific response to restore normal conditions.

hormone-sensitive lipase: an enzyme inside adipose cells that responds to the body's need for fuel by hydrolyzing triglycerides so that their parts (glycerol and fatty acids) escape into the general circulation and thus become available to other cells as fuel. The signals to which this enzyme responds include epinephrine and glucagon, which oppose insulin.

human immunodeficiency virus (HIV): the virus that causes AIDS. The infection progressively destroys the immune system and leaves its victims defenseless against numerous infections.

hunger: the physiological need to eat, experienced as a drive to obtain food; an unpleasant sensation.

husk: the outer, inedible part of a grain; also called the *chaff*.

hydrochloric acid: an acid composed of hydrogen and chloride atoms (HCl). The gastric glands normally produce this acid.

hydrodensitometry: a method of measuring body density in which the person is first weighed and then submerged in water.

hydrogenation: a chemical process by which hydrogens are added to monounsaturated or polyunsaturated fats to reduce the number of double bonds, making the fats more saturated (solid) and more resistant to oxidation (protecting against rancidity). Hydrogenation produces *trans*-fatty acids.

hydrolysis: a chemical reaction in which a major reactant is split into two products, with the addition of a hydrogen atom (H) to one and a hydroxyl group (OH) to the other (from water, H_2O).

hydrolyzed formula: a liquid diet that contains broken-down molecules of protein, such as amino acids and short peptide chains, and is therefore easy to digest and absorb; also called a *monomeric formula*.

hydrophilic: a term referring to water-loving, or water-soluble, substances.

hydrophobic: a term referring to water-fearing, or non-water-soluble, substances; also known as *lipophilic* (fat loving).

hyperactivity: a condition of excessive activity.

hyperammonemia: an elevated blood ammonia level. Normal blood ammonia levels are less than 50 µg/100 ml.

hypercalcemia: high blood calcium. Hypercalcemia may develop from a variety of disorders, including vitamin D toxicity, but it does *not* develop from a high calcium intake.

hypercalciuria: excessive urinary excretion of calcium.

hyperglycemia: elevated blood glucose.

hyperkalemia: an excessive amount of potassium in the blood.

hyperlipidemia: elevated blood lipids.

hyperosmolar hyperglycemia nonketotic coma: coma that occurs in uncontrolled NIDDM precipitated by the presence of hypertonic blood and dehydration.

hyperplastic obesity: obesity due to an increase in the *number* of fat cells.

hypertension: higher-than-normal blood pressure.

hyperthermia: an above-normal body temperature.

hypertonic formula: a formula with an osmolality higher than that of blood serum.

hypertrophic obesity: obesity due to an increase in the *size* of fat cells.

hypertrophy: of muscles, growing larger; an increase in size in response to use.

hypnotherapy: a technique that uses hypnosis and the power of suggestion to improve health behaviors, relieve pain, and heal.

hypoglycemia: an abnormally low blood glucose concentration.

hypothalamus: a brain center that controls

activities such as maintenance of water balance and regulation of body temperature.

hypothermia: a below-normal body temperature.

hypoxemia: lack of oxygen in the blood.

idopathic hypercalciuria: excessive urinary excretion of calcium not related to a known underlying medical condition.

ileocecal valve: the sphincter separating the small and large intestines.

ileostomate: a person who has a surgically formed opening from the ileum to the outside of the body (an ileostomy).

ileum: the last segment of the small intestine.

illness: as used in this book, any medical condition that alters nutrient needs. Not all such conditions are diseases. For example, major surgery is a metabolic stress that can alter nutrient needs though it is not a disease.

imagery: a technique that guides clients to achieve a desired physical, emotional, or spiritual state by visualizing themselves in that state.

imitation food: a food that substitutes for and resembles another food, but is nutritionally inferior to it with respect to vitamin, mineral, or protein content. If the substitute is not inferior to the food it resembles and if it provides an accurate name for itself, it need not be labeled "imitation."

immunity: the body's ability to recognize and eliminate foreign invaders.

implantation: the stage of development in which the zygote embeds itself in the wall of the uterus and begins to develop; occurs during the first two weeks after conception.

inborn error of metabolism: an inherited flaw evident as a metabolic disorder or disease present from birth.

indemnity insurance: traditional insurance that pays a fee for service.

indirect additives: substances that can get into food as a result of contact with foods during growing, processing, packaging, storing, cooking, or some other stage before the foods are consumed; also called *incidental* or *accidental additives*.

indirect calorimetry: the estimation of energy output from measures of the amount of oxygen used and carbon dioxide eliminated.

induration: a raised, hardened area of skin.

inflammatory response: the changes that occur in tissues when they are injured by such forces as blows, wounds, foreign bodies (chemicals, microorganisms), heat, cold, electricity, or radiation.

initiators: factors such as radiation and carcinogens which cause mutations that give rise to cancer.

inorganic: not containing carbon or pertaining to living things.

inositol: a nonessential nutrient that can be made in the body from glucose. Inositol is used in cell membranes.

insulin: a hormone secreted by special cells in the pancreas in response to (among other things) increased blood glucose concentration. The primary role of insulin is to control the transport of glucose from the bloodstream into the cells.

insulin-dependent diabetes mellitus (IDDM): the less common type of diabetes in which the person produces no insulin at all; also known as *type I diabetes* or *juvenile-onset diabetes* (because it frequently develops in childhood), although some cases arise in adulthood.

insulin–like growth factor (IGF-1): somatomedin–C.

insulin reaction: hypoglycemia that results from an overdose of insulin, strenuous physical activity, skipped meals, or inadequate intake of food; also called *insulin shock*.

insulin resistance: the condition in which a set amount of insulin produces a subnormal effect.

intentional additives: additives intentionally added to foods, such as nutrients, colors, and preservatives.

intermittent claudication: severe calf pain caused by inadequate blood supply; it occurs when walking and subsides during rest.

intermittent feeding: delivery of no more than 250 ml of a tube feeding over 30 minutes.

international units (IU): a measure of vitamin activity, determined by such biological methods as feeding a compound to vitamin-deprived animals and measuring growth. This system was used to measure fat-soluble vitamins before direct chemical analysis was possible.

interstitial fluid: fluid between the cells, usually high in sodium and chloride. Interstitial fluid is a large component of *extracellular fluid* (fluid outside the cells), which also includes plasma and the water of structures such as the skin and bones. Extracellular fluid accounts for approximately one-third of the body's water.

intra-abdominal fat: fat stored within the abdominal cavity in association with the internal abdominal organs, as opposed to the fat stored directly under the skin (subcutaneous fat).

intracellular fluid: fluid within the cells, usually high in potassium and phosphate. Intracellular fluid accounts for approximately two-thirds of the body's water.

intractable diarrhea: severe, chronic diarrhea that does not respond to treatment.

intravenous (IV): through a vein.

intrinsic: inside the system.

intrinsic factor: a glycoprotein (a protein with short polysaccharide chains attached) made in the stomach that aids in the absorption of vitamin B_{12}.

invert sugar: a mixture of glucose and fructose formed by the hydrolysis of sucrose in a chemical process; sold only in liquid form and sweeter than sucrose. Invert sugar is used as a food additive to help preserve freshness and prevent shrinkage.

involuntary activities: the component of a person's daily energy expenditure that occurs independently, without conscious will or knowledge—heart beating, lungs breathing, glands secreting, GI tract muscles contracting, and other activities critical to maintaining life.

iodopsin: the light-sensitive pigment of the cones in the retina. Both rhodopsin and iodopsin contain retinal; the protein portions of the pigments differ.

ions: atoms or molecules that have gained or lost electrons and therefore have electrical charges. Examples include the positively charged sodium ion (Na^+) and the negatively charged chloride ion (Cl^-).

iridology: the study of changes in the iris of the eye and their relationships to disease.

iron deficiency: the state of having depleted iron stores.

iron-deficiency anemia: a blood iron deficiency that results in small, pale, red blood cells.

iron overload: toxicity from excess iron.

isotonic formula: a formula with an osmolality similar to that of blood serum (300 mOsm/kg).

IV catheter: a thin tube inserted into a vein through which nutrient solutions or medications can be given directly.

jaundice: yellowing of the skin, due to spillover of the bile pigments *bilirubin* from the liver into the general circulation; also known as *hyperbilirubinemia*. Jaundice may be caused by obstruction of bile passageways, hemolysis, or dysfunctional liver cells.

jejunostomy: an opening in the jejunum made surgically or under local anesthesia through which a feeding tube can be passed.

jejunum: the first two-fifths of the small intestine beyond the duodenum.

Kaposi's sarcoma: a type of cancer rare in the general population but common in people with HIV infection.

kcalorie (energy) control: management of food energy intake.

keratin: a water-insoluble protein; the normal protein of hair and nails. Keratin-producing cells may replace mucus-producing cells in vitamin A deficiency.

keratinization: accumulation of keratin in a tissue; a sign of vitamin A deficiency.

keratomalacia: softening of the cornea seen in severe vitamin A deficiency that leads to irreversible blindness.

kernicterus: the condition of bile pigments invading the brain.

Keshan disease: a heart disease associated with selenium deficiency that is characterized by heart enlargement and insufficiency; the middle layer of the walls of the heart, which are normally composed of muscle tissue, are replaced with fibrous tissue.

keto acid: an organic acid that contains a carbonyl group (C=O).

ketone bodies: the product of the incomplete breakdown of fat when glucose is not available in the cells.

ketonemia: ketones in the blood.

ketonuria: ketones in the urine.

ketosis: an undesirably high concentration of ketone bodies in the blood and urine.

kosher: foods prepared according to Jewish dietary laws.

kwashiorkor: a form of PEM that results from either inadequate protein intake or, more commonly, from severe stress or infections.

lactase: an enzyme that hydrolyzes lactose.

lactase deficiency: a lack of the enzyme required to digest the disaccharide lactose into its component monosaccharides (glucose and galactose).

lactation: production and secretion of breast milk for the purpose of nourishing an infant.

lactic acid: an acid produced from pyruvate during anaerobic metabolism.

lacto-ovo-vegetarians: people who include milk, milk products, and eggs, but exclude meat, poultry, fish, and seafood from their diets.

lactoferrin: a factor in breast milk that binds iron and keeps it from supporting the growth of the infant's intestinal bacteria.

lactose: a disaccharide composed of glucose and galactose; commonly known as milk sugar.

lactose intolerance: a condition that results from inability to digest the milk sugar lactose; characterized by bloating, gas, abdominal discomfort, and diarrhea. Lactose intolerance differs from milk allergy, which is caused by an immune reaction to the protein in milk.

lactovegetarians: people who include milk and milk products, but exclude meat, poultry, fish, seafood, and eggs from their diets.

large intestine (or colon): the lower portion of intestine that completes the digestive process; its segments are the ascending colon, the transverse colon, the descending colon, and the sigmoid colon.

larynx: the voice box.

LBW: see *low birthweight*.

LDL (low-density lipoprotein): the type of lipoprotein derived from very-low-density lipoproteins (VLDL) as cells remove triglycerides from them; composed primarily of cholesterol.

lecithin: one of the phospholipids; a compound of glycerol to which are attached two fatty acids, a phosphate group, and a choline molecule. Both nature and the food industry use lecithin as an emulsifier to combine two ingredients that do not ordinarily mix, such as water and oil.

legal: established by law.

legumes: plants of the bean and pea family. Bacteria in the root nodules of legumes "fix" nitrogen by trapping nitrogen from the air into the soil and then making it a part of the protein in the beans. Thus legumes are rich in high-quality protein compared with other plant-derived foods. Ultimately, the plant leaves more nitrogen in the soil than it takes out (sparing the land). Farmers sometimes plow under legume plants to fertilize the soil.

leukemias: cancers that arise from the white blood cells.

levulose: an older name for fructose.

license to practice: permission under state or federal law, granted on meeting specified criteria, to use a certain title (such as dietitian) and offer certain services. Licensed dietitians may use the initials LD after their names.

life expectancy: the average number of years lived by people in a given society.

life span: the maximum number of years of life attainable by a member of a species.

limiting amino acid: the essential amino acid found in the shortest supply relative to the amounts needed for protein synthesis in the body.

linoleic acid: an essential fatty acid with 18 carbons and two double bonds (18:2).

linolenic acid: an essential fatty acid with 18 carbons and three double bonds (18:3).

lipase: an enzyme that hydrolyzes lipids (fats).

lipids: a family of compounds that includes triglycerides (fats and oils), phospholipids, and sterols.

lipoic acid: a nonessential nutrient.

lipoprotein lipase (LPL): an enzyme mounted on the surface of fat cells (and other cells) that hydrolyzes triglycerides passing by in the bloodstream and directs their parts into the cells, where they can be metabolized or reassembled for storage.

lipoproteins: clusters of lipids associated with proteins that serve as transport vehicles for lipids in the lymph and blood.

liver: the organ that manufactures bile and is the first to receive nutrients from the intestines.

living will: a document signed by a competent adult that specifically states whether the person wishes any heroic measures to be taken in the event of terminal illness or irreversible coma from which the person is not expected to recover.

LPL: see *lipoprotein lipase*.

longevity: long duration of life.

low birthweight (LBW): a birthweight of 5½ pounds (2500 g) or less; indicates probable poor health in the newborn and poor nutrition status in the mother during pregnancy, before pregnancy, or both. Normal birthweight for a full-term baby is 6½ to 8¾ pounds (about 3000 to 4000 g).

low-risk pregnancy: a pregnancy characterized by indicators that make a normal outcome likely.

lumen: the inner open space of a tube or hollow organ (such as the intestine).

lymph: a clear yellowish fluid that resembles blood without the red blood cells; lymph from the GI tract transports fat and fat-soluble vitamins to the bloodstream via lymphatic vessels.

lymphatic system: a loosely organized system of vessels and ducts that convey fluids toward the heart; the GI part of the lymphatic system carries the products of digestion into the bloodstream.

lymphomas: cancers that arise from lymph tissue.

lysosomes: sacs of degradative enzymes.

macroangiopathies: disorders of the large blood vessels, including atherosclerosis.

macrobiotic diets: extremely restrictive diets limited to brown rice, miso soup, sea vegetables, and other traditional Japanese foods; based on metaphysical beliefs and not on nutrition.

macrocytic (or megaloblastic) anemia: large-cell anemia.

magnesium: a cation within the body's cells, active in many enzyme systems.

major minerals: essential mineral nutrients found in the human body in amounts larger than 5 g. The major minerals are calcium, phosphorus, potassium, sodium, chloride, magnesium, and sulfur.

malignant tumors: tumors that multiply out of control, threaten health, and require treatment.

malnutrition: any condition caused by excess or deficient food energy or nutrient intake or by an imbalance of nutrients.

maltase: an enzyme that hydrolyzes maltose.

maltose: a disaccharide composed of two glucose units; sometimes known as *malt sugar*.

managed care: a health care delivery system that is directed at providing quality health care at tolerable costs by coordinating services.

maple sugar: a sugar (mostly sucrose) purified from the concentrated sap of the sugar maple tree.

marasmus: a form of PEM that results from a severe deprivation, or impaired absorption, of energy, protein, vitamins, and minerals.

margin of safety: when speaking of food additives, a zone between the concentration normally used and that at which a hazard exists. For common table salt, for example, the margin of safety is 1/5 (five times the amount normally used would be hazardous).

massage therapy: a healing method in which the therapist manually kneads muscles to reduce tension, increase blood circulation, improve joint mobility, and promote healing of injuries.

mastication: the process of chewing.

matrix: the basic substance that gives form to a developing structure; in the body, the formative cells from which teeth and bones grow.

meat replacement: products formulated to look and taste like meat, fish, or poultry; usually made of textured vegetable protein.

mechanical soft diet: a diet that excludes all foods that are difficult to chew or swallow; also called a *dental soft diet*.

mechanical ventilator: a machine that "breathes" for the person who can't.

medical (or individual) approach: recommendations that urge dietary changes only for people who are known to need them.

medical nutrition therapy: a term introduced by the American Dietetic Association in 1994 to emphasize the role of nutrition in medical care. In this book, the terms *medical nutrition therapy* and *diet therapy* are used interchangeably.

medical record: a continuous written account of a client's health history, diagnosis, therapy, and prognosis.

meditation: a self-directed technique of relaxing the body and calming the mind.

melanomas: cancers that arise from pigmented skin cells.

melatonin: a hormone secreted by the pineal gland believed to help regulate the body's daily rhythms and promote sleep. Proof of safety or effectiveness is lacking.

menadione: a synthetic form of vitamin K.

MEOS (microsomal ethanol-oxidizing system): a system of enzymes in the liver that oxidize not only alcohol, but also several classes of drugs. (The *microsomes* are tiny particles of membranes with associated enzymes that can be collected from broken-up cells.)

metabolism: the sum total of all the chemical reactions that go on in living cells.

metalloenzyme: an enzyme that contains one or more minerals as part of its structure.

metallothionein: a sulfur-rich protein that avidly binds with metals such as zinc.

metastasize: to spread from one part of the body to another.

metastatic calcification: the deposition of phosphorus and calcium salts in soft tissue.

MFP factor: a factor associated with the digestion of meat, fish, and poultry that enhances iron absorption.

micelles: tiny spherical complexes that arise during fat digestion; each carries about 20 fatty acids and/or monoglycerides into intestinal cells.

microalbuminuria: the loss of albumin in the urine in quantities that are greater than normal but not enough to precipitate symptoms.

microangiopathies: disorders of the capillaries.

microcytic hypochromic anemia: small, pale red blood cells common in iron-deficiency anemia.

microvilli: tiny, hairlike projections on each cell of every villus that can trap nutrient particles and transport them into the cells; singular *microvillus*.

milk anemia: iron-deficiency anemia that develops when an excessive milk intake displaces iron-rich foods from the diet.

milliequivalents (mEq): the concentration of electrolytes in a volume of solution. The number of milliequivalents is a useful measure when considering ions, because the number of charges reveals characteristics about the solution that are not evident when expressed in terms of weight.

mineralization: the process in which calcium, phosphorus, and other minerals crystallize on the collagen matrix of a growing bone, hardening the bone.

minerals: inorganic elements; some minerals are essential nutrients required in small amounts.

mineral water: water from a spring or well that typically contains 250 to 500 ppm of minerals. Minerals give water a distinctive flavor. Many mineral waters are high in sodium.

misinformation: false or misleading information.

moderate exercise: activity that can be sustained comfortably for 60 minutes or so.

moderation: in relation to dietary intake, providing enough but not too much of a substance; in relation to alcohol consumption, not more than two drinks a day for the average-sized man and not more than one drink a day for the average-sized woman.

modified or therapeutic diet: a regular diet that is adjusted to meet special nutrition needs. Such diets can be adjusted in consistency, in level of energy and nutrients, in amount of fluid, in number of meals, or by the elimination of certain foods.

modules: formulas or foods that provide a single nutrient and are designed to be added to other formulas or foods to alter nutrient composition; they can also be combined together to create a highly individualized formula.

molasses: the thick brown syrup produced during sugar refining. Molasses retains residual sugar and other by-products and a few minerals; blackstrap molasses contains significant amounts of calcium and iron—the iron comes from the *machinery* used to process the sugar.

molecule: two or more atoms of the same or different elements joined by chemical bonds. Examples are molecules of the element oxygen, composed of two oxygen atoms (O_2), and molecules of the compound water, composed of two hydrogen atoms and one oxygen atom (H_2O).

molybdenum: a trace element.

monoglyceride: a molecule of glycerol with one fatty acid attached.

monosaccharide: a carbohydrate of the general formula $C_nH_{2n}O_n$ that consists of a single ring.

monounsaturated fatty acid: a fatty acid that lacks two hydrogen atoms and has one double bond between carbons—for example, oleic acid.

mouth ulcers: lesions or sores in the lining of the mouth. Certain drugs, radiation therapy, and some disorders, such as oral herpes virus infections, can cause mouth ulcers.

mucosal ferritin: a protein that holds iron in the cell.

mucosal transferrin: a protein that passes iron from the cell on to *blood transferrin*.

mucous membranes: the membranes, composed of mucus-secreting cells, that line the surfaces of body tissues.

mucus: a slippery substance secreted by goblet cells of the GI lining (and other body linings) that protects the cells from exposure to digestive juices (and other destructive agents). (The noun is *mucus*; the adjective is *mucous*.)

multiple daily injections (MDI): delivery of different types of insulin by injection three or more times daily.

muscle endurance: the ability of a muscle to contract repeatedly without becoming exhausted.

muscle strength: the ability of muscles to work against resistance.

muscular dystrophy: a hereditary disease in which the muscles gradually weaken; its most debilitating effects arise in the lungs.

mutation: an alteration in a gene such that an altered protein is produced.

mutual supplementation: the strategy of combining two protein foods in a meal so that each food provides the essential amino acid(s) lacking in the other. Mutual supplementation is the dietary strategy that brings complementary proteins together in a meal.

myoglobin: the oxygen-holding protein of the muscle cells.

NAD (nicotinamide adenine dinucleotide): the main coenzyme form of the vitamin niacin; its reduced form is NADH.

narcotic: any drug that dulls the senses, induces sleep, and becomes addictive with prolonged use.

nasoduodenal: from the nose to the duodenum.

nasoenteric: from the nose to the stomach or intestine. *Nasoenteric feedings* include nasogastric, nasoduodenal, and nasojejunal feedings. Most clinicians use *nasoenteric* to refer to nasoduodenal and nasojejunal feedings only.

nasogastric: from the nose to the stomach.

nasojejunal: from the nose to the jejunum.

natural water: water obtained from a spring or well that is certified to be safe and sanitary. The mineral content may not be changed, but the water may be treated in other ways such as by filtration or ozonization.

naturopathic medicine: a system that integrates traditional medicine with botanical medicine, clinical nutrition, homeopathy, acupuncture, East Asian medicine, hydrotherapy, and manipulative therapy.

nausea: the feeling that one is about to vomit.

nephritis: inflammation of the kidneys.

nephrons: the working units of the kidneys; each consists of a glomerulus and a tubule.

nephropathy: a disorder of the kidneys.

nephrosclerosis: impairment of renal blood flow because of renal artery damage. It can be caused by hypertension or atherosclerosis.

nephrotic syndrome: the complex of symptoms that occur when glomerular function fails; it includes proteinuria and albuminuria.

net protein utilization (NPU): the amount of protein nitrogen that is retained from a given amount of protein nitrogen eaten; a measure of protein quality.

neuron: a nerve cell; the structural and functional unit of the nervous system. Neurons initiate and conduct nerve transmissions.

neuropathy: a disorder of the nerves.

neurotransmitters: chemicals that are released at the end of a nerve cell when a nerve impulse arrives there; they diffuse across the gap to the next cell and alter the membrane of that second cell to either inhibit or excite it.

niacin: a B vitamin. Niacin can be eaten preformed or made in the body from its precursor, tryptophan, one of the amino acids. The active coenzyme forms are NAD (nicotinamide adenine dinucleotide) and NADP (the phosphate form of NAD).

niacin equivalents: the amount of niacin present in food, including the niacin that can theoretically be made from its precursor, tryptophan, present in the food.

night blindness: slow recovery of vision after flashes of bright light at night or an inability to see in dim light; an early symptom of vitamin A deficiency.

nitrates: salts that are converted to nitrites by bacteria.

nitrites: salts added to food to prevent botulism; one example is sodium nitrite, which is used to preserve meats.

nitrogen balance: the amount of nitrogen consumed (N in) as compared with the amount of nitrogen excreted (N out) in a given period of time.

nitrosamines: derivatives of nitrites that may be formed in the stomach when nitrites combine with amines; nitrosamines are carcinogenic in animals.

nocturnal hypoglycemia: hypoglycemia that occurs while a person is sleeping.

noninsulin-dependent diabetes mellitus (NIDDM): the more common type of diabetes that develops gradually and is associated with insulin resistance; also called *type II diabetes* or *adult-onset diabetes*. NIDDM is usually milder than IDDM and progresses more slowly. A type of NIDDM that develops during the teen years has been termed *maturity-onset diabetes in the young* (MODY).

nonnutrients: compounds in foods with no known nutritional value.

nonnutritive sweetners: sweetners that provide no energy.

NPO: an order to give a client nothing orally (including food, beverages, and medications): NPO stands for *nil per os*, which means "nothing by mouth."

nucleotides: nitrogen-containing components of RNA and DNA. Nucleotides can be synthesized in the body and therefore are not essential in the diets of healthy individuals. In severely stressed individuals, however, a dietary source may be beneficial.

nursing bottle tooth decay: extensive tooth decay due to prolonged tooth contact with formula, milk, fruit juice, or other carbohydrate-rich liquid offered to an infant in a bottle.

nutraceuticals: substances that supposedly provide medical and health benefits; a term not recognized by the FDA.

nutrient additives: vitamins and minerals added to improve nutritive value.

nutrient density: a measure of the nutrients a food provides relative to the energy it provides. The more nutrients and the fewer kcalories, the higher the nutrient density.

nutrients: substances obtained from food and used in the body to provide energy and structural materials and to regulate growth, maintenance, and repair of the body's tissues; nutrients may also reduce the risks of some chronic diseases.

nutrition assessment: the evaluation of many factors that influence or reflect nutritional health; the tools used for nutrition assessment include historical information, physical examinations, anthropometric findings, and biochemical analyses.

nutrition care plan: a plan that translates nutrition assessment data into a strategy for meeting a client's nutrient and nutrition education needs.

nutrition care process: an organized approach to nutrition intervention that consists of five steps (assessing, analyzing, planning, implementing, and evaluating). The nutrition care process parallels the *nursing care process* except that it focuses on nutrition concerns.

nutrition screening: the use of routine nutrition assessment procedures to identify people who are malnourished or are at risk for malnutrition.

nutrition status survey: a survey that evaluates people's nutrition status using diet histories, anthropometric measures, physical examinations, and laboratory tests.

nutritional yeast: a preparation of yeast cells grown especially as a nutrient supplement, particularly for vegetarian diets. The type of yeast used is brewer's yeast, not baker's yeast. Different species of yeasts produce different compounds; yeast cells used in brewing produce alcohol, proteins, and B vitamins as they grow. The nutrients are removed from beer and wine in the filtering process. Yeast cells used in baking produce mostly carbon dioxide, which causes bread dough to rise.

nutritionist: a person who specializes in the study of nutrition. Some nutritionists are registered dietitians, whereas others are self-described experts whose training is questionable. In states with responsible legislation, the term applies only to people who have MS or PhD degrees from properly accredited institutions.

nutritive sweeteners: sweeteners that yield energy, including both sugars and sugar alcohols.

obligatory water excretion: the amount of water the body has to excrete each day to dispose of its wastes—about 500 ml, or a pint.

oligopeptide: an intermediate-length string of four to nine amino acids.

oliguria: minimal urine volume.

oliguric phase: the early phase of acute renal failure, when urine volume is reduced.

omega: the last letter of the Greek alphabet (ω), used by chemists to refer to the position of the endmost double bond in a fatty acid.

omega-3 fatty acid: a polyunsaturated fatty acid in which the first double bond is three carbons away from the methyl (CH_3) end of the carbon chain.

omega-6 fatty acid: a polyunsaturated fatty acid in which the first double bond is six carbons from the methyl (CH_3) end of the carbon chain.

omnivores: people who have no formal restriction on the eating of any foods.

opportunistic infections: infections from microorganisms that normally do not cause disease in the general population but can cause great harm in people once their immune systems are compromised (as in HIV infection).

opsin: the protein portion of the visual pigment molecule.

oral antidiabetic agents: drugs taken by mouth to lower blood glucose levels. They include sulfonylureas, metformin, and acarbose. Sulfonylureas are also called *hypoglycemic agents* because they stimulate insulin secretion.

oral rehydration therapy (ORT): the administration of a simple solution of sugar, salt, and water, taken by mouth, to treat dehydration caused by diarrhea.

organic: a substance or molecule containing carbon-carbon bonds or carbon-hydrogen bonds. Some farmers call their produce "organic" if it was grown without manufactured fertilizers and pesticides, but by the definition given here, all foods are organic.

organic halogen: an organic compound containing one or more atoms of a *halogen*—fluorine, chlorine, iodine, or bromine.

orogastric: from the mouth to the stomach. This method is often used to tube feed infants because they breathe through their noses, and tubes inserted through the nose can hinder the infant's breathing.

ORT: see oral rehydration therapy.

orthomolecular medicine: the use of large doses of vitamins to treat chronic disease.

osmolality: the concentration of particles in a solution, expressed as the number of milliosmoles (mOsm) per kilogram.

osmotic diarrhea: diarrhea that results from an increase in the osmolarity of the intestinal contents due to unabsorbed water and electrolytes.

osmotic pressure: the pressure that develops when two solutions of different concentrations are separated by a membrane that permits water, but not the solutes, to cross. Water flows *toward* the side of the membrane on which the solutes are more concentrated.

osteitis fibrosis: a type of renal osteodystrophy that results from hyperparathyroidism and is characterized by kidney stones, decalcification and softening of bones, and, sometimes, formation of cysts and tumors.

osteoblasts: cells that build bone.

osteoclasts: cells that destroy bone during growth.

osteomalacia: a bone disease characterized by softening of the bones; symptoms include bending of the spine and bowing of the legs. The disease occurs most often in adult women.

osteopenia: a metabolic bone disease characterized by reduced bone mass common in preterm infants; also called *rickets of prematurity*.

osteoporosis: a condition of older persons in which the bones become porous and fragile due to a loss of minerals; also called *adult bone loss*.

ostomate: a person who has a surgically formed opening from the bowel to the outside of the body, bypassing the anus.

overnutrition: excess energy or nutrients.

overt: out in the open and easy to observe.

overweight: body weight above some standard of acceptable weight that is usually defined in relation to height (such as the weight-for-height tables).

ovum: the female reproductive cell, capable of developing into a new organism upon fertilization; commonly referred to as an *egg*.

oxidant: a compound (such as oxygen itself) that oxidizes other compounds. Compounds that prevent oxidation are called *anti*oxidants, whereas those that encourage it are called *pro*oxidants.

oxidation: the process of a substance combining with oxygen.

oxidative stress: damage to biological systems caused by free-radical formation.

ozone therapy: the use of ozone gas to enhance the body's immune system.

pagophagia: ice craving.

palatability: pleasing taste. When tasting foods, the tongue presses them against the *palate*, or roof of the mouth.

pancreas: a gland that secretes digestive enzymes and juices into the duodenum.

pancreatic juice: the exocrine secretion of the pancreas, containing enzymes for the digestion of carbohydrate, fat, and protein as well as bicarbonate, a neutralizing agent.

pancreatitis: inflammation of the pancreas.

pantothenic acid: a B vitamin; the principal active form is part of coenzyme A, commonly called "CoA" in metabolism.

parathormone: a hormone from the parathyroid gland that raises blood calcium; also called parathyroid hormone.

parenteral formulas: formulas given by vein.

parenteral nutrition: delivery of nutrient solutions directly into a vein, bypassing the intestines.

pasteurization: a process of heating milk sufficiently to kill many disease-causing microbes commonly transmitted through milk; not a sterilization process. Pasteurized milk retains bacteria that cause milk spoilage. Unpasteurized ("certified" raw) milk transmits many food-borne diseases to people each year.

pathogens: microorganisms or substances capable of producing disease.

pathological stresses: stresses imposed by disease or trauma.

PCM: see *protein-energy malnutrition*.

peak bone mass: the highest attainable bone density for an individual, developed during the first three decades of life.

peer review: a process in which a panel of scientists rigorously evaluates a research study to assure that the scientific method was followed.

PEG: see *percutaneous endoscopic gastrostomy*.

PEJ: see *percutaneous endoscopic jejunostomy*.

pellagra: the niacin-deficiency disease.

PEM: see *protein-energy malnutrition*.

pepsin: a gastric protease.

pepsinogen: a precursor protein that is activated by stomach acid to form the enzyme pepsin.

peptic ulcer: an erosion in the mucous membrane of either the stomach (a gastric ulcer) or the duodenum (a duodenal ulcer). Ulcers may also develop in the mouth, esophagus, and intestines and on the skin.

peptidase: a digestive enzyme that hydrolyzes peptide bonds. *Tripeptidases* cleave tripeptides; *dipeptidases* cleave dipeptides. *Endopeptidases* cleave peptide bonds *within* the chain to create smaller fragments, whereas *exopeptidases* cleave bonds at the *ends* to release free amino acids.

peptide bond: a bond that connects the acid end of one amino acid with the amino end of another, forming a link in a protein chain.

percutaneous endoscopic gastrostomy (PEG): a gastrostomy created under local anesthesia.

percutaneous endoscopic jejunostomy (PEJ): a misnomer that refers to a feeding tube insertion technique in which a feeding tube is guided into the jejunum from a gastrostomy created using a nonsurgical procedure.

peripheral parenteral nutrition: the use of the peripheral veins to provide a solution that meets nutrient needs.

peripheral resistance: resistance to the flow of blood by the vessels at the periphery of the body—the smallest arteries and capillaries.

peripheral veins: the small-diameter veins that bring blood to the extremities (arms and legs).

peripherally inserted central catheter (PICC): a catheter inserted into a peripheral vein and advanced into a central vein.

peristalsis: wavelike muscular contractions of the GI tract that push its contents along.

peritoneal dialysis: a method of eliminating excess fluids and wastes from the blood in kidney failure using the peritoneum as a semipermeable membrane.

pernicious anemia: a blood disorder that reflects a vitamin B_{12} deficiency caused by lack of intrinsic factor and characterized by a deficit of red blood cells, muscle weakness, and neurological disturbances.

peroxidation: the production of unstable molecules containing more than the usual amount of oxygen. Hydrogen peroxide, H_2O_2, for example, may be produced from water, H_2O.

persistence: stubborn or enduring continuance; with respect to food contaminants, the quality of persisting, rather than breaking down, in the bodies of animals and human beings.

persistent vegetative state: exhibiting motor reflexes but without the ability to regain cognitive behavior, communicate, or interact purposefully with the environment.

pesticides: chemicals used to control insects, diseases, weeds, fungi, and other pests on plants, vegetables, fruits, and animals. Used broadly, the term includes herbicides (to kill weeds), insecticides (to kill insects), and fungicides (to kill fungi).

pH: the unit of measure expressing a substance's acidity or alkalinity (pH 7 is neutral). The lower the pH below 7, the stronger the acid. A pH above 7 is alkaline, or base.

pharmacological effect: the body's response to a large dose of a nutrient (two to ten times greater than the RDA) that overwhelms some body system and acts like a drug.

phenylketonuria (PKU): an inborn error of metabolism in which phenylalanine, an essential amino acid, cannot be converted to tyrosine. Alternative metabolites of phenylalanine (phenylketones) accumulate in the tissues, causing damage, and overflow into the urine.

phospholipid: a compound similar to a triglyceride but having choline (or another nitrogen-containing compound) and a phosphate group (a phosphorus-containing salt) in place of one of the fatty acids.

phosphorus: a major mineral found mostly in the body's bones and teeth.

photon: a unit of light energy. Depending on its wavelength, a photon conveys different colors of light.

photosynthesis: the process by which green plants make carbohydrates from carbon dioxide and water using the green pigment chlorophyll to trap the sun's energy.

physiological age: a person's age as estimated from her or his body's health and probable life expectancy.

physiological effect: the body's response to a normal dose of a nutrient (levels commonly found in foods and not exceeding 150 percent of the RDA) that provides a normal blood concentration.

physiological fuel value: the number of kcalories that the human body derives from a food, as contrasted with the kcalories determined by calorimetry.

physiological stresses: stresses that fall within the body's normal and healthy functioning.

phytic acid: a nonnutrient component of plant seeds; also called *phytate*. Phytic acid occurs in the husks of grains, legumes, and seeds and is capable of binding minerals such as zinc, iron, calcium, magnesium, and copper in insoluble complexes in the intestine, which the body excretes unused.

phytochemicals: nonnutrient compounds in plant-derived foods that have biological activity in the body.

pica: a craving for nonfood substances.

pigment: a molecule capable of absorbing certain wavelengths of light, so that it reflects only those that we perceive as a certain color.

PKU: see *phenylketonuria*.

placebo: an inert, harmless medication given to provide comfort and hope; a sham treatment used in controlled research studies.

placebo effect: the healing effect that faith in medicine, even inert medicine, often has.

placenta: the organ that develops inside the uterus early in pregnancy, in which maternal and fetal blood circulate in close proximity so that materials can be exchanged between them. The fetus receives nutrients and oxygen across the placenta; the mother's blood picks up carbon dioxide and other waste products to be excreted.

plaque, atheromatous: mounds of lipid material, mixed with smooth muscle cells and calcium, which develop in the artery walls in atherosclerosis.

plaque, dental: a gummy mass of bacteria that grows on teeth and can lead to dental caries and gum disease.

plasma: the fluid that remains when unclotted blood is centrifuged.

platelets: tiny, disc-shaped bodies in the blood, important in blood clot formation.

point of unsaturation: the double bond of a fatty acid, where hydrogen atoms can easily be added to the structure.

polar: a neutral molecule that has opposite charges spatially separated within the molecule; see Appendix B for more details.

polydipsia: excessive thirst.

polypeptide: many (ten or more) amino acids bonded together.

polyphagia: excessive eating.

polysaccharide: many monosaccharides linked together.

polyunsaturated fatty acid (PUFA): a fatty acid that lacks four or more hydrogen atoms and has two or more double bonds between carbons—for example, linoleic acid (two double bonds) and linolenic acid (three double bonds). A *polyunsaturated fat* is composed of triglycerides containing a high percentage of PUFA.

polyuria: excessive urine production.

portal hypertension: elevated blood pressure in the portal vein caused by obstructed blood flow through the liver.

post term (infant): an infant born after the 42nd week of pregnancy.

postgastrectomy diet: a carbohydrate-controlled diet given to prevent the symptoms of dumping syndrome and hypoglycemia that sometimes follow gastric surgery.

postpartum amenorrhea: the normal temporary absence of menstrual periods immediately following childbirth.

potable water: water that is suitable for drinking.

potassium: the principal cation within the body's cells; critical to the maintenance of fluid balance, nerve transmissions, and muscle contractions.

precursors: substances that precede others; with regard to vitamins, compounds that can be converted into active vitamins; also known as *provitamins*.

preeclampsia: a condition characterized by hypertension, fluid retention, and protein in the urine.

preferred provider organization (PPO): a form of managed care that encourages subscribers to select health care providers from a group that has contracted with the organization to provide services at lower costs.

preformed vitamin A: dietary vitamin A in its active form.

pregnancy-induced hypertension (PIH): high blood pressure that develops in the second half of pregnancy.

preservatives: antimicrobial agents, antioxidants, and other additives that retard spoilage or maintain desired qualities, such as softness in baked goods.

pressure sores: the breakdown of skin and underlying tissues due to constant pressure and lack of oxygen to the affected area; often called *decubitus ulcers* or *bedsores*.

preterm (infant): an infant born prior to the 38th week of pregnancy; also called a *premature* infant.

preventive (or population) approach: recommendations that urge all people to make dietary changes believed to forestall or prevent disease.

primary deficiency: a nutrient deficiency caused by inadequate dietary intake of a nutrient.

proenzyme: the inactive form or an enzyme.

prognosis: the predicted course and outcome of a disease.

promoters: factors that favor the development of cancer once it has begun.

proof: a way of stating the percentage of alcohol in distilled liquor. Liquor that is 100 proof is 50 percent alcohol; 90 proof is 45 percent, and so forth.

protease: an enzyme that hydrolyzes proteins.

protein digestibility: a measure of the amount of amino acids absorbed from a given protein intake.

protein digestibility–corrected amino acid score (PDCAAS): a measure of protein quality assessed by comparing the amino acid balance of a food protein with the amino acid requirements of preschool-age children and then correcting for the true digestibility of the protein; recommended by the FAO/WHO and used to establish protein quality of foods for Daily Value percentages on food labels.

protein efficiency ratio (PER): a measure of protein quality assessed by determining how well a given protein supports weight gain in growing rats; used to establish the protein quality for infant formulas and baby foods.

protein-energy malnutrition (PEM): a deficiency of both protein and energy; the world's most widespread malnutrition problem, including kwashiorkor, marasmus, and instances in which they overlap; also called *protein-kcalorie malnutrition (PCM)*.

protein isolate: a protein that has been separated from a food. Examples include casein from milk and albumin from egg.

protein-losing enteropathy: the intestinal loss of serum proteins.

proteins: compounds composed of carbon, hydrogen, oxygen, and nitrogen atoms, arranged into amino acids linked in a chain. Some amino acids also contain sulfur atoms.

protein-sparing action: the action of carbohydrate (and fat) in providing energy that allows protein to be used for other purposes.

protein turnover: the degradation and synthesis of endogenous protein.

proteinuria: loss of protein in the urine.

prothrombin time: a laboratory test that evaluates the time it takes for blood to clot.

puberty: the period in life in which a person becomes physically capable of reproduction.

public health nutritionist: a dietitian who specializes in public health nutrition.

public water: water from a municipal or county water system that has been treated and disinfected.

PUFA: see *polyunsaturated fatty acids*.

pulmonary: of or pertaining to the lungs.

pureed foods: foods that have been strained and blenderized to a thickened, near-liquid consistency.

purgative: a strong laxative.

purified water: water that has been processed through distillation, deionization, or reverse osmosis and meets U.S. Pharmacopoeia standards for medical and research purposes.

pyelonephritis: an inflammation of the kidneys and bladder.

pyloric sphincter: the circular muscle that separates the stomach from the small intestine and regulates the flow of partially digested food into the small intestine; also called *pylorus* or *pyloric valve*.

pyruvate: pyruvic acid, a 3-carbon compound that, in metabolism, can be derived from glucose, certain amino acids, or glycerol.

radiation: ionizing rays used to sterilize and protect food.

radiation enteritis: damage to the intestine caused by radiation therapy.

radiation therapy: the use of radiation to arrest or destroy cancer cells.

radiolytic products: chemicals formed during the irradiation of food.

randomization: a process of choosing the members of the experimental and control groups without bias.

raw sugar: the first crop of crystals harvested during sugar processing. Raw sugar cannot be sold in the United States because it contains too much filth (dirt, insect fragments, and the like). Sugar sold as "raw sugar" domestically has actually gone through over half of the refining steps.

RBP: see *retinol-binding protein*.

RD: see *registered dietitian*.

RDA: see *Recommended Dietary Allowances*.

RDI: see *Reference Daily Intakes*.

RE (retinol equivalent): a measure of vitamin A activity; the amount of retinol that the body will derive from a food containing preformed retinol or its precursor beta-carotene.

reactive hypoglycemia: hypoglycemia experienced simultaneously with epinephrine-release symptoms one to three hours after a meal; also called *postprandial hypoglycemia*.

rebound hyperglycemia: hyperglycemia resulting from excessive secretion of counterregulatory hormones in response to excessive insulin; also called the *Somogyi effect*.

rebound scurvy: vitamin C deficiency resulting from the sudden withdrawal of excessive doses of vitamin C.

recessive gene: a gene that has no observable effect on an organism as long as it is paired with a normal gene that can produce a normal product. In this case, the normal gene is said to be *dominant*.

recombinant DNA technology: methods of joining (recombining) pieces of the genetic material DNA in order to change the proteins produced by the altered DNA.

Recommended Dietary Allowances (RDA): the amounts of selected nutrients considered adequate to meet the known nutrient needs of practically all healthy people.

rectum: the muscular terminal part of the intestine, extending from the sigmoid colon to the anus.

refeeding syndrome: a set of physiologic and metabolic complications associated with reintroducing adequate nutrition too rapidly for a person with severe PEM. These complications can include malabsorption, cardiac insufficiency, respiratory distress, congestive heart failure, convulsions, coma, and possibly death.

Reference Daily Intakes (RDI): a set of standards for protein, vitamins, and minerals used on food labels as part of the Daily Values; previously known as the U.S. RDA.

reference protein: a standard against which to measure the quality of other proteins.

refined: the process by which the coarse parts of a food are removed. When wheat is refined into flour, the bran, germ, and husk are removed, leaving only the endosperm.

reflux: a backward flow.

reflux esophagitis: the backflow or regurgitation of gastric contents from the stomach into the esophagus, causing inflammation of the esophagus; also called *gastroesophageal reflux*, *gastric reflux*, or *acid indigestion*.

registered dietitian (RD): a dietitian who has graduated from a university or college after completing a program of dietetics that has been accredited by the American Dietetic Association (or Dietitians of Canada), has served in an internship or coordinated program to practice the necessary skills, has passed the association's registration examination, and maintains competency through continuing education. Many states require licensing for practicing dietitians.

registration: with respect to health professionals, listing with a professional organization that requires specific course work, experience, and passing of an examination.

remodeling: the dismantling and re-formation of a structure, in this case, bone.

renal: pertaining to the kidneys.

renal colic: the severe pain that accompanies the movement of a kidney stone from the kidney through the ureter to the bladder.

renal failure: failure of the kidneys to maintain normal function.

renal insufficiency: reduced renal function but not to the degree that requires dialysis or a kidney transplant.

renal osteodystrophy: bone disorders resulting from calcium and phosphorus imbalances in renal disease.

renal reserve: the capacity of the kidneys to function despite loss of some nephrons.

renal threshold: the point at which blood glucose rises so high that the kidneys cannot reabsorb it.

renin: an enzyme secreted by the kidneys in response to a reduced blood flow that triggers the release of the hormone aldosterone from the adrenal glands. Aldosterone, in turn, signals the kidneys to retain sodium and water.

rennin: an enzyme that coagulates milk; found in the gastric juice of cows, but not human beings.

replication: repeating an experiment and getting the same results.

requirement: the amount of a nutrient that will maintain normal biochemical and physiological functions and prevent the development of specific deficiency signs; distinguished from the RDA, which is a recommended and generous allowance that provides for variability among individuals.

residue: whatever remains. In the body, the total amount of material in the GI tract, including dietary fiber and also undigested food, intestinal secretions, bacterial cell bodies, and cells shed from the intestinal mucosa. In agriculture, the amounts of pesticides that remain on or in foods when people buy and use them.

resistant starch: starch that is not absorbed in the small intestine of healthy people.

respiratory acidosis: a condition of too much acid in the blood caused by failure of the lungs to adequately expel carbon dioxide during exhalation.

respiratory distress: a disorder of the lung membranes that results in delayed onset of respiration at birth and difficulty in breathing after birth.

respiratory failure: failure of the lungs to exchange gases; also known as *adult respiratory distress syndrome (ARDS)*.

respiratory quotient (RQ): the ratio of carbon dioxide produced to oxygen consumed. Clinicians used the RQ to estimate total energy needs and the appropriate mix of carbohydrate and fat to meet those needs.

retina: the layer of light-sensitive nerve cells lining the back of the inside of the eye; consists of rods and cones.

retinal: the aldehyde form of vitamin A, active in the eye.

retinoic acid: the acid form of vitamin A.

retinoids: chemically related compounds with biologic activity similar to retinol; metabolites of retinol.

retinol: the alcohol form of vitamin A.

retinol-binding protein (RBP): the specific protein responsible for transporting retinol.

retinopathy: a disorder of the retina.

rheumatic heart disease: heart damage (often affecting the heart valves) that follows rheumatic fever (caused by a systemic bacterial infection).

rhodopsin: the light-sensitive pigment of the rods in the retina; it contains the retinal form of vitamin A.

riboflavin: a B vitamin; the coenzyme forms are FMN (flavin mononucleotide) and FAD (flavin adenine dinucleotide).

rickets: the vitamin D–deficiency disease in children characterized by inadequate mineralization of bone (manifested in bowed legs or knock-knees, outward-bowed chest, and knobs on ribs). A rare type of rickets, *not* caused by vitamin D deficiency, is known as *vitamin D–refractory rickets*.

risk: a measure of the probability and severity of harm.

risk factors: factors associated with an elevated frequency of a disease but not proven to be causal.

rods: the cells of the retina that respond to dim light and convey black-and-white vision.

saccharin: a 0-kcalorie sweetener used in the United States but available in Canada only in pharmacies and only as a sweetener, not as an additive.

safety: a judgment that considers the risks acceptable.

saliva: the secretion of the salivary glands; its principal enzyme begins carbohydrate digestion.

salivary glands: exocrine glands that secrete saliva into the mouth.

salts: compounds composed of a positive ion other than H^+ and a negative ion other than OH^-. An example is sodium chloride (Na^+Cl^-).

sarcomas: cancers that arise from muscle, bone, or connective tissues.

satiety: the feeling of satisfaction and fullness that food brings.

saturated fatty acid: a fatty acid carrying the maximum possible number of hydrogen atoms—for example, stearic acid. A *saturated fat* is composed of triglycerides in which all or virtually all of the fatty acids are saturated.

science of nutrition: the study of the nutrients in foods and of the body's handling of them (including ingestion, digestion, absorption, transport, metabolism, interaction, storage, and excretion). A broader definition includes the study of the environment and of human behavior as it relates to food.

scurvy: the vitamin C–deficiency disease.

secondary deficiency: a nutrient deficiency caused by something other than diet, such as a disease condition that reduces absorption, accelerates use, hastens excretion, or destroys the nutrient.

secondary hypertension: high blood pressure that is caused by a specific disorder such as kidney disease.

secretin: a hormone produced by cells in the duodenum wall. Target organ: the pancreas. Response: secretion of bicarbonate-rich pancreatic juice.

secretory diarrhea: diarrhea that results from an accelerated movement of fluids and electrolytes from the intestinal capillaries into the lumen of the intestine.

sedentary: physically inactive (literally, "sitting down a lot").

segmentation: a periodic squeezing or partitioning of the intestine at intervals along its length by its circular muscles.

selenium: a trace element.

semivegetarians: people who include some, but not all, groups of animal-derived foods in their diets; they usually exclude red meat, but may occasionally include poultry and seafood; sometimes called *partial vegetarians*.

senile dementia: the loss of brain function beyond the normal loss of physical adeptness and memory that occurs with aging.

senile dementia of the Alzheimer's type (SDAT): a degenerative disease of the brain involving memory loss and major structural changes in neuron networks; also known as *primary degenerative dementia of senile onset* or *chronic brain syndrome*, but often simply called *Alzheimer's disease*.

sepsis (or septicemia): the presence of microorganisms or their poisonous products in the bloodstream.

serotonin: a neurotransmitter important in sleep and sensory perception; it is synthesized from the amino acid tryptophan with the help of vitamin B_6.

serum: the watery portion of the blood that remains after removal of the cells and clot-forming material.

set point: the point at which controls are set (for example, on a thermostat). The set-point theory proposes that the body tends to maintain a certain weight by means of its own internal controls.

severe stresses: pathological stresses that rapidly and markedly raise the body's metabolic rate and significantly upset its normal internal balance.

shock: a critical event that occurs when a sudden drop in the blood volume disrupts the supply of oxygen to the tissues and the return of blood to the heart.

short-bowel or short-gut syndrome: severe malabsorption that may occur when the absorptive surface of the small bowel is reduced, resulting in diarrhea, weight loss, bone disease, hypocalcemia, hypomagnesemia, and anemia.

sickle-cell anemia: a hereditary form of anemia characterized by abnormal sickle- or crescent-shaped red blood cells. Sickled cells interfere with oxygen transport and blood flow. Symptoms include hemolytic anemia (red blood cells burst), fever, and severe pain in the joints and abdomen; they are precipitated by dehydration and insufficient oxygen (as may occur at high altitudes).

SIDS: see *sudden infant death syndrome*.

silent heart attack: a heart attack that goes unnoticed.

simple carbohydrates (sugars): monosaccharides and disaccharides.

sitophobia: fear of eating.

SMA (simultaneous multiple analysis): the measurement of several blood components during a single blood test. SMA is followed by a number (for example, SMA-12) that indicates how many tests will be run.

small intestine: a 10-foot length of small-diameter intestine that is the major site of digestion of food and absorption of nutrients; its segments are the duodenum, jejunum, and ileum.

socioeconomic history: a record of a person's social and economic background, including such factors as education, income, and ethnic identity.

sodium: the principal cation in the extracellular fluids of the body, critical to the maintenance of fluid balance, nerve transmissions, and muscle contractions.

soft water: water with a high sodium concentration.

solanine: a poisonous narcotic-like substance present in potato peels and sprouts. Physical symptoms of solanine poisoning include headache, vomiting, abdominal pain, diarrhea, and fever; neurological symptoms include apathy, restlessness, drowsiness, confusion, stupor, hallucinations, and visual disturbances.

solutes: the substances that are dissolved in a solution.

sperm: the male reproductive cell, capable of fertilizing an ovum.

sphincter: a circular muscle surrounding, and able to close, a body opening.

spring water: water originating from an underground spring or well. It may be carbonated or not ("flat" or "still"). Brand names such as "Spring Pure" do not necessarily mean that the water comes from a spring.

standard diet: a *regular diet*—that is, one that includes all foods and meets the nutrient needs of normal, healthy individuals.

standard formula: a liquid diet that contains complete molecules of proteins; also called *intact* or *polymeric formulas*.

starch: a plant polysaccharide composed of glucose that is digestible by human beings.

steatorrhea: fatty diarrhea characteristic of fat malabsorption; stools are loose, foamy, and foul smelling.

sterile: free of microorganisms, such as bacteria.

sterol: a compound composed of C, H, and O atoms arranged in rings, like those of cholesterol, with any of a variety of side chains attached.

stoma: a surgically formed opening, as in a gastrostomy jejunostomy, ileostomy, or colostomy.

stomach: a muscular, elastic, saclike portion of the digestive tract that grinds and churns swallowed food, mixing it with acid and enzymes to form chyme.

stools: waste matter discharged from the colon; also called *feces*.

stress: any threat to a person's well-being; a demand placed on the body to adapt.

stress eating: eating in response to arousal.

stress fractures: bone damage or breaks caused by stress on bone surfaces during exercise.

stress response: the body's response to stress, mediated initially by both nerves and hormones; begins with an *alarm reaction*, proceeds through a stage of *resistance*, and then leads to *recovery* or, if prolonged, to *exhaustion*. This three-stage response has also been termed the *general adaptation syndrome*.

stressor: an environmental element, physical or psychological, that causes stress.

stroke: an event in which the blood flow to a part of the brain is cut off; also called a *cerebrovascular accident* (CVA).

struvite: crystals of magnesium ammonium phosphate.

subclinical deficiency: a deficiency in the early stages, before the outward signs have appeared.

substitute food: a food that is designed to replace another.

subtotal (or partial) gastrectomy: removal of a portion of the stomach.

sucralose: a 0-kcalorie sweetener that is 600 times sweeter than sucrose; FDA approval pending in the United States; approved in Canada.

sucrase: an enzyme that hydrolyzes sucrose.

sucrose: a disaccharide composed of glucose and fructose; commonly known as table sugar, beet sugar, or cane sugar. Sucrose also occurs in many fruits and some vegetables and grains.

sudden infant death syndrome (SIDS): the unexpected and unexplained death of an apparently well infant; the most common cause of death of infants between the second week and the end of the first year of life; also called *crib death*.

sugar alcohols: sugarlike compounds that can be derived from fruits or commercially produced from dextrose; also called *polyols*. Like sugars, sugar alcohols are sweet to taste and yield 4 kcalories per gram, but they are absorbed more slowly and metabolized differently than other sugars in the human body, and are not readily utilized by ordinary mouth bacteria. Examples are *maltitol*, *mannitol*, *sorbitol*, and *xylitol*.

sulfites: salts containing sulfur that are added to foods to prevent spoilage.

sulfur: a mineral present in the body as part of some amino acids.

supplements: pills, liquids, or powders that contain purified nutrients, or foods with purified nutrients added in amounts per serving greater than 50 percent above a standard considered sufficient for all healthy people.

sushi: vinegar-flavored rice and seafood, typically wrapped in seaweed and stuffed with colorful vegetables. Some sushi is stuffed with raw fish; other varieties contain only cooked ingredients.

sustainable: able to continue indefinitely. Here, the term means the use of resources at such a rate that the earth can keep on replacing them—for example, cutting trees no faster than new ones grow and producing pollutants at a rate with which the environment and human cleanup efforts can keep pace, so that no net accumulation of pollution occurs.

syndrome X: the combination of insulin resistance, glucose intolerance, hypertension, elevated blood lipids, and obesity frequently observed in people with cardiovascular disease.

synthetase: an enzyme that enables two or more substances to form a more complex structure.

systemic: affecting the whole body rather than one part or organ system.

systemic inflammatory response syndrome (SIRS): the changes that result from the activation of immune and inflammatory factors during stress.

tachycardia: a rapid heart rate.

TEF: see *thermic effect of food*.

tempeh: a fermented soybean food, rich in protein and fiber.

tension-fatigue syndrome: apparent hyperactivity produced in a child by the combination of lack of sleep, overstimulation, and anxiety.

teratogenic: causing abnormal fetal development and birth defects.

term (infant): an infant born between the 38th and 42nd week of pregnancy.

terminal illness: a progressive, irreversible disease that will lead to death in the near future.

textured vegetable protein: processed soybean protein used in vegetarian products such as soy burgers.

thermic effect of food (TEF): an estimation of the energy required to process food (digest, absorb, transport, metabolize, and store ingested nutrients); also called *diet-induced thermogenesis* (DIT), the *specific dynamic effect* (SDE) of food, or the *specific dynamic activity* (SDA) of food.

thermogenesis: the generation of heat; used in physiology and nutrition studies as an index of how much energy the body is spending.

thiamin: a B vitamin; the coenzyme form is TPP (thiamin pyrophosphate).

thirst: a conscious desire to drink.

thrombosis: the formation of a blood clot that may obstruct a blood vessel, causing gradual tissue death.

thrombus: a blood clot that obstructs a blood vessel or a cavity of the heart.

thrush: a fungal infection of the mouth and esophagus caused by *Candida albicans*; the technical term for this infection is *candidiasis*. Thrush is characterized by a thick white coating of the tongue that alters taste sensations and causes pain on chewing and swallowing.

tocopherol: a general term for several chemically related compounds, most of which have vitamin E activity.

tocopherol equivalents (TE): the units in which vitamin E activity is measured. One TE equals the amount of vitamin E activity in 1 mg of D-alpha-tocopherol.

tofu: a curd made from soybeans, rich in protein and often fortified with calcium; used in many Asian and vegetarian dishes in place of meat.

tolerance level: the maximum amount of a residue permitted in a food when a pesticide is used according to label directions.

total gastrectomy: removal of the entire stomach.

toxicity: the ability of a substance to harm living organisms. All substances are toxic if high enough concentrations are used.

total parenteral nutrition (TPN): the delivery of all nutrient needs by vein.

trabecular bone: the lacy inner structure of calcium crystals that supports the bone's structure and provides a calcium storage bank.

trace minerals: essential mineral nutrients found in the human body in amounts less than 5 g. The trace minerals are iron, iodine, zinc, chromium, selenium, fluoride, molybdenum, copper, and manganese.

trachea: the windpipe; the passageway from the mouth and nose to the lungs.

***trans*-fatty acids:** fatty acids with an unusual configuration around the double bond.

transamination: the transfer of an amino group from one amino acid to a keto acid, producing a new nonessential amino acid and a new keto acid.

transgenic organism: an organism that grows from an embryonic, stem, or germ cell into which a gene is inserted; the organism then carries the new gene in all of its cells.

transient ischemic attack (TIA): a temporary reduction in blood flow to the brain that causes temporary symptoms that depend on the part of the brain that is affected. Some common symptoms include lightheadedness, visual disturbances, paralysis, staggering, numbness, or dysphagia.

translocation: the passage of infectious agents into the body through the intestinal tract.

transnasal: through the nose. A *transnasal feeding tube* is one that is inserted through the nose.

trauma: physical insult to the body that causes tissue damage including fractures, wounds, burns, or surgery.

triglycerides: the chief form of fat in the diet and the major storage form of fat in the body; composed of a molecule of glycerol with three fatty acids attached; also called *triacylglycerols*.

trimester: a three-month period, often used to describe a time during pregnancy.

tripeptide: three amino acids bonded together.

tube feedings: delivering nutrient solutions via a tube into the stomach or intestine.

tubule: a tubelike structure that surrounds the glomerulus and descends through the nephron. A pressure gradient between the glomerular capillaries and the tubule returns needed materials to the blood and moves wastes into the tubule to be sent to the bladder.

tumor: a new growth of tissue forming an abnormal mass with no function; also called a *neoplasm*.

turbinado sugar: sugar produced using the same refining process as white sugar, but without the bleaching and anti-caking treatment; traces of molasses give turbinado its sandy color.

24-hour recall: a record of foods eaten by a person for one 24-hour period.

type I osteoporosis: osteoporosis characterized by rapid bone losses, primarily of trabecular bone.

type II osteoporosis: osteoporosis characterized by gradual losses of both trabecular and cortical bone.

ulcer: an erosion in the topmost, and sometimes underlying, layers of cells in an area; see also *peptic ulcer*.

ulcerative colitis: inflammation and ulceration of the colon; see also *Crohn's disease*.

ultrahigh temperature (UHT) treatment: sterilizing a food by short-time exposure to temperatures above those normally used.

umbilical cord: the ropelike structure through which the fetus's veins and arteries reach the placenta; the route of nourishment and oxygen into the fetus and the route of waste disposal from the fetus.

umbilicus: the scar in the middle of the abdomen that marks the former attachment of the umbilical cord; commonly known as the "belly button."

unavailable carbohydrates: carbohydrates such as fibers that human digestive enzymes cannot break down.

unbleached flour: a tan-colored endosperm flour with texture and nutritive qualities that approximate those of regular white flour.

undernutrition: deficiency of energy or nutrients.

underweight: body weight below some standard of acceptable weight that is usually defined in relation to height (such as the weight-for-height tables).

unsaturated fatty acid: a fatty acid that lacks hydrogen atoms and has at least one double bond between carbons (includes monounsaturated and polyunsaturated fatty acids). An *unsaturated fat* is composed of triglycerides in which some of the fatty acids are unsaturated.

upper safe: the amount of a nutrient that appears safe for *most healthy people* and beyond which there is concern that some people will experience toxicity symptoms.

urea: the principal nitrogen-excretion product of metabolism. Two ammonia fragments are combined with carbon dioxide to form urea.

urea kinetic modeling: a technique used to evaluate dialysis and guide diet therapy that takes into account the kidneys' ability to clear urea and the person's protein catabolic rate.

uremia (or azotemia): abnormal accumulation of nitrogen-containing substances in the blood.

uremic syndrome: the many symptoms that accompany the buildup of toxic waste products in the blood.

uremic frost: the appearance of urea crystals on the skin.

urethra: the tube through which urine from the bladder passes out of the body.

USDA (U.S. Department of Agriculture): the federal agency responsible for enforcing standards for the wholesomeness and quality of meat, poultry, and eggs produced in the United States; conducting nutrition research; and educating the public about nutrition.

uterus: the muscular organ within which the infant develops before birth; the womb.

vagotomy: surgery that severs the nerves to the stomach that stimulate gastric acid secretion.

validity: having the quality of being founded on fact or evidence.

variable: a factor that changes. A variable may depend on another variable (for example, a child's height depends on his age), or it may be independent (for example, a child's height does not depend on the color of her eyes). Sometimes both variables correlate with a third variable (a child's height and eye color both depend on genetics).

variety (dietary): eating a wide selection of foods within and among the major food groups (the opposite of monotony).

vasoconstrictor: a substance that constricts or narrows the blood vessels.

vegans: people who exclude all animal-derived foods (including meat, poultry, fish, eggs, and dairy products) from their diets; also called *pure vegetarians*, *strict vegetarians*, or *total vegetarians*.

vegetarians: a general term used to describe people who exclude meat, poultry, fish, or other animal-derived foods from their diets.

vein: a vessel that carries blood back to the heart.

villi: fingerlike projections from the folds of the small intestine; singular *villus*.

vitamin A activity: a term useful for referring to both the preformed vitamin A and the carotene contents of foods without distinguishing between them.

vitamin B_6: a family of compounds—pyridoxal, pyridoxine, and pyridoxamine; the primary active coenzyme form is PLP (pyridoxal phosphate).

vitamin B_{12}: a B vitamin characterized by the presence of cobalt; the active forms of coenzyme B_{12} are methylcobalamin and deoxyadenosylcobalamin.

vitamins: organic, essential nutrients required in small amounts by the body for health. The water-soluble vitamins are vitamin C and the eight B vitamins: thiamin, riboflavin, niacin, vitamins B_6 and B_{12}, folate, biotin, and pantothenic acid. The fat-soluble vitamins are vitamins A, D, E, and K.

VLDL (very-low-density lipoprotein): the type of lipoprotein made primarily by liver cells to transport lipids to various tissues in the body; composed primarily of triglycerides.

voluntary activities: the component of a person's daily energy expenditure that involves conscious and deliberate muscular work—walking, lifting, climbing, or other physical activity.

vomiting: expulsion of the contents of the

stomach up through the esophagus to the mouth.

water balance: the balance between water intake and output (losses). Water balance = intake − output.

water intoxication: the condition in which body water contents are too high.

water-miscible vitamins: fat-soluble vitamins that readily mix with water and can be absorbed without fat.

wean: to gradually replace one form of feeding with another, such as replacing breast milk or infant formula with semi-solid foods, parenteral nutrition with enteral nutrition, or enteral formulas with table foods.

weight cycling: repeated cycles of weight loss and gain. The weight-cycling pattern is popularly called the *ratchet effect* or *yo-yo effect* of dieting.

well water: water drawn from groundwater by tapping into an aquifer.

Wernicke-Korsakoff syndrome: symptoms commonly seen in malnourished alcohol abusers that are similar to those seen in thiamin deficiency and that can be treated with thiamin supplements.

wheat flour: any flour made from wheat, including white flour.

white flour: an endosperm flour that has been refined and bleached for maximum softness and whiteness.

white sugar: pure sucrose or "table sugar," produced by dissolving, concentrating, and recrystallizing raw sugar.

WHO (World Health Organization): an international agency that has adopted standards to regulate pesticide use among other responsibilities.

whole grain: a grain milled in its entirety (all but the husk), not refined.

whole-wheat flour: flour made from whole-wheat kernels; a whole-grain flour.

wine: an alcoholic beverage made by fermenting grape juice.

xanthophylls: pigments found in plants; responsible for the color changes seen in autumn leaves.

xerophthalmia: progressive blindness caused by vitamin A deficiency.

xerosis: drying of the cornea; a sign of vitamin A deficiency.

Zollinger-Ellison syndrome: marked hypersecretion of gastric acid and consequent peptic ulcers caused by a tumor of the pancreas, which releases gastrin.

zygote: the product of the union of ovum and sperm; so-called for the first two weeks after fertilization.

Index

This index lists primarily topics that received significant mention in the text. Inclusive pages (for example, 53–56) indicate major discussions; pages in **boldface** refer to defined terms; pages in *italics* refer to figures, diagrams, or chemical structures; pages followed by a "t" refer to tables; pages followed by an "n" refer to notes; letter-number combinations (such as C-24) refer to appendixes.

CHAPTER OPENING ELECTRON MICROGRAPHS © Michael Davidson

1 carrot; **36** spinach; **71** green pepper; **101** fructose; **146** olecic acid; **179** hemoglobin; **218** acetyl coA; **256** adenosine triphosphate; **287** litesse; **325** vitamin C; **374** beta carotene; **408** calcium; **449** selenium; **485** capsaicin; **518** leptin; **543** vitamin A; **561** thiamine; **584** folate; **625** growth hormone; **665** serotonin; **694** vitamin B 12; **722** vitamin D; **755** glutamine; **782** arginine; **803** epinephrine; **825** ammonia; **845** glucose; **881** prostaglandin; **909** urea; **933** AZT; **963** vitamin E.

PHOTO CREDITS

xi, xii, xiii, xiv, xv, xvi, xvii, xviii, xix © Michael Davidson, **7** (Top), **12, 36** (Far right), **38, 40, 42, 43, 48, 98, 123, 166, 169, 196, 209, 216, 330, 333, 337** (Bottom), **341, 362, 385, 397, 405** (Left), **424, 430, 455, 461, 468, 505, 570, 572, 573, 636, 645** © Thomas Harm & Thomas Peterson/Quest Photographic Inc.; **2** © Tom McCarthy/PhotoEdit; **3** © Bob Daemmrich/Tony Stone Worldwide; **6** © Felicia Martinez/PhotoEdit; **7** © (Bottom left) Tony Freeman/PhotoEdit; **7** © (Bottom right) David Young-Wolff/PhotoEdit; **9** © Tony Freeman/PhotoEdit; **10** © Christopher Bissell/Tony Stone Worldwide; **14** © Bill Bachman/PhotoEdit; **22** © Michael Newman/PhotoEdit; **29** © Frank Siteman/Tony Stone Worldwide; **32** © Marilynne Herbert; **39** © Rosemary Weller/Tony Stone Worldwide; **41** © Michael Dwyer/Stock, Boston Inc.; **45** © Tony Freeman/PhotoEdit; **50** (Far left) Ray Stanyard; **50** © Felicia Martinez/PhotoEdit; **50** © Michael Newman/PhotoEdit; **51** © Tony Freeman/PhotoEdit; **52** Courtesy of the FDA; **63** © David Simson/Stock, Boston Inc.; **66** © Merritt Vincent/Stock, Boston Inc.; **67** © Felicia Martinez/PhotoEdit; **68** © Michael Newman/PhotoEdit; **69** © Bill Aron/PhotoEdit; **73** © Felicia Martinez/PhotoEdit; **84** From D. W. Fawcett, *The Cell*, 2nd ed. (Philadelphia: Saunders, 1981); **92** © Michael Newman/PhotoEdit; **99** © Jeff Dunn/The Picture Cube Inc.; **103** © David Young-Wolff/PhotoEdit; **116** © David Young-Wolff/PhotoEdit; **117** © Tony Freeman/PhotoEdit; **126** © Felicia Martinez/PhotoEdit; **133** © Sunette Division, Hoechst Celanese Corp.; **145** © Felicia Martinez/PhotoEdit; **148** © Peter Correz/Tony Stone Worldwide; **163** © John Neubauer/PhotoEdit; **164** Ray Stanyard; **165** © Tony Freeman/PhotoEdit; **171** © Felicia Martinez/PhotoEdit; **176** © Mary Kate Denny/PhotoEdit; **188** © Robert Finken/The Picture Cube; **197** © Michael Newman/PhotoEdit; **199** © Alan Oddie/PhotoEdit; **200** Courtesy of Robert S. Goodhard, M.D.; **201** Courtesy of Robert S. Goodhard, M.D.; **219** © Paul Mozell/Stock, Boston; **238** © Michael Newman/PhotoEdit; **245** © Southern Living/Photo Researchers Inc.; **266** © David Young-Wolff/PhotoEdit; **268** © John Bahlik; **272** © Lori Adamski Peek/Tony Stone Worldwide; **273** © David Young-Wolff/PhotoEdit; **274** © David Young-Wolff/PhotoEdit; **278** © Vic Bider/PhotoEdit; **279** (Left) © Michael Newman/PhotoEdit; **279** (Right) © Jonathan Nourok/PhotoEdit; **282** © Phil McCarten/PhotoEdit; **283** © Tony Freeman/PhotoEdit; **284** © Amy G. Etra/PhotoEdit; **285** © Felicia Martinez/PhotoEdit; **289** © Tony Freeman/PhotoEdit; **292** © Frank Whitney/The Image Bank; **293** © AP/Wide World Photos; **305** © David Young-Wolff/PhotoEdit; **315** © Tony Freeman/PhotoEdit; **316** © Michael Newman/PhotoEdit; **320** © Michael Newman/PhotoEdit; **329** © L. V. Bergman & Associates, Inc.; **337** © L. V. Bergman & Associates, Inc.; **341** Peter Chapman/Stock, Boston Inc.; **350** © Martin M. Rotker; **355** © Science Photo Library/Photo Researchers, Inc.; **361** (Top) © L. V. Bergman & Associates; **361** (Bottom) From C. Conn, The Specialties in General Practice, 2nd ed. (Philadelphia: Saunders, 1957); **366** © Tony Freeman/PhotoEdit; **381** © David Farr; **384** © Ken Greer/Visuals Unlimited; **388** Courtesy of Parke-Davis & Company; **390** David Young-Wolff/PhotoEdit; **391** © Daniel Brody/Stock, Boston Inc.; **392** © Tom Prettyman/PhotoEdit; **400** © Mary Kate Denny/PhotoEdit; **405** (Right) © Tom McCarthy/The Picture Cube; **409** © Lawrence Migdale/Stock, Boston Inc.; **421** © David Young-Wolff/PhotoEdit; **437** © Bob Daemmrich/Stock, Boston Inc.; **439** Courtesy of Gjon Mill; **440** With permission from Dempster et al., J. Bone Min. Res I 15–21, 1986; **458** © Martin M. Rotker; **466** © Reproduced with permission of "Nutrition Today" Magazine; **470** © L. V. Bergman & Associates, Inc.; **475** Courtesy of H. Kaplan & V. P. Robbache; **480** © Tony Freeman/PhotoEdit; **486** Bob Daemmrich/Stock, Boston Inc.; **492** © Felicia Martinez/PhotoEdit; **493** © Lawrence Migdale/Photo Researchers, Inc.; **499** © Myrleen Ferguson Cate/PhotoEdit; **500** © George Loun/Visuals Unlimited; **501** © Felicia Martinez/PhotoEdit; **502** © Richard Brown/Tony Stone Worldwide; **503** © Felicia Martinez/PhotoEdit; **506** © Diane Graham-Henry/Tony Stone Worldwide; **507** © Felicia Martinez/PhotoEdit; **512** Smithsonian Photo by Antonio Montaner; **515** © Jeff Greenberg/PhotoEdit; **519** © Mary Kate Denny/PhotoEdit; **526** © Joseph Nettis/Tony Stone Worldwide; **535** © Steve Goldberg/Monkmeyer Press; **536** © Michelle Bridwell/PhotoEdit; **539** © Michael Newman/PhotoEdit; **544** © Mary Kate Denny/PhotoEdit; **545** (Top) © Tony Freeman/PhotoEdit; **545** (Bottom) © Michael Newman/PhotoEdit; **546** © John

Coletti/The Picture Cube; **550** © David Young-Wolff/PhotoEdit; **551** © W & D McIntyre/Photo Researchers, Inc.; **559** © David Young-Wolff/PhotoEdit; **567** © Michael Newman/PhotoEdit; **571** © Felicia Martinez/PhotoEdit; **579** (Top) © David Young-Wolff/PhotoEdit; **579** (Bottom) © William Thompson/The Picture Cube; **581** © Charles Gupton/Stock, Boston Inc.; **587** (Top and bottom left) © Petit, Format/Nestle/Photo Researchers, Inc.; **589** © Michael Newman/PhotoEdit; **590** © Bill Bachman/Stock, Boston Inc.; **591** © David Sams/Stock, Boston Inc.; **598** © Nik Kleinberg/Stock, Boston Inc.; **600** © Leslie Sponseller/Tony Stone Worldwide; **602** © Streissguth, A. P., Clarren, S. K. & Jones, K. L. (1985, July) Natural History of the Fetal Alcohol Syndrome: A ten-year follow-up of eleven patients, Lauret II, 89–92; **603** © George Steinmetz; **606** © Myrleen Ferguson Cate/PhotoEdit; **607** © Harry Wilks/Stock, Boston Inc.; **608** © Myrleen Ferguson Cate/PhotoEdit; **614** © Bob Daemmrich/Tony Stone Worldwide; **615** © Penny Tweedie/Tony Stone Worldwide; **617** © Bob Daemmrich/Stock, Boston Inc.; **618** © Jerry Irwin/Photo Researchers, Inc.; **619** © Diane Lowe/Stock, Boston Inc.; **620** © David Austen/Stock, Boston Inc.; **621** © David Austen/Stock, Boston Inc.; **622** Courtesy of NASA; **626** © C. J. Allen/Stock, Boston Inc.; **630** © Owen Franken/Sygma; **633** (Top) © Mary Kate Denny/PhotoEdit; **633** (Bottom) Courtesy of H. Kamplan and V. P. Rabbach; **637** © Tony Freeman/PhotoEdit; **639** © Anthony Vanelli; **642** © David Young-Wolff/PhotoEdit; **644** © Michael Newman/PhotoEdit; **648** © David Young-Wolff/PhotoEdit; **652** © Phyllis Picardi/Stock, Boston Inc.; **658** © David Young-Wolff/Tony Stone Worldwide; **659** Reproduced by permission of ICI Pharmaceuticals Division, Cheshire, England; **669** © Tom McCarthy/The Picture Cube; **670** © David Young-Wolff/PhotoEdit; **672** © Christopher Brown/Stock, Boston Inc.; **673** © Michael Newman/PhotoEdit; **679** © Bill Bachman/PhotoEdit; **681** © D & I MacDonald/PhotoEdit; **682** © Bill Aron/PhotoEdit; **684** (Top) © Myrleen Ferguson Cate/PhotoEdit; **684** (Bottom) © L. Druskis/Stock, Boston Inc.; **688** © Darrell Gulin/Tony Stone Images; **748** © David Young-Wolff/PhotoEdit; **752** © B. F. King, University of California School of Medicine/BPS; **757** © Charles Gupton/Stock, Boston Inc.; **761** (Top) © Michael Newman/PhotoEdit; **761** (Bottom) Flexiflo® Over–The–Guidewire Nasojeunal Feeding Tube, Courtesy of Ross Products Division, Abbott Laboratories, Columbus, Ohio; **776** (Top, Middle) Felicia Martinez/PhotoEdit; **776** (Bottom) Courtesy of Anderson Benner Associates, from the 3 Dimensional Puree Deluxe Recipe Set: 59 Firefall, Ct., The Woodlands, TX 77380; **779** © Gary Wagner/Stock, Boston; **783** © Mary Kate Denny/PhotoEdit; **784** © David Young-Wolff/PhotoEdit; **794** Courtesy Zevex, Inc.; **797** © Grace Moore/Medichrome/The Stock Shop; **813** © David Young-Wolff/PhotoEdit; **820** © L. O'Shaughnessy/Medichrome/The Stock Shop; **839** © David Young-Wolff/PhotoEdit; **852** © Myrleen Ferguson/PhotoEdit; **857** © Tom McCarty/PhotoEdit; **860** © Tony Freeman/PhotoEdit; **861** © Tony Freeman/PhotoEdit; **865** © Tony Freeman/PhotoEdit; **877** Anne Dowie; **889** © John Greim/The Stock Shop; **891** © Dennis McDonald/PhotoEdit; **900** © Michael Newman/PhotoEdit; **905** © Tony Freeman/PhotoEdit; **922** Anne Dowie; **930** Photo reprinted with permission from *The New England Journal of Medicine*, October, p. 1142, 1992; **934** © Courtesy American Cancer Society; **940** © Jon Riley/Tony Stone Worldwide; **948** © Lauren Goodsmith/The Image Works; **953** © Gary Conner/PhotoEdit; **959** © Amy C. Etra/PhotoEdit.

Acceptable Weight for Height Based on Body Mass Index (BMI)

To determine your acceptable weight range, find your height in the top line. Look down the column below it and find the range represented by the color blue. Look to the left column to see what weights are acceptable for you.

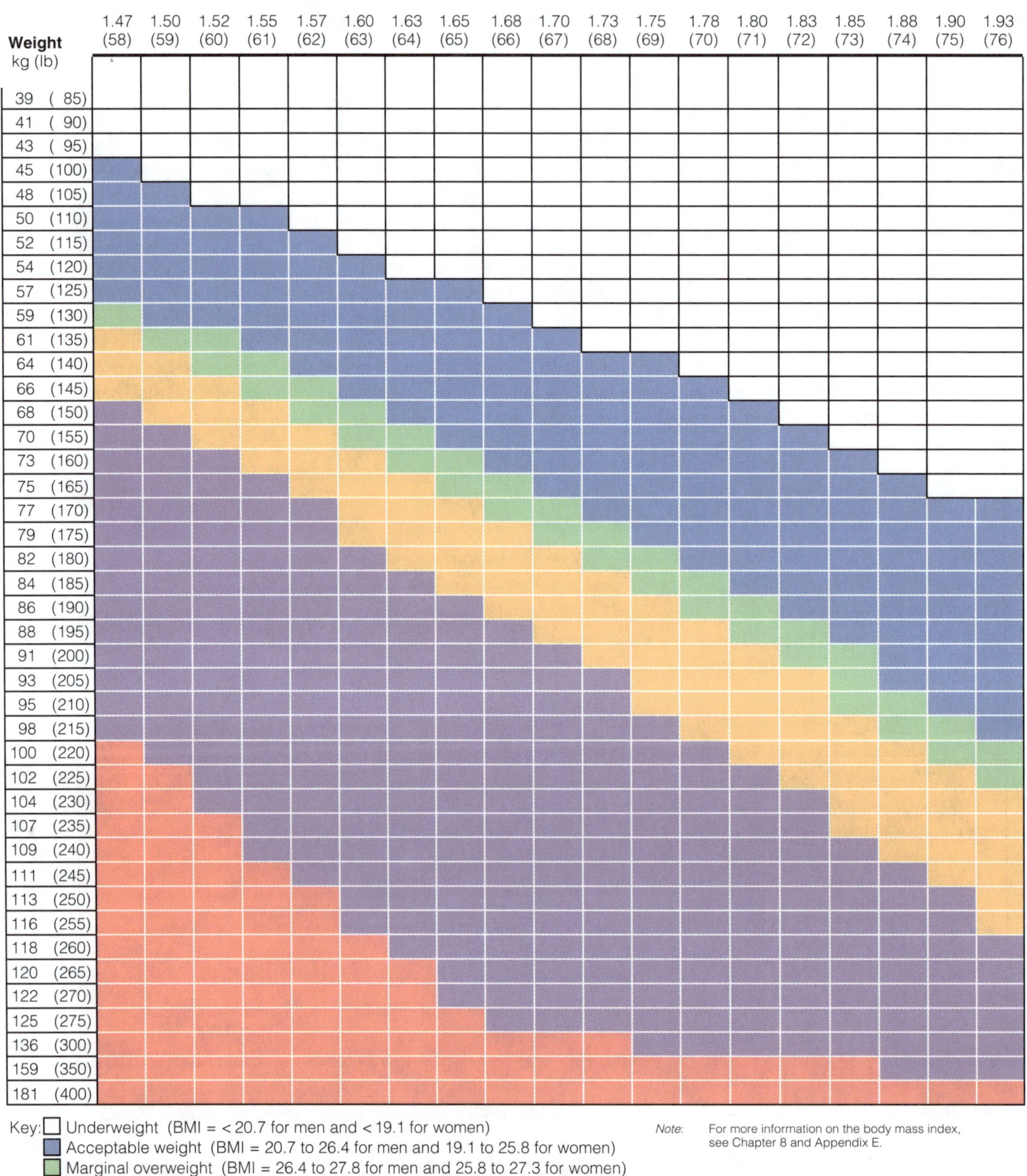

Key:
- ☐ Underweight (BMI = <20.7 for men and <19.1 for women)
- ■ Acceptable weight (BMI = 20.7 to 26.4 for men and 19.1 to 25.8 for women)
- ■ Marginal overweight (BMI = 26.4 to 27.8 for men and 25.8 to 27.3 for women)
- ■ Overweight (BMI = 27.8 to 31.1 for men and 27.3 to 32.2 for women)
- ■ Severe overweight (BMI = 31.1 to 45.4 for men and 32.3 to 44.8 for women)
- ■ Morbid obesity (BMI = >45.4 for men and >44.8 for women)

Note: For more information on the body mass index, see Chapter 8 and Appendix E.

Source: Adapted from M. I. Rowland, A nomogram for computing body index, *Dietetic Currents* 16 (1989): 8–9, used with permission from Ross Laboratories, Columbus, OH 43216.

Acceptable Weight for Height Based on Body Mass Index (BMI)

To determine your acceptable weight range, find your height in the top line. Look down the column below it and find the range represented by the color blue. Look to the left column to see what weights are acceptable for you.

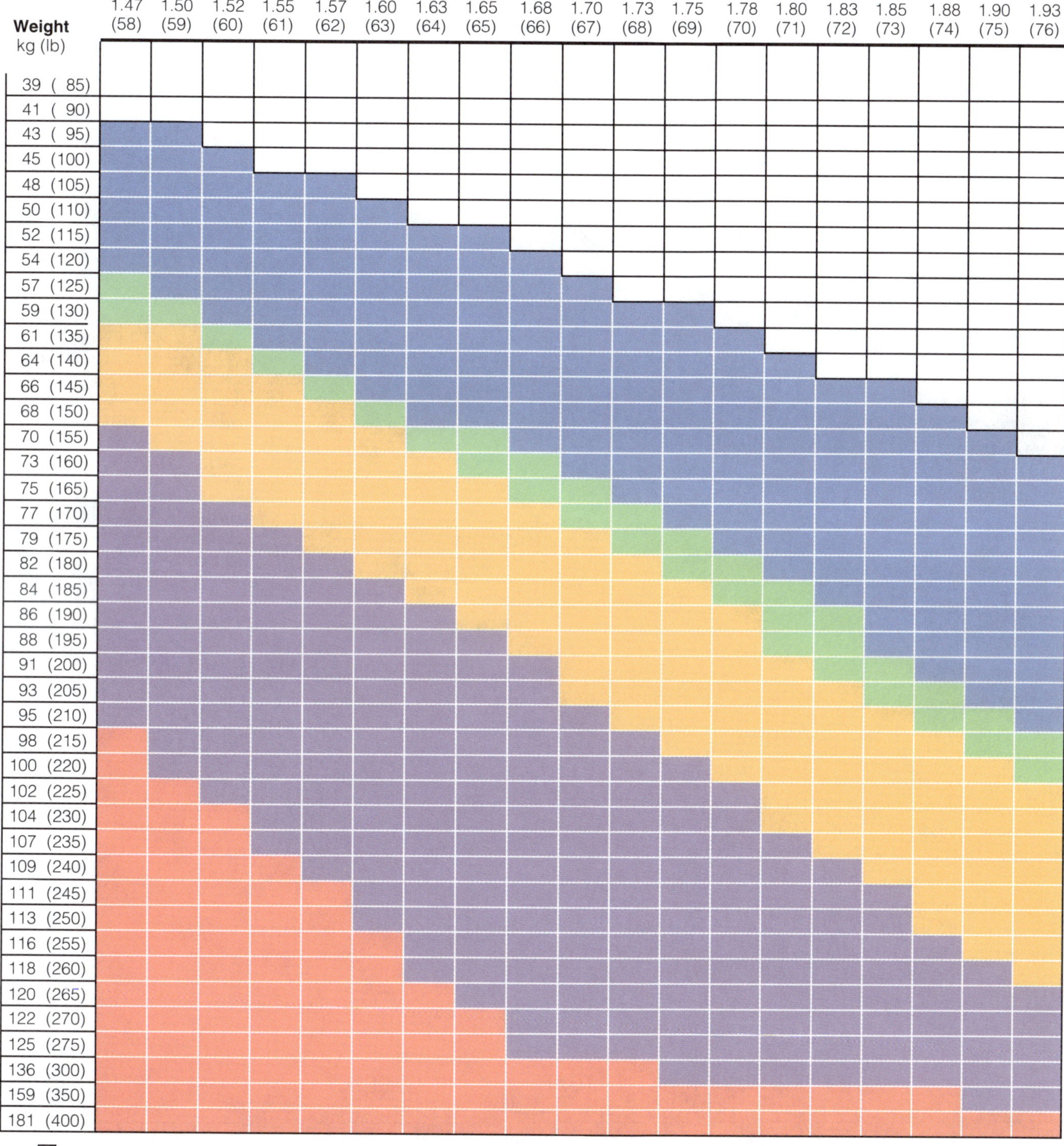

Key:
- Underweight (BMI = <20.7 for men and < 19.1 for women)
- Acceptable weight (BMI = 20.7 to 26.4 for men and 19.1 to 25.8 for women)
- Marginal overweight (BMI = 26.4 to 27.8 for men and 25.8 to 27.3 for women)
- Overweight (BMI = 27.8 to 31.1 for men and 27.3 to 32.2 for women)
- Severe overweight (BMI = 31.1 to 45.4 for men and 32.3 to 44.8 for women)
- Morbid obesity (BMI = >45.4 for men and >44.8 for women)

Note: For more information on the body mass index, see Chapter 8 and Appendix E.

Source: Adapted from M. I. Rowland, A nomogram for computing body index, *Dietetic Currents* 16 (1989): 8–9, used with permission from Ross Laboratories, Columbus, OH 43216. Copyright 1989 Ross Laboratories.